Essentials of
PEDIATRIC INTENSIVE CARE

Essentials of
PEDIATRIC INTENSIVE CARE

Edited by

Daniel L. Levin, M.D.

Professor, Department of Pediatrics, University of Texas Southwestern Medical Center; Medical Director, Pediatric Intensive Care Unit, Children's Medical Center of Dallas; Medical Director, Pediatric Trauma Intensive Care Unit, Parkland Memorial Hospital, Dallas, Texas

Frances C. Morriss, M.D.

Director of Pediatric Anesthesia and Assistant Medical Director, Pediatric Intensive Care Unit, Children's Medical Center of Dallas; Clinical Associate Professor of Pediatrics, University of Texas Southwestern Medical Center, Dallas, Texas

Nick G. Anas, M.D., Editor for Pulmonary

Director, Pediatric Intensive Care Unit; Co-Director, Apnea Diagnostic Center, Children's Hospital of Orange County, Orange, California

Carolanne Capron, R.N., B.S.N., Editor for Nursing

Clinical Nurse Educator, Pediatric Intensive Care Unit, Children's Medical Center of Dallas, Texas

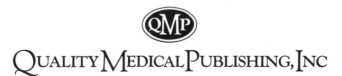

QUALITY MEDICAL PUBLISHING, INC

ST. LOUIS, MISSOURI
1990

PUBLISHER   Karen Berger

EDITOR   Beth Campbell

PROJECT MANAGER   Carolita Deter

MANUSCRIPT EDITOR   Marilyn Wynd

PRODUCTION   Susan Trail, Judy Bamert, Billie Forshee

BOOK DESIGN   Susan Trail

COVER DESIGN   Diane M. Beasley

ILLUSTRATOR   William M. Winn

Quality Medical Publishing, Inc.
2086 Craigshire Dr.
St. Louis, Missouri 63146

Every effort has been made to ensure the accuracy of the drug dosages listed in this book; however, the health care professional is legally responsible for verifying the indications and dosage requirements with the manufacturers' package inserts and is thus advised.

Quality Medical Publishing, Inc., and Mosby-Year Book, Inc., mutually recognize and respect the contribution made by the authors to this work. In this spirit, Quality Medical Publishing, Inc., acknowledges and gratefully accepts the permission to use portions of this work that previously appeared in Mosby-Year Book's *A Practical Guide to Pediatric Intensive Care*.

Printed in the United States of America.

LIBRARY OF CONGRESS CATALOGING-IN-PUBLICATION DATA

Essentials of pediatric intensive care / [edited by] Daniel L. Levin,
    Frances C. Morriss; Nick G. Anas, editor for Pulmonary; Carolanne
Capron, editor for Nursing.
        p.   cm.
    Includes bibliographical references.
    Includes index.
    ISBN 0-942219-03-1
    1. Pediatric intensive care.   I.   Levin, Daniel L. (Daniel Louis),
1943-   . II. Morriss, Frances C. (Frances Connally), 1943-
    [DNLM: 1. Critical Care—in infancy & childhood.   2.   Intensive
Care Units, Pediatric.   WS 366 E78]
RJ370.E84   1990
618.92′0028—dc20
DNLM/DLC
for Library of Congress   90-8858
                                                                CIP

GW/PC/PC
5   4   3   2   1

Section Editors

Nick G. Anas	Pulmonary
Billy S. Arant, Jr.	Nephrology
William M. Belknap	Gastrointestinal
George R. Buchanan	Hematology/Oncology
Carolanne Capron	Nursing
Jay D. Cook	Neurology
David E. Fixler	Cardiology
Charles M. Ginsburg	Poisonings
Katherine Lipsky	Psychosocial Issues
James F. Marks	Endocrine
Charles E. Mize	Metabolic/Nutrition
Frances C. Morriss	Anesthesia
Jane D. Siegel	Infectious Disease
Frederick H. Sklar	Neurosurgery
Ron Somers-Clark	Ethical Issues
Theodore P. Votteler	Surgery
Richard L. Wasserman	Immunology

Contributors

Steven R. Alexander, M.D.
Associate Professor of Pediatrics, Renal Division, University of Texas Southwestern Medical Center; Medical Director of Dialysis and Renal Transplantation, Children's Medical Center of Dallas, Texas

Stephanie Allen, M.S., R.N.
Program Coordinator, Children's Medical Center of Dallas, Texas

Kathy Amoroso, M.D.
Postdoctoral Fellow, Pediatric Rheumatology, Department of Pediatrics, University of Texas Southwestern Medical Center, Dallas, Texas

Nick G. Anas, M.D.
Director, Pediatric Intensive Care Unit; Co-Director, Apnea Diagnostic Center, Children's Hospital of Orange County, Orange, California

Ron J. Anderson, M.D.
President and Chief Executive Officer, Parkland Memorial Hospital, Dallas, Texas

Walter S. Andrews, M.D.
Assistant Professor, University of Texas Southwestern Medical Center; Director, Pediatric Liver Transplant Program, Children's Medical Center of Dallas, Texas

Billy S. Arant, Jr., M.D.
Professor, Department of Pediatrics, University of Texas Southwestern Medical Center; Director of Renal Service, Children's Medical Center of Dallas, Texas

Nancy A. Ayres, M.D.
Assistant Professor of Pediatrics and Medicine and Associate Pediatric Cardiologist, Abercrombie Section of Pediatric Cardiology, Baylor College of Medicine; Director, Echocardiology Laboratory, Texas Children's Hospital of Houston, Texas

Donna E. Badgett, C.R.T.T.
Quality Assurance and Finance Coordinator, Respiratory Therapy, Children's Medical Center of Dallas, Texas

Mary Grandy Baker, R.N., B.S.N., CN II
Staff nurse, Pediatric Intensive Care Unit, Children's Medical Center of Dallas, Texas

Alison B. Ballew, R.N., C.P.T.C.
Manager of Recovery Services, Southwest Organ Bank, Dallas, Texas

Gene A. Basham, R.N., B.S.N.
Pediatric Intensive Care Unit Transport Nurse, Children's Medical Center of Dallas, Texas

Michel Baum, M.D.
Associate Professor of Pediatrics, Section of Nephrology, University of Texas Southwestern Medical Center; Attending, Children's Medical Center of Dallas, Texas

William M. Belknap, M.D.
Assistant Professor of Pediatrics, Director of Gastroenterology and Nutrition, University of Texas Southwestern Medical Center, Dallas, Texas

Donald E. Berry, R.Ph.
Pediatric Intensive Care Unit Pharmacist, Children's Medical Center of Dallas, Texas

Gina Blount, R.N., B.S.N., C.N. III
Staff Nurse, Pediatric Intensive Care Unit, Children's Medical Center of Dallas, Texas

John E. Brimm, M.D.
President, EMTEK Health Care Systems, Tempe, Arizona

Lela W. Brink, M.D.
Assistant Professor, University of Texas Southwestern Medical Center; Medical Director of Transport Services, Children's Medical Center of Dallas, Texas

John G. Brooks, M.D.
Professor of Pediatrics, Strong Memorial Hospital; Director, Pediatric Pulmonology Medicine, Department of Pediatrics, University of Rochester Medical Center, Rochester, New York

Orval E. Brown, M.D.
Associate Professor of Otorhinolaryngology, University of Texas Southwestern Medical Center; Attending, Children's Medical Center of Dallas, Texas

Derek A. Bruce, M.D.
Clinical Associate Professor of Neurosurgery, University of Texas Southwestern Medical Center; Director, International Pediatric Neurosurgical Institute, Humana Hospital of Dallas, Texas

Elizabeth Brunetti-Fyock, R.N., B.S.N.
Senior Pediatric Liver Transplant Coordinator, Children's Medical Center of Dallas, Texas

Lynn M. Butler, R.R.T.
General Care Coordinator for Respiratory Care, Children's Medical Center of Dallas, Texas

H. Steven Byrd, M.D.
Associate Professor, Division of Plastic Surgery, University of Texas Southwestern Medical Center, Dallas, Texas

Carolanne Capron, R.N., B.S.N.
Clinical Nurse Educator, Pediatric Intensive Care Unit, Children's Medical Center of Dallas, Texas

Beth Clark, R.N., B.S.N.
Emergency Room Staff Nurse, Baylor University Medical Center, Dallas, Texas

Dale Coln, M.D.
Director of Pediatric Surgery, Baylor University Medical Center; Clinical Associate Professor of Surgery, University of Texas Southwestern Medical Center, Dallas, Texas

Jay D. Cook, M.D.
Department of Pediatrics, King Faisal Specialist Hospital and Research Center, Riyadh, Saudi Arabia

Marjorie Craft, R.N., C.N. III
Pediatric Intensive Care Unit Transport Nurse, Children's Medical Center of Dallas, Texas

Cynthia Cunningham, M.S., R.D./L.D.
Director of Nutritional Services, Children's Medical Center of Dallas, Texas

M. Douglas Cunningham, M.D.
Professor of Clinical Pediatrics and Neonatology, University of California, Irvine, Medical Center; Medical Director, Infant Special Care Unit, Saddleback Women's Hospital, Laguna Hills, California

William Dammert, M.D.
Clinical Associate Professor of Pediatric Surgery, University of Texas Southwestern Medical Center, Dallas, Texas

Stan L. Davis, M.D.
Clinical Assistant Professor of Pediatrics, Division of Anesthesiology, University of Texas Southwestern Medical Center; Attending, Pediatric Intensive Care Unit, Children's Medical Center of Dallas, Texas

Mauricio R. Delgado, M.D., F.R.C.P.
Assistant Professor of Neurology, University of Texas Southwestern Medical Center; Director of Neurology and Neurophysiology Departments, Texas Scottish Rite Hospital of Dallas, Texas

Patricia T. Driscoll, M.S., J.D.
Attorney at Law; Assistant Professor, Texas Woman's University, Health Care Administration Program, Dallas, Texas

Patti Duer, R.N., B.S.N., C.I.C.
Infection Control Coordinator, Children's Medical Center of Dallas, Texas

Gary Elmore, R.R.T.
Administrative Director of Respiratory Care, Children's Medical Center of Dallas, Texas

Roy D. Elterman, M.D.
Clinical Assistant Professor of Pediatrics and Neurology, University of Texas Southwestern Medical Center, Dallas, Texas

Graham J. Emslie, M.D.
Associate Professor of Psychiatry, University of Texas Southwestern Medical Center; Director, Psychiatry Services, Children's Medical Center of Dallas, Texas

Mary M. Farrell, M.D.
Associate Director, Pediatric Intensive Care Unit, Arnold Palmer Hospital for Children and Women, Orlando, Florida

Elizabeth Farrington, Pharm.D.
Director of Clinical Pharmacy Services, Children's Medical Center of Dallas; Clinical Professor of Pharmacy, University of Texas at Austin, Texas

Timothy F. Feltes, M.D.
Assistant Professor of Pediatrics and Medicine, Baylor College of Medicine; Associate Pediatric Cardiologist, Texas Children's Hospital, Houston, Texas

David E. Fixler, M.D.
Professor of Pediatrics, University of Texas Southwestern Medical Center; Chief, Section of Cardiology, Children's Medical Center of Dallas, Texas

Stephanie M. Ford, R.N., B.S.N., C.C.R.N.
Assistant Director, Pediatric Intensive Care Unit, Children's Medical Center of Dallas, Texas

Cole A. Giller, Ph.D., M.D.
Assistant Professor, Department of Neurosurgery, University of Texas Southwestern Medical Center, Dallas, Texas

Charles M. Ginsburg, M.D.
Professor and Chairman, Department of Pediatrics, Robert L. Moore Chair in Pediatrics, University of Texas Southwestern Medical Center; Chief of Staff, Children's Medical Center of Dallas, Texas

Gary Goodman, M.D.
Associate Director, Pediatric Intensive Care Unit; Medical Director, Pediatric Transport, Children's Hospital of Orange County, Orange, California

Susan A. Gray, R.N.
Pediatric Transplant Coordinator, Children's Medical Center of Dallas, Texas

David M. Habib, M.D.
Assistant Professor of Pediatrics, Division of Critical Care Medicine, Children's Hospital, Charleston, South Carolina

Stephen D. Haid, B.A., C.P.T.C.
Executive Director, Southwest Organ Bank, Dallas, Texas

Katherine A. Hammond, R.N., B.S.N., C.N. II
Staff Nurse, Pediatric Intensive Care Unit, Children's Medical Center of Dallas, Texas

Bill and Cathy Hare
Parents

Mary F. Harris, M.D.
Assistant Professor of Anesthesia, University of Texas Southwestern Medical Center; Director of Anesthesiology, Texas Scottish Rite Hospital of Dallas, Texas

Nancy L. Hatfield, C.R.T.T.
Pulmonary Function Technician, Pulmonary Laboratory, Children's Medical Center of Dallas, Texas

Mary Fran Hazinski, R.N., M.S.N., F.A.A.N.
Departments of Surgery and Pediatrics, Vanderbilt University School of Medicine, Nashville, Tennessee

David A. Hicks, M.D.
Assistant Clinical Professor of Pediatrics, University of California, Irvine; Pulmonologist and Neonatologist, Children's Hospital of Orange County, Orange, California

Lenetta G. Hogue, M.S.W., C.S.W.
Houston, Texas

Pam Holbrook, R.N., M.S.
Pediatric Intensive Care Unit Transport Nurse, Children's Medical Center of Dallas, Texas

Angela R. Holder, LL.M.
Clinical Professor of Pediatrics (Law), Yale University School of Medicine, New Haven, Connecticut

Mary Elaine Jones, Ph.D.
Assistant Professor, University of Texas at Arlington, School of Nursing, Arlington, Texas

Barton A. Kamen, M.D., Ph.D.
Professor of Pediatrics and Pharmacology, Division of Hematology and Oncology, University of Texas Southwestern Medical Center; Burroughs Wellcome Scholar, Clinical Pharmacology, Children's Medical Center of Dallas, Texas

Vicki D. Kelley, B.S., C.C.L.S.
Child Life Specialist, Children's Medical Center of Dallas, Texas

Steven R. Leonard, M.D.
Associate Clinical Professor, University of Texas Southwestern Medical Center; Associate Attending in Cardiothoracic Surgery, Children's Medical Center of Dallas, Texas

Debbie L. LeVasseur, R.N., C.C.T.C.
Renal Transplant Coordinator, Children's Medical Center of Dallas, Texas

Daniel L. Levin, M.D.
Professor, Department of Pediatrics, University of Texas Southwestern Medical Center; Medical Director, Pediatric Intensive Care Unit, Children's Medical Center of Dallas; Medical Director, Pediatric Trauma Intensive Care Unit, Parkland Memorial Hospital, Dallas, Texas

Gretta Liljeberg, R.N., B.S.N.
Staff Nurse, Pediatric Intensive Care Unit, Children's Medical Center of Dallas, Texas

Steven L. Linder, M.D.
Clinical Assistant Professor, Division of Pediatric Neurology, University of Texas Southwestern Medical Center, Dallas, Texas

Dwight Lee Lindholm, M.D.
Postdoctoral Fellow, Pediatric Neurology, Texas Scottish Rite Hospital of Dallas, Texas

Katherine Lipsky, A.C.S.W., C.S.W.-A.C.P.
Director of Social Work, Children's Medical Center of Dallas, Texas

William M. Longworth, Ph.D.
Associate Minister, First United Methodist Church, Fort Worth, Texas

Edward J. Lose, M.D.
Co-Chief Resident, Children's Medical Center of Dallas, Texas

Paul Lubinsky, M.B., Ch.B.
Attending, Critical Care Medicine, Children's Hospital of Orange County, Orange, California

Cindy K. Lybarger, R.N., B.S.N., M.S.N.
Clinical Nurse Specialist, Pediatric Critical Care, Vanderbilt University Medical Center, Nashville, Tennessee

George H. McCracken, Jr., M.D.
Professor of Pediatrics, University of Texas Southwestern Medical Center; Attending, Division of Infectious Disease, Children's Medical Center of Dallas and Parkland Memorial Hospital, Dallas, Texas

Lynn Mahony, M.D.
Assistant Professor of Pediatrics, Division of Cardiology, University of Texas Southwestern Medical Center, Dallas, Texas

Scott C. Manning, M.D.
Assistant Professor of Otorhinolaryngology, University of Texas Southwestern Medical Center; Attending, Children's Medical Center of Dallas, Texas

James F. Marks, M.D., M.P.H.
Associate Professor, Department of Pediatrics, Division of Endocrinology, University of Texas Southwestern Medical Center, Dallas, Texas

Steven R. Mayfield, M.D.
Assistant Professor of Pediatrics and Nutrition, Division of Neonatology, University of Texas Southwestern Medical Center, Dallas, Texas

Charles E. Mize, M.D., Ph.D.
Associate Professor, Department of Pediatrics and Biochemistry, University of Texas Southwestern Medical Center; Director of Clinical Nutrition and Metabolism, Children's Medical Center of Dallas, Texas

Michelle Morris-Copeland, R.N., B.S.N., C.N. III
Cardiac Nurse Educator, Pediatric Intensive Care Unit, Children's Medical Center of Dallas, Texas

Frances C. Morriss, M.D.
Director of Pediatric Anesthesia and Assistant Medical Director, Pediatric Intensive Care Unit, Children's Medical Center of Dallas; Clinical Associate Professor of Pediatrics, University of Texas Southwestern Medical Center, Dallas, Texas

Annette Musselman-Jarvis, R.R.T.
Coordinator of Ambulatory Care, Pulmonary Medicine, Children's Medical Center of Dallas, Texas

Mahmoud M. Mustafa, M.D.
Postdoctoral Fellow, Pediatric Infectious Disease, University of Texas Southwestern Medical Center, Dallas, Texas

John D. Nelson, M.D.
Professor of Pediatrics, Division of Infectious Disease, University of Texas Southwestern Medical Center, Dallas, Texas

Edgar A. Newfeld, M.D., P.A.
Clinical Associate Professor of Pediatrics, Division of Cardiology, University of Texas Southwestern Medical Center, Dallas, Texas

Hisashi Nikaidoh, M.D.
Clinical Associate Professor, University of Texas Southwestern Medical Center; Director of Thoracic Surgery, Children's Medical Center of Dallas, Texas

Lorene S. Nolan, R.N., C.C.R.N.
Clinical Application Specialist, EMTEK Health Care Systems, Tempe, Arizona

P. Pearl O'Rourke, M.D.
Assistant Professor of Pediatrics and Adjunct Assistant Professor of Anesthesia, University of Washington; Director of Pediatric Intensive Care Unit and Associate Director of Respiratory Therapy, Children's Hospital and Medical Center of Seattle, Washington

Mary Orr-McDonald, M.S., R.N., M.S.
Nutrition Clinical Nurse Specialist, Children's Medical Center of Dallas, Texas

Maria Ortega, M.D.
Anesthesiologist, Children's Medical Center of Dallas, Texas

David B. Owen, M.D.
Clinical Instructor, Pediatric Neurology, University of Texas Southwestern Medical Center, Dallas, Texas

Mark Parrish, M.D.
Associate Professor of Pediatrics and Chief, Division of Cardiology, University of California Davis, Sacramento, California

Ronald M. Perkin, M.D.
Associate Professor of Pediatrics and Director, Pediatric Critical Care Medicine, Loma Linda University Medical Center, Loma Linda, California

Murray M. Pollack, M.D.
Professor, Anesthesiology and Pediatrics, and Associate Director, Pediatric Intensive Care Unit, Children's Hospital National Medical Center, Washington, D.C.

Michael L. Ponaman, M.D.
Postdoctoral Fellow, Critical Care Medicine, Children's Medical Center of Dallas; Resident, Anesthesia, Parkland Memorial Hospital, Dallas, Texas

Paul R. Prescott, M.D.
Assistant Professor of Clinical Pediatrics, University of Texas Southwestern Medical Center; Medical Director, Child Abuse and Neglect Program, Children's Medical Center of Dallas, Texas

Richard Quan, M.D.
Assistant Professor of Pediatrics, Section of Gastroenterology/Nutrition, University of Texas Southwestern Medical Center, Dallas, Texas

Raymond P. Quigley, M.D.
Fellow, Division of Pediatric Nephrology, University of Texas Southwestern Medical Center, Dallas, Texas

Donna S. Rahn, R.N., B.S.N., C.N. III
Staff Nurse, Pediatric Intensive Care Unit, Children's Medical Center of Dallas, Texas

Octavio Ramilo, M.D., Ph.D.
Assistant Instructor, Pediatrics and Microbiology, University of Texas Southwestern Medical Center, Dallas, Texas

W. Gary Reed, M.D.
Professor of Internal Medicine and Chief, General Internal Medicine, University of Texas Southwestern Medical Center, Dallas, Texas

Kyoo H. Rhee, M.D.
Clinical Assistant Professor, Pulmonary/Critical Care Medicine, Department of Pediatrics The University of Arizona H.S.C., Tucson, Arizona

W. Steves Ring, M.D.
Professor and Chairman, Thoracic and Cardiovascular Surgery, Department of Surgery, University of Texas Southwestern Medical Center, Dallas, Texas

Lynn E. Rogers, R.N., M.N.
Pulmonary Clinical Nurse Specialist, Children's Hospital of Orange County, Orange, California

James S. Roloff, M.D.
Associate Professor of Pediatrics, Division of Hematology-Oncology, M.S. Hershey Medical Center, Hershey, Pennsylvania

James A. Royall, M.D.
Assistant Professor of Pediatrics, Division of Critical Care Medicine and Division of Pediatric Pulmonology, University of Alabama at Birmingham, Alabama

Richard F. Salmon, L.C.D.R., M.C., U.S.N.R.
Section of Nephrology, Department of Pediatrics, Naval Hospital, Portsmouth, Virgina

Joann M. Sanders, M.D.
Assistant Instructor in Pediatrics, Division of Pediatric Hematology and Oncology, University of Texas Southwestern Medical Center, Dallas, Texas

Mouin G. Seikaly, M.D.
Assistant Professor, Department of Pediatrics, Renal Division, University of Texas Southwestern Medical Center, Dallas, Texas

Kenneth Shapiro, M.D.
Clinical Associate Professor, Department of Neurosurgery, University of Texas Southwestern Medical Center, Dallas, Texas

Valerie Shasteen, R.N., B.S.N.
Assistant Director, Pediatric Intensive Care Unit, Children's Medical Center of Dallas, Texas

Jane D. Siegel, M.D.
Associate Professor, Division of Infectious Disease, University of Texas Southwestern Medical Center, Dallas, Texas

Douglas P. Sinn, D.D.S.
Professor and Chairman, Oral and Maxillofacial Surgery, University of Texas Southwestern Medical Center, Dallas, Texas

Frederick H. Sklar, M.D.
Clinical Associate Professor of Neurosurgery, University of Texas Southwestern Medical Center; Director of Pediatric Neurosurgery, Children's Medical Center of Dallas, Texas

Thomas Smith, M.D.
Associate Professor, Department of Radiology, State University of New York at Stony Brook, New York

Ron Somers-Clark, Th.M.
Director, Department of Pastoral Care, Children's Medical Center of Dallas, Texas

Judy B. Splawski, M.D.
Assistant Professor of Pediatrics, Division of Pediatric Gastroenterology, University of Texas Southwestern Medical Center, Dallas, Texas

Robert H. Squires, Jr., M.D.
Assistant Professor of Pediatrics, Division of Gastroenterology, University of Texas Southwestern Medical Center, Dallas, Texas

Jean Stone, R.N., B.S.N., C.N. III
Pediatric Intensive Care Unit Transport Nurse, Children's Medical Center of Dallas, Texas

Kathy Thomas, R.N., B.S.N., C.N. III
Nursing Recruitment Department, Children's Medical Center of Dallas, Texas

Luis O. Toro-Figueroa, M.D.
Assistant Professor of Pediatrics, Section of Critical Care Medicine, University of Texas Southwestern Medical Center; Attending, Pediatric Intensive Care Unit and Medical Director of Respiratory Care, Children's Medical Center of Dallas, Texas

Gary R. Turner, M.D.
Clinical Assistant Professor of Anesthesia, University of Texas Southwestern Medical Center, Dallas, Texas

Ricardo Uauy, M.D., Ph.D.
Associate Professor of Pediatrics and Human Nutrition, University of Texas Southwestern Medical Center; Attending Physician, Parkland Memorial Hospital and St. Paul Hospital, Dallas, Texas

Daved van Stralen, M.D.
Instructor, Department of Pediatric Emergency Medicine, Loma Linda University Medical Center; Instructor, School of Nursing and School of Allied Health Professions, Loma Linda University; Professor of Emergency Medical Care, Crafton Hills College, Loma Linda, California

Richard L. Vinson, C.R.T.T.
Critical Care Coordinator, Department of Pulmonary Medicine, Children's Medical Center of Dallas, Texas

Theodore P. Votteler, M.D.
Clinical Professor of Surgery and Pediatrics, University of Texas Southwestern Medical Center; Director of Surgical Services, Children's Medical Center of Dallas, Texas

Becky Wade, R.R.T.
Clinical Application Specialist, Criticare Systems, Inc., Dallas, Texas

David C. Waagner, M.D.
Postdoctoral Fellow, Pediatric Infectious Disease, University of Texas Medical Center, Dallas, Texas

David A. Waller, M.D.
Associate Professor of Psychiatry and Pediatrics and Chief, Child and Adolescent Psychiatry, University of Texas Southwestern Medical Center and Children's Medical Center of Dallas, Texas

Elizabeth A. Wanek, M.D.
Postdoctoral Fellow, Pediatric Surgery, University of Texas Southwestern Medical Center, Dallas, Texas

Richard L. Wasserman, M.D., Ph.D.
Director of Pediatric Immune and Infectious Diseases; Assistant Chief of Services of Pediatrics, Baylor Medical Center of Dallas, Texas

Steven Weitman, M.D., Ph.D.
Fellow, Hematology/Oncology, Department of Pediatrics, Children's Medical Center of Dallas, Texas

Linda White, R.N., B.S.N., C.N. I.
Staff Nurse, Pediatric Intensive Care Unit, Children's Medical Center of Dallas, Texas

Penny Williams, M.S., R.N.
CPR Education Specialist, Department of Nursing Education and Research, Children's Medical Center of Dallas, Texas

Naomi J. Winick, M.D.
Assistant Professor, Department of Pediatrics, University of Texas Southwestern Medical Center; Director, Clinical Oncology, Children's Medical Center of Dallas, Texas

Kim Yeakel, R.N., C.N. II
Pediatric Intensive Care Unit Transport Nurse, Children's Medical Center of Dallas, Texas

Maureen Zipkin, R.N., M.M., C.N.A.
Nurse Manager, Multidisciplinary ICU, Children's Hospital, Boston, Massachusetts

Robert Jeffrey Zwiener, M.D.
Assistant Professor of Pediatrics, Department of Pediatrics, Division of Gastroenterology and Nutrition, University of Texas Southwestern Medical Center, Dallas, Texas

To the

Staff
past, present, and future, of the
Pediatric Intensive Care Unit
Children's Medical Center of Dallas

and especially for

Micah, Brendan, Erin, and **Laura**

Foreword

Pediatrics is a specialty whose raison d'être is growth and development. It is altogether fitting, therefore, that one of the specialty's youngest progenies, critical care medicine, has experienced orderly differentiation and exponential growth. In less than two decades the discipline has evolved from a handful of hardworking, dedicated individuals found in specialized areas within hospitals into a true subspecialty that has defined thoughtful guidelines for the education and training of its young and a certification process sanctioned by the American Board of Pediatrics. Contrary to some prognostications and, possibly, wishful thinking by some in the past, pediatric critical care medicine is now firmly established and recognized as an important subspecialty of pediatrics.

The evolution of the discipline has been fascinating. Despite being a very sophisticated, high-tech subspecialty, pediatric critical care medicine is broad spectrum and caring. Pediatric intensivists, in my mind, are a contemporary version of the well-trained generalists of the past who confined their practices to hospitalized patients. Similar to their generic ancestors, critical care specialists must have a broad base of knowledge with expertise and experience in virtually all pediatric and surgical subspecialties and anesthesia as well as an understanding and working knowledge of the more basic disciplines of physiology, pharmacology, biochemistry, and cell biology. The intensivist of today integrates basic biologic principles with the products of the technologic revolution to provide optimal care to his or her patients. The evolution and maturation of the species has been a boon to the critically ill child.

This text promises to be an essential resource for students, postgraduate trainees, and practitioners who care for critically ill infants and children. It is comprehensive, pragmatic, and, most important, usable. This text provides pertinent background information for the reader and covers the important elements of basic pathophysiology in a succinct manner. An especially important feature is that the text contains straightforward algorithms for management of critically ill children. In addition the book contains many useful tables and other information helpful to individuals who want to establish critical areas within their hospitals. All who provide care to critically ill children and their families will find this text to be an invaluable resource.

Charles M. Ginsburg, M.D.

Professor and Chairman
Department of Pediatrics
University of Texas Southwestern Medical Center

Preface

Over the past 20 years the field of intensive care has become firmly established as a medical and nursing subspecialty with its own certifying examinations and college of critical care medicine. Pediatric intensive care has developed in concert with but separate from intensive care for internal medicine and surgery patients. Although 15 years ago there were three or four units with full-time pediatric intensive care services and subspecialty training programs, there are now 46 training programs in the United States and Canada and countless other units have been opened.

In 1976 we published, if not the first text, one of the first texts dealing exclusively with pediatric intensive care and it was very successful, not only because of its quality but also because of the need. Practitioners, residents, nurses, and respiratory therapists all needed a quick, authoritative reference on matters of pathophysiology, specific diseases, monitoring, and equipment and techniques, and that book fulfilled those particular needs. We have undergone a great deal of evolution and development since that time, but even with the increased sophistication of the field and the publication of several other textbooks since then, practitioners are still expressing the same needs.

We have attempted to fulfill those needs with this text. For several reasons it is a completely new book. In addition to adding new material to stay current with developments in the field, we have altered and improved on some of the shortcomings of previous texts. The book has grown larger, not only because we cover more and newer topics but also because we have decided not to eliminate all redundancy from the text and by so doing have made individual sections and chapters more readable.

Because this book is large, we have added the "baby book," which attempts to assemble all the urgent, quick-reference material from the main text in one small, easy-to-carry and easy-to-use pocketbook. We hope that *Essentials of Pediatric Intensive Care: A Pocket Companion* will maximize the benefit of the material presented in the main text.

As Robert Crumley indicates below, the pediatric intensive care unit is a difficult place to work even at the best of times. We hope that this book will aid in making it a better place to work and enhance the care of critically ill children.

We want to acknowledge the enormous contribution of Mrs. Jean Pitzer in assembling this book and making our work, as always, a bit easier.

Daniel L. Levin
Frances C. Morriss

The pediatric intensive care unit is a complex place in which to do ministry. It is a place where reality often cannot be accurately assessed. It is a place of contradictions and paradox. It is a place where prayers seem miraculously answered and where God seems determined to be found. It is a place where many find hope and meaning for their lives and where peoples' deepest fears and agonies are realized.

Robert E. Crumley, M.Div.

Contents

| | | P A R T   III
Specific Diseases and Problems

For Normal Laboratory Values, see the *Pocket Companion*, p. 4.

Essentials of
PEDIATRIC INTENSIVE CARE

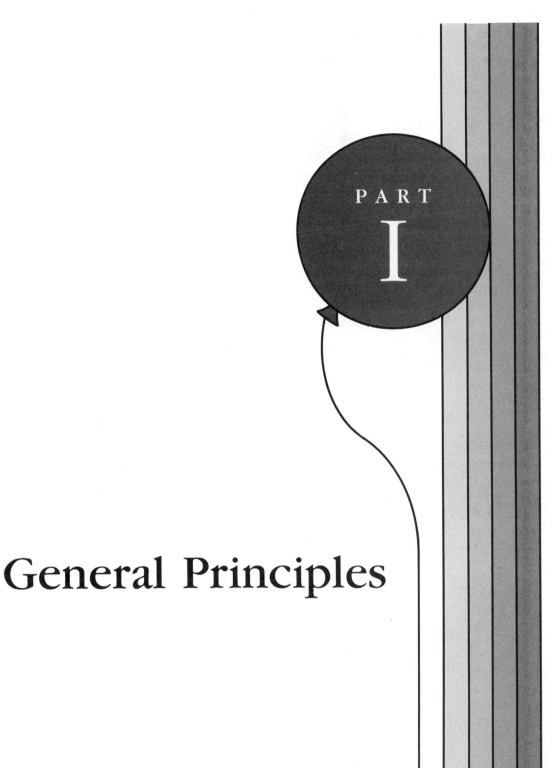

PART

I

General Principles

1 Pediatric Intensive Care

Daniel L. Levin

Pediatric intensive care is a service provided in a unique setting by specially trained professionals intended to improve the chances of young infants and children not only surviving critical illnesses but thriving thereafter. Although the particular illnesses in some cases overlap, many that are seen in either neonatal or adult intensive care units and others are unique to pediatrics. The pathophysiologic responses of neonates, pediatric patients, and adults vary, and the specifics of therapy and management in pediatric patients are quite different in many ways. The pediatric intensive care unit is not, therefore, a place for critically ill small adults or large neonates; its physical character and the nature and training of the personnel who work there make it a highly specialized unit.

Both nursing and medicine have recognized the need for long-term specialized training for the professionals who work in such units. Specific requirements for training and board certification by examination are part of the process of qualifying to participate in the care of critically ill children. Most of us who worked in the first designated pediatric intensive care areas, which had little organization and leadership, and later in well-run units intuitively understood that the presence of full-time nurses and physicians made a difference in care and outcome. Recent studies have shown this to be true. In a pinch, neonatal or adult nurses and doctors can care for pediatric intensive care patients, and many times the results will be satisfactory. The more global view of such practices cannot, however, be condoned since the best care for many pediatric patients can only be provided in units especially designed for them and organized and staffed by pediatric critical care specialists.

Not only is the training of the personnel important but the dedication and availability of the personnel as well. To acquire and maintain expertise in pediatric intensive care the nurses, physicians, and other personnel such as respiratory therapists, radiologists, laboratory technicians, pharmacists, social and child life workers, and pastoral counselors must have continued, not intermittent, exposure to the pediatric intensive care unit and its patients. Someone from every facet of care must be available at all times. For nurses, physicians, and respiratory therapists this means continuous availability in the unit; that is the essence of pediatric intensive care service. Pediatric patients whose conditions are unstable or potentially unstable have little reserve to compensate for untoward physiologic or pathogenic events and may suddenly and dramatically deteriorate. The need for ongoing assessment of their physical state and reassessment of therapeutic efforts is constant. The professionals who need to respond to such changes must be not only specifically trained to do so, but immediately accessible. In teaching institutions this may include pediatric intensive care nurse interns, RN staff, pediatric, anesthesia, and surgical house staff as well as intensive care fellows and attending physicians.

The monitoring of pediatric intensive care patients is presented throughout this book, especially in the last section. The patients are assumed to be critically ill and unstable or potentially unstable, and the monitoring in many cases is both anticipatory and invasive. It is therefore not without significant risk, and although individual techniques may be employed outside of the intensive care unit, the complete description of monitoring presented here is intended for the pediatric intensive care unit patient. In this patient population it is necessary to learn to identify warning signs and to be able to respond to those signs rapidly and effectively to prevent complications, including long-term residua and death. The risks of monitoring must always be balanced against those potential benefits described above.

The physical setting of pediatric intensive care is a very special one designed for patients with a variety of needs and their families as well as for the most efficient functioning of staff. This topic is specifically addressed in Chapter 106.

ADDITIONAL READING

• American Board of Pediatrics Sub-Board of Critical Care Medicine. Eligibility criteria for certification, Chapel Hill, N.C.: 1988.
• Committee on Hospital Care and Pediatric Section of the Society of Critical Care Medicine (Bergeson PS, Holbrook PR). Guidelines for pediatric intensive care units. Pediatrics 72:364-372, 1983.

Grenvik A, Leonard JJ, Arens JF, Carey LC, Disney FA. Critical care medicine. Certification as a multidisciplinary sub-specialty. Crit Care Med 9:117-125, 1981.

Pollack MM, Katz RW, Ruttimann UE, Getson PR. Improving the outcome and efficiency of intensive care: The impact of an intensivist. Crit Care Med 16:11-17, 1988.

Pollack MM, Alexander SR, Clarke N, et al. Comparison of tertiary and non-tertiary intensive care: A statewide comparison. Pediat Res 23(Part 2):234A, 1988.

Task Force on Guidelines Society of Critical Care Medicine. Recommendations for program content for fellowship training in critical care medicine. Crit Care Med 15:971-977, 1987.

Task Force on Guidelines Society of Critical Care Medicine. Recommendations for the qualifications of a director of a fellowship training program in critical care medicine. Crit Care Med 15:977, 1987.

2 Physiologic and Anatomic Differences Between Children and Adults

Mary Fran Hazinski · Daved van Stralen

BACKGROUND

The critically ill child is both physically and physiologically immature and differs from the critically ill adult in several important ways. Everyone caring for the critically ill child must be able to approach the patient at a level appropriate to the child's psychosocial development and level of distress, modifying assessment techniques and interventions accordingly. In addition, equipment utilized must not only be smaller, but it must be designed to serve the unique characteristics of the child's maturing body.

Treatment of the critically ill child must include treatment and support of the family, which necessitates excellent communication among members of the health care team and clear, consistent, and frequent communication with the parents. For further information regarding the psychosocial support of the child and family, the reader is referred to Chapters 96, 97, 99, and 100.

Anyone working in the critical care environment should develop the ability to determine at a glance if the child "looks good" or "looks bad." This determination involves rapid visual evaluation of the child's skin perfusion, hydration, level of activity, responsiveness, and position of comfort. The healthy child will have pink mucous membranes and nail beds and uniform skin color over the trunk and extremities. The child's skin will be warm, peripheral pulses strong, and capillary refill instantaneous (<1 to 2 seconds).

The adult in cardiorespiratory distress will express discomfort and may complain of dyspnea or chest pain. The critically ill or injured child usually acts ill, but this assessment will rely on nonverbal rather than verbal clues. The child in cardiorespiratory distress may grimace or will be unusually irritable or lethargic. The moderately ill infant or child usually does not demonstrate good eye contact, may be irritable when aroused, and often is unable to find a comfortable position. The extremely ill child will be unresponsive to most stimulation and usually demonstrates flaccid muscle tone. A decreased response to painful stimulus is abnormal in the child of any age and usually indicates severe cardiorespiratory or neurologic deterioration.

CARDIOVASCULAR DIFFERENCES
Anatomic Differences

Cardiac location. The heart of the infant, child, and adult is located under the lower third of the sternum. Cardiac compression during resuscitative efforts necessitates compression one fingerbreadth below the nipple line in the infant and one fingerbreadth above the costal-sternal notch in the child and the adult.

Ventricular morphology. During postnatal adaptation to extrauterine life, systemic vascular resistance rises. As a result, the work load of the left ventricle increases, and hypertrophy and hyperplasia of left ventricular myocytes occur during the first 3 to 6 months of life. Left ventricular wall thickness nearly doubles during this time.

Pulmonary vascular resistance falls after birth, and the work load of the right ventricle decreases proportionately. Myocyte growth is slower in the right than the left ventricle during the first months of life,

5

NORMAL HEMODYNAMIC VARIABLES IN CHILDREN

Calculation of systemic vascular resistance (SVR)

$$\text{SVR (in units)} = \frac{\text{Mean arterial pressure} - \text{Mean right atrial pressure}}{\text{Cardiac index}}$$

Normal SVR (in units) in neonates: 10-15 units/m² BSA
Normal SVR (in units) in children: 15-30 units/m² BSA

Calculation of pulmonary vascular resistance (PVR)

$$\text{Pulmonary vascular resistance} = \frac{\text{Mean pulmonary artery pressure} - \text{Mean left atrial pressure}}{\text{Cardiac index}}$$

Normal PVR (in units) in neonates: 8-10 units/m² BSA
Normal PVR (in units) in children: 1-3 units/m² BSA

Normal oxygen consumption

Infants < 2-3 wk of age: 120-130 ml/min/m² BSA
Children > 2-3 wk of age: 150-160 ml/min/m² BSA *or* 5-8 ml/kg/min
Normal arterial oxygen content: 18-20 ml O₂/dl blood

NOTE: To convert units to dynes · sec/cm⁻⁵, change cardiac index to cardiac output in denominator of equation and multiply equation by 80.
BSA = body surface area.

and right ventricular muscle thickness remains the same throughout childhood. Right and left ventricular weights are approximately equal at birth, but the right ventricular/left ventricular weight ratio is only 0.5 to 0.6 by 2 months of age. These changes in right and left ventricular size produce corresponding changes in the infant's ECG. Right ventricular dominance is present during the first months of life, but left ventricular dominance is usually apparent by 3 to 6 months of age. During childhood the P wave duration, PR interval, QRS duration, and QRS magnitudes increase.

Circulating blood volume. The child's circulating blood volume is higher per kilogram body weight than the blood volume of the adult (average 70 to 80 ml/kg). However, the child's absolute blood volume is still small, and relatively small amounts of blood loss may result in critical intravascular volume depletion. For this reason a total of all blood lost or drawn for laboratory analysis (including any neces-

sary "discard" samples) must be recorded on the nursing flow sheet and blood replacement therapy considered (in conjunction with other patient assessment variables) when acute unreplaced blood loss totals 5% to 7% of the child's circulating blood volume. Other patient assessment variables must always be considered (e.g., heart rate, color) as well. Excess blood loss can be virtually eliminated through use of careful sampling techniques.

Physiologic Differences

The differences between neonatal and adult cardiovascular function are largely the result of the transition from fetal to extrauterine circulation. For the most part the hemodynamic changes discussed below are only relevant during the first weeks or months of life. However, cardiopulmonary disease may delay or modify the transition and affect the changes in cardiac function and vascular resistance beyond this time.

Cardiac output. At birth cardiac output is higher per kilogram body weight than during any other time in life, averaging approximately 300 ml/kg/min; cardiac output per kilogram body weight ultimately decreases to 100 ml/kg/min during adolescence and to 70 to 80 ml/kg/min during adult years. Since the child's body weight is small, the child's absolute cardiac output at birth is only approximately 0.6 L/min, but it increases to approximately 6 L/min in the large adolescent or adult male (Table 2-1). The cardiac index throughout childhood is slightly higher than the cardiac index of the adult and is normally 3.5 to 4.5 L/min/m² BSA.

Cardiac output is the product of heart rate and stroke volume. During childhood, heart rate is very rapid and stroke volume is small, so cardiac output is directly proportional to heart rate.

Heart rate. The normal heart rate decreases as the child grows (Table 2-2). Tachycardia provides the most efficient method of increasing cardiac output in a patient of any age, and an increase in heart rate should be observed when the child is active, anxious, or febrile or when cardiorespiratory disease is present. Since, however, the cardiac ouput of the neonate and young infant may be near maximal, an increase in heart rate may only marginally improve cardiac output during early life. In fetal lambs a 40% to 65% increase in heart rate is necessary to improve cardiac output 10% to 20%.

Some slowing of the heart rate should normally be expected when the child is asleep or sedated (Table 2-2). However, a significant fall in heart rate below normal may produce a substantial fall in cardiac output, particularly if cardiorespiratory disease is present. In fetal lambs a fall in heart rate of only 25% can be expected to produce a 20% fall in cardiac output.

Dysrhythmias. In the pediatric patient most dysrhythmias are clinically insignificant; that is, they do not compromise cardiac output or systemic perfusion, and they are not likely to deteriorate into significant dysrhythmias. These insignificant dysrhythmias do not need treatment.

The most common clinically significant dysrhythmias in children are bradycardia and supraventricular tachycardia. The terminal cardiac rhythm in children is most often bradycardia, progressing to asystole. Bradycardia is usually an ominous clinical sign in critically ill or injured children. Slowing of the heart rate may occur as the result of vagal stimulation, and it may be observed in the presence of hypoxemia and acidosis.

Table 2-1 Normal Cardiac Output in Children*

Age	Cardiac Output (L/min)	Heart Rate	Normal Stroke Volume (ml)
Newborn	0.8-1.0	145	5
6 mo	1.0-1.3	120	10
1 yr	1.3-1.5	115	13
2 yr	1.5-2.0	115	18
4 yr	2.3-2.75	105	27
5 yr	2.5-3.0	95	31
8 yr	3.4-3.6	83	42
10 yr	3.8-4.0	75	50
15 yr	6.0	70	85

NOTE: Cardiac index $= \dfrac{\text{Cardiac output}}{\text{m}^2 \text{ BSA}}$

Normal cardiac index in children $= 3.4\text{-}4.5$ L/min/m² BSA

*Reproduced by permission from Hazinski MF. Cardiovascular disorders. In Hazinski MF, ed. Nursing Care of the Critically Ill Child. St. Louis: CV Mosby, 1984, p 90; modified from extrapolation of normal postnatal changes in cardiac output, heart rate, and stroke volume from Rudolph AM. Changes in the circulation after birth. In Congenital Diseases of the Heart. Chicago: Year Book, 1974, p 27.

Table 2-2   Normal Vital Signs in Children

Normal Heart and Respiratory Rate*			
Age	Awake Heart Rate	Sleeping Heart Rate	Respiratory Rate
Infant	120-160/min	80-180/min	30-60/min
Toddler	90-140/min	70-120/min	24-40/min
Preschool	80-110/min	60-90/min	22-34/min
School age	75-100/min	60-90/min	18-30/min
Adolescent	60-90/min	50-90/min	12-16/min

Normal Blood Pressure Ranges†		
Age	Systolic Pressure (mm Hg)	Diastolic Pressure (mm Hg)
Neonate (1 mo)	85-100	51-65
Infant (6 mo)	87-105	53-66
Toddler (2 yr)	95-105	53-66
School age (7 yr)	97-112	57-71
Adolescent (15 yr)	112-128	66-80

*Rates extrapolated from Gillett PC, Garson A, Porter CJ, McNamara DG. Dysrhythmias. In Adams FH, Emmanouilides GC, eds. Moss' Heart Disease in Infants, Children, and Adolescents, 3rd ed. Baltimore: Williams & Wilkins, 1983; and Hazinski MF. Children are different. In Hazinski MF, ed. Nursing Care of the Critically Ill Child. St. Louis: CV Mosby, 1984.
†Blood pressure tables taken from the 50th to 90th percentile ranges of the ages noted; extrapolated from graphs published by Horan MJ (Chairman). Task force on blood pressure control in children. Report of the Second Task Force on Blood Pressure in Children—1987. Pediatrics 79:1, 1987.

Clinically significant ventricular dysrhythmias are unusual in children unless complex congenital heart disease, myocarditis, cardiomyopathy, electrolyte abnormalities, or asphyxia is present. Ventricular dysrhythmias are fairly common in adult patients, however, and the terminal cardiac rhythm in the adult is likely to be ventricular tachycardia or fibrillation.

Myocardial function. Stroke volume is small in the infant and young child, averaging approximately 1.5 ml/kg. During maturation, stroke volume increases from approximately 5 ml in the neonate to approximately 70 to 90 ml in the adolescent (Table 2-1). Ventricular end-diastolic volume increases from approximately 40 ml/m² BSA in infants to approximately 70 ml/m² BSA in children beyond 2 years of age. Infant myocardium actually has a higher ejection fraction than that of the older child.

Most information about developmental changes in myocardial function is based on studies of isolated or nonhuman myocardium; these findings must, therefore, be applied with caution to the human. Newborn lamb myocardium is less compliant and contains a higher water content and less contractile mass than adult sheep myocardium. Fetal animal myocardial fibers shorten less effectively than adult myocardial fibers, and immature canine myocardium demonstrates maximal contractility at smaller end-diastolic volume than the mature dog. Neonatal lambs demonstrate a blunted cardiac output response to volume therapy.

The above research has led to the widespread belief that infants need higher preload (higher ventricular end-diastolic pressure) to maximize cardiac output and may be incapable of increasing stroke volume and cardiac output even with fluid challenges. However, even infant lambs are capable of increasing cardiac output significantly (35% to 70%) in response to volume loading, particularly if systemic vascular resistance is low.

Certainly, by the time the infant is 3 to 8 weeks of age, myocardial response to volume therapy is similar to the response of the adult myocardium, and by 1 to 2 years of age the child's myocardial function is similar to adult myocardial function.

Vascular resistances. At birth, with the conversion from placental to pulmonary oxygenation of the blood, alveolar oxygen concentration increases, and pulmonary vascular resistance begins to fall from 8 to 10 units/m^2 BSA, reaching the "adult" normal levels of 1 to 3 units/m^2 BSA within the first 6 to 8 weeks of life (see p. 6). Right ventricular muscle mass decreases, and a corresponding reduction in right ventricular ECG voltage is seen during infancy.

Even after the normal fall in pulmonary vascular resistance has occurred, the pulmonary vascular bed of the neonate may remain reactive, and reactive pulmonary vasoconstriction may also occur in children with pulmonary hypertension. Reactive pulmonary vasoconstriction is likely to develop as a response to alveolar hypoxia, acidosis, or hypothermia and will produce a rise in pulmonary vascular resistance and an increase in right ventricular afterload.

Systemic vascular resistance and systemic arterial pressure begin to rise with separation of the circulation from the placenta (see p. 6). Normal systemic vascular resistance is 10 to 15 units/m^2 BSA in the infant, 20 to 30 units/m^2 BSA after 12 to 18 months of age, and 30 to 40 units/m^2 BSA during adult years. The rise in systemic vascular resistance corresponds to an increase in left ventricular muscle mass and ECG voltage.

Effect of afterload on myocardial function. In newborn lambs, stroke volume falls dramatically when mild elevations in ventricular afterload are produced. However, human infants seem to be able to maintain normal cardiac output even in the face of moderately elevated afterload (such as that produced by semilunar valve stenosis) unless the increase in afterload is severe or acute.

Response to catecholamines. The development of human adrenergic receptors and the response of normal infants and children to adrenergic receptor stimulation have not been documented. Animal research has demonstrated that cardiovascular parasympathetic innervation and response are virtually the same in all age groups. Sympathetic nervous system innervation to the newborn myocardium is, however, incomplete at birth. Although cardiac adrenergic receptors are present at birth, cardiac norepinephrine levels are lower than adult levels for the first 3 weeks of age. These findings suggest that the neonate will demonstrate a predominance of vagal effects during

the first weeks of life and that cardiac rate and contractile response to endogenous β_1-adrenergic receptor catecholamine stimulation will be limited during this time.

Research regarding response of children to (exogenous) catecholamine administration has yielded contradictory information. Generalization of study conclusions has been impossible since the age and underlying cardiovascular function of the children in each study have varied. It is imperative, therefore, that vasoactive drug administration be titrated at the bedside and the drug selection, dosage, and patient response be carefully and frequently evaluated.

Age-related changes in catecholamine metabolism have not been documented in humans. Excretion of vasoactive drugs will probably be related more to the child's condition than to age, and catecholamine clearance is likely to be prolonged in the presence of hepatic or renal dysfunction in the patient of any age. During catecholamine administration it will be necessary to monitor the patient closely for adverse or toxic effects of each drug, including extreme tachycardia, increased pulmonary artery or wedge pressure, and systemic hypotension.

Historically, higher doses of cardiac glycosides (per kilogram body weight) have been administered to infants than to older children or adults; however, no data exist to support this differential dosage. The volume of distribution of digoxin is larger in infants and children than in adults because much of the drug is stored in skeletal muscle (which constitutes a larger portion of the body mass of the infant than of the adult). However, infant myocardium accumulates digoxin more than adult myocardium, particularly during administration of large "loading" doses of the drug. In addition, digoxin excretion is affected by the glomerular filtration rate, so the half-life of the drug is longest in neonates. For these reasons, premature neonates and infants <12 months of age should receive *lower* digoxin doses per kilogram body weight than children or adults. Caution must be used when administering a digitalis derivative to *premature* neonates since the incidence of clinical toxicity is highest (nearly 30%) in these patients.

PULMONARY DIFFERENCES

The five major components of the respiratory system include (1) the CNS, which serves as the controller of ventilation, (2) the airways, which conduct gas to and from the alveoli, (3) the chest wall that encloses the lungs, (4) the respiratory muscles, and (5) the acinar tissue, which includes the alveolar space and capillaries. Since each of these major components is incompletely developed at birth, newborn respiratory function is inefficient, and the infant is particularly susceptible to respiratory failure.

Anatomic Differences

Central (e.g., carotid body) and peripheral chemoreceptors needed to control ventilation are present at birth, although peripheral chemoreceptors are less numerous in the infant than in the child; all receptors are functional at birth. Developmental changes in control of respiration are discussed in the "Physiologic Differences" section.

Airways. All conducting airways are present at birth, and their numbers do not increase after birth. By contrast, the alveolar epithelial and endothelial layers continue to develop after birth, until 10 to 12 years of age. Thus discrete lung injury early in life may not impair lung development during childhood, and compensatory alveolar growth may occur. However, diffuse neonatal lung injury (e.g., bronchopulmonary dysplasia) may disrupt or delay alveolar growth, resulting in pulmonary dysplasia.

The airway branching pattern is complete at birth, and the airways increase in size and length throughout childhood. Not only are the child's airways smaller than those of the adult, but supporting airway cartilage is not developed until school age. In addition, small airways muscles may be incompletely developed during the first years of life. For these reasons the child's airways are more likely to become obstructed as a result of laryngospasm, bronchospasm, edema, or mucus accumulation. The lack of development of the small airways muscles may render young infants less responsive to bronchodilator therapy than older children.

Closing volume as a percent of total lung volume is higher in infants than it is in healthy adults. There is some evidence that some of the airways remain closed even during normal breathing in the young infant. The significance of this finding is unknown, but it may make the infant more susceptible to atelectasis.

The pediatric larynx is more anterior and cephalad than the adult larynx, and the stiff, cartilaginous epiglottis articulates at a more acute angle with the lar-

ynx than in the adult. Thus the epiglottis may obscure the glottic opening, making intubation difficult. Since the anterior attachment of the vocal cords is below the posterior attachment, a curved endotracheal tube can easily become caught in the anterior commissure, preventing proper advancement of the tube into the trachea. Application of pressure on the cricoid cartilage during intubation will displace the larynx posteriorly and may facilitate intubation.

The pediatric trachea is relatively short, so inadvertent endotracheal tube migration into either mainstem bronchus may easily occur. In addition the orotracheal tube will move with changes in head position—flexion of the neck displaces the tip of the tube further into the trachea and extension of the neck moves the tube further out of the trachea.

The narrowest part of the pediatric larynx (until 8 years of age) is at the cricoid cartilage, whereas the narrowest portion of the adolescent or adult larynx is at the vocal cords. This difference must be considered during selection of the endotracheal tube; the child's endotracheal tube must be smaller than that which will easily pass through the vocal cords and should allow a slight air leak at the level of the cricoid cartilage when approximately 20 cm H_2O positive pressure is provided. Use of a cuffed tube is thought to be contraindicated in children <8 years of age since the cuff may damage the trachea.

During the first 5 to 8 years of age the growth of the child's distal airways is proportionately slower than the growth of the proximal airways, so the distal airways provide proportionally more resistance to airflow than the distal airways of the adult.

Chest wall. The chest wall encloses and supports the lungs. The cartilaginous ribs of the infant and young child are twice as compliant as the bony ribs of the older child or adult. During episodes of respiratory distress the infant's chest wall will retract; this reduces the infant's ability to maintain functional residual capacity or increase tidal volume, and it increases the work of breathing.

The infant's ribs are oriented in a more horizontal direction than in the adult because they articulate linearly with the spinal column and sternum. The infant's chest has less anterior-posterior displacement during inspiration than the adult chest. These factors tend to reduce the mechanical efficiency of respiratory muscle function during the first years of life since intercostal muscles do not have the leverage needed to lift the ribs effectively. As the child grows, the rib articulation changes to a 45-degree angle, and the intercostal muscles are able to elevate the ribs and contribute to chest expansion.

The diaphragm muscles insert horizontally on the inner surfaces of the ribs of the infant instead of obliquely as in the adult. If the infant is placed in the supine position, diaphragm movement may be compromised since diaphragm contraction may well draw the ribs inward rather than expand the chest outward.

Respiratory muscles. The respiratory muscles consist of the muscles of the upper airway, the lower airways, and the diaphragm, and they contribute to expansion of the lung and maintenance of airway patency. The respiratory muscles of the infant and young child may lack tone, power, and coordination; this will reduce respiratory efficiency.

In a patient of any age the diaphragm is the chief muscle of respiration. Anything that impedes diaphragm movement (e.g., abdominal distention) can result in respiratory failure in the young child. In the relaxed state the neonatal diaphragm is located higher in the thorax and has a smaller radius of curvature than the adult diaphragm, reducing the efficiency of diaphragm contraction. If a hemidiaphragm is paralyzed during infancy or early childhood, a type of flail chest results. The flaccid hemidiaphragm will be pulled up into the chest during contraction of the functioning (contralateral) hemidiaphragm, and respiratory failure usually results.

The intercostal muscles are not fully developed until school age, so they act primarily to stabilize the chest wall during the first years of life. Since the intercostal muscles have neither the leverage nor the strength to lift the rib cage, the young child depends on diaphragm function to generate a tidal volume.

Lung tissue. Postnatal pulmonary growth consists of an increase in alveolar size and number, which produces a corresponding increase in alveolar surface area from 2.8 to 32 m² and an increase in lung volume from 200 ml to 2.2 L by 8 years of age. There is a smaller amount of elastic and collagen tissue in the neonatal lung as compared to the adult lung. As a result, liquid or air can easily enter the pulmonary interstitium; this may explain the increased tendency of infants to develop pulmonary edema, pneumomediastinum, pneumothorax, and interstitial emphysema. Reduced elastic fibers contribute to the ten-

dency for small airway collapse. Because elastic recoil of the thorax and lung is low, pleural pressure is nearly atmospheric; this may also contribute to premature airway closure during this age. Elastic fibers increase in number, approaching adult quantities by approximately 4 years of age.

Physiologic Differences

CNS control of breathing. At birth all central (in the ventral brain stem) and peripheral (in the carotid body) chemoreceptors are present and functioning to control respiration, and chemoreceptor response is normal soon after birth. For unknown reasons, however, the premature infant and the neonate may demonstrate a biphasic response to hypoxemia, consisting of a transient hyperpnea followed by hypoventilation. Beyond the neonatal period, control of breathing should resemble that of the adult.

Airways. The airways of the child are significantly smaller than the airways of the adult. Since resistance to airflow is inversely proportional to one divided by the fourth power of the airway radius (resistance to airflow increases exponentially as the radius of the airway is reduced), a small reduction in airway radius from edema or mucus accumulation can produce substantial increases in resistance to airflow. For example, if the infant with a 4 mm trachea has 1 mm of circumferential laryngeal edema or inflammation, the airway radius will be reduced by 50% (from 2 to 1 mm) and resistance to airflow increased 16-fold. If the adult patient with a 10 mm larynx has 1 mm of circumferential edema, the airway radius will be reduced by only 20% (from 5 to 4 mm) and resistance to airflow increased only 2-fold.

The peripheral airways of the adult provide approximately 20% of total airway resistance; these same airways contribute up to 50% of the total airway resistance in children up to 5 years of age. As a result, small airways diseases such as bronchiolitis may result in significant increases in resistance to airflow and severe respiratory distress.

During mechanical ventilation the high peripheral airway resistance and reduced lung compliance of the child must be considered. Not only must adequate inspiratory time be allowed, but adequate exhalation time must be provided or air trapping will develop.

Chest wall. As noted above, the compliance of the infant's chest wall is approximately double the compliance of the chest wall of the adult. Since the infant's lungs are stiff, it may become very difficult for the spontaneously breathing infant to maintain an adequate lung volume even at rest and particularly during periods of respiratory distress.

During effective positive pressure ventilation the infant's compliant chest wall should expand outward easily. If the chest wall does not expand during positive-pressure ventilation, it is likely that the child is not being adequately ventilated.

As the child grows, chest wall compliance decreases, and elastic outward recoil of the rib cage increases because of an increase in chest wall muscle tone. These changes improve the child's ability to maintain functional residual capacity, reducing the likelihood of atelectasis and small airway closure.

Respiratory muscles. Since respiratory muscles of the infant often lack the tone, power, and coordination of the adult respiratory system, respiratory failure is likely to develop during episodes of respiratory distress. Abdominal breathing is normal in infants and young children; typically the abdomen and chest wall rise together during inspiration. Therefore abdominal distention or decreased abdominal wall compliance (such as occurs with gastric distention or peritonitis) can interfere with diaphragm excursion and effective ventilation. Paradoxical abdominal motion during inspiration, with the abdomen protruding outward when the chest retracts inward, may be a sign of severe respiratory distress and will further impair the infant's ability to generate an adequate tidal volume.

The infant with severe respiratory distress will often grunt during exhalation. Grunting results from closure of the glottis during active exhalation, which increases transpulmonary pressure, lung volume, and functional residual capacity. If grunting is observed, ventilatory support should be considered. The effect of grunting is mimicked by provision of continuous positive airway pressure or positive end-expiratory pressure during assisted ventilation.

Lung tissue. During childhood, lung distensibility or compliance (change in lung volume per cm H_2O change in pressure) increases from approximately 4 to 6 ml/cm H_2O in the neonate to approximately 77 ml/cm H_2O in the school-age child. Lung compliance in the adult averages approximately 150 ml/cm H_2O. Since the chest wall is becoming progressively "stiffer" as the lung compliance increases, ventilation becomes more efficient as the child grows.

The relative sizes of lung volumes and capacities remain the same throughout life. The tidal volume averages 6 to 7 cc/kg body weight and constitutes approximately 8% of total lung capacity. Since the absolute tidal volume of the child is small, mechanical ventilators for children must be capable of providing small tidal volumes in short inspiratory times at low pressures. This usually requires use of ventilators with flow characteristics that are different from the ventilators used with adult patients.

NEUROLOGIC DIFFERENCES
Anatomic Differences

At birth, all major structures of the brain and all cranial nerves are developed. As the child grows the brain increases dramatically in size and complexity. During the first years of life the brain achieves more than 90% of the adult number of brain cells, and it triples in weight as a result of the development of fiber tracts, synapses, and myelination. By 2½ years of age the brain has reached 75% of its mature adult weight, and by 6 years approximately 90% of the mature adult brain weight has been achieved.

The cranial nerves and some central neurons are myelinated at birth. At 1 year of age all major nerve tracts are myelinated.

The cranial sutures do not fuse until approximately 16 to 18 months of age. As a result, if there is a gradual increase in intracranial volume during infancy, head circumference may increase. This potential for head expansion will not, however, prevent increased intracranial pressure from developing, particularly if intracranial volume increases acutely.

Normal cerebral blood flow and cerebral perfusion pressure values in infants and children are unknown. Cerebral blood flow has been estimated at 30 to 55 ml blood flow/100 g brain tissue/min, and it is primarily distributed in the temporal and occipital regions during infancy. Adult cerebral blood flow has been measured at 50 ml/100 g brain tissue/min and is distributed preferentially to the frontal lobes of the brain.

The normal volume of CSF production during childhood is unknown, although the average volume of CSF present in the neonatal CNS is estimated at 40 to 50 ml. Normal CSF content varies as the child matures. The normal neonatal CSF may demonstrate 1 to 4 white blood cells (WBCs)/ml and occasional polymorphonuclear leukocytes. However, beyond 6 months of age WBCs are generally absent, and polymorphonuclear leukocytes should not be seen. Protein concentration is generally >90 mg/100 ml in the neonate and ranges from 15 to 40 mg/100 ml beyond 6 months of age.

Physiologic Differences

At birth the infant functions largely at a subcortical level, and most responses are reflexive in nature. Many reflexes are of a primitive nature and will disappear with maturation. The term infant will demonstrate a dominance of flexor tone, and children of all ages will be responsive to touch.

Electrical activity in the brain is incompletely developed at birth. During infancy there is an increase in frequency and amplitude of resting electrical activity. Brief periods of flattening of the EEG have been reported in normal neonates; this observation has led the Task Force on Brain Death Determination in Children to recommend an extended observation period (i.e., 48 hours) for infants 7 days to 2 months of age before brain death is pronounced, although this is controversial.

There is a general perception that survival and recovery following head injury during childhood is better than following head injury during the adult years, and this is attributed to the continued growth of the CNS during early childhood. Although it is not clear that pediatric survival is better than adult survival, most children who do survive serious head injury ultimately make a good to excellent recovery.

The Glasgow Coma Scale is not thought to be useful in predicting outcome following severe cerebral insult in preverbal or intubated children. Since it does not accurately differentiate between survivors and nonsurvivors in the pediatric population, several alternative pediatric scoring systems have been developed.

FLUID AND ELECTROLYTE BALANCE
Anatomic Differences

Water distribution. A major portion of a child's body weight is water, constituting approximately 75% of the full-term infant's weight and approximately 60% to 70% of the weight of the adolescent or adult. During the first months of life most body water is located in the extracellular compartment, and much of this water is exchanged daily. Both the infant and young child have a large surface area/volume ratio; they therefore lose a larger amount of water to the environment through evaporation than does the adult.

Renal development. At birth the neonate possesses the adult complement of nephrons, but only approximately 50% of the nephrons are located in the renal cortex. After birth, however, tubular length and volume and glomerular size increase, and 85% of all nephrons will be located in the cortex.

Renal blood flow accounts for only approximately 5% to 10% of total cardiac output at birth, and only approximately 50% of renal blood flow passes through the cortex because the cortical glomeruli are immature and renal vascular resistance is high. In the older child, approximately 25% of cardiac output passes through the kidneys, and most (80% to 90%) of this blood flow passes through the renal cortex.

Absolute glomerular filtration rate (GFR), as well as GFR in relation to weight or body surface area, is low in the neonate. During the first weeks of life, GFR increases rapidly as the result of the increase in renal blood flow and a decrease in renal vascular resistance. GFR in the neonate averages approximately 2.5 ml/min and rises to approximately 15.5 ml/min in the 6-month-old infant and to approximately 50 ml/min in the preschooler. By adult years GFR has increased to approximately 131 ml/min.

Electrolyte balance. For the most part, maintenance of electrolyte balance is identical in children and adults.

Glucose homeostasis. Hypoglycemia is more likely to develop in infants than in adults. Infants have high caloric needs and low glycogen stores; thus, during episodes of stress, the infant is likely to develop hypoglycemia, whereas the adult may well demonstrate hyperglycemia.

Physiologic Differences

Water distribution. The child's metabolic rate and evaporative losses are higher than those of the adult, so the child has higher maintenance fluid requirements per kilogram body weight. However, since the child's body weight is small, the absolute fluid volume administered to the child will be small. All fluid administered in the PICU must be administered through a volume-controlled infusion pump to enable precise regulation of fluid administration. Maintenance fluid requirements must be calculated for each child and modified by the health care team according to the child's clinical condition (see Chapter 15).

The young child may rapidly become dehydrated or fluid overloaded. It is imperative to keep track of all sources of fluid intake (including oral intake, IV fluids, and all fluids used to flush monitoring lines or administer medications) and all sources of fluid loss (including urine, stool, emesis, and drainage). The critically ill child's fluid balance must be calculated on an hourly basis so that appropriate modifications in therapy may be made as needed.

Renal function. After birth there is a significant increase in renal blood flow and GFR. In addition, an increase in renal cortical blood flow occurs. These changes are associated with a rapid rise in renal sodium reabsorption within the first days of life. Even at birth the kidney is capable of excreting a large volume load, although maximal volume excretion occurs when the GFR increases.

The fetal kidney produces large quantities of urine with a high sodium concentration. During the first 72 hours of life continued renal sodium and water excretion result in a normal weight loss equivalent to approximately 5% to 10% of birthweight. By the end of the first week of life in the term infant there is equilibration between sodium and water intake and excretion. Premature infants, however, may continue to demonstrate sodium wasting for several weeks as the result of immature tubular function and relative aldosterone insensitivity.

The newborn kidney is less capable of excreting a solute load than is the kidney of the older child because of decreased availability of urea and decreased tubular length and responsiveness to antidiuretic hormone (ADH). The neonate utilizes nearly all dietary protein for growth; as a result, less protein is catabolized to urea, and less medullary urea is available in the loop of Henle to concentrate the urine. As the infant's protein intake increases, more urea is available in the urine, and urine osmolality increases. In addition, as the child grows, the tubules lengthen and become more responsive to ADH; for these reasons renal concentrating ability increases.

During the first year of life the kidney has a lower threshold for bicarbonate reabsorption than during any other period of life. The ability to excrete acid is limited during the first weeks of life by the low GFR, so metabolic acidosis may develop rapidly in the infant with increased hydrogen ion production.

Normal minimal urine volume in the well-hydrated infant averages 2 ml/kg/hr, and normal minimal urine volume in the child averages 1 ml/kg/hr.

The well-hydrated adult may only excrete an average of 0.5 ml/kg/hr. Normal urine osmolality is hypotonic with respect to plasma during the first days of life, but it should approach adult values within the first month of life.

Glucose homeostasis. As noted previously, hypoglycemia is likely to occur in critically ill infants. Therefore the infant's serum or heelstick glucose concentration must be closely monitored (hourly or more often if condition and marginal glucose levels indicate). The critically ill infant requires a continuous source of glucose intake to maintain an acceptable serum glucose level; intermittent "bolus" administration of glucose in response to hypoglycemia will only perpetuate wide fluctuations in serum glucose, and therefore a continuous glucose infusion is a preferable method of treatment for hypoglycemia.

GASTROINTESTINAL FUNCTION AND METABOLIC DIFFERENCES
Anatomic Differences

GI system. At birth all structures of the alimentary tract are present, although they increase in size and function during childhood. GI secretory function, enzyme activity, and carbohydrate and fat absorption are similar in the infant and adult. The mucosal barrier within the small intestine epithelium is incomplete in the neonate, so absorption of ingested food antigens may occur during the first weeks of life. In addition the bacterial flora of the GI tract may be a source of bacteremia in the neonate.

At birth the liver synthesizes plasma proteins (except immunoglobulins); stores, synthesizes, and converts carbohydrates; and releases glucose from glucagon, just as in the adult. However, the neonatal liver is immature, and enzymatic synthesis and degradation do not reach adult levels until several weeks of age. Synthesis of vitamin K–dependent clotting factors is reduced significantly at birth, and prothrombin time is often dramatically prolonged on the second or third day of life; this drop in clotting factor levels is prevented by the administration of vitamin K to the neonate.

Nutritional requirements. The child's metabolic rate is higher than that of the adult, so the child's nutritional and caloric needs will also be higher per kilogram body weight than the adult.

Thermoregulation. Infants and young children have a large surface area/volume ratio and decreased insulating subcutaneous fat stores. As a result, they can lose a great deal of heat to the environment through evaporation and radiation. Additional heat loss will occur with the administration of large volumes of room temperature IV or dialysis fluids. The infant cannot shiver to generate heat and will be forced to break down "brown fat," which is located around the kidneys, adrenals, between the scapulae, and around the large thoracic vessels.

Physiologic Differences

GI system. Gastric motility is reduced and gastric emptying is more rapid in the neonate and infant than in the older child, and virtually all neonates have some degree of gastroesophageal reflux.

The neonatal liver is less able to metabolize toxic substances through oxidative detoxification or conjugation than is the liver of the older child or adult. Depression of these activities may result in prolongation of beneficial or toxic effects of drugs or their metabolites.

Conjugation of bilirubin by the newborn liver is less efficient than in older children or adults. During the neonatal period, bilirubin load is increased as the result of more rapid erythrocyte turnover and bilirubin production and enhanced intestinal bilirubin reabsorption. These conditions result in transient hyperbilirubinemia in even normal neonates and more profound hyperbilirubinemia in premature neonates.

Nutritional requirements. The child's maintenance caloric requirements are higher per kilogram body weight than the requirements of the adult. In addition a large portion of the child's caloric requirements are needed for basal metabolism and cell growth. For this reason even the comatose child will need high-calorie nutrition, and the child with cardiorespiratory distress, sepsis, wound healing, or multisystem disease or trauma may well need nearly double the average "maintenance" calories. Caloric requirements will be increased approximately 10%/°C elevation if the temperature is >37° C/day. The highest known caloric requirements occur in burn patients.

Thermoregulation. When the infant is exposed to a cold environmental temperature, endogenous norepinephrine is secreted, stimulating the breakdown of brown fat and release of heat. However, this "nonshivering thermogenesis" is an energy-requiring process and will result in an increase in the infant's oxygen consumption. To eliminate the need for non-shivering thermogenesis, a neutral thermal environment should be provided for the neonate and young infant. A neutral thermal environment is that environmental temperature at which the neonate maintains a rectal temperature of 37° C with the lowest oxygen consumption. The ranges of neutral thermal environment have been experimentally determined for infants of various ages and birth weights (see Chapter 21). Neutral thermal environments can be maintained most efficiently in the PICU through use of overbed warmers; these warmers heat the air surrounding the infant or child, yet allow ready access to the patient for observation or treatment. Such warmers should only be used with servo-controls, so the risk of excessive or inadequate warming and thermal injury is reduced (see Chapter 110), and drafts near the bedside need to be eliminated. Use of radiant warmers will increase evaporative fluid losses in young infants, so fluid administration rate needs to be evaluated accordingly.

IMMUNOLOGIC DIFFERENCES

Neonates are particularly vulnerable to infection for several reasons. Passive immunity is normally conveyed from the mother to the fetus through transmission of immunoglobulins during the last trimester, so the very premature neonate is immunoglobulin-deficient. The neonate has decreased polymorphonuclear leukocyte function and small polymorphonuclear leukocyte storage pools. Neonates also have a decreased ability to synthesize new antibodies, and they cannot make and deliver adequate numbers of phagocytes to sites of infection. Poor nutrition during hospitalization can lead to reduced protein synthesis and further reduction in antibody formation.

Infants have not yet built up their own immunoglobulin stores, and maternal immunoglobulin stores are depleted at approximately 2 to 5 months of age. As a result, infants are less able to phagocytize bacteria or form antibodies, leaving them particularly vulnerable to polysaccharide-carrying bacteria (e.g., *Haemophilus influenzae*) between 4 to 18 months of age. Low immunoglobulin levels also render the infant very susceptible to viral infection. Adult levels of immunoglobulins are achieved at approximately 4 to 7 years of age.

Although there is a widespread perception that children are also more susceptible to infection than adults, the incidence of nosocomial infections in the

PICU is actually lower than the incidence of similar infections in adult ICUs. Nosocomial infections in children are most likely to develop as cutaneous infections, bacteremias, or pneumonias, whereas nosocomial infections in adults are most likely to appear as urinary tract or wound infections.

There is no question that the risk of nosocomial infection increases when the child remains in the PICU for more than 14 days and when the child requires prolonged intubation, arterial or CVP catheterization, or ICP monitoring. Thorough handwashing before and after patient contact is mandatory for every member of the health care team (see Chapter 41).

ADDITIONAL READING

Agostoni E, Mognoni P, Torri G. Relation between changes of rib cage circumference and lung volume. J Appl Physiol 20:1179, 1965.

Aherne W, Hull D. Brown adipose tissue and heat production in the newborn infant. J Pathol Bacteriol 91:223, 1966.

Berman WJ Jr. The relationship of age to the effects and toxicity of digoxin in sheep. In Heymann MA, Rudolph AM (Co-Chairpersons). The Ductus Arteriosus. Report of the Seventy-fifth Ross Conference on Pediatric Research. Columbus, Ohio: Ross Laboratories, 1978.

Bohn DJ, Poirier CS, Edmonds JF, et al. Hemodynamic effects of dobutamine after cardiopulmonary bypass in children. Crit Care Med 8:367, 1980.

Boyden EA. Development and growth of the airways. In Hodson WA, ed. Development of the Lung. New York: Marcel Dekker, 1977.

Brown RB, Hosmer D, Chen HC, et al. A comparison of infections in different ICUs within the same hospital. Crit Care Med 13:472, 1985.

Bruce DA, Schut L. Management of acute craniocerebral trauma in children. Contemp Neurosurg 10:1, 1979.

• Chameides L, ed. Texbook of Pediatric Advanced Life Support. Dallas: American Heart Association, 1988.

Chernick V, Avery ME. The functional basis of respiratory pathology. In Kendig EL, ed. Disorders of the Respiratory Tract in Children. Philadelphia: WB Saunders, 1977.

Clyman RI, Roman C, Heymann MA, et al. How a patent ductus arteriosus affects the premature lamb's ability to handle additional volume loads. Pediatr Res 22:531, 1987.

• Clyman RI, Teitel D, Padbury J, et al. The role of beta-adrenoreceptor stimulation and contractile state in the preterm lamb's response to altered ductus atreriosus patency. Pediatr Res 23:316, 1988.

• Coulter DL. Neurologic uncertainty in newborn intensive care. N Engl J Med 316:841, 1987.

Davis GM, Bureau MA. Pulmonary mechanics in newborn respiratory control. Clin Perinatol 14:551, 1987.

Donn SM, Kuhns LR. Mechanisms of endotracheal tube movement with change of head position in the neonate. Pediatr Radiol 9:39, 1980.

Driscoll DJ. Use of inotropic and chronotropic agents in neonates. Clin Perinatol 14:931, 1987.

Edelman CM Jr., Barnett HL, Troupka V. Renal concentrating mechanisms in newborn infants. J Clin Invest 39:1062, 1960.

Eisenberg M, Bergner L, Hallstrom A. Epidemiology of cardiac arrest and resuscitation in children. Ann Emerg Med 12:672, 1983.

Finholt DA, Kettrick RG, Wagner HR, et al. The heart is under the lower third of the sternum. Am J Dis Child 140:646, 1986.

Freeman JM, Ferry PC. New brain death guidelines in children: Further confusion. Pediatrics 81:301, 1988.

Friedman WF. The intrinsic physiologic properties of the developing heart. In Friedman WF, ed. Neonatal Heart Disease. New York: Grune & Stratton, 1973.

Friedman WF, Pool PE, Jacobowitz D, et al. Sympathetic innervation of the developing rabbit heart. Circ Res 23:25, 1968.

Friss-Hansen B. Body water compartments in children. Pediatrics 28:169, 1961.

Godfrey S. Respiration. In Godfrey S, Baum J. Clinical Pediatric Physiology. Oxford: Blackwell, 1979.

Graham TP Jr., Jarmakani JM, Atwood GF, et al. Right ventricular volume determinations in children. Normal values and observations with volume or pressure overload. Circulation 47:144, 1973.

Harrison VC, de Hesse E, Klein M. The significance of grunt in hyaline membrane disease. Pediatrics 41:549, 1968.

• Hazinski MF. Hemodynamic monitoring of children. In Daily EK, Schroeder JS, eds. Techniques in Bedside Hemodynamic Monitoring, 4th ed. St. Louis: CV Mosby, 1989.

Hogg JC, Williams J, Richardson JB, et al. Age as a factor in the distribution of lower-airway conductance and in the pathologic anatomy of obstructive lung disease. N Engl J Med 282:1283, 1970.

Jansen AH, Chernick V. Onset of breathing and control of respiration. Semin Perinatol 12:104, 1988.

Klopfenstein HS, Rudolph AM. Postnatal changes in the circulation and responses to volume loading in sheep. Circ Res 42:839, 1978.

Kirsch JR, Traystman RJ, Rogers MC. Cerebral blood flow measurement techniques in infants and children. Pediatrics 75:887, 1985.

Liebman J, Plonsey R. Electrocardiography. In Adams FH, Emmanouilides GC, eds. Moss' Heart Disease in Infants, Children and Adolescents, 3rd ed. Baltimore: Williams & Wilkins, 1984.

McBride JT, Wohl MEB, Strieder DJ, et al. Lung growth and airway function after lobectomy in infancy for congenital lobar emphysema. J Clin Invest 66:962, 1980.

Menon RK, Sperling MA. Carbohydrate metabolism. Semin Perinatol 12:157, 1988.

Milliken J, Tait GA, Ford-Jones EL, et al. Nosocomial infections in a pediatric intensive care unit. Crit Care Med 16:233, 1988.

Morray JP, Tyler DC, Jones TK, et al. Coma scale for use in brain-injured children. Crit Care Med 12:1018, 1984.

Muller NI, Bryan AC. Chest wall mechanics and respiratory muscles. Pediatr Clin North Am 26:503, 1979.

Orlowski J. Optimum position for external cardiac compression in infants and young children. Ann Emerg Med 15:667, 1986.

Park MK. Use of digoxin in infants and children, with specific emphasis on dosage. J Pediatr 108:871, 1986.

Perkin RM, Levin DL, Wcbb R, et al. Dobutamine: A hemodynamic evaluation in children with shock. J Pediatr 100:977, 1982.

Portnoy JM, Olson LC. Normal cerebrospinal values in children: Another look. Pediatrics 75:484, 1985.

Robatham JL. Maturation of the respiratory system. In Shoemaker WC, Thompson WL, Holbrook PR, eds. Textbook of Critical Care, 2nd ed. Philadelphia: WB Saunders, 1988.

Roberts RJ. Drug Therapy in Infants: Pharmacologic Principles and Clinical Experience. Philadelphia: WB Saunders, 1984.

Robillard JE, Nakamura KT, Matherne GP, et al. Renal hemodynamics and functional adjustments to postnatal life. Semin Perinatol 12:143, 1988.

Romero TE, Friedman WF. Limited left ventricular response to volume overload in the neonatal period: A comparative study with the adult animal. Pediatr Res 13:910, 1979.

Romero T, Covell J, Friedman W. A comparison of pressure-volume relations of the fetal, newborn and adult heart. Am J Physiol 222:1285, 1972.

Rowlatt UF, Rimoldi HJA, Lev M. The quantitative anatomy of the normal child's heart. Pediatr Clin North Am 10:499, 1963.

Rudolph AM. Fetal circulation and cardiovascular adjustments after birth. In Rudolph AM, ed. Pediatrics, 18th ed. East Norwalk, Conn.: Appleton & Lange, 1986.

Rudolph AM. The changes in the circulation after birth. Circulation 41:343, 1970.

Rudolph AM, Heymann MA. Cardiac ouput in the fetal lamb: The effects of spontaneous and induced changes of heart rate on right and left ventricular ouput. Am J Obstet Gynecol 124:183, 1976.

Sarff LD, Platt LH, McCracken GH Jr, et al. Cerebrospinal fluid evaluation in neonates: Comparison of high-risk neonates with and without meningitis. J Pediatr 88:473, 1976.

Schreiber MD, Meymann MA, Soifer SJ. Increased arterial pH, not decreased $PaCO_2$ attenuates hypoxia-induced pulmonary vasoconstriction in newborn lambs. Pediatr Res 20:113, 1986.

Shelley HJ. Carbohydrate reserves in the newborn infant. Br Med J 1:273, 1964.

Spotnitz WD, Sponitz HM, Truccone NJ, et al. Relation of ultrastructure and function. Sarcomere dimensions, pressure-volume curves, and geometry of the intact left ventricle of the immature canine heart. Circ Res 44:679, 1979.

• Task Force on Brain Death Determination in Children. Guidelines for the determination of brain death in children. Pediatrics 80:298, 1987.

Thornburg KL, Morton MJ. Filling and arterial pressures as determinants of RV stroke volume in the sheep fetus. Am J Physiol 244:H656, 1983.

Tooley WH. Lung growth in infancy and childhood. In Rudolph AM, ed. Pediatrics, 18th ed. East Norwalk, Conn.: Appleton & Lange, 1986.

Walsh CK, Krongrad E. Terminal cardiac electrical activity in pediatric patients. Am J Cardiol 51:557, 1983.

Wilson CB. Immunologic basis for increased susceptibility of the neonate to infection. J Pediatr 108:1, 1986.

Younkin D, Delivoria-Papadopoulos M, Reivich M, Jaggi J, et al. Regional variations in human newborn cerebral blood flow. J Pediatr 112:104, 1988.

• Zaritsky A, Chernow B. Use of catecholamines in pediatrics. J Pediatr 105:341, 1984.

Zaritsky A, Lotze A, Stull R, et al. Steady-state dopamine clearance in critically ill infants and children. Crit Care Med 16:217, 1988.

Zuccarello M, Facco E, Zampieri P, et al. Severe head injury in children: early prognosis and outcome. Childs Nerv Syst 1:158, 1985.

3 Admission Procedures

Donna S. Rahn

BACKGROUND

Patients admitted to a pediatric intensive care unit (PICU) may vary in age from the newborn infant just a few hours old to teenagers approaching adulthood. Their illnesses are as varied as their ages and involve all major organ systems. The one thing they all have in common is that they are critically ill and are dependent on the expertise and knowledge of the medical team to get them through their crises. Patients may come from the operating room following surgery and need close observation by a staff skilled in caring for their particular needs. Patients may also be transferred from the wards and need more aggressive care and closer supervision than can be provided on the ward, or they may come from another hospital that was unable to care for them. All patients admitted to the PICU have specific problems; an initial, thorough assessment is imperative to identify and treat these specific problems early, thoroughly, and aggressively.

The initial assessment is the basis of all further observations and is relied on throughout the hospital stay as a basis for comparison to later observations. Early observations, best noted by the admitting nurse, must be recorded accurately and completely through charting. Recording of the basic assessment and initial data is necessary for proper management of the patient and demonstrates the success or failure of that management by noting changes from the information recorded initially. Medications, fluid calculations, and placement of various catheters rely on the accuracy of the nurse in obtaining and charting the patient's weight and body measurements (e.g., frontal-occipital head circumference, abdominal girth, chest, length or height, shoulder to umbilicus measurement). The admission routines are performed as quickly and thoroughly as the patient's condition will allow. Patients admitted under emer-

gency conditions will need more immediate attention with a brief assessment to identify the most critical needs, followed by a complete assessment once the patient is stabilized. A thorough assessment can identify problems not related to the admitting diagnosis and can alert the health care team to other unrecognized or potential problems.

The PICU nurse and physician must rely on their instincts as well as the physical data in caring for the critically ill child. Physical data can be interpreted as critical or not, depending on the overall assessment of the patient. The health care specialists at the bedside need to look at the patient, review the entire process, and rely on past experiences to realize how sick these children really are. When children become ill, their condition tends to deteriorate quite rapidly until medical attention intervenes to slow down or stop the process. Therefore, when patients are scheduled for admission to the PICU, all necessary preparation must be completed before their arrival.

PREPARING FOR ADMISSION

The most important initial task is to prepare for the patient's arrival at the PICU. Having become familiar with all available information about the patient, the admitting nurse can prepare for the admission. The nurse must anticipate the patient's needs and have all necessary equipment available and in good working order for any emergency situation that might arise on arrival or shortly thereafter.

Once the patient is accepted for admission to the unit, the nurse must set up the patient care area. The appropriate size bed, Isolette, or radiant warmer is acquired. A cardiac-respiratory monitor with capability for pressure readings is checked for proper functioning, along with an oxygen saturation monitor and a Dinamapp (noninvasive automatic blood pressure device), when available. Essential emergency resuscitation equipment must be at all bedsides: for example, anesthesia bag and appropriate size mask for hand ventilation; suction and appropriate size catheters; tonsil suction; oxygen; and IV equipment, including infusion pump and tubing. A crash cart (including emergency medications), a procedure cart for intubation and/or cutdowns, a thoracentesis tray, and a defibrillator must be immediately available. A scale for weighing the patient must be at the bedside, and respiratory therapy is notified to have, when indicated, a mechanical ventilator available. Possible procedures need to be anticipated and any necessary supplies collected: for example, nasogastric or feeding tube; bladder catheterization set; transducers for pressure lines (arterial or central venous pressure); and/or lumbar puncture tray. The bedside drawers are stocked with a stethoscope and appropriate size blood pressure cuff as well as necessary equipment for routine care. The necessary paperwork is assembled for the admission routines: nurse's assessment and narrative notes; medication and graphic records; physician orders; and respiratory therapy records.

ADMISSION ASSESSMENT

On arrival the patient must be assessed for any distress or other problems that must be taken care of immediately. If the child seems to be stable, the vital signs need to be taken at once. Vital signs must include heart and respiratory rates, systemic arterial blood pressure, temperature, and capillary refill. After vital signs are measured, the patient can be transferred to the scales. When a patient is being weighed, every precaution must be taken to provide adequate

---

ESSENTIAL BEDSIDE ITEMS

Alcohol swabs	Betadine swabs	Lancets
Band-Aids	Cotton balls	Temperature probe pasties
Electrodes	Tape measures	Finger cots
Rubber bands	Safety pins	Adhesive remover
Syringe adapters	Injection caps	Hematocrit tubes
Tape	Dextrostix	Blood specimen tubes
Labstix	Lubricant packets	Syringes
Needles	Tongue blades	Cotton-tip applicators
Stethoscope	Blood pressure cuff	Manometer

ADMISSION ROUTINES

Weight	Specific gravity
Temperature	Suction
Heart rate	Measurements (for infants <1 mo old and/or <2500 g)
Respiratory rate	Frontal-occipital
Blood pressure	Abdominal girth
Dextrostix	Length
Hematocrit	Chest
Bag for urinalysis	Shoulder-umbilicus
Labstix	

NURSING

PAGE E

DATE ___ / ___ / ___

TIME	NEURO							CARDIAC				RESPIRATORY			
	PUPILS		COMA SCORE				FONT	ACTIV	HEART SOUNDS	PERIPH PULSES	CAPIL REFILL	COLOR LIPS/NAILS	RESP QUALITY	BREATH SOUNDS	
	L	R	E	V	M										

CODES

NEURO

Pupils

± REACTS SLOWLY
+ REACTS
‡ REACTS BRISKLY
– NO REACTION

Coma Score

E O 4 — SPONTANEOUSLY
Y P 3 — TO SPEECH
E E 2 — TO PAIN
S N 1 — NONE
    0 — CLOSED BY SWELLING

V R 5 — ORIENTED
E E 4 — CONFUSED, EASILY AROUSED
R S 3 — INAPPROPRIATE
B P   WORDS, CRIES TO STIMULUS
A O 2 — INCOMPREHENSIBLE
L N   SOUNDS
S 1 — NONE
E 0*— ETT, TRACH

M R 6 — OBEYS COMMANDS
O E 5 — LOCALIZE PAIN
T S 4 — WITHDRAWS IN
O P   RESPONSE TO PAIN
R O 3 — FLEXION TO PAIN
N 2 — EXTENSION TO PAIN
S 1 — NONE
E   USUALLY RECORD
    BEST ARM RESPONSE

Mod. Infant Coma Score

V R 5 — COOS, BABBLES
E E 4 — IRRITABLE; CRIES
R S 3 — CRIES TO PAIN
B P 2 — MOANS TO PAIN
A O 1 — NONE
L N
S
E

M 6 — NORMAL SPONTANEOUS
O E   MOVEMENTS
T S 5 — WITHDRAWS TO TOUCH
O P 4 — WITHDRAWS TO PAIN
R O 3 — ABNORMAL FLEXION
N 2 — ABNORMAL EXTENSION
S 1 — NONE
E

Fontanel

S — SOFT   Fr — FIRM
F — FLAT   Fl — FULL
D — DEPRESSED B — BULGING

Activity

SA — SPONTANEOUSLY ACTIVE,
    MOVES ALL EXTREMITIES
AS — ACTIVE WITH STIMULATION
I — IRRITABLE
J — JITTERY
S — SEIZURE*
↓ — DECREASED ACTIVITY
↑ — INCREASED ACTIVITY
N — NO RESPONSE

CARDIAC

Heart Sounds

S — STRONG
R — REGULAR
I — IRREGULAR
M — MURMUR
D — DISTANT

RESPIRATORY

Color

P — PINK
W — PALE
D — DUSKY
C — CYANOTIC

Respiratory Quality

N — EASY, UNLABORED
S — SHALLOW
R — RETRACTIONS
F — NASAL FLARING
P — PERIODIC
A — APNEIC
IP — IN PHASE

Breath Sounds

= — EQUAL
↓ — DECREASED
C — CLEAR
CO — COARSE
CR — CRACKLES
WH — WHEEZES
W — WET
A — AbSENT

SUCTIONING

Airway

NT — NASAL TRACHEAL TUBE
OT — ORAL TRACHEAL TUBE
T — TRACHEOSTOMY
H — HALO
F — FACE TENT
M — MIST TENT

Secretion Color

C — CLEAR
W — WHITE
Y — YELLOW
T — TAN
G — GREEN
B — BLOODY

Consistency

T — THIN
TH — THICK
F — FROTHY

G. I.

Abdomen

S — SOFT
F — FLAT
R — ROUNDED
FM — FIRM
D — DISTENDED

Bowel Sounds

+ — PRESENT
– — ABSENT
↑ — HYPERACTIVE
↓ — HYPOACTIVE

NG Color

C — CLEAR
G — GREEN
Y — YELLOW
CG — COFFEE GROUND
OB — OLD BLOOD
BR — BRIGHT RED
A — ANTACID

G. U.

Urine Source

D — DIAPER
F — FOLEY
UB — URINE BAG
O — OTHER*

Color

C — CLEAR
W — PALE
Y — YELLOW
A — AMBER
O — ORANGE
B — BLOODY

Clarity

C — CLEAR
CL — CLOUDY
S — SEDIMENT

OTHER

Skin Integrity

W — WARM   P — PETECHIAE
C — COOL   R — RASH
M — MOIST   S — SCALY
D — DRY   O — OTHER*

Skin Turgor

E — ELASTIC
TA — TAUT
TN — TENTING

Edema

P — PITTING
N — NON-PITTING

Muscle Tone

A — APPROPRIATE
F — FLACCID
E — EXAGGERATED

Patient Turned

R — RIGHT SIDE
L — LEFT SIDE
P — PRONE
S — SUPINE

* See Nurses Notes

*SEE NURSES NOTES

Fig. 3-1 PICU nursing flow sheet for nursing assessment. (Courtesy Children's Medical Center of Dallas.)

ASSESSMENT

SUCTION — CATHETER SIZE ___				G.I.				G.U.			OTHER						R.N. INIT
AIRWAY	AMOUNT	COLOR / SECRET	CONSIST	ABDOMEN	BOWEL SOUNDS	NG	COLOR	URINE SOURCE	COLOR	CLARITY	SKIN INTEG	SKIN TURGOR	EDEMA	MUSCLE TONE	PATIENT TURNED		R.N. INIT

DAILY EQUIPMENT/CARE CHECKLIST

	07 to 14	15 to 22	23 to 06
C-R MONITOR, ALARMS ON			
SYRINGE PUMPS			
BLANKETROL			
MONATHERM			
GOMCO			
PHOTOTHERAPY LIGHTS			
DINAMAP / DOPPLER			
TRANSDUCERS IN USE			
CT TO SUCTION			
EXTERNAL PACEMAKER			
ISOLETTE, OHIO, CLINITRON			
MONITORS $TcPO_2$			
$TcPCO_2$			
O_2SAT			
END TIDAL CO_2			
EGGCRATE MATTRESS			
IV FLUID CHECKS			
IV SITE CHECKS			
BED CHECKS			
ISOLATION / TYPE _____			
HOB ↑			
RESTRAINTS ARMS			
LEGS			
HEAD			
IV PUMP / TUBING			
TRANSDUCER DOME Δ			
DRESSING Δ — CENTRAL LINE			
WOUND			
FOLEY CARE			
ORAL CARE			
TRACH CARE			
BATH / LINEN Δ			
ROM / PT			
PARENT CONTACT C / V			

IV SITE CONDITION
N—PATENT, INFUSING WELL   H—HARD
R—RED   BL—BLANCHED
E—EDEMATOUS   RS—RED STREAKS
D—DRSG., DRY, INTACT

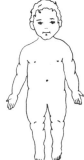

oxygen and ventilatory support; then he needs to be transferred to the PICU bed. The cardiac monitor must be attached, with alarm limits set for each patient and the alarms turned on. Any tubes or catheters must be checked to make certain they are adequately secured and patent. Apply the oxygen saturation monitor, when available. In many situations restraints may need to be placed on the patient's hands and/or feet to prevent the child from removing any invasive lines, drains, or the endotracheal tube. The restraints need to be placed with caution, being careful not to make them too tight but secure enough to serve their purpose.

If an emergency situation presents itself at the time of admission, the child must be placed on the PICU bed immediately. The weight and vital signs can be taken after the critical problems are resolved and the patient is more stable.

A complete assessment must be documented accurately and completely on the nursing records (Fig. 3-1). When symptoms or findings cannot be explained either by codes or by check marks, they need to be described in detail in a nursing narrative. The following are items to be included on every assessment; those that are starred (*) must be done immediately, whereas the others can wait until the patient is stabilized.

Cardiac system

* *Temperature:* Take the axillary temperature of infants who weigh less than 2500 g, are less than 1 month of age, or have GI bleeding. Obtain the rectal temperature of larger infants and children, especially those who have had cardiac surgery or neurosurgery.
* *Heart rate:* Obtain rate for 1 full minute by auscultation over precordium, assess strength and regularity, and listen for possible murmurs.
* *Blood pressure:* Determine value (with cuff two thirds the size of the upper arm) by auscultation, palpation, or Dinamapp. Include arterial systolic, diastolic, and mean blood pressure when available.

Pulses: Palpate pulses in all four extremities for strength and regularity.

Capillary refill: Count number of seconds it takes color to return after pressing on skin or nail beds.

Venous access: Observe condition of present IV line or assess possible IV sites.

Respiratory system

* *Respiratory rate:* Count for 1 full minute, assessing respiratory effort; observe for distress, nasal flaring, grunting, retractions, audible wheezing, and chest asymmetry.
* *Color:* Note color of skin, lips, mucous membranes, and nail beds.
* *Breath sounds:* Auscultate for bilateral air movement; note any wheezes, crackles, or coarseness. If patient is intubated, make certain the endotracheal tube is taped securely and confirm position of tip of tube by chest roentgenogram.
* *Secretions:* Suction nose, mouth, pharynx, and endotracheal tubes when necessary, assuring patency of airway; note color and consistency of secretions when suctioning is done.

Gastrointestinal system

Abdomen: Inspect for distention; auscultate for presence or absence of bowel sounds; check placement of nasogastric tube (inject 3 cc of air in nasogastric tube while listening over stomach with stethoscope); palpate for tightness or tenderness.

Drainage: Empty stomach contents with a feeding tube or nasogastric tube (use NG tube if it is going to be left in for continuous drainage); note the position of any surgically placed drains (Hemovac or Jackson-Pratt drains, chest tubes, peritoneal dialysis catheter); note color, consistency, and quantity of all drainage; perform Hematest reading on drainage when any bleeding is suspected.

Stool: When stool is present, describe color, consistency, and amount; check for presence of blood when bleeding is a possibility.

Genitourinary system

Urine: Verify with transport team when the patient last voided. When necessary, place urine collection bag on patient to secure a sample for a urinalysis; also check urine with a Labstix and measure specific gravity. Note color, clarity, odor, and quantity.

Bladder: Whether or not a bladder catheter is in place, palpate bladder for fullness, notifying physician of any distention.

Neurologic system

* *Level of consciousness:* Determine alertness, awareness, and response to painful stimuli (nonpurposeful vs. purposeful).

* *Pupils:* Observe pupils with a bright light and determine their responsiveness and size.
* *Activity:* Note movement and strength of extremities; also note any jitteriness or irritability.
* *Seizures:* Observe and describe any seizure activity; note areas affected by the seizure, eye deviation, length of time seizure lasts, and response to any interventions.

Joints: Chart any contractures or immobilized limbs.

Integument

Skin: Observe the skin for rashes, bruises, petechiae, wounds, or areas of breakdown. Document the patient's skin temperature, skin turgor, muscle tone, and any edema noted.

Measurements for infants (Fig. 3-2)

Frontal-occipital head circumference (FOC): Measure daily to detect any increase in size, ruling out hydrocephalus.

Abdominal girth (AG): An increase in size is one of the first signs of necrotizing enterocolitis in infants. In older children it denotes abdominal distention relative to intra-abdominal problems.

Length (HC): Use heel-to-crown measurement to determine the proper length of a nasotracheal tube (length $\times$ 0.21 + 1 cm).

Shoulder-umbilicus (SU): Use this measurement when an umbilical artery catheter is to be placed; the proper length of the catheter from tip to point of exit from abdomen = SU $\times$ 0.65.

Chest circumference: This measurement should be approximately the same size as the FOC.

Laboratory tests on admission

Hematocrit: Obtain as a baseline value on the newly admitted patient or on the postoperative patient. Chart whether the sample was from a heelstick or centrally obtained (from a catheter or venipuncture).

Dextrostix: This reading determines the glucose homeostasis of the patient; it is imperative to perform this test on infants under the age of 6 months and

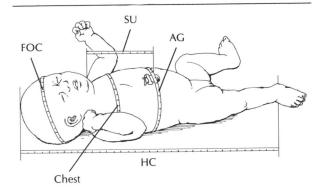

Fig. 3-2 Drawing of infant showing correct placement for measuring: *FOC*, frontal-occipital circumference; chest; *SU*, shoulder-umbilicus; *AG*, abdominal girth; *HC*, heel-crown.

on anyone suspected of being hypoglycemic or hyperglycemic (e.g., coma, seizures). If the Dextrostix value is less than 45 mg/dl, an IV line must be started immediately to raise the serum glucose; use a dextrose solution and continue checking the Dextrostix every half hour until the value is greater than 45 mg/dl in infants or greater than 90 mg/dl in older children.

Other laboratory values will be ordered by the physician based on the patient's condition. Anticipate drawing laboratory samples and have blood tubes readily available, along with supplies with which to obtain the samples.

ADDITIONAL READING

Alspach JG, Williams SM. Core Curriculum for Critical Care Nursing. Philadelphia: WB Saunders, 1985.

Hazinski MF. Nursing Care of the Critically Ill Child. St. Louis: CV Mosby, 1984.

Silver HK, Kempe CH, Bruyn HB. Handbook of Pediatrics. Los Altos, Calif.: Lange, 1975.

Whaley LF, Wong DL. Nursing Care of Infants and Children. St. Louis: CV Mosby, 1979.

4 Intensive Care Monitoring and Daily Care

Donna S. Rahn

BACKGROUND

Once admitted to the PICU, the patient will need close, constant supervision and monitoring by both nurse and physician. Highly sophisticated equipment has aided the health care profession in monitoring and caring for the critically ill child. The information supplied by the most up-to-date equipment must be recorded in order to communicate that information to all members of the health care team. Patient data are primarily communicated through charting, and the chart serves as a means of notifying all who are responsible for caring for the patient of the pertinent clinical observations and measurements. The nursing records are one of the most valuable tools for maintaining a current record of the routines and daily activities of the patient. Routine monitoring is a must for all patients. These routine activities can disclose important information that might alert the caretakers of an impending problem, thus preventing serious complications. Regardless of the severity of the patient's problem, constant monitoring of all intensive care patients is of the utmost importance in helping them return to a state of wellness.

An ongoing assessment of the PICU patient must be done simultaneously with constant monitoring. A comprehensive assessment, as described in Chapter 3, must be documented in the patient's chart at least daily by the patient's primary physician and by each nurse directly caring for the patient. The assessment continues throughout the day every time vital signs are taken, a medication is given, a dressing is changed, or the patient is turned or fed. All changes noted in the patient's condition must be documented and/or reported to the appropriate persons.

Despite the critical illness of all PICU patients, some need more monitoring and care than others. Daily care (i.e., tracheostomy, oral or bladder catheter care, dressing changes, bath, etc.) must be charted along with any equipment used by the patient (see Fig. 3-1). Charting this information communicates to other health team members the care given, provides documentation of compliance with hospital policy and procedure, and supports patient charges.

All PICU patients need to be on a cardiac-respiratory monitor with alarm settings appropriate for their age and illness (see Appendix). With few exceptions (see Chapter 7) every patient is weighed daily unless deemed a potentially unsafe procedure by medical personnel. The frontal-occipital circumference (FOC) is measured daily on infants <6 months of age and/or those suspected of having hydrocephalus. The abdominal girth (AG) is measured just above the umbilicus every 8 hours on infants susceptible to necrotizing enterocolitis (NEC) and abdominal distress and daily on other infants <6 months of age (Fig. 4-1; see also Fig. 3-2).

VITAL SIGNS

Recording vital signs documents the status of the patient at that time. In the critically ill patient vital signs are taken every 1 to 2 hours and any time there is a significant change. In the chronic and/or more stable patient, vital signs may need to be taken every 4 hours. Vital signs to be recorded include the following:

Temperature: Record the patient's temperature and site obtained (i.e., axillary, rectal, oral). Include the radiant warmer bed temperature and the skin temperature of those infants placed in radiant warmers (see Chapters 3, 110, and 111).

Apical pulse and respiratory rate: Count both the pulse and respiratory rate for 1 full minute and record.

Blood pressures: Record the cuff systemic arterial blood pressure with each set of vital signs in addition to the direct arterial blood pressure (when available). This ensures a baseline value for comparison when the arterial catheter is discontinued. Other pressures included in each set of vital signs, when monitored, include central venous blood pressure (CVP) or right atrial blood pressure (RAP), pulmonary arterial blood pressure (PAP), pulmonary capillary wedge pressure (PCWP), left atrial blood pressure (LAP), and intracranial pressure (ICP). All transducers must be calibrated at least every 8 hours for high-pressure lines (i.e., arterial pressure) and every 4 hours for low-pressure lines (i.e., RAP, CVP, LAP), making certain the transducer is at the proper level when being calibrated (see Chapters 108, 114 to 116, and 118).

RESPIRATORY ASSISTANCE

Simultaneous recording of respiratory assistance with vital signs and when obtaining a blood gas and pH is beneficial for the practitioners when evaluating the patient's respiratory status and/or changes that were made or need to be made. Important ventilator settings to be recorded include expired tidal volume (V_T) or peak inflating pressure, positive end-expiratory pressure (PEEP) or continuous positive airway pressure (CPAP), and the ventilator rate. The fraction of inspired oxygen (Fio_2) must be recorded as well as the method of delivery (i.e., ventilator, face tent, halo). All oxygen saturation, transcutaneous Po_2 and Pco_2, and end-tidal CO_2 values are recorded with vital signs, blood gas sampling, and/or with any significant changes (see Chapters 120 to 123 and 128).

LABORATORY VALUES

Laboratory values are obtained from either an arterial catheter or puncture, heelstick, fingerstick, or venipuncture. Recording the method of sampling is important in evaluating the laboratory result; that is, a potassium level sampled by a heelstick may result in a hemolyzed specimen with a higher than normal value. Common laboratory values that are routinely drawn on the critically ill child include the following.

Hematocrit (Hct): Acquire a spun Hct every 8 hours on the critically ill patient, any patient who necessitates increased blood drawing, and the patient with suspected or confirmed bleeding. In a less critically ill child an Hct will be spun once a day and once 4 hours after transfusion in a patient receiving blood.

Total serum protein (TSP): Check TSP levels in any patient receiving a large volume of human serum albumin or one that is losing a substantial volume of protein through excessive drainage from surgical wounds or drains. Once the Hct has been spun down and read, empty the serum onto the urine refractometer and use the serum solids meter to read the TSP. This can be done on request of the physician with Hct measurements.

Glucose: A Dextrostix or Chemstrip test must be done on any patient <6 months every 8 hours during the critical phase of illness and at least once a day when the patient's condition is stable. Frequent glucose determinations are also needed in any patient experiencing glucose intolerance and those receiving continuous insulin infusion (see Chapter 54), total parenteral nutrition (TPN) (see Chapter 149), or peritoneal dialysis (see Chapter 145).

Electrolytes: Serum electrolytes must be measured as often as the patient's condition demands. Children on IV fluids only must have electrolytes (Na, K, Cl, CO_2, Ca, PO_4) measured at least daily. Any patient who is critically ill, in renal or liver failure, receiving diuretics, or has abnormal values may need to have levels checked as often as every 2 to 4 hours (refer to chapters relating to the specific disease entity or situation for guidelines).

Hemogram (CBC): Sample blood for a CBC on all new medical and surgical patients on arrival at the PICU, on patients suspected of infection, and those receiving immunosuppressive therapy. Patients with documented or suspected bleeding must have an Hb and Hct drawn frequently.

BUN/creatinine: In general, check BUN and creatinine levels in all patients receiving TPN and renal toxic agents (i.e., aminoglycosides) and patients with renal disease or suspected renal impairment. Draw sample for BUN level on all postoperative heart patients and patients admitted for dehydration/hypovolemia (Fig. 4-1).

Text continued on p. 30.

WEIGHT_____ – ____

+ ____

FOC_____

DATE ____ / ____ / ____   AG_____   _____   _____

PAGE A

T I M E	TEMP		APICAL PULSE	RESP	PRESSURES						
	BED / SKIN	PT / SITE			CUFF	ART	MEAN	CVP			

VITAL SIGNS

RESPIRATORY ASSISTANCE

PEAK / V_T	CPAP / PEEP	RATE	FiO$_2$	Tc PO$_2$ / O$_2$ SAT	Tc PCO$_2$ / ET CO$_2$

® TRANSDUCERS RECALIBRATED

Fig. 4-1 PICU nursing flow sheet. (Courtesy Children's Medical Center of Dallas.)

Children's Medical Center of Dallas

PEDIATRIC INTENSIVE CARE UNIT
DEPARTMENT OF NURSING
PATIENT DATA RECORD

PAGE B

BLOOD GASES				
pO_2	pCO_2	pH	Δ	HCO_3 / O_2 SAT

LAB VALUES												
							HEMOGRAM				
HCT / TSP	CS / DXT	Na^+ / K^+	Cl^- / CO_2	GLUC	Ca^+	BUN / CREAT	WBC	RBC	Hgb / Hct	PLTS	OTHER

	BLOOD PRODUCTS	
	PRODUCT	AMT
07		
08		
09		
10		
11		
12		
13		
14		
T		
15		
16		
17		
18		
19		
20		
21		
22		
T		
23		
24		
01		
02		
03		
04		
05		
06		
T		

Continued.

IV SOLUTIONS

A _____ _____   E _____ _____
B _____ _____   F _____ _____
C _____ _____   G _____ _____
D _____ _____   H _____ _____

PAGE C

ALBUMIN		INTRAVENOUS FLUIDS															ARTERIAL			IV FLUSH	IV MEDS
%	AMT	SOLN	RATE	AMT	SOLN	RATE	AMT	SOLN	RATE	AMT	SOLN	RATE	AMT	SOLN	RATE	AMT		
07																			
08																			
09																			
10																			
11																			
12																			
13																			
14																			
T																			
15																			
16																			
17																			
18																			
19																			
20																			
21																			
22																			
T																			
23																			
24																			
01																			
02																			
03																			
04																			
05																			
06																			
T																			

TOTALS		BLOOD PROD. / ALB	IV FLUIDS	ENTERAL	NUTRITION			DRAINAGE	BLOOD	EMESIS	STOOL	URINE
	14						14					
	22				CAL/KG/24°		22					
	06				INTAKE ML/KG/24°		06					
	T				OUTPUT ML/KG/24°		T					

Fig. 4-1, cont'd PICU nursing flow sheet.

DATE ____ / ____ / ____

INTAKE   OUTPUT   PAGE D

ENTERAL FEEDINGS						OTHER					STOOL					URINE				
DIET	ORAL	TUBE	RESID	ANT-ACID				BLOOD	EMESIS		AMT	COLOR	TYPE/CONST	pH/HEME		AMT	SP GRAV	pH	LAB STIX	
																				07
																				08
																				09
																				10
																				11
																				12
																				13
																				14
																				T
																				15
																				16
																				17
																				18
																				19
																				20
																				21
																				22
																				T
																				23
																				24
																				01
																				02
																				03
																				04
																				05
																				06
																				T

TIME	TISS	PSI
___		
___		
___		

RN INIT	NAME	RN INIT	NAME

STOOL

COLOR
B—BROWN   Y—YELLOW
G—GREEN   BLD—BLOODY

TYPE/CONSISTENCY
S—SOFT   M—MECONIUM
F—FORMED   FR—FROTHY
SDY—SEEDY   C—CONSTIPATED
W—WATERY   L—LOOSE

INTAKE

Blood products: Record the blood product and the amount given on an hourly basis. Vital signs must be obtained prior to starting the blood product, after 15 minutes, and hourly throughout the infusion.

Albumin: Record the amount of albumin and label with the percent (i.e., 5% or 25%) being given.

IV fluids: Label each IV source (i.e., PIV, CVP, PA line) and document the solution with all additives in the fluid. Record both the rate of the IV infusion and the amount that is infused each hour. Many small patients are unable to handle any excess fluids; therefore it is important to record all IV flushes and medications that are given so that they may be incorporated into the 24-hour fluid intake volume.

Enteral feedings: Record the type of diet or fluids the patient is taking as well as the amount the child received in the appropriate column, either oral or tube (i.e., gastrostomy, nasogastric, or oral gastric tube). Measure the amount of gastric residual prior to each feeding when tube feedings are being used or when an infant is not tolerating his/her oral formula. Document all antacids given, but do not count it in the 8- or 24-hour totals for fluid intake.

OUTPUT

Other: Many patients have sources of fluid loss that are not common to all patients but must be recorded (i.e., nasogastric tubes, chest tubes, surgical drains, intraventricular drains, or special bladder or kidney catheters). Note both the source and amount of drainage, documenting whether the drain is connected to suction or to gravity drainage. Record the amount of all blood samples from each patient. This reminds the physician of the quantity of blood the patient is losing and may be used as transfusion criteria when accompanied by a drop in the Hb and Hct. Document the patient's having any emesis by estimating and charting the amount.

Stool: Chart whether the stool is small, medium, or large. For patients with watery stools or diarrhea, measure and record the weight of the diaper to aid in keeping track of fluid loss. Chart the color, type, and/or consistency of the stool. For patients with suspected bleeding, perform a Hematest or guaiac analysis on the stool and record the results. For patients experiencing diarrhea due to enteral feedings, get a Testape and/or pH reading on the specimen and chart the results.

Urine: Chart hourly measurements for patient with bladder catheters and weigh infant's diapers (1 g of increased weight equals 1 ml of fluid) to monitor urine output. In the critically ill patient obtain and record specific gravity, pH, and Labstix levels (testing protein, glucose, ketones, blood) every 8 hours or on a daily basis for the more stable, less critically ill patient.

Monitoring 8-hour totals for both patient intake and output enables the nurse and physician to maintain a close watch on the patient's progress and alerts them to impending problems. The 24-hour totals and caloric intake provide an overall look at the patient, helping the medical staff determine the course of treatment.

ADDITIONAL READING

Alspach JG, Williams SM. Core Curriculum for Critical Care Nursing. Philadelphia: WB Saunders, 1985.

Hazinski MF. Nursing Care of the Critically Ill Child. St. Louis: CV Mosby, 1984.

Silver HK, Kempe CH, Bruyn HB. Handbook of Pediatrics. Los Altos, Calif.: Lange Medical, 1975.

Whaley LF, Wong DL. Nursing Care of Infants and Children. St. Louis: CV Mosby, 1979.

5 The Pediatric Risk of Mortality and the Therapeutic Intervention Scoring System

Murray M. Pollack · Carolanne Capron

BACKGROUND

General principles of severity of illness assessment can be applied to all patients in the PICU. Severity of illness assessment emphasizes the natural course of disease rather than specific physiologic mechanisms of disease and recovery. When physicians and nurses can characterize disease in a prognostically meaningful way (i.e., mortality risk), clinical care can be improved because clinically meaningful information has been added. This information will also help answer concerns raised by new social pressures such as quality assurance and cost containment. Physicians and nurses commonly use severity of illness assessment methods, including the Apgar score for newborns, Trauma Score and Injury Severity Scale for trauma victims, and Glasgow Coma Scale for head-injury patients. Now severity of illness assessment methods applicable to all pediatric intensive care patients are available.

Despite the clinical importance of assessing severity of illness, there have been few efforts to understand and teach severity of illness assessment. Studies have documented that physicians at all levels of training are not adept at assessing severity of illness. For example, one study documented that 41% of physician predictions of death and 23% of predictions of survival were incorrect.

This chapter will present the general principles of severity of illness assessment applicable to all pediatric intensive care patients. In general there are two clinically relevant approaches to severity of illness assessment. The physiologic approach is based on the observation that the amount and extent of phys-

iologic dysfunction is related to the patient's mortality risk. The best pediatric mortality risk predictor using the physiologic approach is the *Pediatric Risk of Mortality* (PRISM) score. The therapeutic approach is based on the observation that amount of therapy needed for patient care is related to the amount of physiologic instability and therefore mortality risk. The Therapeutic Intervention Scoring System (TISS) is the best example of the therapeutic approach.

Before proceeding, the reader needs to understand the meaning of mortality risk. A high mortality risk does not mean a patient will die, only that the probability of death is high. If a patient's mortality risk is 50%, then half of all patients with that mortality risk will die. If the mortality risk is 10%, then only 1 of every 10 patients with that risk will die. Except for brain death, there is no absolute predictor of death available at this time. Ethical decisions involving the withdrawal or limiting of care should not be based only on these predictors. Mortality risk predictors, however, help determine which patient is sicker than perceived or which is healthier than thought.

PHYSIOLOGIC APPROACH TO SEVERITY OF ILLNESS ASSESSMENT

In the 1970s physicians realized that a patient's mortality risk was related to the maximum number of organ systems that had failed. In adult medicine this became known as the "rule of 3's." The mortality rate for one organ system failure was 30%, for two organ system failures was 60%, for three organ system failures was 90%, and for four or more organ system failures was 100%. Fortunately the organ system fail-

ure mortality predictions for children are more optimistic than those for adults. Large studies of pediatric patients have defined the following mortality
risks:

No. of Failed Organ Systems	Mortality Rate
0	<0.5%
1	1%
2	10%
3	50%
≥4	75%

The definition of organ system failure in these
studies was either physiologic dysfunction that indicated organ system failure (e.g., creatinine >2.0
mg/dl for renal failure or coma for CNS failure) or
the use of therapies that would change the physiologic variables but, without which, the patient would
have physiologic dysfunction indicating organ system
failure (e.g., mechanical ventilation for respiratory
failure or dialysis for renal failure). It is also clear
that the above chart is most applicable to the number
of simultaneous organ system failures. Therefore, if
a patient has two simultaneous organ system failures,
the general mortality risk is approximately 10%.
Other principles of severity of illness assessment are
evident from the multiple organ system failure
(MOSF) data. First, mortality risk is not simply an
additive computation as originally described in adult
medicine. That is, the mortality risk of three simultaneous organ system failures (50%) is much worse
than the mortality risk from two simultaneous failures
(10%) plus one nonconcurrent failure (1%) or the
mortality risks from three nonconcurrent organ system failures. There is a synergistic effect, with additional organ system failures making the mortality risk
much higher. Second, the mortality risk of an organ
system failure is clearly related to the availability of
successful therapy. For example, cardiovascular failure is relatively easy to treat with fluids and vasoactive
agents, but the therapy for CNS failure is still nonspecific support. Therefore, although the multiple
organ system approach helps define general categories of mortality risk, it is not independent of diagnosis. Finally, the data are convincing that mortality
risks for children are different than for adults, and
pediatricians should not use adult medicine data for
mortality risk predictions for children.

As a direct outgrowth of the MOSF investigations,
we now recognize that within the context of modern

pediatric intensive care the extent of physiologic dysfunction is directly related to the mortality risk. This
is the important conceptual advance that led to the
development of modern pediatric intensive care
prognostic methods.

The initial pediatric efforts led to the Physiologic
Stability Index (PSI). The PSI comprises 34 variables
and 75 predefined, abnormal variable ranges. The
absolute PSI score could be used to determine a
relative mortality risk. By using a logistic equation
that weighs each organ system differently, accurate
mortality risk predictions can be computed.

Fortunately the PSI has been simplified. The new
predictor is the PRISM score, which has only 14 variables and 23 variable ranges (Table 5-1). The PRISM
score will enable either accurate mortality risk prediction for individuals or provide a relative scale for
severity of illness. The PRISM score was developed
from 1415 patients and has now been validated on
over 1700 patients in eight PICUs. Its performance
was excellent in all PICUs. The observed numbers
of survivors and deaths in mortality risk categories
were accurately predicted. The performance is not
changed in major patient classification categories or
the diagnostic categories of cardiovascular, neurologic, respiratory, or miscellaneous diseases.

Computation of the PRISM score is easy. For PICU
mortality predictions based on the first PICU day, the
worst recorded physiologic abnormality is scored.
The bedside vital sign sheet, laboratory reports, and
any other official written documents are used. Data
that are not in the medical record or obtained prior
to the patient's PICU admission are not used. The
time period for scoring in all of our studies has been
the admission day. The admission day is defined as
at least 8 hours; if <8 hours of observation are recorded on the admission day, the data are combined
with all the next day's data. Therefore the admission
day is composed of at least 8 hours but <32 hours
of observation. The admission day may correspond
to the calendar day or may correspond to the PICU's
vital sign sheets (i.e., 7 A.M. to 7 A.M.). Studies are
currently being conducted to further standardize this
time period. Until this has been accomplished, this
time period works exceptionally well because most
physiologic instability for most patients occurs in the
first 4 hours of PICU stay.

For each physiologic variable a point total is provided that directly reflects the contribution of that
instability to mortality risk. For example, a systolic

arterial blood pressure of 60 mm Hg in a child (<12 months) is worth 6 points. If a systolic arterial blood pressure of 70 mm Hg was also recorded, it is not used since a more abnormal variable is available. Fixed, dilated pupils are worth the maximum of 10 points. Only one entry per physiologic variable is allowed. Variables that are not measured in the rou-

tine course of intensive care are not required to be measured; therefore extra tests are not required.

The total PRISM score will give a relative scale of severity of illness. A more precise estimate of mortality risk can be computed from the following equations:

$$\text{Probability (PICU death)} = \exp(R)/[1 + \exp(R)]$$

Table 5-1   PRISM Score

Variable	Age Restrictions and Ranges		Score
Systolic blood pressure (mm Hg)	Infants: 130-160	Children: 150-200	2
	55-65	65-75	2
	>160	>200	6
	40-54	50-64	6
	<40	<50	7
Diastolic blood pressure (mm Hg)	All ages: >110		6
Heart rate (bpm)	Infants: >160	Children: >150	4
	<90	<80	4
Respiratory rate	Infants: 61-90	Children: 51-90	1
	>90	>90	5
	Apnea	Apnea	5
Pao_2/Fio_2*	All ages: 200-300		2
	<200		3
$Paco_2$†	All ages: 51-65		1
	>65		5
Glasgow Coma Scale score‡	All ages: <8		6
Pupillary reactions	All ages: Unequal or dilated		4
	Fixed and dilated		10
PT/PTT	All ages: 1.5 × control		2
Total bilirubin (mg/dl)	>1 month: >3.5		6
Potassium (mEq/L)	All ages: 3.0-3.5		1
	6.5-7.5		1
	<3.0		5
	>7.5		5
Calcium	All ages: 7.0-8.0		2
	12.0-15.0		2
	<7.0		6
	>15.0		6
Glucose	All ages: 40-60		4
	250-400		4
	<40		8
	>400		8
Bicarbonate§	All ages: <16		3
	>32		3

*Cannot be assessed in patients with intracardiac shunts or chronic respiratory insufficiency. Requires arterial blood sampling.
†May be assessed with capillary blood gases.
‡Assessed only if there is known or suspected CNS dysfunction. Cannot be assessed in patients during iatrogenic sedation, paralysis, anesthesia, etc. Scores <8 correspond to coma or deep stupor.
§Use measured values.

where R = 0.207*PRISM − 0.005*age (months) − 0.433*operative status − 4.782. The operative status is scored as 1 if the admission day is postoperative or 0 if not postoperative. The mortality risk may be computed on a hand-held calculator or the PICU may already have programmed its personal computer to make the calculations. When a nonoperative patient of 30 months is used as a standard, the following are the mortality risks corresponding to PRISM scores:

PRISM Score	Mortality Risk (%)
3	1.3
6	2.4
9	4.4
12	8.0
15	13.9
18	23.0
21	35.8
24	50.9
27	65.9
30	78.2

The PRISM score also allows an expansion of some of the clinical principles of assessing severity of illness. First, the worst physiologic instability during a time period is most important. Clearly, only one episode of severe hypotension is enough to result in the death of a patient or severe injury. Second, not all physiologic instability is equivalent. Physicians are relatively successful at treating some types of physiologic instability; therefore the contributions of easy-to-treat physiologic instabilities are less than other hard-to-treat instabilities. Third, the significance of variable abnormality pertains to its ability to directly reflect the severity of the underlying disease (i.e., Glasgow Coma Scale, pupillary reactions, Pao_2/Fio_2), its ability to stimulate disease in other organ systems via mediator release or other pathophysiologic mechanisms (i.e., systolic arterial blood pressure, diastolic arterial blood pressure), or its ability to reflect systemic processes (i.e., glucose, prothrombin time, partial thromboplastin time). Finally, the predictor confirms the basic principle of intensive care to maintain physiologic stability.

The PRISM score may also be used as a daily assessment of physiologic stability. Changes in the score reflect the processes of disease and recovery. An increasing score is characteristic of a patient with worsening disease, whereas an improving score is characteristic of a recovering patient.

Health care professionals must remember when using this or any other prognostic score that mortality risks are based on population data. The individual patient may have an underlying disease that is relatively lethal even without physiologic instability. For example, patients with bone marrow failure, even if they are physiologically stable when admitted to the PICU, have a relatively high mortality risk. Patients with end-stage neuromuscular disease may be relatively stable while receiving mechanical ventilation. However, if mechanical ventilation is withdrawn, the physiologic instability may be severe. Predictors do not substitute for clinical judgment. However, by using the predictor with other clinically relevant information, the individual patient's care can be improved.

THERAPEUTIC APPROACH TO SEVERITY OF ILLNESS ASSESSMENT

Prior to the modern methods based on physiologic instability, physicians used the "amount" of therapy to estimate severity of illness. Methods that rely on therapeutic data are based on the belief that disease processes for all conditions follow common pathophysiologic pathways and the severity of dysfunction of these pathways can be assessed by the amount of therapy received by patients for support. The TISS is the most commonly used of these assessment methods. Table 5-2 shows the TISS score with the pediatric modifications and explanations we have made to allow more realistic use in the pediatric population.

TISS assigns points of 1, 2, 3, and 4 to 76 therapeutic and monitoring care modalities. The points reflect both the invasiveness and complexity of the interventions. For example, a pulmonary artery catheter is given 4 points, and arterial catheter is given 3 points, a CVP catheter is given 2 points, and a single IV catheter is given 1 point. The point total reflects the "amount" of the therapy and therefore can serve as a relative scale of severity of illness.

Some special comments will help the reader to use the TISS. First, many parameters reflect similar therapies. For example, controlled ventilation with or without positive end-expiratory pressure (PEEP), intermittent mandatory ventilation (IMV), continuous positive airway pressure (CPAP), spontaneous respiration via endotracheal tube, and supplemental oxygen via mask or nasal cannulas all pertain to methods of delivering airway support. There are two criteria for input and output, peripheral IV catheters,

Table 5-2 Therapeutic Intervention Scoring System (TISS) With Pediatric Adaptations*

Variable	Explanation	Variable	Explanation
4 points		Active (IV) diuresis for fluid overload or cerebral edema	
Cardiac arrest ± countershock within 48 hr		Active therapy for metabolic alkalosis	
Controlled ventilation (±PEEP)	1	Active therapy for metabolic acidosis	
Controlled ventilation with muscle paralysis	1	Emergency thora-, para-, and peri-cardiocenteses	
Balloon tamponade of varices		Anticoagulation (first 48 hr)	
Continuous arterial infusion	2	>2 IV antibiotics	
Pulmonary artery catheter		Phlebotomy for volume overload	
Atrial ± ventricular pacing		Therapy of seizures or encephalopathy (within 48 hr of onset)	
Hemodialysis (unstable patient)		Complicated orthopedic traction	9
Peritoneal dialysis			
Induced hypothermia	3	*2 points*	
Pressure-activated blood transfusion	4	CVP catheter	10
G-suit		≥2 peripheral IV catheters	
ICP monitor (any method)		Hemodialysis (stable)	
Platelet transfusion		Fresh tracheostomy (within 48 hr)	
Intra-aortic balloon assist		Spontaneous respiration via tracheotomy or ET tube	
Emergency operative procedure (within past 24 hr)	5	GI feedings	
Lavage of GI bleeding		Replacement of excess fluid losses	11
Emergency endoscopy or bronchoscopy		Parenteral chemotherapy	
≥2 continuous vasoactive drug infusions		Hourly neurologic vital signs	12
		Multiple dressing changes	
3 points		Pitressin infusion (IV)	
Central parenteral nutrition			
Pacemaker standby		*1 point*	
Chest tube(s)		ECG monitoring	
IMV or assisted ventilation		Hourly vital signs	12
CPAP		1 peripheral IV catheter	
Concentrated potassium infusion (>60 mEq/L)		Chronic anticoagulation	
Naso- or orotracheal intubation	6	Standard input/output	
Blind intratracheal suctioning	7	<5 stat studies/shift	
Strict input/output	8	Scheduled IV medications	
>4 ABG, bleeding, or stat studies/(any) shift		Routine dressing changes	
>20 ml/kg of blood products/24 hr		Standard orthopedic traction	
Bolus (unscheduled) IV medication		Tracheostomy care	13
1 continuous vasoactive drug infusion		Decubitus ulcer care	
Continuous antiarrhythmia infusions		Urinary catheter	
Cardioversion for arrhythmia		Supplemental oxygen (mask or nasal cannulas)	
Hypothermia blanket		≤2 IV antibiotics	
Arterial catheter		Chest physiotherapy	
Acute digitalization (within 48 hr)		Extensive wound care	
Cardiac output determination		GI decompression	
		Peripheral parenteral nutrition	

KEY: 1, Patient has no spontaneous respiratory rate; 2, excluding arterial infusions to keep catheters patent; 3, active effort to keep temperature <33° C; 4, pump, bag, or manual pressure for rapid delivery; 5, therapeutic only (exclude diagnostic); 6, act of intubation only; 7, nonintubated patient; 8, includes efforts such as diaper weights to record every shift for I/O; 9, Stryker frame, etc.; 10, excluding parenteral nutrition catheters; 11, requires specific replacement orders; 12, any 2 hr consecutively; 13, after first 48 hr.

*Modified from Keene AR, Cullen DJ. Therapeutic intervention scoring system: Update 1983. Crit Care Med 11:1-3, 1983. © by Williams & Wilkins.

antibiotics, IV nutrition, wound care, orthopedic traction, *stat* blood tests, hemodialysis, and pacemakers. Only the highest point total for care modalities that are designed for the identical purpose should be scored even if more than one was provided. For example, a patient may receive controlled ventilation, IMV, CPAP without IMV, and supplemental oxygen after extubation all on the same day. Only the controlled ventilation should be scored since it has the highest point total. Also, some relatively common care practices are not included in the TISS score. We use comparable scores to reflect this deficiency. Continuous arteriovenous hemofiltration is scored as hemodialysis (unstable or stable). An exchange transfusion and membrane oxygenation are scored as 4 points.

Unfortunately, unlike the severity of illness scores previously described, the TISS score is influenced by many factors. First, it has been clearly shown that the disease itself will influence the TISS points. For example, surgical patients often return from the operating room with numerous monitoring catheters placed intraoperatively to monitor physiologic events in the operating room. Many of these patients have low mortality risks and the catheters are not necessary for postoperative care. Medical patients with the same low mortality risks would not have had these catheters placed because they would create additional risk. Second, there has never been an attempt to objectively determine the appropriate point totals for the therapeutic modalities. The point totals assigned to the care modalities were subjectively assigned over 10 years ago. Third, institutional practices clearly influence TISS point totals. For example, some PICUs rely heavily on arterial catheters for blood pressure monitoring and blood drawing, whereas other PICUs rely on noninvasive methods and venipunctures. Our studies clearly show that for a given mortality risk (determined by physiologic instability methods), different institutions deliver TISS points in an amount that may differ by as much as 75% for any given mortality risk. Finally, an institutionally independent mortality predictor has never been determined from the TISS score.

If the TISS score has these drawbacks, why is it still in use? First, the score is an excellent, standardized, bookkeeping method of tracking the use of therapeutic modalities in PICUs. Second, when used with other methods of directly measuring physiologic instability, it can provide valuable data. This is especially true of studies of cost containment because the TISS care items can be classified into monitoring and therapeutic and PICU and non-PICU techniques. Third, even though TISS directly measures very little, it indirectly measures many facets of intensive care. TISS points have been used as indices of nurse and physician manpower needs for patient care and to reflect cost of care.

An area for recording both the PRISM (PSI) and TISS may be incorporated into the patient data record to be calculated and followed by the physician on a daily basis. (An example of such charting can be found in the section on patient documentation.) The inclusion of assigned scores in patient rounds provides an excellent training mechanism for the physician within the "teaching" institution.

The severity of illness scales discussed must not be confused with the nursing-focused patient classification systems. The majority of patient classification systems are utilized for predicting nurse staffing patterns based on validated time studies of provided nursing care. A correlation may be evident between the two systems because the higher acuity patient needs increased nursing time. If available, the severity of illness score may be utilized for estimating potential care needs on patients transferring into the PICU. This may necessitate the incorporation of the scale into any transfer or transport report forms utilized by the institution.

ADDITIONAL USES FOR SEVERITY OF ILLNESS ASSESSMENT

The current social pressures on medicine have created a need to use severity of illness assessment methods in ways that may not be familiar to house officers, nurses, and even intensivists. However, the social climate makes it important to conceptually understand these methods.

The Joint Commission on Accreditation of Healthcare Organizations (JCAHO) recently emphasized that quality assurance methods should assess outcome. The PRISM score enables the computation of mortality risks for each patient in the PICU. By adding these risks together, an expected number of deaths (and survivors) can be computed. These expected outcomes can be statistically compared to the observed numbers of survivors and nonsurvivors. If the PICU is functioning well, the numbers should be in close agreement. If the PICU is not, the number of deaths will be significantly higher than expected. This type of quality assurance approach is appropriate for many reasons. First, physicians and nurses deserve credit for their "saves" as well as the deaths. Traditional methods such as morbidity and mortality conferences emphasize only the bad outcomes. Second, it is always difficult to "see the forest through the trees" in hospital areas as complex as the PICU. This methodology enables the evaluation of a PICU's performance over a long period of time. Third, it is now known that all PICUs do not function with the same quality. Physicians must assess their outcomes in an objective manner to know when improvement is needed.

Another important new social pressure is cost containment. Health care costs are approaching 15% of the gross national product. Stabilization or reduction of intensive care costs resulting in significant savings for individuals can be aided by severity of illness assessment methods. These methods have allowed us to calculate efficiency rates for PICUs. About half of all PICUs have efficiency rates of less than 80%. These institutions could reduce costs by increasing PICU efficiency.

ADDITIONAL READING

Keene AR, Cullen DJ. Therapeutic Intervention Scoring System: Update 1983. Crit Care Med 11:1-3, 1983.

Pollack MM. Prognostics—State of the Art. In Critical Care: State of the Art, vol 8. Fullerton, Calif.: Society of Critical Care Medicine, 1987, pp 209-222.

Pollack MM, Ruttimann UE, Getson PR. The Pediatric Risk of Mortality (PRISM) score. Crit Care Med 16:1110-1116, 1988.

• Pollack MM, Getson PR, Ruttimann UE, et al. Efficiency of intensive care. A comparative analysis of eight pediatric intensive care units. JAMA 258:1481-1486, 1987.

• Pollack MM, Ruttimann UE, Getson PR, et al. Accurate prediction of pediatric intensive care mortality. N Engl J Med 316:134-139, 1987.

Pollack MM, Ruttimann UE, Glass NL, et al. Monitoring patients in pediatric intensive care. Pediatrics 76:719-724, 1985.

Pollack MM, Yeh TS, Ruttimann UE, et al. Evaluation of pediatric intensive care. Crit Care Med 12:376-383, 1984.

Wilkinson JD, Pollack MM, Glass NL, et al. Mortality associated with multiple organ system failure and sepsis in the PICU. A multi-institutional study. J Pediatr 11:324-326, 1987.

Yeh TS, Pollack MM, Ruttimann UE, et al. Validation of a physiologic stability index for use in critically ill infants and children. Pediatr Res 18:445-451, 1984.

Yeh TS, Pollack MM, Holbrook PR, et al. Assessment of pediatric intensive care—Application of the therapeutic intervention scoring system. Crit Care Med 10:497-500, 1982.

6 Drug Monitoring and Pharmacokinetics

Steven Weitman · Elizabeth Farrington · Donald E. Berry ·
Barton A. Kamen

BACKGROUND

Therapeutic drug monitoring is based on the concept that pharmacologic response of many drugs correlates better with the blood concentration of drug than with the dosage. The dose of most drugs relates somewhat to the intensity of pharmacologic effects, but this relationship may vary widely due to interpatient differences in absorption, distribution, metabolism, and elimination of drugs. Therefore standard dosages may not always produce predictable drug concentration.

For certain drugs, studies in patients have provided information on the plasma concentration range that is effective and safe in treating specific diseases; that is, within this range, the desired effects of the drug are seen. Below this range the therapeutic benefits are not realized; above it, toxicity may occur. There are no absolute boundaries for each drug that separate subtherapeutic, therapeutic, and toxic drug concentrations. Variability in a patient's response is influenced by both pharmacodynamic and pharmacokinetic factors. Individual differences in drug metabolism, elimination, and absorption will affect therapeutic response. In addition, the altered physiologic status associated with disease states can change pharmacodynamics directly or by influencing pharmacokinetics.

Determination of plasma/fluid drug concentrations to optimize a patient's drug therapy is known as therapeutic drug monitoring (TDM). The potential advantages of TDM are the maximization of therapeutic drug benefits and the minimization of toxic drug effects. For a TDM assay to be clinically useful, however, several criteria must be met. First, the assay method must be specific, sensitive, precise for the intended range of drug concentrations, and able to measure active metabolites if they make a significant contribution to the overall pharmacologic effect of the drug or to differentiate between the drug and its inactive metabolites. Second, a relationship must be established between the drug concentration and its pharmacologic effect. Third, information on the absorption, distribution, metabolism, and rate of elimination must be available. These pharmacokinetic variables determine the sample collection time, the clinical interpretation of drug concentrations, and the means for adjusting dosage regimens based on plasma drug concentrations.

Measuring drug levels is time consuming and expensive. Before routine monitoring of drug levels can be justified, the indications for doing so must be carefully considered. The general indications for drug monitoring are as follows:

1. When a wide interpatient variation in drug plasma levels results from a given dose (particularly important in children, in whom differences in body weight and metabolic rate are great)
2. When saturation kinetics occur, causing a steep relationship between dose and plasma level within the therapeutic range (phenytoin)
3. When the drug has a narrow therapeutic index; that is, when therapeutic doses are close to toxic doses (aminoglycoside antibiotics, digoxin)
4. When the drug's desired pharmacologic effects cannot be assessed readily by other simple means (e.g., blood pressure measurement in

patients taking antihypertensive medications) or the usual response is hidden (anticonvulsants in the paralyzed patient)

5. When symptoms occur that might be the result of toxicity or undertreatment of the underlying disease
6. When prognosis and management are related to blood levels after acute overdose (acetaminophen, barbiturates, ethanol)
7. When GI, hepatic, or renal disease is present, causing a disturbance of drug absorption, metabolism, and excretion
8. When a drug-drug interaction is suspected
9. During clinical trials of new drugs to establish therapeutic and toxic ranges

A word of caution needs to be sounded, however, since there is always the danger of treating the plasma level rather than the patient. With a number of drugs, measurement of the plasma level is invaluable, but it is no substitute for careful clinical assessment of the patient's response. A plasma level that falls outside the appropriate therapeutic range may not warrant a dosage adjustment if, on clinical grounds, a patient has shown satisfactory response to therapy without evidence of toxicity.

BASIC PHARMACOKINETICS

Clinical pharmacokinetics defines the relationship between the dose administered and the concentration of drug reached in the plasma. A basic knowledge of pharmacokinetic principles is needed to properly order and interpret drug concentrations and calculate dosage regimens based on the concentrations obtained. Without an understanding of these principles, drug concentration monitoring can be ineffective, a waste of time and money, and possibly harmful to the patient. Definitions and terms used are as follows.

Bioavailability

Bioavailability of a drug is the percentage of the dose reaching the systemic circulation as unchanged drug following administration by any route. It is calculated by multiplying the dose administered (D) by a bioavailability factor (F). The bioavailability of parenterally administered drugs is considered to be 100% (i.e., F = 1.0); however, for a drug administered orally, bioavailability may be less than 1. This usually results from incomplete absorption or a large first-pass phenomenon.

Plasma Concentration

Unless otherwise noted, the plasma concentration (Cp) of a drug is the total amount of drug (i.e., drug bound to plasma proteins plus the drug that is unbound or free) in the plasma. Since only the unbound portion is pharmacologically active, Cp may only be an indirect reflection of the concentration of active drug available.

Two major plasma proteins are responsible for approximately 95% of all drug binding: albumin (acidic drugs) and α_1-acid glycoprotein (basic drugs). Some disease states are associated with decreased plasma proteins (renal failure, hepatic cirrhosis, hepatitis, burns, malnutrition, and stress/trauma) or with decreased binding of drugs to plasma proteins (hyperbilirubinemia, hyperuremia, drug interactions). Changes in the binding characteristics of a drug could affect pharmacologic response to the drug; thus a lower plasma concentration than usual will give the desired therapeutic effect. In addition, signs of drug toxicity may be seen within the therapeutic range. α_1-Acid glycoprotein is known to rise in short- and long-term inflammation, malignancy, stress, and various hematologic conditions. Its rise will cause increased binding of basic compounds such as lidocaine and quinidine. Therefore, when interpreting plasma drug concentrations, one must consider altered protein binding and whether the fraction of free-drug concentration is altered. For drugs that are highly protein bound (>90%), minor changes in protein binding can have a substantial effect.

Volume of Distribution

The volume of distribution (V_d) relates the amount of drug in the body to the concentration of drug (Cp) in the blood or plasma. This volume does not necessarily refer to an identifiable physiologic volume but to the fluid volume that would be needed to account for all the drug in the body. A small V_d implies that the drug is largely retained within the vascular compartment, whereas a large V_d implies distribution throughout the total body water or sequestration in certain tissues. It is calculated by dividing the drug dose (D) by the Cp of the drug at 0 time (Fig. 6-1).

$$V_d \ (ml/kg) = \frac{Dose}{\substack{Concentration \ of \ drug \\ in \ plasma \ at \ 0 \ time}} = \frac{D \ (mg/kg)}{Cp0 \ (mg/ml)}$$

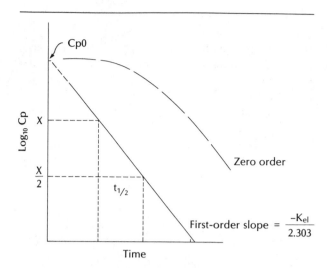

Fig. 6-1   First-order kinetics, half-life, and elimination rate constant. The dashed line represents a theoretical zero-order reaction. Note that there is little change in plasma value as a function of time at high drug concentration in a zero reaction. The slope of the line is proportional to $-K_{el}$.

Cp0 is obtained by extrapolating Cp to 0 time to obtain apparent plasma concentration. Remember if the drug is not given parenterally, the dose delivered to the body will be modified by F (bioavailable fraction), that is, $F \times D$.

Loading Dose

The V_d plus a predetermined (desired) target Cp allows us to calculate a milligram per kilogram loading dose (LD) using the equation:

$$LD \ (mg/kg) = \frac{Cp \times V_d}{F}$$

when $F = 1$,

$$LD \ (mg/kg) = Cp \ (mg/ml) \times V_d \ (ml/kg)$$

The rate at which a loading dose can be given depends on several factors: (1) drug toxicity (i.e., how large is Cp before one sees signs of toxicity), (2) where the drug is active (i.e., in plasma or in tissue), (3) rate of equilibration of the drug into various body compartments (see next section), and (4) degree of plasma protein binding (e.g., diazoxide).

Compartments

Many drugs act as if the body were a single fluid compartment. In some cases a two-compartment model may be more accurate (Fig. 6-2). The first compartment is the rapidly equilibrating volume, usually made up of blood and those organs with high blood flow. This is referred to as the initial volume (V_i). The second compartment takes a longer time to equilibrate with a drug and is referred to as the tissue volume (V_t). The sum of these two volumes is equal to the V_d. Drugs are assumed to enter into and be eliminated from V_i.

Because of the time needed for drug distribution into the V_t, a rapidly administered dose calculated on the basis of $V_d = (V_i + V_t)$ can result in an initial Cp larger than predicted because of the smaller V_i of distribution. For drugs that exert their effects on target organs located in V_i such as lidocaine, the loading dose needs to be administered at a slow enough rate to allow for drug distribution into V_t, or the total loading dose needs to be given in small increments so that the Cp in V_i does not reach a toxic concentration.

Half-Life and Elimination Constant

Measuring the drug Cp is generally the only convenient way to obtain data to express pharmacokinetic variables. Since most drugs are eliminated in an exponential fashion (first-order elimination), a semilogarithmic plot of Cp vs. time (Fig. 6-1) yields a straight line. The half-life ($t_{1/2}$) is the time it takes for the Cp to decrease by 50%. The $t_{1/2}$ is related to the elimination constant (K_{el}). Specifically, $t_{1/2} = 0.693/K_{el}$. Therefore the elimination constant $K_{el} = 0.693/t_{1/2}$. Since $t_{1/2}$ for a given drug is often known or easy to obtain, this relationship is useful in understanding the concepts of clearance and calculations of steady-state plasma concentration (Cp_{ss}, see p. 41) and loading dose (see above).

As noted, most drugs show first-order clearance from the plasma. First-order elimination occurs when the amount of drug eliminated from the body is directly proportional to the amount of drug in the body. The fraction of a drug in the body eliminated over a given time remains constant. This concept is different from zero-order elimination, where the amount of drug eliminated for each time interval is constant, regardless of the amount of drug in the body. In these instances a small increment in dose can result in a

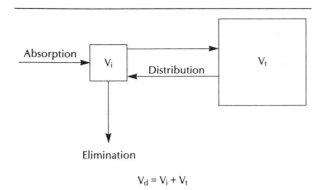

Fig. 6-2 Two-compartment model.

$$V_d = V_i + V_t$$

$$Cp_{ss} = \frac{F \times Dose}{Cl \times T}$$

when $F = 1$,

$$Cp_{ss} = \frac{Dose}{Cl \times T} \qquad (1)$$

where T = time interval between doses.

Since $Cl_p = V_d \times K_{el}$ and $K_{el} = 0.693/t_{1/2}$, if Cl_p is not known but V_d and $t_{1/2}$ are:

$$Cl = V_d \frac{0.693}{t_{1/2}} \qquad (2)$$

Thus for IV drug administration:

$$Cp_{ss} = \frac{Dose}{V_d \dfrac{0.693}{t_{1/2}} \times T}$$

more profound rise in Cp. Virtually all drug biotransformation, renal tubular secretion, and certain biliary secretion processes involve enzyme or carrier systems. These systems are capable of being saturated if enough drug is administered resulting in zero-order kinetics. Ethanol shows zero-order elimination at such low Cp that it easily accumulates and causes its well-known side effects. Depending on the dose, phenytoin, theophylline, and salicylic acid can be eliminated according to first-order kinetics; however, slight increases may "oversaturate" metabolic clearance and result in a switch to zero-order kinetics.

Clearance

Clearance (Cl) is the pharmacokinetic variable that accounts for drug loss from the body. It is a representation of the ability of the body to eliminate a drug. Clearance is expressed as volume of blood (or plasma) cleared of drug per unit time. In fact, it is defined as the product of V_d and K_{el}.

$$Cl = V_d \times K_{el}$$

Total drug clearance occurs by two major routes: renal and hepatic (metabolic and/or biliary elimination). These routes are assumed to be independent and additive ($Cl_t = Cl_h + Cl_r$). Therefore in a patient with renal or hepatic failure or both, changes in total clearance can be estimated. This adjusted clearance value can then be used to estimate the maintenance dose.

Applying the definition for Cl with previously noted equations generates several useful equations.

Remember when using these equations, units must match (e.g., if $t_{1/2}$ is in minutes, T must be in minutes, not hours). To calculate a dose rate to maintain a specific Cp_{ss}:

Dose rate (mg/kg/time) =
$$Cp_{ss} \times Cl \ (mg/ml \times ml/kg/time)$$

Dose rate determines absolute Cp_{ss}, whereas $t_{1/2}$ determines time to achieve Cp_{ss}.

HELPFUL HINT: Goodman and Gilman's *The Pharmacologic Basis of Therapeutics* has an extensive appendix of pharmacokinetic data (e.g., K_{el}, $t_{1/2}$) that will facilitate use of any or all of the equations.

PLASMA SAMPLING

To obtain useful drug concentrations, a plan for plasma sampling must consider the route of administration, dosage form, dosing schedule, and pharmacokinetic variables of the drug. Proper interpretation of the drug concentrations can only be made if the dose, dosage form, administration times, and sampling time are accurately documented. Without this information, the drug concentrations obtained can be useless or even dangerously misleading.

The timing of the sample must be as close to steady state as possible to assess the efficacy of the current dosage regimen. Blood drawn less than two half-lives after beginning a new drug regimen will allow determination of V_d, but not the clearance. Therefore the steady-state concentration cannot be predicted nor can a maintenance dose be calculated. This is true even if a loading dose is given. However, a sample drawn before two half-lives can be useful in some patients to avoid excessive drug accumulation by holding the next scheduled dose if the concentration is too high or show a loading dose is needed if the concentration is too low. To obtain information about a drug's Cp$_{ss}$, the sample must not be drawn before three to four half-lives have elapsed (i.e., 87.5% to 92.5% equilibrium reached). NOTE: According to the same principle, it will take four half-lives to eliminate >90% of the drug in the plasma.

The timing of the sample must also take into consideration the time of dosing and the route of administration. Enough time must be allowed for a drug to distribute from the plasma compartment to its site of action, which may be in the tissues of a specific organ. If a drug concentration is obtained prior to completion of this distribution phase, it may be significantly higher than expected, and an incorrect adjustment in dosage might be made. For most IV drugs, a sample taken at least 1 hour after the infusion is

Table 6-1   Therapeutic Drug Monitoring

Drug	Route	Timing of Blood Samples	Therapeutic Range	Toxic Level
Amikacin	IV	pk: 30 min after 30-min infusion tr: IBTND	pk: 20-35 μg/ml tr: 1-10 μg/ml	>35 μg/ml >10 μg/ml
Gentamicin	IV	Same as above	pk: 5-12 μg/ml tr: 1-2 μg/ml	>12 μg/ml >2 μg/ml
Tobramycin	IV	Same as above	pk: 5-12 μg/ml tr: 1-2 μg/ml	>12 μg/ml >2 μg/ml
Vancomycin	IV	pk: 1 hr after 1-hour infusion tr: IBTND	pk: 20-50 μg/ml* tr: 5-10 μg/ml	>80 μg/ml
Theophylline	IV	30 min after 20- to 30-min infusion; any time during continuous infusion	Asthma: 10-20 μg/ml Neonatal apnea: 5-10 μg/ml	>20 μg/ml
	PO	pk: Uncoated tablet or liquid, 2 hr after dose; slow-release tablet (Theo-Dur), 4 hr after dose tr: IBTND		
	PR	pk: rectal solution 2 hr after dose tr: IBTND		
Digoxin	IV/PO	pk: 4 hr after IV dose; 6 hr after PO dose tr: IBTND	0.8-2.0 ng/ml	>2 ng/ml
Phenytoin	IV	pk: 4 hr after injection tr: IBTND	Adult, child: 10-20 μg/ml Neonate/preterm to 12 wk: 6-14 μg/ml	>20 μg/ml
	PO	pk: 12 hr after dose tr: IBTND		
Phenobarbital	IV	pk: 1 hr after injection tr: IBTND	15-45 μg/ml	>70 μg/ml
	PO	pk: 8-12 hr after dose tr: IBTND		
Lidocaine	IV	>8 hr after start of continuous infusion	2-5 μg/ml	>5 μg/ml

pk = peak; tr = trough; IBTND = immediately before the next dose.
*Depending on assay.

complete will avoid the initial distribution phase. Two commonly used drugs are exceptions to this rule. Aminoglycosides may be sampled for peak concentrations 30 minutes after the infusion is complete, and after an IV dose of digoxin, a concentration must not be drawn for at least 4 hours because of its very long distribution phase. Drugs administered by continuous infusion do not have an appreciable distribution phase and drug concentrations may be drawn at any time once Cp_{ss} has been achieved.

Care must be taken not to obtain the blood sample for determination of drug concentration from the same IV line through which the drug is administered. Even if the line is flushed, enough drug may still be present to contaminate the sample, causing a falsely elevated plasma level measurement.

For most drugs administered orally, the distribution phase will be shorter than the absorption phase, so blood sampling may be done at any time after absorption is complete, usually 1 to 2 hours. Digoxin, again an exception, has a very long distribution phase after oral administration and cannot be sampled sooner than 6 hours after an oral dose.

Table 6-1 shows the correct sampling times for some commonly monitored drugs.

PLASMA DRUG CONCENTRATION INTERPRETATION

To interpret serum drug concentrations, one must take into account all available clinical information. Therapeutic ranges have been established for many drugs, but these are average values to guide dosing and may not apply to all patient situations. Many factors affect a patient's response to a given concentration of drug at its site of action. Some patients with a seemingly subtherapeutic or toxic drug concentration may receive an adequate therapeutic effect without significant toxicity. Other patients may develop tolerance to a drug after prolonged administration and will need to be maintained at a concentration higher than the normal therapeutic limit. Therapeutic ranges of plasma drug concentrations may need to be altered if synergistic or antagonistic drugs are administered at the same time. Changes in drug protein binding or the existence of pharmacologically active metabolites must also be considered in any interpretation of serum drug concentrations. Recommended therapeutic ranges of drugs are guidelines for dosing. Patient condition and clinical response

must also be considered in the total management of each patient's pharmacotherapy.

Unexpected high or low drug concentrations observed in some patients can be caused by several physiologic factors. In addition one must always consider that an inappropriate dosage might have been given, either from an incorrect drug order, misinterpretation of an order, or an error in administration. Malabsorption of an orally administered drug in a patient with decreased GI motility due to surgery, drugs, or disease will result in reduced concentrations. Changes in bioavailability can occur when drug formulations are changed, yielding unexpected variations in plasma drug concentrations.

With many drugs being administered concurrently to the critically ill patient, the possibility of drug-drug interactions must always be considered. The concentration of one or both of the drugs in question can be affected, and the change in level can be either an increase or decrease. Altered plasma drug concentrations can be a result of modification of intestinal absorption of one drug by another, competition for plasma protein-binding sites, or changes in hepatic metabolism and/or renal excretion of one or both of the drugs. Drugs given intravenously may also be incompatible when mixed together, chemically inactivating the drugs, with or without an obvious physical reaction taking place.

The presence of renal or hepatic disease can decrease the elimination or metabolism of many drugs to varying degrees. Ignoring changes in these organ functions can lead to accumulation of drug with potentially fatal results.

The effects of altered protein binding must be considered in the interpretation of concentrations of any drugs that demonstrate significant binding. In disease states with decreased plasma proteins (i.e., hypoalbuminemia) or decreased binding of drugs to plasma proteins (i.e., uremia), the drugs that are usually highly protein bound have a larger percent of unbound drug in the plasma. As a result, a greater pharmacologic effect can be expected for a given concentration of drug in the plasma, and a lower drug concentration than normal will be needed to obtain the desired therapeutic effect without significant toxicity.

Once plasma drug concentrations have been obtained and interpreted, a decision must be made whether the dosage is appropriate or not. If a change in dosage is needed, in most cases it can be done by making a change in the maintenance dose proportional to the change in steady-state plasma concentration desired. In critical situations where a more exact calculation of dosage is needed, a set of serum drug concentrations can be used to determine individual pharmacokinetic parameters that can then be used for a more precise estimate of that patient's drug dosing regimen.

PEDIATRIC PHARMACOKINETICS

Children are not "scaled down adults." Growth rate exceeds that found in adults, body proportions are different, and metabolic capabilities are not identical (see Chapter 2). For example, a newborn's head circumference is nearly 40% that of an adult, but the weight (3.5 kg) is approximately 5% that of an adult. The surface-to-volume relationship in infants and adults is so different that in children <1 year of age (or about 10 kg in weight), dosing based on square meters may result in an overdose. Specifically, if a dose for a given drug is in drug/square meters for a child or adult and the patient is <10 kg, to calculate a drug/kilogram dose divide the square meter dose by 30 (a 1 m² child is approximately 30 kg), then multiply by the infant's weight (in kilograms). These and other considerations of growth and development are reviewed below.

Since pharmacokinetics involves drug absorption, distribution, metabolism, and eventually elimination of the parent compound and metabolites and significant differences between the adult and pediatric populations exist regarding these variables, age-dependent alterations in drug pharmacokinetics and ultimately pharmacodynamics are commonly seen. If these differences are not appreciated, needless drug toxicity or ineffective therapy may result.

Absorption

Absorption following oral administration is largely influenced by gastric acidity and motility. Alterations in gastric pH will alter drug ionization and therefore ease of membrane transport. Gastric motility affects duration of exposure and time to reach absorptive surfaces. In comparison to metabolism and excretion, prediction of absorption based on the patient's age and drug structure is difficult. It is known that gastric contents at birth are relatively neutral, with a pH in the range of 6 to 8, but within the first 24 hours it falls to values of 1 to 3, until at day 8 to 10 of life

there is practically no acid secretion. Infants after the newborn period have a relative achlorhydria; gastric acid secretion increases with the development of gastric mucosa and reaches adult values by 3 years of age. This relative achlorhydria accounts for the increased bioavailability of penicillin and ampicillin in newborns and delayed absorption of phenytoin and phenobarbital. In general, drugs that are not acid labile show equivalent bioavailability in infants and children. Acetaminophen, digoxin, and sulfonamides are well absorbed in children of all ages. Gastric motility also fluctuates with age; it is unpredictable and irregular. In general, gastric emptying time is prolonged (up to 6 to 8 hours), reaching adult levels at 6 to 8 months. Since many factors influence oral drug absorption, it is difficult to predict absorptive capacity.

The ratio of surface area to body weight is higher in neonates than in adults. Therefore, given an equal application per area of skin, the percutaneous absorption is greater than in an adult when based on body weight. Toxicity has resulted from increased absorption of many drugs, including corticosteroids and hexachlorophene, producing growth retardation and encephalopathy, respectively.

The disease state may also affect efficiency of drug absorption. Diarrhea and gastroenteritis in children usually result in reduced absorption of ampicillin, penicillin, isoniazid, and nalidixic acid. A malabsorption syndrome may also reduce digoxin and penicillin absorption, producing decreased steady-state levels. This may result from a decreased transit time and insufficient exposure to absorptive surfaces. Hyperthyroidism may also reduce transit time, decreasing bioavailability, whereas hypothyroidism produces an opposite affect.

Distribution

Drug distribution is affected by many factors, including percentages of body water/fat, plasma proteins, and blood distribution. All of these factors change rapidly postnatally and are followed by a more gradual change to adult levels.

As the percentage of total body weight, the approximate total body water falls from 87% and 77% in the premature and full-term neonate, respectively, to 73% at 3 months, 59% at 1 year, and 55% by adulthood. The extracellular water falls from 45% of total body weight in the full-term neonate to 33% at 3 months, 28% at 1 year, and 20% in the adult. The percentage of total body weight that is adipose tissue increases from 0.5% at 5 months' gestation to 12% to 16% in the full-term neonate. Adipose tissue continues to increase very rapidly in the first year. In general, there tends to be an increased V_d for most water-soluble drugs and a decreased V_d for lipid-soluble drugs in neonates. Because of the expanded V_d, for a given serum concentration the amount of drug in body tissues of a neonate may be larger than in older children and adults. Therefore drugs that are distributed in the extracellular space usually require a higher dose per kilogram body weight in small children than adults. Since extracellular fluid volume is almost linearly correlated to body surface area, dosages based on square meters may be more comparable to adult levels. This relationship does not exist in low-weight patients (<10 kg) or children with markedly abnormal body habitus. Plasma protein binding, which determines proportion of pharmacologically active free drug, also varies with age. In general, plasma protein binding is decreased in children, especially in the neonate because of qualitative and quantitative differences in albumin compared with adults. This persists until approximately 1 year of life. Fatty acid concentrations that compete with protein-bound drugs are also increased after birth. Both decreased plasma protein binding and increased fatty acid concentrations may produce toxicity from excess free drug and may, in part, explain the floppy baby syndrome associated with benzodiazepine administration.

Metabolism

Drug metabolism alters a drug's chemical structure, usually producing a water-soluble metabolite for renal or biliary excretion. Age-related changes in metabolism may frequently necessitate changes in dosing regimens. Hydroxylating activity and conjugation with glucuronic acid appear to be the two metabolic pathways that are most defective at birth, whereas sulfate and glycine conjugation and dealkylation activities are close to the adult pattern. Drug metabolism is slowest from birth to about 2 months and most rapid from 2 months to 3 years, followed by a gradual decrease in metabolic rates to adult levels at puberty. Age-dependent dosage adjustments are best illustrated with theophylline. A nearly 10-fold variation in theophylline dosage occurs depending on the patient's age. This age-dependent biotransformation has been observed with several drugs, including phenytoin, phenobarbital, digoxin, carbamazepine, and valproic acid. Dosages must be adjusted based on information available in the current literature and monitoring of drug levels.

The prolonged half-life of chloramphenicol in newborns was partially responsible for the gray baby syndrome seen in the 1950s. The decreased capacity for glucuronidation of chloramphenicol led to accumulation of the parent drug and circulatory collapse manifested by an ashen gray, cyanotic appearance.

Elimination

Renal excretion is the primary route for elimination of most drugs from the body. Unlike hepatic metabolism, excretion of most drugs by the kidney achieves adult capacity early in life, although, during the first 2 weeks to 30 days of postnatal life, renal excretion is markedly prolonged. Usually after 30 days the half-life of most drugs eliminated by the kidney is comparable to adult values. These observations have resulted in adjusting of dosing regimens to avoid toxicity, which is especially true for antibiotics, including cephalosporins and penicillins. To avoid concentration-dependent toxicity, dosage adjustment in a patient's early months is necessary for most aminoglycosides.

ADDITIONAL READING

Benet LZ, Massoud N, Oambertoglio JG. Pharmacokinetic Basis for Drug Treatment. New York: Raven Press, 1984.

• Clark B, Smith DA. An Introduction to Pharmacokinetics. Oxford: Blackwell, 1981.

• DiPiro JT, Blouin RA, Pruemer JM. Concepts in Clinical Pharmacokinetics. Bethesda: American Society of Hospital Pharmacists, 1988.

Evans WE, Oellerich M, eds. Therapeutic Drug Monitoring Clinical Guide. North Chicago: Abbott Laboratories, 1984.

Evans WE, Schentag JJ, Jusko WJ. Applied Pharmacokinetics: Principles of Therapeutic Drug Monitoring. Spokane: Applied Therapeutics, 1980.

Morselli PL. Clinical pharmacokinetics in neonates. Clin Pharmacokinet 1:81-98, 1976.

Rane A, Wilson JT. Clinical pharmacokinetics in infants and children. Clin Pharmacokinet 1:2-24, 1976.

Steward CF, Hampton EM. Effect of maturation on drug disposition in pediatric patients. Clin Pharm 6:548-564, 1987.

Winter ME. Basic Clinical Pharmacokinetics. Spokane: Applied Therapeutics, 1988, pp 5-67.

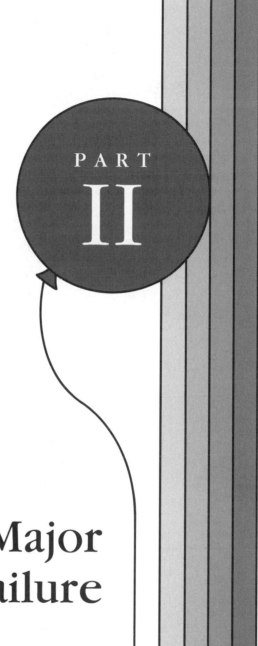

PART
II

General Major
System Failure

7 Increased Intracranial Pressure

Kenneth Shapiro · Cole A. Giller

BACKGROUND AND PHYSIOLOGY

A wide variety of intracranial and systemic abnormalities lead to intracranial hypertension, with processes as diverse as toxic encephalopathies, infections, neoplasia, and vascular disease having intracranial hypertension as a common end point. The mechanism by which intracranial hypertension occurs in each of these processes can differ and can involve both the systemic effects of the disease process as well as direct alterations of brain physiology. Although practical matters may dictate that the clinician respond to each of these conditions by a stereotyped treatment of intracranial hypertension, a clear understanding of the mechanisms causing elevated ICP can lead to an approach directed to the cause of intracranial hypertension in each situation and can improve the outcome. While this statement seems straightforward, all too often a child harboring an acute traumatic epidural hematoma has been treated by prolonged osmotic diuresis because that is the conditioned response to treating intracranial hypertension. In this simple example the appropriate lifesaving treatment is evacuation of the epidural hematoma.

This chapter outlines the mechanisms by which ICP becomes elevated and presents a plan for the appropriate and timely treatment of the causes of intracranial hypertension in individual patients.

Normal Intracranial Pressure

The upper limit of normal ICP is given as 15 mm Hg. Transient events such as coughing, straining, and suctioning raise pressure considerably above this level. Once these events pass, pressure will return spontaneously to 15 mm Hg or below. However, this limit of 15 mm Hg holds for adults and older children.

Only inferential data have been gathered to document the normal upper limits of ICP in infants and toddlers. The upper limits of normal are below 10 mm Hg during infancy but unknown in toddlers.

Neural tissue itself is remarkably resistant to the direct effects of pressure. High ICP affects the function of nervous tissue by reducing cerebral blood flow. To characterize this further, consider the concept of cerebral perfusion pressure (CPP), which is the difference between mean systemic arterial blood pressure and mean ICP (CPP = MAP − ICP). When the CPP falls below 40 to 50 mm Hg, ischemia occurs secondary to decreased cerebral blood flow. This relationship has been shown in both experimental and clinical settings. However, the effective CPP in children and infants has not been documented. Moreover, it is not known what minimal effective CPP is needed at a local level to adequately perfuse injured brain. Because the metabolic demands of immature brain may be less than the needs of the fully developed brain, a lower CPP may be tolerated in immature subjects.

Because of these factors most believe that ICP must be kept below 15 or 20 mm Hg. Additional support for this notion can be marshaled from the descriptors of ICP-volume relationships. Many studies show that the relationship between volume added to the neural axis and the resulting rise of ICP is not linear. ICP-volume relationships in experimental settings are described by a sigmoid-shaped curve. The hyperbolic portion of this curve depicts the relationship between ICP and volume added to the neural axis in clinical settings. At relatively low ICPs small increments of volume produce relatively modest changes in ICP. As successive incremental additions occur, the pressure-volume curve becomes more vertical so that pressure rises relatively abruptly as volume is added. The point at which this pressure-volume curve becomes more vertical depends on the size of the neural axis as well as on the status of ICP-volume relationships in individual patients. Smaller children have what appears to be a tighter or less compliant pressure-volume relationship based solely on the reduced volume of the neural axis compared to adults. Similarly, patients who have already had changes in their ICP-volume relationships as a result of cerebral edema, for example, can have steeper ICP-volume relationships even though their ICPs are normal.

Factors Governing Intracranial Pressure Dynamics

In most settings the neural axis is bound by rigid bony coverings (the skull and the spinal column), which do not allow significant changes in volume to occur without changing the pressure. Even in small children with unfused calvarial sutures and open anterior fontanelles, the rapidity with which changes occur within the neural axis does not allow for the storage of significant volumes without changing ICP. The Monro-Kellie doctrine embraces these principles and states that the container of the neural axis forms a rigid box in which craniospinal-intradural volumes are nearly constant. Since the components of the volumes contained within the neural axis, that is, brain parenchyma, CSF, and blood, are essentially incompressible, any change in one of these components requires a reciprocal change in the others to maintain a relatively constant ICP. When an extraneous volume (such as a hematoma) is added, the three components previously described must diminish in volume in order for ICP to remain stable. Thus the rapidity of volumetric changes and the ability to produce reciprocal changes in the other components will determine the pressure status within the neural axis.

The largest constituent of the neural axis is the brain, which constitutes approximately 80% of total intracranial volume. The brain can respond to volume changes by undergoing compression, dislocation, or shift. The ability of the brain to accommodate mass lesions depends on the rapidity with which the mass enlarges. By compressing the brain and reducing its local water content, relatively large masses can be accommodated, but this takes significant periods of time. CSF represents another 10% of neural axis volume. Because the ability to absorb CSF can be enhanced greatly, some have estimated that between 30% and 70% of total compensatory reserve for volume exchange can occur through the mechanism of increased CSF absorption. This occurs as the brain is compressed by dislocating fluid from the compressed ventricle and forcing it further along the path of the CSF outflow. Once the CSF spaces have been compressed, this compartment can obviously no longer serve as a means of buffering intracranial mass. Finally, intracranial blood volume constitutes the remainder. Because most blood resides on the venous or capacitance side, many believe that this component can most readily respond to rapid changes in intracranial volume. Although this mechanism is intuitively logical, buffering via the venous capacitance system has not been documented.

MONITORING
Signs of Intracranial Hypertension

The clinical symptoms of elevated ICP are many and varied. As indicated above, the time course of the development of ICP will often dictate the clinical symptoms. When processes develop over several days or weeks, the clinical manifestations include intermittent headaches, which are often severe enough to produce screaming or crying. Since the rise of ICP may be intermittent, these headaches may be transient and occasionally associated with transient visual loss or even episodic changes in the level of consciousness. When these transient episodes occur, they are suggestive of waves of intracranial hypertension or plateau waves. In these cases headaches may last for 15 to 20 minutes and may be associated with pallor and obtundation.

The confirmatory clinical findings of increased ICP include a sixth nerve palsy when ICP is diffuse or a third nerve palsy when there is transtentorial herniation. In chronic settings, papilledema may be found, but clinical experience shows that intracranial hypertension may exist in the absence of papilledema. Especially in children less than 10 years of age, slowly evolving processes associated with elevated ICP will produce separation of the calvarial bones at the sutures and may often not be associated with papilledema. Obviously the presence of a full and tense anterior fontanelle clearly indicates elevated ICP in infants or some toddlers.

When a patient is awake and becomes progressively more obtunded in the face of these clinical symptoms or signs of increased ICP, the pressure likely is continuing to increase. However, in a patient already obtunded the only way to recognize changes in ICP is to monitor it.

Measurement of Intracranial Pressure

The cornerstone for effectively treating intracranial hypertension is the continuous monitoring of ICP. The treatment of ICP is analogous to treating systemic hypertension: without knowing the pressure and its response to therapy, it cannot be determined whether treatment has been effective.

The techniques of monitoring ICP are outlined in Chapter 118. In general the components needed to effectively monitor ICP consist of an interface with the intracranial compartment; a monitor that displays the waveform from this monitoring device to ensure that the information is derived from a functioning device; a means of recording the pressure; and an alarm system to alert the PICU staff to abrupt changes in pressure. The most common pitfall encountered in measuring ICP and assessing the effectiveness of treatment is the lack of a hard copy to correlate the temporal response of ICP to treatment. Since intracranial hypertension needs to be treated according to the absolute pressure in each patient and not according to a cookbook approach, the inability to determine whether treatment has been effective or must be accelerated has led to ineffective treatment and poor outcome.

In theory the component responsible for intracranial hypertension is the one that must be treated. Although this conceptual approach is ideal, in practice it cannot always be achieved. However, for purposes of discussion the following sequence will be used.

Cerebrospinal fluid

When CSF accumulates, such as in hydrocephalus, the pressure that occurs following its accumulation can be lowered either by decreasing its formation or by drainage of CSF. In most situations a ventricular catheter must be inserted to drain CSF. Often this is part of the monitoring system used to measure ICP. Since CSF forms at approximately 0.3 ml/min, considerable reduction in ICP can be achieved by intermittent or continuous drainage of CSF. When hydrocephalus is documented on a CT scan, CSF drainage is the most effective means of controlling ICP.

The situation that leads to the development of hydrocephalus will often dictate the mechanism of treatment. Thus, if hydrocephalus occurs with a pos-

terior fossa brain tumor, temporary treatment of ICP by ventricular drainage can be effective, but ultimately the brain tumor must be removed. Removal of CSF can also be accomplished by spinal drainage. However, this must be done only under close neurosurgical supervision and after documenting that the CSF spaces of the supertentorial compartment communicate with the spinal subarachnoid space.

The production of CSF can be decreased by using agents that affect the sodium-potassium pump of the choroid plexus. Transient effects from acetazolamide and furosemide have been documented. Corticosteroids can also decrease CSF production.

Although all of these pharmacologic means of manipulating ICP have a place in the management of ICP, the time course for their effectiveness often dictates their application. Thus, when a rapid decrease in ICP is needed, these drugs are usually not effective. When chronic modification of ICP is required and one has the clinical luxury of time, then these drugs can be employed.

When used, the preferred corticosteroid is dexamethasone. This can be given in a loading dose of 0.2 mg/kg or more and then repeated at a dose of 0.1 to 0.4 mg/kg every 6 to 8 hours. Because of the danger of inducing Cushing's or stress ulcers, gastric acidity needs to be lowered concurrently if possible. Normally the effect of these drugs is not seen for at least 24 hours, and their administration must be carefully titrated to the cause and duration of intracranial hypertension. Since their effect in the setting of head injuries is controversial, many physicians do not use corticosteroids in head-injured patients. The effects from corticosteroids must be titrated to the individual patient. In some settings, after cerebral edema peaks at approximately 72 hours, they can be slowly tapered over 3 to 7 days. When the steroid is tapered, the patient must be observed carefully for rebound effects.

Cerebral blood volume

Increases of cerebral blood volume can raise ICP. When cerebral venous return is impaired, cerebral venous congestion occurs and ICP rises. The most rapid lowering of ICP can be achieved by proper positioning of the patient. Placing a patient with his head higher than his heart to avoid jugular obstruction encourages cerebral venous return and lowers ICP. Another way of lowering cerebrovascular outflow resistance is achieved serendipitiously by monitoring ICP in children. Because sedation or paralysis must be induced in order to maintain ventilatory control, intrathoracic pressure decreases and promotes cerebrovenous return.

The cerebral vasomotor tone directly affects the volume of blood within the cerebral vasculature. The precapillary cerebral arterioles are exquisitely sensitive to changes in pH, $Paco_2$, and Pao_2. By ensuring adequate oxygenation and maintaining relative hypocarbia, cerebral blood volume can be reduced. With $Paco_2$ between 20 to 60 mm Hg, cerebral blood flow is almost linearly related to $Paco_2$. By relative hyperventilation, $Paco_2$ can be diminished, thus diminishing cerebral blood volume. Experimental studies show that cerebral vasodilatation occurs after 6 hours of hyperventilation. However, repeated clinical experience shows that the effects of hyperventilation can be sustained for days. Brief periods of extreme hyperventilation often abort plateau waves in patients already hyperventilated. Theoretically, lowering $Paco_2$ below 20 mm Hg should diminish cerebral blood flow to the point where the brain becomes ischemic. When extreme hyperventilation is needed, a catheter may be inserted in the jugular bulb to measure the arteriovenous oxygen difference and determine whether ischemia is occurring (i.e., no O_2 extraction).

To facilitate hyperventilation and maintain ventilatory control, either heavy sedation or muscular paralysis must be employed (see Chapters 129 and 130).

Brain volume

When increased brain bulk is caused by a process that is not discrete and cannot be removed surgically, other measures are necessary. Corticosteroids have been shown to reduce cerebral edema in many settings. These agents can be used at relatively high doses to stabilize the production of edema. Often, when used in the presence of a brain tumor, steroids will markedly reduce edema. In other settings where there is increased water within the brain, osmotic diuretics such as glycerol or mannitol can be employed. Usually mannitol (0.25 to 1.0 g/kg/dose) is given intravenously. Mannitol is confined to the intravascular compartment and draws out excess brain water and thus reduces the bulk of the brain tissue. One of the effects of osmotic dehydration is a hyperosmolar state that can be deleterious in itself. When osmotic agents are used, especially when they are given more often than every 6 hours or when

they have been given for a prolonged period of time, serum osmolality and electrolytes must be carefully monitored. Since these patients who are being treated with osmotic diuresis are also under a two thirds maintenance fluid regimen, central venous blood pressure and urine output need to be monitored to maintain euvolemia. In addition a bladder catheter must be inserted and osmotic diuresis instituted.

When these treatment modalities fail to control ICP, many physicians have employed barbiturates to reduce cerebral metabolic demands and lower ICP. High-dose barbiturate therapy appears to help control ICP more effectively in children than in adults. Because these agents cause many systemic complications, careful monitoring must be used.

TREATMENT

Since a combination of factors will cause intracranial hypertension in many patients, a stepwise approach to the treatment of intracranial hypertension is usually needed. As indicated above, the treatment of ICP can only be performed when ICP is known. Thus all patients treated by the sequence outlined below must have an indwelling continuous ICP monitor. As indicated in Chapter 118, this monitor will also permit draining of CSF if needed. When a patient fails the first level of treatment, the treatment must be advanced to the next level of therapeutic intensity.

Initially the patient must undergo endotracheal intubation and sedation (see Chapters 127 and 129). Neuromuscular blockade with vecuronium (see Chapter 130) must also be used for controlled hyperventilation to maintain $Paco_2$ below 30 mm Hg. When ICP exceeds 15 to 20 mm Hg, hyperventilation should be increased, lowering $Paco_2$ to 25 mm Hg. If this fails to maintain ICP below 15 mm Hg, osmotic dehydration with mannitol is introduced. The dosage of mannitol varies: some have demonstrated a response with doses as low as 0.25 g/kg/dose, but the generally accepted dose is 0.5 to 1.0 g/kg/dose. This is given as a rapid IV infusion and should lower ICP within 30 minutes to an hour after infusion. Although many administer mannitol at preset intervals, mannitol is best given when ICP exceeds 15 mm Hg. Thus mannitol may be needed as infrequently as 8 to 10 hours or as often as every 4 to 6 hours. As the frequency of the administration of mannitol increases, close sampling of electrolytes and serum and urine osmolalities is critical. Concomitant administration of furosemide (1 mg/kg IV) has been shown by some to be useful in this setting. Others use dexamethasone, although its efficacy for intracranial hypertension following head injury has not been demonstrated.

When mannitol must be given more frequently than every 4 hours or when serum osmolalities become excessive, advancement to barbiturate therapy can be considered. Other indications for advancing to barbiturates include ICPs exceeding 20 mm Hg for several hours, peaks of pressure exceeding 30 mm Hg for 1 hour, or peaks of pressure exceeding 40 mm Hg for brief periods of time.

During the initiation of barbiturate therapy the therapies enumerated above continue. Usually pentobarbital is the barbiturate of choice. This can only be given in a PICU setting with either a central venous blood pressure catheter (see Chapter 114) or a Swan-Ganz catheter (see Chapter 116) placed to monitor the status of circulating blood volume. One must be prepared to treat systemic hypotension with cautious volume loading or the addition of vasopressors such as dopamine, as needed. A loading dose of 10 mg/kg of pentobarbital is given over 30 minutes, followed by a 5 mg/kg dose every hour for the next 3 hours. A maintenance dose of 1 mg/kg/hour can be adjusted to maintain the serum barbiturate level in the range of 3 to 4 mg/dl. The end points of this treatment include an isoelectric EEG, marked systemic arterial hypotension, and failure to control intracranial hypertension.

Treatment continues at this level until ICP can be maintained below 15 or 20 mm Hg for a period of at least 48 hours. When a patient has been advanced to barbiturate control of intracranial hypertension, this drug must be slowly tapered over the next several days. Should the ICP rebound, loading doses of barbiturates can be given and barbiturate therapy begun again. If the ICP stabilizes following the withdrawal of barbiturates, the next drug added (i.e., mannitol) can then slowly be tapered. Again this must occur over several days under close observation to ensure that the ICP does not rebound. Similarly, hyperventilation can be withdrawn after discontinuing the mannitol while continuing to monitor ICP.

In the approach outlined above the intracranial hypertension of at least 80% of patients can be managed successfully. Whether the management of intracranial hypertension will be associated with a favorable outcome depends primarily on the process caus-ing the intracranial hypertension (e.g., patients with intracranial hypertension caused by head injuries without evidence of brain parenchyma injury may have a better outcome compared to those with intracranial hypertension caused by diffuse infectious processes).

ADDITIONAL READING

Braakman R, Schouten HJA, Blaauw-Van Dishoeck M, et al. Megadose steroids in severe head injury: Results of a prospective double-blind clinical trial. J Neurosurg 58:326-330, 1983.

Bruce DA. Treatment of intracranial hypertension. In Section of Pediatric Neurosurgery of the American Association of Neurological Surgeons, eds. Pediatric Neurosurgery: Surgery of the Developing Nervous System. New York: Grune & Stratton, 1982, pp 265-276.

• Bruce DA, Alavi A, Bilaniuk L, et al. Diffuse cerebral swelling following head injuries in children: The syndrome of "malignant brain edema." J Neurosurg 54:170-178, 1981.

• Eisenberg HM, Frankowski RF, Contant CF, et al. High-dose barbiturate control of elevated intracranial pressure in patients with severe head injury. J Neurosurg 69:15-23, 1988.

Marshall LF, Smith RW, Shapiro HM. Outcome with aggressive treatment in severe head injuries. II. Acute and chronic barbiturate administration in the management of head injury. J Neurosurg 50:26-30, 1979.

Marshall LF, Smith RW, Rauscher LA, et al. Mannitol dose requirements in brain-injured patients. J Neurosurg 48:169-172, 1978.

Miller JD. Barbiturates and raised intracranial pressure. Ann Neurol 6:189-192, 1979.

Muizelaar JP, Lutz HA III, Becker DP. Effect of mannitol on ICP and CBF and correlation with pressure autoregulation in severely head injured patients. J Neurosurg 61:700-706, 1984.

Muizelaar JP, Van Der Pool HG, Li Z, et al. Pial arteriolar vessel diameter and CO_2 reactivity during prolonged hyperventilation in the rabbit. J Neurosurg 69:923-927, 1988.

Shapiro K, Marmarou A. Clinical applications of the pressure-volume index in treatment of pediatric head injuries. J Neurosurg 56:819-825, 1982.

Ward JD, Becker DP, Miller JD, et al. Failure of prophylactic barbiturate coma in the treatment of severe head injury. J Neurosurg 62:383-388, 1985.

Welch K. The intracranial pressure in infants. J Neurosurg 52:693-699, 1980.

• Wilkinson HA, Rosenfeld S. Furosemide and mannitol in the treatment of acute experimental intracranial hypertension. Neurosurgery 12:405-410, 1983.

8   Altered Mental Status

Steven L. Linder

BACKGROUND AND PHYSIOLOGY

Since the days of ancient Greece men have recognized that normal behavior depends on intact brain function. An altered state of consciousness is a reduction in neuronal function resulting from disruption of the cerebral cortical or brain stem integrity. An altered state of consciousness combined with reduced capacity of arousal to visual, auditory, and tactile stimuli has been arbitrarily divided into four categories: lethargy, obtundation, stupor, and coma. With *lethargy,* the primary defect is one of attention. The patient can communicate verbally but is easily distracted, has memory problems, and drowsiness is prominent. This problem can be seen with toxic and metabolic disorders as well as with any structural lesion that affects the cerebral hemispheres. With *obtundation,* attention is blunted and the patient is less responsive to auditory or visual stimuli but still can communicate. With *stupor,* the patient can only be aroused by vigorous stimulation and intelligible speech is lost. With *coma,* the patient is completely unresponsive with no noted speech and no reactions to external stimuli. The patient will exhibit no spontaneous movement and will lie with his eyes closed.

The integrity of the cerebral hemispheres and the subcortical structures in the diencephalon, midbrain, and upper pons can be altered by conditions that depress the function of the cerebral hemispheres, such as supratentorial mass lesions. Examples of these problems are tumor, infarction, brain abscess, and hemorrhage. The patient may also have a subtentorial lesion that will depress the ascending reticular activating system. This system, located in the brain stem, is responsible for arousal of the patient. Problems involving this area are often related to trauma, tumor, and hemorrhage into the posterior fossa. Metabolic disorders can also depress the hemispheres and/or brain stem function. Problems can be caused by any of the above lesions affecting the ascending reticular activating system or both cerebral hemispheres. A unilateral cerebral lesion will cause coma if increased intracranial pressure compromises the contralateral structure. However, unilateral lesions normally do not compromise consciousness.

Four important pathophsyiologic responses may help describe the functional level of involvement. These responses may change rapidly and care must be taken to understand and evaluate these changes. Changes may involve the patterns of respirations, size and reactivity of the pupils, spontaneous and induced eye movements, and motor response (Table 8-1).

Respiratory Patterns

Control of the respiratory center is located in the lower pons and medulla. These centers are connected with the cortical centers of the frontal lobe. The different patterns of breathing have been described for years. Even for a well-trained observer, however, it is difficult to differentiate these patterns and often they overlap. These patterns can change dramatically, so when examining the patient it is best to provide a description utilizing pictures of the patient's respiratory status so that the other examiners will be able to determine if there has been a clinical change. Disruption of the medullary center leads to an erratic breathing pattern, termed ataxic. The patient will have intermittent gasping, and almost all of these patterns are associated with apnea. With lesions in the pons, the patient may have normal breathing; however, they also may have periods when there is a cessation of respiratory effort on inspiration. This pattern has been called apneustic breathing. Lesions in the midbrain will cause marked hyperventilation with forced inspiration and expiration, which is termed central neurogenic hyperventilation. If there is destruction of the pathways from the frontal lobes to the brain stem, there will be a breathing pattern characterized by crescendo-decrescendo periods fol-

Table 8-1   Reflex Responses in Altered States of Consciousness*

Level of CNS Lesion	Level of Consciousness	Pupillary Size and Reactivity	Oculocephalic, Oculovestibular Reflexes	Respiratory Pattern	Motor Responses
Thalamus	Lethargy, stupor	Small, reactive	Increased or decreased	Cheyne-Stokes	Normal posture, tone slightly increased
Midbrain	Coma	Midpositioned, fixed	Absent	Central neurogenic hyperventilation	Decorticate
Pons	Coma	Pinpoint	Absent	Eupnea or apneustic breathing	Decerebrate, flaccid
Medulla	Coma	Small, reactive	Present	Ataxic breathing	Flaccid

*Reproduced by permission from Morriss FC, Cook JD. Altered states of consciousness. In Levin DL, Morriss FC, Moore GC, eds. A Practical Guide to Pediatric Intensive Care, 2nd ed. St. Louis: CV Mosby, 1984, p 31.

lowed by periods of apnea, which has been described as Cheyne-Stokes breathing. These breathing patterns can be extremely confusing to the observer and rapidly change, especially when dealing with metabolic or toxic encephalopathy.

Pupillary Responses

The size of the pupils and their reactivity are determined by the interaction of the parasympathetic (constrictors) and the sympathetic (dilators) fibers. Abnormal pupillary size and reaction often will help differentiate metabolic disturbances from structural lesions. Even in some of the most severe metabolic problems, the pupillary response is maintained to some degree. It may be so slight as to require a magnifying glass to actually see the pupil reacting. Unfortunately certain pharmacologic agents taken either orally or instilled locally can abolish these responses, and a careful drug history is necessary to make certain this is not the case. Any time a drug is instilled directly into the eye it is mandatory that a note be written in the chart and taped to the bed regarding the date, time, and medication used.

The pupillary response to structural lesions depends on the size and location of the lesion. Cerebral lesions and lesions at the level of the thalamus do not typically influence pupillary response, except mass lesions. With involvement of the hypothalamus and pathways caudal to the hypothalamus (including cervical abnormalities), the patient will have small, reactive pupils that may be slightly asymmetric. Lesions in the midbrain will disrupt both the parasympathetic and sympathetic fibers, resulting in midpo-

sitioned and fixed pupils. This is also the region where the third cranial nerve arises from the brain stem, and compromise of the nerve by the expanding mass lesion will cause an ipsilateral third nerve palsy with a pupil that is dilated and nonreactive to light. This abnormality is one of the signs seen with transtentorial herniation. Lesions in the pons will spare the parasympathetic fibers, and thus the pupil will be extremely small and pinpoint. The size of the pupils is similar to that seen with metabolic encephalopathy but can be differentitated from it since the pupils will not dilate with stimulation of the ciliospinal reflex. This reflex is elicited by producing a painful stimulus in the region of the neck; if the reflex pathway is intact, the pupils will dilate. Lesions in the medulla will cause small, reactive pupils since the sympathetic chain has been disrupted, but the parasympathetic chain remains intact.

Eye Movement

The ocular motor system is under the control of the cerebral hemisphere and brain stem. Voluntary control is lost during coma and replaced by brain stem reflexes, known as the oculocephalic reflex (doll's eyes) and oculovestibular reflex (cold calorics). Care must be taken during oculocephalic reflex testing of critically ill patients since most often they are intubated and passive movement of the head can change the position of the endotracheal tube and cause respiratory embarrassment. It is best to test this reflex in the horizontal plane because, when intracranial pressure is increased, vertical compression of the neck can cause depression of the cervical medullary junction, exacerbating increased ICP. In the normal doll's eyes response, the patient's eyes will deviate to the opposite side the head is turned, and this reflex persists as long as there is an intact brain stem to the level of the pons. At times this test is difficult to perform because of the equipment attached to or near the patient. In addition, the test results can be equivocal. If this is the case, the oculovestibular or cold caloric test can be done. Cold calorics are performed by placing 1 to 2 ml of ice water into the patient's external ear canal with his head tilted at a 15-degree angle. If the patient's brain is functioning at the pontine level, the eyes deviate slowly to the side of the stimulus and there is no nystagmoid component. The mnemonic COWS (cold opposite, warm same) is used to remember this normal response. The reflex is seen with an intact cerebral hemisphere and is lost when the patient has significant alteration of consciousness. Often this can be helpful when dealing with a hysterical patient who presents with an altered state of consciousness. Abnormalities and functions of cranial nerves III and VI can be easily established with this test and, if abnormal, are diagnostic of brain stem dysfunction. Dysfunction can be structural, metabolic, or toxic.

Motor Responses

Structural lesions can lead to localized weakness that can be easily missed. Muscle strength, tone, and deep tendon reflexes may not be equal on both sides, and it can be difficult to examine a patient because of multiple IV lines and dressings, but it is necessary to document minor asymmetries for early medical or surgical treatment. *Decorticate* posturing (flexion of the upper extremities with extension of the lower extremities) is seen with involvement of the cortex and subcortical white matter with preservation of brain stem structures. *Decerebrate* posturing (extension of the arms and legs with rigidity) denotes cortical disease with brain stem involvement at the level of the pons. Both of these abnormalities can be seen with increased ICP and herniation syndrome. It may also be seen in a metabolic disturbance, especially anoxia or liver dysfunction. Rarely the patient will have an unusual form of seizures that mimic either decorticate or decerebrate posturing. These two forms are important to define and observe for changing patterns since they can help localize intracranial abnormalities. The patient may present with no mus-

cle tone and thus will be flaccid, which is seen in both metabolic encephalopathy and abnormalities of the cervical medullary junction (especially high in the cervical cord). Pathologic involvement of these regions will present with none of the previously described motor difficulties. However, the patient will lie in a nonresponsive, flaccid state but will have primitive reflex withdrawal to painful stimuli since spinal reflexes are normally intact. With this type of clinical problem it is imperative to make certain you are not dealing with a treatable structural lesion at the cervical medullary junction.

MONITORING AND LABORATORY TESTS

Coma scales have been developed to help follow the patient's clinical course. A scale appropriate for children must emphasize the cerebral function as well as brain stem reflexes, and the tests must be easily done, reproducible, and cause no harm. In the past we have utilized the Glasgow Coma Scale as well as the Cornell Coma Scale; recently the Cornell Coma Scale has been modified by Vannucci. The major difference between Vannucci's scale and the coma scale below is the absence of corneal reflex testing. Corneal reflex testing can be extremely helpful at times, but repeated minor insults may cause extensive corneal damage; consequently, they cannot be done on a regular basis unless there is some question about the patient's clinical state that cannot be determined by routine testing.

Neurologic coma profile

1. *Eye opening*
   Spontaneous
   To verbal stimulus
   To noxious stimulus
   None
2. *Pupillary reaction*
   Present
   Asymmetric
   Absent
3. *Spontaneous eye movements*
   Orienting
   Roving
   Abnormal
   None
4. *Oculocephalic (doll's eye) responses*
   Normal
   Tonic conjugate
   Minimal or dysconjugate
   None

5. *Oculovestibular (caloric) responses*
   Normal (nystagmus)
   Tonic conjugate
   Minimal or dysconjugate
   None
6. *Respiratory pattern*
   Regular
   Irregular (describe type of breathing pattern at this time)
   Absent
7. *Skeletal muscle tone*
   Normal
   Rigidity
   Flexor
   Extensor
   Flaccidity
8. *Motor responses*
   Purposeful
   Withdrawal
   Flexion
   Extension
   None
9. *Deep tendon reflexes*
   Normal
   Increased
   Asymmetric
   Absent

Laboratory testing includes Dextrostix and blood glucose, BUN, serum electrolytes, calcium, ammonia, and amylase as well as blood and urine for toxins. Renal metabolic variables must be monitored closely since the syndrome of inappropriate antidiuretic hormone (SIADH) secretion is common. Liver function studies are necessary during the diagnostic period and also when the patient is having frequent seizure activity.

TREATMENT

The main goal in treatment of patients with altered states of consciousness is preservation of cerebral function while establishing the diagnosis and correcting treatable problems. It is necessary to maintain adequate oxygenation, cerebral blood flow, and glucose homeostasis. Except for anticonvulsants, all medications that affect the CNS must be discontinued. Increased ICP needs to be treated aggressively. Patients may have seizures that can be difficult to control. Manifestations of the seizures will depend on the area where the seizure focus developed. Once a patient is electively paralyzed for mechanical venti-

lation the motor component of seizure activity is lost, and thus frequent EEGs and, even more optimal, continuous EEG monitoring may be necessary for documentation of persistent seizure activity. If at all possible it is best to stop the seizures by using standard medications such as phenytoin, phenobarbital, and lorazepam. Unfortunately, if the seizures cannot be controlled by routine medications, it may be necessary to utilize pentobarbital to put the patient into a pharmacologically induced coma. When using pentobarbital-induced coma, continuous EEG monitoring and frequent assessment of pentobarbital levels are necessary. During this time period care must be taken not to overlook subtle infections and electrolyte and acid-base abnormalities. Blood glucose levels need to be kept in the range of 100 to 150 mg/dl, and serial blood gases and pH determinations must be performed because cerebral blood flow depends in part on the level of PCO_2, which needs to be in the range of 24 to 26 mm Hg. Either elevated levels of PCO_2 >30 mm Hg or levels <22 mm Hg will decrease cerebral blood flow and can further compromise CNS function. The patient's airway must be protected since the patient's gag or cough responses can be absent.

Multiple medications are often used, and unfortunately the blood levels may be misleading because of drug-drug interactions. In addition, if the patient has underlying liver or renal disease, the serum albumin may drop dramatically, altering protein binding and changing the "normal" blood level. The laboratory normally measures the "bound" material, but the active ingredient that penetrates the brain is "free." In an extremely ill patient with a low serum albumin who is on anticonvulsant medication, the "normal" range may not be truly normal and the free level in the brain may be high (see Chapter 6). This is further complicated by drug-drug interactions that can further change the drug binding. Under these circumstances an understanding of the different anticonvulsants being used and their effect on the patient's serum albumin is mandatory. The serum albumin must be kept in a normal range and the physician needs to use the least number of drugs possible to control the seizures (see Chapter 9).

When dealing with a compromised patient, extreme care must be taken to prevent damage to other organ systems that ultimately can cause further CNS dysfunction. The following are brief, general points:

1. Maintain cardiovascular and respiratory systems at optimal levels; try to keep laboratory values in ranges to provide optimal cerebral blood flow and decreased ICP (see Chapter 7).
2. Correct glucose, acid-base, as well as fluid and electrolyte abnormalities; observe for SIADH (see Chapter 57). Monitor liver function studies, including albumin.
3. Maintain temperature stability.
4. Treat increased ICP aggressively and avoid fluctuations in ICP by minimizing unnecessary manipulation of the patient. If indicated, utilize ICP monitoring (see Chapter 7).
5. Continue use of anticonvulsant medication until the patient has recovered from the insult, at which time logical decisions can be made as to long-term therapy. Keep the medications as simple as possible.
6. Continue assessment to find the etiology of the patient's underlying problem with constant monitoring of all extracranial systems.
7. Be alert to early signs of infectious processes.

ADDITIONAL READING

Plum F, Posner J. The Diagnosis of Stupor and Coma. Philadelphia: FA Davis, 1980.

• Tinsdall RSA. Evaluation and treatment of the comatose patient. In Rosenberg R, ed. Current Treatment of Neurological Disease. New York: Spectrum Publications, 1977.

• Young RSD, Vannucci RC. Diagnosis and Management of Coma in Children. Neurologic Emergencies in Infancy and Childhood. New York: Harper & Row, 1984, pp 123-143.

9 Status Epilepticus

Mauricio R. Delgado

BACKGROUND AND PHYSIOLOGY

Status epilepticus is one of the most common neurologic emergencies encountered in children. Between 15% and 25% of children diagnosed as having epilepsy prior to 15 years of age present at some time with status epilepticus. Status epilepticus is defined as any situation where a patient has more than two seizures without fully recovering consciousness between seizures or has a continuous seizure for more than 30 minutes. Status epilepticus is distinct from serial seizures, in which consciousness is regained between episodes. Serial seizures, however, not infrequently evolve into status epilepticus, and for this reason they need to be treated aggressively.

There are as many types of status epilepticus as there are types of epileptic seizures. Status epilepticus can be classified based on the current international classification of seizures as follows:

Generalized
    Convulsive
        Tonic-clonic
        Tonic
        Clonic
        Myoclonic
    Nonconvulsive
        Absence
        Atonic
Partial
    Simple (without alteration of consciousness)
    Complex (with alteration of consciousness)

Both simple and complex partial status epilepticus may be convulsive or nonconvulsive, depending on the presence or absence of predominant motor features. The various types of status epilepticus show considerable differences. A generalized convulsive status has a more serious prognosis than absence status and a different treatment approach is needed. Alternatively, some types of convulsive status epilepticus are more localized to one side of the body (i.e., unilateral status seen in infants in association with hyperthermia resulting in hemiplegia) and theoretically would be classified as partial; however, they share some features with generalized convulsive status epilepticus, including the same type of sequelae as in the generalized status. Continuous simple partial seizure (without alteration of consciousness) has been termed epilepsia partialis continua.

The most common form of status is generalized convulsive status epilepticus; the seizures are tonic-clonic. Pure tonic status epilepticus is seen occasionally in children (Lennox-Gastaut syndrome), whereas pure clonic status epilepticus usually occurs in infants and young children. Generalized convulsive status epilepticus represents the greatest threat to life, with a mortality rate of approximately 10% and morbidity rate of 20% to 50%.

Status epilepticus can be either cryptogenic (idiopathic) or symptomatic (when a specific etiology is known). Febrile seizures, because of their frequency, are probably a major cause of cryptogenic status epilepticus in young children. Approximately one third of all cases of status epilepticus in children will be cryptogenic and two thirds symptomatic. One third of the symptomatic cases will be caused by an acute CNS infection and 40% to 50% will have a chronic encephalopathy of some type. Trauma, metabolic disorder, electrolyte disturbance, acute anoxia, and intoxication (i.e., theophylline, piperazine, tricyclic antidepressants) are other less frequent causes of status epilepticus. In exceptional cases, brain tumors are the cause of status epilepticus occurring in children.

Intercurrent infections, sleep deprivation, and especially anticonvulsant drug withdrawal are the main precipitating factors of status epilepticus in children with epilepsy. Status epilepticus may cause neuronal cell damage by mechanisms that are still not clearly understood.

Direct
    Underlying cause of status
    Seizure activity itself
Indirect (systemic effects)
    Hyperthermia
    Hypotension
    Hypoxia
    Hypoglycemia

Damage to the CNS may be caused by the acute insult precipitating the status or by the direct and/or indirect systemic effects that status epilepticus may have on the CNS. The cerebral cortex, limbic structures, and cerebellum are particularly vulnerable. Significant autonomic manifestations such as tachycardia, hyperpnea, hypersecretion, and mydriasis occur during generalized convulsive seizures. As the seizures persist, fever, systemic arterial hypertension followed by hypotension, and respiratory depression may occur.

Hyperthermia. Hyperthermia is a complication of generalized convulsive status epilepticus as a result of sustained motor activity. In experimental primates, hyperthermia is the only variable other than duration of the status that is correlated with residual CNS damage.

Cardiovascular changes. Increased catecholamine concentrations may have special consequences for cardiovascular function. The prominent vasoconstriction that occurs during generalized seizures is due to the elevated concentrations of norepinephrine. The increase in pulmonary and systemic vascular resistance causes systemic, pulmonary, and left atrial hypertension and is probably responsible for the 50% drop in cardiac output that is observed during the initial 5 to 10 minutes of status. Pulmonary arterial and left atrial blood pressures return to normal after 15 to 30 minutes and systemic arterial blood pressure after 60 minutes of status. Hypotension may then follow. The mechanisms for the decline in blood pressure despite sympathetic activation are as yet undefined. Hypotension can compromise cerebral blood flow, which depends on systemic arterial blood pressure. Decreased cerebral blood flow in the presence of increased metabolic rate in the brain may result in neuronal death and permanent neurologic sequelae. Cardiac dysrhythmia may occur as well, and this may have implications for the sudden unexplained death seen in epileptic patients. All vascular responses to seizures are eliminated by transection of the cervical spinal cord in experimental animals,

documenting the neural mediation of these vascular pressure changes.

Hypoxia. Respiratory system dysfunction and failure accompany the disturbances of the cardiovascular system. Apnea, hyperventilation, Cheyne-Stokes respirations, excessive oral-bronchial secretions, possible aspiration of stomach contents, and pulmonary congestion can result in systemic and cerebral hypoxia. The latter may contribute to further brain damage in particularly susceptible areas such as the limbic system (hippocampus) and the cerebellum.

Acidosis. Lactate production due to excessive muscle activity causes a profound fall in blood pH. Lactate is rapidly metabolized after cessation of the seizure activity and the acidosis resolves within 1 hour. A variable respiratory contribution to the acidosis is seen in many patients. The risk of neuropathologic damage during status is independent of the degree of lactic acidosis in the absence of cardiac failure. Thus routine correction of metabolic acidosis in status is of questionable value.

Hyperkalemia. During status hyperkalemia may occur, increasing the risk of cardiac dysrhythmia. Hyperkalemia may be due to muscle necrosis during the sustained motor activity noted in convulsive status epilepticus. However, recent investigators have reported hyperkalemia in paralyzed animals and postulate an alpha-adrenergic mechanism.

Myoglobinuria. Increased muscle activity during convulsive status epilepticus (especially if associated with hyperthermia) may cause rhabdomyolysis, with subsequent myoglobinuria that may produce renal failure.

Hypoglycemia. Initial elevation of blood glucose levels is due to the high levels of epinephrine. However, hypoglycemia occurs 30 minutes after the onset of status.

Cerebral blood flow and ICP. The elevation of the mean systemic arterial blood pressure causes an increase in the cerebral perfusion pressure, which in combination with a paralyzed cerebral autoregulation produces an increase in cerebral blood flow of 200% to 600% of control values. The increased ictal cerebral perfusion pressure persists for 40 minutes and subsequently falls to control values even though status continues and catecholamine concentrations remain high. Despite the significant increase in cerebral blood flow, there is only a brief, slight rise of 7 to 20 mm Hg in the ICP. By the end of the first 15 minutes of seizure activity, the ICP returns to normal.

Pulmonary edema. Repetitive rather than single seizures may produce pulmonary edema. It has been found in at least one third of patients who died during status. The pulmonary edema is neurogenic in origin since this complication does not occur in experimental animals who had cervical cord transection. The pulmonary edema is independent of hypoxia and airway obstruction. The effect of generalized seizures on fluid flux in the lung is the result of a neurally mediated pressure gradient and not a sympathetic alteration of pulmonary capillary permeability.

Neuronal damage. Experimental studies have amply confirmed that seizure activity can produce neuronal damage. The neuropathologic condition produced in animal models by prolonged, induced seizures is partly due to the systemic changes associated with the seizures. However, brain damage is also seen in animals with prolonged convulsions, even when systemic changes are prevented. This suggests that persistent seizure activity may itself produce CNS damage. When seizure activity is sustained, the capacity of the cell to sequester or extrude calcium is exceeded, and mitochondrial swelling occurs, leading to cell death.

MONITORING AND LABORATORY TESTS

Although brain damage can occur in the absence of systemic abnormalities, fever, hypoglycemia, hypotension, and hypoxia occurring during status epilepticus can increase the neuronal damage. Failure to recognize and treat these systemic abnormalities quickly will result in neuronal damage or death.

The following steps need to be taken in order to properly assess and manage the patient with status epilepticus. Remember that time is of the essence and that assessment and therapy are done simultaneously.

- Assess and monitor cardiorespiratory function by respiratory rate, type of respiration, presence of cyanosis, systemic arterial blood pressure, ECG, and Sao_2. Monitor body temperature.
- Identify the type of seizure activity present (generalized, focal, etc.) since this will have both prognostic and therapeutic implications. Note the time of onset of the seizure.
- Take a short history and perform a neurologic and general physical examination to seek any clues that might indicate an etiology for the status (Med-Alert bracelet, head injury, etc.).
- Obtain blood for complete blood count, electrolytes, calcium, magnesium, glucose, BUN, creatinine, arterial blood gas and pH, toxicology screen, and antiepileptic drug levels. Since prolonged seizures may cause hypoglycemia, it is important to continue to monitor serum glucose.
- Bacterial and viral cultures of CSF, blood, nasopharynx, etc. need to be done if clinically indicated. A complete septic workup must be done in neonates who present with status epilepticus.
- Perform EEG monitoring in cases of questionable seizures, nonconvulsive status epilepticus, and paralysis.
- Continuous monitoring of vital signs and frequent assessment of neurologic status (see Chapter 4) need to be performed during and after the status is controlled and until the patient becomes stable.

TREATMENT

The treatment of status epilepticus necessitates a team approach within an emergency department or PICU. Although antiepileptic drugs are essential for treating status epilepticus, systemic consequences of prolonged seizure activity must be recognized and treated. Support of vital functions, cessation of seizure activity, and identification and treatment of etiologic and precipitating factors are the main goals of treatment in status epilepticus.

Supportive Treatment

Protect the patient from injury. Place the patient in a slight Trendelenburg position with the head turned to one side to facilitate drainage of oral secretions or vomit and prevent aspiration. Do not restrain the patient since this may cause fractures or soft tissue injuries.

Secure an airway and support respiration if necessary. Establish an IV line. Two lines are preferred: one with 0.9% sodium chloride solution, in the event drugs such as phenytoin or diazepam are used, and the second to administer substances such as glucose and pyridoxine. However, starting an IV solution is not always easy, especially in small children. If only one IV line is used, do not mix phenytoin with dextrose since it may precipitate and reduce its effect. Obtain the blood sample for laboratory tests indicated above.

Administer IV glucose in case of hypoglycemia. Give a trial dose of 50% glucose, 1 to 2 ml/kg IV (or

2 to 4 ml/kg of 25% glucose). Thiamine, 100 mg IV, should precede the glucose administration in patients suspected of alcoholism.

Additional Treatment

In addition, when treating such patients, the physician must:

- Administer pyridoxine, 100 mg IV (particularly in infants)
- Treat hypotension if present
- Control hyperthermia

Pharmacologic Treatment

There is no general agreement regarding the pharmacologic treatment of status epilepticus. Antiepileptic drugs that are commonly used in pediatrics for the control of status epilepticus include diazepam, lorazepam, phenobarbital, phenytoin, and paraldehyde (Table 9-1).

Although the IV route is preferred, there are some instances when the rectal route is necessary because of the difficulty in starting an IV line. Diazepam, lorazepam, paraldehyde, and valproate can all be given rectally. Start with lorazepam or diazepam at the dose indicated below. Paraldehyde is the second choice. Use valproate for a patient already taking this drug orally or having absence status.

Benzodiazepines

Diazepam. This drug enters the brain rapidly. Unfortunately its antiepileptic effect is often temporary because of its rapid redistribution to other tissues, and administration of another long-acting antiepilep-

tic drug is necessary. Most types of status respond to this drug. The usual dose is 0.2 to 0.4 mg/kg delivered as a single bolus. The dose may be repeated after 10 to 20 minutes, to a maximum of 5 mg in children less than 5 years of age and 10 mg in older children. Larger doses may be given but must not be administered unless ventilatory support can be provided. Diazepam and its metabolite *N*-desmethyl diazepam have relatively long half-lives. Therefore accumulation of this drug and potential toxicity may occur with repeated doses. The drug must be given slowly at a rate of 1 to 2 mg/min. Rectal administration of 0.5 to 0.75 mg/kg may be used if an IV line is not established. Diazepam must not be administered intramuscularly because of its irregular and slow absorption. Toxic side effects of diazepam include respiratory depression and rarely cardiocirculatory depression. Previous administration of barbiturates significantly increases the risk of respiratory depression.

Lorazepam. This potent benzodiazepine is chemically similar to oxazepam and equally effective as diazepam in the treatment of status epilepticus. However, it has a longer duration of action because of the less extensive peripheral tissue uptake, allowing clinically effective concentrations in the brain to persist for much longer after a single dose. When effective, it can prevent the recurrences of seizures for 2 to 72 hours. The usual latency of onset of effective action is under 3 minutes despite the fact that the peak effect of lorazepam occurs 45 to 60 minutes after IV administration. Another important difference is that lorazepam has lower protein binding than

Table 9-1   Drugs Used in the Treatment of Status Epilepticus

Medication	Route	Dose	Infusion Rate	Cautions
Diazepam	IV	0.2-0.4 mg/kg (max. dose: 5 mg <5 yr; 10 mg >5 yr)	1-2 mg/min	Respiratory depression
	Rectal	0.5-0.75 mg/kg		
Lorazepam	IV	0.05 mg/kg (may repeat ×3)	1 mg/min	Respiratory depression
	Rectal	?		
Phenytoin	IV	18-20 mg/kg (may dilute in saline solution)	1 mg/kg/min	Hypotension; cardiorespiratory failure
Phenobarbital	IV	10-20 mg/kg	2 mg/kg/min	Respiratory depression
Paraldehyde	Rectal	0.3 ml/kg (dilute with mineral or vegetable oil)		Do not use if respiratory or liver failure is present

diazepam. The free fraction of lorazepam in plasma is six times that of diazepam, allowing a higher rate of transfer of the drug to protein-free body compartments such as the CSF. It may depress respiratory function less than diazepam when used in combination with other drugs such as barbiturates. Although the optimal dosage has not yet been clearly established, several authors have used an initial dose of 0.05 mg/kg given at 1 mg/min with the dose repeated up to three times if necessary.

Phenytoin

Alone or in combination with a benzodiazepine, phenytoin is the drug of choice in the treatment of status according to several authorities. It may be even more effective than benzodiazepines for the control of partial status epilepticus. It can be used safely in infants and children. It has the advantage of not altering the level of consciousness as much as other anticonvulsant drugs. It is the drug of choice in patients with seizures secondary to head trauma. A loading IV dose of 18 to 20 mg/kg is recommended. It must be given at a rate no faster than 1 mg/kg/min because of the risk of cardiorespiratory depression and arrest associated with fast administration. Systemic arterial blood pressure and ECG monitoring is important during its administration. The drug must never be mixed with IV solutions that contain glucose because it will form crystals. Peak brain levels of the drug will be reached in 15 to 60 minutes. Intravenous phenytoin can be used even if the patient is on chronic phenytoin treatment and has therapeutic levels.

Phenobarbital

Phenobarbital remains the drug of choice for treatment of status epilepticus in neonates. An IV loading dose of 20 mg/kg will achieve serum concentrations above 16 μg/ml. It can be mixed with the usual IV solutions. Sedation is common and in combination with diazepam frequently leads to respiratory depression.

Paraldehyde

Paraldehyde controls convulsive status epilepticus in a high proportion of patients even when other agents fail. It is more effective in generalized than in partial status. The rectal route is the most popular because of its easy administration and rapid absorption. A dose of 0.3 ml/kg diluted in two volumes of mineral or vegetable oil is usually effective. The buttocks need to be held together for at least 20 minutes after administration to prevent expulsion of the drug. Since paraldehyde can dissolve plastics, it is recommended that plastic tubing or syringes not be exposed to paraldehyde. The drug is metabolized in the liver and excreted by the lungs, with a small amount excreted unchanged by the kidneys; therefore it must be administered with caution in patients with significant pulmonary disease. IV administration is not recommended since cardiorespiratory depression, apnea, coughing, pulmonary edema, and thrombophlebitis have been reported.

General anesthesia

When the antiepileptic drugs mentioned above fail, general anesthesia is indicated. Unfortunately few guidelines are available regarding the depth and duration of the anesthesia. Some authors recommend the use of halothane, whereas others use thiopental. Thiopental is given in a continuous IV drip with control of ventilation and neuromuscular blockade, and the response to therapy is monitored by continuous EEG recording.

Thiopental is used in sufficient doses to produce burst-suppression EEG tracings.

A maintenance dose of antiepileptic drugs can be started 12 hours after the loading dose.

ADDITIONAL READING

• Aicardi J. Status epilepticus. In The International Review of Child Neurology Series. Epilepsy in Children. New York: Raven, 1986, pp 240-259.

Crawford TO, et al. Lorazepam in childhood status epilepticus and serial seizures: Effectiveness and tachyphylaxis. Neurology 37:190-195, 1987.

Delgado-Escueta AV, et al. Management of status epilepticus. N Engl J Med 306:1337-1340, 1982.

Delgado-Escueta AV, et al. Status epilepticus. Adv Neurol 34:1-551, 1983.

Dreifuss FE, et al. Proposal for revised clinical and electroencephalographic classification of epileptic seizures. Epilepsia 22:489-501, 1981.

• Holmes GL. Status epilepticus. Diagnosis and management of seizures in children. Philadelphia: WB Saunders, 1987, pp 262-276.

Lockman LA. Status epilepticus. In Morselli CE, et al., eds. Antiepileptic drug therapy in Pediatrics. New York: Raven, 1983.

Simon RP. Physiologic consequences of status epilepticus. Epilepsia 26(Suppl):S58-S66, 1985.

10   Respiratory Failure

Nick G. Anas

BACKGROUND AND PHYSIOLOGY

Respiratory failure is the inability to maintain gas exchange at a rate that matches the body's metabolic demands. Although respiratory failure may be defined simply in terms of blood gas tension abnormalities, the institution of appropriate therapy depends on determining the pathophysiologic mechanism responsible for the derangement, that is, either hypercapnia or hypoxemia or both. Throughout this discussion respiratory failure is considered in terms of three mechanisms: (1) inadequate alveolar ventilation, (2) mismatching of alveolar ventilation and pulmonary perfusion, and (3) abnormal diffusion of gases at the alveolar capillary interface. The goal in the management of the patient with respiratory failure is to ensure adequate gas exchange and oxygen delivery to vital organ systems. Equally important to achieving blood gas homeostasis is providing sufficient blood flow (i.e., cardiac output and distribution) and maximizing the capacity for gas exchange (i.e., hemoglobin content). These aspects of the management of cardiorespiratory diseases are presented in Chapter 12. Finally, as with all disorders, respiratory failure is a condition created by the interaction of external influences and a vulnerable host. The high frequency of respiratory failure in the pediatric population is explained by these host factors: (1) small and collapsible airways, (2) an unstable chest wall, (3) inadequate collateral ventilation for alveoli, (4) poor control of the upper airway, particularly during sleep, (5) the tendency for respiratory muscles to fatigue, (6) reactivity of the pulmonary vascular bed, and (7) an inefficient immune system.

Physiology of Gas Exchange
Alveolar ventilation

Alveolar ventilation depends on CNS input and the function of both the respiratory pump (i.e., peripheral nerves, intercostal and accessory muscles, dia-phragm, rib cage) and the lung. The lung can be divided functionally into conducting airways, the trachea and bronchi, and the alveoli. The conducting airways are referred to as anatomic dead space since the air in these spaces does not participate in gas exchange. This differs from physiologic dead space (VD), which comprises areas of abnormal lung where ventilation-perfusion ($\dot{V}/\dot{Q}$) mismatch prevents normal gas exchange. Tidal volume (VT) is the amount of air inspired in a single breath and includes both the anatomic dead space volume and the alveolar volume. The VT generated is a function of effort, airways resistance (Raw), alveolar compliance (C), and chest wall elasticity. The product of VT and respiratory rate is the minute ventilation (VE); subtracting VD (dead space volume × respiratory rate) from the VE yields alveolar ventilation (VA). The relationship of arterial CO_2 tension (PaCO$_2$) to VA is inverse and is described by the equation:

$$\text{Paco}_2 = \frac{\dot{V}\text{co}_2}{\text{VA}}$$

where $\dot{V}$co$_2$ represents CO_2 production. Thus hypercapnic respiratory failure can occur as a result of either increased CO_2 production or decreased VA, the latter condition being the problem much more commonly encountered in the PICU. From this discussion possible causes of a reduction of VA resulting in hypercapnic respiratory failure (PaCO$_2$ >55 mm Hg) include reduced CNS input, inadequate neuromuscular transmission of this input, respiratory muscle fatigue or failure, rib cage instability, increased VD, increased airways resistance, or reduced alveolar compliance (Table 10-1).

Ventilation-perfusion matching

The adequacy of $\dot{V}/\dot{Q}$ matching is determined by the composition of alveolar O_2 and CO_2 and the degree to which VA and pulmonary perfusion are balanced.

Alveolar gas is a mixture of nitrogen (PAN_2), oxygen (PAO_2), carbon dioxide ($PACO_2$), and water (PAH_2O). The difference in O_2 tension between the inspired gas and alveolar gas is a function of Dalton's law (i.e., the total pressure exerted by a gas mixture is equal to the sum of the pressures of the individual gases). Since the total pressure of the gas mixture equals the barometric pressure (PB), the partial pressure of inspired O_2 (PIO_2) is the product of the fractional concentration of O_2 (FIO_2) and the PB. If it is assumed that the inspired and alveolar nitrogen concentrations are identical, the PAO_2 will differ from the PIO_2 by the partial pressures exerted by CO_2 (the product of metabolism) and by water (PH_2O), the result of humidification of gases in the upper airway. The $PACO_2$ value is a function of the respiratory exchange quotient (R), which is the ratio of CO_2 production to O_2 consumption (normally about 0.8, meaning that more O_2 is consumed than CO_2 is produced during the metabolic process). Therefore:

$$PAO_2 = FIO_2 \times (PB - PH_2O) - PACO_2/R$$

Assuming complete diffusion of blood gases at the alveolar-capillary interface, the alveolar gas tensions should be identical to those measured in arterial blood, also making this equation clinically useful since arterial blood gas tensions are measured easily. For CO_2 assume this to be true, and therefore substitute $PaCO_2$ for $PACO_2$ in the above equation. A difference exists between the alveolar and arterial O_2 ($A\text{-}aDO_2$); however, this value is 10 to 20 mm Hg and is explained by venous admixture due to anatomic

---

EQUATIONS USEFUL IN DETERMINING THE STATE OF GAS EXCHANGE

Alveolar ventilation

1. $VA = VE - VD$

2. $VE = VT \times RR$

3. $VD = \dfrac{PaCO_2 - PetCO_2}{PaCO_2}$

4. $PaCO_2 = \dfrac{\dot{V}CO_2}{VA}$

Ventilation-perfusion matching

1. $PAO_2 = [FIO_2 \times (PB - PH_2O)] - PaCO_2/R$

2. $A\text{-}aDO_2 = PAO_2 - PaO_2$

3. $\dot{Q}s/\dot{Q}t = \dfrac{CcO_2 - CaO_2}{CcO_2 - C\bar{v}O_2}$

4. $CO_2 = [1.34 \,(g\ Hb)\,(SaO_2)] + [PO_2 \times (0.003\ ml\ O_2/100\ ml\ blood/mm\ Hg)]$

5. $C\bar{v}O_2 = CaO_2 - \dot{V}O_2/CO$

Diffusion

1. $V_{gas} = DL(PA - PC)$

KEY

$A\text{-}aDO_2$ = alveolar-arterial oxygen difference
CaO_2 = arterial O_2 content
CcO_2 = capillary O_2 content
CO = cardiac output
CO_2 = O_2 content of blood
$C\bar{v}O_2$ = mixed venous O_2 content
DL = conductance of alveolar membrane
FIO_2 = fraction of inspired O_2
Hb = hemoglobin concentration
$PaCO_2$ = arterial CO_2 tension
PaO_2 = arterial O_2 tension
PA = alveolar gas pressure
$PACO_2$ = alveolar CO_2 tension
PAO_2 = alveolar O_2 tension
PB = barometric pressure
PC = pulmonary capillary gas pressure
$PetCO_2$ = end-tidal CO_2 tension
PH_2O = water vapor pressure
$\dot{Q}s/\dot{Q}t$ = shunt fraction
R = respiratory quotient difference
RR = respiratory rate
SaO_2 = O_2 saturation
VA = alveolar ventilation
$\dot{V}CO_2$ = CO_2 production
VD = dead space ventilation
VE = minute ventilation
$\dot{V}O_2$ = O_2 consumption
VT = tidal volume

shunts through the bronchial and thesbian circulation systems. Abnormalities in gas exchange that occur as a result of changes in the composition of alveolar gas include a reduced FiO_2 (e.g., high altitude), an increased $PaCO_2$ (i.e., conditions of hypoventilation), or alterations in the respiratory exchange ratio (e.g., increased CO_2 production from excessive glucose metabolism). All of these causes of respiratory failure will be characterized by hypercapnia ($PaCO_2$ >55 mm Hg) and by hypoxemia (PaO_2 <50 mm Hg) with a normal A-aDO_2.

In addition to the composition of alveolar gas the adequacy of gas exchange is determined by the balance of ventilation and pulmonary perfusion. In the normal lung, the $\dot{V}/\dot{Q}$ ratio is affected by gravity; in the standing position the base of the lung has a $\dot{V}/\dot{Q}$ of 0.6, whereas the apex has a $\dot{V}/\dot{Q}$ value of 3.0. For the purposes of patient management, however, it can

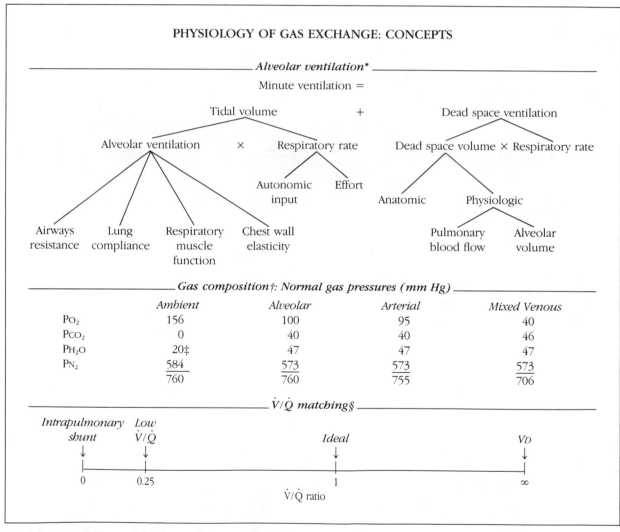

PHYSIOLOGY OF GAS EXCHANGE: CONCEPTS

——————————— *Alveolar ventilation** ———————————

Minute ventilation =

Tidal volume   +   Dead space ventilation

Alveolar ventilation   ×   Respiratory rate   Dead space volume × Respiratory rate

Autonomic   Effort   Anatomic   Physiologic
input

Airways   Lung   Respiratory   Chest wall   Pulmonary   Alveolar
resistance   compliance   muscle   elasticity   blood flow   volume
                          function

——————————— *Gas composition†: Normal gas pressures (mm Hg)* ———————————

	Ambient	*Alveolar*	*Arterial*	*Mixed Venous*
PO_2	156	100	95	40
PCO_2	0	40	40	46
PH_2O	20‡	47	47	47
PN_2	584	573	573	573
	760	760	755	706

——————————— *$\dot{V}/\dot{Q}$ matching§* ———————————

Intrapulmonary   *Low*
shunt $\dot{V}/\dot{Q}$ *Ideal* V_D

↓   ↓   ↓   ↓

0   0.25   1   ∞

$\dot{V}/\dot{Q}$ ratio

*Physiologic determinants of alveolar ventilation.
†Composition of gases provides data necessary to calculate alveolar-arterial oxygen gradient, percent intrapulmonary shunt, and oxygen delivery and consumption.
‡Dependent on relative humidity.
§Graphic representation of the spectrum of ventilation-perfusion disorders.

Table 10-1   Examples of Pathophysiologic Conditions Resulting in Respiratory Failure

Physiologic Abnormality	Anatomic Correlate	Clinical Correlate
Hypercapnia		
Reduced alveolar ventilation	CNS inhibition	Coma, status epilepticus, narcotic administration
	Impaired peripheral nervous system function	Spinal cord trauma, botulism, Guillain-Barré syndrome
	Respiratory muscle failure	Muscular dystrophies
	Respiratory muscle fatigue	Excessive work of breathing, shock states
	Upper airway obstruction	Croup, foreign-body inhalation, tracheomalacia, pharyngeal hypotonia
	Reduced lung compliance	Pulmonary edema, fibrosis
	Increased airways resistance	Asthma, cystic fibrosis
	Increased chest wall compliance	Flail chest
	Disrupted pleural space	Pneumothorax, pleural effusions
Increased dead space ventilation	Reduced pulmonary blood flow	Pulmonary hypertension syndromes, decreased cardiac output
	Alveolar overdistention	Asthma
Increased CO_2 production	Increased metabolic rate	Burns
	Altered respiratory quotient	Excessive glucose administration
Hypoxemia		
Intrapulmonary shunting		
With increased PVR	Widespread alveolar flooding with pulmonary vascular obliteration	Adult respiratory distress syndrome
Without increased PVR	Local alveolar flooding	Lobar pneumonia
Low $\dot{V}/\dot{Q}$ match		
With increased PVR	Bronchospasm with increased pulmonary artery tone	Meconium aspiration syndrome
Without increased PVR	Alveolar flooding	Cardiogenic pulmonary edema
Intracardiac shunting		
With increased PVR	Right to left shunting with increased pulmonary artery tone	Endocardial cushion defect
Without increased PVR	Right to left shunting without pulmonary vascular disease	Pulmonic stenosis with ventricular septal defect
Hypoventilation	Reduced alveolar ventilation	Upper airway obstruction
Diffusion impairment	Increased interstitial space	Fibrosis
Reduced $P\bar{v}O_2$	Increased O_2 extraction	Cardiogenic shock

PVR = pulmonary vascular resistance; $P\bar{v}O_2$ = mixed venous O_2 tension.

be assumed that the overall $\dot{V}/\dot{Q}$ match is ideal (i.e., $\dot{V}/\dot{Q} = 1$). Conditions that alter ideal situations do so largely either by reducing V_A (e.g., pulmonary edema, atelectasis) or by reducing pulmonary blood flow (e.g., pulmonary embolus). The extreme example of reduced ventilation $\dot{V}/\dot{Q}$ (i.e., $\dot{V}/\dot{Q} = 0$) is defined as intrapulmonary shunting; the extreme of reduced perfusion is defined as V_D (i.e., $\dot{V}/\dot{Q} = \infty$). In most clinical disorders of $\dot{V}/\dot{Q}$ balance the $\dot{V}/\dot{Q}$ ratios span these extreme values and are limited by protective reflexes (e.g., hypoxic vasoconstriction in areas of reduced ventilation). Respiratory failure as a result of $\dot{V}/\dot{Q}$ mismatch therefore is manifested by hypoxemia with an increased A-aD_{O_2} (i.e., >20 mm Hg). The extent to which regions of $\dot{V}/\dot{Q}$ mismatch produce hypoxemia depends on the size of the low $\dot{V}/\dot{Q}$ regions, the degree to which ventilation is reduced in these regions, and the amount of pulmonary perfusion (i.e., the effectiveness of hypoxic vasoconstriction).

The percent of intrapulmonary shunt is determined by the ratio of the shunted flow ($\dot{Q}s$) to the total flow ($\dot{Q}t$) or cardiac output. $\dot{Q}s/\dot{Q}t$ is calculated by comparing the O_2 content in the arterial, mixed venous, and pulmonary capillary beds while breathing 100% O_2 and is obtained by utilizing this equation:

$$\dot{Q}s/\dot{Q}t = \frac{C_{CO_2} - Ca_{O_2}}{C_{CO_2} - C\bar{v}_{O_2}}$$

where C_{CO_2}, Ca_{O_2}, and $C\bar{v}_{O_2}$ represent the O_2 content in the capillary, arterial, and mixed venous beds, respectively. The O_2 content of blood is the sum of that amount bound to hemoglobin and that amount dissolved in blood. One gram of hemoglobin can combine with 1.34 ml O_2, and therefore the total amount of bound O_2 is as follows: 1.34 ml O_2/g Hb × g Hb × %Hb saturated with O_2 (Sa_{O_2}). Because 0.003 ml O_2 is dissolved in 100 ml blood/mm Hg P_{O_2}, the total amount of O_2 dissolved is as follows: (0.003 ml O_2/100 ml blood/mm Hg) × P_{O_2} in millimeters of mercury. Therefore the total O_2 content = [1.34 × g Hb × Sa_{O_2}] + [0.003 × Pa_{O_2}]. This calculation of the shunt fraction thus requires the determination of O_2 saturation in three vascular beds; the pulmonary capillary bed is assumed to be 100% saturated, whereas the systemic arterial and mixed venous (pulmonary artery) O_2 saturation values can be measured.

The degree of hypoxemia in low or zero $\dot{V}/\dot{Q}$ states also depends on the cardiac output and the body's oxygen consumption.

The Fick equation states that

$$CO = \frac{O_2 \text{ consumption}}{Ca_{O_2} - C\bar{v}_{O_2}} \quad or$$

$$C\bar{v}_{O_2} = Ca_{O_2} - \frac{O_2 \text{ consumption}}{CO}$$

Any condition that reduces the mixed venous O_2 tension (e.g., reduced CO) or increases O_2 consumption (e.g., increased metabolic rate) will worsen hypoxemia in the presence of $\dot{V}/\dot{Q}$ imbalance. Finally, hypocapnia (Pa_{CO_2} <35 mm Hg) occurs in conditions characterized by low or zero $\dot{V}/\dot{Q}$ balance because hypoxemia is a stimulus to increase V_E; thus it is common for the patient with hypoxemic respiratory failure from low $\dot{V}/\dot{Q}$ matching to present with hypocapnia as long as the respiratory muscles can sustain the state of hyperventilation.

Increased V_D occurs when pulmonary perfusion is reduced relative to V_A. This may occur as the result of pulmonary vasoconstriction (e.g., pulmonary hypertension in the newborn), obliteration of small vessels in the pulmonary arterial bed (e.g., adult respiratory distress syndrome), or multiple pulmonary emboli (e.g., secondary to endocarditis). The calculation of V_D requires the determination of the end-tidal CO_2 tension (Pet_{CO_2}) and the arterial CO_2 tension (Pa_{CO_2}) and is represented by the equation:

$$V_D = \frac{Pa_{CO_2} - Pet_{CO_2}}{Pa_{CO_2}}$$

Diffusion

The third determinant of gas exchange is the ability of O_2 and CO_2 to diffuse across the alveolar-capillary membrane. Diffusion through tissues is described by Fick's law, which states that the rate of transfer of a gas through a sheet of tissue is proportional to the tissue conductance and the difference in gas concentration between the two sides. Thus:

$$\text{Gas flow} = D_L \times (P_A - P_C)$$

where D_L is the conductance of the alveolar-capillary membrane, P_A is the alveolar gas pressure, and P_C is the pulmonary capillary gas pressure (see p. 65). The conductance of the membrane in turn is proportional to its cross-sectional area and directly related to the blood volume in the pulmonary capillary bed. As a rule abnormal diffusion sufficient to cause a blood gas tension abnormality is likely only when at least two of three possible stresses in the diffusion equation are present: (1) decreased Pa_{O_2}, which reduces the driving pressure; (2) increased thickness of the alveolar-capillary membrane, which increases the resistance to diffusion (e.g., interstitial edema or fibrosis); or (3) either a reduction in the cross-sectional area of the pulmonary capillary bed (e.g., adult respiratory distress syndrome) or reduced time for red blood cell loading in the capillary bed (e.g., states of increased cardiac output).

MONITORING AND LABORATORY TESTS

Management of respiratory failure begins with determination of etiology and institution of monitoring designed to follow the course of the disease process and the adequacy of therapy. The diagnosis is made and the cause of respiratory failure is determined by physical examination, by the interpretation of arterial blood gases and pH and chest roentgenogram, and by using the equations outlined on p. 65 to best determine the mechanism responsible for impaired gas exchange.

The following symptoms, signs, and warnings of respiratory failure are nonspecific, but they are useful for predicting the course and therefore urgency of further evaluation and therapy.

Hypercapnia

Headache
Drowsiness, coma
Sweating
Tachycardia, hypertension
Peripheral vasodilation
Apnea
Excessive work of breathing, shortness of breath
Stridor, wheezing
Paradoxical chest wall–abdominal motion
Reduced air entry by auscultation
Asymmetric air entry by auscultation

Hypoxemia

Cyanosis
Confusion, agitation, restlessness
Shortness of breath
Sweating
Tachycardia, hypertension, dysrhythmias

Bradycardia, hypotension (particularly in association with evidence of pulmonary hypertension and/or shock)
Peripheral vasoconstriction
Rales by auscultation
Murmur by auscultation

Obtain arterial blood gases and pH. The diagnosis of acute respiratory failure can be made when the Pa_{CO_2} >55 mm Hg (assuming there is no preexisting lung disease resulting in chronic CO_2 elevation) or the Pa_{O_2} <50 mm Hg (assuming there is no cyanotic congenital heart disease).

The interpretation of arterial blood gas values is shown below: Analysis of the pH and bicarbonate levels will aid in this assessment by demonstrating the presence of chronic CO_2 elevation, metabolic acidemia or alkalemia, or hypocapnia (Pa_{CO_2} <35 mm Hg) in response to hypoxemia, metabolic acidosis, or disorders that primarily increase $\dot{V}E$ (e.g., increased intracranial pressure).

Obtain a chest roentgenogram and check for abnormalities that necessitate immediate intervention (e.g., pneumothorax or malposition of an endotracheal tube in a previously intubated patient). Further diagnostic tests and therapy will be guided by the findings on the chest roentgenogram. If they are available, compare current films to previous films.

Measure the Pa_{O_2} and calculate the $A\text{-}aD_{O_2}$; recall that hypoxemia with a normal $A\text{-}aD_{O_2}$ results from hypoventilation, whereas an increased $A\text{-}aD_{O_2}$ results from either $\dot{V}/\dot{Q}$ mismatch or a diffusion abnormality. Begin continuous measurement of O_2 saturation (Sa_{O_2}) using pulse oximetry. Recall that the relationship of Sa_{O_2} and Pa_{O_2} is expressed by the sigmoid-shaped O_2 dissociation curve (Fig. 10-1). When using continuous oximetry, remember Sa_{O_2} may be constant over a wide range of Pa_{O_2} values (flat portion of the curve) or may drop precipitously with relatively little change in Pa_{O_2} (steep portion of curve). Furthermore, the Sa_{O_2} for any given Pa_{O_2} value depends on the position of the curve, which may move left or right as indicated in the figure.

Begin continuous monitoring of the patient (both by physical examination and bedside technology). Special attention to the following parameters is mandatory: level of consciousness, respiratory rate and effort, patency of the upper airway, color, and peripheral perfusion. Available monitors include indwelling arterial catheters, continuous pulse oximetry, transcutaneous Pao_2 and $Paco_2$ electrodes, end-tidal CO_2 samples, as well as chest wall impedance leads to monitor respiratory rate and to assess qualitatively the depth of respiration. Serial assessment of arterial blood gases, pH, and hemoglobin concentration may be indicated. Construct a bedside flow sheet to follow the patient's course and response to therapy continuously.

If a pulmonary artery catheter is placed, calculate the $\dot{Q}s/\dot{Q}t$, measure the $P\bar{v}o_2$, determine both O_2 delivery ($CO \times Cao_2$) and O_2 consumption [$CO \times$ ($Cao_2 - C\bar{v}o_2$)], and evaluate both pulmonary artery blood pressure and pulmonary vascular resistance (see Chapter 12).

If a patient needs mechanical ventilation and is receiving a constant tidal volume, determine both static and dynamic lung compliance (see Chapter 128). Perform bedside pulmonary function tests if possible (see Chapter 125). Obtain sputum for Gram's stain and culture if clinically appropriate to do so. Reassess the patient after any therapeutic maneuver in order to determine the response to intervention and to guide further therapy.

INTERPRETATION OF ARTERIAL BLOOD GASES

Elevated $Paco_2 \rightarrow$ Diagnosis: Hypoventilation $\rightarrow$ Further diagnostics necessary
Normal $Paco_2 \rightarrow$ Diagnosis: Adequate ventilation
Reduced $Paco_2 \rightarrow$ Diagnosis: Hyperventilation
    Reduced $Pao_2 \rightarrow$ Administer 100% O_2
        $Pao_2 < 100$ mm Hg $\rightarrow$ Diagnosis: Shunt $\rightarrow$ Further diagnostics necessary
        $Pao_2 > 100$ mm Hg $\rightarrow$ Diagnosis: Low $\dot{V}/\dot{Q}$ match or diffusion disturbance $\rightarrow$ Further diagnostics necessary
    Normal $Pao_2 \rightarrow$ Evaluate pH/bicarbonate
        Bicarbonate reduced $\rightarrow$ Diagnosis: Metabolic acidosis $\rightarrow$ Further diagnostics necessary
        Bicarbonate normal $\rightarrow$ Primary hyperventilation $\rightarrow$ Further diagnostics necessary

---

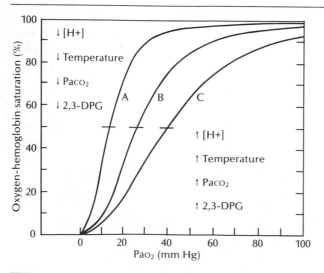

Fig. 10-1 Oxygen-hemoglobin saturation curve. *A,* Shift of curve to left resulting in reduced O_2 dissociation from hemoglobin; the effect is increased O_2 saturation for any given Pao_2 value. *B,* Oxygen-hemoglobin saturation curve. Note the flat portion of the curve where a reduction in Pao_2 has little effect on O_2 saturation and the steep portion where a reduction in Pao_2 significantly diminishes O_2 saturation. *C,* Shift of curve to right (with factors responsible for the phenomenon) resulting in increased O_2 dissociation from hemoglobin; the effect is a reduced O_2 saturation for any given Pao_2 value. (Reproduced by permission from Levin DL, Morriss FC, Moore GC. A Practical Guide to Pediatric Intensive Care, 2nd ed. St. Louis: CV Mosby, 1984.)

TREATMENT

Once the abnormality of gas exchange is determined (hypercapnia, hypoxemia, or both) and the likely pathophysiologic mechanism is ascertained, therapy of respiratory failure can be instituted rationally. The methods for increasing V_A, administering O_2, improving lung volume, and increasing pulmonary blood flow as well as the management of specific disorders are outlined in Chapters 12, 126, 127, and 128. Tables 10-2 and 10-3 provide a summary of the goals and treatments available for physiologic disorders that present with either hypercapnia and/or hypoxemia.

Table 10-2   Management of Hypercapnia

Physiologic Disorder	Goal	Treatment
Central apnea	Increase V_A	Assisted ventilation, theophylline, caffeine, doxapram
Obstructive apnea	Airway control	Endotracheal intubation, oropharyngeal or nasopharyngeal suctioning, racemic epinephrine
Increased airways resistance	Bronchodilators	Beta-adrenergic agonists, steroids, theophylline
Increased dead space ventilation	Improve pulmonary blood flow	Vasodilators, induced alkalosis, heparin, urokinase/streptokinase, reduced PEEP, inotropes
Reduced lung compliance (low lung volume)	Correct lung volume	PEEP, diuretics, assisted ventilation, high-frequency oscillation
Respiratory muscle fatigue	Rest muscles	Assisted ventilation
	Improve muscle function	Beta-adrenergic agonists, theophylline
Inability to cooperate with assisted ventilation	Synchronize breathing	Sedation, pharmacologic neuromuscular paralysis

Table 10-3   Management of Hypoxemia

Physiologic Disorder	Goal	Treatment
Low $\dot{V}/\dot{Q}$	Treat hypoxemia	$\uparrow FiO_2$
	Correct lung volume	PEEP, diuretics, bronchodilators, surfactant replacement
Intrapulmonary shunt	Convert shunt to low or normal $\dot{V}/\dot{Q}$	PEEP, diuretics, bronchodilators
Intracardiac shunt		
Ductus arteriosus–dependent lesions	Maintain patency of ductus	PGE_1 infusion
Tetralogy of Fallot	Relax pulmonary infundibulum	Morphine sulfate, propranolol
Hypoventilation	Increase V_A	Assisted ventilation, intubation, racemic epinephrine
Increased dead space ventilation	Improve pulmonary blood flow	Vasodilators, induced alkalosis, inotropes
	Bypass pulmonary circuit	Extracorporeal membrane oxygenation
Diffusion disturbance	Increase alveolar O_2	$\uparrow FiO_2$
	Reduce resistance to diffusion	Diuretics, steroids

ADDITIONAL READING

• Alonzo GG, Dantzker DR. Respiratory failure, mechanisms of abnormal gas exchange, and oxygen delivery. Med Clin North Am 67:557, 1983.

Dantzker DR. The influence of cardiovascular function on gas exchange. Clin Chest Med 42:149, 1983.

Dantzker DR, Brook CJ, DeHart P, et al. Ventilation-perfusion distributions in the adult respiratory distress syndrome. Am Rev Respir Dis 120:1039, 1979.

Newth CJL. Recognition and management of respiratory failure. Pediatr Clin North Am 26:617, 1979.

Nichols DG, Rogers MC. Developmental physiology of the respiratory system. In Rogers M, ed. Textbook of Pediatric Intensive Care. Baltimore: Williams & Wilkins, 1987, p 83.

• Perkin RM, Anas NG. Pulmonary hypertension in pediatric patients. J Pediatr 105:511, 1984.

Redding GJ, Morray JP, Rea C. Respiratory failure in childhood. In Morry J, ed. Pediatric Intensive Care. Norwalk, Conn.: Appleton & Lange, 1987, p 107.

• Roussos C, Macklem PT. The respiratory muscles. N Engl J Med 307:786, 1982.

West JB, Dollery CT, Narmark J. Distribution of blood flow in isolated lung: Relation to vascular and alveolar pressures. J Appl Physiol 19:713, 1964.

Zapol WM, Snider MT. Pulmonary hypertension in severe acute respiratory failure. N Engl J Med 296:476, 1977.

11 Congestive Heart Failure

Mark Parrish

BACKGROUND AND PHYSIOLOGY

The physiologist defines congestive heart failure as an inability of the heart to pump sufficient blood to meet the needs of the body. However, the clinician defines heart failure in terms of the signs and symptoms it produces (i.e., tachypnea, tachycardia, edema, cardiomegaly). Circulatory and hormonal compensatory mechanisms produce the majority of these symptoms. Inadequate cardiac output stimulates certain compensatory mechanisms, including elevated circulatory catecholamines, antidiuretic hormone, and aldosterone. These hormones produce the classic signs and symptoms of congestive heart failure (tachycardia, fluid and salt retention, increased oxygen consumption, failure to thrive).

Four factors determine the cardiac output. These are (1) preload, (2) afterload, (3) contractility, and (4) heart rate. Preload can be thought of as the volume of blood filling the ventricle during diastole and is often estimated clinically with the ventricular filling pressure. Afterload is the resistance against which the ventricle must eject blood and is usually estimated by the systemic or pulmonary vascular resistance. Contractility refers to the strength of myocardial contraction, independent of the effects of preload and afterload. Clinical estimates of contractility are either cumbersome to perform or are moderately inaccurate due to our inability to separate the influences of preload and afterload. Nevertheless, left ventricular contractility is often estimated clinically with the shortening fraction (from the echocardiogram) or the ejection fraction (from radionuclide imaging or cineangiography).

Aberrations of preload, afterload, contractility, and heart rate occur with congestive heart failure. Fig. 11-1 illustrates how some of these factors interact in patients; several important clinical lessons about congestive heart failure can be learned from studying this figure. It is difficult to increase cardiac output in

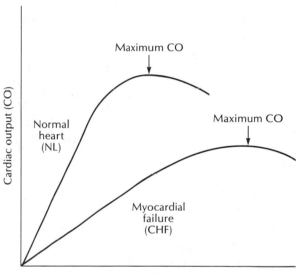

Observations: NL vs. CHF
1. Patients with CHF require higher filling pressure to achieve their maximum CO
2. Curve shifted to left (more favorable output/filling pressure relationship) by:
   a. Positive inotropic stimulation (digoxin, catecholamines, etc.)
   b. Afterload reduction (vasodilation)
3. Curve shifted to right by:
   a. Worsening contractility
   b. Immaturity of myocardium
   c. Hypertrophy of myocardium

Fig. 11-1 Relationship of ventricular filling pressure and cardiac output in patients with congestive heart failure and those with normal hearts. (Modified from Mason DT. Regulation of cardiac performance in clinical heart disease. Am J Cardiol 32:439, 1973.)

patients with congestive heart failure by increasing filling pressure. In comparison to normal hearts, each increment of cardiac output in patients with myocardial failure requires a very large increment in ventricular filling pressure. Acceptable capillary hydrostatic pressures are quickly exceeded, and systemic and/or pulmonary edema results. Furthermore, the output/filling pressure curve for immature and hypertrophied hearts is unfavorably shifted to the right compared with normal hearts. This means that many infants and children with myocardial failure have greater difficulty than adults in responding favorably to increases in ventricular filling volume.

The cardiac output/filling pressure relationship can be improved (shifted to the left) by stimulating contractility. Unfortunately children may again be at a disadvantage, since the immature myocardium appears to have less contractility reserve and is less responsive to the usual positive inotropic drugs than the adult heart. The cardiac output/filling pressure relationship can also be improved by reducing ventricular afterload. Differences in the response of the immature and adult myocardium to changes in afterload have not been well studied.

Congestive heart failure in children is precipitated by congenital or acquired heart disease that adversely affects preload, afterload, contractility, or heart rate. Table 11-1 lists some of the specific cardiac diseases seen in children and indicates how they disrupt the normal cardiac output.

MONITORING AND LABORATORY TESTS

Evaluation of critically ill patients with congestive heart failure has three goals. First, studies may be performed to investigate the etiology of the heart failure. Second, one may wish to evaluate the patient for any complicating features of the heart failure, such as a secondary pneumonia, or electrolyte disturbance. Third, continuous or periodic monitoring will be necessary to assess the effects of treatment.

If the etiology of congestive heart failure is unclear from the history and physical examination, certain laboratory investigations may be necessary to establish a cause for the condition. Many of the structural heart defects listed in Table 11-1 can be diagnosed correctly from the physical examination, with a little assistance from electrocardiograms and chest roentgenograms. If the diagnosis remains obscure after these simple studies, a cardiology consultant may recommend echocardiography or cardiac catheteriza-

tion. Sometimes evaluation of the patient reveals decreased ventricular function with no evidence of structural congenital heart disease. In this case the patient may have heart failure due to myocardial disease (cardiomyopathy or myocarditis). Numerous studies can be performed to investigate the cause of myocardial disease, including serum chemistries, triiodothyronine (T_3), levothyroxine (T_4), thyroid-stimulating hormone (TSH), viral titers, carnitine levels, and myocardial biopsies. However, these studies are frequently unrevealing, and a specific etiology for myocardial failure cannot be identified in a large number of patients.

Certain studies need to be performed routinely in patients with severe congestive heart failure to evaluate complicating features (Table 11-2). Many of the studies need to be repeated daily, if not more frequently, in patients with severe congestive heart failure.

Continuous or intermittent monitoring of circulatory physiology can facilitate therapeutic decision making. Table 11-3 lists some physiologic variables and how they are monitored. In patients with severe congestive heart failure it is quite helpful to monitor all of these variables. For example, a patient who deteriorates clinically will usually demonstrate a reduction in oxygen transport to the tissues. This worsening oxygen transport may be due to a decreased arterial oxygen saturation (deterioration in pulmonary status), decreased cardiac output, or anemia. If the cardiac output is decreased, this may be due to decreasing preload, increasing afterload, worsening contractility, or a change in the cardiac rhythm. When we understand the factors involved in a patient's deterioration, we can devise specific therapies to ameliorate the problem.

TREATMENT

Treatment for congestive heart failure falls into one of two cateogries: cure or palliation. Sometimes congestive heart failure can be cured if the failure is caused by a specific structural defect or a dysrhythmia. However, it is not the purpose of this chapter to discuss the surgical treatment of congenital heart defects or the medical treatment of dysrhythmias. Instead, the focus is on the numerous therapies that palliate congestive heart failure.

Medical palliation of congestive heart failure has two goals: to decrease the oxygen consumption of the body and to improve oxygen delivery to the tis-

Table 11-1 Cardiac Diseases Presenting as Congestive Heart Failure in Children

Defect/Disease	Primary Effect
Congenital problems	
Left-to-right shunts	Excessive pre-load
Ventricular septal defect	
Atrial septal defect	
Patent ductus arteriosus	
Atrioventricular canal	
Aortopulmonary window	
Absent pulmonary valve	
Obstruction	Excessive afterload
Coarctation of aorta	
Aortic stenosis	
Pulmonic stenosis	
Mitral stenosis	
Cyanotic defects	Excessive pre-load
Truncus arteriosus	
Transposition of great arteries with ventricular septal defect	
Total anomalous pulmonary venous drainage	
Hypoplastic left heart	
Dysrhythmias	
Tachyarrhythmias—ventricular or supraventricular tachycardia	Excessive heart rate
Bradycardia—complete heart block or sick sinus syndrome	Inadequate heart rate
Acquired problems	
Hypertension	Excessive afterload
Myocarditis	Inadequate contractility
Dilated cardiomyopathy	Inadequate contractility
Hormonal or electrolyte disturbances (hypothyroidism, hypocalcemia, hypoglycemia, hypomagnesemia)	Inadequate contractility
Rheumatic heart disease	Excessive pre-load
Ischemic or hypoxic cardiac injury	Inadequate contractility

Table 11-2 Laboratory Studies in Patients With Congestive Heart Failure

Complicating Feature	Laboratory Test
Anemia	Complete blood count
Dysrhythmias	Electrocardiogram
Electrolyte disorders	Electrolytes, Ca, Mg, PO_4
Hepatic failure	Serum transaminases, prothrombin time, partial thromboplastin time, alkaline phosphatase
Hypoglycemia	Serum glucose
Hypoxia	Arterial blood gas and pH
Metabolic alkalosis/acidosis	Arterial blood gas and pH
Pericardial effusion	Chest roentgenogram, echocardiogram
Renal failure	Blood urea nitrogen, creatinine
Sepsis/pneumonia	Cultures, chest roentgenogram, urinalysis

Table 11-3 Monitoring Circulatory Physiology

Physiologic Feature	Monitoring Method
Cardiac output	Fick method: O_2 consumption/ (Arterial − Venous O_2 content)*
	Thermodilution method (measures pulmonary blood flow)
	Skin temperature
Oxygen transport	Cardiac output × Arterial O_2 content
Heart rate and rhythm	Continuous oscillographic monitor
Preload	Central venous pressure
	Pulmonary capillary wedge pressure
	Chest roentgenogram (heart size)
Afterload	Systemic vascular resistance: (Arterial − Venous pressure)/ Cardiac output
	Pulmonary vascular resistance: (Pulmonary artery − Pulmonary wedge pressure)/Cardiac output
Contractility	Echocardiogram: left ventricular shortening fraction
	Radionuclide ventriculogram: ventricular ejection fraction

*O_2 content = Saturation × Hemoglobin × 1.34 ml oxygen/g hemoglobin.

sues. A conceptual scheme for treating heart failure is outlined below.

Decrease systemic oxygen consumption

Bed rest
Sedation and/or paralysis
Mechanical ventilation
Optimize nutrition
Homeothermic environment and antipyretics

Improve oxygen transport

Increase arterial oxygenation
    Respirations (ventilation, inspired oxygen, continuous positive airway pressure)
    Decrease pulmonary edema (diuresis)
    Increase hemoglobin concentration (transfusion)
    Increase cardiac output
        Preload (increase with volume infusion, decrease with diuresis and salt restriction)
        Decrease afterload (vasodilators)
        Increase contractility (positive inotropic drugs)
        Heart rate (convert dysrhythmia, slow or increase sinus rate with positive inotropic drugs)

The patient's oxygen consumption can be decreased by prescribing bed rest and sedation. In severely ill patients who need mechanical ventilation, paralytic agents may be helpful in further decreasing oxygen consumption. See Chapters 129 and 130 for appropriate dosages for sedatives and paralytic agents. Oxygen consumption may be decreased by improving the patient's nutritional status. Malnourished infants with congestive heart failure have greater oxygen demands than those who receive adequate nutritional support. To gain weight, infants with congestive heart failure usually require 130 to 150 calories/kg/day. Maintaining an optimal thermal environment will also reduce the patient's oxygen consumption. Thus it is important to treat fever with antipyretics and provide good external warmth for small infants.

Most therapies for congestive heart failure are aimed at improving oxygen transport to the tissues. As noted in Table 11-3, oxygen transport is determined by three factors: arterial oxygen saturation, hemoglobin concentration, and cardiac output. Therefore measures that improve the patient's effective ventilation, arterial oxygen saturation, and hematocrit need to be the first steps in treating congestive heart failure. If the hematocrit is less han 40% in an infant with severe congestive heart failure, packed red blood cells are slowly transfused.

Drug therapy for congestive heart failure attempts to improve the cardiac output/filling pressure relationship. Since the cardiac output is determined by preload, afterload, contractility, and heart rate, effective drug therapy influences one of these factors. Diuretics are often the clinician's first choice for improving preload. Table 11-4 lists several diuretic agents and their dosages. When acute diuresis is needed, IV administration of the diuretic is usually preferred. Diuresis is often more rapid and effective when the drug is delivered intravenously. Furosemide is one of the most potent and commonly used diuretics. However, chronic use of this drug causes numerous electrolyte and metabolic problems, including hypokalemia, hypochloremia, metabolic alkalosis, and urinary calcium loss. Furosemide is usually given in conjunction with spironolactone or potassium chloride to ameliorate some of the complications. If the diuretic effect of furosemide alone is inadequate, additional natriuretic effect can be achieved occasionally by adding metolazone to the therapeutic regimen. This must be done cautiously since severe sodium, potassium, or water depletion may result. One alternative to the use of a diuretic is to attempt to restrict sodium and fluid intake. Water intake may be reduced to 60% to 80% of maintenance levels. However, in patients with chronic heart failure, fluid intake must sometimes be increased above the usual maintenance levels in order to deliver sufficient calories to the patient.

Cardiac output can also be improved by decreasing ventricular afterload. If the systemic vascular resistance is high, vasodilation is a particularly effective treatment. However, if systemic vascular resistance is low, vasodilation may produce severe hypotension, decrease coronary artery perfusion, and cause myocardial ischemia. When elevated pulmonary vascular resistance is the cause of heart failure, vasodilators must be used with extreme caution. Attempts to produce pulmonary vasodilatation also may cause systemic hypotension and death. When treating severe pulmonary hypertension with vasodilators, pulmonary arterial blood pressure, systemic arterial blood pressure, and cardiac output need to be closely monitored. See Chapter 12 for recommended doses of vasodilators. For acute vasodilation, we have found nitroprusside to be very effective. If high dosages are used or if the treatment is used for more than 48 hours, serum thiocyanate levels need to be monitored to assess potential toxicity. For chronic vasodilation, an angiotensin-converting enzyme inhibitor such as captopril can be used. Captopril may cause hyperkalemia when used with spironolactone, so that serum potassium levels need to be monitored. For the pharmacologic treatment of pulmonary hypertension, alpha-adrenergic blocking agents such as chlorpromazine or tolazoline can be used.

Sometimes cardiac output can be improved in children by increasing the contractile strength of the

Table 11-4 Diuretics

Drug	Dose
Chlorothiazide (Diuril)	PO = 20-40 mg/kg/day (bid dosing)
Ethacrynic acid (Edecrin)	IV = 0.4-1.0 mg/kg/day PO = 10-20 mg/kg/day (qid dosing)
Furosemide (Lasix)	IV, IM, or PO = 1-4 mg/kg/day (qd or bid dosing)
Hydrochlorothiazide (Hydrodiuril)	PO = 2-4 mg/kg/day (bid dosing)
Spironolactone (Aldactone)	PO = 1-4 mg/kg/day (qd or bid)
Metolazone (Zaroxolyn)	PO = 0.05-0.1 mg/kg/day (qd dosing)

Table 11-5 Digoxin

Age Group	Oral Loading Dose*	Maintenance Dose†
Premature infant	15-30 μg/kg	6-8 μg/kg/day
Newborn	30-40 μg/kg	8-10 μg/kg/day
Children	40 μg/kg	10-14 μg/kg/day

Maximum loading dose = 1000 μg; maximum maintenance dose = 500 μg/day.

NOTE: For IV dose reduce to two thirds of oral dose; for patients with myocarditis, reduce dose by 20%; in renal failure, use serum levels to adjust maintenance dose. Clearance of digoxin is decreased and dose must be reduced in hypothyroidism or if quinidine, verapamil, or amiodarone are being given.

*Loading dose is usually given in three divided doses—½ of total initially, ¼ of total after 6 to 8 hours, remaining ¼ of total after another 6 to 8 hours.

†Maintenance dose is usually divided into two doses and given twice/day.

heart. See Chapter 12 for doses of IV drugs that enhance cardiac contractility. In addition to its positive inotropic effect, each drug has additional characteristics that influence the clinician's choice of therapeutic agent. For example, isoproterenol, amrinone, and milrinone (not approved by the FDA for use in children at this time) are potent vasodilators. All of the agents listed increase heart rate and may cause dysrhythmias, but epinephrine and isoproterenol are particularly potent in this regard. The agents that increase heart rate and contractility (epinephrine, norepinephrine) also markedly increase myocardial oxygen consumption, whereas those agents that cause systemic vasodilation (amrinone and milrinone) do not appear to affect myocardial oxygen consumption to the same degree. Dopamine is often chosen because of its ability to selectively increase renal blood flow. Epinephrine is sometimes chosen because it is highly effective in increasing systemic arterial blood pressure, although this increase may occur at the expense of increasing systemic vascular resistance. Unfortunately there is little information available in children to support choosing one drug over another. Clinical and laboratory data suggest that isoproterenol and dopamine are effective stimulants of contractility in children, although the renal receptors for dopamine may mature relatively late. Experimental data also indicate amrinone may paradoxically decrease the contractile strength of the immature heart. All of these IV drugs may have diminished efficacy when used for prolonged periods.

For long-term stimulation of cardiac contractility, digoxin is used. Digoxin may be combined with other intravenous positive inotropic agents in patients with severe congestive heart failure. Digoxin must be used with extreme caution in patients with decreased renal function or hypokalemia. Table 11-5 describes the recommended doses for digoxin.

ADDITIONAL READING

Artman M, Graham TP. Congestive heart failure in infancy: Recognition and management. Am Heart J 103:1040-1055, 1982.

Artman M, Parrish MD, Graham TP. Congestive heart failure in childhood and adolescence: Recognition and management. Am Heart J 105:471-480, 1983.

Friedman WF, George BL. New concepts and drugs in the treatment of congestive heart failure. Pediatr Clin North Am 31:1197-1227, 1984.

12   Shock

Ronald M. Perkin · Daniel L. Levin

BACKGROUND AND PHYSIOLOGY

Shock is an acute, complex abnormality of hemodynamic function in which sufficient amounts of nutrients, especially oxygen, are not delivered to meet the needs of tissues. In this context the shock state may be viewed as a state of acute cellular oxygen deficiency, most commonly from a limitation of blood flow or oxygen delivery. However, in some instances a limitation of oxygen utilization may contribute to the deficiency.

Delivery of oxygen is a direct function of the cardiac index (CI) and the arterial content (Cao_2):

$$O_2 \text{ delivery (ml/min/m}^2) = \\ CI \text{ (L/min/m}^2) \times Cao_2 \text{ (ml/dl)} \times 10 \text{ (dl/L)}$$

Reduced oxygen content, seen in anemia, poor arterial oxygen saturation, or both, will induce an even greater dependency on cardiac output to maintain oxygen delivery. Inadequate oxygen delivery is usually the result of an absolute reduction in cardiac output, but occasionally increased oxygen requirements, as seen in fever, sepsis, or trauma, may result in circulatory failure at a normal cardiac output. If a relatively "inadequate" cardiac output is allowed to continue, even though it may be significantly increased above normal, cellular anoxic damage eventually becomes evident.

If, for any reason, oxygen delivery does not meet cellular metabolic requirements, various compensatory mechanisms are activated; shock is the clinical syndrome that is a manifestation of compensation for the acute cellular oxygen deficiency. Therefore the exact cardiorespiratory pattern manifest during shock depends on the complex interaction of host and illness over time. The precipitating event initiates a state of circulatory failure, and these circulatory problems are modified or augmented by complex neuroendocrine activity; products of cellular breakdown; altered metabolism; vascular mediators; and individual host factors such as blood volume status, nutritional state, and myocardial competence. Because of the multiple factors involved, the cardiorespiratory pattern will vary considerably as the shock state evolves.

Because of its progressive nature, shock may be divided into three phases: compensated, uncompensated, and irreversible. In compensated shock, vital organ function is maintained by intrinsic compensatory mechanisms. The common denominator in this early stage is not low blood flow; flow is usually normal or increased unless it is limited by preexisting hypovolemia or myocardial dysfunction. More often blood flow is uneven or maldistributed in the microcirculation. Nonspecific measurements such as systemic arterial blood pressure, pulse rate, and cardiac output do not differentiate between the normal state and compensated shock states despite the important underlying physiologic derangements in compensated shock.

When shock progresses to the uncompensated phase, the cardiovascular system is no longer efficient and perfusion is marginal in small vascular beds even though compensatory mechanisms exist. In the end, the abnormalities of the circulation become self-sustaining, and further compensatory mechanisms may even worsen the progression and self-sustaining nature of the shock state. Toxic cellular products are made that further interfere with normal cardiac function and vasomotor adjustment. Arterioles may not regulate blood flow in the capillaries and may allow vasodilation in some vessels but at the same time allow vasoconstriction in others. This sluggish flow pattern allows platelet adhesion and coalescence of red blood cells, and in concert with the high level of endogenous catecholamines, may produce detrimental chain reactions in both the coagulation and kinin systems. As cellular function in various capillary beds deteriorates, abnormalities become demonstrable in all organ systems.

The terminal or irreversible phase of shock indicates damage has occurred in key organs such as the heart or brain of such magnitude that death occurs even if therapy can return cardiovascular functions to normal levels.

Hypovolemic Shock

Hypovolemic shock represents the most common form of shock. It occurs when there is such a profound decrease in the circulating blood volume that there is inadequate ventricular filling, which results in a severely decreased cardiac output.

Hypovolemic shock can occur secondary to loss of blood, plasma, or fluid and electrolytes. Blood can be lost by obvious, visible, external bleeding or by concealed internal bleeding such as into body cavities or into the gastrointestinal tract. Plasma loss may occur from burn-related, denuded skin or from third-space shifts, as seen in peritonitis or bowel obstruction. Profound fluid loss may occur from the gastrointestinal tract because of vomiting or diarrhea; renal salt and water losses or profuse sweating also can produce hypovolemia if fluid replacement is inadequate.

In addition to these forms of absolute hypovolemia, in which there is actual loss of blood or fluid, relative hypovolemia also may occur. Decreased vascular resistance may follow CNS or spinal cord injury or inappropriate drug therapy and can lead to intravascular blood pooling and decreased venous return to the heart. Therefore hypovolemic shock is best defined as a sudden decrease in the intravascular blood volume relative to the vascular capacity to the extent that effective tissue perfusion cannot be maintained.

Physiologic mechanisms of the body compensate for the loss of intravascular fluid in children in the same way that they do in adults. Acute losses of 10% to 15% of the circulatory blood volume are well tolerated and in healthy children are easily compensated. Activation of peripheral and central baroreceptors produce an outpouring of catecholamines, resulting in tachycardia and peripheral vasoconstriction, which are usually adequate to support the blood pressure with little or no evidence of hypotension. An acute loss of 25% or more of the circulating blood volume, however, frequently results in a clinically

apparent hypovolemic state that necessitates immediate and aggressive management.

The most reliable indicators of early, compensated hypovolemic shock in children are persistent tachycardia, cutaneous vasoconstriction, and diminution of the pulse pressure. The best clinical evidence of decreased tissue perfusion is skin mottling, prolonged capillary refill, and cool extremities. Systemic arterial blood pressure is frequently normal, the result of increased systemic vascular resistance. Neurologic status is normal or only minimally impaired.

With continued loss of blood volume or with delayed or inadequate blood volume replacement, the intravascular fluid losses surpass the body's compensatory abilities and decompensated phases appear. The pronounced systemic vasoconstriction and hypovolemia produce ischemia and stagnant hypoxia in the visceral and cutaneous circulations. Altered cellular metabolism and function occur in these areas, resulting in damage to blood vessels, kidneys, liver, pancreas, and bowel. Stroke volume and cardiac output are decreased and patients are hypotensive, acidotic, lethargic or comatose, and oliguric or anuric. Arterial blood pressure falls only after compensations are exhausted, which may occur long after the precipitating event and after severe reduction in cardiac output. Terminal phases of hypovolemic shock are characterized by myocardial dysfunction and widespread cell death.

Cardiogenic Shock

Cardiogenic shock is defined as an abnormal condition in which cardiac dysfunction is responsible for failure of the cardiovascular system to deliver sufficient metabolic requirements to meet the needs of the tissues. The common element is depressed cardiac output, which in most cases results from decreased myocardial contractility. Although implicit in any definition of cardiac failure is impairment of the heart's ability to maintain its pumping function, a growing body of evidence has shown that heart failure and its clinical expression may be produced by different, although interdependent, mechanisms that govern the process of myocardial relaxation. Impaired relaxation changes the pressure-to-volume ratio during diastole and increases left ventricular pressure at any volume. This is hemodynamically unfavorable since increased left ventricular diastolic pressure will be transmitted to the lungs, resulting in dyspnea and perhaps pulmonary edema. Additionally, increased diastolic stiffness may limit cardiac output by reducing ventricular filling. Diastolic properties of the ventricle appear to be the first to become abnormal in patients with ischemic heart disease or disorders associated with ventricular hypertrophy. Therefore, when approaching a patient with cardiogenic shock, it is important to characterize both diastolic and systolic function since therapy designed to improve systolic function alone may further impair myocardial relaxation.

A common cause of cardiogenic shock in children is impaired cardiac performance following intracardiac surgery, and this type of shock is associated with significant morbidity and mortality in the early postoperative period. Other clinically important causes of cardiogenic shock in children are dysrhythmias, drug intoxication, hypoxic/ischemic episodes, acidosis, hypothermia, metabolic derangement (hypoglycemia, myopathies), extrinsic inflow or outflow obstructions (tension pneumothorax, tension pneumopericardium, pericardial effusion with tamponade), severe congestive heart failure secondary to congenital heart disease, and myocardial dysfunction secondary to blunt chest injury.

Blunt injuries to the heart are more common in the child than in the adult. Blunt cardiac injury can cause myocardial contusion, myocardial concussion, aneurysm, septal defects, chamber rupture, valvular rupture, and damage to the pericardium. Each of these entities has separate presentations, although the lesions are often concurrent. Careful cardiac evaluation must be done in every pediatric trauma patient.

In patients in shock, cardiac function can be depressed due to causes other than direct myocardial insult. Myocardial dysfunction is frequently a late manifestation of shock of any etiology. Although the cause of myocardial dysfunction as a late manifestation of shock is not completely understood, the following mechanisms have been proposed: (1) specific toxic substances released during the course of shock that have a direct cardiac depressant effect; (2) myocardial edema; (3) adrenergic receptor dysfunction; (4) impaired sarcolemmal calcium flux; and (5) reduced coronary blood flow resulting in impaired myocardial systolic and diastolic function.

As opposed to hypovolemic shock, compensatory responses can have deleterious effects in patients with cardiogenic shock. Compensatory responses are nonspecific, not precisely set, and in patients with

cardiogenic shock they may contribute to the progression of shock by further depressing cardiac function. For example, as pump function deteriorates and cardiac output decreases, systemic vascular resistance increases in order to maintain circulatory stability. However, the increase in afterload adds to the heart's work load and further decreases pump function. Therefore in cardiogenic shock a negative feedback system is established in which ventricular dysfunction is exacerbated by neurohumoral vasoconstrictive mechanisms and vice versa. Because of the self-perpetuating cycle, compensated phases of cardiogenic shock may not be observed, and frequently only one cardiorespiratory pattern, in varying degrees of severity, is observed. The patients are tachycardic, hypotensive, diaphoretic, oliguric, and acidotic. Extremities are cool and mental status is altered. Hepatomegaly, jugular venous distention, rales, and peripheral edema may be observed. Cardiac output is depressed and elevations in central venous blood pressure, pulmonary capillary wedge pressure, and systemic vascular resistance are observed.

Cardiogenic shock in childhood represents a diagnostic and therapeutic challenge largely because of the myriad etiologies in this age group. Diagnosis is facilitated by a careful history and physical examination as well as chest radiography, electrocardiography, and echocardiography. Echocardiography is useful not only for diagnosing congenital cardiac malformations but also for quantifying chamber size and estimating cardiac function; sequential echocardiograms can be helpful in evaluating response to therapy.

Septic Shock (Distributive Shock)

Abnormal distribution of blood in the microcirculation can lead to extreme deficiencies in perfusion of the tissue beds. Abnormal distribution may have many causes, including vasomotor paralysis, increased venous capacitance, or physiologic shunting past capillary beds. There are many causes of shock due to abnormal distribution of blood flow in children, including anaphylaxis, sepsis, CNS injury, and drug intoxication (barbiturates, smooth muscle relaxants, antihypertensive medications, tranquilizers).

Septic shock continues to be a major cause of death despite careful monitoring, aggressive surgery, and the use of specific antibiotic therapy. Septic shock comprises a cascade of metabolic, hemodynamic, and clinical changes resulting from invasive infection and the release of microbial toxins in the bloodstream. Historically, a distinction was made between the clinical findings and the type of invading microorganism. However, on closer analysis it became apparent that the systemic response was independent of the type of invading organism (bacteria, virus, fungus, rickettsia); rather it was a host-dependent response. Septic shock is a constellation of signs and symptoms that reflects multiple organ system derangements at the subcellular level. It is difficult to differentiate septic shock from sepsis without shock arbitrarily because each appears to represent a different stage in the spectrum of sepsis.

In comparison to other forms of shock the pathophysiology of septic shock is markedly different. The pathogenesis of septic shock remains controversial and is probably multifactorial in origin. Because of the multiple factors involved, the clinical pattern and presentation of septic shock may vary a great deal and depends on the dynamic interplay of the invading organism, elapsing time, and host status (Fig. 12-1). In addition to the organism and its toxins, a network of mediators and activators interact to produce the septic syndrome. The mediators and activators may include autonomic discharge of catecholamines;

products of specific cells such as macrophages, granular leukocytes, and platelets; products of activated protein cascade systems (complement, coagulation); endogenous vasodilators and vasoconstrictors; and yet-to-be characterized myocardial and vascular depressant factors. Sepsis in a previously healthy patient should be readily correctable. However, septic shock only occasionally presents as a community-acquired disease. Rather, hospitalized patients are at greatest risk of developing septic shock. This population includes seriously ill surgical and medical patients who are likely to be debilitated or immunodeficient. They may have a variety of invasive devices and are often receiving antibiotic therapy.

Abnormal hemodynamic responses constitute a primary hallmark of septic shock. The early stages consist of a hyperdynamic state characterized by an elevated cardiac output, a decreased systemic vascular resistance, a widened pulse pressure, episodic hypotension, and warm extremities on physical examination. In this hyperdynamic state the syndrome can also be recognized by the presence of high fever, mental confusion, and hyperventilation with hypocapnia and respiratory alkalosis. Although these patients are typically tachycardic and tachypneic, the

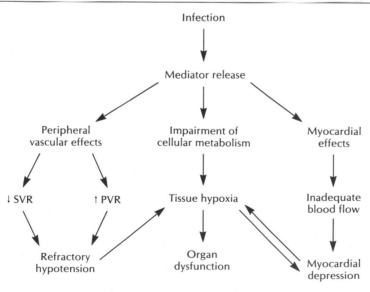

Fig. 12-1 Factors in the pathogenesis of septic shock. (SVR = systemic vascular resistance; PVR = pulmonary vascular resistance.)

vital signs and clinical examination may not reflect the severity of disease. Close neurologic examination, however, usually shows that the patients are confused or hallucinating; this is a valuable, but often neglected, clinical clue.

If sepsis is unchecked and uncorrected, steady deterioration in cardiovascular performance occurs, characterized by a decline in cardiac output, hypotension, and metabolic acidosis. Hypotension occurs even with a normal or elevated cardiac output. One fundamental abnormality in patients with septic shock is an altered relationship of systemic vascular resistance and cardiac output. The patient's status deteriorates when cardiac compensation for diminishing systemic vascular resistance is lost. Some patients die from refractory hypotension as a result of a very low systemic vascular resistance. The progression from high to low cardiac output may happen quickly (in minutes or hours) or slowly over days. The lower the cardiac output, the more likely it is that progressive lactacidemia will terminate in a fatal outcome. Often infants present with a hypodynamic picture, probably because of limited cardiac reserve. Such an ill-appearing infant presents a diagnostic challenge because the differential diagnosis is extensive. However, these infants must be considered to have sepsis and quickly managed as such.

Survival in septic shock has been related to the host's ability to establish and maintain a hyperdynamic cardiovascular state. In early stages, hypovolemia or myocardial dysfunction resulting from preexisting or intercurrent ventricular disease can blunt or eliminate the hyperdynamic response to sepsis. Several factors may contribute to hypovolemia, which commonly occurs in septic shock. Increased microvascular permeability, arteriolar and venular dilation with subsequent peripheral pooling of intravascular blood volume, inappropriate polyuria, and poor oral intake all combine to result in a reduced effective circulating blood volume. Fluid loss secondary to fever, diarrhea, vomiting, or sequestered third-space fluid also contributes to the hypovolemia.

In some patients without complicating preexisting heart disease a *relative* depression in left ventricular contractility exists even in early stages. The cause of depressed contractility in septic shock is not immediately apparent. Diffuse myocardial edema, the inhibitory effects of a myocardial depressant factor, adrenergic receptor dysfunction, and impaired sarcolemmal calcium flux have all been proposed. In patients who survive, this myocardial depression is transient, lasting for 1 to 4 days, and then myocardial function returns to normal.

Although right ventricular failure is uncommon in critically ill septic patients, subtle and potentially important changes in right ventricular function do oc-

---

DIFFERENTIAL DIAGNOSIS OF THE SEPTIC-APPEARING INFANT

Infections

Meningitis
Bacterial sepsis
Viral infection
Urinary tract infection

Cardiac

Dysrhythmias
   Supraventricular tachycardia
   Atrioventricular block
Congenital heart disease
Pulmonary hypertension
Cardiomyopathies
   Myocarditis
   Infiltrative disease

Metabolic

Electrolyte disturbances
Hypoglycemia
Inborn errors of metabolism

Gastrointestinal

Intestinal obstruction or ischemia
Gastroenteritis with dehydration
Vomiting

Miscellaneous

Child abuse, shaken child syndrome
Anemia
Hepatic failure, Reye's syndrome

cur. Impedance to right ventricular ejection may be increased as a consequence of an elevated pulmonary vascular resistance and mean pulmonary arterial blood pressure. Humorally mediated pulmonary vasoconstriction, microembolic occlusion of the pulmonary vasculature, structural changes in pulmonary arteriolar smooth muscle with protracted lung injury, and the use of positive end-expiratory pressure all contribute to an increase in pulmonary arterial blood pressure. Regardless of mechanism, the occurrence of pulmonary hypertension in septic patients has demonstrable effects on right ventricular performance that potentially can limit the hyperdynamic state necessary to ensure tissue oxygen delivery.

Septic shock is a syndrome characterized by abnormal use of oxygen. Although sepsis is a well-known hypermetabolic stress associated with increased oxygen demands, deterioration during the septic process characteristically shows a fall in oxygen consumption during a period when cardiovascular function and oxygen delivery remain increased. This reduction in oxygen consumption is the result of decreased oxygen extraction and reflects a severe impairment of oxidative metabolism at a time of major metabolic and physiologic stress. The pathophysiology of inadequate oxygen consumption in septic shock is still unclear. The most widely accepted theories to account for this oxygen debt are the redistribution of blood flow, with a consequent decrease in nutrient capillary flow, and the development of a cellular metabolic blockade at the mitochondrial level such that delivered oxygen cannot be used. More likely a spectrum of abnormalities exists. In early stages, flow-dependent oxygen consumption is observed and a high cardiac output allows the required oxygen consumption to be maintained. As the septic shock state progresses, a failure of central venous hemoglobin desaturation occurs. The arteriovenous oxygen content difference becomes inappropriately low for the existing level of cardiac output. As this phenomenon continues, the total body oxygen consumption falls despite large volumes of oxygen delivered to the periphery. Progressive deterioration in oxygen consumption and oxygen extraction portends a poor prognosis for septic shock patients.

In addition to oxygen, impaired use of other metabolic substrates has been demonstrated in septic shock. The septic event appears to hinder sequentially the utilization of glucose, then fat, and finally protein as energy sources. Late stages of septic shock are characterized by abnormalities in energy availability and substrate utilization. The exact process responsible for these abnormalities is not known; however, the overall metabolic picture is consistent with a progressive inhibition of substrate entry into the Krebs cycle. Multiple system organ failure is the result of this progressive peripheral energy deficit (see Chapter 22).

Sequelae of Shock

Multiple organ failure, progressive organ failure, and sequential organ failure describe complications that may occur after circulatory dysfunction has lasted for prolonged periods. Common sequelae include respiratory failure, renal failure, hepatic dysfunction, pancreatic ischemia, disseminated intravascular coagulation, gastrointestinal hemorrhage, immunologic dysfunction, alterations in mental status, and a host of endocrinologic problems. Although in the past attention has focused on the purely cardiovascular aspects of the shock syndromes, there is an increasing awareness of the importance of other organ system problems, which may become the limiting factors to overall treatment success. Therapy and monitoring must therefore be directed not only to restoration of cardiovascular status but also toward support of vital organ systems.

The lung is sensitive to the shock state, and respiratory failure develops rapidly and frequently can be the cause of death. These patients have increased extravascular lung water, which is caused by two mechanisms: hydrostatic edema, produced by elevation of pulmonary microvascular blood pressure, or permeability edema (adult respiratory distress syndrome), in which there is damage to the alveolar epithelium and the pulmonary capillary endothelium. Because of cellular damage, pulmonary capillaries become permeable and proteinaceous fluid leaks into both the interstitium and alveoli. Resultant changes in alveolar compliance and flooding lead to a significant alteration in ventilation-perfusion relationships with increased shunt and venous admixture. Although the exact mechanism of pulmonary injury is unclear, numerous factors probably contribute (see Chapter 35).

Constant surveillance of respiratory status and efforts to correct hypoxemia and acidosis need to be priorities in management. In addition, patients in shock, with or without hypoxemic respiratory failure, will have increased work of breathing. However, because of decreased or redistributed cardiac output, respiratory muscle blood flow may be limited to levels less than those necessary to support the increased work of breathing. Respiratory muscle fatigue may then occur, leading to acute respiratory failure and circulatory collapse. This complication can be prevented by early initiation of mechanical ventilation.

Progressive azotemia, with or without oliguria, may occur in association with any of the shock syndromes. It is best to think of the shock-related renal failure syndromes as a continuum from acute prerenal failure, through classic acute tubular necrosis, to the extreme of cortical necrosis. Although the precise mechanisms involved in the production of renal failure are unclear, diminished renal perfusion due to persistent vasospasm with reduced glomerular filtration rate, enhanced distal exchange site activity secondary to increased aldosterone production, and increased free-water absorption caused by elevated antidiuretic hormone activity all seem to be operative. These mechanisms, however, do not completely account for the oliguria of acute renal failure, and they certainly do not provide a satisfactory basis for understanding the nonoliguric renal failure syndrome that is often seen in septic shock. Nevertheless, prevention of renal failure and subsequent complications associated with peritoneal dialysis, ultrafiltration, and hemodialysis are of paramount importance.

Hypoperfusion and local hypoxia may produce profound liver, gut, and brain dysfunction in shock patients. The precise mechanisms involved are not well defined but presumably relate to deficient energy and substrate availability for the cells.

Multiple endocrinologic problems may arise and complicate the management of children in shock. Included in these are problems with fluid, electrolytes, and mineral balance. Severe abnormalities of calcium homeostasis can occur in the course of any acute hemodynamic deterioration. Marked decreases in serum ionized calcium levels have been reported in conditions associated with inadequate tissue perfusion, regardless of etiology.

Sustained decreases in ionized calcium have been associated with depressed myocardial function, tachycardia, hypotension, acidosis, cyanosis, temperature instability, and alterations in mental status. For these reasons, therapeutic intervention is justified when serum ionized calcium levels fall below normal.

MONITORING AND LABORATORY TESTS

Most patients in shock need aggressive monitoring and management that can be invasive and risky. Some patients, however, may have a specific, immediately remediable cause of shock such as paroxysmal atrial tachycardia with congestive heart failure, or hypovolemia due to diarrhea that rapidly responds to fluid administration. These latter patients may not need the full extent of monitoring; however, in many patients shock is not immediately reversed and extensive and invasive monitoring is needed.

For the cardiovascular system, frequent physical examinations including assessment of skin (color, temperature, capillary refill), mental status (restless, anxious, agitated, or depressed consciousness), pulse (rate, quality, rhythm), respiration (rate, depth), and hourly urine output. In addition, arterial blood gas tensions and pH are obtained initially and every 1 to 2 hours. Systemic arterial blood pressure is monitored continually, making note of the arterial pressure waveform and pulse pressure. Also CVP is monitored continuously. Echocardiography may need to be done to determine anatomy, to estimate ventricular function and volume, and to exclude pericardial effusions. If readily available, measurement of arterial lactate concentration is useful as an indicator of the severity of perfusion failure and is often used as a prognostic guide.

Occasionally in order to evaluate perfusion failure most accurately and to define appropriate interventions, variables that relate to oxygen transport must be determined. These include cardiac output, hemoglobin concentration, arterial oxygen saturation, and mixed venous oxygen saturation. Measurement of these variables can be obtained by using a thermodilation pulmonary artery catheter (Table 12-1).

For other systems, renal and liver function tests are monitored frequently, coagulation status checked initially and as necessary, and electrolyte and mineral status monitored frequently.

TREATMENT

Since shock is a clinical syndrome reflecting inadequate tissue oxygenation, therapeutic efforts, in addition to treatment of the primary underlying process, involve optimizing and maintaining oxygen delivery. However, if the patient has hypotension and is in a decompensated state, the primary goal of therapy must be to increase the mean systemic arterial blood pressure so the perfusion to the core circu-

Table 12-1 Derived Values From Pulmonary Artery Catheterization*

Variable	Formula	Normal Range
Hemodynamic		
Stroke index	$SI = CI/hr$	30-60 ml/m²
Cardiac index	$CI = CO/BSA$	3.5-5.5 L/min/m²
Systemic vascular resistance index	$SVRI = \dfrac{79.9\,(MAP - CVP)}{CI}$	800-1600 dyne · sec/cm⁵/m²
Pulmonary vascular resistance index	$PVRI = \dfrac{79.9\,(MPAP - PCWP)}{CI}$	80-240 dyne · sec/cm⁵/m²
Oxygen transport		
Arterial oxygen content	$Cao_2 = (Hb)(1.34)(\%sat) + (Pao_2)(0.003)$	17-20 ml/dl
Mixed venous oxygen content	$C\bar{v}o_2 = (Hb)(1.34)(\%sat) + (P\bar{v}o_2)(0.003)$	12-15 ml/dl
Oxygen content difference	$A\text{-}vDo_2 = Cao_2 - C\bar{v}o_2$	3-5 ml/dl
Oxygen availability	$O_2\ avail = Cao_2 \times CI \times 10$	550-650 ml/min/m²
Oxygen consumption	$\dot{V}o_2 = CI \times A\text{-}vDO_2 \times 10$	120-200 ml/min/m²

HR = heart rate; BSA = body surface area; MAP = mean arterial blood pressure; MPAP = mean pulmonary arterial blood pressure; PCWP = pulmonary capillary wedge pressure.
*Modified from Katz AM, Pollack M, Weibley R. Pulmonary artery catheterization in pediatric intensive care. Adv Pediatr 30:169, 1984. Reproduced with permission from Year Book.

lation is maintained. If allowed to continue, hypotension itself will result in multiple organ system failure.

Once systemic arterial blood pressure is stabilized, therapeutic efforts are directed to increasing oxygen supply, decreasing oxygen demands, and correcting metabolic abnormalities. Prior to discussing measures to improve oxygen supply, efforts to reduce oxygen requirements may be important in therapy. This is especially true in young infants in whom the myocardium may be functioning effectively but is still unable to provide adequate blood flow and oxygen to meet systemic tissue demands. If a therapy that improves cardiac output also increases oxygen demand in the face of a limited supply, the benefits of increasing cardiac output and oxygen delivery may be offset by the increased myocardial oxygen consumption.

An appreciation of oxygen supply and demand is paramount in managing children in cardiorespiratory distress. Frequent heroic attempts are made to increase cardiac output and oxygen delivery in shock patients, but little attention is directed to decreasing oxygen requirements. The benefits gained by reducing oxygen needs with assisted ventilation, allaying anxiety, and maintaining an optimal ambient environment may be dramatic.

Oxygen supply is optimized by maintaining arterial oxygen saturation, by correcting anemia, and by efforts aimed at increasing cardiac output and systemic blood flow. Improvement of the cardiac output involves manipulation of the four major determinants of ventricular performance: heart rate, preload, afterload, and contractility. The interrelationships of these factors are expressed schematically in Fig. 12-2.

Cardiac output is defined as the volume of blood ejected by the ventricle (stroke volume) times the number of ejections per minute (heart rate). Heart rate is controlled by both adrenergic and cholinergic receptor systems. Heightened adrenergic activity such as is seen with increased endogenous or exogenous circulating catecholamines will increase heart rate. A reduction in heart rate occurs with an increase in vagal tone as a reflex response following hypertension or with severe hypoxemia. An increase in heart rate produces an increase in cardiac output provided that diastolic ventricular filling is adequate. Reduction in heart rate may decrease cardiac output if augmentation of stroke volume does not occur.

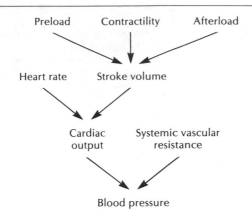

Fig. 12-2 Interrelationships of the factors determining cardiac output and blood pressure.

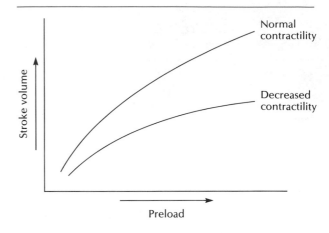

Fig. 12-3 Frank-Starling curve.

Therapy of shock, regardless of etiology, must include measures to optimize heart rate and to prevent dysrhythmias. A number of factors seen in children in shock may predispose them to cardiac dysrhythmias.

Etiologies of dysrhythmias

Myocardial injury or infarction
Myocarditis
Hypoxia
Acidosis, alkalosis
Electrolyte imbalance
Temperature instability
Drug intoxication or side effect
Blood volume changes
Pain, fear, anxiety
Mechanical stimulation or irritation

Stroke volume is governed by ventricular preload, afterload, and contractility. The ventricular preload of either ventricle is represented by the degree of stretch at end-diastole or the end-diastolic volume. An increase in preload will increase the work output of the heart according to the familiar Frank-Starling mechanism (Fig. 12-3). Venous return to the heart is the principal determinant of preload, and changes in circulating blood volume and venous capacitance most directly influence venous return. An absolute or relative blood volume deficit is often a primary component of shock syndromes; therefore the pos-

sibility of hypovolemia must be considered and efforts made to restore an effective circulating blood volume. It is important to realize that ventricular preload may not be accurately represented by measurements of end-diastolic pressure such as CVP or pulmonary wedge pressure. The relationship between end-diastolic pressure and end-diastolic volume describes the compliance characteristics of the respective ventricle. Unfortunately the relationship is not linear and is altered by both disease processes and common therapeutic modalities.

Contractility is the inherent capacity of the myocardium to function as a pump. Change in contractility (inotropic state) of the heart is an alteration in cardiac performance that is independent of changes resulting from variations in preload or afterload. When loading conditions remain constant, an improvement in contractility will augment cardiac performance (positive inotropic effect), whereas a depression in contractility will lower cardiac performance (negative inotropic effect). Although difficult to measure, contractility may be viewed as the heart's ability to generate a stroke volume at any given end-diastolic pressure or volume, as illustrated in Fig. 12-3. Negative influence on myocardial contractility occurs with severe hypoxia, hypocalcemia, hypoglycemia, or acidosis and may significantly reduce stroke volume and cardiac output.

Ventricular afterload defines the resistance against

which the ventricle contracts or the tension the ventricle must develop in ejecting the stroke volume. It is closely related to the vascular resistance and the ventricular radius; with an increase in vascular resistance, afterload increases, stroke volume decreases, and the work of the myocardium increases.

Hypovolemic Shock

Initial treatment of the child in hypovolemic shock is similar regardless of etiology (Fig. 12-4). Therapy begins with establishing adequate oxygenation and ventilation. Oxygen must always be the first drug administered. Once the airway is established (may require trachael intubation) and the patient is adequately ventilating, measures to restore an effective circulating blood volume need to begin. Placement of a large, secure IV catheter for rapid volume replacement is the single most important maneuver in reestablishing the circulation. Central venous catheterization is infrequently necessary during initial resuscitation unless the central circulation offers the only available access for a large IV catheter.

Volume resuscitation

Available fluids. Volume resuscitation includes the use of crystalloid and/or colloid solutions as well as blood (Table 12-2). Crystalloids are electrolyte-containing solutions distributed throughout the body due to their chemical composition and tonicity. Isotonic solutions (lactated Ringer's solution, 0.9% sodium chloride) are distributed to the extracellular space because of the cellular sodium-potassium pump. Hypotonic solutions have a proportion of water not associated with sodium and are therefore distributed uniformly throughout the entire body water. Hypertonic solutions (i.e., sodium concentrations in excess of 180 mEq/L) increase serum osmolality and therefore induce movement of water from the intracellular into the extracellular space. Hypotonic crystalloid solutions are not given in the early phases of fluid resuscitation of patients in shock.

Colloids used in the treatment of patients in shock include plasma, prepared plasma fractions, and synthetic plasma substitutes. Colloid solutions have large molecules that are generally restricted to the intravascular compartment, exerting an oncotic effect on the distribution of water. In so doing, iso-oncotic solutions, including 5% albumin, fresh frozen plasma, or plasma protein fractions, result in a greater plasma

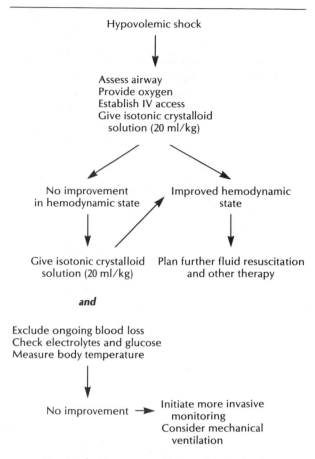

Fig. 12-4   Treatment of hypovolemic shock.

expansion than isotonic crystalloid solutions when the same volume of fluid is infused. Hyperoncotic solutions such as 25% albumin move fluid into the vascular compartment from the interstitial space.

Modern plasma expanders such as the dextrans, hydroxyethyl starch, stroma-free hemoglobin, and perfluorochemical (PFL) emulsions are available for intravascular volume replacement. Each is a colloid fluid with potential for excellent plasma volume expansion. Each has unique pharmacologic properties and, as a result, unique advantages and disadvantages. Stroma-free hemoglobin solutions and PFL emulsions not only expand the plasma volume but can transport additional volumes of oxygen as well.

Since the 1960s a controversy has existed regarding the fluid resuscitation of the shock patient. The

Table 12-2   Crystalloid-Colloid Solutions Available for Volume Resuscitation

Type	Description-Composition	Comment
Crystalloid (isotonic)		
Normal saline solution	0.9% sodium chloride in water Sodium, 154 mg/L Chloride, 154 mg/L Osmolality, 308 mOsm/L	Inexpensive No risk of hepatitis transmission Potential fluid overload due to retention Possible hyperchloremic metabolic acidosis
Lactated Ringer's solution	Sodium, 130 mEq/L Potassium, 4 mEq/L Calcium, 2.7 mEq/L Chloride, 109 mEq/L Lactate, 27 mEq/L	Lactate conversion requires aerobic metabolism
Colloid		
Human plasma	Uncoagulated, unconcentrated plasma Contains all plasma proteins, including albumin Contains clotting factors	Expensive Risk of viral hepatitis and other viral infections
Plasma protein fraction (e.g., Plasmanate)	5% solution of human plasma proteins in normal saline solution Contains albumin, α- and β-globulins Sodium, 130-160 mEq/L Potassium, 1-2 mEq/L	Low risk of hepatitis Osmotically equivalent to plasma Numerous side effects: hypotension, hypersensitivity Deficient in clotting factors
5% albumin	Albumin, 50 g/L Sodium, 130-160 mEq/L	*Rare* transmission of virus
25% albumin	Contains albumin and globulins, 250 g/L Sodium, 130-160 mEq/L Osmolality, 1500 mOsm/L	Extreme care must be used when giving 25% albumin solutions
Low molecular weight dextran	10% solution of glucose polysaccharides with average molecular weight of 40,000 in normal saline solution or glucose water	Low risk of anaphylactic reactions May prolong bleeding time
High molecular weight dextran	6% solution of glucose polysaccharide with molecular weight of 70,000 in normal saline solution or glucose water	Alters urine specific gravity and urine osmolality
Hydroxyethyl starch (hetastarch)	6% solution containing synthetic polymar of hydroxethyl starch in normal saline solution (osmolality, 310 mOsm/L)	Less expensive than albumin solutions Potential for causing coagulopathy Elevates serum amylase No danger of virus transmission Data demonstrating safe administration to children is limited

controversy centers around the decision to administer crystalloid fluids or colloid fluids. The principal theoretical objection to resuscitation with crystalloid solution is that infusion of salt solution without albumin promotes development of interstitial pulmonary edema by lowering colloid osmotic pressure. In addition an increase in capillary membrane permeability leads to fluid distribution, with little of the crystalloid solution remaining in the intravascular compartment. However, several experimental and clinical studies do not substantiate this concern.

The principal theoretical reason for using colloid solutions is the maintenance of colloid oncotic pressure and the increase in oxygen-carrying capacity (in the case of blood administration). It is argued that resuscitation with colloid solution will maintain a near-normal plasma colloid oncotic pressure and minimize formation of interstitial pulmonary edema. However, the actual importance of maintaining a normal plasma oncotic pressure in protecting the lung from edema has yet to be established.

Fluid selection. The choice of fluid depends on the nature of the loss. The early correction of hypovolemia is the major factor preventing the later complications of shock. Crystalloid solutions, being readily available, can be used in initial volume resuscitation. As far as oxygen-carrying capacity is concerned, it reaches its maximum at a hematocrit of 30% to 35% with normovolemic hemodilution and decreases rapidly when the hematocrit exceeds 40% because of blood viscosity–induced reductions in cardiac output and tissue perfusion. In all likelihood, uncomplicated, promptly treated hypovolemic shock does not lead to a significant pulmonary capillary injury and leak. However, severe, prolonged hypovolemic shock, traumatic shock with extensive soft tissue injury, and burn shock may produce significant damage to the pulmonary capillary membrane. Sepsis complicating hypovolemic shock may also seriously impair capillary integrity. Therefore, once systemic arterial blood pressure and urine output have been restored, a drastic reduction in volume administration in the absence of demonstrable ongoing fluid losses is usually recommended. At this point maintenance of preload and hemodynamic function with the administration of colloid is indicated.

In summary, it seems likely that the controversy about whether crystalloid or colloid is the preferable

solution to use in shock resuscitation is largely artificial and that a combination of crystalloid and colloid will be needed to produce both an effective restoration of blood volume and an improvement in tissue perfusion.

Amount of fluid. The amount of fluid needed to reestablish an effective circulating blood volume depends on both the amount lost (deficit) and the rate of ongoing loss. Since the capacitance of the vascular space is expanded and cellular membrane function is abnormal, the total amount of fluid given to a patient in shock often exceeds the total volume lost. Enough fluid needs to be given so that it can cross the microcirculation, consistently elevate the CVP, and therefore provide an adequate cardiac filling pressure. An adequate filling pressure, however, only ensures that this one component of cardiac performance has been provided. It does not ensure adequate normal distribution of blood flow for perfusion of tissue beds or that the patient's myocardium has the functional reserve to respond appropriately with an increased stroke volume to the volume of fluid administered. In patients with hypovolemic shock uncomplicated by myocardial dysfunction, fluid resuscitation can precede as indicated in Fig. 12-4.

Fluid resuscitation is initiated using isotonic crystalloid solutions. The first fluid infusion (20 ml/kg) must be administered rapidly and the heart rate, pulse pressure, systemic arterial blood pressure, peripheral perfusion, quality of mentation, and volume of urine output need to be monitored. Improvement in these measurements can be expected if the blood volume loss is in the 20% range; under these conditions, a rapid response to resuscitation can be anticipated. Maintenance fluid administration can then be initiated and vital signs monitored. The appropriate maintenance fluid to be used depends on the measurements of the serum electrolytes, total protein, and hematocrit.

If hypotension persists after the first fluid infusion is completed, a second infusion of 20 ml/kg can be started. If improvement, as manifested by increased systemic arterial blood pressure, increased pulse pressure and peripheral perfusion, adequate urine output (0.5 to 1.0 ml/kg/hr), and decreased metabolic acidosis, does not occur after two infusions of isotonic crystalloid solution, more aggressive monitoring and therapy are clearly indicated. Patients in profound hypovolemic shock will need frequent or continuous monitoring of heart rate, systemic arterial blood pressure, arterial blood gases and pH, central venous blood pressure, and urinary output.

In the case of hemorrhagic hypovolemia, blood must be obtained and transfused if hypotension persists despite early crystalloid infusions; either the initial hemorrhage was massive or rapid ongoing losses persist. The possibility of occult intrathoracic or intraabdominal bleeding must be considered.

It is uncommon for children with nonhemorrhagic hypovolemic shock to be unresponsive to 40 ml/kg of crystalloid solution, and if this occurs, they must be evaluated for complicating factors. Causes of unresponsive shock include unrecognized pneumothorax or pericardial effusion, intestinal ischemia (volvulus, intussusception), sepsis, myocardial dysfunction, adrenocortical insufficiency, and pulmonary arterial hypertension.

The first approach to further diagnosis of patients remaining in shock is establishing a central venous catheter for measurement of right atrial blood pressure and placing a bladder catheter. Central venous blood pressure in infants and children needs to be measured by a pressure transducer rather than water manometry, which produces a falsely high reading from poor equilibration at rapid heart rates. In the hypotensive patient a central venous blood pressure of less than 10 mm Hg can be carefully augmented by fluid infusion until that level of preload is reached. If there is no improvement in systemic arterial blood pressure, peripheral perfusion, or urine output, cardiogenic causes of circulatory failure must be considered. Arterial blood gases and pH, hematocrit, serum electrolytes, glucose, and calcium must be reevaluated. Correction of acidosis (pH <7.20), hypoxemia, or metabolic derangement is essential. Blood and other appropriate sites must be cultured and broad-spectrum parenteral antibiotic coverage begun if sepsis is suspected.

Shock persisting in the face of central venous blood pressures exceeding 10 mm Hg is an indication for placing a flow-directed thermodilution pulmonary artery catheter. NOTE: Central venous blood pressure is not strictly an indication of circulating blood volume nor does it demonstrate the functional efficiency of the left ventricle. The left and right sides of the heart may function disparately and fail independently. Although disparate ventricular function appears to be less common in children than in adults,

it has been observed to occur in shock, regardless of etiology. In such patients, synchronous monitoring of pulmonary capillary pressure and central venous blood pressure is necessary. Pulmonary capillary pressure has been shown to accurately reflect left atrial blood pressure and the mean left ventricular diastolic blood pressure in acute cardiac diseases and other critical illnesses. However, there are several factors that can affect the pulmonary capillary pressure, including heart rate, preload, afterload, pericardial or pleural pressure, diastolic properties of the left ventricle, and the left ventricular inotropic state.

Because of the multiplicity of factors that affect preload measurements, the best use of these measurements is to to assess the changes in these values that occur with fluid challenge. Utilized this way the measurement of central venous blood pressure and pulmonary capillary pressure allows detection of limitation in cardiac competence and therefore provides an important guide for volume replacement. Fluid administration must be discontinued when ventricular filling pressure rises without evidence of improvement in cardiovascular performance.

Acid-base balance

Metabolic acidosis is a common disturbance in shock and is most frequently the result of inadequate tissue perfusion and the accumulation of acid products of anaerobic metabolism. Metabolic acidosis is usually corrected as oxygenation of tissues and renal function improve; therefore the logical treatment is restoration of blood volume and peripheral circulation. Occasionally acidosis may be so severe that pH correction is necessary before tissue perfusion can be restored. Acidemia exerts a pernicious effect on the cardiovascular system. Reduction in arterial and intracellular pH causes depression of myocardial contractility, decreased responsiveness to catecholamines, inhibition of glycolysis and other key metabolic pathways, and increased pulmonary vascular resistance. Correction is indicated in serious metabolic acidosis (arterial blood pH <7.20), particularly when the acidosis arises from the loss of bicarbonate from the body. Given the restraints of the relationship among arterial Pco_2, bicarbonate concentration, and hydrogen ion concentration, as the serum bicarbonate concentration falls below 10 mEq/L, the degree of blood acidification greatly accelerates.

Sodium bicarbonate is usually chosen as the alkali for management of systemic acidosis. Emergency therapy is given as 1 to 2 mEq/kg of body weight. Further doses need to be based on measurement of blood pH and bicarbonate concentration. Potential complications of bicarbonate administration include paradoxical acidification of spinal fluid, impaired delivery of oxygen to the tissues, increased carbon dioxide production that can aggravate acidemia by increasing arterial Pco_2, increased lactic acid production, hypokalemia, hypocalcemia, hypernatremia, and hypertonicity.

In some patients use of another buffer, trishydroxymethyl-aminomethane (THAM), may be preferable, although it has the disadvantages of causing respiratory depression, hypoglycemia, and hyperkalemia. Recent reports demonstrate that newer agents, dichloroacetate and carbicarb, can have positive metabolic and hemodynamic effects in patients with lactic acidosis. Such drugs would be beneficial in the management of circulatory failure, and further investigation is warranted.

Cardiovascular-pulmonary system

Attempts must be made to correct dysrhythmias. Blood volume replacement usually corrects tachycardia. Bradycardia and irregular rhythms may result from multiple causes (see p. 86). Investigation and treatment must be prompt.

Intravascular blood pressures respond to volume replacement except when cardiac failure or other complications exist, as described previously. Inotropic agents may be needed, and further investigation is necessary (i.e., chest roentgenogram, echocardiogram, hematocrit and electrolyte measurements, abdominal ultrasonogram) when volume replacement alone does not improve the patient's condition.

Intubation and mechanical ventilation must be considered in children with altered neurologic status or when oxygen costs of breathing are high (i.e., exaggerated respiratory rates, presence of pulmonary edema). Observe the patient for the development of respiratory failure (elevation of $Paco_2$ with respiratory acidosis) and institute appropriate management when it occurs (see Chapter 10).

Other therapeutic considerations

Since moderate increases or decreases in temperature increase metabolic demands and oxygen consumption, normothermia must be maintained.

Renal failure. Prompt and adequate restoration of plasma volume and treatment of ventricular dysfunc-

tion are needed to prevent renal failure. If fluid replacement is adequate but oliguria persists, mannitol and/or furosemide can be tried in an attempt to convert oliguric renal failure to nonoliguric renal failure (see also Chapter 14). Low-dose dopamine infusion may also be helpful in improving renal blood flow and function. Failure of these measures to induce a diuresis confirms the diagnosis of established renal failure, and meticulous measures must be taken to control fluid, electrolyte, and acid-base balances. Ultrafiltration or dialysis is available and can be used when appropriate indications exist (see Chapters 145, 146, and 148). Although oliguria in shock is more likely to lead to concern and investigation than is polyuria, the latter may be just as important and as potentially lethal. Adequate urine output is occasionally associated with inadequate circulatory blood volume and/or renal function. These patients will need appropriate fluid therapy and electrolyte, mineral, and glucose control. If renal failure exists, drugs excreted by the kidney must be eliminated or the dosages adjusted.

Hepatic and gastrointestinal dysfunction. The survival of patients in severe shock can be affected by hepatic dysfunction due to shock; therefore maintaining circulation to maintain liver function and prevent hepatocellular damage is important to therapy. Liver function studies need to be performed, and if dysfunction exists, drugs metabolized by the liver must be given carefully. The stomach must be emptied and kept evacuated with a nasogastric tube. Measures to prevent stress ulceration and erosive gastritis need to be instituted. Provision of nutrition is critical and must be started as soon as possible; once started it must be monitored closely (see Chapter 149).

Cardiogenic Shock

The general supportive and pharmacologic measures employed in the treatment of severe congestive heart failure or cardiogenic shock are listed on p. 92. These measures are designed to increase tissue oxygen supply, decrease tissue oxygen requirements, and correct metabolic abnormalities.

Volume expansion and correction of mechanical problems (e.g., pneumothorax) may enhance cardiac function temporarily, but pharmacologic agents are usually necessary to improve cardiac function. Drugs with the capability to restore or augment myocardial contractility and/or improve cardiac output will restore and maintain blood flow. Knowledge of both

---

GENERAL PRINCIPLES IN THE TREATMENT OF SEVERE CONGESTIVE HEART FAILURE OR CARDIOGENIC SHOCK

Minimize oxygen demands
    Normalize temperature
    Provide sedation
    Correct anemia
    Consider mechanical ventilation
Maximize oxygen delivery
    Control rhythm disturbances
    Optimize vascular volume
        Careful fluid infusion
        Diuretics for vascular congestion
    Improve contractility
        Provide oxygen
        Ensure ventilation
        Correct metabolic abnormalities
        Provide inotropic drugs
    Reduce afterload
        Sedation, pain relief
        Correct hypothermia
        Appropriate use of vasodilators
Exclude the presence of congenital cardiac defects

---

the exact hemodynamic disturbance and of the pharmacologic properties is essential in choosing the proper drugs.

Proper utilization of the various vasoactive drugs listed in Table 12-3 often requires the presence of an indwelling arterial catheter, central venous catheter, and thermodilution catheter. These monitoring devices allow the generation of data that will characterize the hemodynamic state, direct appropriate therapy, and allow for evaluation of the response to therapy. There is neither a best drug nor a standard drug dose for patients in shock; instead therapy must be continually adjusted to the patient's response.

Most of these agents are given as continuous IV infusion, and a secure, centrally placed catheter must be used. A second catheter, which may be peripheral, needs to be available for switching the infusion in case of malfunction of the primary catheter. An infusion pump must be used and the infusion can never be interrupted since the half-life of the drugs may be only minutes. Rapid administration of these drugs can be fatal. Thus the catheter must never be flushed. All drug infusions need to be carefully labeled with drug name, concentration, and diluent.

Myocardial contractility: Inotropic agents. Although catecholamines are the most potent positive inotropic agents available, unfortunately their effects are not limited to inotropy. In addition they possess both chronotropic properties and complex effects on vascular beds of the various organs of the body. The choice of a particular agent depends as much on the state of the circulation as it does on the condition of the myocardium. Manipulation of the side chain of the catecholamine molecule has yielded synthetic catecholamines with greater propensity to activate one receptor or another. The available catecholamines are norepinephrine, epinephrine, isoproterenol, dopamine, and dobutamine. These catecholamines have been used extensively in infants and children, but the dose-response relationships have not been fully investigated. Therefore their effects must be carefully observed.

In children with cardiogenic shock, in whom maximal inotropic support is necessary and peripheral vasoconstriction is deleterious, isoproterenol or dobutamine may be indicated. In children under 1 year of age, isoproterenol may be the inotrope of choice because of the direct relationship between heart rate and cardiac output and because dobutamine appears to be a less effective inotrope in this age group and may produce undesirable effects on the pulmonary vascular bed. However, inotropic agents utilized in an attempt to improve cardiac output may do so at the cost of increasing myocardial oxygen demand; this may result in or intensify myocardial ischemia and lead to worsening myocardial function. In children older than 1 year, dobutamine is the preferred drug. Although dopamine has activity on both alpha and beta receptors, particularly at high doses, it is unique as a stimulator of dopaminergic receptors. Renal and mesenteric flows are increased by dopaminergic stimulation. Since dobutamine lacks salutary dopaminergic effects on the kidneys, a combination of low renal-effective doses of dopamine with dobutamine is frequently used in children with cardiogenic shock.

Digitalis glycosides are able to augment myocardial contractility, but because of a narrow therapeutic to toxic range, its use in patients with cardiogenic shock should be delayed.

Newer drugs, amrinone and milrinone, belong to a class of nonglycoside, nonsympathomimetic ino-

Table 12-3   Commonly Used Cardiovascular Drugs in Shock Syndromes

Drug	Dose (μg/kg/min)	Comment
Inotropic agents		
Norepinephrine (α-adrenergic)	0.05-1.0	Most frequently used for profound hypotension not responding to fluid or other inotropic drugs.
Epinephrine (α- and β-adrenergic)	0.05-1.0	Dose-related response; higher doses cause vasoconstriction. Useful in maintaining cardiac output and blood pressure in patients unresponsive to dopamine or dobutamine.
Isoproterenol (β-adrenergic)	0.05-0.5	Indicated in bradycardia unresponsive to atropine; as an inotrope if increase in heart rate is not excessive; may be helpful in reactive pulmonary hypertension.
Dopamine (α-, β-, and dopaminergic)	1-20	Cardiovascular effects are complex and dose related. Specific peripheral effects are useful when low-dose infusion can restore cardiovascular stability and improve renal function.
Dobutamine (α- and β-adrenergic)	1-20	Racemic mixture whose overall activity is due to the sum of the individual stereoisomers. Positive inotropic effect with minimal changes in heart rate or systemic vascular resistance.
Amrinone	1-10	Initial bolus infusion may be required. Limited data available in children.
Vasodilators		
Nitroprusside	0.05-8	Balanced arterial and venous dilator. May result in thiocyanate or cyanide toxicity.
Phentolamine	1-20	Causes dilation of arterial and venous beds. Indirect inotropic effect may cause compensatory tachycardia.
Nitroglycerine	0.5-20	Venous dilator. Dose not well established for infants and children.

tropic agents. They appear to act via a potent and selective inhibition of phosphodiesterase. Intravenous administration of amrinone increases cardiac output and reduces cardiac filling pressures and systemic vascular resistance with minimal effect on the heart rate and systemic arterial blood pressure at low doses in adult patients. Amrinone may serve a role as a second-line, short-term therapy for severe, refractory congestive heart failure. Data are not available to provide recommendations for use of amrinone in children.

Afterload reduction: Vasoactive drugs

As discussed earlier, compensatory mechanisms that initially compensate for a fall in output of the failing heart, some vasoconstrictive and others leading to salt and water retention, in time become a major part of the problem. The kidney's response to a decrease in cardiac output leads to expansion of extracellular fluid volume and ultimately to circulatory congestion

and edema. The vasoconstriction will raise aortic impedance, which, while tending to maintain perfusion pressure in the face of declining cardiac output, eventually impairs ventricular function. It therefore becomes the rationale of treatment to counteract those physiologic responses to the decline in cardiac function with, for example, the use of vasodilators to oppose systemic vasoconstriction, angiotensin-converting enzyme inhibitors to block the renin-angiotensin system, and diuretics to prevent or reverse abnormal fluid retention.

A large number of vasodilators, representing several different pharmacologic classes, have been shown to improve cardiac performance and lessen clinical symptoms by means of arterial and venous smooth muscle relaxation. Arterial relaxation should result in an increase in ejection fraction, an increase in stroke volume, and a decrease in end-systolic left ventricular volume. There is some evidence to suggest that some vasodilator drugs may produce an acute increase in left ventricular compliance. Since left ventricular end-diastolic volume is the most important determinant of stroke volume, an increase in stroke volume would occur at a comparatively lower level of filling pressure if compliance were increased. However, the principal mechanism by which vasodilators improve cardiac function is by decreasing left ventricular outflow resistance; thus these agents are likely to be more effective when systemic vascular resistance is elevated. Alternatively, venous relaxation should shift blood into the periphery and reduce right and left ventricular diastolic volume, with attendant beneficial effects on pulmonary and systemic capillary pressure. This, in turn, ought to be reflected in decreased edema, reduced myocardial wall stress, and improved diastolic perfusion of the myocardium.

For treatment of cardiogenic shock, IV vasodilators with a rapid onset of action and short half-life are preferred. The commonly used vasodilator agents are sodium nitroprusside, nitroglycerin, and phentolamine (Table 12-3). Although these vasodilator drugs produce similar qualitative hemodynamic effects, the quantitative hemodynamic responses vary. Therefore the random choice of a vasodilator agent for treatment of left ventricular dysfunction is inappropriate; selection of such an agent needs to be made according to its principal hemodynamic effects and in relation to the specific hemodynamic abnormalities in individual patients. Factors that increase systemic vascular resistance such as hypothermia, acidosis, hypoxia, pain, and anxiety must be treated prior to considering vasodilator drugs.

The use of vasodilators in shock is generally limited to situations in which cardiac dysfunction is associated with elevated ventricular filling pressures, elevated systemic vascular resistance, and normal or near-normal systemic arterial blood pressure. The usefulness of vasodilators in the treatment of ventricular dysfunction provides two pharmacologic means of improving cardiac output in shock syndromes: inotropic drugs and vasodilators. Occasionally the combination of vasodilator and inotropic therapy results in hemodynamic improvement not attainable with either drug alone.

The thin-walled right ventricle has been obscured by its muscular neighbor, the left ventricle. However, there is a growing awareness that right ventricular dysfunction often plays a pivotal role in some of the most frequently encountered and important cardiopulmonary disorders in children, including congenital heart disease, adult respiratory distress syndrome, bronchopulmonary dysplasia, and other chronic pulmonary disorders. The ability of the right ventricle to respond to increased pulmonary vascular resistance seen in these situations often determines outcome. Measures to decrease pulmonary vascular resistance have therefore become more common in the treatment of many seriously ill pediatric patients. However, the use of vasodilators in the treatment of pulmonary hypertension is a complex subject with confusing and conflicting results reported in the literature. Therefore pharmacologic reduction of pulmonary vascular resistance must be attempted only in the fully monitored patient.

A number of congenital cardiac defects may present in severe congestive heart failure and cardiogenic shock. Diagnosis of these defects is critical since surgery is often needed before hemodynamic stability can be achieved.

Septic Shock

Primary therapeutic goals for initial treatment of septic shock are rapid reversal of perfusion failure and identification and control of the infection.

The removal or control of microorganisms is the single most important principle of treatment. Antibiotic treatment is appropriate in patients with circulatory shock whenever an infectious etiology is suspected. Before broad-spectrum antibiotic therapy is initiated, blood, urine, and samples from other potentially infected sites must be sent for culture and antibiotic-susceptibility testing.

Improved patient survival is unlikely if the source of infection is not eradicated. Surgical drainage of closed-space infections is mandatory, and a vigorous search for the infection's site is indicated in patients unresponsive to appropriate antibiotic therapy.

Cardiovascular support

The primary goal in the initial management of septic shock is to restore hemodynamic stability. Interruption of the natural pathophysiologic progression of septic shock by controlling cardiopulmonary variables may improve the outcome. Every effort to enhance oxygen delivery to the tissues must be made. Maximizing cardiac output and arterial oxygen content while minimizing oxygen requirements are fundamentals of management. Many studies indicate that normal ranges of cardiopulmonary variables are not necessarily optimal for children in septic shock. Establishing a hyperdynamic state, because of the high oxygen requirements and the failing oxygen extraction, may improve survival. Although maximizing cardiac output appears to be important, efforts to decrease oxygen requirements may play a role in management. The increased work of breathing commonly found in patients with shock can increase tissue oxygen consumption substantially. This problem can be overcome by using assisted ventilation and administering paralytic and/or sedative medications. Extremes in body temperature also increase oxygen requirements; therefore efforts to maintain normothermia must be made.

Volume resuscitation is the first therapeutic measure for decreased cardiac output. Early and effective expansion of the circulating blood volume may enhance oxygen delivery and prevent progression of the septic shock state. Central venous access must be obtained and fluid administration started. Patients in septic shock have an enormous fluid requirement caused primarily by peripheral vasodilation and capillary leak. In some patients, blood volume restoration on the basis of central venous blood pressure measurements alone may be deleterious. Disparate ventricular function, abnormalities in ventricular compliance, and elevated pulmonary vascular resistance may make central venous blood pressure unreliable and preclude appropriate volume replacement. Placement of a thermodilution pulmonary artery catheter may be indicated in children who demonstrate a sluggish response to fluid infusion, have signs of pulmonary edema with normal central venous blood pressure, or show clinical or echocardiographic evidence of myocardial dysfunction.

Debate continues regarding the use of crystalloid or colloid solutions in restoring intravascular volume in the presence of septic shock. Isotonic crystalloid solution may be used initially if it increases the blood volume and cardiac output; however, there is evidence that colloid solutions expand blood volume more effectively in these patients.

Although fluid administration and antimicrobial therapy remain the cornerstones of the therapeutic approach to sepsis and septic shock, patients often need inotropic agents and/or vasoactive drugs. Myocardial depression may complicate septic shock and prevent the development of optimal cardiac output despite adequate intravascular volume. Optimal cardiac output is best judged by obtaining any or all of the following objective criteria: a state in which oxy-

gen consumption is not flow dependent, an appropriate level of existing oxygen consumption, and absence of metabolic acidosis. In most cases, meeting these criteria requires that cardiac output be maintained at greater than normal values.

Dopamine is frequently the initial inotropic agent of choice in septic shock because of its beta-adrenergic effects in the myocardium, its alpha-adrenergic effects in the peripheral vasculature, and its selective dopaminergic effects on renal and splanchnic vascular beds. If myocardial function is decreased and systemic vascular resistance is elevated, the combined use of dobutamine and low-dose dopamine may be helpful.

Patients with profound hypotension and myocardial depression may not respond to large amounts of dopamine or dobutamine. In these cases, epinephrine or norepinephrine needs to be added. Unfortunately use of these potent vasoconstrictors may not lead to an increase in systemic vascular resistance and systemic arterial blood pressure. Sepsis-induced abnormalities in adrenergic function (e.g., alpha-adrenergic receptor down regulation) and peripheral vascular adrenergic action depression may account for this poor response. New nonadrenergic inotropic agents (milrinone, amrinone) may find a place in the treatment of septic shock when severe myocardial failure is resistant to adrenergic agents.

Electrolyte abnormalities, metabolic acidosis, hypocalcemia, hypophosphatemia, and hypoglycemia may be present in septic shock and must be treated. Correction of these biochemical aberrations helps optimize myocardial function.

Vasodilator drugs may be indicated in treatment if systemic vascular resistance is elevated in the face of adequate volume resuscitation and appropriate inotropic therapy.

Multiorgan support

Shock, regardless of etiology, is a multiorgan system disease. Several complications of septic shock may arise despite antibiotic therapy and cardiovascular support. Renal failure, liver dysfunction, coagulopathy, CNS dysfunction, and respiratory failure have all been described and must be anticipated.

Sepsis is recognized as a leading cause of adult respiratory distress syndrome (ARDS). The mortality of patients with septic ARDS in many reported series ranges from 80% to 90%. The therapy of patients with

ARDS complicating shock is disappointing. However, positive end-respiratory pressure (PEEP) in conjunction with mechanical ventilation has been shown to improve respiratory function. PEEP must be carefully used so that adverse effects on cardiac output and tissue oxygen delivery do not occur. Treating hypovolemia in patients who also have ARDS is particularly difficult because the choice of fluid and the level of pulmonary capillary wedge pressure may lead to increased accumulation of extravascular lung water. Glucocorticoids, fibronectin, anticoagulants, and other experimental therapies have undergone trials in the therapy of ARDS. To date, there is no conclusive evidence of improved survival with any of these agents (see Chapter 35).

Even in the absence of ARDS, shock may be augmented by hypoventilation caused by respiratory muscle fatigue. Hyperventilation in the early stages of shock, coupled with respiratory muscle ischemia from hypoperfusion, may result in profound interference with respiratory muscle function. This may result in inadequate minute ventilation, worsening of systemic acidosis, and respiratory arrest. Mechanical ventilation reverses these changes.

Nutrition

It has long been recognized that septic patients develop protein-calorie malnutrition as a principal manifestation of the mediated metabolic response. In patients who were previously malnourished or remain hypermetabolic, this rapidly developing malnutrition is believed to contribute to morbidity and mortality. However, the abnormalities in intermediary metabolism described earlier make the provision of an adequate level of metabolic support challenging. The septic process, in some unknown way, triggers a progressive sequential fuel failure. In early stages the ability to use glucose as an energy source is limited, and fat is increasingly relied on as an energy source.

In this stage a balanced fuel mixture, including low quantities of glucose with lipid constituting at least 30% to 40% of the calories, and a complete amino acid profile should be used. Parenteral nutrition needs to be begun as soon as cardiovascular stability is achieved. In the late stages of sepsis, triglyceride intolerance develops and there is an inability to clear standard long-chain fat load. At this point branched-chain amino acids (BCAA) are used preferentially as a fuel source because of the abnormalities in glucose and fat utilization. As a result the

body autocannibalizes its skeletal muscle protein to obtain adequate amounts of BCAA fuel substrate. Fat administration must then be adjusted on the basis of repeated assessment of fat tolerance, and the use of BCAA-enriched solution may be better than a balanced amino acid solution. The mechanism for fat intolerance may be due in part to an absolute or relative carnitine deficiency. Carnitine administration in this setting may be useful.

Recent studies suggest an advantage to enteric feeding, when it is possible, because the first passage of substrate from the gut is to the liver and also involves activation of normal pancreatic hormone regulation. However, there are many instances in which sepsis occurs and effective bowel function cannot be maintained. Under these circumstances, parenteral nutrition is a necessity.

Experimental therapies

Corticosteroids. There are many potential mechanisms for the possible beneficial actions of steroids in sepsis and shock, but most remain unproved. The most straightforward benefit of steroids would be the demonstration that sepsis and shock has produced hypoadrenalism and that replacement of adrenal corticosteroids was necessary. Although this explanation is reasonable, it does not justify the large doses of steroids advocated in the recent literature. The rationale for the use of steroids in septic shock has included the ability of these drugs to stabilize lysosomal and cell membranes, to inhibit complement-induced granulocyte and platelet aggregation, to improve myocardial performance, to modulate the release of endogenous opiates, to reverse metabolic defects involving the heart and liver, to decrease products of arachidonic acid metabolism, to prevent oxygen radical–mediated cell damage, and to decrease red blood cell oxygen affinity. Potential adverse effects include superinfection, electrolyte disturbances, hyperglycemia, gastrointestinal bleeding, psychosis, and dysrhythmias. Recent studies have not shown steroids to be efficacious in the management of septic shock. Moreover, the data suggest a greater mortality in steroid-treated patients. On the basis of this information the use of high-dose corticosteroids provides no benefit in the treatment of severe sepsis and septic shock and should not be used.

Opiate antagonists. Much interest has been generated regarding the role of naloxone in the treatment of septic shock. Naloxone is an antagonist of endogenous opiates, a group of peptides that are reported to be a pathophysiologic mediator of hypotension during sepsis. Animal studies using naloxone have shown improvement in cardiovascular function and reversal of hypotension. Use of naloxone in human subjects has not consistently confirmed animal studies, and serious adverse reactions have occurred. Use of naloxone in septic shock cannot be advocated at this time.

Other investigational therapies. A number of pharmacologic agents and other therapies have been evaluated as adjunctive treatment in sepsis and septic shock. Such modalities of therapy include a multitude of drugs that inhibit arachidonic acid metabolism and the formation of thromboxanes, prostaglandins, and leukotrienes; exchange transfusion and plasmapheresis; white blood cell infusions; passive immunotherapy; toxic oxygen scavengers; inhibitors of myocardial depressant factors; and fibronectin administration. Although these therapies may have significant potential therapeutic usefulness, further study is needed.

ADDITIONAL READING

Appelbaum A, Blackstone EH, Douchoukos NT, Kirklin JW. Afterload reduction and cardiac output in infants early after cardiac surgery. Am J Cardiol 39:445-451, 1977.

Artman M, Parrish MD, Graham TP. Congestive heart failure in childhood and adolescence: Recognition and management. Am Heart J 105:471-480, 1983.

Aubier M, Trippenbach T, Roussos C. Respiratory muscle fatigue during cardiogenic shock. J Appl Physiol 51:499-508, 1981.

Ayres SM. SCCM's new horizons on sepsis and septic shock. Crit Care Med 13:864-866, 1985.

Bonadio WA, Losek JD. Infants with myocarditis presenting with severe respiratory distress and shock. Pediatr Emerg Care 3:110-113, 1987.

Calvin JE, Driedger AA, Sibbald WJ. Does the pulmonary capillary wedge pressure predict left ventricular preload in critically ill patients? Crit Care Med 9:437-443, 1981.

Cohn JN. Treatment by modification of circulatory dynamics. Hosp Pract 19:37-52, 1984.

Dibbald WT, Calvin JE, Holliday RL. Concepts in the pharmacologic and nonpharmacologic support of cardiovascular function in critically ill surgical patients. Surg Clin North Am 63:455-482, 1983.

Friedman WF, George BL. Treatment of congestive heart failure by altering loading conditions of the heart. J Pediatr 106:697-705, 1985.

Green TP. Therapeutic approach to the failing heart. Pediatr Ann 14:304-311, 1985.

Groenveld ABJ, Bronsveld W, Thijs LG. Hemodynamic determinants of mortality in human septic shock. Surgery 99:140-152, 1986.

• Katz AM. A physiologic approach to the treatment of heart failure. Hosp Pract 22:117-148, 1987.

Kouchoukos NT, Karp RM. Management of the postoperative cardiovascular patient. Am Heart J 92:513-531, 1976.

Levine TB. Role of vasodilators in the treatment of congestive heart failure. Am J Cardiol 55:32A-35A, 1985.

Luce JM. Pathogenesis and management of septic shock. Chest 91:883-888, 1987.

Oakley CM. Clinical decisions in the cardiomyopathies. Hosp Pract 20:41-60, 1985.

• Parker MM, Parillo JE. Septic shock—hemodynamics and pathogenesis. JAMA 250:3324-3327, 1983.

Perkin RM, Anas NG. Nonsurgical contractility manipulation of the failing circulation. In Swedlow DB, Raphaely RG, eds. Cardiovascular Problems in Pediatric Critical Care. New York: Churchill Livingstone, 1986, pp 229-256.

• Perkin RM, Levin DL. Shock in the pediatric patient. J Pediatr 101:319-332, 1982.

• Perkin RM, Levin DL. Shock in the pediatric patient. J Pediatr 101:163-169, 1982.

Pollack MM, Fields AJ, Ruttimann UE. Sequential cardiopulmonary variables of infants and children in septic shock. Crit Care Med 12:554-559, 1984.

Ross J. The failing heart and the circulation. Hosp Pract 18:151-168, 1983.

Shippy CR, Appel PL, Shoemaker WC. Reliability of clinical monitoring to access blood volume in critically ill patients. Crit Care Med 12:107-112, 1984.

Shoemaker WC. Pathophysiology and therapy of shock syndromes. In Shoemaker WC, Thompson WL, Holbrook PR, eds. Textbook of Critical Care. Philadelphia: WB Saunders, 1984, pp 52-72.

Siegal JH, Cerra FB, Coleman B. Physiological and metabolic correlations in human sepsis. Surgery 86:163-189, 1979.

Tenzer ML. The spectrum of myocardial contusion: a review. J Trauma 25:620-627, 1985.

Veterans administration systemic sepsis cooperative study group. Effect of high-dose glucocorticoid therapy on mortality in patients with clinical signs of systemic sepsis. N Engl J Med 317:659-665, 1987.

Wiles JB, Cerra FB, Siegel JH, Border JR. The systemic septic response: Does the organism matter? Crit Care Med 8:55-60, 1980.

Witte MK, Hill JH, Blumer JL. Shock in the pediatric patient. Adv Pediatr 34:139-174, 1987.

• Zaritsky A, Chernow B. Use of catecholamines in pediatrics. J Pediatr 105:341-350, 1984.

Zimmerman JL, Dietrich KA. Current perspectives on septic shock. Pediatr Clin North Am 34:131-163, 1987.

13 Anaphylaxis

Frances C. Morriss

BACKGROUND AND PHYSIOLOGY

Anaphylaxis is a life-threatening allergic reaction of the immediate hypersensitivity type that is characterized by a generalized systemic response and can be fatal. The incidence of drug-induced anaphylaxis in hospitalized patients is 1:2700. Allergic reactions are produced by immunologic mechanisms and have several characteristics: (1) previous exposure to a particular antigen, (2) interaction of the antigen with specific antibodies and/or effector cells, and (3) an amnestic response or the occurrence of the same reaction when that particular antigen is reintroduced. Not all immune reactions produce anaphylaxis; Table 13-1 classifies the various immune reactions. Systemic reactions resembling anaphylaxis may be produced by nonimmune mechanisms that result in the release of the same mediators that cause immediate hypersensitivity reactions. Such reactions are referred to as anaphylactoid and cannot be differentiated clinically from antibody-mediated reactions.

Antigens are foreign molecules that on entering an organism can stimulate an immune response, including the production of protein macromolecules that can bind specific antigens. Such proteins, known as antibodies, are produced after transformation of B-cell lymphocytes; they share a common but not identical structure that facilitates recognition and binding of a wide range of antigens. Protein antibodies, known as immunoglobulins, are synthesized by lymphocytes and plasma cells throughout the body and are secreted into blood, saliva, and other body fluids. In addition antibodies are bound to cellular membranes of mast cells. There are five types of immunoglobulins:

1. IgG, a serum antibody that activates complement and is the major antibody involved in host defense mechanisms
2. IgE or reagin, the antibody responsible for type I hypersensitivity reactions
3. IgD, a lymphocyte antibody that acts as a membrane receptor
4. IgM, a serum antibody stimulated by carbohydrate antigens and capable of fixing complement
5. IgA, a secretory antibody located on mucosal surfaces and involved in protection against pathogens

Anaphylaxis occurs when a polyvalent antigen binds two or more IgE molecules located on mast cell or basophil surface membranes. Deformation of these receptors on the cell membrane initiates a calcium- and energy-dependent cell activation resulting in the release of primary mediators from intracellular storage granules and the synthesis of secondary mediators. Table 13-2 lists primary and secondary mediators of anaphylaxis and their physiologic actions. Histamine is the best known primary mediator; two types of histamine receptors (H_1 and H_2) are located throughout the vascular system, tracheobronchial tree, myocardium, gastric mucosa, and mast cells. The initial hypotension and cutaneous symptoms seen in anaphylactic reactions are attributed to the action of histamine. Histamine release may also occur with:

1. Activation of the complement cascade through IgM or IgG—antigen interactions (e.g., cardiopulmonary bypass, radiographic contrast agents, transfusion reactions)
2. Activation of blood coagulation system
3. Activation of fibrinolytic systems
4. Nonantibody-mediated interactions resulting in kinin production (e.g., endotoxin exposure)
5. Pharmacologically initiated degranulation of mast cell histamine (e.g., hyperosmotic agents, neuromuscular blocking agents, protamine, antibiotics, narcotics, thiopental)

The other preformed mediators appear to facilitate recruitment of additional inflammatory agents, promote tissue destruction, and inhibit coagulation and fibrin deposition.

Table 13-1   Gell and Coombs' Classification of Immunologic Reactions*

Reaction	Synonyms	Antibody	Chemical Mechanism	Examples
Type I	Immediate hypersensitivity	IgE	Antigen binds to IgE on the surface of mast cells and basophils with release of mast cell products	Anaphylaxis Cutaneous wheal and flare Extrinsic asthma
Type II	Cytotoxic	IgG IgM	IgG and IgM bind antigen on cell membranes; complement is activated with liberation of anaphylatoxins and cellular destruction	Transfusion reactions Hemolytic anemia Rh disease
Type III	Immune	IgG	IgG and IgM bind antigen in fluid phase and deposit in small blood vessels; complement is activated with cellular destruction	Serum sickness Glomerulonephritis
Type IV	Delayed hypersensitivity Cell-mediated immunity	Not involved	Sensitized thymus-derived lymphocytes bind antigen and release effectors known as lymphokines	Contact dermatitis Tuberculin immunity

*From Levy JH. Anaphylactic Reactions in Anesthesia and Intensive Care. Boston: Butterworth, 1986, p 4.

The synthesized mediators, arachidonic acid metabolites, platelet-activating factor, and kinins, have multiple effects; the inflammatory response is generally enhanced and increased capillary permeability and bronchospasm are facilitated.

An anaphylactic reaction occurs within 2 to 20 minutes of injection of the antigen, which is usually a pharmacologic agent, and may involve the cardiovascular, respiratory, gastrointestinal, and cutaneous systems. Physiologic manifestations (Table 13-3) may vary from mild to severe in any system, and a wide range of symptoms may be exhibited by various individuals exposed to the same antigen. An allergic history is often absent. Such reactions may be difficult to recognize in the patient who is anesthetized or sedated and intubated; in a study of 227 such patients cardiovascular collapse was the most common feature in 97%, the most severe feature in 68%, and the only manifestation in 5%. Other common features included vasodilation and cardiac dysrhythmias; bronchospasm and cutaneous signs were not as reliably recognized. When anaphylactic reactions have occurred in patients undergoing hemodynamic monitoring, decreases in systemic arterial blood pressure, systemic vascular resistance (often the most profound change), pulmonary capillary wedge pressure, pulmonary vascular resistance, and left ventricular end-diastolic volume have been demonstrated; stroke volume, ejection fraction, and cardiac output have been increased. Increased cardiac output may result from sudden afterload reduction and increased inotropy from histamine. In addition histamine release and hypotension stimulate the sympathetic nervous system to increase adrenergic output. Decreased cardiac output may occur, however, as a result of dysrhythmias, decreased coronary perfusion, pulmonary arterial hypertension, and hypoxia, and irreversible shock may supervene. Hypotension is sustained by action of secondary mediators that cause increased capillary permeability and subsequent loss of significant fraction of the intravascular volume. Airway problems include upper airway obstruction from laryngeal edema and lower airway obstruction from bronchial smooth muscle constriction, mucosal edema, and increased mucus production. These changes are reversible but can be severe enough to contribute to hemodynamic instability, particularly with respect to right ventricular function. Persistence of severe bronchospasm may result from continued stimulation of secondary mediators (leukotrienes, prostaglandins). In a PICU setting a nonparenteral route of antigen administration is unlikely; however, in this instance development of symptoms may be delayed by several hours. Table 13-4 lists pharma-

Table 13-2   Mediators of Anaphylaxis

Mediators	Site	Action
Primary (preformed)		
Histamine	Mast cell and basophil storage granule	H_1 receptors: bronchoconstriction, increased capillary permeability, coronary artery vasoconstriction, promotion of prostaglandin production, enhanced neutrophil migration H_2 receptors: increased gastric acid secretion, pulmonary arterial vasodilation, positive chronotropy and inotropy, T-cell lymphocyte inhibition
Heparin	Pulmonary and cutaneous mast cell storage granules	
Eosinophilic chemotactic factor	Mast cell storage granules	Eosinophil migration to site of reaction
Neutrophilic chemotactic factor	Mast cell storage granules	Polymorphonuclear neutrophil migration, promotes and prolongs inflammatory response
Enzyme mediators (neutral proteases, acid hydrolases, peroxidases)	Mast cell and basophil storage granules	Suppresses coagulation; recruit mediators to amplify inflammatory processes
Secondary (synthesized) *Arachidonic acid metabolites*		
Cyclooxygenase products Prostaglandin D_2	Mast cells	Increased migration of neutrophils, bronchoconstriction, inhibition of enzyme release, enhanced microvascular permeability
Prostaglandin E_1	Mast cells, neutrophils	Bronchodilates, blocks antigen-induced histamine release; vasodilates, stimulates lymphocyte differentiation and inhibits lymphokine antibody production
Prostaglandin F_2	Mast cells, macrophages	Vasoconstriction, bronchoconstriction
Thromboxane A_2	Mast cells, platelets, neutrophils	Platelet aggregation, vasoconstriction (particularly of pulmonary artery), bronchoconstriction
Prostacyclin	Pulmonary mast cells	Increased microvascular permeability
Lipoxygenase products* Leukotriene B_4	Mast cells	Prolongs bronchoconstriction by promoting edema, neutrophil migration, and increased mucus production
Leukotriene C_4	Pulmonary mast cells, neutrophils	Bronchoconstriction
Leukotriene D_4		Small airways constriction, pulmonary vasoconstriction, increases microvascular permeability
Platelet-activating factor	Mast cells	Platelet and neutrophil activation and aggregation, increases capillary permeability
Kinins (bradykinin, prekallikrein)	Pulmonary mast cells	Increases capillary permeability, vasodilation

*Slow-reacting substance of anaphylaxis.

Table 13-3   Physiologic Manifestations of Anaphylaxis

System	Subjective Complaint	Symptom	Measured Variable
Cardiovascular	Dizziness	Disorientation	
	Retrosternal pressure	Tachycardia	
		Dysrhythmia	ST-T wave abnormalities
			AV conduction abnormalities
			Ventricular fibrillation
		Cardiovascular collapse	Decreased BP
			Decreased SVR
			Increased CO
			Decreased filling pressure (PWP)
			Increased Hct
		Cardiac arrest	Increased PVR
Respiratory	Sneezing	Rhinitis	
	Nasal stuffiness	Cough	
	Wheezing	Bronchospasm	Increased airways resistance
	Dyspnea	Stridor	
	Chest discomfort	Laryngeal edema	
		Pulmonary edema	
		Cyanosis	Decreased Pao_2
			Increased $Paco_2$
Gastrointestinal	Nausea	Emesis	
	Cramping	Diarrhea	
		Angioedema of bowel	
Cutaneous	Itching	Flushing	
	Burning	Urticaria	
	Tingling	Perioral or periorbital edema	

NOTE: In the intubated and sedated or anesthetized patient sudden cardiovascular collapse may be the only manifestation of anaphylaxis.

Table 13-4   Agents Implicated in Anaphylactic and Anaphylactoid Reactions*

Anesthetic drugs		*Other agents*	
Induction agents	Muscle relaxants	Antibiotics	Colloid volume expanders
Cremophor-solubilized	Succinylcholine	Cephalosporins	Albumin
drugs	Gallamine	Penicillin	Dextrans
Barbiturates	Alcuronium	Vancomycin	Protein fractions
Ketamine	Pancuronium	Blood products	Hydroxyethyl starch
Etomidate	*d*-Tubocurarine	Cryoprecipitates	Cyclosporine
Local anesthetics	Metocurine	Fresh frozen plasma	Drug additives
Para-aminobenzoic ester	Atracurium	Packed red blood cells	Mannitol
agents	Narcotics	Platelets	Methylmethacrylate (bone
	Meperidine	Whole blood	cement)
	Morphine	Chymopapain	Protamine
			Radiographic contrast medium

*Reproduced, with permission, from Levy JH. Anaphylactic Reactions in Anesthesia and Intensive Care. Stoneham, Me.: Butterworth Publishers, 1986, p 9.

cologic agents associated with immediate life-threatening reactions, both immune and nonimmune mediated.

MONITORING

Invasive monitoring of hemodynamic variables is highly recommended because of the potential severity of cardiovascular symptoms. In addition to the usual noninvasive monitoring (see Chapter 4) during and after antigen administration, a central venous and pulmonary arterial catheter will allow periodic determination of central venous pressure (CVP), pulmonary arterial pressure (PAP), pulmonary wedge pressure (PWP), pulmonary vascular resistance (PVR), systemic vascular resistance (SVR), and cardiac output (CO) and direct assessment of treatment modalities, particularly as these are changed (see Chapter 116). Direct intra-arterial systemic blood pressure measurements are needed to monitor potentially unstable perfusion and to provide access for arterial blood gas and pH determinations. In addition continuous ECG monitoring is needed to assess for dysrhythmias and signs of myocardial ischemia such as decreased coronary perfusion. A bladder catheter must be placed to monitor urine output; an output of less than 0.5 ml/kg/hr suggests inadequate volume expansion. All usual ventilatory variables need to be monitored if the patient is treated with mechanical ventilation (Sao$_2$, peak, mean, and end-expiratory pressures, expired tidal volume, Fio$_2$, frequency of ventilation, and end-tidal carbon dioxide tension). Resuscitative equipment, including a source of oxygen and airway support, must be immediately available.

Laboratory evaluation needs to include serial hematocrit determinations to assess the degree of hemoconcentration that has been shown to correlate well with loss of intravascular volume. Obtain a 12-lead ECG to diagnose potential myocardial damage from hypotension, coronary vasoconstriction, or dysrhythmias. All patients must have a chest roentgenogram to determine the degree of interstitial edema and air trapping, to assess placement of the endotracheal tube and vascular catheter, and to evaluate ongoing fulminant pulmonary edema. Clotting variables, BUN, creatinine, and serum electrolyte determinations may be useful as well as serial theophylline determinations if an aminophylline infusion is needed.

TREATMENT

Treatment of anaphylactic reactions must be directed at inhibition of mediator release or synthesis, blockade of the tissue receptors for these mediators, and treatment of physiologic effects of mediators. If possible, infusion of all suspected antigens must be stopped to prevent further involvement of mast cells and basophils. Start 100% inspired oxygen and secure the airway; intubate the patient's airway immediately if either stridor, indicating the onset of laryngeal edema, or facial angioneurotic edema occurs. Even if there are no overt signs of pulmonary involvement, ventilation-perfusion abnormalities can persist for several hours. Immediately initiate vigorous volume expansion to correct hypotension, which is most likely secondary to loss of intravascular volume (up to 37%) through capillary leak and not secondary to myocardial depression. Replacement must be rapid and should not be discontinued if pulmonary edema develops. Pulmonary edema indicates pulmonary vascular leak comparable to the increase in systemic vascular permeability; volume replacement should continue with careful hemodynamic monitoring and airway support. Large IV catheters in the upper extremities or placement of a central venous catheter provides the best access for rapid intravascular expansion. Crystalloid (lactated Ringer's or 0.9% NaCl solutions) or colloid solutions may be used; colloids are more appropriate in infants and patients with known cardiac dysfunction, particularly those with decreased cardiac reserve. The major pharmacologic agent used is epinephrine, which has both α- and β-adrenergic agonist properties. Of particular importance are dilation of bronchial smooth muscle and peripheral vasoconstriction, which treat two of the major disturbances of the reaction (bronchoconstriction and vasodilation). In addition epinephrine increases myocardial contractility and rate (positive inotropy and chronotropy) and inhibits release of mediators from activated mast cells and basophils, preventing degranulation, by stimulating the production of cyclic adenosine 3',5'-monophosphate. Administer epinephrine intravenously if possible, or in the case of cardiac arrest administer the drug through an endotracheal tube; subcutaneous or intramuscular administration results in erratic or low drug absorption, particularly if perfusion to the injection site is compromised. Primary and adjuvant therapy for anaphylaxis is summarized in Table 13-5.

Table 13-5   Management of Anaphylaxis

Therapy	Rationale	Monitor
Initial		
Discontinue antigen administration	Prevent mast cell recruitment and further mediator release	
Secure airway—intubate if necessary, increase Fio_2 to 1.0	Treat $\dot{V}/\dot{Q}$ mismatch, bronchospasm, pulmonary capillary leak (pulmonary edema)	Sao_2, mean and peak pressures, breath sounds, arterial blood gases
Initiate rapid volume expansion (if hypotensive), 0.9% NaCl or lactated Ringer's, 20-50 ml/kg or 5% albumin, 10-20 ml/kg	Replace intravascular volume lost from incompetent capillaries (up to 37% of estimated blood volume)	Noninvasive BP, direct arterial pressure, CVP, capillary refill, urinary output, pulmonary wedge pressure, cardiac output, SVR, mental status
Epinephrine (IV if possible) Initial bolus: 0.5 to 1.0 μg/kg and prn infusion: 0.01 to 0.05 μg/kg/min (titrate dose to effect) Cardiac arrest: 10 μg/kg/IV or per endotracheal tube	α- and β-Agonists counteract vasodilation and bronchoconstriction; positive inotropy; inhibits mediator release from mast cell granules	All cardiovascular parameters and integrity of infusion site; persistent unresponsive hypotension suggests inadequate volume replacement
Adjuvant		
Antihistamines Diphenhydramine, 0.5 to 1.0 mg/kg IV	H_1-receptor antagonist (will not prevent symptoms after histamine release)	
Cimetidine, 5 mg/kg IV	H_2-receptor antagonist (use only if bronchospasm is absent and hypotension persists)	
Aminophylline infusion: 5 to 6 mg/kg bolus followed by 0.5 to 0.9 mg/kg/hr	Treatment of persistent bronchospasm (bronchodilation by inhibition of phosphodiesterase); hemodynamic function must be stable	Serum level; airway pressures, arterial blood gases, Sao_2, ECG
Corticosteroids Hydrocortisone, 0.25 to 1.0 g IV	Attenuation of late-phase reactions produced by inflammatory cells	
Methylprednisolone, 35 mg/kg IV	Inhibition of complement-induced neutrophil aggregation; inhibition of lysosome enzyme release	
Airway assessment (particularly prior to extubation)	Airway edema may persist after hemodynamic stability occurs	Endotracheal tube leak, direct laryngoscopy to visualize upper airway
Other catecholamine infusions Isoproterenol, 0.01 to 0.1 μg/kg/min, titrated to effect	β-Agonist: treatment of persistent bronchospasm, effects additive to aminophylline	Continuation ECG, arterial blood gases, Sao_2, end-tidal CO_2
Norepinephrine, 0.5 to 0.1 kg/min, titrated to effect	α-Agonist	All hemodynamic variables
Dopamine, 2 to 5 μg/kg/hr	May treat persistent oliguria after volume expansion	All hemodynamic variables

Secondary drugs that may be helpful include antihistamines, aminophylline, corticosteroids, and other catecholamines such as isoproterenol, norepinephrine, and dopamine. Antihistamines will *not* prevent symptoms caused by histamine once degranulation and release of that agent have occurred. Administration of H_2 antagonist may be effective, but there is no direct clinical evidence for its use. The beneficial effects of steroids may require hours to days to occur, so they are not useful just before administration of antigen. The addition of other catecholamines depends on how the course of the reaction proceeds; invasive hemodynamic monitoring allows specific α- and β-agonists to be chosen to correct such persistent problems as increased pulmonary artery blood pressure, decreased systemic vascular resistance, or bronchospasm. Diuretics are not useful in treating pulmonary edema, which occurs secondary to increased capillary permeability and not cardiac dysfunction. Potentiation of volume deficit occurs after administration of a diuretic. Mechanical ventilation offers a better method of treatment.

Immediate resuscitation of the patient experiencing anaphylaxis must be followed by ongoing monitoring and evaluation of possible complications such as renal dysfunction, disseminated intravascular coagulation, cerebral hypoxia, coronary ischemia, or persistent laryngeal edema in a PICU or comparable care situation. Late responses to antigen may develop with recurrence of symptoms 12 to 24 hours after the initial episode. All types of agents (antibiotics, radiographic contrast media, foods, insect venom) have been responsible for ongoing reactions; all agents suspected of causing the reaction must be withheld until the patient is completely recovered. Once the patient has recovered, every effort must be made to identify the antigen responsible for the reaction; the patient may need to be referred to an allergist for specific testing. The patient should wear a Medi-Alert bracelet to identify that he is at risk. Patients with known risk factors such as a specific identified allergy, multiple drug allergies, or a history of asthma, atopy, or angioneurotic edema may need to receive prophylactic treatment prior to necessary antigen exposure (Table 13-6). The purpose of pretreatment is not to prevent the reaction but to modify and attenuate the host response to mediators, and more especially to histamine, which is responsible

Table 13-6   Pharmacologic Prophylaxis of Anaphylaxis

Anaphylactic Reactions		Anaphylactoid Reactions	
Regimen	Rationale	Regimen	Rationale
Diphenhydramine, 0.5 to 1 mg/kg q6h for 24 hr before exposure	H_1-receptor antagonist	Diphenhydramine, 0.5 to 1 mg/kg IM or PO 1 hr before exposure	H_1-receptor antagonist
Cimetidine, 5 mg/kg PO q6h for 24 hr before exposure	H_2-receptor antagonist		
Prednisone, 0.5 mg/kg PO q6h for 24 hr before exposure	Attenuation of late inflammatory reactions; potentiates β-agonists; increases vascular epithelial integrity; decreases substrate availability for cyclooxygenase and lipooxygenase pathways	Prednisone, 0.5 mg/kg PO 13, 7, and 1 hr before exposure or methylprednisolone for reactions involving complement activation (transfusion related, protamine)	Attenuation of late inflammatory reactions; potentiates β-agonists; increases vascular epithelial integrity; decreases substrate availability for cyclooxygenase and lipooxygenase pathways
Hydrocortisone, 2.5 mg/kg IV q6h	See above	Ephedrine, 0.5 to 1 mg/kg PO 1 hr before procedure	α- and β-Agonists

for most of the immediate symptoms. When an antigen known to cause a hypersensitivity reaction is to be given, the patient must be in an area where resuscitative equipment, including an oxygen source, is immediately available. Blood pressure, ECG, and oxygen saturation monitoring should be started before antigen administration and continued for several hours afterward. The antigen should be administered as slowly as possible or in incremental doses to allow evaluation for possible untoward effects. Antigen administration must be stopped as soon as any sign suggestive of adverse reactions appears.

ADDITIONAL READING

Ahmed T, Oliver W. Does slow-reacting substance of anaphylaxis mediate hypoxic pulmonary vasoconstriction? Am Rev Respir Dis 127:566-571, 1983.

Fisher MM. Clinical observations on the pathophysiology and treatment of anaphylactic cardiovascular collapse. Anaesth Intensive Care 14:17-21, 1986.

• Levy JH. Anaphylactic Reactions in Anesthesia and Intensive Care. Boston: Butterworth, 1986.

Radermacker M, Gustin M. An in vivo demonstration of the antianaphylactic effect of terbutaline. Clin Allergy 11:79-86, 1981.

14 Acute Renal Failure

Raymond P. Quigley · Steven R. Alexander

BACKGROUND

Acute renal failure (ARF) is a syndrome that is characterized by a sudden and often reversible deterioration in the kidneys that affects their ability to maintain homeostasis of body fluids. Retention of nitrogenous wastes such as urea and creatinine is a consistent feature of ARF but oliguria is not. ARF may occur with or without diminished urine output. Nonoliguric forms of ARF are common in adult patients, accounting for up to 50% of reported cases in series published after 1970. Nonoliguric ARF has been described less frequently in pediatric patients, but this may reflect only the reluctance of pediatricians to suspect ARF in patients whose urine output is not decreased.

Pathophysiology

The pathogenesis of ARF remains poorly understood despite more than 30 years of intense investigation. Some of the confusion probably results from the fact that ARF is a *syndrome* that arises from many different etiologies. The heterogeneity of ARF pathophysiology is evident in the different laboratory models that have been used to study the syndrome, many of which are capable of producing ARF via different pathogenetic mechanisms. There are, however, several features common to the major ARF experimental models that probably play a role in the pathophysiology of many cases of ARF in human patients. A brief review of some basic principles of normal renal physiology may be a helpful introduction to a discussion of several of the prevailing theories of ARF pathogenesis.

The formation of urine occurs in two steps. Glomerular filtration begins the process, and tubular function (reabsorption and secretion) completes it. The fluid volumes handled by this system each day are enormous. In a typical 15 kg child (BSA = 0.7 m²) with a normal glomerular filtration rate (GFR) of 100 ml/min/1.73 m², the kidneys produce nearly

60 L of glomerular filtrate each day. The amount of glomerular filtrate produced every 30 minutes is approximately equal to the entire circulating blood volume of the child. Under normal conditions more than 98% of this filtrate is reabsorbed, yielding a final daily urine volume of about 800 ml (2 L/1.73 m²/day).

The processes of glomerular filtration and tubular reabsorption are closely linked by an intricate regulatory mechanism that is only partially understood. It is generally held that the key regulatory process involves the delivery of filtered NaCl to the macula densa of the distal nephron. When the GFR increases in response to an increase in glomerular blood flow, NaCl delivery to the macula densa is also increased. A feedback loop is formed through the macula densa to the juxtaglomerular cells of the afferent arteriole, resulting in an increase in vascular tone, a decrease in blood flow to the glomerulus, and a fall in the GFR. At this lower GFR delivery of NaCl to the macula densa is decreased, and, via the same feedback loop, relaxation of afferent arteriolar tone produces a corresponding increase in glomerular blood flow and a return to a higher GFR. Thus glomerular and tubular functions remain balanced. The mechanism(s) responsible for the maintenance of glomerular-tubular balance is (are) undoubtedly more complex, but the details remain controversial and have been incompletely described.

The healthy proximal tubule is capable of reabsorbing about 85% of the sodium filtered by the glomerulus. In the syndrome of ARF the cells of the proximal tubule are injured, for example, by ischemia or a toxic substance, and solute reabsorption becomes less efficient. An inappropriate increase in the delivery of solutes to the distal nephron results. The increased amount of NaCl reaching the macula densa no longer reflects glomerular blood flow and GFR. A further reduction in the GFR occurs in response to the increase in distal NaCl delivery, but the injured proximal tubule continues to deliver inappropriate amounts of NaCl to the distal nephron despite the falling GFR. A breakdown in the feedback control mechanism develops, consisting of decreasing glomerular blood flow, decreasing GFR, and persistently elevated distal NaCl delivery from the injured proximal tubule. As much as 50% of the reduction in GFR seen in ARF may be caused by these perturbations in normal glomerular-tubular balance.

From the perspective of the organism as a whole, however, the abrupt fall in GFR that occurs in ARF can be considered a highly successful, protective response to proximal tubule cell injury. If GFR were maintained at normal levels despite the inability of the injured proximal tubule cells to reabsorb filtered solutes, the rate at which solutes and fluid would be lost from the body could result in circulatory collapse in a matter of hours.

There are several other factors that are thought to contribute to the decreased GFR of ARF. One of the most consistent findings on pathologic examination of kidneys in animal models of ARF and in renal biopsies from patients with ARF is the formation of casts blocking the tubular lumina. These casts are formed when proximal tubule cells become necrotic and slough off the basement membrane into the lumen of the tubule. Partial or complete obstruction of the tubule by a cast decreases the flow of tubular fluid, causing intratubular pressure to rise and GFR to fall. The location of casts in the tubules of animal models of ARF is highly variable, which may explain why casts are not seen in every ARF biopsy specimen.

The backflow of fluid through the damaged tubular basement membrane is another mechanism thought to contribute to the decrease in effective GFR seen in patients with ARF. This phenomenon has been demonstrated in both animal models and patients with ARF using radiolabeled substances of varying molecular weights. Other factors that may contribute to the decrease in GFR but have been less well demonstrated include occlusion of nephrons by interstitial edema, redistribution of renal blood flow from outer cortical to juxtamedullary nephrons, and altered glomerular capillary permeability. (Readers interested in a more complete discussion of these and other proposed pathogenetic mechanisms should consult Bonventre, Leaf, and Malis; Gaudio and Siegel; and Levinsky cited at the end of this chapter.)

Incidence and Common Etiologies

In developing countries ARF is a common pediatric disorder that occurs most often as a complication of infectious diarrhea, dehydration, bronchopneumonia, and sepsis. In North America and Western Europe ARF is more likely to be encountered in neonates who survive perinatal asphyxia and shock, in infants and young children who undergo surgery for congenital heart disease, in children with multiple organ system failure of any etiology, and in children with hemolytic-uremic syndrome (HUS). The clinical settings in which ARF should be suspected are as follows:

1. First 24 hours postoperatively, especially after cardiac surgery
2. Following any episode of shock
3. In neonates with perinatal asphyxia, hypotension, or severe respiratory distress syndrome (RDS)
4. Following multiple trauma, severe burns, or crush injuries
5. During chemotherapy for lymphoproliferative tumors
6. Following an IV contrast study, especially in a marginally hydrated, diabetic, or nephrotic child
7. Following severe transfusion reactions
8. In patients receiving aminoglycoside antibiotics, especially if other nephrotoxic agents are present
9. In children with preexisting chronic renal disease who develop an acute illness of any kind
10. In renal transplant recipients who develop any illness

Mortality

Mortality rates remain disturbingly high among patients with ARF. Since the introduction of dialysis to clinical medicine over 30 years ago, published series of adult patients show that the ARF mortality rate has remained around 50%. Nonoliguric forms of ARF in adults and neonates are associated with lower mortality rates. Mortality rates among children with ARF have been reported to range from 33% to 100%, with the highest mortality rate occurring in postoperative patients.

It is frequently claimed that the persistently high mortality rates seen in ARF reflect the severity of the underlying clinical problems that led to the development of ARF. It is also argued (usually by nephrologists) that, while overall mortality has changed little in several decades, improvements in critical care have resulted in an ARF patient population that is much older and sicker in the case of adults, and much younger (e.g., premature infants weighing 500 g) and sicker in the case of pediatric patients. While this may be true, the fact remains that ARF can be a particularly lethal complication of many medical and surgical conditions in patients of all ages.

Classification and Differential Diagnosis

It is both traditional and clinically useful to attempt to classify all patients with ARF into one of three large categories: prerenal, postrenal, or "intrinsic" renal failure. Although no attempt has been made to present an exhaustive differential diagnosis, most of the conditions commonly encountered in pediatric ARF patients are listed below.

Renal hypoperfusion (i.e., prerenal failure, functional azotemia)

1. Absolute decrease in intravascular volume
   a. Dehydration
   b. Hemorrhage
   c. Third space losses (nonmeasured fluid losses) bowel surgery, intestinal infarction, peritonitis, nephrotic syndrome, acute pancreatitis
   d. Burns
2. Relative decrease in intravascular volume
   a. Septic shock
   b. Anaphylaxis
   c. Ganglionic blocking agents and vasodilating antihypertensive medications
3. Decreased cardiac output
   a. Congestive heart failure
   b. Cardiac tamponade
   c. Tension pneumothorax
4. Renal vascular obstruction
   a. Renal artery embolus
   b. Aortic thrombosis

Obstructive uropathy (i.e., postrenal failure)

1. Urethral obstruction
   a. Foreign body
   b. Obstructed bladder catheter
   c. Congenital urethral valves (posterior and anterior)
   d. Stricture following urethral instrumentation
   e. Perineal trauma with urethral injury
   f. Calculus
   g. Clots
   h. Ectopic ureterocele
   i. Prostatic hypertrophy in adults; in children, rarely caused by prostatic cancer (e.g., sarcoma botryoides)
2. Bladder outlet obstruction
   a. Neoplasm
   b. Calculus
   c. Functional (e.g., neurogenic bladder, narcotics)
3. Ureteral obstruction (rarely a cause of ARF, except when only one kidney or a renal transplant is present)
   a. Clots
   b. Calculi (e.g., oxalosis, cystinuria, hyperuricemia)
   c. Necrotizing papillitis (sickle cell disease, diabetes)
   d. Extraureteral mass (chronic granulomatous disease)
   e. Stenosis following ureteral surgery or instrumentation
   f. Congenital ureteropelvic junction or ureterovesical obstruction
   g. Iatrogenic or traumatic ligation or compression of the ureters
   h. Ureteroceles
   i. Infection with strictures

"True" (intrinsic) renal failure

1. Nephrotoxins
   a. Bismuth, mercury, gold, lead, cadmium, platinum
   b. Ethylene glycol, gasoline ingestion
   c. Carbon tetrachloride
   d. Aminoglycoside antibiotics, aspirin ingestion, therapy with other nonsteroidal anti-inflammatory agents, and a multitude of additional nephrotoxic drugs
   e. IV contrast agents
   f. Uric acid (tumor lysis products)
   g. Hemoglobinuria, myoglobinuria, rhabdomyolysis
   h. Cyclosporin
   i. Captopril and other angiotensin converting enzyme inhibitors in children with diminished renal blood flow caused by aortic coarctation, bilateral renal artery stenosis, renal transplant artery stenosis, or severe intravascular volume depletion
2. Intravascular coagulation
   a. Hemolytic-uremic syndrome
   b. Septic shock
   c. DIC of any etiology
3. Diseases of the kidney and blood vessels
   a. Acute poststreptococcal glomerulonephritis
   b. Rapidly progressive (crescentic) glomerulonephritis
   c. Acute interstitial nephritis (postinfectious or hypersensitivity in origin)
   d. Renal venous thrombosis

e. Systemic diseases with renal manifestations (e.g., systemic lupus erythematosus, polyarteritis)

f. As a complication of any primary renal disease (e.g., minimal change nephrotic syndrome, focal glomerulosclerosis, membranoproliferative glomerulonephritis)

g. Renal transplant rejection

4. Circulatory insufficiency producing the syndrome of acute tubular necrosis (also known as acute vasomotor nephropathy)

   a. Shock
   b. Perinatal asphyxia, profound hypoxia, acidosis
   c. Following cardiac surgery
   d. Following prolonged prerenal azotemia of any etiology

5. Congenital disorders

   a. Polycystic kidney disease
   b. Renal hypoplasia, dysplasia
   c. Congenital nephrotic syndrome
   d. Renal agenesis (Potter's syndrome)

6. Infections

   a. Severe acute pyelonephritis (rare)

7. Tumors

   a. Tumor cell infiltrates (acute lymphocytic leukemia, acute myelogenous leukemia)
   b. Uric acid nephropathy from tumor cell lysis
   c. Wilms' tumor with associated glomerulopathy

8. Severe, prolonged electrolyte disorders

   a. Hypernatremia
   b. Hypercalcemia

> ## CLINICAL FEATURES OF ARF
>
> Azotemia (serum creatinine level increases by 0.5 to 1.5 mg/dl/day, depending on the muscle mass of the child)
>
> Hypervolemia, leading to circulatory congestion, pulmonary edema, and peripheral edema
>
> Hyperkalemia
>
> Metabolic acidosis
>
> Hyponatremia, often as a consequence of the continued administration of relatively hypotonic fluids in the oliguric patient
>
> Systemic arterial hypertension
>
> Anemia (dilutional at first, then from frequent blood sampling and marrow suppression)
>
> Hyperphosphatemia
>
> Hypocalcemia
>
> Uremic encephalopathy, seen with rapid increases of BUN to high levels (100 to 150 mg/dl)
>
> Increased bleeding time resulting from platelet dysfunction seen with high BUN (>100 mg/dl)
>
> Toxic effects of many drugs given at usually safe dosages, especially digitalis preparations, aminoglycosides, and phenothiazines
>
> Oliguria (defined as urine output <1 ml/kg/hr), if not present from the onset of ARF, may occur at any time during the course of the disorder

---

"Prerenal failure" is the term primarily used to describe conditions involving renal hypoperfusion, either on the basis of hypovolemia or cardiac (pump) failure. Postrenal failure includes all forms of obstructive uropathy. Intrinsic renal failure includes those conditions in which renal dysfunction occurs as a consequence of renal cell injury that is not correctable by improvement in renal perfusion or relief of urinary tract obstruction.

Common Clinical Manifestations

The syndrome of ARF has protean manifestations that may appear suddenly and progress rapidly to life-threatening degrees. Commonly encountered clinical features are listed. These conditions rarely develop simultaneously, but all patients with ARF should be considered at risk to develop any of these conditions. The clinical management of each of these problems is reviewed later in this chapter.

Diagnosis of Prerenal, Postrenal, and Intrinsic Renal Failure
The initial workup

In the typical clinical setting it is frequently necessary to determine whether a patient who has newly discovered azotemia and oliguria has suffered prerenal, postrenal, or intrinsic ARF. Early diagnosis is important because both renal hypoperfusion and obstructive uropathy are potentially reversible, and each can lead to intrinsic renal failure if allowed to persist long enough. The first order of business in such situations is to determine whether the observed oliguria and azotemia reflect an appropriate response to decreased renal perfusion or an acutely obstructed urinary tract. Clinical judgment based on a thorough history and physical examination will occasionally resolve the issue, but in the typically complex PICU patient additional diagnostic maneuvers are usually required. The following approach to the early evaluation of the child with ARF has been generalized and should be modified to fit the individual clinical situation.

History and physical examination. Search diligently for possible causes of ARF. Is the urinary catheter obstructed? Is the bladder distended? Are any of the conditions known to be associated with intrinsic ARF (see p. 107) present in this patient?

Urine sample. Insert a urinary catheter using strict aseptic technique, and obtain a urine sample to send for the following studies: urinalysis, sodium, creatinine, osmolality, and culture.

Sonography. Obtain a sonogram of the abdomen and pelvis to rule out obstructive uropathy. *Do not obtain an intravenous pyelogram.* Contrast media are potent nephrotoxins in this setting and may also precipitate circulatory overload. A radionuclide renal scan adds little to the initial evaluation and in most centers requires transporting a very sick patient to the nuclear medicine department. Alternatively, sonography may be performed at the bedside in the PICU.

Blood studies. Send blood samples for the following studies: BUN, creatinine, sodium, potassium, chloride, total CO_2 (or venous or arterial blood gases), ionized calcium, phosphorus, uric acid, total serum protein, osmolality, magnesium, and CBC (including red blood cell morphology, WBC count, and differential and platelet counts). Additional studies may be indicated in specific clinical situations (e.g., blood cultures in suspected sepsis or PT, PTT, fibrinogen, and fibrin split products in suspected DIC).

Renal failure index (RFI) and fractional excretion of sodium (FE$_{Na}$). Calculate the RFI and FE$_{Na}$ using the following formulas:

$$RFI = \frac{Urine\ sodium}{Urine\ creatinine/serum\ creatinine}$$

$$FE_{Na} = \frac{(Urine\ sodium/serum\ sodium) \times 100}{Urine\ creatinine/serum\ creatinine}$$

These calculations are based on studies obtained acutely on a spot urine sample, and they provide insight into renal tubular response to various physiologic stresses. The healthy nephron responds to inadequate perfusion by increasing the reabsorption of filtered sodium, thereby lowering urine sodium concentration and reducing urine volume. Creatinine concentration rises in the urine disproportionately to the rise in serum creatinine since glomerular filtration and tubular secretion of creatinine are maintained in the healthy tubule despite falling renal blood flow. The RFI and FE$_{Na}$ in such prerenal patients will be low (<2.5 in neonates and <1.0 in older pediatric patients and adults) because the urine sodium concentration is low (the numerator) and the ratio of urine to serum creatinine concentration is high (the denominator). The opposite conditions prevail in patients with intrinsic renal failure and obstructive uropathy where renal tubular cell injury results in diminished tubular function (i.e., higher urine sodium concentration and lower urine to plasma creatinine concentration ratio).

Neither the RFI nor the FE$_{Na}$ can be used to evaluate a patient who has recently received a diuretic because diuretics spuriously increase urine sodium concentration. The RFI and FE$_{Na}$ may also be misleading in early cases of acute postinfectious glomerulonephritis and HUS in which the RFI and FE$_{Na}$ often suggest prerenal failure, despite severe intrinsic renal injury and the absence of any potential for response to maneuvers designed to increase renal perfusion.

Representative values for RFI, FE$_{Na}$, and other indices of renal function obtained from studies performed in adults and neonates with prerenal and intrinsic ARF are listed in Table 14-1. The RFI and the FE$_{Na}$ are the most useful of these indices in patients who have not recently received diuretics. The use of the RFI and FE$_{Na}$ in children beyond the newborn period has not been systematically studied, but for most clinical purposes the adult reference values given in Table 14-1 appear adequate for pediatric patients beyond 4 to 6 weeks of age (postconceptional age >44 to 46 weeks). Note that the higher RFI and FE$_{Na}$ seen in neonates with prerenal azotemia reflect the relative inefficiency with which the kidney of a newborn conserves sodium in response to renal hypoperfusion. Sodium conservation is particularly difficult for premature infants whose postconceptional age is <32 weeks. In these infants the RFI and FE$_{Na}$ are helpful only if <2.5; higher values may only reflect renal immaturity rather than intrinsic renal failure.

Free-water clearance (C$_{H_2O}$). Oliguric patients are often given diuretics before any attempt is made to define the cause of the oliguria. When this occurs,

Table 14-1   Urinary Diagnostic Indices in ARF

	Prerenal Azotemia		Intrinsic ARF	
	Adults/Children	Neonates	Adults/Children	Neonates
U_{Na} (mEq/L)	<20	<30	>50	>50
U_{osm} (mOsm/kg H_2O)	>500	>350	<300	<300
RFI	<1	<2.5	>1	>2.5
FE_{Na}	<1	<2.5	>1	>2.5
C_{H_2O}*	−25 to −180 ml/hr/1.73 m^2 BSA		−15 to +15 ml/hr/1.73 m^2 BSA	

RFI = renal failure index = $\dfrac{U_{Na}}{(U/P)\ \text{creatinine}}$; FE_{Na} = fractional excretion of sodium = $\dfrac{(U/P)\ Na \times 100}{(U/P)\ \text{creatinine}}$; C_{H_2O} = free-water clearance (see text for formula).

*The C_{H_2O} has not been studied in neonates.

the RFI and FE_{Na} usually cannot be used to separate prerenal from intrinsic renal failure. The C_{H_2O} is a diagnostic index of renal function that is independent of urine sodium concentration and reflective of renal tubular concentrating capacity. A precise 2-hour urine collection is obtained to measure urine osmolality and volume. C_{H_2O} is calculated as follows:

$$C_{H_2O} = [UO\ (ml/hr)] - \frac{[UO\ (ml/hr)] \times [U_{osm}]}{S_{osm}}$$

where UO = measured hourly urine output over at least 2 hours; U_{osm} = urine osmolality; and S_{osm} = serum osmolality.

Studies in adult ICU patients have shown the C_{H_2O} to be an accurate indicator of renal functional status when serial studies are obtained. In these patients who were recovering from cardiac surgery a C_{H_2O} of −15 ml/hr or less predicted a good response to measures designed to increase renal perfusion (e.g., a fluid challenge or an increase in inotrope infusion rate). When C_{H_2O} was between −15 ml/hr and +15 ml/hr, either the patient was in perfect fluid balance, needing neither concentration nor dilution of the urine, or the patient was developing intrinsic renal failure. Loss of the ability to concentrate and dilute the urine in response to changes in renal perfusion is a common feature of intrinsic renal failure, leading to the characteristic isosthenuria of renal failure. Alterations in renal sodium and chloride reabsorption produced by diuretics such as furosemide do not influence the handling of free water by the distal

nephron in response to changes in renal perfusion. Therefore the C_{H_2O} can be used in patients who have received diuretics.

The use of the C_{H_2O} as an index of renal function in critically ill pediatric patients has not been studied systematically. Disorders of antidiuretic hormone secretion and other factors perversely influencing urine osmolality may invalidate the C_{H_2O} in some patients. In our center, when we have used the C_{H_2O} to assess renal function in oliguric pediatric patients who have recently received diuretics, we have found a C_{H_2O} of −25 to −180 ml/hr/1.73 m^2 BSA to be indicative of prerenal azotemia. A C_{H_2O} of −15 to +15 ml/hr/1.73 m^2 BSA has been associated with intrinsic renal failure and has been predictive of unresponsiveness to volume or inotropes.

MONITORING AND LABORATORY TESTS
Intake and Output

Strict intake and output records and frequent weights are mandatory. An indwelling urinary catheter must be removed from the oligoanuric patient as soon as possible to reduce the risk of urinary tract infection (UTI). Precise measurement of minimal urine output is of little benefit and is far outweighed by the increased risk of UTI associated with indwelling urinary catheters.

Frequent laboratory tests are necessary in all patients with ARF who are being managed conservatively without dialysis or continuous arteriovenous hemofiltration (CAVH). Serum electrolytes, including total CO_2, need to be measured every 6 to 8 hours.

BUN, creatinine, calcium (preferably the ionized fraction), phosphorus, magnesium, uric acid, venous or arterial blood gases, pH, and CBC need to be measured every 12 to 24 hours. Blood gases and pH allow interpretation of mixed acid-base disorders; these measures are most helpful in patients who also have respiratory dysfunction with retention of CO_2, and should be monitored more frequently in these patients. Measurement of the creatinine clearance is usually of little value early in the course of ARF when renal function is changing rapidly. In the stable nonoliguric patient creatinine clearance may be helpful as an estimate of GFR that can be used to adjust medication dosages. Creatinine clearance substantially overestimates GFR in patients with reduced renal function. An average of the urea and creatinine clearances probably gives a better estimate of GFR at levels <50% of normal.

TREATMENT
PICU Care With Pediatric Renal Replacement Therapy Capability

Because of the high mortality rates associated with ARF, all pediatric patients with ARF need to be treated in an intensive care setting in a facility capable of rapid institution of acute renal replacement therapy in pediatric patients. Acute renal replacement therapy capability optimally includes the ready availability of peritoneal dialysis (see Chapter 145), hemodialysis (see Chapter 146), and CAVH (see Chapter 148). At a minimum the facility must be capable of performing acute peritoneal dialysis in pediatric patients. If the appropriate renal replacement therapy is unavailable, *early* consideration must be given to transferring the patient to a tertiary pediatric nephrology center *before* the need to do so becomes an emergency.

Treatment of the Underlying Cause of ARF

A thorough search must be made for the underlying cause of ARF in each patient, and appropriate treatment undertaken concurrently with treatment of the ARF syndrome.

Medication Dosage Adjustment

A complete review of medications must be made with adjustment of regimens to reflect the patient's decreased GFR. Recommendations for adjustments to commonly used medications in children with renal failure have been published by Trompeter. Drugs that are highly nephrotoxic (e.g., aminoglycoside anti-

biotics) must be avoided whenever an equally effective but less nephrotoxic alternative is available. When drugs that are excreted predominantly by the kidneys are administered, frequent blood levels must be taken to guide therapy.

Conversion of Oliguric to Nonoliguric ARF

Nearly one third of adult patients with oliguric ARF can be "converted" to the nonoliguric form of ARF by the administration of furosemide. Nonoliguric ARF is easier to manage and has been shown to be associated with a lower mortality rate in adults and neonates. IV furosemide can be given in individual doses of 1 mg/kg, 2 mg/kg, and a maximum of 4 mg/kg, the dose being advanced at 1-hour intervals until diuresis is achieved or the maximum 4 mg/kg dose has been given. Administering larger doses of furosemide or continuing attempts to convert to nonoliguric ARF beyond these three recommended doses are not likely to be successful and incur increased risks of furosemide nephro- and ototoxicity. Mannitol has also been used effectively in this setting; however, the risk of acute circulatory overload is high when mannitol is used unsuccessfully in the oliguric patient. Furosemide appears safer than mannitol and equally effective, although a systematic comparison of the two agents in pediatric patients has not been made.

Fluid Therapy

Precise management of fluid therapy is a hallmark of successful ARF treatment. Inadequate fluid restriction in the oliguric patient can rapidly precipitate the need for renal replacement therapy. Although every patient must be considered individually, the following general suggestions may be helpful:

1. If the patient is clinically dehydrated, a *cautious* attempt to restore near-normal intravascular volume is indicated. The CVP must be closely monitored in such patients. Small doses (5 ml/kg) of an isotonic fluid (either 0.9% NaCl solution or isotonic mixtures of NaCl and $NaHCO_3$ in the severely acidotic patient) can be given slowly, using the CVP as a guide. Although strict guidelines cannot be given, it is probably wise to avoid pushing the CVP beyond 4 to 6 cm H_2O in the oliguric ARF patient. Fluid therapy for the dehydrated patient with ARF is often given in conjunction with the attempt to convert to nonoliguric ARF using furosemide.

2. Fluid therapy for patients who are clinically eu-

volemic is designed to precisely replace ongoing fluid losses. Total fluid intake should be equal to the insensible water losses plus all measured fluid losses (e.g., urine, stool, nasogastric tube drainage, chest tube drainage, emesis). It is advisable to use conservative estimates of insensible losses, for example, 30 to 35 ml/100 kcal/24 hr. Ideally the euvolemic patient's weight will remain unchanged or will decrease by <1% each day. Recorded intake and output and the observed change in weight over 24 hours can be used to revise estimates of insensible losses on a daily basis.

3. The management of the patient with fluid overload varies according to the severity of the overloaded state. Hypertension and congestive heart failure are the most dangerous consequences of fluid overload. Hypertension alone may be managed with antihypertensive drugs, but congestive heart failure, with or without hypertension, mandates rapid fluid removal with dialysis or CAVH. If the patient is clinically stable and only mildly overloaded, and if there is some fluid output in addition to insensible losses, it is theoretically possible to achieve euvolemia without dialysis or CAVH by severely restricting fluid intake. This approach is not recommended beyond 24 to 48 hours. Such severe fluid restriction results in the patient receiving grossly inadequate nutrition, which further accelerates the hypercatabolic state of ARF.

Sodium

Patients with oliguric or nonoliguric ARF need only enough sodium to replace ongoing losses. Urinary sodium losses can be large in nonoliguric patients. It is often helpful to monitor urine sodium concentration in these patients daily, using a 4- to 6-hour pooled urine sample to reduce the influence of fluctuations in urine sodium concentration seen in spot urine samples. Oliguric patients lose little sodium and readily become sodium overloaded, which leads to edema formation, aggravates hypertension, and increases the risk of circulatory congestion.

Patients with ARF frequently present with moderate degrees of dilutional hyponatremia, which is the result of continued administration/intake of hypotonic fluids (IV or PO) in the presence of unrecognized oliguric ARF. These patients do not have a sodium deficit and will correct slowly if free water is appropriately restricted. Severe and/or symptomatic hyponatremia (i.e., serum [Na] <125 mEq/L) in

the oliguric, hypervolemic patient should be treated with dialysis or CAVH. Similar recommendations apply to oliguric hypernatremic patients (e.g., serum [Na] >150 mEq/L). In both settings conservative fluid management techniques usually will not correct the serum sodium abnormalities in the appropriate time period (over approximately 48 hours) because the patient is oliguric. Nonoliguric patients with abnormal serum sodium concentrations can usually be treated without dialysis or CAVH. For the majority of patients with serum sodium concentrations in the normal range it is frequently preferable to administer all sodium as sodium bicarbonate. Such patients often need substantial base therapy, and when given as sodium bicarbonate, more than enough sodium is provided. It may be necessary to measure sodium concentration in urine, gastric fluid, and other fluid losses to more precisely adjust administered sodium. It may also be important to consider the sodium contributions of certain medications such as ticarcillin that contain large amounts of sodium.

Management of Complications of ARF
Fluid overload/congestive heart failure
See the preceding discussion.

Hyponatremia, hypernatremia
See the preceding discussion.

Hyperkalemia
Of the metabolic derangements that occur during ARF, hyperkalemia is the most life threatening because it can induce cardiac dysrhythmias. Before reviewing the effects of potassium on the heart it may be helpful to review some fundamentals of potassium homeostasis.

Potassium homeostasis. Potassium is the second most abundant cation in the body. The adult body contains about 3500 mEq (50 mEq/kg) of potassium, which is distributed between the intracellular and extracellular fluids. Most potassium is intracellular, where the concentration ranges from 140 to 150 mEq/L. Only about 2% of the body's potassium is in the extracellular fluid, where the concentration is tightly regulated at 4 to 5 mEq/L. Healthy individuals are in potassium balance (i.e., the daily intake of potassium [about 1.5 to 2.5 mEq/kg] is equal to the amount excreted). The kidneys are responsible for excretion of 90% to 95% of ingested potassium, with the gastrointestinal tract excreting the remainder.

The manner in which the renal system handles potassium is complex. First, potassium is freely filtered by the glomerulus and appears in the initial tubular fluid at almost the same concentration as in the serum. Thus the daily filtered load of potassium is about 600 mEq/1.73 m² BSA. Most of the filtered potassium is reabsorbed in the proximal tubule, and the remainder (15% to 20%) is reabsorbed in the loop of Henle. By the time the tubular fluid reaches the distal nephron, almost all of the filtered potassium has been reabsorbed. Thus renal excretion of the daily potassium load is a *secretory* process that takes place in the distal tubule and collecting duct.

Cells in the distal nephron secrete potassium in two steps. First, potassium is actively transported into the cell from the extracellular fluid across the basolateral cell membrane by a process driven by the enzyme Na-K-ATPase, which is located on the membrane. The activity of this enzyme maintains the high intracellular concentration of potassium and keeps intracellular sodium concentration low. Potassium exits the distal tubule cell via channels in the apical membrane leading into the tubular lumen. The electrochemical gradient favoring passive diffusion of potassium out of the cell is maintained by the high intracellular potassium concentration and the negative electrical potential within the lumen of the distal nephron. This lumen negative potential is maintained by the high conductance of sodium across the apical cell membrane into the cell and the low intracellular concentration of sodium that results from Na-K-ATPase activity on the basolateral cell membrane.

Perturbations in renal potassium excretion occur when one or more of the above mechanisms is disturbed. Proximal tubule reabsorption of potassium can be inhibited by carbonic anhydrase inhibitors such as acetazolamide; osmotic diuretics such as mannitol, glycerol, and glucose; and chronic acidosis. These same factors also increase potassium excretion by increasing the distal delivery of sodium and fluid. Although the secretion of potassium by the distal tubule is regulated in part by aldosterone, which acts by stimulating Na-K-ATPase activity, it is the delivery of sodium and fluid that most profoundly affects distal tubule potassium handling. Increased distal delivery of fluid increases potassium secretion by keeping the luminal potassium concentration low, thereby maintaining a large chemical gradient for potassium diffusion into the luminal fluid. The kaliuretic effect of increased distal fluid delivery is independent of distal sodium delivery and may be the primary mechanism responsible for the kaliuresis that accompanies the use of most diuretics, including drugs with primary sites of action in all segments of the nephron (e.g., thiazides, furosemide, and many others). These diuretics also increase distal sodium delivery, which results in increased potassium secretion in exchange for sodium reabsorption.

Two classes of diuretic agents that *do not* produce a distal kaliuresis are sodium channel blockers such as amiloride and triamterene and aldosterone antagonists such as spironolactone. Sodium channel blockers act by reducing apical sodium conductance out of the luminal fluid, thereby decreasing potassium diffusion across the apical cell membrane into the luminal fluid. Aldosterone antagonists can markedly diminish distal Na-K-ATPase activity by blunting the stimulatory effects of aldosterone. Diuretics in these two potassium-sparing classes of drugs must be avoided in patients who have even mild degrees of renal insufficiency.

Although the renal handling of potassium is closely regulated by several different mechanisms, the response of these renal mechanisms to changes in extracellular fluid potassium concentration is slow, taking hours to days. A modest IV or oral potassium load will increase the serum potassium concentration by <1 mEq/L, yet only about one half of the administered potassium appears in the urine within 6 hours. The bulk of the potassium load is quickly transported into cells as a result of the actions of two hormones, insulin and epinephrine. The minute-to-minute regulation of potassium homeostasis is accomplished not by the kidneys, but by these hormones acting on large cell populations (e.g., muscle, liver). The ability to maintain extracellular fluid potassium concentration within such a narrow range (i.e., ±0.5 mEq/L) despite highly variable potassium intake can only be explained by invoking these nonrenal regulatory mechanisms.

The effects of insulin on potassium transport into cells, primarily muscle and liver, are independent of insulin's effects on glucose transport. Hyperkalemia is a potent stimulus for insulin release. The infusion of an insulin antagonist, somatostatin, results in an increase in serum potassium concentration by as much as 0.6 mEq/L as the effects of basal insulin secretion are inhibited. If somatostatin is given with a potassium load, serum potassium concentration increases dramatically. Epinephrine also stimulates potassium uptake by liver and muscle cells. This action can be inhibited by a nonspecific β-receptor blocking agent such as propranolol, by specific β_2-receptor blockade, and by α-receptor stimulation. When the modulating effects of epinephrine on potassium homeostasis are blunted by β_2-receptor blockade or α-receptor stimulation, serum potassium concentration will rise.

A third hormone, aldosterone, plays an important role in potassium homeostasis. Aldosterone has been shown to directly stimulate potassium secretion by both the kidney and the colon, and aldosterone may act similarly at additional nonrenal sites.

Potassium homeostasis is also influenced by disorders of acid-base status and tonicity. When a patient becomes acutely hypertonic, water moves from the intracellular (ICF) to the extracellular fluid (ECF) space. Convective transport (i.e., solvent drag) results in the simultaneous movement of intracellular solutes into the ECF, and since potassium is the most abundant intracellular cation, modest degrees of hypertonicity can deliver substantial amounts of potassium to the ECF.

The effects of acid-base disorders on potassium homeostasis are complex and controversial. A complete discussion of this subject is beyond the scope of this text, but the main factors involved can be summarized as follows: In general, acute acidemia results in a shift of potassium ions from the ICF to the ECF space. Classically it has been taught that serum potassium concentration rises by about 0.5 mEq/L for each 0.1 unit decrease in the arterial pH. However, observed changes in serum potassium concentration vary widely, depending in part on the origin of the acid load. Retention of CO_2 (i.e., respiratory acidosis) is associated with an increase in serum potassium concentration of only 0.1 to 0.3 mEq/L for each 0.1 pH unit change. Infusion of inorganic acids such as hydrochloric acid produces the most dramatic increase in serum potassium concentration, but this form of experimental metabolic acidosis has limited clinical relevance. When metabolic acidosis results from increased concentrations of organic acids (e.g., lactic acid, β-OH butyric acid), serum potassium concentration rises less predictably. The blunted effects of organic acidemia are probably caused by the permeability of the cell membrane to many organic acids. As a result, the complete organic acid molecule can accompany the influx of protons (i.e., hydrogen ions) into the cell, relieving potassium ions of the

obligation to leave the cell to maintain electrochemical balance.

Renal response to acidosis is also variable, depending on the origin and the duration of the acidemic state. Acute acidemia inhibits distal nephron potassium secretion and potentially participates in the acute development of *hyper*kalemia. Chronic acidemia has the opposite effect—the transport of filtered solutes and water by the proximal tubule is inhibited, and the resulting increase in distal delivery of sodium and fluid causes a net increase in potassium secretion that may contribute to the development of *hypo*kalemia. The effects of organic acidosis on renal potassium handling can also be confusing. When the load of filtered anion (e.g., lactate, β-OH butyrate) exceeds the reabsorptive capability of the nephron, increased amounts of both sodium and potassium are lost in the urine as accompanying cations.

Disturbances of potassium homeostasis in ARF. From the previous discussion of normal potassium homeostasis it should be no surprise that oliguric acute renal failure is often complicated by hyperkalemia. Potassium secretion by the kidney is severely limited in ARF, not only by ischemic or toxic injury to distal tubule cells, but by the drastic reduction in the delivery of fluid to the distal nephron. The inability of the acutely failing kidney to excrete acid leads to acute acidosis, which contributes to the development of hyperkalemia by inhibiting distal tubule potassium secretion and by shifting potassium from the ICF to the ECF compartment. Restoration of adequate urine output and correction of acidosis are both important elements in the prevention and treatment of the hyperkalemia of ARF.

Cardiac effects of hyperkalemia. Hyperkalemia is a life-threatening complication of ARF because of the increased risk of cardiac dysrhythmias that accompanies elevated serum potassium concentrations. The electrical potential difference (PD) between the intracellular fluid and the surrounding interstitial fluid is determined by the concentrations of all of the ions residing inside and outside of the cell, and by the differential permeability of the cell membrane to those ions. At rest, excitable cells such as neurons and cardiac myocytes have a high permeability to potassium and a low permeability to sodium. The PD across the cell membrane can be calculated for potassium from the Nernst equation:

$$PD = -60 \log \frac{(K^+ \text{ inside})}{(K^+ \text{ outside})}$$

Under normal resting conditions

$$PD = -60 \log (140/4)$$
$$= -92.6 \text{ mV}$$

The actual measured PD is about -90 mV, which corresponds with the high resting membrane permeability to potassium. ICF and ECF sodium concentrations are the inverse of the potassium concentrations, which would give a PD of about $+90$ mV if the membrane were permeable to sodium at rest. However, the resting cell membrane permeability to sodium is almost zero, which explains why the resting PD is determined predominantly by the differential potassium concentrations.

When the cardiac cell receives a signal to contract, cell membrane sodium permeability increases, resulting in an increase in cell PD toward zero. As the cell PD increases, it reaches a point known as the "threshold potential" (about -60 mV) where the action potential is triggered, causing the cell to contract and sending the signal on to the next cell. Hyperkalemia increases the risk of cardiac dysrhythmias because the increase in serum potassium concentration shifts the myocardial cell resting PD toward the threshold potential and thus renders the cell more easily triggered. For example, when the serum potassium concentration rises to 8.0 mEq/L, the resting PD becomes

$$PD = -60 \log (140/8)$$
$$= -74 \text{ mV}$$

When the resting potential is this close to the threshold potential, the myocardium is said to be "irritable" and is clearly at risk to develop aberrant depolarization foci and disordered conduction of the normal depolarization signal. Initial treatment of life-threatening levels of hyperkalemia needs to be directed at stabilization of the myocardium with calcium, and to a lesser extent with sodium, in an attempt to prevent dysrhythmias.

ECG abnormalities in hyperkalemia. The ECG is a sensitive indicator of potassium's effect on the heart. Continuous ECG monitoring is essential in all patients with ARF. Typical ECG changes associated with different degrees of hyperkalemia are shown in Fig. 14-1. As the potassium concentration rises, the T waves become tall and peaked. At higher potassium levels the P interval becomes prolonged and P waves may disappear altogether as atrial standstill develops. QRS complexes widen and the PR intervals become

irregular. Finally, ventricular tachycardia that leads to ventricular fibrillation or to asystole is a terminal event. Representative serum potassium concentrations shown with each ECG abnormality in the figure must be considered only approximate and are unlikely to apply directly to any given patient. The sequence of ECG abnormalities associated with rising serum potassium levels generally follows that shown in Fig. 14-1, but the potassium levels at which specific ECG abnormalities occur vary widely from patient to patient.

Treatment of hyperkalemia

1. *Stabilize the myocardium.* Give *calcium chloride,* 0.2 to 0.3 ml/kg of a 10% $CaCl_2$ solution intravenously. Monitor therapy by following serum ion-

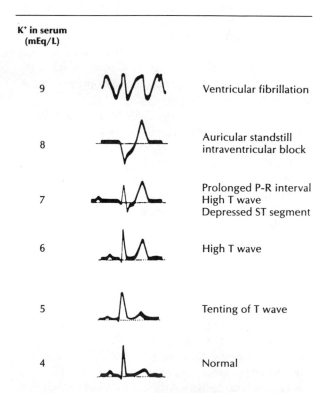

K+ in serum (mEq/L)

9	Ventricular fibrillation
8	Auricular standstill intraventricular block
7	Prolonged P-R interval High T wave Depressed ST segment
6	High T wave
5	Tenting of T wave
4	Normal

Fig. 14-1   Representative ECG changes caused by increasing degrees of hyperkalemia. Serum potassium levels are approximate and in the individual patient may not correlate directly with the ECG abnormalities shown. (From Kjellstrand CM, Davin TJ, Matas AJ, Buselmeier TJ. Postoperative acute renal failure: Diagnosis, etiologic and symptomatic treatment and prognosis. In Najarian JS, Delaney JP, eds. Clinical Surgical Care. New York: Grune & Stratton, 1977, p 309.)

ized calcium levels, preferably after each dose. Frequently the salutory effects of IV calcium are almost immediately registered on the ECG.

Some authorities have recommended *hypertonic saline solution* in this setting, but the myocardial stabilizing effects of IV sodium can be as readily obtained from an infusion of $NaHCO_3$, which has the additional benefits noted below.

2. *Promote movement of potassium into cells.* Increase the pH of the acidotic patient. The most rapid treatment for hyperkalemia in the acidotic patient is *hyperventilation;* however, the decrease in serum potassium level seen with acute increases in pH resulting from decreases in Pco_2 may be less than that seen with comparable improvements in pH obtained with IV $NaHCO_3$.

Sodium bicarbonate can be effective in the patient who can tolerate the volume load and in whom hyperventilation has been used to a maximum degree. $NaHCO_3$ will have little effect on the hyperkalemic patient who is not also acidotic, and its use in this setting may lead to an "overshoot" metabolic alkalosis, especially in oliguric patients unable to excrete the administered $NaHCO_3$. Patients with coexisting respiratory failure usually should not be given $NaHCO_3$ because the increase in CO_2 production that results from the addition of bicarbonate to the patient with metabolic acidosis may actually worsen acidosis when the additional CO_2 cannot be excreted by the lungs.

Insulin plus *hypertonic dextrose* is the most potent therapy for temporary treatment of hyperkalemia. The recommended dose of regular insulin is 1 unit/ 4 g of dextrose in older infants and children, and 1 unit/8 to 12 g of dextrose in neonates (who are at greater risk for hypoglycemia). It is convenient to prepare 100 ml aliquots of D_{25} to which have been added 6 units of regular insulin. This mixture can be given in 1 to 2 ml/kg doses by slow IV push. *Remember* that the effects of IV insulin frequently extend several hours after the hypertonic dextrose has been consumed, resulting in delayed hypoglycemia. Frequent fingerstick tests to monitor blood glucose level are required during and for several hours after infusions of insulin and dextrose.

3. *Remove potassium from the patient. Sodium polystyrene sulfonate resin* (Kayexalate) is most often given as a retention enema at a dose of 1 g/kg in a 20% sorbitol suspension. When this dose is retained for at least 1 hour the serum potassium concentration usually decreases by about 1 mEq/L. Kayexalate enemas are only useful in the stable patient who has an intact gastrointestinal tract and who has shown no signs of dysrhythmia or other evidence of cardiac toxicity. Hypernatremia and hypertension are potential complications of Kayexalate since sodium is delivered to the patient in equimolar amounts with the potassium that is removed. Kayexalate may be given via nasogastric tube.

Exchange transfusion has been used as an emergency treatment for life-threatening hyperkalemia in neonates, in whom dialysis can be difficult to initiate promptly in some centers. To avoid adding to the patient's potassium burden, only washed packed red blood cells resuspended in fresh frozen plasma must be used. The potassium concentration of the blood preparation to be used in the exchange transfusion should be <5.0 mEq/L, which should be confirmed before the procedure is started. A double blood volume exchange has been recommended.

Dialysis is the most effective treatment for hyperkalemia. To be most effective, peritoneal dialysis must be instituted early because potassium clearance rates by the peritoneal membrane are limited by the limitations on dialysate flow rates inherent in the peritoneal dialysis system (see Chapter 145). Hemodialysis removes potassium from the patient much more efficiently than all other available treatment modalities. Hemodialysis is the treatment of choice in patients with life-threatening levels of hyperkalemia (see Chapter 146).

CAVH is a relatively new form of renal replacement therapy that can be an effective treatment for hyperkalemia, but only if large volumes of filtrate are removed during the procedure (see Chapter 148). CAVH is not the treatment of choice for life-threatening hyperkalemia. In situations where CAVH is planned, it is preferable to begin with 1 or 2 hours of hemodialysis to rapidly restore serum potassium concentration to normal, then follow with CAVH to maintain the potassium level in the normal range. Modifications of the standard CAVH procedure (e.g., high-flow predilution CAVH and CAVHD [continuous arteriovenous hemodiafiltration]) are more effective at removal of potassium than standard CAVH. These techniques are also discussed in Chapter 148.

Choice of therapy for hyperkalemia. The treatment of hyperkalemia in the patient with ARF must be individualized to each clinical situation. Unstable patients with high serum potassium levels (>7 mEq/

L) and ECG evidence of myocardial toxicity represent medical emergencies of the most severe type, demanding immediate therapy. All such patients must receive calcium chloride and insulin plus dextrose, and most will also benefit from sodium bicarbonate. However, these therapies should be used primarily to buy time in which to prepare for emergency dialysis. Many stable patients who have only mildly elevated serum potassium concentrations (6.0 to 6.5 mEq/L) and who do not have ECG evidence of cardiac toxicity can be effectively treated with Kayexalate. However, if renal function does not return promptly in these patients, dialysis is virtually inevitable. Efforts should be made to begin dialysis *before* hyperkalemia reaches life-threatening levels and *before* there is ECG evidence of cardiac toxicity. This can only be accomplished if all of the potential contributing factors in each case are considered in the decision to institute dialysis. For example, in the child with HUS (see Chapter 52) dialysis needs to be considered early in the course because hemolysis may occur rapidly, resulting in sudden increases in potassium levels. Improvements in the safety and effectiveness of dialysis and other renal replacement therapies in most pediatric renal centers have allowed earlier institution of treatment for hyperkalemia in patients with ARF in an effort to anticipate and therefore avoid this potentially lethal complication. Such an aggressive approach to hyperkalemia in patients with ARF is highly recommended.

Metabolic Acidosis

The kidney provides primary mechanisms for excretion of acid and generation of bicarbonate required to maintain normal acid-base balance. Patients with ARF rapidly develop severe metabolic acidosis as a consequence of impaired renal acid excretion. Severe acidemia results in depression of myocardial contractility and decrease in peripheral vascular resistance. Hypotension and ventricular fibrillation are potential consequences of severe acidemia. Splanchnic venoconstriction has also been reported with metabolic acidosis, which may lead to rapid development of pulmonary edema when compounded by depressed myocardial contractility and too-rapid administration of IV fluids.

The most effective emergency treatment for severe metabolic acidosis in the intubated patient is *hyperventilation*. Sodium bicarbonate may also be given,

but it must be given slowly (see below) because many oligoanuric patients are intolerant of the acute expansion of intravascular volume that occurs as a consequence of rapid IV bicarbonate therapy. In patients with mixed respiratory (i.e., CO_2 retention) and metabolic acidosis, the routine use of bicarbonate is not recommended; these patients need to be treated with dialysis or CAVH.

It is possible to calculate an initial treatment dose of sodium bicarbonate for severely acidemic patients (i.e., patients with bicarbonate or total CO_2 [tCO_2] levels <15 mEq/L) as follows:

1. The target serum tCO_2 level for the initial dose of IV sodium bicarbonate is 15 mEq/L.
2. Calculate the initial "deficit" by subtracting the patient's measured tCO_2 from 15 mEq/L.
3. Estimate the acute volume of distribution (V_d) of IV sodium bicarbonate as follows:

$$V_d \text{ (bicarbonate, acute)} = (\text{Wt [kg]}) \times 0.3$$

4. Total bicarbonate dose needed to raise the patient's tCO_2 to 15 mEq/L is calculated as:

$$\text{Total bicarbonate dose} = (15 - [\text{patient's } tCO_2]) \times (\text{Wt [kg]}) \times 0.3$$

Give one half of the calculated correction dose during the first hour of therapy and the remainder over the ensuing 3 hours. Repeat measurements of blood pH or serum tCO_2 (hourly during acute sodium bicarbonate therapy) to allow adjustments to be made to reflect changing conditions. EXAMPLE: 10 kg infant with tCO_2 = 9 mEq/L:

$$(15 - 9) \times 10 \times 0.3 = 18$$

Administer 9 mEq $NaHCO_3$ during the first hour, then 3 mEq/hour for 3 more hours; monitor therapy with hourly blood pH determinations.

Patients with ARF who are more stable usually need supplemental bicarbonate therapy during conservative management. A dose of 1 to 3 mEq $NaHCO_3$/kg/day is usually sufficient to maintain normal acid-base status in such patients.

Hyperphosphatemia

Hyperphosphatemia can be difficult to treat in the oliguric patient because oral phosphate binders such as aluminum hydroxide or calcium carbonate are able to remove only small amounts of phosphate directly from the patient. Oral phosphate binders are primarily effective at binding dietary phosphate before it can be absorbed by the patient. Thus severe hyperphosphatemia can only be treated with dialysis or CAVH. Fortunately most pediatric patients tolerate very high phosphate levels (e.g., 10 to 12 mEq/L), although seizures from hypocalcemia have been reported with severe hyperphosphatemia.

Hypocalcemia

Hypocalcemia occurs in concert with and largely as a result of hyperphosphatemia. Hypocalcemia can be difficult to treat in the presence of severe hyperphosphatemia. It is probably prudent to attempt to maintain a low-normal serum ionized calcium level in these patients by administering small IV doses of one of the parenteral calcium preparations. Metastatic calcification may be occurring whenever the product of the serum calcium and phosphorus concentrations exceeds 70.

Hypocalcemia may persist despite normalization of serum phosphorous concentration. Patients with ARF are resistant to the action of parathyroid hormone, which is often elevated. In patients with ARF associated with crush injuries, lightning or other high-voltage electrical injuries, or any cause of severe muscle damage, profound hypocalcemia may develop early in the course of the disease as calcium is deposited in necrotic muscle tissue. *Hypercalcemia* may be a serious late complication in such patients as calcium is mobilized from muscle tissue; aggressive dialysis using calcium-free dialysate is usually necessary to manage hypercalcemia in this setting.

Hypertension

Medical therapy of hypertension is often necessary in the oliguric ARF patient. Recommendations for antihypertensive therapy may be found in Chapter 53. Antihypertensive drug dosage regimens need to be adjusted to reflect decreased GFR. Some authorities caution against the use of captopril and other angiotensin-converting enzyme inhibitors in patients with ARF, but this has not been studied in children.

Hypermagnesemia

Severe/symptomatic hypermagnesemia probably occurs only when patients with ARF are treated with magnesium-containing antacids or total parenteral nutrition. Dialysis or CAVH must be used to treat symptomatic hypermagnesemia.

Hyperuricemia

Hyperuricemia frequently accompanies ARF, but symptomatic gout is a rare complication. The use of a xanthine oxidase inhibitor such as allopurinol is usually not indicated.

Nutrition therapy

Nutrition therapy is an easily overlooked but essential element of the successful management of ARF. Efforts must be made to provide adequate nonprotein calories; 45 to 55 kcal/kg/day is a reasonable goal. Protein must be restricted to prevent rapid increases in BUN, phosphorus, and acidosis. Patients with a creatinine clearance of <10 ml/min/1.73 m^2 should receive only 0.5 g protein/kg/day; up to 1 g/kg/day may be given to patients with better clearances. Minimal dietary potassium should be given, usually <600 mg/day. Dietary sodium is usually limited to <1 g/day, especially in hypertensive patients.

Patients receiving TPN may have larger protein intakes if a preparation of all essential amino acids is used. Give a total amino acid preparation until the BUN is >50 mg/dl, then switch to a preparation of all essential amino acids.

Nutritional therapy is much easier in nonoliguric patients and patients receiving dialysis or CAVH. The opportunity to provide complete nutrition in the oliguric patient is one of the most compelling arguments in favor of early institution of renal replacement therapy. However, the postulated beneficial effect of early full nutritional support on ARF mortality rates has not been demonstrated conclusively.

Indications for renal replacement therapy

The time to initiate renal replacement therapy, dialysis or CAVH, like the choice of therapeutic modality, depends on the individual circumstances involved. Each of the renal replacement therapies currently available to the pediatric nephrologist is discussed in a subsequent chapter. The most commonly encountered indications for renal replacement therapy in patients with ARF are as follows:

1. Volume overload, often complicated by hypertension and/or congestive heart failure
2. Hyperkalemia (e.g., $[K+] >7.0$ mEq/L)
3. Acidosis unresponsive to conservative measures
4. Uremic encephalopathy
5. Bleeding, if caused by uremia

6. Hypocalcemia and hyperphosphatemia severe enough to cause hypocalcemic seizures (uncommon)
7. Severe hyponatremia or hypernatremia
8. Severe azotemia (BUN >150 mg/dl)
9. Removal of fluid so that optimal nutrition, transfusions, and other therapies may be given to the oligoanuric patient

A more complete discussion of the indications for each therapeutic modality in the setting of ARF is included in Chapters 145, 146, and 148.

ADDITIONAL READING

Bonventre JV, Leaf A, Malis CD. The nature of the cellular insult in ischemic acute renal failure. In Brenner BM, Lazarus JM, eds. Acute Renal Failure, 2nd ed. New York: Churchill Livingstone, 1988, pp 3-44.

Brown RS. Renal dysfunction in the surgical patient: Maintenance of the high output state with furosemide. Crit Care Med 7:63-68, 1979.

Brown RS, Babcock R, Talbert J, et al. Renal function in critically ill postoperative patients: Sequential assessment of creatinine, osmolar and free water clearance. Crit Care Med 8:68-72, 1980.

Ellis EN, Arnold WC. Use of urinary diagnostic indices in renal failure in the newborn. Am J Dis Child 136:615-617, 1982.

Feld LG, Springate JE, Fildes RD. Acute renal failure. I. Pathophysiology and diagnosis. J Pediatr 109:401-408, 1986.

Fildes RD, Springate JE, Feld LG. Acute renal failure. II. Management. J Pediatr 109:567-571, 1986.

• Gaudio KM, Siegal NJ. Pathogenesis and treatment of acute renal failure. Pediatr Clin North Am 34:771-787, 1987.

Levinsky NG. Pathophysiology of acute renal failure. N Engl J Med 296:1453-1458, 1977.

Mathew OP, Jones AS, Jones E, et al. Neonatal renal failure: Usefulness of diagnostic indices. Pediatrics 65:57-60, 1980.

Miller TR, Anderson RJ, Linas SL, et al. Urinary diagnostic indices in acute renal failure: A prospective study. Ann Intern Med 89:47-50, 1978.

Rigden SPA, Barratt TM, Dillon MJ, et al. Acute renal failure complicating cardiopulmonary bypass surgery. Arch Dis Child 57:425-430, 1982.

• Stapleton FB, Jones DP, Green RS. Acute renal failure in neonates: Incidence, etiology and outcome. Pediatr Nephrol 1:314-320, 1987.

• Trompeter RS. A review of drug prescribing in children with end-stage renal failure. Pediatr Nephrol 1:183-194, 1987.

15 Mineral and Glucose Requirements and Abnormalities

Ronald M. Perkin · Daniel L. Levin

BACKGROUND AND PHYSIOLOGY

Water, the largest single component of the body, is expressed as a proportion of total body weight (80% in intrauterine life and early infancy and decreasing gradually during the first 6 to 12 months to approximately 60% to 65%). It remains fairly constant at about 65% after the age of 12 months.

Body water is divided into intracellular fluid (ICF) and extracellular fluid (ECF), although this is a simplification of its complex distribution since each space is divisible into several subspaces differing in their water content. In this chapter the term "intracellular water," or ICF, is used to mean the total amount of water within all the cells of the body; "extracellular water," or ECF, includes the water in the interstitial spaces and in plasma. There is a gradual increase in the ICF and a decrease in the ECF with growth.

Adequate levels of water and electrolytes, which are normally lost through the kidneys, skin, respi-

Table 15-1 Fluid, Mineral, and Glucose Requirements: Maintenance*

Element	Body Weight	Amount	Example
Water	For each kg ≤10 kg	100 ml/kg/24 hr	4 kg infant: 400 ml/24 hr
	For each kg, 11-20 kg	Add 50 ml/kg/24 hr	14 kg infant: 1200 ml/24 hr
	For each kg >20 kg	Add 20 ml/kg/24 hr	24 kg child: 1580 ml/24 hr
Electrolytes			
Sodium (Na)		3-4 mEq/kg/24 hr	4 kg infant: 16 mEq/24 hr
Potassium (K)		2-3 mEq/kg/24 hr	4 kg infant: 12 mEq/24 hr
Chloride (Cl)		3-4 mEq/kg/24 hr	4 kg infant: 16 mEq/24 hr
Calcium (Ca)		50-200 mg/kg/24 hr	4 kg infant: 200-800 mg/24 hr
Magnesium (Mg)		0.35-0.45 mEq/kg/24 hr	4 kg infant: 1.4-1.8 mEq/24 hr
Phosphate (PO_4)†		3-10 mg/kg/24 hr (0.1-0.2 mmol/kg/24 hr)	4 kg infant: 12-40 mg/24 hr
Glucose		200-400 mg/kg/hr (4-6 mg/kg/min glucose utilization)	4 kg infant: 400-1600 mg/hr

NOTE: Add 10% for infants receiving bilirubin phototherapy; add 20% for infants placed in radiant warmers; add or subtract 12% for each degree centigrade above or below, respectively, rectal temperature of 37.8° C. Most infants do not need maintenance Na, K, and Cl during the first 24 hr of life. However, they frequently do need Ca during the first 24 hr of life.

*Modified by permission from Levin DL, Morriss FC, Moore GC. A Practical Guide to Pediatric Intensive Care, 2nd ed. St. Louis: CV Mosby, 1984, p 94.

† See text.

ratory tract, and GI tract, must be maintained. Water exchange is part of cellular metabolism and can be related to metabolic rate more than to simple indicators of body size. If activity is minimal and there are no abnormal thermal and other losses, an acceptable estimate of maintenance water require-

ments can be made according to the method outlined in Table 15-1. These calculations assume relatively normal renal function (i.e., of every 100 ml of resting water requirement, approximately 55 ml will be excreted by the kidneys). Fluid requirements in newborn infants may be greater, depending on the in-

Table 15-2 Compositions of Common Parenteral Fluid Solutions*

Solution	Solute	Concentration (g/100 ml)	pH	Ionic Concentration (mEq/L)					Calculated Osmolality (mOsm/L)
				[Na⁺]	[K⁺]	[Ca⁺⁺]	[Cl⁻]	[Lactate]	
Dextrose in water									
5.0%	Glucose	5	4.7	—	—	—	—	—	250
10.0%	Glucose	10	4.6	—	—	—	—	—	505
Saline									
0.45% (hypotonic)	NaCl	0.45	5.3	77	—	—	77	—	155
0.90% (isotonic)	NaCl	0.9	5.3	154	—	—	154	—	310
Dextrose in saline									
2.5% in 0.45%	Glucose	2.5							
	NaCl	0.45	4.9	77	—	—	77	—	280
5.0% in 0.20%	Glucose	5.0							
	NaCl	0.20	4.6	34	—	—	34	—	320
5.0% in 0.45%	Glucose	5.0							
	NaCl	0.45	4.6	77	—	—	77	—	405
5.0% in 0.90%	Glucose	5.0							
	NaCl	0.90	4.6	154	—	—	154	—	560
Polyionic	Lactate	0.31							
Lactated Ringer's (RL)	NaCl	0.60	6.3	130	4	3	109	28	275
	KCl	0.03							
	CaCl₂	0.02							
Dextrose in polyionic									
2.5% in ½ RL	Glucose	2.5							
	Lactate	0.155							
	NaCl	0.30	5.1	65	2	1.5	54	14	265
	KCl	0.015							
	CaCl₂	0.01							
4.0% in modified RL	Glucose	4.0							
	Lactate	0.062							
	NaCl	0.12	5.0	26	0.8	0.5	22	5.5	280
	KCl	0.006							
	CaCl₂	0.004							
5.0% in RL	Glucose	5.0							
	Lactate	0.31							
	NaCl	0.60	4.7	130	4	3	109	28	515
	KCl	0.03							
	CaCl₂	0.02							
5% albumin	Albumin	5.0	6.9	154	1		154	—	310
(Plasmanate)	NaCl	0.9							

*From Perkin RM, Levin DL. Common fluid and electrolyte problems in the pediatric intensive care unit. Pediatr Clin North Am 27:567-586, 1980.

fant's maturity, the method of providing warmth, and the ambient humidity.

The type of replacement fluid to be used varies. Generally, if any mineral is not depleted or overloaded and renal function is adequate, a maintenance solution can provide the necessary electrolytes and glucose as shown in Table 15-1.

The commonly used maintenance requirements

Table 15-3 Concentrated Solutions for Addition to Infusion Fluids*

Solution	mg/ml	mEq/ml	mOsm/ml
50% glucose	500	—	2.53
3% sodium chloride	30	0.513	1.0
5% sodium chloride	50	0.855	1.7
15% sodium chloride	150	2.5	5.0
8.4% sodium bicarbonate	84	1.0	2.0
20% potassium chloride	149	2.0	4.0
10% calcium gluconate	100	0.46	0.7
10% calcium chloride	100	1.36	2.0
10% magnesium sulfate	100	0.8	0.4
50% magnesium sulfate	500	4.0	2.0

EXAMPLES:

Desired solution	*Formula*
3.5% dextrose in 0.45% sodium chloride solution	7 ml 50% dextrose 43 ml sterile water 50 ml 0.9% sodium chloride solution
10% dextrose in 0.225% sodium chloride solution	70 ml 10% dextrose 6 ml 50% dextrose 25 ml 0.9% sodium chloride solution
15% dextrose	87.5 ml 10% dextrose 12.5 ml 50% dextrose

*From Perkin RM, Levin DL. Common fluid and electrolyte problems in the pediatric intensive care unit. Pediatr Clin North Am 27:567-586, 1980.

assume that water and minerals are not being excreted in large amounts via the kidney or extrarenal routes such as the GI tract. Such losses do occur commonly during many diseases, and these patients need careful attention as to the content and volume of the losses so that adequate replacement can be made. In critically ill patients, especially in those with multiorgan system failure, each component of the IV solution, including water and glucose, must be calculated independently. Standardized IV solutions that provide the necessary concentrations of minerals and glucose are available (Table 15-2). Individual mixtures of the indicated amounts of concentrated solutions may be necessary in patients who have complex imbalances (Table 15-3). Specific abnormalities of fluid, mineral, and glucose balance are discussed below.

Disorders of Osmolality

Osmotic forces affect the distribution of water between the intracellular and extracellular compartments. Although almost impermeable to most solutes, cell membranes are freely permeable to water. Thus ICF and ECF osmolality equalizes due to water shifts even though they have different solute compositions. Each compartment has one major solute restricted primarily to that compartment, which acts to hold water within the compartment. For example, sodium salts (extracellular osmoles), potassium salts (intracellular osmoles), and the plasma proteins (intravascular osmoles) help to maintain the volumes of the extracellular, intracellular, and intravascular spaces, respectively.

Osmolality of a solution results from the number of solute particles per kilogram in that space of water. Sodium salts, glucose, and urea are the primary extracellular osmoles; therefore the plasma osmolality and intracellular fluid osmolality can be approximated by the following formula:

$$\text{Plasma osmolality} = 2 \times [\text{Na}] + \frac{[\text{Glucose}]}{18} + \frac{[\text{BUN}]}{2.8}$$

where [Na] = serum sodium concentration, [Glucose] = serum glucose concentration, and [BUN] = blood urea nitrogen.

Hypo-osmolality (hyponatremia)

Since the serum sodium concentration is the main determinant of the plasma osmolality, hypo-osmolality usually reflects hyponatremia. The etiology, diagnosis, and therapy of hypo-osmolality are shown in Fig. 15-1. Hyponatremia can be caused by water retention or sodium loss or both; therefore ECF volume may be low, normal, or high. When renal function is normal, analysis of urine sodium concentration may be helpful in determining the etiology of the hyponatremia. As osmolality decreases, a gradient for osmolality develops across the blood-brain barrier, and water moves into the brain. This is responsible for the symptoms of hypo-osmolality and hyponatremia, although the degree of symptoms depends on the etiology, magnitude, and acuteness of the condition. As the serum sodium decreases to <125 mEq/L, nausea, vomiting, muscular twitching, lethargy, and obtundation occur; when the serum sodium concentration is <115 mEq/L, the more severe symptoms of seizures and coma develop.

True hyponatremia must be differentiated from pseudo- or factitious hyponatremia. Factitious hyponatremia occurs when hyponatremia is generated by a redistribution of water between ECF and ICF as a consequence of the addition of nonpermeate solutes such as glucose or mannitol to the ECF. Diabetes mellitus is the leading cause of factitious hyponatremia in children. The true serum sodium in these patients can be estimated by adding 1.6 mEq/L of sodium to the measured serum sodium for each increase above normal of 100 mg/dl of blood sugar.

Pseudohyponatremia is a falsely low serum sodium concentration occurring because of the replacement of serum water by lipid, protein, or both. Sodium salts are dissolved in the percentage of serum that is water (usually 90% to 93%); however, the determination of serum sodium concentration is per-

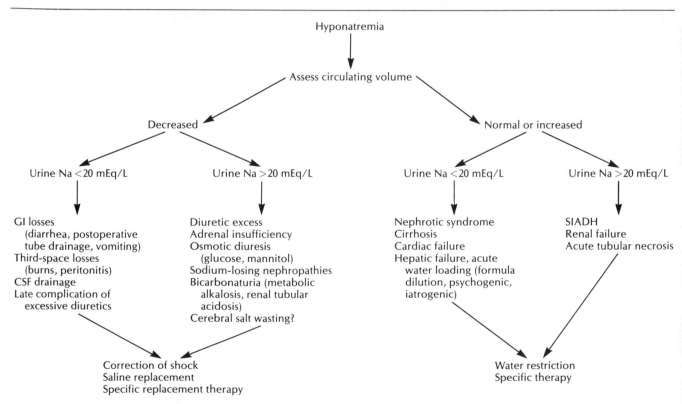

Fig. 15-1 Hyponatremia. Differential diagnosis and approach to therapy. (From Perkin RM, Levin DL. Common fluid and electrolyte problems in the pediatric intensive care unit. Pediatr Clin North Am 27:567-586, 1980.)

formed on a diluted aliquot of serum. Therefore a sodium concentration of 135 mEq/L of serum in a serum that has a water content of 90% would represent a concentration of 150 mEq/L of serum water (135/0.9). In hyperlipidemia or hyperproteinemia the lipids or proteins may occupy a significant volume of the serum, so that the percentage of serum that is water is reduced. If the water content is reduced to 75% of hyperproteinemic serum, then a sodium concentration of 150 mEq/L of serum water would correspond to a sodium concentration per liter of hyperproteinemic serum of 112.5 mEq (150 × 0.75). Hyponatremia in these instances would not reflect an electrolyte abnormality or diminished effective osmolality of the water of the serum.

Hyponatremia with hypovolemia. Patients with hyponatremia and hypovolemia may lose fluid through renal or extrarenal routes. Extrarenal losses most commonly occur via the GI tract (i.e., diarrhea or vomiting) but may be attributed to other disorders, including burns, pancreatitis, or peritonitis. Sodium and water conservation are the normal kidney responses to these hypovolemic states; thus a hypertonic urine with a sodium concentration <10 mEq/L would be expected. Adrenal insufficiency may be present in a patient with hyponatremia and hypovolemia whose urine sodium concentration is >20 mEq/L, particularly if the serum potassium concentration is increased. The salt-losing form of congenital adrenal hyperplasia is a common cause of hyponatremia with hypovolemia in the infant and young child (see Chapter 55). Acute infection with hemorrhage into the adrenal glands (see Chapter 12), inadequate replacement of adrenocorticosteroids in patients on adrenocorticosteroids, and inappropriate tapering of steroid doses are other possible etiologies.

Hyponatremia with normal volume or hypervolemia. Hypervolemic hyponatremia occurs most commonly in edema-forming conditions when the net retention of water exceeds that of sodium. Two clinical settings may be associated with hypervolemic hyponatremia: (1) edema-generating disorders such as cirrhosis, heart failure, and nephrosis in which the urinary concentration of sodium is often <10 mEq/L and (2) advanced acute or chronic renal failure in which the urinary sodium may be variable but usually exceeds 20 mEq/L.

The syndrome of inappropriate secretion of antidiuretic hormone (SIADH) must be considered in patients with hyponatremia who have neither contraction of ECF volume nor expansion to the point of clinical edema. A concentrated urine despite hyponatremia is characteristic of patients with SIADH; their urinary sodium concentration parallels their sodium intake and is usually >20 mEq/L. The most common error in recognizing SIADH is failure to realize that the urine osmolality need only be inappropriately elevated and the urine is not maximally concentrated (see also Chapter 57).

Hyperosmolality

Hypertonic states are characterized by elevated concentrations of ECF solutes and net ICF volume depletion. When hypertonicity develops rapidly, osmolality equalizes, primarily because of water movement out of cells. Cell volume may be protected by the brain cells because of their ability to generate new solute intracellularly (i.e., idiogenic osmoles). The identity of these idiogenic osmoles and the speed with which they develop are functions of the cause and time course of hypertonicity. When hypertonicity develops too rapidly, idiogenic osmoles may not form quickly enough to prevent permanent brain damage or death from intracellular volume depletion. The speed at which idiogenic osmoles can be removed or inactivated is unknown; therefore, as hypertonicity is corrected, an overly rapid replacement by infusion of hypotonic solutions may cause cerebral edema and scizures, which may result in long-term neurologic sequelae or death.

Hypertonicity occurs with many different etiologies (Fig. 15-2). Although hypernatremia is a common and most frequently discussed cause of hyperosmolality, hyperosmolality can occur independently of hypernatremia and be just as harmful to the CNS. Solutes that increase serum osmolality include urea, glucose, glycerol, galactose, mannitol, and various alcohols including ethanol and methanol. Increases in blood urea or alcohols that distribute equally throughout most of the body water (permeate solutes) lead to hyperosmolality without internal rearrangement of water, whereas the addition of nonpermeate solutes such as sugars to the ECF does influence the distribution of water between ECF and ICF with depletion of intracellular water.

Hypovolemic hypernatremia

Hypotonic fluid loss. Hypovolemic hypernatremia can be generated by either loss of water alone or by

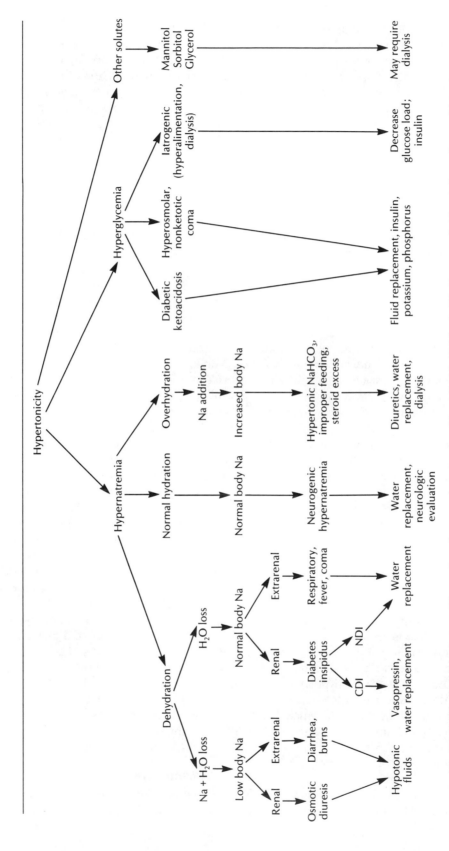

Fig. 15-2 The hypertonic state. Diagnosis and approach to therapy. (From Perkin RM, Levin DL. Common fluid and electrolyte problems in the pediatric intensive care unit. Pediatr Clin North Am 27:567-586, 1980.)

the loss of hypotonic fluid. The most common mechanism in children is the loss of hypotonic fluids, usually from gastroenteritis. Such losses are often aggravated by increases in insensible water loss through the lung or skin and by the simultaneous ingestion of relatively hypertonic fluids.

Hypernatremia in infancy is a true medical emergency since the developing brain is highly susceptible to either permanent damage or death. Clinical detection of hypernatremic dehydration can be difficult, however, because plasma volume is maintained by the movement of water from cells; 10% to 15% of the patient's body weight can be lost before evidence of dehydration is detectable by clinical examination. Most patients, however, have symptoms referable to the CNS. If they are arousable, patients tend to be irritable; however, depression of the sensorium is characteristic and varies from lethargy to coma; some patients have seizures. The symptoms can be related to the movement of water out of the brain cells along the osmotic gradient created by the elevation in plasma osmolality. The severity of neurologic symptoms is related to both the degree and the rate of rise in plasma osmolality.

Primary water loss. A surprisingly large water loss can occur through the lungs during marked hyperventilation and through the skin when environmental temperature is high and humidity low. Abnormal water balance occurs through the kidneys if there is a defect in the production or release of antidiuretic hormone (central diabetes insipidus) (see Chapter 58) or if there is a defect in the renal response to antidiuretic hormone (ADH), called nephrogenic diabetes insipidus (NDI).

NDI is either a congenital or acquired disorder in which hypothalamic function and ADH release are normal, but the kidney's ability to concentrate urine is reduced because of diminished or absent renal responsiveness to ADH. Renal disease, electrolyte disturbances (e.g., hypercalcemia, hypokalemia), sickle cell disease, and the use of some drugs are examples of acquired NDI. NDI caused by hypernatremia may be corrected with cautious water replacement; long-term therapy is usually not necessary, particularly in patients with a reversible defect or without polyuria.

Osmotic diuresis can cause hypertonicity, whether the solute is permeable (e.g., urea) or impermeable (e.g., glucose, mannitol) since urine osmolality approaches isotonicity during brisk osmotic diuresis.

Since the solute causing the diuresis constitutes a considerable fraction of urine solute, the remaining electrolyte concentration of the urine must be hypotonic relative to body fluids. Hypotonic urine losses may lead to hypertonicity in patients infused with urea or mannitol for treatment of cerebral edema and in patients with hyperglycemia and glycosuria.

Hypernatremia with normal hydration. The absence of ECF volume depletion, a normal capacity to release endogenous ADH, and a normal renal response to ADH define neurogenic hypernatremia. Two types of neurogenic hypernatremia are known; both are related to hypothalamic disorders that cause thirst deficit (hypodipsia) and/or osmoreceptor insensitivity. These two types can be distinguished by their response to forced water intake. In one type forced water intake returns the plasma osmolality to normal; in the other water loading is ineffective (i.e., essential hypernatremia).

Hypernatremia with overhydration. Hypernatremia with overhydration is usually related to iatrogenic or accidental causes. Severe hypernatremia can occur as a result of the acute ingestion or infusion of hypertonic sodium solutions, as seen in infants given feedings with high sodium concentrations or in infants given sodium bicarbonate intravenously. Rapid and massive increases in sodium draw water into the vascular space, resulting in an increase of sodium and water but a greater increase in sodium than water, and may cause cerebral bleeding, pulmonary edema, and systemic arterial hypertension.

Hyperglycemia. Hyperglycemia is a commonly observed clinical condition. Rapid development of hyperglycemia is unusual, except when it occurs in a hospitalized patient (e.g., during peritoneal dialysis [see Chapter 145] or during total parenteral nutrition [TPN] [see Chapter 149]). Most episodes of hyperglycemia take at least a few days to develop and result in glycosuria so that these patients, in addition, will have sodium and water loss due to an osmotic diuresis. Diabetic ketoacidosis (DKA) (see Chapter 54) and hyperglycemic, nonketotic coma are the two symptomatic, hyperglycemic syndromes. Although the latter has been well documented in adults, it appears to be rare in children.

Disorders of Potassium Balance

Potassium's location is almost entirely intracellular, unlike sodium, which is located almost entirely in the ECF; potassium functions in the regulation of a variety of cell functions. The absolute quantity of potassium present and the ratio of the intracellular potassium concentration to the extracellular potassium concentration are important because they affect the resting membrane potential of nerve and muscle cells (see Chapter 14). Hypokalemia elevates the resting potential and hyperpolarizes the cell membrane, making it more resistant to depolarization. With hyperkalemia the membrane potential is lowered, making the cell more excitable and reducing its ability to repolarize. Despite potassium's effects on the resting potential, the effect of hypokalemia or hyperkalemia can still be variable; two factors are responsible for this variability: the speed with which the change occurred and ions other than potassium, including calcium, magnesium, sodium, and hydrogen, that also affect membrane excitability.

Hypokalemia

Causes of hypokalemia include decreased intake, increased movement into the intracellular compartment (e.g., correction of acidosis, alkalosis, administration of insulin), increased urine losses (e.g., hyperaldosteronism, loop diuretics, renal tubular acidosis), and increased GI losses (e.g., vomiting, diarrhea, continuous GI suction). Symptoms of hypokalemia are related to its effects on skeletal and smooth muscle, renal function, and cardiac conduction. Muscle weakness, diminished or absent bowel sounds, and abdominal distention (ileus) are typical findings on physical examination. Polyuria and polydipsia can result from impairment of the kidney's ability to concentrate urine. Typical changes in the ECG produced by hypokalemia include ST segment depression, decreased T wave amplitude, increased height of the U wave, and prolongation of the QU interval; these findings are primarily caused by delayed ventricular repolarization. As potassium depletion becomes more severe, P wave amplitude increases, the PR interval becomes prolonged, and the QRS complex widens. A variety of dysrhythmias may also be observed, which are intensified in both frequency and severity in patients taking digitalis.

Hyperkalemia

Causes of hyperkalemia are increased intake, increased movement into the extracellular space (acidosis, tissue catabolism, cell destruction), and impaired renal excretion (renal failure, adrenal insuf-

ficiency). Effects of hyperkalemia are limited to muscle weakness and abnormal cardiac conduction, the latter being the more dangerous feature. Prominent manifestations are found on the ECG (see Fig. 14-1). Peaked, narrow T waves and a shortened QT interval, reflecting more rapid repolarization (with serum potassium levels of 6.5 mEq/L) are the earliest changes. With increasing potassium concentration the QRS complex widens and merges with the T wave to produce a sine-wave pattern, followed by ventricular fibrillation or standstill (at potassium concentrations ≥9 mEq/L). Hypocalcemia, hyponatremia, acidosis, and a rapid elevation in the serum potassium concentration enhance the cardiac toxicity of hyperkalemia.

Disorders of Calcium Balance

Calcium is the skeleton's most prevalent element and a significant cofactor for neural transmission, enzyme activity, blood coagulation, and other cellular functions. Abnormalities of calcium metabolism are seen more frequently in neonates than in older children and adolescents.

Hypocalcemia

Hypocalcemia is an uncommon endocrine emergency with multiple etiologies. Defined as a total serum calcium concentration <8 mg/dl or an ionized serum calcium level of <3.5 mg/dl, hypocalcemia in the PICU is most frequently seen in newborn infants, particularly those who are products of complicated pregnancies (e.g., infants of diabetic mothers), and newborns with hyperbilirubinemia, respiratory distress, asphyxia, or cerebral injuries. Hypoparathyroidism, pancreatitis, sepsis, hypomagnesemia, renal tubular acidosis, renal failure, and parathyroid surgery, thyroidectomy, or any other surgical procedure in the neck are other etiologies seen in PICU patients. A number of drugs may either bind calcium or impair parathyroid function, resulting in hypocalcemia. Infants with DiGeorge's syndrome will have hypocalcemia that quickly changes to hypercalcemia with calcium administration and just as quickly returns to hypocalcemia. Hypocalcemia may occur also with massive transfusions due to ultimate binding of calcium. Symptoms of hypocalcemia include irritability, tremor, laryngospasm, twitching, and seizures. Infants may be lethargic, feed poorly, vomit, and have symptoms easily confused with sepsis. Hypotension, congestive heart failure, renal failure, and a prolonged QT interval may all result from hypocalcemia.

Serum protein (or albumin) and arterial pH influence ionized calcium levels. Alkalosis decreases ionized calcium, whereas the total serum calcium remains unchanged. Occasionally patients with chronic hypocalcemia do not develop symptoms unless they become alkalotic through vomiting, hyperventilation, or alkali ingestion. Conversely, when serum proteins are low, total serum calcium will decrease but ionized calcium levels are frequently normal.

Hypercalcemia

Hypercalcemia (>14 mg/dl) is less frequently observed in the PICU. Cancer patients and patients who have undergone prolonged immobilization are most likely to be hypercalcemic.

A high ionized calcium level suppresses nerve conduction and may be manifested by a shortened refractory period, slowed conduction, and a greater likelihood of ventricular ectopy developing. With reduced neural excitability and transmission in brain tissue, an alteration in sensorium develops, varying from drowsiness when the serum calcium level approaches 14 mg/dl to stupor and coma if it increases further. In the GI tract, similar changes can cause constipation, anorexia, nausea and vomiting, and abdominal pain.

Whatever its etiology, hypercalcemia will worsen when patients are immobilized or dehydrated. Since even mild hypercalcemia impairs renal tubular function and promotes water loss, serum calcium increases further in patients who cannot maintain normal hydration.

Other Common Disorders

Hypomagnesemia

Hypomagnesemia is defined as a serum concentration <1.5 mEq/L. Magnesium is an essential element for numerous enzymatic reactions involving transphosphorylation, carbohydrate metabolism, protein synthesis, and activation of adenosine triphosphate. Serum magnesium concentration is also important in determining membrane excitation; both magnesium and calcium depletion lead to increased neuronal excitability and enhanced neuromuscular transmission. Hypomagnesemia, especially when associated with digitalis administration, can contribute to disturbances in cardiac rhythm. ECG changes seen with hypomagnesemia include a prolonged PR interval, wide QRS complexes, ST segment depression, and low T waves.

Hypomagnesemia can be due to intestinal losses because of diarrhea, nasogastric suctioning, or malabsorption; renal losses from diuretics, hyperaldosteronism, and diabetes; and insufficient administration in patients on TPN. A variety of drugs may also affect magnesium homeostasis.

Hypermagnesemia

Hypermagnesemia is usually iatrogenic and may occur from too large a dose of magnesium in a patient with normal renal function or from normal doses of magnesium and/or magnesium-containing antacids in patients with abnormal renal function. Physiologic consequences of hypermagnesemia include decreased nerve induction and weakness as well as prolongation of the effects of neuromuscular blocking agents.

Hypophosphatemia

In children the concentration of inorganic phosphate in serum varies between 4.0 and 7.0 mg/dl (1.3 to 2.3 mmol/L). In adults the concentration in serum varies between 2.7 to 4.5 mg/dl (0.9 to 1.5 mmol/L). Phosphorus' role in muscle, nervous system, and red blood cell function is essential, as is its contribution to the intermediary metabolism of carbohydrate, protein, and fat and to the body's entire apparatus of generating and storing energy. Severe hypophosphatemia (<1.0 mg/dl) can result from inadequate administration to patients on TPN, nutritional recovery after starvation, treatment of DKA, the combination of phosphate-binding antacids with dialysis, and the anabolic-diuretic state that follows severe burns. Muscle weakness, acute respiratory failure, altered myocardial performance, hemolytic anemia, diminished phagocytosis, platelet dysfunction and hemorrhage, hepatocellular damage, and neurologic abnormalities including seizures, tremors, and coma are all consequences of severe hypophosphatemia. Correction of these problems is usually rapid with administration of phosphate; a positive correlation exists between the amount of phosphate administered and the serum inorganic phosphate levels measured.

MONITORING AND LABORATORY TESTS
(see also Chapters 4 and 5)

Input and output records must be completed hourly, including an estimate of stool volume (by weight use

Table 15-4 Fluids, Minerals, and Glucose: Correction of Deficits*

Element	Deficit	Dose			Example (4 kg infant)		
Water†	5% (mild)	Maintenance plus maintenance × 0.5			400 ml + 200 ml = 600 ml		
	10% (moderate)	Maintenance plus maintenance × 1.0			400 ml + 400 ml = 800 ml		
	15% (severe)	Maintenance plus maintenance × 1.5			400 ml + 600 ml = 1000 ml		
Electrolytes		*Hypotonic*	*Isotonic*	*Hypertonic‡*	*Hypotonic*	*Isotonic*	*Hypertonic*
		(mEq/kg/24 hr)			(mEq/kg/24 hr)		
Sodium (Na)		10-12	8-10	2-4	40-48	32-40	8-16
Potassium (K)§		8-10	8-10	0-4	32-40	32-40	0-16
Chloride (Cl)		10-12	8-10	2-6¶	40-48	32-40	8-24
Calcium (Ca)		200 mg/kg/24 hr divided, by slow IV push every 3-4 hr (as gluconate)			=133 mg every 4 hr		
Magnesium (Mg)		0.8 mEq/kg/24 hr in 3 divided doses, by slow IV push			=1.1 mEq every 8 hr		
Phosphate (PO_4)		5-10 mg/kg (0.15-0.33 mmol/kg) IV over 6 hr (initial dose, then repeat measurement)			=20-40 mg over 6 hr		
Glucose		Increase by 100 mg/kg/hr repeatedly until serum glucose is 90 mg/dl (may desire higher concentrations, e.g., in Reye's syndrome)					

*Modified by permission from Levin DL, Morriss FC, Moore GC. A Practical Guide to Pediatric Intensive Care. St. Louis: CV Mosby, 1984, p 96.

†Usually the first half of correction is carried out in the first 8 hr, and the second half of correction is carried out over the next 16 hr. If the patient is hypotensive or in shock, immediately give 0.9% sodium chloride or lactated Ringer's solution, 20 ml/kg. Repeat this until systemic arterial blood pressure, capillary filling, and urinary output are restored (see Chapter 12).

‡Patients with hypertonic dehydration may develop cerebral edema and seizures with rapid correction of water deficit. Correct such patients slowly over 48 to 72 hr. Never give such a patient fluid without some salt content (usually these patients are acidotic, and sodium bicarbonate can be added to D_5W to correct acidosis and provide some salt). This will help prevent cerebral edema from developing.

§Potassium at a concentration ≦80 mEq/L at a rate ≦0.3 mEq/kg/hr.

¶Balance indicates excess at the beginning of treatment.

1 g as equivalent to 1 ml). Check the clinical signs every hour in severely dehydrated patients and every 4 to 8 hours in less ill patients. These signs include skin turgor, eyes (moisture, turgor), anterior fontanelle fullness, mucous membrane hydration, heart rate (continuously), capillary refill, and systemic arterial blood pressure (continuously). In addition to urine and serum sodium, potassium, and chloride measure the urine and serum calcium, magnesium, and phosphates and osmolality when appropriate. Large volumes of output from nasogastric tubes, drains, and stool may need to be periodically checked for sodium and potassium content. In severely ill patients measure blood urea nitrogen and serum creatinine at least every day until they are normal.

Obtain arterial blood-gas tensions and pH determinations initially in all patients and every 4 hours if abnormal.

TREATMENT

The components of fluid, mineral, and glucose therapy must be calculated separately using the guidelines given in Table 15-4.

Disorders of Osmolality

Hypo-osmolality (hyponatremia)

Hyponatremia with hypovolemia. The goal is to expand the ECF volume with salt-containing solutions (see Chapter 12). Enough fluid needs to be given for both maintenance requirements and deficit fluids. The adequacy of replacement must be evaluated by both physical examination and laboratory data.

The underlying disease must also be treated and attempts made to control ongoing losses. When shock is present, first give 0.9% sodium chloride solution rapidly, 10 to 20 ml/kg IV over 10 to 20 minutes, and repeat this dose until systemic arterial blood pressure is restored and urine is produced or until the CVP is 10 to 12 mm Hg or pulmonary capillary wedge pressure is >16 mm Hg. Patients with adrenal insufficiency may need glucose, potassium, and adrenocorticosteroid replacement (see Chapter 55).

Acute severe symptomatic hyponatremia is a medical emergency: use hypertonic saline solution (3% to 5%). However, because overuse of hypertonic saline solution can result in the complications of congestive heart failure or cerebral hemorrhage, be careful to use only enough hypertonic saline solution to correct the serum sodium to a level of 120 to 125 mEq/L. The amount of hypertonic saline solution

needed can be calculated using the following formula:

$$mEq\ Na = (0.60)\ (body\ weight\ in\ kg)\ (125 - Na)$$

where Na = serum sodium concentration in mEq/L and 0.6 is the Na compartment of the body.

Hyponatremia with normal volume or hypervolemia (dilutional syndromes). Direct therapy at maximal improvement of the underlying disorder. Because total body sodium is normal or even elevated, efforts to increase serum sodium through saline administration will only result in further expansion of the ECF volume and may worsen the clinical status of the patient. First attempt to decrease the total body water by severe fluid restriction (50% of maintenance). Note that many drugs (e.g., antibiotics) contain significant amounts of sodium. Excess body sodium needs to be concomitantly treated by sodium restriction and judicious use of loop diuretics. For further treatment of SIADH, see Chapter 57.

Hyperosmolality

Hypernatremia. In hypernatremia with dehydration secondary to water loss in excess of sodium loss from enteric disease, a large water deficit may be present, but rapid correction of the hypernatremia with water can result in cerebral edema, seizures, and death. Therefore use the approach outlined in Fig. 15-3. The most important initial assessment is the adequacy of intravascular volume. Once the intravascular volume abnormality has been corrected, proceed cautiously in correcting water deficits. If the patient shows initial neurologic improvement and later deteriorates, cerebral edema must be suspected even if serum sodium concentrations and osmolality remain greater than normal. Administration of water must be stopped, and osmotherapy with hypertonic saline solution or mannitol needs to be begun and continued until signs of cerebral edema (i.e., seizures or depressed level of consciousness) are no longer observed.

For treatment of primary water loss, see Chapter 58. For treatment of patients with essential hypernatremia, that is, hypernatremia with normal hydration, chlorpropamide has been successful in lowering the plasma sodium concentration toward normal. Since patients with hypernatremia with overhydration are volume-expanded, the administration of water to lower the serum sodium concentration can aggravate the problem. First remove excess sodium.

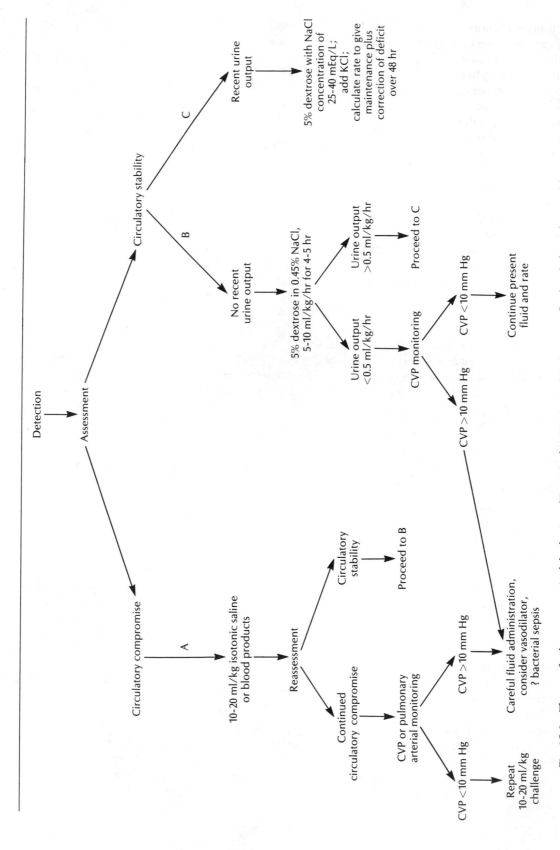

Fig. 15-3   Therapy for hypernatremic dehydration. (From Perkin RM, Levin DL. Common fluid and electrolyte problems in the pediatric intensive care unit. Pediatr Clin North Am 27:567-586, 1980.)

When renal function is normal, the sodium load may be excreted rapidly in the urine by inducing sodium and water diuresis with diuretics and replacing the urine output with water. In patients with poor renal function or in infants, peritoneal dialysis is usually needed.

Hyperglycemia. Direct therapy toward each of the metabolic disturbances that may be present in the hyperglycemic patient, including hyperosmolality, ketoacidosis, potassium imbalance, and volume depletion. Since absolute or relative insulin deficiency is responsible for most of these problems, the administration of insulin and volume repletion are the mainstays of therapy (see Chapter 54).

Hypertonicity due to solutes other than glucose or sodium. If renal function is poor and sugar too slowly metabolized, dialysis may be necessary to remove the solute and the excessive ECF (e.g., mannitol).

Disorders of Potassium Balance
Hypokalemia

Potassium replacement is the principal therapy. It is usually given intravenously, but if time and the patient's condition permit, the slower oral route may be safer. One must always treat the underlying condition.

Carefully calculate the rate of administration of potassium as well as the concentration of potassium in IV solutions. Cells have a limited rate at which they can restore their potassium content; therefore rapid administration of potassium is potentially dangerous even in patients who are severely potassium depleted and may result in fatal dysrhythmias. Always monitor the ECG continuously when giving potassium intravenously and measure serum potassium concentration frequently. Usually infusion rates <0.3 mEq/kg/hr and concentrations <80 mEq/L are adequate for replacement and are safe. Greater amounts can be given more rapidly, but it is dangerous to do so and the benefits to the patient need to be weighed against the risks. Infusions of highly concentrated potassium are irritating and may cause thrombophlebitis. When patients are alkalotic, potassium must be replaced as the chloride salt since chloride depletion usually accompanies potassium depletion. When patients are acidotic and hypokalemic, serum potassium levels at normal pH are even lower and correcting pH before giving potassium may make the serum potassium dangerously, even fatally low.

Hyperkalemia (see also Chapter 14)

True potassium levels >7 mEq/L and/or ECG changes such as a widened QRS complex, heart block, or ventricular dysrhythmias are an emergency. Therapy includes diluting the ECF, creating a chemical antagonism to the membrane effect of potassium by administering sodium bicarbonate and calcium gluconate, increasing the cellular uptake of potassium by the use of glucose infusion and insulin, and removing potassium from the body by the use of potassium-exchange resins or dialysis. Always remember to diagnose and treat the underlying disease to prevent further episodes of hyperkalemia (Table 15-5).

Disorders of Calcium Balance
Hypocalcemia

Use 10% calcium gluconate (100 mg/ml); give 2 ml/kg IV as an initial dose while monitoring the cardiac rate for evidence of bradycardia during infusion. Start replacement therapy with 200 mg/kg/24 hr IV, divided 6 times per day; measure serum calcium every 12 hours and increase maintenance dose as indicated (see Table 15-1) to maintain total serum calcium to at least 8 mg/dl or ionized calcium >3.5 mg/dl. Calcium chloride may be used in cases of very acute decreases in calcium with decreased cardiac output. Use 10 to 20 mg/kg IV by slow push with ECG monitoring.

Hypercalcemia

Patients with hypercalcemia often have had anorexia, nausea, and vomiting for some time prior to recognition, and severe dehydration and oliguria may be present. Therefore first rehydrate the patient with IV fluids. Hypokalemia frequently occurs concomitantly with hypercalcemia and will also need treatment. If patient immobilization is the cause, mobilization and weight bearing, if possible, are effective therapy.

Reduction of the serum calcium by decreasing or eliminating dietary sources of calcium and vitamin D is simple but usually of no help in the acute situation. Administration of corticosteroids results in inhibition of calcium-absorptive mechanisms from the GI tract but also is of little help in the acute situation.

Because renal calcium clearance is a linear function of sodium clearance, urinary excretion of calcium can be increased by increasing urinary excretion of sodium. Use large amounts of sodium chloride solutions. If congestive heart failure or renal failure

Table 15-5   Treatment of Hyperkalemia*

Modality	Dose	Mechanism*	Comments
Calcium gluconate (10%)	0.5-1.0 ml/kg IV	2	Give in 2-5 minutes with ECG monitoring; the immediate improvement in ECG is a transient effect since there is no change in serum potassium concentration
Glucose	0.5-1.0 g/kg IV	1, 3, ±4	Give as IV infusion over 15-30 minutes; follow glucose levels; insulin 0.1 unit/kg SQ or IV may be required; effect begins in 1 hour, transient duration
Sodium bicarbonate	1.5-2.0 mEq/kg IV	1, 2, 3	Give over 5-10 minutes; effect begins in 30-60 minutes, transient duration
Sodium chloride	Isotonic solution (0.9%): 10 ml/kg IV or 3%:3 ml/kg IV	1, 2, ±3	More effective if patient is hyponatremic; transient effect
Sodium polystyrene sulfonate (Kayexalate)	0.5-1.0 g/kg per rectum (PR) or PO via NG tube	4	Give with sorbitol (70%)

1 = ECF expansion; 2 = antagonism to membrane effect; 3 = increased cellular uptake; 4 = removal of potassium from body; ± = may or may not.

*From Perkin RM, Levin DL. Common fluid and electrolyte problems in the pediatric intensive care unit. Pediatr Clin North Am 27:567-586, 1980.

Table 15-6   Therapeutic Parenteral Phosphorus Preparations*

Preparation	Composition	pH	mOsm/kg H_2O	Phosphate (mmol/ml)	Phosphorus (mg/ml)	Sodium (mEq/ml)	Potassium (mEq/ml)
Neutral sodium phosphate	10.07 mg Na_2HPO_4 + 2.66 mg NaH_2PO_4 − H_2O/ml	7.35	202	0.09	2.8	0.16	0
Neutral sodium potassium phosphate	11.5 mg Na_2HPO_4 + 2.58 mg KH_2PO_4/ml	7.40	223	0.1	3.1	0.16	0.02
Sodium phosphate	142 mg Na_2HPO_4 + 276 mg NaH_2PO_4 − H_2O/ml	5.70	5580	3.0	93	4	0
Potassium phosphate	236 mg K_2HPO_4 + 224 mg KH_2PO_4/ml	6.60	5840	3.0	93	0	4.4

*From Perkin RM, Levin DL. Common fluid and electrolyte problems in the pediatric intensive care unit. Pediatr Clin North Am 27:567-586, 1980.

is not present, diuresis can be initiated with 0.9% sodium chloride solution and continued until the CVP reaches 10 mm Hg. Follow the initial infusion with infusion rates that maintain the CVP at this level. When this treatment alone is not effective, also give furosemide 1 to 2 mg/kg. Furosemide is known to promote natriuresis and calciuresis even without the intermediate sodium chloride infusion. Ethylenediaminetetraacetic acid (EDTA) (15 to 50 mg/kg IV over 4 to 6 hours) increases urinary excretion of calcium by forming filterable soluble complexes that are not reabsorbed by the renal tubule. Peritoneal dialysis can be performed regardless of renal function and success depends solely on the calcium gradient established across the peritoneum. Bone resorption also can be decreased or bone formation increased with corticosteroids, mithramycin, calcitonin, and phosphate administration. The onset of action of a single dose of calcitonin (3 to 6 IU/kg) is rapid, occurring within hours. When repeated at 4- to 8-hour intervals, calcitonin produces a 1 to 4 mg/dl decrease in serum calcium.

Other Common Disturbances
Hypomagnesemia

For hypomagnesemia give 0.2 mEq/kg magnesium sulfate intramuscularly (deep in a large muscle) or intravenously every 6 hours. When IV administration is used, dilute the dose in a volume given over several hours to avoid systemic arterial hypotension.

Hypophosphatemia

Inorganic phosphate usually exists in serum as a mixture of two valence states, with an average valence of 1.8 at pH 7.4. Variations in serum pH are common and will alter the molar ratio and average valence of phosphate ions; therefore the use of milliequivalents or milliequivalents per liter is confusing and may lead to large dosage errors. In contrast, the concentrations of phosphate ion in millimoles (mmol) and elemental phosphorus in milligrams (mg) are constant and independent of pH in therapeutic solutions as well as in serum; therefore these terms are preferable. Each millimole of phosphate contains 31 mg of elemental phosphorus. Maintenance requirements (i.e., hyperalimentation) for phosphorus are a dose of 0.1 to 0.2 mmol/kg/24 hr (3 to 10 mg/kg/24 hr). For patients with DKA, in whom hypophosphatemia is common, approximately 20 mEq/L of potassium replacement in IV solutions may be given as the phosphate salt (Table 15-6).

Recommendations for correcting low serum inorganic phosphate levels <1 mg/dl are not possible in a given patient since neither the size of the body deficit nor the response to phosphorus therapy can be predicted. Therefore select an initial dose that will correct the severe hypophosphatemia while minimizing side effects. Hazards associated with administration of phosphate include hyperphosphatemia, leading to hypocalcemia and metastatic deposition of calcium phosphate; hypotension; hyperkalemia from excessive quantities of potassium phosphate; and dehydration and hypernatremia related to the osmotic diuretic effect of filtered phosphate. When phosphorus is given rapidly, side effects are greater; therefore we recommend cautious rates of administration and low initial doses. An initial dose of 5 to 10 mg/kg (0.15 to 0.33 mmol/kg) can be given intravenously over 6 hours. Calcium supplements may be needed for hypocalcemia, but the addition of calcium to phosphate-containing solutions or administration through the same IV tubing causes precipitation and must be avoided.

Hypoglycemia

Give patients with hypoglycemia (<45 mg/dl) either $D_{25}W$, 2 ml/kg IV, or $D_{10}W$, 5 ml/kg IV (i.e., 0.5 g/kg). Be careful to maintain IV glucose administration with either D_5W or $D_{10}W$ thereafter to avoid reactive hypoglycemia that can follow the administration of large amounts of glucose.

Glucose in a high concentration is a potent sclerosing agent and a secure large-bore IV catheter is mandatory. The umbilical vein is an inappropriate route for concentrated glucose infusion since liver damage is a common consequence.

ADDITIONAL READING

Arieff AI, Guisado R. Effects on the central nervous system of hypernatremic and hyponatremic states. Kidney Int 10:104-116, 1976.

Baumgart S, Engle WD, Fox WW, Polin RA. Effect of heat shielding on convective and evaporative heat losses and on radiant heat transfer in the premature infant. J Pediatr 99:948-956, 1981.

Berl T, Anderson RJ, McDonald KM, et al. Clinical disorders of water metabolism. Kidney Int 10:117-132, 1976.

Burch GE, Giles TD. The importance of magnesium deficiency in cardiovascular disease. Am Heart J 94:649-657, 1977.

• Chernow B, Zaloga GP. SCCM—Ions for society members (sulfate, chloride, calcium, magnesium). In Shoemaker WC, ed. Critical Care—State of the Art, vol 5. Fullerton, Calif.: Society of Critical Care Medicine, 1984, pp V(K) 1-43.

Feig PA, McCurdy DK. The hypertonic state. N Engl J Med 197:1444-1454, 1977.

Finberg L. Hypernatremic (hypertonic) dehydration in infants. N Engl J Med 289:196-198, 1973.

Goldsmith RS. Treatment of hypercalcemia. Med Clin North Am 56:951-960, 1972.

Haddon JE, Cohen DL. Understanding and managing hypernatremic dehydration. Pediatr Clin North Am 21:435-441, 1974.

Hochman HI, Grodin MA, Crone RK. Dehydration, diabetic ketoacidosis and shock in the pediatric patient. Pediatr Clin North Am 26:803-824, 1979.

Holliday MA. Maintenance therapy in emergencies. In Pascoe DJ, Grossman M, eds. Quick Reference to Pediatric Emergencies, 3rd ed. Philadelphia: JB Lippincott, 1984.

Kleeman CR, Fichman MP. The clinical physiology of water metabolism. N Engl J Med 277:1300-1307, 1967.

Knochel JP. The pathophysiology and clinical characteristics of severe hypophosphatemia. Arch Intern Med 137:203-220, 1977.

Levinsky NG. Management of emergencies—hyperkalemia. N Engl J Med 274:1076-1077, 1966.

Loeb JN. The hyperosmolar state. N Engl J Med 290:1184-1187, 1974.

Mendelssohn S, Rothschild J. Differential diagnosis of hyponatremia. In Swartz AB, Lyons H, eds. Acid-Base and Electrolyte Balance. New York: Grune & Stratton, 1977, pp 149-164.

Noguchi M, Eren N, Tsang RC. Parathyroid hormone in hypocalcemic and normocalcemic infants of diabetic mothers. J Pediatr 97:112-114, 1980.

• Perkin RM, Levin DL. Common fluid and electrolyte problems in the pediatric intensive care unit. Pediatr Clin North Am 27:567-586, 1980.

Robson AM. Parenteral fluid therapy. In Vaughan VC III, McKay AJ, eds. Nelson's Textbook of Pediatrics, Philadelphia: WB Saunders, 1975.

Root AW, Harrison HE. Recent advances in calcium metabolism. II. Disorders of calcium homeostasis. J Pediatr 88:177-199, 1976.

Rose BD. Clinical physiology of acid-base and electrolyte disorders. New York: McGraw-Hill, 1977.

Suki WN, Yium JJ, Miaden MV, et al. Acute treatment of hypercalcemia with furosemide. N Engl J Med 283:836-840, 1970.

Surawicz B. Relationship between electrocardiogram and electrolytes. Am Heart J 73:814-830, 1967.

Weil WB, Baile MD, eds. Fluid and Electrolyte Metabolism in Infants and Children: A Unified Approach. New York: Grune & Stratton, 1977, pp 151-199.

Winters RW, ed. The Body Fluids in Pediatrics. Boston: Little, Brown, 1973.

16   Acute Hepatic Failure

William M. Belknap

BACKGROUND AND PHYSIOLOGY

Fulminant hepatic failure (FHF) is defined as liver dysfunction evidenced by incorrectable coagulopathy, jaundice, and encephalopathy occurring together in an illness of less than 8 weeks' duration. FHF is caused by massive destruction of liver tissue following one of several insults. In the United States the most common cause of FHF is acute viral hepatitis; the second is drug toxicity, principally from acetaminophen overdosage.

Causes of FHF in infants and children

1. *Infections*
   Viral hepatitis
      Hepatitis A
      Hepatitis B
      Hepatitis non-A, non-B
      Hepatitis delta (in hepatitis B patients only)
   Systemic viral infections with liver involvement (NOTE: Prominent in infancy)
      Herpes virus
      Enterovirus (echovirus)
      Epstein-Barr virus
      Cytomegalovirus
      Adenovirus
   Rickettsia
      Coxiella burnetti
2. *Drugs, toxins*
   Acetaminophen
   Valproic acid
   Isoniazid
   Halothane
   Amanita phalloides (mushroom ingestion)
   Phenytoin (hypersensitivity)
   Carbon tetrachloride
   Tetracycline
   Other drugs, miscellaneous agents
3. *Hypoxia, ischemia*
   Cardiogenic shock
   Sepsis and shock
   Heatstroke
   Budd-Chiari syndrome
4. *Metabolic disease* (NOTE: Prominent in infancy)
   Galactosemia
   Hereditary fructose intolerance
   Cystic fibrosis (infancy)
   Tyrosinosis
5. *Neoplasia*
   Metastatic disease to the liver
   Erythrophagocytic syndrome

Rather than simply an isolated condition of critical liver dysfunction, FHF is acutally a syndrome in which liver destruction quickly results in secondary disease in multiple other organ systems.

Complications of FHF

Encephalopathy
Cerebral edema
Coagulopathy
   Hepatic
   Disseminated intravascular coagulation
Hypotension
Defective ventilation
   Hypoxemia
   Hypocapnia
Pulmonary edema
Electrolyte imbalance
Acid-base disturbance
Renal dysfunction
Hypoglycemia
Cardiac dysfunction (dysrhythmias)
Pancreatitis
Infections (immunocompromised host)
Portal hypertension
Aplastic anemia

Organ failure, most notably in the CNS as cerebral edema progressing to brain death, occurs commonly. The overall mortality rate is exceedingly high—approximately two thirds of pediatric patients die. The prognosis in the individual patient is proportional to the stage of hepatic encephalopathy (Table 16-1); of patients exhibiting stage IV encephalopathy, 5% at

Table 16-1   Acute Hepatic Encephalopathy*

Stage	Description	Mentation	Tremor†	EEG
I	Prodrome	Euphoria, occasional depression, confusion; slow mentation, offset; disordered speech; sleep pattern reversal	Slight	Normal
II	Impending coma	Stage I signs amplified; sleepy; inappropriate behavior, combative; loss of sphincter control	Present (readily elicited)	Generalized slowing
III	Stupor	Rousable, but generally asleep; incoherent speech; marked confusion	Present (if patient cooperates)	Abnormal
IV	Coma	Responds to pain only or no response	Absent (usually)	Abnormal (marked)

*Modified from Jones EA, Schafer DF. Fulminant hepatic failure. In Zakim D, Boyer TD, eds. Hepatology: A Textbook of Liver Disease. Philadelphia: WB Saunders, 1982, pp 415-45.
†Asterixis.

most can be expected to survive. If hepatic encephalopathy can be prevented or minimized, complete clinical resolution and hepatic regeneration can be anticipated. Therefore prompt identification of this syndrome and admission to the PICU with early, rigorous adherence to the principles of intensive supportive care are always indicated. Moreover, the pediatric clinician may expect to encounter the entire possible diagnostic spectrum causing this disease.

Patients presenting with FHF have generally exhibited clinical symptoms for less than 2 weeks. The parent will state that the illness began with general malaise, loss of appetite, or vomiting. These symptoms are usually followed by jaundice; the most ominous finding, however, is a change in the patient's mental status. This may occur as fatigue or excessive sleepiness, reversal of day/night sleep pattern, or more overt signs and symptoms (Table 16-1). Physical examination may be limited to jaundice and signs of encephalopathy. Body size and habitus are normal, the liver may be small or not palpable, and ascites is generally absent. This is in contrast to chronic liver disease presenting in acute decompensation where one or more of the following conditions are usually present: short stature, arachnoid habitus, enlarged liver that is firm or nodular, splenomegaly, ascites, spider angiomas, or finger clubbing. Physical findings may be few in either instance.

Multiple laboratory abnormalities are found in patients with FHF and reflect the level of liver destruction and the secondary multisystem complications.

Common laboratory abnormalities in FHF

1. *Liver*
   Hypoglycemia (marked)
   Conjugated hyperbilirubinemia
   AST and ALT increased
   Prothrombin time increased
   Partial thromboplastin time increased
   Fibrinogen decreased
   Ammonia increased
   Altered serum amino acids
2. *Hematologic* (may be normal)
   Thrombocytopenia
   Leukopenia
   Anemia
   Aplastic anemia
3. *Renal, electrolyte*
   Prerenal azotemia
   Hypokalemia
   Hypophosphatemia
   Hyponatremia

Hypocalcemia
Hypomagnesemia
Renal failure (acute tubular necrosis or hepato-
renal syndrome)
4. *Acid-base*
Respiratory alkalosis (early)
Metabolic alkalosis
Metabolic acidosis (marked liver failure)
Respiratory acidosis (cerebral edema, pneumonia)

Hypoglycemia from decreased gluconeogenesis is common and immediate identification is critical. Hyperammonemia often results from cessation of urea synthesis; although it quantitatively reflects the degree of liver dysfunction, it often does not correlate to the level of encephalopathy. Patients with FHF are prone to acute gastrointestinal bleeding, most commonly from the stomach or duodenum. Renal function may be impaired and is an important variable to follow carefully because deterioration may be subtle. Pulmonary edema, atelectasis, or pneumonia need to be identified or excluded in all such patients on presentation. Congestive heart failure or cardiogenic shock from other causes may precipitate FHF; otherwise cardiac dysfunction may occur secondarily in patients in the form of dysrhythmia. The circulation exhibits a wide pulse pressure like that occurring in major arteriovenous shunting. Hypotension may ensue, prompting multiple fluid challenges that may inadvertently lead to volume overload and pulmonary edema. Invasive monitoring, as outlined below, is always indicated. Sepsis is a major concern because patients with FHF have altered immune function and are prone to invasive bacterial infection. Intervention with broad-spectrum antibiotics needs to be considered early. This is particularly true in patients who need the most intensive care with intravascular catheters and other forms of mechanical monitoring and support devices that necessitate invasive procedures. An acute onset of glucose intolerance or rapidly falling serum calcium may herald the onset of pancreatitis. Bone marrow hypoplasia or complete aplasia may occur in hepatic failure caused by hepatitis viruses. CNS complications, however, are most likely to determine the ultimate patient outcome because cerebral edema will lead to brain stem herniation and death.

When chronic liver disease first presents, it may simulate the acute syndrome described above. In contrast to acute disease, however, the underlying illness has existed for several months or years and cirrhosis is usually present. The capacity for hepatic regeneration does not exist, and the outcome differs from hepatic failure caused by acute liver disease. Such patients may present with ascites, bleeding, or encephalopathy as the first sign of liver disease. Patient response to therapy will vary with the diagnosis and the cause of acute decompensation. Any of the causes of acute liver disease may be superimposed on chronic disease to produce abrupt liver failure. Because early consideration of liver transplantation may be necessary, high clinical suspicion and early diagnosis are also necessary. This is especially crucial in Wilson's disease (hepatolenticular degeneration caused by abnormal copper metabolism), for patients

---

**EXAMPLES OF CHRONIC LIVER DISEASE
WHOSE FIRST PRESENTATION MAY
SIMULATE ACUTE LIVER DISEASE**

α_1-Antitrypsin deficiency
Wilson's disease
Chronic active hepatitis
    Autoimmune ("lupoid")
    Hepatitis B
    Hepatitis delta (hepatitis B patients only)
    Hepatitis non-A, non-B
Tyrosinosis
Chemotherapy-induced hepatotoxicity

**MECHANISMS OF ACUTE
DECOMPENSATION IN CHRONIC
LIVER DISEASE***

Common	*Less frequent*
Infection	Acute viral hepatitis
Peritonitis	Drug toxicity
Gastrointestinal bleeding	Liver infarction
Hepatorenal syndrome	Hepatoma
Protein overloading	Portal vein thrombosis
Inappropriate diuretic therapy	

*Liver disease may not have been suspected.

ACUTE HEPATIC FAILURE IN WILSON'S DISEASE

Clinical	*Laboratory*
Change in mental status	High serum copper
Jaundice	Low serum ceruloplasmin
Disease unsuspected	High urine copper
Noncompliance with therapy	Renal tubular dysfunction
Cirrhosis	Hemolysis, marked
	Low serum transaminases
	Very low serum alkaline phosphatase
	Conjugated hyperbilirubinemia
	Coagulopathy

---

may present with a unique syndrome of multisystem failure. Liver transplantation is probably the only option in such patients because the vast majority of them either have failed or will fail to respond to medical management.

A very rare form of liver disease occurs as subacute liver failure or submassive necrosis. The degree of liver damage is significant, but is not sufficient to produce failure. This disease is more indolent and may persist for months. Hepatic encephalopathy may not occur, and multiple organ failure syndrome may not follow. An example is cholestatic hepatitis that may occur in hepatitis A virus infection. Although laboratory abnormalities may persist for several weeks to several months, the overall prognosis for submassive necrosis is better than for FHF.

Patients with FHF from acute hepatitis or drug toxicity are within a clinically large spectrum of infants and children presenting with hepatic dysfunction and a change in mental status. Congenital or acquired metabolic encephalopathies such as Reye's syndrome, medium-chain fatty acyl coenzyme A (acyl-CoA) dehydrogenase deficiency, systemic carnitine deficiency, and urea cycle enzyme deficiencies are examples. In contrast to true FHF the pathophysiologic response does not involve necrosis and destruction of the liver. Rather, metabolic by-products act as mediators to produce encephalopathy, or the condition itself may involve the brain. Hyperammonemia is the primary or major mediator for encephalopathy

in these cases. The metabolic diseases listed on p. 137 are true causes of acute hepatic failure. They differ from these entities in that a specific metabolite acts as a destructive hepatotoxin, the accumulation of which results in hepatic necrosis sufficient to produce liver failure.

In patients with acute hepatic failure the disease needs to be identified early and aggressive, intensive supportive care instituted to minimize morbidity and mortality. Intensive care remains the optimal clinical modality to minimize morbidity and mortality.

MONITORING AND LABORATORY TESTS

On identification of the patient with FHF, prompt institution of intensive supportive care and monitoring are indicated:

Monitoring

1. Vital signs and cardiovascular function (see Chapter 4)
   a. Temperature
   b. Respiratory rate
   c. Heart rate and rhythm
      Monitor
      12-lead ECG
   d. Blood pressures (see Chapters 108, 114, 115)
      Systemic arterial catheter
      Central venous catheter
2. Encephalopathy
   a. Quantify neurologic deterioration (Table 16-2)
   b. Define and/or quantify cerebral edema (head CT)
   c. Electroencephalogram (Table 16-1)
3. Monitor gastric contents for blood and pH
4. Urine output
   a. Urinary catheter
   b. Strictly document output
   c. Desired output: 1 ml/kg/hr
5. Systemic oxygenation (O_2 saturation)
6. Perfusion
7. Clinical hepatic deterioration
   a. Shrinking liver size
   b. Evolution of ascites
8. Stool
   a. Check for occult or gross blood
   b. Character (acid, carbohydrate content)

The goals of monitoring and laboratory testing are to determine (1) specific quantification of the level of hepatic dysfunction; (2) the presence or absence of gastrointestinal bleeding; (3) the presence of sepsis; (4) renal function and electrolyte status; (5) acid-base status; (6) respiratory function and oxygenation;

Table 16-2   Glasgow Coma Scale to Identify Patients at Risk for Developing Fatal Cerebral Edema*†‡§

Eye Opening		Best Motor Response		Best Verbal Response	
Spontaneous	4	Obeys commands	6	Oriented	5
To sound	3	Localizes	5	Confused	4
To pain	2	Flexion: normal	4	Inappropriate	3
Never	1	Flexion: abnormal	3	Incomprehensible	2
		Extension	2	None	1
		No response	1		

*From Teasdale G, Jennett B. Assessment of coma and impaired consciousness. A practical scale. Lancet 2:81-84, 1974.
†Patients classified by best response. (Spontaneous activity, loud calling, standardized pain stimulus represents ·continuum of clinical observation.)
‡Grade II: E4, M6, V5.
Grade III: E4-3, M6-5, V4-3.
Grade IV: E2, M4, V3 to E1, M1, V1.
§Highest risk: E1, M3-1, V1. Follow pupillary light reflex, oculovestibular response. If abnormal, monitor intracranial pressure if feasible and administer mannitol.

(7) blood pressure, circulation, and cardiac rhythm; and (8) the level of encephalopathy and the presence or absence of cerebral edema.

Laboratory tests
(obtain daily unless otherwise noted)

1. *Liver function*
   Gluconeogenesis: Serum glucose, Dextrostix (q 4 to 6 hr)
   Coagulation: Prothrombin time, partial prothrombin time, fibrinogen, fibrin degradation products, serial factor VII assays
   Urea synthesis: Arterial blood ammonia
   Excretory function: Bilirubin (total, conjugated)
   Transaminases (AST, ALT)
   Quantitative plasma amino acids
   Alkaline phosphatase, γ-glutamyl transpeptidase
   Total protein, albumin, prealbumin
   Uric acid
2. *Assessment of other organ function (daily to q 4 to 6 hr)*
   Renal: BUN, creatinine, urinalysis, fractional excretion of sodium
   Pulmonary: Arterial blood gases and pH; chest roentgenogram for suspected pneumonia, edema
   Electrolytes: Sodium, potassium, chloride, bicarbonate, phosphate, calcium
   Hematologic: Complete blood count, platelet count, differential count
   Pancreas: Amylase, lipase
   Cardiac function: Chest roentgenogram, ECG, monitoring of rhythm

3. *Diagnosis of etiology (obtain on admission)*
   Hepatitis serology
      Hepatitis A IgM
      Hepatitis B surface antigen and antibody, antibody to core antigen (both IgG and IgM), delta antibody in patients with known hepatitis B infection
   Other viruses
      Urine for cytomegalovirus (CMV)
      CMV serology
      Epstein-Barr virus serology (specify)
      Viral cultures
   Drugs, toxins
      Acetaminophen level
      Urine and serum for drug and toxin screens
   Metabolic (infants)
      Urine for reducing substances
      Erythrocyte galactose-1-phosphate uridyl transferase
      Quantitate urine and serum amino and/or organic acids
   Differentiate from chronic liver disease with acute decompensation
      Serum copper, ceruloplasmin, 24-hr urine for copper (Wilson's disease)
      Serum α₁-antitrypsin level (α₁-antitrypsin deficiency)
      Antinuclear antibody, antismooth muscle antibody (autoimmune hepatitis)
   Liver biopsy (if coagulopathy allows)
      Pattern of injury
      Diagnosis

Bone marrow
  Cases of hypoplastic or aplastic anemia
  Erythrophagocytic syndrome
4. *Investigate for sepsis*
  Blood culture
  Urine culture and urinalysis
  Chest roentgenogram
  Repeat all the above (high index of suspicion for sepsis and the early use of broad-spectrum antibiotic therapy are ideal)

Careful and repeated physical examination for the presence of such prognostic features as ascites, peripheral edema, and progression of neurologic signs and symptoms (Table 16-2) helps to prevent complications or allows early intervention to avoid further progression.

TREATMENT

Early admission of all patients with FHF to the PICU must be considered; clearly, all patients at or above stage II encephalopathy need this care. Specific therapy for treatable conditions must be instituted as rapidly as possible, as in the case of acetaminophen toxicity (see Chapter 77). In metabolic diseases such as galactosemia or fructosemia the removal of the offending dietary sugar will markedly enhance the patient's chances for survival. These points are essential because there is otherwise a frustrating general inability to treat FHF other than through the principles of good, problem-oriented, intensive care management. The principles of intensive care include prevention of hypoglycemia and gastrointestinal bleeding (or aggressive treatment on identification), treatment of hepatic encephalopathy and sepsis, proper ventilation, maintenance of perfusion, and careful attention to the limits for nutritional support during the stages of this syndrome.

Therapy for FHF

1. *Hypoglycemia*
   IV glucose, 8 to 12 mg/kg body weight/min.
   Maintain blood glucose at >130 mg/dl but below renal threshold to avoid glycosuria.
   Spare catabolism of somatic musculature.
2. *Fluid and electrolyte balance*
   Water: 60 to 80 ml/kg/day (a relative restriction).
   Sodium: 1 to 2 mEq/kg/day.
   Potassium: 3 to 6 mEq/kg/day as *minimum*.
   Phosphate: 1 to 2 mmol/kg/day.

3. *Coagulation*
   Routine correction of hepatic coagulopathy with large volumes of fresh frozen plasma or blood factor concentrates is *not* advocated; short-term coverage for liver biopsy or the placement of central venous catheters or arterial catheters is preferable.
   IV vitamin K, 2.5 to 10 mg/day.
4. *Hepatic encephalopathy*
   Protein restriction: 0.5 to 1 g/kg body weight/day.
   Purge gastrointestinal tract.
     Lactulose, 1 ml/kg body weight/dose, 3 to 6 times/day.
     Maintain loose, acid stool and regular stool output.
   Neomycin: 125 to 500 mg, 4 times/day via NG tube.
   Avoid use of hypnosedatives (barbiturates accelerate encephalopathy).
   Treat cerebral edema (see Chapter 7). (NOTE: Not suggested in the absence of intracranial pressure monitor.)
   Decision to ventilate artificially is for the following:
     Hypoventilation
     Airway management
   Management for increased intracranial pressure
5. *Gastrointestinal bleeding*
   Nasogastric tube: Gentle lavage, drug administration, gravity drainage.
   Prophylactic antacids, 0.5 ml/kg q 4 hr via NG tube.
   Cimetidine at a lower dose, 20 mg/kg/day divided into four doses. Monitor serum drug levels whenever possible.
   Monitor gastric contents for ambient pH and presence of blood.
6. *Sepsis*
   Include both coverage for *Staphylococcus aureus* if invasive catheters are in place and sufficient gram-negative enteric bacteria coverage with a broad-spectrum, later generation cephalosporin.
   Fungemia: Amphotericin B
7. *Respiration:* May need ventilatory support.
   Paralysis and ventilation for increased intracranial pressure (see Chapter 7).
   Respiratory failure (centrally mediated).
8. *Renal function:* Avoid diuretics.
9. *Cardiovascular:* Maintain systemic arterial blood pressure by avoiding hypovolemia; inotropic agents usually ineffective.
10. *Nutrition* (parenteral)
    Energy: 50 to 60 kcal/kg/day
    Protein: 0.5 to 1 g/kg/day (restriction)
      Avoid aromatic amino acid-containing solutions
      Branched-chain amino acid supplementation may be useful.

Fat: Essential fatty acids in fresh frozen plasma and small dosages of supplemental IV lipid. Avoid inducing metabolic acidosis, do not use intravenous lipid if serum triglycerides exceed 180 mg/dl.

A daily attempt to correct the coagulopathy with specific coagulation factors or fresh frozen plasma is not advocated. Instead, episodic coverage is utilized during invasive procedures. Plasmapheresis to correct the hepatic coagulopathy may be used instead of massive coagulation factor or fresh frozen plasma replacement for invasive procedures or in preparation for orthotopic liver transplantation. It is strongly suggested that only centers with a large aggregate experience with plasmapheresis on protocol use this modality; the episodic use of this procedure is almost certain to result in a therapeutic misadventure. Systemic hypotension with rapid acceleration of multiple organ failure syndrome, platelet aggregation, and sepsis are all strongly possible when using plasmapheresis in patients with FHF.

Extracorporeal hepatic assist devices have not enhanced overall survival in FHF patients and are not, therefore, generally advocated. The intensive care specialist should have strong reservations regarding use of such modalities as charcoal hemoperfusion based on the most recent available data.

Liver transplantation has been successful in patients with FHF. Specific indications for this procedure, however, have not been established, and consultation from a transplant center is necessary. Evaluation must be immediate; prognosis must be estimated before considering transplantation. All patients with a persistent very low factor VII (<8%) level in the presence of stage II or greater encephalopathy need to be considered. Transplantation has not been generally advocated in cases of FHF from systemic viral infections; this issue is undergoing reevaluation, and successful transplantations have been reported. Thus careful identification of both etiology and specific definition of the level of encephalopathy are essential before liver transplantation is considered.

The approach outlined above will usually permit early identification of this syndrome and specific diagnosis of etiology. Early implementation of appropriate monitoring and therapy may permit survival in certain cases in a disease complex where the mortality rate remains unacceptably high. In the future specific pharmacologic agents that will allow attenuation of the process of liver necrosis may be available. Such agents will theoretically permit hepatic regeneration while sparing the effects of progressive hepatic encephalopathy. Further information regarding the role of and specific indications for hepatic transplantation may soon be available.

ADDITIONAL READING

Acute liver failure in infants. In Alagille D, Odievere M. Liver and Biliary Tract Disease in Children. New York: John Wiley, 1979, pp 94-101.

• Jones EA, Schafer DF. Fulminant hepatic failure. In Zakim D, Boyer TD, eds. Hepatology. A Textbook of Liver Disease. Philadelphia: WB Saunders, 1982, pp 415-445.

O'Grady JG, Gimson AES, O'Brien CJ, Pucknell A, Hughes RD, Williams R. Controlled trials of charcoal hemoperfusion and prognostic factors in fulminant hepatic failure. Gastroenterology 94:1186-1192, 1988.

• Psacharopoulos HT, Mowat AP, Daires M, Portmann B, Silk DBA, Williams R. Fulminant hepatic failure in childhood. An analysis of 31 cases. Arch Dis Child 55:252-258, 1980.

Reily CA. Acute hepatic failure in children. Yale J Biol Med 57:161-184, 1984

Russell GJ, Fitzgerald JF, Clark JH. Fulminant hepatic failure. J Pediatr 111:3134-3219, 1987.

Fulminant hepatic necrosis and hepatic coma. In Silverman A, Roy CC. Pediatric Clinical Gastroenterology. St. Louis: CV Mosby, 1983, pp 655-674.

Williams R, ed. Fulminant hepatic failure. Semin Liver Dis 6:97-173, 1986.

17 Acute Metabolic Crises in the Newborn

Charles E. Mize

BACKGROUND AND PHYSIOLOGY

Major metabolic pathways in the life of a cell may be disrupted by acquired disease such as bacterial sepsis (see Chapter 42) or by genetic errors of metabolism. The clinical manifestations of acquired and inborn metabolic disorders of the cell may be identical. The extent of cellular insult generally dictates the severity of clinical expression.

Cellular metabolic disruption in a patient needing PICU care most often reflects a disruption in key substrate flow or flux in one of the pathways important to energy production and utilization. If anaerobic or aerobic energy transduction for normal cellular metabolism is interrupted or significantly slowed, the normal balance of anabolic and catabolic steps can be seriously affected; this is reflected in imbalanced body fluid ion or substrate handling. Inborn defects in both cytoplasmic (e.g., glycolysis defects) and mitochondrial metabolism (e.g., urea cycle, carboxylase, or oxidase/dehydrogenase defects) can present similarly and, of utmost importance, may coexist with acquired septic disease. Neonatal Reye's syndrome (see Chapter 27) may be the clinical presentation of an underlying defect in the urea cycle or mitochondrial oxidase (the latter leading to clinical organic aciduria); the syndrome may also mimic an herbal alkaloid tea ingestion, a severe adenoviral systemic infection, or a salicylate-sensitized *Haemophilus influenzae* infection.

EARLY CLINICAL CLUES TO PEDIATRIC METABOLIC DISEASE

Overwhelming neonatal illness	Seizures
Sepsis (real or apparent)	Chronic hiccoughs
	Hypotonia
Coma	Unusual odor
Vomiting/pyloric stenosis	Minor malformation
Dermatosis	

EARLY CLUES TO METABOLIC DISEASE

Vomiting

Organic acidemia syndromes
Galactosemia
Hyperglycinemia

Unusual odors

Disease	Odor
Isovaleric acidemia	Sweaty feet
Maple syrup urine disease	Maple syrup
Multiple carboxylase deficiency	Tom cat's urine

Lethargy or coma

Urea cycle defects
Disorders of propionate metabolism
Transient hyperammonemia of the newborn
Isovaleric acidemia
Glutaric aciduria
Pyroglutamic acidemia
Lactic acidemias
Nonketotic hyperglycinemia
Homocystinuria syndromes

The variability of clinical expression of inherited metabolic disease is based on the extent of genetic deficiency coupled with exogenous insult. Early clues to these problems encompass vomiting, unusual odors of urine, breath, or skin gland secretions, and lethargy, if not more severe obtundation or coma. Insidious clues to pediatric metabolic disease include mental retardation, failure to thrive, ectopia lentis, recurrent vomiting, muscle weakness, osteomalacia, and dysostosis multiplex. Further, even occasionally chronic, clues to a metabolic disorder may be evident, but are more difficult to diagnose. CNS disorders that may evolve during a clinical course need to be considered and investigated because encephalopathy can be associated with any one of several pediatric metabolic abnormalities, as outlined below:

1. Severe interruption of substrates
   a. Glucose
   b. Oxygen
   c. Gluconeogenic precursors
   d. Phosphocreatine
2. Biochemical agent excess
   a. Lactate
   b. Cyclic AMP
   c. Phospholipids
   d. Free protons
   e. ADP
   f. NADH
   g. Calcium
   h. Polyunsaturated fatty acids
3. Selective factors
   a. Deficits of acetylcholine, catechols, serotonin, or dehydrogenase activities (pyruvate or fatty acyl-CoA)
   b. Ammonia intoxication
   c. Bilirubin intoxication
   d. Thiamin deficiency

The consequences of metabolic defects may be categorized clinically as:

1. Asymptomatic and without consequence (metabolic variants)
2. Asymptomatic except for accidental circumstances (including pharmacogenetic disorders)
3. Mild to moderate severity
4. Severe to lethal expression

Within this framework it is useful to remember that intermittent or episodic disease can be a clinical hallmark of inborn errors. Acquired insult such as infection may produce a stress to which the infant whose base of metabolic flux is only marginally sufficient cannot adequately respond.

The preceding discussion demonstrates that various aberrations may reflect metabolic derangements of acquired or genetic metabolic disorders; however, it is clearly not necessary for more than one of these observations to be present to diagnose a metabolic disease. Such laboratory clues may become apparent at different times in the clinical evolution of continuing cellular metabolic insult. The clinician must be alert to changes in clinical status that may reflect any of the potentially changing laboratory modulations that underlie progression or regression of cellular metabolic disruption.

MONITORING AND LABORATORY TESTS

The clinician must be attentive to the combination of clinical and laboratory clues. Initial and periodic monitoring is necessary to determine the clinical severity of these metabolic disorders.

Attention directed to possible genetic aberrations leading to early infancy mimicry of sepsis or metabolic collapse can be initiated in the earliest moments of PICU care. A laboratory workup should be initiated at the same time to determine acquired causes of metabolic disruption of parenchymal organ functions and/or coupled cardiovascular aberrations. The earliest pre-intervention samples of body fluids may provide the greatest bias for diagnostic data directly pertinent to diagnosis. This is an opportune time in PICU decision making to direct that separate samples of blood, plasma, or urine should be held for analysis. Laboratory evaluation is crucial because urine and blood sequential data often reveal clues to neonatal metabolic disease.

An initial workup to determine the possibility of genetic metabolic disease presenting with the above clinical or laboratory clues should include:

1. Quantitative serum amino acid analysis
2. Blood lactate (venous or arterial), pH and base deficit, electrolytes (including bicarbonate estimation), glucose, phosphorus, ammonia, prothrombin time, and bilirubin (total and direct)
3. Blood and/or urine toxicology analytic screen
4. Urinary reducing substances (glucose and non-glucose) and ketone bodies
5. Quantitative urine carnitine (free and acylated) analysis
6. Quantitative urine organic acid and orotic acid analytic screen

---

LABORATORY CLUES OF NEONATAL METABOLIC DISEASE

Hypoglycemia	Hypoprothrombinemia
Neutropenia	Metabolic acidosis (including lactic acidosis)
Hyperammonemia	Hyperbilirubinemia
Hyperuricemia	Urinary reducing agents
Blood electrolyte aberrations	Urinary ketone bodies

GENERAL PRINCIPLES OF THERAPY FOR CELLULAR METABOLIC DISRUPTION

Nonspecific initial metabolic-based therapy may benefit a metabolic derangement resulting from septic shock or an inherited defect. Diagnosis of the derangement and ultimately specific therapy to correct it are often aided by nonroutine monitoring (special laboratory data).

Maintenance of adequate substrate flow to parenchymal tissues must be provided exogenously by balanced water, ion, nitrogen, and caloric support to the maximal extent the patient can tolerate. Enteral nutritional control is certainly possible and may be desirable because high caloric density can be achieved in relatively constrained fluid volume (see Chapter 150). If this is not possible, total parenteral nutritional control needs to be considered early in the course of evaluation and treatment (see Chapter 149). Amino acid or protein restriction (1 to 1.5 g/kg/day) may be indicated early in nutritional control until a diagnosis can be confirmed and may lead to potential institution of directed dietary or special disease-specific therapy.

When body fluid concentrations of specific substances such as ammonia are so elevated that they enhance the risk for secondary complications or metabolic events detrimental to further metabolic recovery, early attempts must be directed toward providing an external means of removing the offending material(s). For example, if blood ammonia reaches a level potentially responsible for neurologic obtundation, coma, or seizure potentiation, immediate peritoneal dialysis must be seriously considered (see Chapter 145). Specific therapy for acute hyperammonemia includes consideration of a nominal amount of supplemental oral or intravenous arginine (1 mmol/kg/day) to help enhance flux through the urea cycle and sodium benzoate (200 to 500 mg/kg/day) to enhance nitrogen excretion in the form of benzoylglycine (hippuric acid). The literature also suggests use of supplemental sodium phenylacetate to enhance nitrogen excretion in a number of hyperammonemic syndromes that are associated with urea cycle defects, separately or in combination with sodium benzoate. Significant metabolic acidosis syndromes will necessitate parenteral sodium bicarbonate for attempted compensation of the acidosis, to the extent to which sodium ion tolerance allows this alkalinizing compound to be given.

If severe muscular weakness, especially skeletal or cardiac, is associated with carnitine wasting in metabolic oxidase/dehydrogenase deficits, administer supplemental carnitine (100 to 200 mg/kg/day initially in four divided doses and adjust doses thereafter) to enhance carnitine tissue availability.

ADDITIONAL READING

- Fernandes J, Tada K, Saudubray JM. Inherited Metabolic Disease: Diagnosis and Treatment. Berlin: Springer-Verlag, 1989.

  McKusick VA. Mendelian Inheritance in Man, 8th ed. Baltimore: The Johns Hopkins University Press, 1988.

- Nyhan WL, Sakati NO. Diagnostic Recognition of Genetic Disease. Philadelphia: Lea & Febiger, 1987.

  Scriver CR, Beaudet AL, Sly WS, Valle D. The Metabolic Basis of Inherited Disease, 6th ed. New York: McGraw-Hill, 1989.

18 Bowel Failure

Richard Quan

BACKGROUND AND PHYSIOLOGY

The term "failure" refers to a situation in which the primary functions of an organ cease and a pattern of complications ensues. The main functions of the bowel include secretion, digestion, and absorption, all of which depend on normal gut motility to transfer gut contents to the appropriate site. The major func-

tions of the bowel are interrelated so that impairment of one process can cause dysfunction in another. The term "gut failure" or "bowel failure" has been used to describe situations in which enteral nutrition is not absorbed because of decreased absorptive surface area, as in short bowel syndrome. Here the term "bowel failure" is also used to describe pathophysiologic conditions that disturb *more than one* gut function and that are potentially *life threatening*. For this reason diagnosis and the decision to commit the patient to surgical or nonsurgical management are the major challenges in the intensive care setting.

Evaluation of bowel failure begins with the patient history and physical examination. Unfortunately the clinical signs and symptoms (abdominal pain, abdominal distention, vomiting, diarrhea) are very similar in many abdominal diseases, especially early in their presentation. The keys to diagnosis are a thorough understanding of the pathophysiology of the clinical signs, an appreciation of the natural history of abdominal diseases, and experience in diagnosis. This process often requires a team effort involving the surgeon, radiologist, and pediatric gastroenterologist. The decision for immediate surgical intervention involves weighing the likelihood of spreading infection, life-threatening bleeding, and/or permanent loss of bowel. When supportive measures do not suffice, a laparotomy is diagnostic as well as therapeutic.

Bowel failure often has components of intestinal obstruction, vascular insufficiency, and infection. A discussion of the pathophysiology of obstruction and vascular insufficiency follows. Infection is discussed in other texts.

Intestinal Obstruction

Acute intestinal obstruction is usually divided into mechanical obstruction of the intestinal lumen and paralytic ileus, in which there is a lack of peristaltic

---

> **MECHANISMS OF BOWEL FAILURE***
>
> *Intestinal obstruction*
>
> Mechanical (intraluminal, extrinsic)
> Functional (ileus, Hirschsprung's disease)
>
> *Critical loss in length of bowel*
>
> Necrosis (necrotizing enterocolitis, infarction)
> Congenital
>
> *Critical loss in bowel mucosal lining*
> *(total villus atrophy)*
>
> Infection (rotavirus, enteropathogenic *Escherichia coli, Giardia*)
> Ischemia (shock, postcardiac surgery)
> Antineoplastic therapy (radiation, chemotherapy)
> Graft vs. host disease
>
> *Excessive loss of body protein through bowel*
>
> Protein-losing enteropathy (cow's milk protein enteropathy, Ménétrier's disease, lymphangiectasia, inflammatory bowel disease)
> Congestive heart failure (congenital heart disease, myocarditis)
> Constrictive pericarditis

*Bowel failure may occur as a primary disorder or as a secondary complication in a patient with a major cardiac, pulmonary, neoplastic, or infectious disease.

Table 18-1   Causes of Intestinal Obstruction

Mechanical Obstruction		Paralytic Ileus	
Intraluminal	**Extrinsic**	**Abdominal Conditions**	**Systemic Conditions**
Atresia or stenosis	Malrotation	Hirschsprung's disease	Trauma
Pyloric stenosis	Volvulus	Intestinal pseudo-obstruction	Shock
Foreign body	Hernia	Severe gastroenteritis	Sepsis
Meconium	Annular pancreas	Perforation of viscus	Hypokalemia
Medications	Duplication cysts	Peritonitis	Drugs
Cholestyramine	Adhesions/bands	Pancreatitis	Diabetic acidosis
Antacid	Tumor	Necrotizing enterocolitis	
Kaolin	Granulomatous process	Toxic megacolon	
Intussusception			
Parasitic infection			

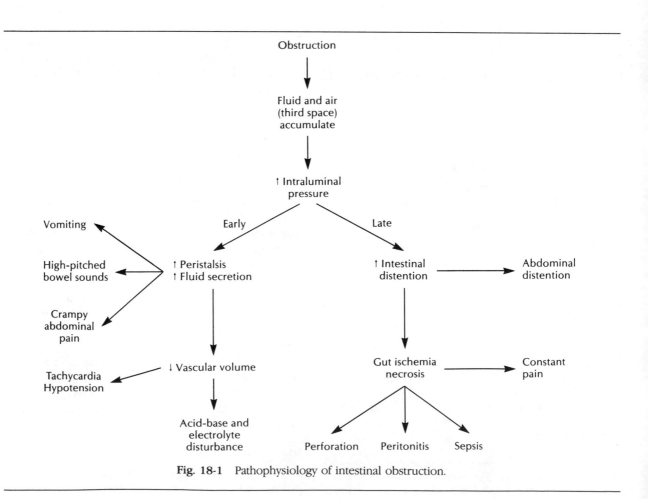

Fig. 18-1   Pathophysiology of intestinal obstruction.

activity and intestinal tone. Common causes are listed in Table 18-1.

When mechanical obstruction occurs, the chain of events diagrammed in Fig. 18-1 occurs. Intestinal secretions and air accumulate in areas proximal to the obstruction and pressure increases in the lumen. The bowel is stimulated to try to clear the fluid and air by increasing peristalsis and actively secreting more fluid. Proximal obstruction often results in vomiting and high-pitched bowel sounds, whereas these signs are less prominent in distal obstruction. Both vomiting and the accumulation of intestinal fluid decrease intravascular volume. Later, peristalsis decreases, and the intestine becomes distended with loss of tone, resulting in further fluid accumulation and abdominal distention. The obstructed bowel becomes edematous and may weep fluid into the peritoneum, further exacerbating fluid accumulation or "third spacing." If the pressure within the bowel persists, areas of bowel become ischemic, necrotic, and may perforate and/or leak bacteria into the peritoneum. This sequence eventually results in fever, tachycardia, peritonitis, hypoproteinemia, hypotension, and death from septic shock.

Alternatively, paralytic ileus is an inhibition of movement in an intestine that is capable of peristalsis. In general adrenergic stimulation inhibits contractile activity; conversely, an adrenergic receptor blocker increases it. However, the exact pathophysiology of the different causes of ileus is not well understood. As intestinal peristalsis is inhibited, the lumen accumulates air and fluid and the bowel distends. This results in decreased vascular volume, third spacing, and electrolyte disturbances as in mechanical obstruction. However, unlike mechanical obstruction, paralytic ileus rarely results in intestinal ischemia and necrosis, especially if adequately decompressed.

Vascular Insufficiency

The vascular supply to the intestine normally undergoes extensive variation in resistance and flow, which is regulated by intrinsic mechanisms. During low-flow states the intestine is able to extract a greater proportion of oxygen to prevent ischemia. This fact plus the extensive intercommunication of arteries makes primary intestinal infarction a relatively rare event. Still it is important to examine intestinal blood supply in patients in the intensive care setting because intestinal ischemia may accompany embolus,

vascular anomalies, or any significant cardiovascular collapse. Acute interruption of the blood supply of the intestine causes an initial spasm of intestinal muscle manifested by severe, colicky periumbilical pain. Gut paralysis and distention follow, with rushes present on auscultation; the bowel sounds rapidly become hypoactive or absent. Shortly thereafter the bowel wall becomes necrotic, allowing bacterial invasion. Serous exudate and blood accumulate in the intestinal lumen, bowel wall, and peritoneal cavity; symptoms of peritonitis such as distention, tenderness, and abdominal rigidity follow. The rates of morbidity and mortality from the complications of intestinal ischemia are clearly very high. A high index of suspicion and rapid action by the intensive care team are needed to prevent a poor outcome.

MONITORING AND LABORATORY TESTS

The initial evaluation of bowel failure needs to be directed toward diagnosis and support. A list of suggested laboratory investigations includes:

> Complete, differential, and platelet counts
> Electrolytes
> Arterial pH
> BUN, creatinine
> Liver function studies
> Serum amylase, lipase
> Stool guaiac
> Stool smear for leukocytes
> Stool culture for enteric pathogens
> Stool for ova and parasites
> Serum total protein, albumin
> Urinalysis, culture
> Abdominal roentgenograms (flat, upright, lateral)
> Blood cultures

Other studies used to evaluate bowel failure include:

> Barium studies
> Abdominal ultrasonography
> Abdominal CT scan
> Abdominal MRI
> Arteriography
> Endoscopy
> Peritoneal lavage (blood, amylase)

Plain abdominal roentgenograms may be useful in differentiating mechanical from paralytic obstruction or suggesting a particular diagnosis (i.e., "double-bubble" of duodenal obstruction). Typical roentgenographic changes of mechanical obstruction include dilated loops of bowel with air-fluid levels proximal to the obstruction. Both the large and small bowel are dilated in paralytic ileus.

If a mechanical obstruction is likely, the site of obstruction must be defined by barium studies or laparotomy. Endoscopic procedures are useful in individual situations but are not obtained routinely. Other studies are helpful when certain diagnostic possibilities are being entertained, but are often of no value when used in a blind fashion. When the diagnosis is in doubt, repeated abdominal examinations and roentgenograms are imperative until a clear diagnosis can be made.

TREATMENT

A primary consideration in the treatment of bowel failure is correction of fluid, electrolyte, and acid-base disturbances. Therapeutic approaches to these problems are detailed in Chapters 12 and 15. Points to consider in the management of bowel failure are as follows: (1) protein losses into the gut can be large and albumin or plasma may be needed to treat depleted intravascular volume; (2) initially, a metabolic alkalosis occurs secondary to vomiting, but later sepsis and starvation ketosis cause metabolic acidosis; and (3) marked intravascular volume depletion causes profound hypotension when general anesthesia is administered or during surgery.

As part of supportive therapy, insertion of nasogastric tubes with low, intermittent suction will decrease intraluminal pressure and abdominal distention. Decompression will not work in some patients, even with patent tubes. In such a situation more definitive therapy cannot be delayed. Other tubes may not work because they are misplaced or plugged; periodic checks of position, function, and output of all tubes are necessary.

Use of weighted Miller-Abbott tubes can cause gastric outlet obstruction; a separate gastric tube may be needed to decompress the stomach. If a tube is to be left in place for a significant period of time a larger double-lumen tube may be preferable to a single-lumen tube, which tends to become obstructed.

Initiation of appropriate antibiotic coverage is a major component of therapy because the bowel is an important barrier against the external environment. The obstructed bowel provides a perfect culture medium for bacteria. Thus a break in the barrier caused by perforation or ischemia quickly leads to sepsis and shock. Broad-spectrum antibiotic coverage must be considered early in the treatment of bowel failure. This must include coverage for common enteric organisms as well as *Staphylococcus* and anaerobic organisms. When selecting antibiotic combinations, the possible synergistic toxic effects of medications and the history of exposure to antibiotic-resistant organisms must be taken into consideration. In general a penicillin or cephalosporin, an aminoglycoside, and an "anaerobic" antibiotic such as clindamycin or metronidazole are utilized.

Nutrition support or replacement of the lost organ function must be initiated early just as ventilatory support must be given to a patient with respiratory failure. In bowel failure the gut is often unable to digest and absorb nutrients. When treatment guidelines are established any large requirements for appropriate macronutrient or micronutrient supplementation need to be taken into account (see Chapters 74, 149, and 150 for a detailed discussion of enteral/parenteral nutrition).

ADDITIONAL READING

Kerner JA Jr, ed. Manual of Pediatric Parenteral Nutrition. New York: John Wiley, 1983.

Silverman A, Roy CC. Intestinal obstruction of infancy and childhood. Pediatric Clinical Gastroenterology, 3rd ed. St. Louis: CV Mosby, 1983, pp 105-128.

Sleisenger MH, Fordtran JS. Gastrointestinal Disease: Pathophysiology, Diagnosis, and Management, 3rd ed. Philadelphia: WB Saunders, 1983, pp 308-319.

19 Disseminated Intravascular Coagulation and Other Acquired Bleeding Disorders

James S. Roloff

BACKGROUND AND PHYSIOLOGY

The commerce of the body depends on the timely and efficient transport of metabolic substrate and product as well as systemic communication. The infrastructure responsible for these essential tasks is a dynamic, multicellular complex of tubes, valves, pressure regulators, and pump, that is, the cardiovascular system. The vessels, like any ducted system, demand constant upkeep to ensure integrity and patency. Added to these stresses is the necessity of elasticity and movement. Like man-made pipelines maintained by monitoring and repair, the vascular system capitalizes on a number of biophysical and biochemical components to guarantee continuous traffic flow throughout the body. Components of this "maintenance" system must be comprehensive in scope, that is, ready for any sort of break or clog, yet efficient, using minimal components that are readily available and/or replenishable. It must be rapidly responsive to demand, yet manageable and able to be modulated easily as needed. This process needs to be limited to the site of damage and must protect all components of itself. It must provide not only this immediate responsiveness, but also facilitate long-term repair and healing. Although both coagulation and dissolution play intertwining roles, this process is referred to as hemostasis. And, instead of being static, awaiting a traumatic event, the hemostatic system proves to be a dynamic process of clot formation and clot re-moval as well as intermittent "plugging" techniques for minor breeches of vessel walls. At the molecular level the biochemical and biophysical parts of the system comprise proteolysis, exocrine release, biologic surface utilization (for both adhesion and spatial geometry), and cofactor modulation. Regulation by promoters and inhibitors at multiple steps from both within and outside the network finely tunes the entire process. Macroscopically the system can be divided into three components: vascular, cellular, and fluid (biochemical) (Fig. 19-1). The initial response to traumatic rupture of a vessel is its spasmodic contraction, followed by the formation of a so-called platelet plug. Subsequently the fluid component contributes to the construction of a system of scaffolding (the fibrin clot), which is stabilized (cross-linked), and eventually removed (fibrinolysis) with healing.

Dividing hemostasis into these three parts proves to be artificial since each component has a striking interdependence on the other two. This sequence is chosen primarily because of the temporal relationship of activation. The vascular response is immediate, with platelet responses following in a matter of seconds. Activation of the coagulation factors, primarily because of their multistep nature and the need for adequate concentrations available to affect subsequent steps, takes place over a matter of minutes. Formation of a stable clot able to contract and reappose the edges of a vascular breech may take minutes

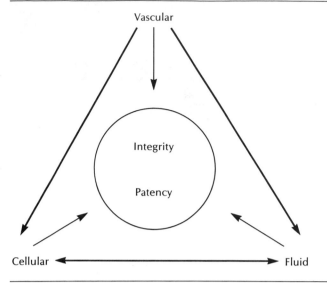

Fig. 19-1 All three components of hemostasis influence one another to maintain the integrity and patency of the vascular system.

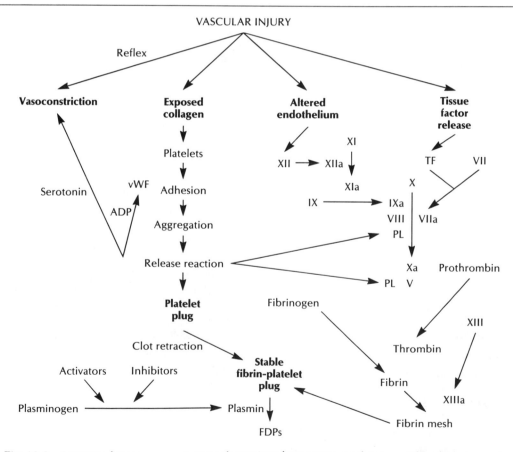

Fig. 19-2 Any vascular injury may initiate the various hemostatic mechanisms. The ultimate product is the stable fibrin plug, which then must be removed. Fluid factors are expressed by Roman numerals, that is, IX and XIIIa (for activated forms); PL = phospholipid; ADP = adenosine diphosphate; vWF = von Willebrand factor; TF = tissue factor; FDPs = fibrin degradation products. (Modified from Lusher JM. Diseases of coagulation: The fluid phase. In Nathan DG, Oski FA, eds. Hematology of Infancy and Childhood, 3rd ed. Philadelphia: WB Saunders, 1987.)

to hours. Recruitment of fibroblasts and phagocytic cells for healing as well as the digestion of the fibrin clot span hours to days.

Mechanisms of Hemostasis (Fig. 19-2)
Vascular phase

The vascular component is the least well characterized of all hemostatic mechanisms. Two separate roles of vessel function are recognized. Mechanical constriction of the vessel may be an immediate abortive attempt to reduce blood loss through the break and is mediated by local factors and enhanced by platelet-released products. In contrast, at a later point, accelerated blood flow (possibly for delivery of needed substrate and removal of excessive amounts of activated coagulation factors) as well as capillary dilatation and increased permeability (again mediated in part by locally generated hemostasis products) takes place. In addition the basement membrane and other subvascular elements, particularly collagen, along with the endothelial cells lining the vessels, play integral roles in the initiation and modulation of the other components of hemostasis.

Cellular phase

The platelet (actually an anuclear fragment of megakaryocyte cytoplasm) represents a unique package of biochemical and biophysical elements that interplay in a multifaceted and complex role to maintain the integrity of the vascular system. Formation of the "platelet plug" is the initial step (Fig. 19-3). Adhesion of the platelet occurs on blood vessel injury. This is mediated by a fluid factor, von Willebrand factor (vWF), and a specific site on the platelet surface. Adhesion is followed by a change of platelet shape from the normally rounded form to one of extended projections. These platelets coalesce and spread to span the region of injury. Concomitantly, platelets release various activators, particularly adenosine diphosphate (ADP), from cytoplasmic granules ("storage pool"), resulting in neighboring platelets being activated and aggregating on the spreading sheet to form the "plug." Fibrinogen spans the interplatelet gap to link them to one another. Platelets provide much of the lipoprotein "surface" and other factors used by the fluid components of hemostasis and also become entrapped in the developing fibrin mesh. This latter phenomenon is important since actinlike proteins within platelets contract, pulling the fibrin mesh tightly together, retracting the clot. Addition-

ally, platelet granules may act as transport bodies for coagulant components, including fibrinogen, F V, and vWF, among others (Table 19-1). Platelets affect not only mechanical plugging, but also release of several factors that regulate vascular reactivity, and this is paralleled by release of similar biochemical products from the vessel wall. The prostaglandin-thromboxane family mediates these reactions. Adequate numbers of platelets as well as platelets that function normally are necessary for an intact hemostatic system.

Fluid phase

Fluid factors may be divided into several categories. A linked cascade of enzymes utilizing trypsinlike proteolysis is the backbone of clot formation and removal. Throughout phylogony, nature has seen fit to address need by using paradigms of biologic function. In hemostasis this reliance on sets of common patterns can be found in the combined use of vascular, cellular, and fluid factors. Enzyme precursors, termed proenzymes or "zymogens," are modified either by conformational (shape) changes or actual cleavage of a portion of the proenzyme to an active form (protease), which in turn can act on substrates (other zymogens or cofactors) in other portions of the cascade, usually, but not exclusively, "downstream." This reaction sequence can be enhanced by "cofactors" that either further modulate conformation or actually cleave additional components of the enzyme to produce even more active forms of the protease. Also, they may provide enhanced attachment for additional substrate. These cofactors, too, can be conformationally or enzymatically modified to become more effective in their role. With regard to enhanced attachment, cofactors facilitate topologic juxtaposition of components of the cascade. In a parallel fashion, inhibitors "down-regulate" the cascade activity, again by conformational and cleavage mechanisms but also by complex formation with the target factor. This multistep sequence allows modulation (both up and down) of the chemical reactions. Thus a small "signal" can be amplified to such degree as to form a structurally sound clot, yet the entire process can be contained at the local area of vascular damage.

The components of the cascade are grouped into substeps with "typical" collections of participants: target zymogen, cofactors, and a surface and a cleaving enzyme (Table 19-2). Each of the zymogens, as well as enzymes, are equipped uniquely to attach closely

Table 19-1   Characteristics of Fluid Factors

Factor	Type*	Concentration in Plasma (μg/ml)	Synonym	Vitamin K Dependent	Site of Synthesis†	Biologic Half-Life (hr)	% Required for Normal Hemostasis
Fibrinogen	S	15-30	F I	−	L	72-120	100 mg/dl
Prothrombin	Z	100	F II	+	L	60-106	30-40
F V	C	10	Proaccelerin	−	L,E,M	12-36	30-40
F X	Z	10-12	Stuart (Prower) factor	+	L	24-60	30-40
F VII	Z	1	Proconvertin	+	L	4-6	30-40
Tissue factor	C		Thromboplastin	−	—	—	—
F VIII:C	C	0.05-1	Antihemophilic factor A	−	L,E,M	10-14	30-40
vWF	C	10	vWF	−	L,E,M	—	—
F IX	Z	4-5	Christmas factor; antihemophilic factor B	+	L	18-30	30-40
F XI	Z	4-6	Plasma thromboplastin antecedent; antihemophilic factor C	−	L	120-168	20
F XII	Z	30	Hageman factor	−	L	52-60	None
F XIII	Z		Fibrin-stabilizing factor	−	L	72-168	1
Prekallikrein	Z	15-50	Fletcher factor	−	L	—	None
Protein C	Z,I	4	—	+	L	—	
Protein S	C	35	—	+	L	—	
High molecular weight kininogen	C	70-90	Fitzgerald factor	−	L	—	None
Plasminogen	Z	200	—	−	L		
Plasminogen activator(s)	Z		—	−	L,E		
Urokinase	Z		—	−	E		
AT-III	I	150	AT-III heparin cofactor	−	L		
α₂-Plasmin inhibitor	I	70	Antiplasmin	−	L		
α₂-Macroglobulin	I	2.5	—	−	L		

*S = substrate; Z = zymogen; C = cofactor; I = inhibitor.

†L = liver; E = endothelium; M = megakaryocyte/platelet.

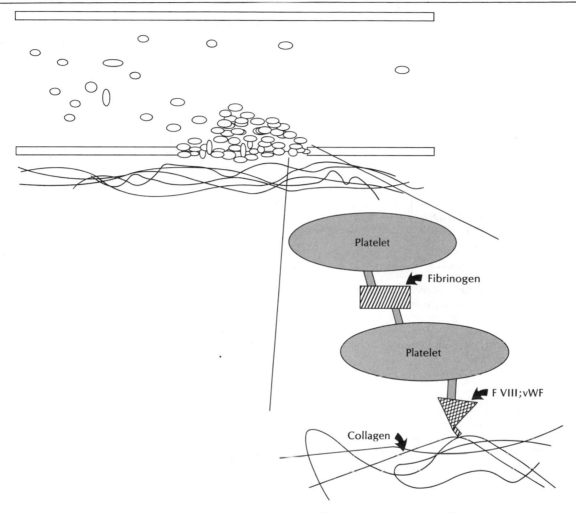

Fig. 19-3   Platelet plug formation is initiated by the adhesion of platelets to collagen mediated by vWF. Platelets then begin to aggregate, mediated by fibrinogen, and become caught in the developing fibrin mesh.

Table 19-2   Paradigms for Reactions of Fluid Phase Components

Enzyme	Zymogen/Cofactors/Surface	Product
F XIIa	F XI/HMWK/collagen	F XIa
F XIa	F IX/Ca^{+2}/ −	F IXa
F IXa	F X/F VIII:C(a); Ca^{+2}/PL	F Xa
"Injury" of tissue	F VI + TF/Ca^{+2}/PL?	F Xa
F Xa	Prothrombin (F II)/F V; Ca^{+2}/PL	Thrombin

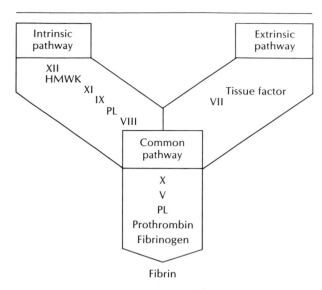

Fig. 19-4 Normal fluid phase components of the cascade may be organized into the intrinsic, extrinsic, and common pathways. (Modified from Wintrobe MM, Lee GR, Boggs DR, Bithell TC, Foerster J, Athens JW, Lukens JN, eds. Clinical Hematology, 8th ed. Philadelphia: Lea & Febiger, 1981.)

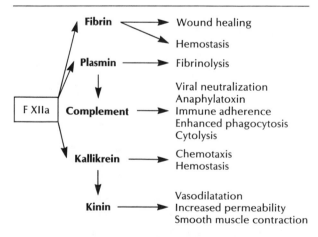

Fig. 19-5 Activated F XII (F XIIa) mediates many biologic reactions, only some of which are directly involved with hemostasis. Many of the phenomena illustrated are speculative. (From Wintrobe MM, Lee GR, Boggs DR, Bithell TC, Foerster J, Athens JW, Lukens JN, eds. Clinical Hematology, 8th ed. Philadelphia: Lea & Febiger, 1981.)

enough to one another as well as to a reaction surface for the reaction to occur. They often utilize similar or even identical mechanisms (probably reflecting a common genetic origin). An example is the multiply carboxylated "vitamin K–dependent" factors: F II,* F VII, F IX, and F X. All these reactions lead to the formation of thrombin, the pivotal product of the fluid portion of hemostasis. A division into two routes to thrombin formation has been described, although they are not meant to be considered independent of one another.

The so-called intrinsic system begins with a conformational change of F XII by exposure to collagen or basement membrane (Fig. 19-4). This leads to formation of F XIIz, which then cleaves F XI to its activated form, F XIa. High molecular weight kininogen (HMWK) acts as cofactor for F XIIa action on other zymogens as well as a source of bradykinin. Additional products of F XIIa include kallikrein and plasmin (Fig. 19-5). F XIa interacts with the next zymogen/cofactor: F IX/Ca^{+2} (a surface is not required here). This in turn produces F IXa, the interactant for a third group of reactants: F X/F VIII:C; Ca^{+2}/PL producing F Xa. The alternative "extrinsic system" varies slightly on this theme. A glycoprotein, tissue thromboplastin, or so-called tissue factor (TF) borne by most nonvascular tissues as well as the vascular endothelium and leukocytes, but in a "crypted" (hidden) form, complexes with F VII (here not requiring a surface) and through simple conformational changes there results F VIIa. The complex F X/Ca^{+2}/PL is the target of F VIIa; F X is converted to F Xa. Production of F Xa, the confluence point of these two tributaries, leads into the main ("common") pathway also acting on a similar theme: prothrombin/F V; Ca^{+2}/PL. Thrombin is generated, which is the crucial product of the entire cascade. Thrombin has several unique features separating it from the other vitamin K–dependent factors. Instead of remaining attached to a surface it is solubilized and released into the environment of the developing hemostatic unit. Left untethered, the thrombin could precipitate a pro-

---

*Throughout this chapter procoagulants (zymogens) will be written "FY," whereas activated factors (enzymes) will be called "FYa." The "Y" will be any of the traditional Roman numerals (e.g., F IX). Exceptions include thrombin (F IIa), fibrinogen (F I), etc. (see Table 19-1). Cofactors, too, exhibit parallel characteristics and function, e.g., F V and F VIII:C.

found effect on regional and systemic clotting mechanisms. It has been estimated that there is enough thrombin produced in a small clot to thrombose the entire body in a matter of a few seconds. Clearly, regulatory mechanisms must exist to localize thrombin's effect and prevent its causing systemic damage. The primary target of thrombin activity is fibrinogen, a large linear protein with the unique capacity of being polymerized electrostatically and then covalently cross-linked to form a structural net (the fibrin clot). Thrombin affects the initial cleavage of fibrinogen, resulting in an "unstable" polymer of fibrin, but also activates F XIII to F XIIIa, which can chemically connect these fibrin strands to form the stable three-dimensional mesh. Thrombin also can increase cofactor activity (particularly F V and F VIII:C).

Regulatory proteins of thrombin act by "sheathing" the molecule. This is accomplished by several factors, the most important of which is antithrombin III (AT-III) under the influence of heparin. AT-III also modifies other enzyme activities, including F IXa, F Xa, F XIa, and F XIIa. Other regulatory cofactors include protein C, which inhibits F V and F Va as well as F VIII:C and F VIII:Ca. Protein S enhances protein C inhibition. Additional regulatory factors include α_2-antiplasmin and α_2-macroglobulin. The latter is a nonspecific binder inhibitor that may provide a sequestered "pool" of activated coagulation factors. Regulation also includes removal of activated coagulant factors and reaction products, primarily by the liver and other reticuloendothelium system (RES) components.

Fibrinolysis acts by regular cleavage of the fibrin net. This normally is targeted to cross-linked fibrin and is mediated by plasmin, which is the cleavage product of the zymogen plasminogen. Plasminogen is usually interwoven into the fibrin net and so it remains localized. With slow activation of plasminogen, the fibrin net will be disassembled over a period of time. Activation of plasminogen results from various "plasminogen activators" (PAs) found in tissue and plasma. The plasma PAs are mediated by F XIIa, whereas tissue PAs include endothelium-based enzymes (tissue plasminogen activator [TPA] and urokinase) and poorly characterized enzymes found in specific organs. The endothelium activators likely play the most important role in normal clot dissolution. Extensive organ damage may result in

excessive plasmin production as a consequence of activator release. With pathologic fibrinolysis, uncross-linked fibrin strands and even fibrinogen may be digested. As mentioned above, α_2-antiplasmin controls plasmin activity. The products of these reactions, so-called fibrin degradation (or split) products (FDPs or FSPs), are cleared by the liver. In excess, FDPs may interact with sites usually reserved for fibrin or fibrinogen and compromise many hemostatic processes.

Acquired Abnormalities in Hemostasis

A congenital abnormality in hemostasis usually represents a single lesion in the complex network. The effect, albeit clinically significant, often can be handled by correcting the singular abnormality. Acquired abnormalities often involve multiple factors being compromised, resulting in a panoply of clinical manifestations and consequences demanding multiple therapeutic maneuvers.

Disseminated Intravascular Coagulation

Disseminated intravascular coagulation (DIC) is a constellation of abnormalities in hemostasis in which the integrity of the hemostatic balance is compromised by an overly zealous production and/or destruction of the formed clot (Fig. 19-6). Mediated by many different factors, DIC, instead of being a disease, is actually a syndrome characterized by excessive utilization of coagulation factors (both cellular and fluid) that exceeds the replenishment capacity of the organism and results in either the formation of an excessive amount of thrombus or excessive bleeding secondary to the failure of clot formation. The usual events that precede the onset of clinically significant hemostatic failure are massive or unrestrained activation of the hemostatic processes. These can be classified into several large groups. Leading these are infections. Many bacterial processes elicit activating factors initiating the intrinsic system. Additionally, endothelial damage and/or tissue damage may further augment intrinsic stimulation as well as activate the extrinsic pathway. Normally this would result in the formation of a localized clot, but if excessive amounts of stimulus occur, generalized clotting may result, even in the distant vasculature. Intravascular fibrin strands can contribute to mechanical red cell destruction (microangiopathic hemolytic anemia). Additionally, clotting cascade activation may have a secondary and even tertiary effect, involving the fibrinolytic as well as vasoactive (kallikrein and complement) systems. This results in the formation of fibrinolytic proteins, vasoconstriction, and other detrimental processes. With excessive activation, fibrinolysis, acting first on formed fibrin, may extend its effect, catabolizing fibrinogen. FDPs interfere with normal hemostasis. As fibrinogen stores are depleted, the body compensates in an attempt to continue to form fibrin, particularly with continued stimulus from thrombogenic factors (e.g., uncontrolled infection). This results in many factors being totally consumed. Platelets are rapidly utilized in an attempt to "plug" bleeding sites. Those factors have a very short half-life, or those slowly synthesized are not able to be replenished quickly enough. Subsequently the ability to form a clot is ablated and the patient has an overall failure in clot formation, leading to dis-

seminated bleeding. If for some reason the fibrinolytic network is not activated or fails, the excessive stimulus can result in extensive thrombosis, with small vessels being particular targets. Gangrenous necrosis may result.

The basic therapeutic approach is not simply to correct the abnormality(ies) by replenishing factor(s), although this is an appropriate component of treatment (see below), but to address the etiology of the initiator of clotting (i.e., correct the underlying disorder). Once this has been accomplished, subsequent hemostatic corrections may be undertaken without throwing coagulation components into a "large hole." Another tenant in the approach to DIC is to repair first the weakest link in the chain of coagulation. If fluid factors have failed through excessive consumption, transfusing with appropriate

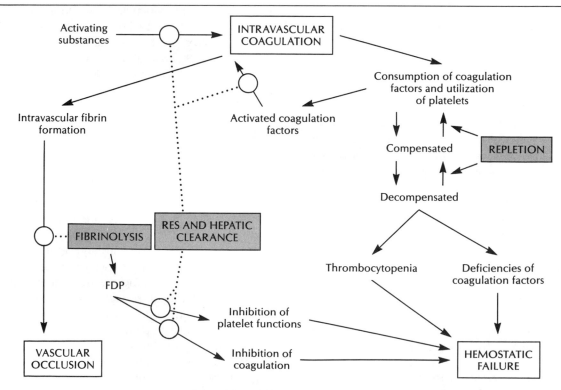

Fig. 19-6 The pathogenesis of DIC. Compensatory mechanisms are in screened blocks. (From Wintrobe MM, Lee GR, Boggs DR, Bithell TC, Foerster J, Athens JW, Lukens JN, eds. Clinical Hematology, 8th ed. Philadelphia: Lea & Febiger, 1981.)

plasma components containing the deficient factor(s) is indicated. If the patient is thrombocytopenic and the bleeding appears to reflect deficiency of platelets, platelet transfusion is in order. (NOTE: Thrombocytopenia is often slow to disappear after DIC. Without clinical bleeding, platelet transfusions are usually not needed.) Heparin has been advocated by some. In theory, its use attempts to "block" consumption of coagulant factors by inhibiting several cascade reactions. Convincing efficacy data have not appeared and use of heparin remains controversial. On occasion, several component needs may have to be addressed. Therapy has to be tailored to the clinical as well as laboratory information available.

Acquired Abnormalities of Platelets

Examining the characteristics of abnormalities involving the cellular component of hemostasis, the platelet is obviously a primary role player. Both quantitative and qualitative abnormalities are recognized, but some clinical conditions have abnormalities in both.

FACTORS ASSOCIATED WITH DIC*

Injury to endothelial cells and/or activation of intrinsic system

Gram-negative sepsis
Gram-positive sepsis
Rocky Mountain spotted fever
Fungal infections
Protozoal infections
Viruses
Angiography
Prolonged hypotension
Severe acidosis
Diabetic ketoacidosis
Hypoxemia
Polycythemia and stasis
Intrauterine growth retardation
Cavernous hemangioma
Lymphangioma

Tissue injury with liberation of tissue thromboplastin activity and activation of the extrinsic system

Obstetric complications
    Abruptio placentae
    Amniotic fluid embolism
    Dead twin fetus
    Eclampsia and preeclampsia
Brain injury
Surgical procedures: cardiopulmonary bypass
Trauma
Extensive burns

Heat stroke
Rhabdomyolysis
Drowning
Necrotizing enterocolitis
Neoplasms
    Acute promyelocytic leukemia
    Acute nonlymphocytic and acute lymphocytic leukemia
    Solid tumors

Direct activation: F II, F X

Snake venom

Red blood cell, platelet, or immunologic injury

Intravascular hemolysis
    Incompatible RBC transfusion
    Severe erythroblastosis fetalis
Antigen-antibody reactions
    Renal transplant reactions

RES injury with decreased clearance of activated coagulation factors

RES hypofunction
Hepatic disease

Miscellaneous

Congenital deficiency of anticoagulants (e.g., protein C deficiency)
Types II and IV hyperlipidemias
F IX replacement therapy

*Modified from Stuart MJ, Kelton JG. The platelet: Quantitative and qualitative abnormalities. In Nathan DG, Oski FA, eds. Hematology of Infancy and Childhood, 3rd ed. Philadelphia: WB Saunders, 1987.

Quantitative abnormalities of platelets

Thrombocytopenia. Factitious abnormalities in platelet enumeration are probably more common than is appreciated. The normal platelet count for children ranges from 150,000 to 450,000/mm³. Since these counts are often determined by electronic counting devices, statistical errors may creep into the determination and account for false data. This can be compounded by the effect of the anticoagulant used (EDTA), the presence of agglutinins that are active at room temperature, and "satellitism," in which platelets adhere to other cellular components of the blood. Examination of the peripheral blood smear should be used as a means of substantiating true thrombocytopenia.

Thrombocytopenia can be asssigned to one of three mechanisms: (1) increased destruction exceeding the capacity of replacement, (2) primary failure of production, or (3) sequestration.

Increased destruction. The increased destruction of platelets can be mediated either by immune or nonimmune mechanisms. The classic example of immune thrombocytopenia in children is so-called acute idiopathic (?immune) thrombocytopenic purpura (ITP). Seen in all ages of pediatric patients, it peaks between the ages of 2 and 5 years. There is an equal incidence between boys and girls and no racial differences. The medical history often reports a viral infection within 2 to 3 weeks of the onset of spon-

---

ACQUIRED QUANTITATIVE ABNORMALITIES IN PLATELETS*

Destructive thrombocytopenia

Primary platelet consumption
  Immune
    Idiopathic thrombocytopenic purpura
    Drug-induced thrombocytopenia
    Infection-induced thrombocytopenia
    Posttransfusion purpura
    Autoimmune or lymphoproliferative disorders
    Neonatal immune thrombocytopenia
    Allergy and anaphylaxis
    Posttransplant thrombocytopenia
  Nonimmune
    Chronic microangiopathic hemolytic anemia and thrombocytopenia
    Hemolytic uremic syndrome
    Thrombotic thrombocytopenic purpura
    Catheters, prostheses, or cardiopulmonary bypass
    Congenital or acquired heart disease
Combined platelet and fibrinogen consumption
  DIC
  Kasabach-Merritt syndrome
  Other causes of local consumption coagulopathy
Miscellaneous
  Specific to the neonate
    Phototherapy
    Perinatal aspiration syndromes

Persistent pulmonary hypertension
Rhesus alloimmunization
Following exchange transfusion
Polycythemia
Metabolic acidosis
Glomerular disease
Preeclampsia
Fatty acid–induced thrombocytopenia

Impaired or ineffective production

Metabolic disorders
  Methylmalonic acidemia
  Ketotic hyperglycinemia
  Holocarboxylase synthetase deficiency
  Isovaleric acidemia
Aplastic anemia
Marrow infiltrative processes
Drug- or radiation-induced; following bone marrow transplantation
Nutritional deficiency states (iron, folate, or vitamin B_{12})

Sequestration

Hypersplenism
Hypothermia

---

*Modified from Stuart MJ, Kelton JG. The platelet: Quantitative and qualitative abnormalities. In Nathan DG, Oski FA, eds. Hematology of Infancy and Childhood, 3rd ed. Philadelphia: WB Saunders, 1987.

taneous bruising. It is presumed antibodies are generated that become associated with platelets. These children not uncommonly are brought to the attention of the physician because physical abuse is suspected. A careful history should reveal no other associated abnormalities that might suggest either a congenital immune etiology (such as the Wiscott-Aldrich syndrome) or familial thrombocytopenia. Physical examination is important to establish the nature and extent of bleeding as well as any associated signs that might suggest alternative etiologies. The presence of mucous membrane purpura (so-called wet purpura) should alert the physician to the increased potential for catastrophic CNS bleeding. The presence of lymphadenopathy and/or hepatosplenomegaly would suggest a marrow-based hematologic abnormality. Laboratory values are often characterized by a profound thrombocytopenia, commonly less than 20,000/mm³, with an otherwise benign peripheral smear. Occasionally the patient may demonstrate a mild increase in mean red cell volume and reticulocyte count, particularly if there has been any substantial bleeding. Various therapeutic approaches have been considered, although none is clearly determined to be absolutely appropriate. Since this process is self-limited, it has been argued that intervention is unnecessary. However, a concern derives from the potential risk of life-threatening bleeding (particularly into the CNS) as well as from compromise of day-to-day activities. Patients often will have a spontaneous remission within 2 to 6 weeks of diagnosis. Pharmaceutical intervention has been advocated by some. This has ranged from the use of corticosteroids to immunosuppressive chemotherapy. A recent development is the use of intravenous immunoglobulin (IVIgG). The RES is thought responsible for clearance of immunoglobulin-tagged platelets. Administration of IVIgG potentially "blockades" the RES, diminishing the removal of the platelets. However, this has proved an expensive and only temporizing process. Therapy must be chosen based on the clinical needs of the patient. In cases of life-threatening bleeding, administration of platelets may be appropriate prior to surgical intervention (see below). Giving platelets in less significant settings is to no avail since exogenous platelets, like the intrinsic platelets, are susceptible to immunologic removal. Splenectomy has been performed in emergency circumstances. Following splenectomy for acute ITP commonly there is a dramatic rise in platelet numbers

and arrest of bleeding. The platelet count after splenectomy sometimes exceeds 1 million/mm³, but eventually returns to lower values (although often above the normal range). This transient thrombocytosis is not associated with excessive risk of thrombosis and does not require therapeutic intervention. By definition patients with "acute" ITP recover in less than 6 months. "Chronic" ITP in children is defined similarly to the acute form except that it lasts beyond 6 months. It is often associated with other autoimmune diseases, and thus a comprehensive workup of the immune system is indicated. Girls exceed boys in incidence, probably reflecting the higher frequency of autoimmune disease in females. This disease usually is treated with immunosuppression, often with steroids or IVIgG followed by splenectomy. Splenectomy usually is withheld for younger children because of the risks of sepsis after splenectomy. One curious variation of this theme is the so-called Evans syndrome, which is an autoimmune process involving not only platelets but red cells. Coombs' (direct antibody) test is positive in this condition. It has been recognized that individuals with Evans' syndrome are more prone to long-term consequences associated with significant bleeding and ultimately life-threatening complications. Immunosuppression is the indicated therapy. Other immunologically induced thrombocytopenias include the interaction with drugs, either by affecting platelet antigens so that immunologic surveillance removes these abnormal platelets or by functioning as a hapten.

In the context of transplantation of organs the presence of thrombocytopenia may in fact reflect the overall rejection phenomenon. However, thrombocytopenia is sometimes seen in individuals who are not undergoing rejection. Clearly, in the context of bone marrow transplantation, thrombocytopenia may reflect the rejection of the marrow (as well as slow or incomplete engraftment). Immune complexes seen in allergy and associated diseases have been incriminated as causative of thrombocytopenia. However, this has been incompletely investigated. A variety of other immune diseases have been associated with thrombocytopenia.

A major category of decreased platelet numbers is seen with transfusions in which alloimmunization or isoimmunization (in the newborn) occurs. In spontaneous alloimmunization (a rare event), autoantibodies are the likely cause, although this has not been completely established. Transfusion of

DRUGS REPORTED TO CAUSE IMMUNE THROMBOCYTOPENIA

Acetaminophen	Ethchlorvynol	Phenoximide
Acetazolamide	Fenoprofen	Phenylbutazone
Acetylsalicylic acid (aspirin)	Gold salts	Phenyldimethylisopropylpyrozolone
Actinomycin D	Heparin	Procainamide
Allylisopropylcarbamide	Hydrochloroquin	Propylthiouracil
Antazoline	Hydrochlorothiazide	Quinidine
Carbamazepine	Imipramine	Quinine
Centalin	Isoniazid	Rifampin
Cephalothin	Levodopa	Sodium valproate
Chlorazepam	Lidocaine	Streptomycin
Chloroquine	Meprobamate	Sulfamethazine
Chlorothiazide	Methicillin	Sulfathiazole
Chlorpheniramine	Methyldopa	Sulfisoxazole
Chlorpromazine	Novobiocin	Sulfonamide
Chlorpropamide	Organic arsenicals	Tetracycline
Desipramine	Oxyphenbutazone	Tolbutamide
Diazepam	Para-aminosalicylic acid	Trimethoprim-sulfamethoxazole
Digitoxin	Penicillin	
Diphenylhydantoin	Phenothiazine	

large amounts of platelets may result in development of transfusion alloantibodies, limiting effectiveness of subsequent transfusions. Single-donor platelet sources or even HLA-matched donors may provide palliation in some patients. Isoimmune thrombocytopenia is seen in the newborn period in which (as in Rhesus [Rh] immunization) the platelet antigen–negative mother is immunized by the platelet antigen–positive platelets from the fetus. IgG antibodies develop and then are passed to the fetus transplacentally. Another circumstance in which the fetus may be affected by maternal antibodies is when the mother has developed an IgG autoantibody (as in chronic ITP), which is passed across the placenta. The process is often self-limited in the child. Therapy is usually not indicated, although transfusion of maternal platelets (for isoimmune, not autoimmune, disease) may arrest significant bleeding.

Infections, including bacterial, viral, and parasitic, have been implicated in immune thrombocytopenia. Although possibly related to the presence of DIC, bacterial infection is believed occasionally to induce excessive amounts of immunoglobulin that may bind to the platelet, leading to increased removal. Additional mechanisms may play a role in the thrombocytopenia associated with bacteremia. Viruses, too, are incriminated with direct as well as immune-mediated mechanisms for thrombocytopenia. Protozoa, particularly malaria, have been incriminated as causative agents as well. IgG generated against the malarial organism has been found to co-bind with the parasite and platelet, with subsequent removal of both.

Decreased numbers of platelets can result from nonimmune mechanisms as well. Hemolytic-uremic syndrome (HUS) and thrombotic thrombocytopenic purpura (TTP) are classic examples. Current theory holds that an unidentified plasma factor(s) is missing or is inhibited, resulting in a thrombotic process, with the kidney the "target" for damage in HUS and the CNS in TTP. Both platelet numbers and function may be abnormal. Microangiopathic hemolytic anemia is commonly a part of HUS. Plasma transfusion or plasmapheresis has an ameliorating effect on these processes.

Thrombocytopenia has been seen in individuals with cyanotic congenital heart disease (CCHD). Usually these individuals have elevated hematocrit levels.

The associated aberrant rheology may result in not only stasis but local coagulation. This has not been clearly established, however. Hemostatic mechanisms seem to be quite variable from patient to patient. Some kinetic studies have substantiated that platelet survival is diminished and likewise functional abnormalities have been described in CCHD, although clinical bleeding is usually not appreciated. One cautionary note is that in the presence of an elevated hematocrit, factitious prolongation of the coagulation studies (activated partial thromboplastin time, prothrombin time) may occur. Adjustment must be made for the amount of anticoagulant in the collection vessel. "Naturally" occurring valvular heart disease has been associated with thrombocytopenia. This is probably a function of increased consumption as well as activation of platelets.

The presence of foreign bodies in the circulation (venous catheters, prosthetic valves, etc.) provides a ready site for platelet adhesion and aggregation with subsequent consumption. This may be seen to evolve shortly after the placement of the foreign material and slowly correct with time. Obviously the activation by these devices of the whole hemostatic network can play a role in consumption of platelets (DIC). In patients placed on extracorporeal circulation not only can consumption of platelets be identified, but sequestration and dilution may play roles as well. As will be mentioned below, platelet function may be affected so that even with correction to normal numbers, bleeding may remain a problem.

Like DIC, the giant hemangioma syndrome (of Kasabach-Merritt) is associated with thrombocytopenia. This is believed to represent a localized intravascular coagulation (LIC) resulting from the low flow through the cavernous hemangiomatous tissue. There also appear to be abnormalities in the endothelium that provide stimulation for platelet adhesion and aggregation.

Additional causes of destructive thrombocytopenia can include glomerular disease such as glomerulonephritis, but exactly what the mechanism is for this loss of platelets into the glomeruli is unclear. Both immunologic factors as well as platelet activation by abnormal vascular lesions have been suggested. The platelet also may play a role in the actual pathogenesis of the glomerular damage.

Premature neonates have been noted to have thrombocytopenia, often attributed to DIC or immune mechanisms. With exchange transfusion, thrombocytopenia is certainly to be expected. Additionally, bacterial sepsis may play a role. Thrombocytopenia is not uncommonly seen in respiratory distress syndrome and necrotizing enterocolitis. Phototherapy, too, has been incriminated as causative of thrombocytopenia. The specific mechanism here is unclear, although aberrations of platelet chemistry and morphology have been described. In the polycythemic newborn (as in CCHD), thrombocytopenia can occur (see Chapter 38). Hyperlipidemia has been associated with thrombocytopenia, although careful studies have not reproduced the finding consistently. Preeclampsia has been associated with thrombocytopenia, possibly the result of vascular endothelial damage and elevated amounts of maternal immunoglobulin. Activation of the platelets is seen as well. It is of interest that thrombocytopenia is not uncommonly seen in infants born of mothers who are preeclamptic and thrombocytopenic. This is thought to reflect consumption of platelets as well as immunologic and vascular abnormalities in the newborn.

Decreased production. Decreased numbers of platelets can be found in individuals in whom actual production is impaired. This would be seen in the various bone marrow failure syndromes such as aplastic anemia, leukemia, or drug-induced suppression from either cancer chemotherapy or radiation or drugs such as chloramphenicol. Also poor or slow engraftment after bone marrow transplantation may cause low platelet counts.

Sequestration. Not only can abnormalities in numbers of platelets result from increased removal or decreased production, but also from sequestration of platelets. If for any reason the spleen becomes overly effective or enlarged, platelets may be trapped or pooled. There is often an associated decrease in red cell and white cell numbers. Usually there is no associated bleeding. Splenectomy often results in recovery of the platelet count to the normal range. As pointed out on p. 161, thrombocytosis follows splenectomy, although usually counts return to normal or slightly elevated values. Occasionally, with severe cooling of the body (<25° C), platelet counts may fall. This is thought to represent an aggregation in the circulation of platelets. It appears to be reversible with warming.

Thrombocytosis. Quantitative abnormalities in platelets also include excessive numbers. These can be classified as either primary or secondary. Primary

CAUSES OF THROMBOCYTOSIS IN INFANCY AND CHILDHOOD*

Primary or autonomous thrombocytosis

Myeloproliferative syndromes
  Essential thrombocythemia
  Polycythemia vera
  Chronic myelogenous leukemia
  Myeloid metaplasia
  5q- syndrome

Secondary or reactive thrombocytosis

Inflammatory disease
  Acute infections
  Acute rheumatic fever
  Rheumatoid arthritis
  Ankylosing spondylitis
  Ulcerative colitis
  Regional enteritis
  Celiac sprue
  Tuberculosis
  Sarcoid
  Chronic hepatitis
  Chronic osteomyelitis
Drug-induced
  Epinephrine
  Vinca alkaloids
  Therapy for iron deficiency or vitamin B_{12} deficiency
  Passively addicted neonates

Immune disorders
  Collagen vascular disorders
  Graft-vs.-host disease
  Nephrotic syndrome
Hematologic disorders
  Iron deficiency
  Vitamin E deficiency
  Chronic hemolytic anemias and hemoglobinopathies
  "Rebound" following thrombocytopenia
Neoplasms
  Lymphomas
  Hodgkin's disease
  Neuroblastoma
  Hepatoblastoma
  Other childhood solid tumors
  Carcinomas
Surgical or functional asplenia
Miscellaneous
  Following hemorrhage or GI blood loss
  Following surgery
  Following exercise
  Caffey's disease
  Kawasaki syndrome

*Modified from Stuart MJ, Kelton JG. The platelet: Quantitative and qualitative abnormalities. In Nathan DG, Oski FA, eds. Hematology of Infancy and Childhood, 3rd ed. Philadelphia: WB Saunders, 1987.

CLINICAL CONDITIONS REPORTED ASSOCIATED WITH ACQUIRED QUALITATIVE ABNORMALITIES IN PLATELETS

Antiplatelet antibodies
Asthma, allergic rhinitis
Chronic hemodialysis
Diabetes mellitus
DIC
Drug exposure (e.g., see p. 166)
Essential fatty acid deficiency
Extracorporeal circulation
Fructose-1,6-diphosphate deficiency
Glycogen storage disease (type I)

Heart disease, congenital and valvular
Hemoglobinopathies (SS) and thalassemia
Hemophilia A
Hepatic disease
Homocystinuria
HUS
Hyperlipoproteinemia (type II)
Infections
Leukemia (acute and chronic)

Myelofibrosis
Myeloproliferative disorders
Paraproteinemia
Pernicious anemia
Platelet storage
Polycythemia vera
Renal transplant rejection
Renal disease
Scurvy
Uremia

thrombocytosis is associated with the myeloproliferative disorders, abnormalities rare in children. It is usually associated with a qualitative defect in platelet function as well. The problems associated with this can include both thrombosis and bleeding. Secondary thrombocytosis can result from inflammation, drugs, immune factors, other blood diseases, neoplasms, the absence of the spleen, as well as miscellaneous disorders. Generally hemostatic therapy is not indicated in most of these disorders.

Qualitative abnormalities of platelets: Thrombocytopathies

Components of platelet function include adhesion, aggregation, activation, secretion, and platelet coagulant interaction. Abnormalities in platelet function can be acquired. One large group of children who develop platelet dysfunction are those who are uremic. The uremia (or other plasma factors) has a direct effect on the platelet, although accompanying fluid coagulation abnormalities may play a role in clinical bleeding. Several mechanisms have been suggested, including abnormalities in the platelet–vascular wall interaction through prostaglandins. Unfortunately transfusion of normal platelets does not correct the lesion, as the exogenous platelets acquire the same abnormality. Cryoprecipitate or desmopressin complex (DDAVP) may have transient benefit. Effective dialysis may prove beneficial as well. Liver disease may have an associated qualitative platelet abnormality. This possibly relates to decreased synthesis by the liver of cofactors integral in platelet function as well as impaired clearance of coagulation products, specifically FDPs seen in the production of fibrin and its removal. FDPs may interfere with the aggregation of platelets, since fibrinogen interacts with the proteins of the platelet surface in order to produce aggregation. The use of DDAVP, which releases stored vWF, has been suggested for clinical bleeding. The role of vWF in platelet function is described elsewhere. Extracorporeal circulation as well as congenital and acquired cardiac lesions (as described above) may result not only in decreased platelet numbers but also exhaustion of platelet components by prolonged activation. Administration of normal platelets should temporarily correct a bleeding problem.

Myeloproliferative disorders have been associated with a derangement of platelet function as well as platelet numbers. This is a rare disease and the underlying process must be dealt with in order to correct the lesion. The use of aspirin or other platelet-active agents may prove of some therapeutic value to these patients (see below). Aspirin, however, has been noted to actually cause bleeding in some patients with myeloproliferative disorders. The more common leukemias have also been associated with thrombocytopathies. Although usually found in acute, nonlymphocytic leukemia, acute lymphocytic leukemia has been described as having an associated platelet dysfunction. Along with leukemia chemotherapy, treatment with platelet transfusion is needed for bleeding.

Drugs have an association of impairment of platelet function, probably by affecting several metabolic systems, including arachidonic acid metabolism. A classic agent is a nonsteroidal anti-inflammatory, aspirin. Aspirin acetylates the enzymes of the prostaglandin system, rendering platelets incapable of producing intrinsic metabolities. This results in a partially impaired hemostasis system, aggravating any concomitant hemostatic lesion such as thrombocytopenia. Antibiotics, too, have been noted to contribute to platelet dysfunction. Semisynthetic penicillins in particular are incriminated, along with the cephalosporins. Additional drugs affecting platelet function are listed below.

Qualitative lesions of platelets may result in "hypercoagulability" or increased chance of thrombosis. This is more a theoretic concept and very difficult to characterize. No common laboratory tests clearly define this entity. It has been seen in various settings.

Acquired Abnormalities of Fluid Factors

The other major category of acquired hemostatic abnormalities is that involving disorders in the fluid phase of hemostasis. These include (1) abnormalities in fluid factor synthesis, (2) hepatic disease, DIC, and inhibitors. One of the most common is vitamin K deficiency seen in the newborn. As pointed out above, vitamin K is an integral part of the carboxylation of several of the hemostatic factors (F II, F VIII, F IX, F X, and proteins S and C). Carboxylation is an integral component in adhesion to substrates and surfaces. The newborn infant often is deficient in vitamin K at the time of delivery. Unsupplemented, the child may develop a significant hemostatic problem shortly after birth. Beyond the newborn period, vitamin K is absorbed from the gut. Any circumstance in which vitamin K is not made available, either

---

DRUGS REPORTED TO CAUSE QUALITATIVE ABNORMALITIES IN PLATELETS

Amantadine	Glyceryl guaiacolate	Phenylbutazone
Aspirin	Heparin	Promethazine
Carbamazepine	Ibuprofen	Propranolol
Clofibrate	Indomethacin	Sodium valproate
Dextran and related agents	Nitrofurantoin	Sulfinpyrazone and related forms
Diphenhydramine	Papaverine	Sulindac
Diphenylhydantoin	Penicillins (ampicillin, carbenicil-	Tricyclic antidepressants
Dipyridamole	lin, mezlocillin, nafcillin, peni-	Vincristine
Ethanol	cillin G, piperacillin, ticarcillin)	

---

through malabsorption, inadequate diet, or antibiotic therapy modifying gut flora, may result in an acquired dysfunction of the coagulation factors and subsequent bleeding. Drugs, too, can produce an aberration in vitamin K metabolism. Coumarin impedes vitamin K–modulated carboxylation. The clinical presentation is of massive bleeding from virtually all sites of trauma as well as mucous membranes. Rapid, dramatic recovery is seen with administration of vitamin K. Anticoagulants, too, such as heparin, have been found on occasion to affect the amount of coagulation factor present.

Liver disease is associated with acquired coagulation abnormalities. As pointed out in Table 19-1, F V, F VII, F IX, F X, F XI, F XII, F XIII, fibrinogen, prothrombin, prekallikrein, and high molecular weight kininogen are all synthesized by the liver. In addition, AT-III and proteins S and C as well as many of the inhibitors of fibrinolysis are of hepatic origin. Any derangement in the liver's capacity to synthesize one or several of these may result in significant hemostatic failure. Treatment is replacement of the diminished factor(s). Various plasma products contain several of the factors synthesized by the liver (Table 19-3). Hepatic clearance of activated factors as well as those that impair platelet function such as FDPs also may cause hemostatic problems.

Congenital heart disease has been associated with a loss of coagulation factors. This has been reported in both cyanotic and acyanotic lesions. In the cyanotic lesion the patient is often polycythemic and therefore has a problem with increased viscosity, possibly resulting in decreased flow and associated coagulation consumption. Renal failure, too, is associated with a

consumption of one or several of the hemostatic factors in addition to platelets. Nephrotic syndrome has been associated with urinary loss of the smaller coagulation factors as a part of the global proteinuria. These can include not only several of the procoagulants, but also AT-III and plasminogen, which might result in thrombosis.

Autoanticoagulants occasionally occur. These include the "lupus-like anticoagulant" described in normal children. Also antibodies directed against specific coagulant factors are seen in individuals with congenital deficiency of the native factor, for example, hemophilia A (F VIII:C deficiency) following exposure to exogenous (antigenic) factor concentrates. Diagnosis requires incubation studies of the patient's plasma with normal (factor-containing) plasma. Titers of inhibition (Bethesda units) are used to estimate the degree of immunologic response. In this clinical circumstance use of "activated" coagulant concentrates appears to have some benefit.

Acquired Abnormalities of Vascular Function

An additional abnormality should be mentioned in passing, the "vascular purpuras." These are associated with neither quantitative nor qualitative abnormalities of platelets nor fluid phase abnormalities, but probably represent a defect in vascular function such as a vasculitis with extravasation. The typical pediatric example is Schönlein-Henoch purpura.

Approach to the Bleeding Patient

As in most clinical conditions, obtaining a complete history (including drug history) and family history and performing a comprehensive physical exami-

CLINICAL CONDITIONS OR DISEASES THAT MAY BE ASSOCIATED WITH A "HYPERCOAGULABLE" STATE IN CHILDREN*

Acute peripheral arterial insufficiency
Arteriovenous shunts
Cancer
Cardiomyopathy, atrial fibrillation, mitral valve prolapse
Catheters
Chronic valvular heart disease
Cigarette smoking
Contraceptive therapy (estrogens)
Crohn's disease
Deep vein thrombosis
Diabetes mellitus
Diet high in saturated fats
DIC
Glomerular disease
Heparin therapy
Homocystinuria

HUS
Hyperbetalipoproteinemia type II
Hypercholesterolemia
Hypothermia
Intravenous therapy with clotting factor (especially F IX deficiency)
Kawasaki syndrome
Liver disease
Lupus anticoagulant
Myeloproliferative syndromes
Nephrotic syndrome
Nutritional deficiencies (vitamin E, selenium)
Oxygen toxicity
Placental insufficiency syndromes
Plasminogen and plasminogen-activator abnormalities

Postoperative state (especially cardiopulmonary and orthopedic)
Prosthetic devices in circulation
Preeclampsia
Pregnancy
Prosthetic devices in circulation
Protein C and S deficiencies
Renal allograft rejection
Sickle cell anemia
Snake venoms
Stasis
Streptokinase or coumarin therapy
TTP
Ulcerative colitis
Vasculitis
Ventriculojugular shunts

*Modified from Stuart MJ, Kelton JG. The platelet: Quantitative and qualitative abnormalities. In Nathan DG, Oski FA, eds. Hematology of Infancy and Childhood, 3rd ed. Philadelphia: WB Saunders, 1987.

Table 19-3   Coagulation Factors Contained in Various Plasma Products[1]

Plasma Products[2]	Plasma Fibrinogen	II/VII/IX/X	V/VIII:C	XI/XII	XIII	AT-III	Platelets
Plasma	+	+	(+)[3]	+	+	+	+/−[4]
FFP	+	+	(+)	+	+	+	−
Factor VIII:C	+	−	+ +	−	−	−	−
Porcine and bovine VIII:C	−	−	+ +[5]	−	−	−	−
Cryoppt	+ +[6]	−	+ +	−	−	−	−
PCC	−	+ +	−	−	−	−	−
APCC	−	+ +[7]	−[7]	−	−	−	−
Platelets	(+)	(+)	(+)	(+)	(+)	(+)	+ +

[1]All plasma products should be suspect for transmission of blood-borne infectious agents. Some products such as cryoprecipitate may have a reduced risk; commercial products prepared in ways that reduce or even eliminate some or all such risks may be available.
[2]Plasma = fresh plasma; FFP = fresh frozen plasma; VIII:C = F VIII:C concentrate; Cryoppt = cryoprecipitate; PCC = prothrombin complex concentrate (vitamin K–dependent factors); APCC = activated prothrombin complex concentrate; platelets = platelet concentrate.
[3]Parentheses indicate variable amounts of factor in the product.
[4]+/− indicates some products may or may not have the indicated factor.
[5]Porcine and bovine F VIII:C concentrates have uses limited only for patients developing inhibitors to human F VIII:C concentrate.
[6]Cryoprecipitate contains approximately 200 to 250 mg/bag.
[7]Activated vitamin K–dependent factors are used to bypass F VIII:C inhibition.

nation can help dissect out the cause of bleeding. In the context of a negative family history, acquired bleeding disorders need to be considered. Like normal hemostasis described previously, bleeding disorders may be classified clinically into large categories, for example, bleeding problems involving the vascular system or platelets vs. those involving the fluid phase. Characteristically, patients with vessel-platelet abnormalities have associated petechiae and superficial ecchymoses as well as bleeding from minor cuts and mucous membranes. In contrast, fluid hemostasis abnormalities are associated with deep-seated bleeding, often involving hematomas or bleeding into the gastrointestinal tract. Joints also may be subject to bleeds in the latter group. There is, however, such intermixing of all hemostatic mechanisms that acquired abnormalities may result in an overlap of many of these clinical findings. In the newborn period, abnormalities in bleeding may be associated with infection (DIC) or the lack of vitamin K (hemorrhagic disease of the newborn). Of note, excessive bleeding from the umbilical stump is characteristic of congenital F XIII deficiency. Many of the underlying factors associated with DIC, as with other acquired abnormalities, may not be apparent readily and a careful diagnostic examination may be needed.

MONITORING AND LABORATORY TESTS

Fortunately evaluation of the hemostatic mechanisms in children can be accomplished easily by the following coagulation screening tests:

> Platelet count (CBC)
> Bleeding time, template
> Prothrombin time (PT)
> Activated partial thromboplastin time (aPTT)
> Thrombin time (TT)
> Fibrinogen quantitation
> Fibrin degradation products (FDPs)
>
> NOTE: Normal values should be established in newborns and children by each individual laboratory.

Remembering the major divisions of the hemostatic mechanism, one can assess systematically the various components and with some degree of speed come to an adequate conclusion and then choose therapy. Evaluation of the vascular and platelet components may be accomplished by a platelet count and a template bleeding time (the only in vivo measure of platelet function). Thrombocytopenia alone will re-

sult in a prolonged bleeding time. Thus this test can only be used to evaluate platelet function when platelet numbers are normal. Determination of platelet numbers (along with a complete blood count and examination of the peripheral smear) may reveal information to help sort out the cause of bleeding. For example, microangiopathic changes of the red cell (schistocytes) or abnormal white cells (leukemic blasts) give a clue to an underlying abnormality. Occasionally bone marrow examination may be needed. Fluid hemostatic mechanisms may be evaluated with a select group of screening tests. The aPTT and the PT, along with the TT and the quantitation of plasma fibrinogen, provide an adequate beginning of assessment (Fig. 19-7). As shown in the accompanying figures, each of these tests evaluates portions of the cascade and appraises the possible sites of abnormality (Fig. 19-8). Additional tests that may prove of value include assessment of FDPs; evaluation of excessive heparin effect with reptilase time (reptilase directly converts fibrinogen to fibrin [like thrombin] but is not affected by the AT-III/heparin inhibitor); quantitation of individual factors; evaluation of inhibition of any of the factors (autoantibodies); and the euglobulin lysis test (testing for excessive fibrinolysis). Usually these are used when specific questions are raised and are not necessary in the initial evaluation or choice of therapy.

THERAPY

Various therapies can be used for correcting hemostatic failure. Drugs and plasma factors available for clinical use are listed in Table 19-4. Selection hinges on specific component needs supplemented by the information generated by the clinical setting.

Except in the context of increased destruction, platelet transfusions are usually effective in arresting bleeding secondary to thrombocytopenia or abnormal function of platelets. One unit of random donor platelets should raise the platelet count by 10,000 to 15,000/mm³. Resorting to single-donor (platelet pheresis) platelets or HLA-matched platelets is reserved for unique situations where allo- or isoimmunization creates the clinical problem. Unfortunately this still may not be effective. As pointed out above, the exogenous platelets may acquire the same lesion as intrinsic platelets in the context of continued activation, removal, or damage.

Administration of coagulation factors depends on

the particular needs and circumstances of the patient. If a specific factor is needed, such as F VIII:C or F IX, commercial concentrates are available. Fresh frozen plasma (FFP) contains multiple factors, although in small concentrations. Volume overload is the limiting consequence of the use of FFP. Of note, cryoprecipitate contains high concentrations of F VIII:C, fibrinogen, and vWF and variable amounts of F XIII. Approximately 100 units of F VIII:C activity is found in each bag of cryoprecipitate. Less commonly APCC, which contains several activated factors, is used. This therapy is reserved for individuals who have developed F VIII:C inhibitors. Investigational agents such as AT-III concentrates and coagulation factors cloned from DNA are still not available for routine clinical use.

Drugs that may find use in the treatment of a patient with a bleeding disorder include epsilon aminocaproic acid (EACA), which inhibits plasminogen activation, as does tranexamic acid. DDAVP, an analog of arginine vasopressin, effects release of vWF and F VIII from the endothelial cells. The effect lasts for approximately 12 hours. Subsequent administration of DDAVP may not effect as dramatic a response, probably reflecting depletion of stores of F VIII activity. Heparin activates AT-III in plasma, which

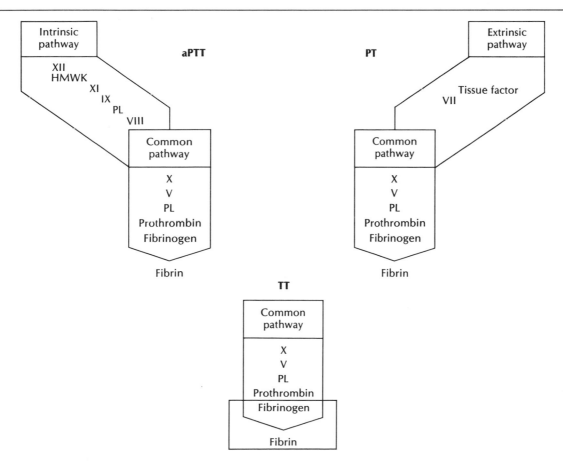

Fig. 19-7 Various laboratory screening tests are used to evaluate the components of the fluid phase cascade. (Modified from Wintrobe MM, Lee GR, Boggs DR, Bithell TC, Foerster J, Athens JW, Lukens JN, eds. Clinical Hematology, 8th ed. Philadelphia: Lea & Febiger, 1981.)

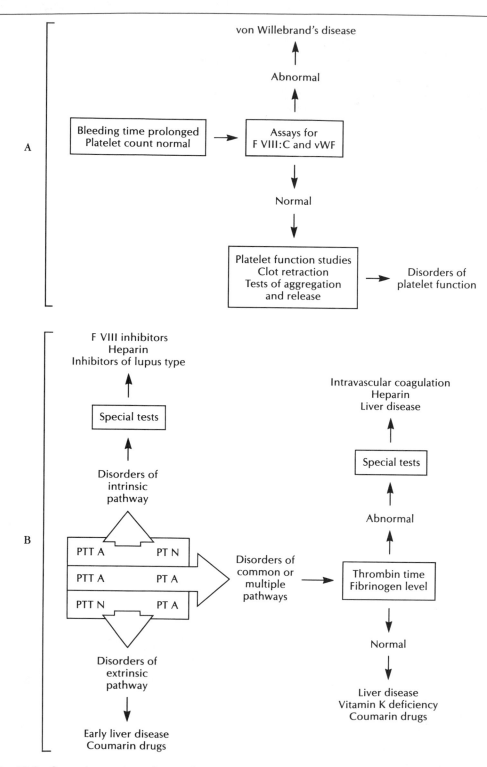

Fig. 19-8 Screening tests can be used to narrow the possibilities of acquired hemostatic failure. **A,** Platelet-vascular abnormalities. **B,** Fluid phase abnormalities. (NOTE: "N" and "A" relate to normal and abnormal values, respectively, of the PT and PTT.) (From Wintrobe MM, Lee GR, Boggs DR, Bithell TC, Foerster J, Athens JW, Lukens JN, eds. Clinical Hematology, 8th ed. Philadelphia: Lea & Febiger, 1981.)

Table 19-4   Therapeutic Agents for Use in Hemostatic Failure

Agent	Dose
Plasma factors	
Platelets	10,000-15,000/mm³/unit
FFP	10 ml/kg
F VIII	0.5% F VIII:C activity/unit/kg
Cryoppt	~100 units F VIII:C activity/bag
PCC (F IX)	1% F IX activity/unit/kg
APCC	75 units/kg of F IX to bypass F VIII:C inhibitor
Drugs	
EACA*	300 mg/kg PO (loading), then 100 mg/kg PO divided q 6 hr; maximum 24 g/day
Tranexamic acid*	100 mg/kg/day PO divided q 6 hr
DDAVP	0.3 μg/kg IV; repeat 1-2 times q 12 hr
Heparin	100 units/kg IV or SC, q 4 hr *or* 100 units/kg IV or SC (loading), then 25 units/kg by continuous infusion
Vitamin K	5-10 mg IV; 0.5 mg/kg to counteract coumarin
Protamine sulfate	1-1.5 mg/100 units of heparin
Aspirin	10 mg/kg/day
Dipyridamole	1.5 mg/kg/day

*Concomitant administration of PCC is not recommended.

will interfere with activated proteases of the hemostatic cascade, particularly thrombin. Coumarin compounds interfere with the production of vitamin K–dependent factors, resulting in a decrease in each of these procoagulants. Because F VII has a short half-life, the PT best reflects the effect of coumarin therapy. Protamine sulfate reverses the effect of heparin, and vitamin K in large amounts can reverse the effect of coumarin.

ADDITIONAL READING

Nathan DG, Oski FA, eds. Hematology of Infancy and Childhood, 3rd ed., Philadelphia: WB Saunders, 1987.
   Chap. 39: Rosenberg RD. Physiology of coagulation: The fluid phase.
   Chap. 40: Handin RI. Physiology of coagulation: The platelet.
   Chap. 41: Lusher JM. Diseases of coagulation: The fluid phase.
   Chap. 42: Stuart MJ, Kelton JG. The platelet: Quantitative and qualitative abnormalities.
Wintrobe MM, Lee GR, Boggs DR, Bithell TC, Foerster J, Athens JW, Lukens JN, eds. Clinical Hematology, 8th ed. Philadelphia: Lea & Febiger, 1981.

20 Immunologic Disorders

Richard L. Wasserman

BACKGROUND AND PHYSIOLOGY

Immunologic emergencies in the PICU setting are rare. In virtually all situations the secondary effect of immunodeficiency (i.e., infections) sends the patient to the PICU. This chapter will consider situations in which the patient is known to be immunodeficient or in which immunodeficiency should be suspected.

In addition to the normal mucocutaneous barriers, four elements make up the host defense system: humoral antibody, cell-mediated immunity, phagocytic cells, and complement.

barriers The normal anatomy of mucocutaneous tissues that prevent microbial invasion.

humoral antibody Immunoglobulins that are active against extracellular pathogens.

cell-mediated immunity Killer lymphocytes that are directed against intracellular and eukaryotic pathogens (fungus and parasites). Required for recovery from viral infection.

phagocytic cells Granulocytes and macrophages/monocytes that are needed for the response to bacteria and fungi.

complement Serum proteins that act with or without antibody to enhance phagocytosis and antimicrobial activity.

Antibody functions primarily against extracellular pathogens such as bacteria. Patients with antibody deficiency are subject to sinopulmonary infections from routine organisms such as pyogenic cocci and *Haemophilus influenzae*. Intact cell-mediated immunity is required for recovery from viral infections and fungal and parasitic disease. Patients with cell-mediated immune defects are often infected with unusual organisms such as *Pneumocystis;* they experience unusually prolonged and severe courses of routine viral infections such as viral pneumonitis or gastroenteritis. Varicella may be fatal in these patients. Phagocytic function is important in the defense

against most bacteria and fungus. Patients who are neutropenic or have functional abnormalities of granulocytes experience deep tissue infections caused by *Staphylococcus aureus* and gram-negative rods. Fungal infections, particularly *Candida* and *Aspergillus,* can also be major problems. Complement deficiencies are the least common immunodeficiencies. Deficiency of any of the terminal components of the classic pathway (C5 through C9) is associated with recurrent meningococcemia and meningococcal meningitis. Deficiency of the early components tends to be associated with milder recurrent infections with bacteria and fungus. Deficiency of C3 is usually fatal during the first year of life. The categories of host defense disorders and the infections seen in patients with those problems are summarized below.

barrier defects Bacterial infections with pyogenic cocci or gram-negative bacteria or rods and occasionally fungus. Located at the site of the defect.

antibody deficiency Most commonly sinopulmonary infection with gram-positive cocci and *Haemophilus influenzae.* Unusual susceptibility to disseminated and CNS enteroviral disease.

cellular immune defects Severe defects usually present early. Fungal and viral infections result, especially pneumonia or chronic diarrhea.

phagocytic cell defects Bacterial and fungal infections of the sinopulmonary tract and deep tissue as well as superficial abscesses. Staphylococcal and gram-negative infections are especially important.

complement defects Recurrent meningococcemia and bacterial and fungal infections.

Immunodeficiency must be suspected in any patient with a history of infection outside the range of normal. Persistent interstitial pneumonitis or even an apparent viral pneumonia with clinically persistent pulmonary findings in children less than 1 year of age should be investigated immediately for T-cell dysfunction. It is crucial to diagnose T-cell deficiency rapidly because many infections are untreatable in the absence of some T-cell function. Other infections suggestive of immunodeficiency, particularly of the cell-mediated immune system, are persistent candidiasis unresponsive to standard therapy; chronic diarrhea, particularly with a persistently positive Rotazyme or other test for enteric virus; and systemic fungal infection without other predisposing risk factors. Recurrent or multiple superficial or deep abscesses should suggest the possibility of a granulocyte disorder. Recurrent focal pneumonias occur in patients with either hypogammaglobulinemia or granulocyte disorder.

MONITORING AND LABORATORY TESTS

Patients with known immunodeficiency seldom need immunologic testing during an acute illness. Occasionally it is useful to measure an IgG level in a patient with known hypogammaglobulinemia who is receiving gamma globulin replacement therapy at the time of an acute illness to determine if the gamma globulin dose needs to be increased. Other measures of the immune system are not useful in immediate patient management.

If cell-mediated immunodeficiency is suspected, it is important to make the diagnosis as rapidly as possible. Absolute total lymphocyte count (normal >2500/mm³) and T-cell marker studies (e.g., T3, T4, T8) are usually available in 24 to 48 hours but are seldom definitive. Delayed hypersensitivity skin testing using diphtheria/tetanus toxoid and *Candida* antigen would be useful in children over 1 year of age, but significant primary cell-mediated immune dysfunction seldom presents after 12 months of age. The most useful screening test for clinically important T-cell dysfunction is a phytohemagglutinin (PHA) stimulation test. Unfortunately this assay requires about 7 days to complete.

Suspected immunoglobulin deficiency needs to be evaluated by measuring IgA, IgG, and IgM initially, although a more extensive evaluation of the humoral immune system may be necessary to define the defect. Disorders of phagocytic cell numbers will be obvious from the complete blood count, but a functional disorder requires measurement of cell movement (i.e., chemotaxis) as well as phagocytosis and the ability to kill ingested organisms. Chemotaxis and chemiluminescence or nitroblue tetrazolium (NBT) assays usually can be completed within 48 hours. A

CH$_{50}$ assay is the best test for screening complement deficiency. If a terminal complement component is deficient, causing increased susceptibility to meningococcemia, the result will be 0. Any result other than 0 or normal must be interpreted in light of the degree of acute inflammation and possible complement consumption occurring at the time the sample was drawn.

TREATMENT

Initial management of infection in immunodeficient patients is always focused on the infection itself. Those patients in whom a diagnosis has been made may also receive specific immunologic therapy. In the acute situation the replacement therapies available for immunodeficiency are gamma globulin for IgG deficiency, granulocyte transfusion for a defect of neutrophil numbers or function (see Chapter 140), and fresh frozen plasma for the replacement of complement. Gamma globulin must always be administered if IgG is deficient. This may occur as a pure IgG deficiency, as part of a panhypogammaglobulinemia (common variable hypogammaglobulinemia), or as a component of combined immunodeficiency in which there is a T-cell defect as well. Granulocyte transfusions are discussed elsewhere and will not be considered here. Although no data support the use of complement replacement in complement-deficient patients, it is reasonable to assume that providing a source of complement to a patient known to be deficient at the time of an acute meningococcal infection may be helpful. Three specific immunologic therapies are available for the acute management of infection in immunodeficient patients:

1. *Gamma globulin*
   Indicated for IgG deficiency
   Routine dose is 200 to 500 mg/kg q 4 weeks
   Acute dose is 400 to 1000 mg/kg; may be repeated daily if indicated
2. *Fresh frozen plasma*
   Possibly useful in complement deficiency
   Usual dose is 10 to 20 ml/kg; may be repeated after 1 to 2 hours during septic shock resulting from meningococcemia in complement-deficient patients
3. *Granulocyte transfusion*
   Useful in patient with neutropenia or neutrophil functional defect.
   Dose in neonates is 0.5 to 1 × 10⁹ granulocytes/kg of recipient weight. Dose in older children is 1 unit.

A sample order for the administration of gamma globulin to a child with humoral antibody deficiency who weighs 20 kg follows:

1. Administer IV gamma globulin, 8 g, as a 3% solution (30 mg/ml)
2. Begin infusion at:
   10 ml/hr for 15 min
   20 ml/hr for 15 min
   40 ml/hr for 15 min
   60 ml/hr for 15 min
   80 ml/hr for 15 min
3. Then, if temperature increases >1° C over baseline or heart rate increases >20% over baseline or respiratory rate increases >25% over baseline, slow the infusion to 5 ml/hr and page the attending physician.

ADDITIONAL READING

Liechtenstein LM, Fauci AS, eds. Current Therapy in Allergy, Immunology and Rheumatology. Toronto: BC Decker, 1985.

Nelson JD, ed. Current Therapy in Pediatric Infectious Disease, vol 2. Toronto: BC Decker, 1988.

21 Abnormalities in Temperature Regulation

Lela W. Brink

BACKGROUND AND PHYSIOLOGY

The maintenance of thermal equilibrium depends on the intact functioning of numerous body systems and their appropriate interaction with the environment. Although abnormalities of thermal regulation are frequently associated with underlying disease states in critically ill patients, primary problems of temperature regulation generally result from exposing the patient to abnormal environmental conditions. Isolated disorders of temperature control in the CNS are unusual.

Man, a homoiothermic (warm-blooded) animal, has a complicated neural and neuroendocrine control system that is designed to maintain a constant core temperature despite changes in environmental temperature or level of activity. Heat exchange with the environment follows a thermal gradient: the change in temperature (ΔT) reflects the net heat flux plus endogenous heat production.

$$\Delta T^\circ = (T_b - T_e) + \text{Heat production}$$

where T_b = body temperature and T_e = environmental temperature.

Mechanisms of Heat Exchange

Heat exchange is a bidirectional process involving the transfer of heat between an object and its environment. There are four mechanisms of heat transfer: evaporation, conduction, convection, and radiation. The rate of heat transfer depends on the temperature gradient ($T_b - T_e$), body surface area and mass, ambient humidity, rate of airflow, and the intact responses of the organism to environmental changes.

Evaporation

Evaporation refers to the loss of heat that accompanies vaporization of a liquid from the body surface. Heat is lost at a rate of 0.58 kcal/g of water evaporated. Evaporative heat losses are characterized as insensible (i.e., losses other than from sweating through the skin or losses from the respiratory tract) or sensible (i.e., losses from sweating through the skin). For this reason infants with a large ratio of body surface area to mass and a relatively high total body water content may have greater heat loss for their size than older children or adults.

Conduction

Conduction refers to the transfer of heat between two objects along a temperature gradient. For example, this type of exchange takes place between the surface of the body and an adjacent solid object or between the body and the air that is in immediate contact with the body.

Convection

Convection refers to the loss of heat to air moving over an exposed body surface. Heat is exchanged by conduction and the newly warmed air is continuously replaced with unwarmed air. This process can rapidly increase the rate of heat loss.

Radiation

Radiation refers to the transfer of heat by infrared rays. The body has several mechanisms for altering the rate of heat exchange. Skin and subcutaneous tissues are the body's natural insulation, with fat conducting heat at only one third the rate of other tissues. The blood supply to these tissues is regulated by arterioles in the cutaneous vascular plexus. Arteriolar dilation or constriction occurs as an autonomic response to stimuli influencing both central and peripheral receptors. Regulation of cutaneous blood flow limits the delivery of core temperature blood to the body surface. Sympathetic stimulation elicits massive cutaneous vasoconstriction, minimizing cutaneous blood flow and conductive heat loss. Conversely, vasodilation in response to an elevated core temperature can accelerate heat loss. In addition to these mechanisms thermal stimuli can elicit an array of behavioral responses ranging from altering activity to seeking a change in environment. The addition of clothing minimizes convective heat losses by trapping an insulating layer of air next to the body surface.

Mechanisms of Heat Production

Heat production is the sum of basal metabolism and shivering and nonshivering thermogenesis. Each of these mechanisms of calorogenesis responds to different endogenous and exogenous stimuli.

Basal metabolic rate

Basal metabolic rate (BMR) refers to heat produced in a resting metabolic state in a neutral thermal environment where no net heat transfer is occurring between the organism and its environment. Alterations in BMR occur slowly as a result of acclimatization or a change in neuroendocrine stimuli.

Shivering thermogenesis

Shivering thermogenesis provides a rapid response to a cold stimulus perceived by spinal cord receptors. The uncontrolled rapid contraction of skeletal muscle can produce a 4-fold increase in heat production, a 2-fold increase in oxygen consumption, and a 6-fold increase in metabolic rate. Heat loss by convection is also increased by the increased muscle activity.

Nonshivering thermogenesis

Nonshivering thermogenesis refers to metabolic heat production in excess of BMR and not as a result of shivering. This can involve lipolysis, the breakdown of both brown and white fat; glycogenolysis, primarily in muscle and liver; and hydrolysis of ATP; or it can result indirectly from gluconeogenesis. Brown fat is the most potent and probably the most important source for thermogenesis in small infants.

Temperature Control Mechanisms

Receptor sites are located centrally in the preoptic region of the anterior hypothalamus and peripherally in the skin, viscera, and spinal cord. Afferent pathways from peripheral receptors ascend via the lateral spinothalamic tract via synaptic relays in the reticular activating system and the posterolateral or ventrolateral nuclei of the thalamus before ascending to the preoptic region of the anterior hypothalamus. Cor-

Table 21-1 Hypothalamic Responses to Change in Temperature

Stimulus	Effector	Response
Cold stimulus (temp.)	Peripheral sympathetic pathways	Vasoconstriction
	Release of neuroendocrine hormones	Basal metabolic rate
	Stimulation of adrenal medulla	Catecholamine release (epinephrine + norepinephrine)
	Stimulation of hypothalamic primary motor center for shivering	Shivering
	Circulating catecholamines	Lipolysis white + brown fat (chemical thermogenesis)
Heat stimulus (temp.)	Eccrine sweat glands	Evaporative heat loss
	Stimulation of peripheral parasympathetics (and inhibition of central sympathetics)	Vasodilation
	Inhibition of central sympathetic centers	Basal metabolic rate

tical connections mediate conscious temperature sensation.

Hypothalamic temperature receptors exist both in the anterior (preoptic) and posterior hypothalamus. Receptors in the preoptic region respond to local temperature changes, whereas those in the posterior portion modulate signals transmitted from peripheral temperature receptors and integrate input from osmoreceptors and baroreceptors (Table 21-1).

The hypothalamus is the central control mechanism that ensures thermal homeostasis. The hypo-thalamus monitors its own temperature, continually comparing it to a given set point temperature.

A complex interaction exists between peripheral and central receptors and neural and neuroendocrine effectors (Fig. 21-1). A discrepancy between set point temperature and the temperature of hypothalamic central receptors or the temperature of hypothalamic central receptors and the temperature sensed by spinal cord or peripheral receptors activates a feedback response aimed at eliminating this discrepancy. Long-term temperature changes such as

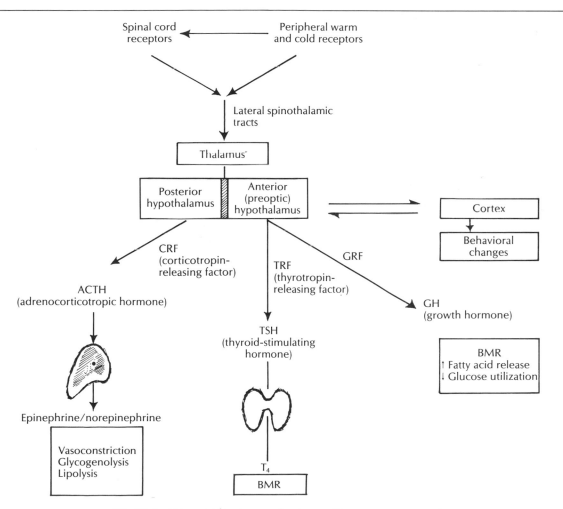

Fig. 21-1 Neuroendocrine mechanisms of temperature control.

any environmental change or long-standing physiologic change may result in a resetting of the hypothalamic set point.

HYPOTHERMIA

Although many schema exist for the classification of hypothermia, from a clinical viewpoint it is best to consider any temperature below 35° C significant. Temperatures below this level are different enough from the usual anterior hypothalamic set point that thermoregulatory control mechanisms are triggered, resulting in shivering thermogenesis and a generalized catecholamine release. Sympathetic neural responses trigger an increased cardiac output, tachypnea, tachycardia, increased oxygen consumption, and a marked cutaneous vasoconstriction (Fig. 21-2).

Etiology

Mild hypothermia (core temperatures of 32° to 35° C) is seen frequently in children admitted to the PICU

secondary to exposure to a relatively cold environment. These children generally have a relatively large body surface area, relatively poor nutritional reserve, and frequently have impaired cardiac, renal, hepatic, and endocrine function. Most patients in the PICU have impaired behavioral, neural, and endocrine responses resulting from their physical and physiologic states. Neuroendocrine responses are frequently impaired by pharmacologic agents. For example, phenothiazines and barbiturates act centrally to depress the anterior hypothalamic response to cold. Phenothiazines and neuromuscular blockers impair shivering thermogenesis. Vasodilators increase heat loss and inhibit the cutaneous vasoconstrictor response affecting temperature stability. Long-term use of vasopressors depletes catecholamine reserves and alters receptor function, thus impairing the responses of the peripheral vasculature.

Moderate to severe hypothermia occurs frequently in patients presenting with histories of trauma, ex-

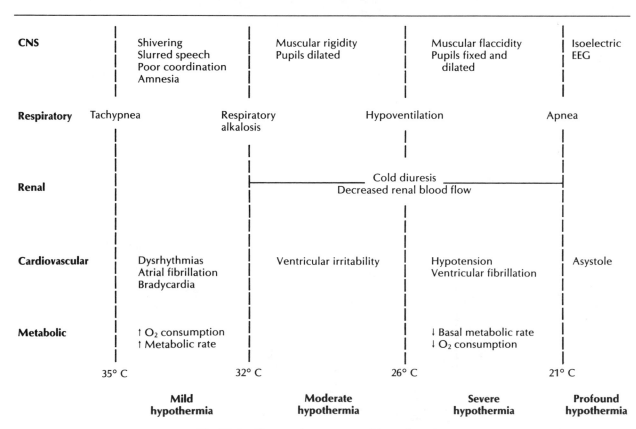

Fig. 21-2   Signs and symptoms of hypothermia.

posure, submersion injury, toxic ingestion, or shock.

Neonates are at greatest risk for severe hypothermia immediately after birth. The infant has a large body surface area, is wet, and has an enormous potential for conductive and evaporative losses. It is imperative to dry the neonate immediately, assist circulation as needed, and place the child in a neutral thermal environment.

Any patient with a suggestive history or unexplained altered sensorium needs to be evaluated for hypothermia by measuring a central temperature.

Monitoring and Laboratory Tests

Accurate temperature measurement and core temperature monitoring are essential for diagnosing hypothermia (see Chapter 111). An electronic thermometer can measure lower temperatures than other types of thermometers. A mercury thermometer that has an inappropriate scale or has not been shaken down low enough could cause the clinician to overlook the existence of hypothermia. Apparent but not actual hypothermia may be measured by axillary temperatures, especially in low perfusion states. Oral and esophageal temperatures may appear falsely high if warmed inspiratory gases are being used. In general continuous monitoring of central (esophageal, rectal, or pulmonary arterial blood) tempera-

ture is indicated in moderate to severe hypothermia or in states of low peripheral perfusion.

Once the diagnosis of hypothermia is established and continuous core temperature monitoring is instituted, a systematic evaluation of risk factors (Table 21-2) and potential complications needs to be made. ECG monitoring is essential because of the significant dysrhythmias noted secondary to myocardial irritability. Close monitoring of systemic arterial blood pressure and frequent evaluation of acid-base status, electrolytes, and glucose make placement of a peripheral arterial catheter a helpful adjunct in the patient with severe hypothermia.

MONITORING AND LABORATORY TESTS FOR HYPOTHERMIA

Core temperature
    Esophageal, rectal, pulmonary arterial blood
Intake and output (NG tube, bladder catheter)
ECG
BP (arterial catheter)
Laboratory values
    CBC with platelets
    Electrolytes, serum osmolarity
    Serum glucose
    BUN, serum creatinine
    Liver function test
    Amylase
CVP
    If cardiovascular instability exists
Swan-Ganz catheter
    If cardiovascular instability exists

Table 21-2 Risk Factors for Hypothermia

Etiology	Mechanism
Exposure	Increased heat loss, especially
Trauma	conductive heat loss (wet
Drownings	clothes or immersion) or
Accidents	convective losses (wind)
CNS depression	
Head injury	Direct central effect on thalamic temperature centers
Stroke, tumor, or infection	
Pharmacologic	
Narcotics	CNS depression and vasodilation
Barbiturates	CNS depression
Phenothiazines	α-Adrenergic block, impaired shivering thermogenesis, set point
Endocrine abnormalities	
Hypoglycemia	Impaired thermogenesis or BMR,
Hypothyroidism	poor metabolic response to cold
Hypopituitarism	Impaired hypothalamic response to cold
Spinal cord transection	Interrupted sensory afferents; inability to sense cold impairs central reflex and behavioral responses
Skin disorders	
Erythroderma	Increased transdermal water and
Erythroderma bullous	heat losses
Stevens-Johnson syndrome	
Burns	

Because evaluation of arterial blood gases is complicated by the difference in CO_2 solubility and oxygen dissociation curve characteristics (curve is shifted to the left) at low temperatures, a decision must be made to employ correction curves or utilize values on rewarmed specimens. When a specimen is drawn from a hypothermic patient and warmed to 37° C, the solubility of CO_2 decreases, resulting in a higher $PaCO_2$ and lower pH than exists in the patient. PaO_2 values should be corrected for temperature because warming the blood increases the solubility of oxygen and results in PaO_2 values significantly higher than in the patient.

To correct PaO_2 the following equation applies:

$$PaO_2 \ (Tc) = PaO_2 \ (37° \ C) - (37° - Tc) \ (0.072)$$

where Tc is the core temperature.

Pathophysiology

The immediate sympathetic response to a cold stimulus is followed by a temperature-dependent biphasic response.

At temperatures from 30° to 35° C shivering thermogenesis is initiated, resulting in an intense heat production and a marked increase in both oxygen consumption and metabolic rate. Hepatic and muscular glycogenolysis may result in a transient hyperglycemia, whereas catabolism of fat may lead to ketosis. Metabolic acidosis occurs secondary to lactate production, and compensatory respiratory alkalosis is seen. These changes peak at 34° to 35° C, and as core temperature falls below 30° C, nonshivering thermogenesis occurs. Heat production decreases and metabolic rate falls below basal requirements.

After the phase of shivering thermogenesis, total body metabolism (oxygen consumption) is proportionately reduced with progressive hypothermia. There is a 6% fall in oxygen consumption per degree centigrade. The extent of reduction of metabolism varies in each organ system even if core temperature was reduced uniformly. At normothermia oxygen consumption is highest in the kidney, which is the organ most rapidly affected by hypothermia.

Cardiovascular changes occur secondary to hypothermia. After an initial tachycardia secondary to catecholamine response, a decrease in cardiac conductivity and automaticity and an increase in refractory period occur during the phase of shivering thermogenesis. Atrial fibrillation is common at core temperatures below 34° C, whereas more severe bradydysrhythmias are noted with cooling. First-degree atrioventricular block is common below 30° C, whereas third-degree block occurs below 20° C. These may be refractory to treatment until rewarming occurs.

Characteristic ECG changes are also noted. Below 33° C an increasingly prominent "J" point elevation is evident (Fig. 21-3). With temperature-associated dysrhythmias, ECG findings may accurately identify the severity of hypothermia.

Changes in respiration are less characteristic. An initial tachypnea occurs secondary to the cold stimulus. Compensatory alkalosis may occur in response to shivering thermogenesis, but below 30° C hypoventilation is marked. With progressive cooling a central apnea supervenes.

Renal responses to cold stimuli have been characterized as "cold diuresis." This phenomenon includes a good urine output despite a marked decrease in renal blood flow and glomerular filtration rate. This is believed to be secondary to a defect in tubular reabsorption of water, and diuresis may persist despite systemic hypotension, dehydration, and hyperosmolarity.

CNS abnormalities, including confusion and behavioral changes, occur with mild to moderate hypothermia. Progressive levels of stupor and coma follow, and below 26° C flaccidity, unresponsiveness, and fixed dilated pupils are present. This hypothermic state can be protective to the CNS by reducing metabolic and oxygen demands. This will, of course, depend on the degree and duration of hypothermia, underlying disease processes, cardiopulmonary status, and prior or concomitant use of medications. Brain death cannot be diagnosed in the hypothermic patient because effects on the CNS (e.g., flaccidity, fixed dilated pupils, isoelectric EEG) and metabolism (e.g., decreased cerebral metabolic rate, oxygen demands, cerebral blood flow) so closely mimic the clinical criteria for death. Rewarming to a temperature >35° C is recommended before evaluating for brain death.

Because nerve conduction is markedly slowed in the hypothermic patient, conventional monitoring of neuroparalysis with a nerve stimulator may be inaccurate and may reflect cold effects rather than adequate pharmacologic neuromuscular blockade.

The marked decrease in metabolic rate seen in moderate to severe hypothermia results in decreased

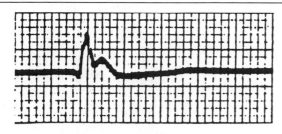

Fig. 21-3   J point elevation (lead I) hypothermia.

oxygen consumption (decrease of 6% per degree Celsius) and affects the rate of chemical reactions (a decrease of 50% for each 10° C fall in temperature). Although it is known that drug clearance is generally decreased secondary to reduced cardiac output, dehydration, slowed hepatic metabolism, decreased glomerular filtration, and abnormal tubular filtration and reabsorption, it is difficult to predict drug levels or effect in hypothermic patients. Anesthetic requirements are decreased with moderate hypothermia, and the effects of barbiturates are exaggerated. Both barbiturates (secondary to their CNS depressant effect) and phenothiazines (because of their alpha-adrenergic blocking effects) potentiate hypothermia. The inotropic dose of digitalis glycosides is reduced, but the toxic dose is increased. The myocardium becomes more sensitive to potassium-induced arrest and calcium-induced dysrhythmias. The cardiotonic effects of catecholamines are enhanced in mild to moderate hypothermia but depressed at temperature levels below 26° C.

Hematologic abnormalities, including a rising hematocrit (secondary to a cold diuresis), may occur below 30° C, resulting in a hyperviscous, hypercoagulable state. Neutropenia may increase susceptibility to infection and thrombocytopenia may exacerbate coagulopathies.

Treatment
General

Initial stabilization is aimed at preventing further heat loss. The removal of wet clothing, sheltering of the victim, and providing cover are simple ways to achieve this goal. The patient needs to be transported with care, especially when hypothermia is moderate to severe, because of the risks of life-threatening dys-

rhythmias. Once hospital transport is accomplished and cardiac monitoring is instituted, fluid resuscitation needs to be initiated. Severe peripheral vasoconstriction in a hypovolemic patient makes placement of a central venous catheter desirable. The physician must be aware that the myocardial instability of hypothermia may result in dysrhythmias that are difficult to treat. As stated previously, dysrhythmias may not respond to conventional therapy until rewarming is completed, at which time spontaneous conversion to a normal rhythm may occur.

Bretylium (5 to 10 mg/kg) may be preferable to lidocaine (1 mg/kg) in the treatment of patients with ventricular dysrhythmias. Bretylium may decrease the risk of fibrillation and increase the success of cardioversion.

Rewarming

Passive external rewarming is the slowest, least invasive method of rewarming available. It requires prevention of further heat loss and relies on endogenous thermogenesis to restore body temperature. With this technique alone the body temperature usually rises by only 0.4° C/hr.

Active external rewarming involves the application of conductive and radiant warming devices. Hot water bottles, heating pads, and warm blankets can be applied to the body surface or radiant warmers may be used. These techniques are most commonly used in mild hypothermia, but their application in more severe cases is controversial. Even though use of external rewarming techniques has been reported to be successful even in cases of profound hypothermia, the mortality rate is high. Problems with external rewarming include the following: (1) control of the rate of rewarming is poor, (2) peripheral vasodilation may cause shock secondary to blood flow redistribution, (3) acidosis may worsen secondary to mobilization of acid from the hypoperfused periphery, and (4) poorly perfused peripheral areas may suffer burns.

Active central rewarming includes a number of techniques that give a reliable rate of rewarming but, in general, are more invasive. The risk vs. benefit of such procedures must be considered.

Warming (heating) of inspired gases can be achieved safely using gases heated to 42° to 44° C by cascade humidifiers. Temperatures greater than 46° C are associated with mucosal burns. A temperature rise of 1° C/hr can be achieved with this technique.

IV infusions have been heated to 37° to 43° C to expedite rewarming. Infusions need to be thermocontrolled, for example, through use of a blood warmer, because superheating may induce massive hemolysis.

Gastric lavage either directly or via a gastric balloon can be used to introduce large volumes of warmed sodium chloride solutions centrally. If direct irrigation is used, an unknown amount of water and electrolyte may be absorbed. Irrigation of the bladder with sterile solutions has also been suggested. Solutions should be heated to no greater than 46° C.

Peritoneal dialysis with 0.9% sodium chloride or dialysate warmed to 38° to 43° C can be used with brief (15 minute) dwells or by continuous lavage using dual-catheter placement. A rise in temperature of 4° C/hr can be achieved.

Placement of arterial and venous cannulas permits external warming of blood by either continuous hemodialysis or partial arteriovenous bypass. In patients with severe cardiovascular collapse, bypass with rewarming using a membrane oxygenator permits cardiovascular support and nearly complete control of acid-base balance.

Open chest and mediastinal lavage are rarely indicated. Controversy exists over the relative indications for each of the above techniques as well as the optimal rate of rewarming. No studies have been performed to assess the relative merits of these types of lavage in various age groups.

HYPERTHERMIA

Hyperthermia refers to a core body temperature above normal. Hyperthermia becomes clinically significant when core temperatures exceed 40° C.

Etiology

Etiologies of hyperthermia are multiple, but some of the most common are:

1. Excessive heat load: Elevated environmental temperatures, especially in the face of high humidity, or a closed environment that limits convection currents
2. Alterations in metabolic rate secondary to underlying physiologic abnormalities (e.g., thyrotoxicosis, pheochromocytoma) or pharmacologic therapy (e.g., exogenous hormonal therapy, amphetamines)
3. Lack of acclimatization limiting the body's response to heat
4. CNS injury secondary to lesions in the anterior hypothalamus or elsewhere that affects the body's response to central stimuli
5. Spinal cord injury impeding signal processing from peripheral and spinal cord receptors
6. Dermal abnormalities that destroy receptor sites, prevent conductive heat losses, or impair the normal sweat gland response (e.g., scleroderma ichthyosis or burn sequelae)
7. Pharmacotherapeutics: Phenothiazines, barbiturates, myocardial depressants, and exogenous hormonal therapy or amphetamines

Pathophysiology

Hyperthermia occurs whenever there is a net positive heat balance secondary to increased environmental temperatures, increased endogenous heat production, or decreased heat elimination.

Fever

Fever commonly causes increased core temperature, but because thermoregulatory control mechanisms remain intact, fever should be distinguished from other hyperthermic disorders. During fever the thermoregulatory set point of the anterior hypothalamus is elevated in response to release of pyogenic substances. Fever is accompanied by increased hypothalamic levels of serotonin, prostaglandin E_1, prostaglandin E_2, and cyclic adenosine monophosphate. Since normal thermoregulatory responses exist during fever, a patient will shiver to raise the core temperature to the new set point level.

The hypermetabolic state that exists with fever is rarely life threatening, and temperatures do not generally rise over 41° C unless other factors impair the thermoregulatory control mechanisms.

Treatment. The treatment of fever has become a controversial subject. It is believed that fever may be an element of the body's defense system, perhaps decreasing the rate of replication of the invading organism. Fever is often treated to effect patient comfort and to reverse the physiologic consequences of fever (i.e., the increased metabolic rate, the increased water loss) that may be harmful to the patient. Certain patients may not tolerate fever well and for example the cardiac patient may not tolerate the tachycardia of temperature elevation and the croup patient may not tolerate the physiologic tachypnea. Fever should also be treated in any case where a condition may impair the normal thermoregulatory control system.

Modes of treatment generally employed to control fever include passive and active external cooling and pharmacotherapeutics. Removing clothing and other barriers to heat loss are simple maneuvers that facilitate heat dissipation. Active cooling with cold baths or ice tubs is generally contraindicated because marked vasoconstriction may occur, and the peripheral sensation of rapid cooling may elicit a shivering thermogenesis that can raise the core temperature. Facilitating conductive, convective, and evaporative heat loss short of shivering may be useful.

Aspirin and corticosteroids are effective in blocking the febrile response at the hypothalamic level. The risks of using aspirin as an anticoagulant, its tendency to irritate the GI tract, and its association with Reye's syndrome have made it less popular as an antipyretic. Corticosteroids are generally avoided because they inhibit the normal inflammatory response (masking symptoms and impeding host defenses) and because of their side effects, including GI hemorrhage.

Acetaminophen has actions similar to aspirin as an antipyretic but generally has a shorter duration of action than aspirin and fewer side effects. The usual dosage is 10 to 15 mg/kg/dose. An overdose may lead to potentially fatal hepatic necrosis (see Chapter 77).

Chlorpromazine in doses of 0.5 to 1 mg/kg acts as a depressant at the level of the anterior hypothalamus, decreasing the body's ability to maintain a set point temperature. The body temperature therefore becomes more like that of the environment. Chlorpromazine also inhibits shivering thermogenesis and has been used in this manner as an adjunct to cooling therapies.

Hyperthermic Syndromes

Hyperthermic syndromes reflect disorders of temperature control. The most common of these is heat stroke, but malignant hyperthermia and the neuroleptic malignant syndromes must also be considered in the appropriate clinical settings (see Chapter 60).

Heat stroke is characterized by temperatures >41° C and an absence of normal thermoregulatory controls. Heat stroke may be classified as exertional or classic (Table 21-3). Exertional heat stroke occurs in previously healthy individuals performing strenuous exercise with mild to moderate elevations in environmental temperature or humidity. Classic heat stroke occurs in the very young or very old in patients

Table 21-3 Characteristics of Heat Stroke

	Exertional	Classic
Elevated environmental temperature	Common	Common
Predisposing illness	Rare	Common
Occurrence	Sporadic	Heat waves
Sweating	Initially profuse	Minimal/absent
Rhabdomyolysis	Common	Rare
Lactic acidosis	Common	Rare
Renal failure	Common	Sometimes

with underlying physical or psychiatric disorders or in patients whose normal responses (physical or behavioral) are impaired.

Etiology

Predisposing factors to heat stroke can be divided between those involving increased heat production and those involving impaired heat loss. For this reason patients with increased metabolic rate (i.e., those with fever or hyperthyroidism or those taking amphetamines) are at increased risk for heat stroke. Patients who are unable to alter their environment, most often infants, the elderly, the physically handicapped, or those with altered levels of consciousness from any cause, are at increased risk. Paraplegics and quadriplegics who have altered sensation and impaired mobility are frequent victims of heat stroke.

Acclimatization is the adaptive process the body undergoes in response to a temperature stress to increase heat tolerance. It is characterized by increased cardiac output (to improve peripheral circulation and heat dissipation) and increased aldosterone production (expanding extracellular volume and decreasing sodium losses in sweat). Unacclimatized patients are at increased risk for heat stresses.

Other patients at risk for heat stroke include those with decreased cardiac reserve, for example, those with underlying cardiovascular pathology and those receiving pharmacologic myocardial depressants such as β-adrenergic blocking drugs. Any process that decreases intravascular volume also adversely affects heat adaptation. This includes dehydration, whether

RISK FACTORS FOR HEAT STROKE

States of increased heat production

Exercise
Fever
Drug effects: Amphetamines, hallucinogens
Drug toxicity: Aspirin, thyroid hormone
Thyrotoxicosis
Pheochromocytoma

States of decreased heat elimination

High environmental temperature and humidity
Decreased cardiovascular functioning
Dehydration or hypovolemia
Skin disorders: Scleroderma, ichthyosis, scarring
Anhydrosis or hypohydrosis
Drug effects: Anticholinergics, phenothiazines, alcohol, diuretics, laxatives, β-adrenergic blockers
CNS disorders
    Tumors
    Infection
    Stroke
    Spinal cord injury

Table 21-4   Monitoring and Laboratory Tests for Hyperthermia

Test	Condition Tested
WBC	Infection
Hb/Hct	Hemoconcentration
Platelet count	Platelet consumption, disseminated intravascular coagulation (DIC)
BUN/creatinine	Dehydration, renal function
Creatine phosphokinase	Rhabdomyolysis
Arterial blood gases and pH	Acidosis
Electrolytes	Hypokalemia, fluid shifts
Liver function tests	Liver dysfunction—hepatic necrosis (ALT, AST, gamma glutamyl transferase)
PT/PTT	Disseminated intravascular coagulation (if elevated, evaluate fibrinogen, fibrin degradation products)
Toxicology	If drug ingestion possible/suspected
T$_4$, TSH	If clinically indicated
Glucose	Hypoglycemia

secondary to illness, diuretic or laxative therapy, or water deprivation.

Electrolyte imbalance may adversely affect myocardial function. Hypokalemia may also decrease muscle function and impair sweat production.

Evaporative losses from sweat and saliva may be affected by numerous drugs, including anticholinergics (atropine) and drugs with anticholinergic properties (phenothiazines, butyrophenones, and antiparkinsonism agents).

Skin disorders such as scleroderma and ichthyosis impede heat transfer and may affect sweat production. Scarring from burns frequently involves the dermal tissues that incorporate the sweat glands. Patients with cystic fibrosis also are at risk for hyperthermia secondary to abnormal sweat production.

Diagnosis

The diagnosis is suggested by the history and physical examination and confirmed by a core temperature greater than 41° C. The patient will usually present with neurologic impairment ranging from disorientation to stupor or coma. The differential diagnosis includes severe infection, CNS disorders, and endocrinopathies.

Laboratory evaluation

When a patient presents with suspected heat stroke, physical examination and laboratory studies must assess the target organ systems (Table 21-4). There is a high risk for multiple organ system failure with its attendant high morbidity (see Chapter 22).

Pathophysiology

An increase in core temperature above a critical maximum level (usually 42° C) is a direct cellular toxin affecting mitochondrial and enzyme function and membrane stability. Physiologic sequelae of hyperthermia such as dehydration, hypoxemia, and metabolic acidosis can adversely affect organ function as well.

The cardiovascular response to heat stress is increased cardiac output secondary to an increase in stroke volume and a decrease in systemic vascular resistance. If the intravascular volume is decreased, whether secondary to preexisting dehydration or intercurrent volume loss secondary to sweating, hypotension may occur secondary to high-output failure.

CNS symptoms (disorientation, combativeness, obtundation) may result from a direct thermal effect on the brain or secondary to compromised cerebral perfusion, cerebral edema, and hemorrhage. Seizures are common, and cerebellar ataxia may reflect the area's sensitivity to temperature change.

Rhabdomyolysis is seen in exertional heat stress and predisposes to acute renal failure (see Chapter 14). Hypovolemia-induced acute tubular necrosis also occurs.

GI ulcerations secondary to stress and/or ischemia are common. Hepatotoxicity appears to result from a direct thermal effect. Hepatic necrosis and cholestasis may not be present until 2 or 3 days after the insult.

Hemoconcentration secondary to dehydration increases the risk of cerebral infarction. Platelet dysfunction can be seen alone or with DIC. A coagulopathy may result from hepatic dysfunction alone or as part of a more generalized process.

Hypoglycemia may occur and frequently complicates exertional heat stroke. Adrenal insufficiency may be secondary to infarction of the adrenal cortex.

Adult respiratory distress syndrome and myocardial dysfunction may complicate the pulmonary picture.

Monitoring and Laboratory Tests

Monitoring cardiovascular function and intravascular volume status is essential. Hourly intake and output and aggressive fluid replacement therapy are essential because there is a potential for renal failure. Continuous core temperature monitoring is necessary, and central blood temperature may be most accurate during active cooling therapies. Frequent laboratory assessment of hematocrit, pH (determined by arterial blood gases), electrolytes, and renal and liver functions is indicated for 48 to 72 hours after the insult.

Invasive monitoring with indwelling arterial and central venous catheters or a Swan-Ganz catheter may be indicated in patients with underlying disease processes or intercurrent organ failure.

Treatment

Initial treatment of hyperthermia is aimed at rapid cooling and then at assessment and treatment of complications. Cooling techniques commonly used include the following:

Surface cooling utilizes evaporative and convective heat loss by wetting the skin and blowing fans across the body. *Direct cooling* by immersing the body in ice water or packing the body in ice is advocated by many authors. Cardiovascular monitoring is difficult, and these patients are at risk for sudden cardiovascular collapse. *Central cooling* employs the use of peritoneal, gastric, or bladder lavage with sodium chloride iced to 9° to 20° C. Fluid shifts may be significant and electrolyte status must be monitored. Hemodialysis or cardiopulmonary bypass with external cooling is rarely indicated. *Chlorpromazine* has been suggested as a pharmacologic adjunct to surface cooling and direct cooling but is rarely indicated. It acts centrally as a depressant to the hypothalamus and inhibits shivering thermogenesis.

Cooling processes need to be discontinued when the core temperature falls below 39° C.

ADDITIONAL READING

Curley FJ, Irwin R. Disorders of temperature control: Part I. Hyperthermia. Intensive Care Med 1:5-14, 1986.
• Curley FJ, Irwin R. Disorders of temperature control: Part III. Hypothermia. Intensive Care Med 1:270-288, 1986.
• Danzl D. Hyperthermic syndromes. Am Fam Physician, 37:157-162, 1988.
Guyton AC. Textbook of Medical Physiology. Philadelphia: WB Saunders, 1986.
Matz R. Hypothermia: mechanisms and countermeasures. Hosp Pract 1:45-71, 1986.
Wong KC. Physiology and pharmacology of hypothermia [medical progress]. West J Med 138:227-232, 1983.

22 Multiple Organ System Failure

Luis O. Toro-Figueroa

BACKGROUND

Multiple organ system failure (MOSF) is defined as the failure of at least two organs 3 to 10 days after the initial event. The initial event may or may not be resolved. This clinical entity accounts for 97% of the deaths in pediatric critical care units.

The literature describing MOSF in pediatric patients is very limited. Only two articles address the entity, both by Wilkinson, Pollack, and associates in 1986 and 1987. Most of the present knowledge is described in the adult surgical literature, making it difficult to compare MOSF in pediatric patients.

Several events have been reported to trigger MOSF. Whereas some of these are the most common causes for admission to a PICU, others are only seen in the adult patient population. The incidence in adult patients varies according to the population studied. An incidence of 6% has been reported in patients who have had emergency surgery and 55% in patients with intra-abdominal sepsis. MOSF was implicated in 24% of the patients admitted to a PICU. An incidence

of 40% has been reported in children with adult respiratory distress syndrome (ARDS). The overall mortality rate in adults with MOSF varies from 8.2% to 18%, and in pediatric patients an overall mortality of 7.5% to 11% has been reported.

The number of organ systems affected is associated with higher mortality rates. In pediatric patients, one, two, three, and four or more organ systems affected are associated with a mortality of 1%, 11% to 26%, 50% to 62%, and 75% to 88%, respectively. Patients admitted to a PICU without MOSF had an overall mortality rate of 0.3%, whereas the overall mortality rate of patients admitted with MOSF was 54%. Of the patients who died in the PICU, 97% had MOSF. Patients with nonsimultaneous MOSF had a lower mortality rate than those with simultaneous MOSF when the same number of organ systems were involved. The mortality rate of the nonsimultaneous MOSF group was similar to that of the group with simultaneous MOSF when the same number of organ systems were involved simultaneously (e.g., a patient

---

EVENTS REPORTED TO TRIGGER MOSF

Advanced age	GI bleeding	Poor nutrition
Alcoholism	Intra-abdominal infection	Sepsis
Atherosclerotic cardiovascular disease	Liver cirrhosis	Shock
Burns	Malignancy (specifically cachexia)	Splenectomy
Chronic renal failure	Multiple transfusions	Steroids
Diabetes mellitus	Neurologic trauma	Vascular procedure
Emergency surgery (specifically abdominal)	Pancreatitis	Others
	Polytrauma	

with three organs failing, but only two failing simultaneously, has the same mortality rate as a patient with a total of two organs failing simultaneously). It is believed that the maximum number of organ systems failing may be the most appropriate indicator of severity of illness.

The incidence of specific organ system failure in pediatric patients is respiratory, 88%; cardiovascular, 44%; neurologic, 24%, hematologic, 24%; and renal, 5%. There are no reports on the incidence of failure of the hepatic or gastrointestinal systems, although they definitely can be involved. The low incidence of renal involvement may relate to the high values used as criteria for entry. No specific combination of organ system involvement was found to be associated with a higher rate of mortality.

PATHOPHYSIOLOGY

No single primary mechanism that accounts for the events of MOSF has been determined. Dysfunction probably occurs at the cellular level, and several theories implicate different pathogenic mechanisms. The following mechanisms have been described by different authors: (1) generalized cellular insult, (2) immune complex deposition, (3) endotoxins, (4) sepsis, (5) macrophage/Kupffer cell secretory products, and (6) redox imbalance.

Generalized Cellular Insult

MOSF has been associated with a generalized cellular injury in the postoperative period (Fig. 22-1). The initial damage to the cell may not be clinically apparent because of significant physiologic reserve, and this may account for the delay in onset of MOSF after the initial event. During this delay period some compensatory hemodynamic events have been observed. Increased cardiac output, oxygen delivery, and oxygen consumption have been documented in patients in the postoperative period who survived ARDS.

Oxidative substrate availability depends on the degree of severity of illness and the magnitude of the surgical procedure and may become inadequate as energy expenditure increases. A dependence on glucose metabolism as a result of a decrease in circulation and uptake by tissues of free fatty acids and ketones has been demonstrated. As glucose intake decreases in the postoperative period, glycogen becomes the next source of energy and hepatic stores are depleted quickly. Gluconeogenesis from protein and lipid breakdown becomes the major source of

energy. Protein breakdown gluconeogenesis may account for the clinical picture of insulin-resistant hyperglycemia. During muscle protein breakdown branched-chain amino acids (BCAA) are preferentially oxidized, and availability of BCCA constitutes the rate-limiting step in the synthesis of cellular protein.

As muscle protein breakdown increases, hepatic protein synthesis increases by using the newly available amino acids. Anesthesia and laparotomy increase skeletal protein degradation by 66%, but the addition of sepsis only increases degradation slightly. Hepatic protein synthesis, however, increases by 42% in uncomplicated surgical procedures and by 164% in cases complicated by sepsis. Albumin may also be a source of amino acids for hepatic protein synthesis. The low content of isoleucine in albumin necessitates a high utilization rate of albumin, and this may account for the hypoalbuminemia seen in postoperative critically ill patients.

Immune Complex Deposition

Immune complexes, which were previously implicated in renal and idiopathic pulmonary disease, have been implicated as playing a role in the pathophysiology of MOSF. Immunoglobulin deposits in the pa-

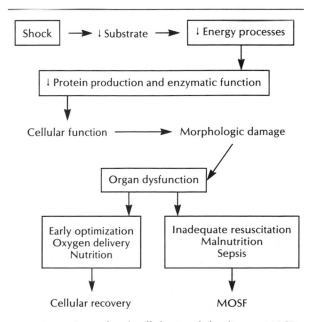

Fig. 22-1   Generalized cellular insult leading to MOSF.

tients' livers and less frequently in their lungs were demonstrated. A rabbit model with peritonitis induced by cecal perforation demonstrated a high frequency of immune complex deposits in kidneys and livers and occasional deposits in the lungs.

Anaphylatoxin (C4a and C3a) elevations have been demonstrated in 44 trauma patients with infection, and the high levels correlated with MOSF.

Endotoxins

Endotoxins from the cell wall of the gram-negative bacteria stimulate monocytes and neutrophils, which are then activated and adhere to the endothelium and endothelial basement membrane. The activated monocytes and neutrophils release cytokines that cause cellular inflammatory and metabolic responses. Neutrophil and platelet adherence proteins have been described in cellular injury. These adherence proteins are expressed when they are stimulated by a number of mediators. The use of monoclonal antibodies to these adhesion proteins has shown that minimal homology exists between these two adherent proteins and cross-reactivity is not a tendency.

Endothelial cell adhesion is less well understood. Endothelial cells may be stimulated by interleukin-1 (IL-1), lipopolysaccharides (LPS), or tumor necrosis factor (TNF). After stimulation the endothelial cells synthesize and express a number of secondary factors: (1) endothelial-leukocyte-adhesion molecules (ELAMs), (2) TNF, (3) tissue plasminogen activator 1, and (4) granulocyte macrophage–colony-stimulating factor (GM-CSF). These secondary factors cause an inflammatory process.

The role of platelets in neutrophil-endothelial cell injury is unclear. Platelets contain substances that inhibit superoxide anion generation, chemotaxis, and degranulation by neutrophils. Platelets also enhance neutrophil adherence to endothelial cells in the presence of inflammatory mediators. The major end point of the neutrophil and platelet–endothelial cell injury is oxidant mediated.

Sepsis

Bacterial sepsis plays a role in MOSF, but it is not well understood. The rate of mortality for adult patients with MOSF and sepsis varies from 58% to 100%. The only pediatric reports state a mortality rate of 47% in patients who have MOSF with or without sepsis. When early- and late-onset sepsis are compared, the rate of mortality (57% vs. 33%, respectively) in pediatric patients with MOSF and sepsis has no significant statistical difference.

It has been postulated that sepsis increases metabolic requirements, alters microcirculation of blood flow, alters mitochondrial function, alters cellular nutrition, and makes nutritional support more difficult in the postoperative adult patient.

Macrophage/Kupffer Cell Secretory Products

Two mechanisms of hepatic injury have been described: a primary mechanism that would cause injury when tissue is well perfused and a secondary mechanism when there is prolonged and profound tissue hypoperfusion. This primary mechanism is believed to be mediated by macrophages and Kupffer cells and to be responsible for hepatic injury in MOSF.

Increased cardiac output and oxygen delivery have been demonstrated in patients preceding MOSF. Changes in energy charge and the oxireduction state in the hepatic mitochondria and cytoplasm have been shown in association with increases in ketone body production in the absence of hypoperfusion. Kupffer cell hyperplasia, macrocyte infiltration, and perinfiltrative focal hepatocyte necrosis have been documented in patients with liver failure. Hypertrophy and hyperplasia of Kupffer cells have been demonstrated in cholestatic jaundice and acute viral hepatitis. There is intimate contact between Kupffer cells and hepatocytes in the hepatic sinusoidal wall. The macrophage's potential for causing cytotoxicity has been well documented, especially in tumor cell lines. Kupffer cells and macrophages have similar phagocytic and secretory properties. Macrophage-mediated cytotoxicity is discriminate in nature, and its effect is profound when prior stimulation has occurred. The discriminate nature of the injury includes a nonimmunologic target cell specificity for injured or abnormal cells, prolonged intimate contact, and some alteration of their lipid structure cell membrane. This mechanism may play a role in the delayed onset of MOSF.

Many stimulants are known to enhance the cytotoxic effect of macrophages on target cells when macrophages are exposed prior to injury. Bacille Calmette-Gúerin, *Corynebacterium parvum,* starch, glucan, phytohemagglutinin, and thyoglycolate are known stimulants. Glucan decreases the half-time removal rate of particles by Kupffer cells, whereas methylpalmitate increases it. Methylpalmitate has been shown to prevent galactosamine-induced acute fulminant hepatic insufficiency.

Direct phagocytosis of hepatocytes by macrophages or Kupffer cells cannot be implicated as the cause of organ dysfunction. Extracellular mediators are more likely responsible. These mediators are active oxygen intermediates, neutral proteases, acid hydrolases, prostaglandins, and IL-1. Neutral proteases include plasminogen-activating factor, collagenase, and elastase. Isolated hepatocytes pretreated with dexamethasone inhibited release of plasminogen-activating factor and increased survival of hepatocytes. IL-1 has been shown to release acute-phase reactants and depress albumin synthesis even though hepatocellular necrosis does not occur. This mechanism is an example of nonlethal target cell dysfunction and not of target cell lysis. Target cell dysfunction and not lysis may be the primary mechanism for hepatic failure in MOSF. Intestinal hypoperfusion may also play a role in the hepatic injury of MOSF by causing release of mediators into the portal venous system.

It has been demonstrated that nonparenchymal rat liver preparations containing 35% to 40% Kupffer cells did not affect hepatocyte protein synthesis and neither did endotoxin by itself. When hepatocytes were exposed to both simultaneously, there was a significant decrease in hepatocyte protein synthesis with no change in microscopic morphology or ability to exclude trypan blue. This evidence supports the concept of modulation of organ function.

In summary, a stimulus (i.e., bacteria, endotoxin, antigen-antibody, lymphokine, activated complement) stimulates the effector cell (macrophage or Kupffer cell), which releases cell injury mediators (activated oxygen intermediates, IL-1, protaglandins, lysosomal enzymes) that affect the hepatocyte (target cell) and cause death or modulation of function (dysfunction).

Redox Imbalance

The alteration of systemic oxygen utilization has been implicated as the common cellular insult in patients with uncontrolled infections. Functional and ultrastructural abnormalities in the liver mitochondria as well as a decrease in ATP and decline in oxygen delivery have been demonstrated experimentally. ATP, magnesium, and glucose restore ATP in liver tissue of animals with experimental bacterial peritonitis. Two mechanisms were suggested: the direct repletion of ATP and the enhancement of altered nutrient capillary blood flow by direct vasoactive influences.

The blood ketone body ratio (acetoacetic acid/β-hydroxybutyric acid), which reflects hepatic mitochondrial redox potential, was studied in a group of critically ill patients. It is postulated that a decrease in this ratio is consistent with hepatic energy deficit caused by an inhibition of the turnover rate of the Krebs cycle and by mitochondrial impairment. Patients with ratios <0.4 and ≥ 0.25 had a higher incidence of MOSF. Patients with a ratio <0.25 developed biventricular failure and died. All patients with ratios of 0.4 to 0.25 and above became fully alert with hepatic support measures. There was a positive correlation of the molar ratio of BCAAs to aromatic amino acids with blood ketone body ratio; a negative correlation between blood ketone body ratio and alanine, proline, phenylalanine, and tyrosine was observed. Two mechanisms were postulated to account for the decrease in blood ketone body ratio: enhancement of β-oxidation of fatty acids and inhibition of the electron transport system. Excess production of NADH may be responsible for the enhancement of β-oxidation of fatty acids. This preferential oxidation of fatty acids in hepatic mitochondria has been demonstrated in partially hepatectomized rabbits. In these rabbits the blood ketone body ratio fell to 0.4, which is consistent with a partial impairment of glucose utilization. Inhibition of election transport may be due to hypoxia, hypotension, or mitochondrial impairment secondary to energy-substrate block. Mitochondrial impairment is the most likely mechanism responsible for ratios <0.4.

A decreasing blood ketone body ratio indicates progressive reduction in intramitochondrial NAD^+/NADH. This reduction in redox potential inhibits citrate synthase, which determines the turnover rate of the Krebs cycle. Glutamate, α-ketoglutaric acid, pyruvate, and isocitrate dehydrogenases are NAD^+ dependent and therefore are inhibited by the same mechanism. Amino acids are inhibited from entering the Krebs cycle, therefore increasing serum levels.

Inhibition of pyruvate dehydrogenase prevents pyruvate entrance into the Krebs cycle, resulting in inhibition of glucose oxidation. Reduced hepatic glucose utilization results in clinical hyperglycemia. When there is a prolonged hepatic energy deficit, there is a decrease of the blood ketone body ratio

Table 22-1   Criteria for Failure of Specific Organ Systems*

Organ System	Criteria
Cardiovascular	MAP <40 mm Hg (infants <12 mo) MAP <50 mm Hg (children ≥12 mo) HR <50 bpm (infants <12 mo) HR <40 bpm (children ≥12 mo) Cardiac arrest Continuous vasoactive drug infusion for hemodynamic support
Respiratory	RR >90/min (infants <12 mo) RR >70/min (children ≥12 mo) Pao_2 <40 torr (in absence of cyanotic heart disease) Pao_2 >65 torr $Paco_2/Fio_2$ <250 torr Mechanical ventilation (>24 hr if postoperative) Tracheal intubation for airway obstruction or acute respiratory failure
Neurologic	Glasgow Coma Scale <5 Fixed, dilated pupils Persistent (>20 min) ICP >20 torr or requiring therapeutic intervention
Hematologic	Hemoglobin <5 g/dl WBC <3000 cells/mm³ Platelets <20,000/mm³ Disseminated intravascular coagulopathy (PT >20 sec or aPPT >60 sec in presence of positive FSP assay)
Renal	BUN >100 mg/dl Serum creatinine >2 mg/dl Dialysis
Gastrointestinal	Blood transfusions >20 ml/kg in 24 hr because of GI hemorrhage (endoscopic confirmation optional)
Hepatic	Total bilirubin >5 mg/dl and SGOT or LDH more than twice normal value (without evidence of hemolysis) Hepatic encephalopathy ≥grade II

FSP = fibrin split products; HR = heart rate; LDH = lactic dehydrogenase; MAP = mean arterial pressure; PT = prothrombin time; aPTT = activated partial thromboplastin time; RR = respiratory rate.

*From Wilkinson JD, Pollack MM, Glass NL, Kanter RK, Katz RW, Steinhart CM. Mortality associated with multiple organ system failure and sepsis in pediatric intensive care unit. J Pediatr 111:324-328, 1987.

to <0.25, which cannot be reversed by hepatic support and leads to death.

CLINICAL PICTURE

MOSF usually has a delayed onset of 3 to 10 days after the triggering event (see p. 186). Although diagnostic criteria vary from author to author, Table 22-1 shows one set of criteria used to identify organ failure in pediatric patients. Some of these criteria may be too exclusive, thereby lowering the incidence of that particular organ failure. For example, renal failure requires one of these criteria: BUN >100 mg/dl, serum creatinine >2 mg/dl, or dialysis. These criteria would fail to identify some pediatric patients as having renal failure.

Pediatric MOSF has no specific sequence of failure. The incidence of specific pediatric organ system failure was listed earlier. There are no significant differences between the overall mortality for a group of patients and any specific combination of system failure within a group.

Patients with nonsimultaneous MOSF had a lower mortality rate than the group as a whole. In children the maximum number of simultaneous MOSFs is a simple reliable indicator of severity of illness and mortality. Even though this may be an indicator, it is not sensitive enough to be used as a discriminating tool to withhold therapy.

MONITORING AND LABORATORY TESTS

Because of the delayed onset of MOSF, monitoring is essential for at least 10 days beyond the critically ill period. Baseline and subsequent functions of the organ systems that need to be monitored are as follows:

Pulmonary

Arterial blood gases and pH
Change in ventilatory requirements
Pulmonary function tests
Chest roentgenogram

Cardiovascular

Vital signs and capillary refill
Hemodynamic measurements
    Cardiac index
    Preload and afterload
ECG
Cardiac enzymes
Echocardiography

Neurologic

Complete examination
EEG
ICP monitoring

Hematologic

Hemoglobin and hematocrit
WBC with differential
Platelet count
PT and PTT
Fibrinogen and fibrin split products

Renal

Urine output
BUN and creatinine
Fractional excretion of sodium
Free-water clearance
Drug levels

Metabolic

Acid-base status
Serum glucose
Lactate and pyruvate levels
Serum and urine amino acids
Blood ketone ratio
Oxygen consumption
CO_2 production

Hepatic

Transaminases
PT and PTT
Drug levels
Ammonia

Other gastrointestinal

Amylase
Enteric feeding tolerance

TREATMENT

Presently MOSF is not treated as a primary entity; therefore therapeutic modalities are based on current state-of-the-art resuscitation for each individual organ. Individual organ resuscitation is addressed in other chapters of this book.

New therapeutic approaches must be developed if morbidity and mortality from this syndrome is to be reduced. These therapeutic interventions must be targeted at reversing the primary entity and preventing damage at the cellular level.

MOSF is probably the end result of a combination of the previously discussed pathophysiologic mechanisms; therefore no one specific therapeutic modality will have a dramatic impact. Most likely a com-

Table 22-2   Specific Measures for Therapeutic Intervention in Patients with MOSF

Therapy	Postulated Mechanism of Action
Corticosteroids	Prevent immune complex deposits
	↓ Plasminogen activator factor
BCAAs	Facilitate gluconeogenesis
	↓ Endogenous protein breakdown
Lipids	Facilitate gluconeogenesis
	Prevent lipid catabolism
Carnitine supplementation	Enhance fatty acid transport from cytoplasm to mitochondria
Monoclonal antibodies against neutrophil adherence proteins	Blocks endothelial receptors
Manipulation of granulocyte–colony-stimulating factor	Blocks neutrophil adherence
Deacylation of O-specific side-chain lipopolysaccharides	Neutrophils lose their adherence properties
Methylpalmitate	Increases half-time removal of particles by Kupffer cells
Manipulation of colonic content	Prevents mediator release into portal system
ATP-Mg-glucose complex	Restores ATP deficit
Antioxidant scavenger systems	Protects against tissue injury due to oxygen radicals

bination of therapeutic interventions will minimize cell and organ dysfunction.

General therapeutic measures include (1) prevention of further cellular injury by optimizing oxygen delivery to meet demand, (2) provision of adequate oxidative substrate for energy metabolism, (3) prevention of repetitive insults to decrease prior stimulation and sensitization of effector cells, which increases cytotoxicity, and (4) early intervention and reversal of the triggering event to decrease the ability of macrophages to develop target cell specificity, prevent alteration of the lipid membrane structure, and decrease contact time of effector and target cells. Potential specific therapeutic measures are listed in Table 22-2.

Until further research provides us with safe and clinically applicable therapeutic modalities, the clinician must continue to support each failed organ individually. A rational approach would include adequate oxygen-substrate delivery to meet cellular demands, preventing further cellular injury, and the resolution of the initial triggering event in a prompt and definite manner.

ADDITIONAL READING

Al-Tuwaijri A, Akdamar K, Godiwals T, DiLuzio N. Inhibition of galactosamine (GaIN) induced hepatitis by methyl palmitate induced macrophage suppression. In Liehr H, Grun M, eds. The Reticuloendothelial System and the Pathogenesis of Liver Disease. Amsterdam: Elsevier, 1980.

Bartlett RH, Dechert RE, Mault JR, Ferguson SK, Kaiser AM, Erlandson EE. Measurement of metabolism in multiple organ failure. Surgery 92:771-779, 1982.

Baue AE. Multiple, progressive, or sequential systems failure. Arch Surg 110:779-781, 1975.

Baue AE. Recovery from multiple organ failure. Am J Surg 149:420-421, 1985.

Borzotta AP, Polk HC. Multiple system organ failure. Surg Clin North Am 63:315-336, 1983.

Carrico CJ, Meakins JL, Marshall JC, Dry D, Maier RV. Multiple organ failure syndrome. Arch Surg 121:196-208, 1986.

Cerra FB, Siegel JH, Border JR, Peters DM, McMenamy RR. Correlations between metabolic and cardiopulmonary measurements in patients after trauma, general surgery and sepsis. J Trauma 191:621-629, 1979.

• Cerra FB, Siegel JH, Border JR, Wiles J, McMenamy RR. The hepatic failure of sepsis: Cellular versus substrate. Surgery 86:409-422, 1979.

Clowes GHA, O'Donnell TF, Blackburn GL, Maki TN. Energy metabolism and proteolysis in traumatized and septic man. Surg Clin North Am 56:1169-1184, 1976.

Eiseman B, Sloan R, Hansbrough J, McIntosh R. Multiple organ failure: clinical and experimental. Am Surg 46:14-19, 1980.

• Faist E, Baue AE, Dittmer H, Heberer G. Multiple organ failure in polytrauma patients. J Trauma 23:775-787, 1983.

Ferluga J, Schorlemmer HU, Baptista LC, Allison AC. Production of the complement cleavage product, C3a, by activated macrophages and its tumorolytic effects. Clin Exp Immunol 31:512-517, 1978.

Fry DE, Pearlstein L, Fulton RL, Polk HC. Multiple system organ failure. Arch Surg 115:136-140, 1980.

• Goris RJA, Boekholtz WKF, van Bebber IPT, Nuytinck JKS, Schillings PHM. Multiple-organ failure and sepsis without bacteria. Arch Surg 121:897-901, 1986.

Goris RJA, te Boekhorst TPA, Nuytinck JKS, Gimbrere JSF. Multiple-organ failure. Arch Surg 120:1109-1115, 1985.

Heideman M, Hugli TE. Anaphylatoxin generation in multisystem organ failure. J Trauma 24:1038-1043, 1984.

Hyers TM, Gee M, Andreadis NA. Cellular interactions in the multiple organ injury syndrome. Am Rev Respir Dis 125:952-953, 1987.

• Keller GA, West MA, Cerra FB, Simmons RL. Macrophage-mediated modulation of hepatic function in multiple-system failure. J Surg Res 39:555-563, 1985.

• Keller GA, West MA, Cerra FB, Simmons RL. Multiple systems organ failure. Ann Surg 201:87-95, 1985.

Knaus WA, Draper EA, Wagner DP, Zimmerman JE. Prognosis in acute organ-system failure. Ann Surg 202:685-693, 1985.

Madge RD, Fath JJ, Cerra FB. Metabolic basis of multiple system organ failure. Lancet 1:514, 1986.

Maetani S. Nishikawa T, Hirakawa A, Tobe T. Role of blood transfusion in organ system failure following major abdominal surgery. Ann Surg 203:275-281, 1986.

Manship L, McMillin RD, Brown JJ. The influence of sepsis and multisystem and organ failure on mortality in the surgical intensive care unit. Am Surg 50:94-101, 1984.

Marshall WB, Dimick AR. The natural history of major burns with multiple subsystem failure. J Trauma 23:102-105, 1983.

Mela L, Bacalzo LV, Miller LD. Defective oxidative metabolism of rat liver mitochondria in hemorrhagic and endotoxin shock. Am J Physiol 220:571-577, 1971.

Miller DF, Irvine RW. Jaundice in acute appendicitis. Lancet 1:321-323, 1969.

Miller DJ, Keeton FR, Webber BL, Saunders SJ. Jaundice in severe bacterial infection. Gastroenterology 71:94-97, 1976.

Nishijima SK, Takezawa J, Hosotsubo KK, Takahashi E, Shimada Y, Yoshiya I. Serial changes in cellular immunity of septic patients with multiple organ-system failure. Crit Care Med 14:87-91, 1986.

Norton LW. Does drainage of intraabdominal pus reverse multiple organ failure? Am J Surg 149:347-350, 1985.

Nuytinck JKS, Goris RJA, Redl H, Schlag G, van Muster PJJ. Posttraumatic complications and inflammatory mediators. Arch Surg 121:886-890, 1986.

• Ozawa K, Aoyama H, Yasuda K, Shimahara Y, Nakatani T, Tanaka J, Yamamoto M, Kamiyama Y, Tobe T. Metabolic abnormalities associated with postoperative organ failure. Arch Surg 118:1245-1251, 1983.

• Pfenninger J, Gerber A, Tschappeler H, Zimmermann A. Adult respiratory distress syndrome in children. J Pediatr 101:352-357, 1982.

Pine RW, Wertz MJ, Lennard ES, Dellinger EP, Carrico CJ, Minshew BH. Determinants of organ malfunction or death in patients with intra-abdominal sepsis. Arch Surg 118:242-249, 1983.

Pittiruti M, Siegel JH, Sganga G, Coleman B, Wiles CE, Belzberg H, Wedel S, Placko R. Increased dependence of leucine in posttraumatic sepsis: Leucine/tyrosine clearance ratio as an indicator of hepatic impairment in septic multiple organ failure syndrome. Surgery 98:378-387, 1985.

• Royall JA, Levin DL. Adult respiratory distress syndrome in pediatric patients. 1. Clinical aspects, pathophysiology, pathology, and mechanisms of lung injury. J Pediatr 112:169-180, 1988.

Seglen PO, Solheim AE, Grinde B, Gordon PB, Schwarze PE, Gjessing R, Poli A. Amino acid control of protein synthesis and degradation in isolated at hepatocytes. Ann NY Acad Sci 349:1-17, 1980.

Siegel JH. Cardiorespiratory manifestations of metabolic failure in sepsis and the multiple organ failure syndrome. Surg Clin North Am 63:379-399, 1983.

Soyka LF, Hunt WG, Knight SE, Foster RS. Decreased liver and lung drug-metabolizing activity in mice treated with *Corynebacterium parvum*. Cancer Res 36:4425-4428, 1976.

Tanner A, Keyhani A, Reiner R, Holdstock G, Wright R. Proteolytic enzymes released by liver macrophages may promote hepatic injury in a rat model of hepatic damage. Gastroenterology 80:647-654, 1981.

Tilney NL, Bailey GL, Morgan AP. Sequential system failure after rupture of abdominal aortic aneurysms: An unsolved problem in postoperative care. Ann Surg 178:117-122, 1973.

Van Way CW, Monaghan T, Jones TN. Elevated pulmonary vascular resistance in patients dying from multiple organ failure. Am Surg 501:477-479, 1985.

Vermillion ST, Gregg JA, Baggenstoss AH, Bartholomew LG. Jaundice associated with bacteremia. Arch Intern Med 124:611-618, 1969.

Wahren J, Denis J, Desurmont P, Eriksson LS, Escoffier J-M, Gauthier AP, Hagenfeldt L, Michel H, Opolon P, Paris JC, Veyrac M. Is intravenous administration of branched chain amino acids effective in the treatment of hepatic encephalopathy? A multicenter study. Hepatology 3:475-480, 1983.

Waxman K. Postoperative multiple organ failure. Crit Care Clin 3:429-440, 1987.

• Wilkinson JD, Pollack MM, Ruttimann UE, Glass NL, Yeh TS. Outcome of pediatric patients with multiple organ system failure. Crit Care Med 14:271-274, 1986.

• Wilkinson JD, Pollack MM, Glass NL, Kanter RK, Katz RW, Steinhart CM. Mortality associated with multiple organ system failure and sepsis in pediatric intensive care unit. J Pediatr 111:324-328, 1987.

23 Cardiopulmonary Arrest

Penny Williams · Mary M. Farrell

BACKGROUND AND PHYSIOLOGY

Cardiopulmonary arrest in the infant or child is a unique problem that requires special techniques, diverse equipment, and skilled personnel. Cardiac arrest in children has various causes; however, respiratory conditions are by far the most common. Sudden infant death syndrome (SIDS) and near-drowning are the two leading respiratory conditions that precede cardiac arrest in children. Respiratory failure results in hypoxemia and acidosis, which eventually lead to cardiac arrest. Of all the dysrhythmias associated with cardiac arrest, asystole accounts for 78%, bradydysrhythmias account for 12%, and ventricular dysrhythmias account for the remaining 10%. Because the term "children" designates an entire spectrum of ages up to 18 years, age-related differences in pharmacology and physiology present a special problem in pediatric cardiopulmonary arrest situations.

The mortality for out-of-hospital arrests is 97% compared to 85% for in-hospital arrests, in either case a poor outcome. The outcome of cardiac arrest in children is related to the initial rhythm, being poorest with asystole and best with ventricular dysrhythmias.

THE CHILD AT RISK

Accidents are the leading cause of death in children. Since the majority of these situations are preventable, attention must be given to producing a safe and protected environment for the child. Children in the PICU are always at risk of cardiopulmonary arrest because of the relative instability of their condition. Conditions that pose the greatest risk are:

1. Upper airway obstruction: Croup, epiglottitis, suffocation, foreign body, strangulation
2. Lower airway obstruction: Pneumonia, severe asthma, aspiration, smoke inhalation, pulmonary edema, pneumothorax
3. Unstable cardiovascular status: Shock, dysrhythmias, hemorrhage, inflammatory cardiac disorders
4. CNS disorder: Meningitis, encephalitis, anoxia, near-miss SIDS
5. Artificial airways since respiratory sufficiency depends on airway patency
6. Postoperative period since general anesthetics or sedation may blunt reflexes

Hospitalized children are often subjected to various stressful procedures that place them at additional risk. Situations that may precipitate a cardiopulmonary arrest include:

1. Procedures requiring sedative medications that may depress respirations
2. Procedures that may cause bradycardia from vagal stimulation: Suctioning, passing of a nasogastric tube, rectal temperatures, intubation, manipulation of airway
3. Procedures that may cause bradycardia from Valsalva's maneuvers: Lumbar puncture, painful procedures, patient restraint
4. Decreasing respiratory support to patient by decreasing FIO_2, weaning from the ventilator, extubation
5. Chest physiotherapy (CPT) that can mobilize secretions and cause airway obstruction
6. Oral feedings in patients whose coordination of breathing and swallowing is absent, creating the risk of aspiration

MONITORING

Although stressful procedures are often necessary, even when patients are unstable, early recognition of signs and symptoms of deterioration may prevent a full cardiopulmonary arrest. Such signs include:

1. Change in level of consciousness and response to stimuli
2. Change in cardiovascular status, including bradycardia and poor peripheral perfusion
3. Change in respiratory status, including cyanosis, apnea, and altered respiratory pattern
4. Changes noted in noninvasive routine monitoring of ECG, pulse oximeter, and transcutaneous oxygen and carbon dioxide values

TREATMENT OF CARDIAC ARREST
Basic Life Support

In the arrest victim, basic life support externally supports the circulation and ventilation through the process of cardiopulmonary resuscitation (CPR). There are two theories postulating the mechanism of blood flow during CPR. The cardiac pump theory holds that direct compression of the heart between the sternum and the spine results in an increase in pressure within the ventricles, forcing blood out the aorta and pulmonary artery. The thoracic pump theory holds that chest compressions increase intrathoracic pressures, resulting in blood flow through the great vessels. The cardiac pump theory is believed to be the more plausible one in pediatrics because of the small chest size in these patients.

For the purpose of basic life support an infant is defined as younger than 1 year of age, and a child is defined as between the ages of 1 and 8 years. These are guidelines only, and in a health care setting you often come in contact with children whose sizes differ from the norm. Judgment needs to be exercised in choosing the technique that will produce the best result.

1. *Determine unresponsiveness or respiratory difficulty.* Gently shake the child to determine level of unconsciousness or assess the child for degree of respiratory difficulty.
2. *Call for help.*
3. *Position the child.* Gently move the child to a flat surface, positioning the child on his back while supporting the head and neck.
4. *Open the airway.* Perform a head-tilt/chin-lift procedure to pull the tongue and soft tissues away from the posterior pharynx. With the hand closest to the head, tilt the head back, and with the fingers of the other hand placed on the bony prominence of the lower jaw, lift the chin upward. Care must be

taken not to press on the soft tissues under the chin; this could obstruct the airway.

5. *Establish the presence of apnea.* Place your ear close to the mouth and nose of the patient and look for chest movement; listen and feel for expired air.

6. *Provide artificial ventilation.* (a) Maintain head-tilt/chin-lift and make a seal by placing your mouth over the mouth of the patient, occluding the nose with either your mouth or by pinching the nose (in children). (b) Administer two slow breaths, 1.0 to 1.5 seconds each, with a pause after each breath so the rescuer can take a breath of fresh air. The volume of air administered needs to be that which makes the chest rise slightly.

7. *Assess circulation.*

INFANT: Palpate the brachial pulse in the infant. The brachial pulse is located on the medial aspect of the upper arm between the elbow and shoulder. Palpate the pulse by placing the thumb on the outside of the arm and the index and middle fingers on the inside of the arm, pressing gently toward the bone.

NOTE: The precordial area is not a reliable means of assessing circulation. The presence or absence of the precordial impulse may be mistaken for the presence or absence of a pulse, and an erroneous decision may be made about the need for CPR.

CHILD: Palpate the carotid pulse in the child. While maintaining head-tilt with one hand, use the other hand to palpate the carotid artery located in the groove between the trachea and the neck muscles.

8. *Call for additional help.*

9. *If a pulse is present and breathing is absent, perform rescue breathing.*

INFANT: 20 times/min, or one breath every 3 sec
CHILD: 15 times/min, or one breath every 4 sec

If no pulse is palpated, begin external chest compressions.

INFANT: Place in horizontal position on a firm surface. If the shoulders of the infant lift off the hard surface when performing a head tilt, either place a towel under the shoulders to make a hard surface or place the hand not performing the compressions under the shoulders. Head-tilt is then maintained by the weight of the head and a slight lift of the shoulders.

The location for chest compressions is one fingerbreadth below the intermammary line (Fig. 23-1). Locate an imaginary line between the nipples. Place the index finger of the hand closest to the feet of the infant just under the intermammary line over the sternum. Lift the index finger and use the index and ring fingers to compress the chest.

NOTE: Because of the difference in the size of rescuers' hands and each infant's chest, a careful assessment must be made to avoid pressing on the xiphoid process.

Depth of compressions is 0.5 to 1.0 inch.
Rate of compressions is 100 times/min.

An alternate method of performing chest compression in the neonate and small infant is a side-by-side thumb placement on the sternum with the fingers circling the torso (Fig. 23-2). The thumbs are positioned just below the nipple line. In the very small infant the thumbs may need to be placed on top of each other to avoid excessive pressure on the ribs.

CHILD: To locate the area for chest compressions place the hand closest to the feet of the patient on the lower margin of the rib cage. Follow the rib cage with the middle finger to the notch where the ribs meet the sternum. Place the middle finger in the notch and index finger next to the middle finger. Visually note the placement of the index finger. Lift that hand and place the heel of that hand next to where the index finger was visually noted. Perform compressions with the heel of one hand on the sternum (Fig. 23-3).

NOTE: When visually noting the placement of the index finger, you may find it helpful to estimate the distance from the index finger to the intermammary line. This will aid in guiding you where to place the heel of your hand with initial and subsequent cycles.

Depth of compressions is 1.0 to 1.5 inches.
Rate of compressions is 80 to 100 times/min.

10. *Coordinate compressions and rescue breathing.* External chest compressions must always be performed in combination with rescue breathing. In the infant and the child a ratio of 5 compressions to 1

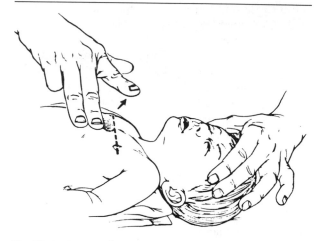

Fig. 23-1   Finger placement for infant chest compressions. (From American Heart Association. Instructor's Manual for Basic Life Support. Dallas: The Association, 1987, p 67. Reproduced with permission. Copyright American Heart Association.)

breath is given. At the end of every fifth compression the rescuer pauses to give a slow ventilation, 1.0 to 1.5 sec/breath.

INFANT: After the end of every fifth compression the rescuer leaves the fingers in light contact with the chest while lowering his head to give a ventilation. The airway is maintained by a head-tilt or by the weight of the head and slight lift of the shoulders.

CHILD: After the end of every fifth compression the rescuer lifts the heel of the hand from the chest and performs a head-tilt/chin-lift for ventilating. The hand closest to the feet is then visually placed in the proper location on the chest for each round of compressions.

Advanced Life Support

Once additional help has arrived at the scene, the most senior person (usually a physician) is designated to take charge. Responsibilities need to be assigned to the people present to avoid confusion and duplication of work. All of the following steps must be carried out simultaneously.

Basic life support

Continue mouth-to-mouth ventilation and closed-chest cardiac compressions.

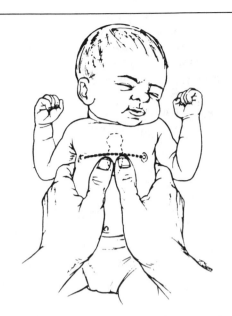

Fig. 23-2 Alternate method for performing infant chest compressions. (From American Heart Association. Standards and guidelines for cardiopulmonary resuscitation [CPR] and emergency cardiac care [ECC]. JAMA 255:2972, 1986. Copyright 1986, American Medical Association.)

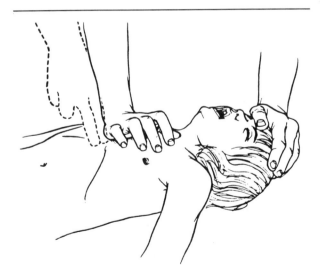

Fig. 23-3 Hand placement for chest compressions on a child. (From American Heart Association. Instructor's Manual for Basic Life Support. Dallas: The Association, 1987, p 67. Reproduced with permission. Copyright American Heart Association.)

Establish and maintain effective ventilation

Mouth-to-mouth ventilation provides 16% to 17% oxygen; therefore supplemental oxygen must be used in all arrest situations. Place artificial airways, either oropharyngeal or nasopharyngeal. Oropharyngeal airways are useful in maintaining airway patency in the unconscious child. They cannot be used in the conscious child since they may stimulate laryngospasm or vomiting and aspiration. In the conscious child a nasopharyngeal airway is better tolerated. A proper fitting face mask needs to be applied over the child's mouth and nose to ensure an airtight seal. Next it can be attached to a bag-valve device. Resuscitation bags must be self-inflating with a reservoir to permit delivery of 100% oxygen. Elective endotracheal intubation must be performed by the most experienced staff member. Ventilation and cardiac compressions may be interrupted for 30 seconds during intubation. If the patient becomes bradycardic (<80 bpm), bag-valve-mask ventilation must be resumed.

Ensure that bilateral breath sounds and adequate chest expansion are present. Institute oxygen saturation monitoring as soon as possible.

Vascular access and volume expansion

Establish IV access through the peripheral, central, or intraosseous routes. The largest and most easily accessible vein is the preferred choice. The central venous route provides more rapid onset and higher peak drug concentration.

Volume expansion is instituted by starting an IV infusion with crystalloid solution (0.9% sodium chloride, lactated Ringer's solution) or colloid (5% albumin, blood, Plasmanate). The volume of the infusion will vary in individuals depending on the cause of the arrest (septic shock, hypovolemia, cardiogenic shock).

Obtain serum Na, K, Cl, Ca, blood glucose, BUN levels.

Cardiac monitoring and treatment of dysrhythmia

1. Establish ECG monitoring.
2. Palpate central pulses (femoral, carotid, or brachial).
3. Measure systemic arterial blood pressure using a cuff of appropriate size.
4. Obtain arterial blood gas and pH determination.

5. Confirm the presence of a dysrhythmia on the ECG monitor and provide appropriate treatment (Table 23-1).
6. Defibrillation.
   a. Recommended energy dose is 2 watt-sec or joules/kg.
   b. Use a paddle of adequate size, which is 4.5 cm in diameter for infants and 8.0 cm in diameter for children.
   c. Apply electrode paste or cream to the paddles and place them over the chest wall, one at the apex and one at the base of the heart (Fig. 23-4).
   d. Ensure that no one is in contact with the patient or the bed.
   e. If defibrillation is not successful, double the energy level and defibrillate again.

Table 23-1   Treatment of Dysrhythmias

Type of Dysrhythmia	Treatment*
Asystole	
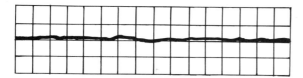	
Rate: Complete absence of any ventricular electrical activity P waves: In some cases P waves may be seen	CPR Epinephrine, 0.01 mg/kg IV Atropine, 0.02 mg/kg IV NaHCO₃, 1 mEq/kg IV if cardiac arrest is prolonged
Sinus bradycardia	
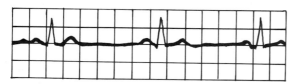	
Rate: Less than 60 bpm Rhythm: Regular P waves: Upright QRS: Following each P wave	Atropine, 0.02 mg/kg IV Consider pacing
Electromechanical dissociation	
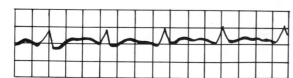	
Rate: Pulse weak or absent Rhythm: Electrical activity present	Epinephrine, 0.01 mg/kg IV Consider NaHCO₃, 1 mEq/kg IV

J = joule.
*The basis of treatment presumes that the dysrhythmia is continuing.

Table 23-1   Treatment of Dysrhythmias—cont'd

Type of Dysrhythmia	Treatment

Premature ventricular contractions (multifocal, bigeminy, or >5/min)

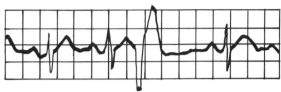

Rate: Varies

Rhythm: Irregular

P waves: Obscured

QRS: Wide and bizarre; ST segment and T wave in direction opposite QRS

Lidocaine, 1 mg/kg IV

Lidocaine infusion at 20 to 40 μg/kg/min

Ventricular tachycardia

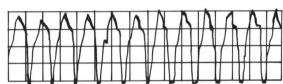

Rate: Close to normal to >400 bpm

Rhythm: Usually regular

P waves: Often not recognizable

QRS: Wide

Lidocaine, 1 mg/kg IV

Synchronized cardioversion 0.5 to 1.0 J/kg

Lidocaine infusion at 20 to 40 μg/kg/min

Ventricular fibrillation

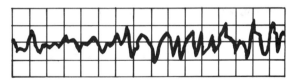

Rate: Rapid; usually too disorganized to count

Rhythm: Irregular; waveforms vary in size and shape

QRS: No P wave, QRS, ST segment, or T wave

Defibrillation, 2 J/kg

Defibrillation, 4 J/kg

Defibrillation, 4 J/kg

Epinephrine, 0.01 mg/kg

Supraventricular tachycardia

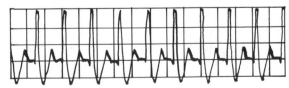

Rate: >230 bpm

Rhythm: Regular

P waves: May be difficult to see

Synchronized cardioversion 0.5 to 1.0 J/kg

NOTE: Verapamil is not recommended in pediatric resuscitation

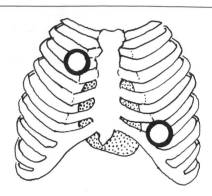

Fig. 23-4 Paddle placement sites for defibrillation. One paddle on the upper right chest below the clavicle and the other to the left of the left nipple in the anterior axillary line (below and slightly lateral to the cardiac apex). Paddles should not be placed over the sternum. (From Moloney-Harmon P. Managing Pediatric Emergencies: Cardiopulmonary Arrest. Baltimore: Resource Applications, 1984.)

Pharmacologic support

This is probably one of the most difficult parts of pediatric advanced life support (PALS) since drug dosages vary with the weight of the child. If the child's exact weight is unknown, it must be estimated. Precalculated drug sheets can be referred to quickly in the event of an arrest to help prevent medication errors. Computer programs can be established so that the patient's weight is the only information needed to generate a drug sheet (Fig. 23-5). Epinephrine, atropine, and lidocaine can be given via the endotracheal route when there is a delay in establishing vascular access. The same dosages as recommended for IV administration can be used, but these drugs must be diluted in 2 to 3 ml of 0.9% sodium chloride solution. Administration is via endotracheal tube, preferably using a syringe connected to a small nasogastric tube with the tip at or below the carina. The following drugs are used most frequently in cardiac arrest:

Epinephrine is an endogenous catecholamine with α- and β-adrenergic properties used in asystole and profound bradycardia with absent pulses (electromechanical dissociation). It may also convert fine ventricular fibrillation into coarse ventricular fibrillation. (Dose: 0.01 mg/kg of 1:10,000 solution.) Dose may be repeated at 5-minute intervals.

Atropine is used to treat bradycardia accompanied by poor perfusion or hypotension. (Dose: 0.02 mg/kg.) A minimum dose of 0.1 mg can be used since less than this may give rise to paradoxical bradycardia. Dose may be repeated at 5-minute intervals. The maximum dose is 1 mg in a child and 2 mg in an adolescent.

Lidocaine is used in the treatment of ventricular ectopy. (Dose: 1 mg/kg IV.)

Bretylium is used in the treatment of ventricular tachycardia and ventricular fibrillation unresponsive to lidocaine or cardioversion. (Dose: 5 mg/kg IV by rapid infusion.)

Calcium chloride is no longer recommended in asystole or electromechanical dissociation. It is used in the treatment of documented hypocalcemia, hyperkalemia, hypermagnesemia, and overdose with calcium-channel blocking agents. (Dose: 20 mg/kg.) The dose may be repeated one time in 10 minutes. Further doses must be based on calcium deficiencies.

Sodium bicarbonate is used in the treatment of metabolic acidosis accompanying cardiac arrest. Since respiratory conditions are the most common cause of cardiac arrest, ventilation is a prime consideration. Bicarbonate may be given in a dose of 1 mEq/kg in prolonged cardiac arrest. Doses may be repeated at 10-minute intervals. Further doses of bicarbonate must be based on arterial blood gas and pH interpretations using the formula 0.3 × kg of body weight × base deficit. If arterial blood gases and pH are not available, a dose of 0.5 mEq/kg can be given. Administration of sodium bicarbonate must be followed by infusion of 0.9% sodium chloride solution flushes since sodium bicarbonate may inactivate catecholamines and precipitate with calcium salts.

Glucose must be administered in the event of hypoglycemia documented by Chemstrip. (Dose: 0.5 to 1.0 g/kg IV.)

Catecholamine infusions in children can be prepared using the rule of six (Table 23-2).

NOTE: Sufficient 0.9% sodium chloride solution flush must be administered to ensure entry of medications into the central circulation. No more than 2 to 5 ml of flush can be administered after each dose of medication to prevent overhydration of the patient.

Postresuscitation stabilization

After adequate ventilation and stable cardiac rhythm are ensured, the child must be transported to the PICU for further management. Placement of nasogastric tube, bladder catheter, arterial catheter, and central venous catheter may be needed. Repeat arterial blood gas and pH determinations, serum electrolytes, and chest roentgenogram must be obtained. Currently most brain resuscitative therapy protocols are experimental; therefore attention to the details

of good support is of paramount importance. The goals of therapy are good oxygenation, ventilation, perfusion, systemic arterial blood pressure, normal temperature, normal glucose level, and prevention of electrolyte imbalance and seizures.

PICU CPR DRUG CALCULATIONS

Name: Smith, Baby Boy   Weight (kg):   10

RESUSCITATIVE MEDICATIONS

Drug/Strength	Dosage	Calculated Dose
Sodium bicarbonate (1 mEq/ml)	1 mEq/kg IV; may repeat in 10 min	10.0 mEq (10.0 ml)
Epinephrine, 1:10,000 (0.1 mg/ml)	0.01 mg/kg IV or ET; repeat every 5 min	0.10 mg (1.00 ml)
Calcium chloride, 10% (100 mg/ml)	20 mg/kg IV; may repeat in 10 min	200.0 mg (2.00 ml)
Atropine sulfate (0.1 mg/ml syringe)	0.02 mg/kg IV or ET; may repeat in 5 min	0.20 mg (2.00 ml)
Lidocaine, 2% cardiac (20 mg/ml)	1 mg/kg IV or ET, then 0.5 mg/kg every 10 min	10.00 mg (0.50 ml) 5.00 mg (0.25 ml)
Dextrose, 25% (250 mg/ml)	500 mg/kg IV 2 ml/kg	5000 mg (20.0 ml)

PROCEDURES

Method	Dosage	Calculated Dose
Defibrillation	2-4 watt-sec/kg	20 to 40 watt-sec
Cardioversion	0.2-1 watt-sec/kg	2 to 10 watt-sec

IV DRIPS

Drug/Strength	Dosage Range	Concentration Formula	Calculated Concentration
Dopamine (40 mg/ml)	2-20 μg/kg/min	6 mg/kg/100 ml at 1 ml/hr = 1 μg/kg/min	60.0 mg/100 ml (1.50 ml/100 ml)
Isoproterenol (0.2 mg/ml)	0.1-1 μg/kg/min	0.6 mg/kg/100 ml at 1 ml/hr = 0.1 μg/kg/min	6.0 mg/100 ml (30.0 ml/100 ml)
Nitroprusside (50 mg/vial)	0.5-8 μg/kg/min	6 mg/kg/100 ml at 1 ml/hr = 1 μg/kg/min	60.0 mg/100 ml
Epinephrine (1 mg/ml ampule)	0.1-1 μg/kg/min	0.6 mg/kg/100 ml at 1 ml/hr = 0.1 μg/kg/min	6.0 mg/100 ml (6.0 ml/100 ml)
Dobutamine (250 mg/vial)	5-15 μg/kg/min	6 mg/kg/100 ml at 1 ml/hr = 1 μg/kg/min	60.0 mg/100 ml
Lidocaine (20 mg/ml)	20-50 μg/kg/min	120 mg/100 ml at 1 ml/kg/hr = 20 μg/kg/min	120 mg/100 ml

Physician Signature

Fig. 23-5 Sample precalculated drug sheet. (Courtesy Children's Medical Center of Dallas.)

Table 23-2 Equation for the Preparation of Catecholamine Infusions

Drug	Preparation	Dose
Isoproterenol Epinephrine Norepinephrine	0.6 × body weight (kg) is mg added to diluent to make 100 ml	1 ml/hr delivers 0.1 μg/kg/min titrated to effect
Dopamine Dobutamine	6 × body weight (kg) is mg added to diluent to make 100 ml	1 ml/hr delivers 1.0 μg/kg/min titrated to effect
Lidocaine	120 mg in 100 ml of D_5W at 1 ml/kg/hr = 20 μg/kg/min	20 to 50 μg/kg/min

---

RESUSCITATION EQUIPMENT

Drugs

Sodium bicarbonate
  10 ml prefilled syringe (1 mEq/ml) (2)
  50 ml vial (1 mEq/ml) (1)
Epinephrine
  10 ml prefilled syringe (0.1 mg/ml) (2)
  1 ml ampule (1 mg/ml) (1)
Calcium chloride: 10 ml prefilled syringe (100 mg/ml) (2)
Atropine: 10 ml prefilled syringe (0.1 mg/ml) (2)
Benadryl: 1 ml ampule (1)
Calcium gluconate: 10 ml ampule (2)
Dextrose 50%: 50 ml vial (2)
Dilantin: 2 ml ampule (2)
Digoxin: 1 ml ampule (2)
Isuprel: 5 ml ampule (2)
Lidocaine: 10 ml prefilled syringe (2)
Narcan: 1 ml ampule (2)
Valium: 2 ml ampule (2)
Versed: 2 ml ampule (2)
Dopamine: 5 ml ampule (2)
Lasix: 2 ml ampule (2)
Potassium chloride: 10 ml vial (2)
Methylprednisolone: 2 ml vial (125 mg) (2)
Heparin: 10 ml vial (1000 units/ml) (2)
0.9% sodium chloride solution: 10 ml vial (nonpreservative) (4)

IV equipment

Lactated Ringer's solution, 250 ml (1)
5% dextrose, 250 ml (1)
5% dextrose in 0.45% sodium chloride, 250 ml (1)
0.9% sodium chloride solution, 250 ml (1)
IV Solusets (microdrip and maxidrip) (2)
Extension tubing (2)
Three-way stopcocks (4)
T-connectors
Latex tourniquet
Alcohol and Betadine swabs
IV catheter (catheter-over-needle), 24 to 16 gauge
Winged needle device, 21 to 25 gauge
Armboards, small and large
Adhesive tape, 1/2" to 2"

Suction/NG

Bulb syringe
Tonsil-suction tip
Suction catheters, tip sizes 6.5 to 16F
Feeding tube (size 8 F)
Catheter adapter
50 ml syringe
Lubricating jelly
Adhesive tape, 1"

Airway

1 L hyperinflation bag
Oxygen flowmeter
Oxygen face masks, sizes neonate to large adult
Oral airways, 40 to 100 mm
Magill forceps, child and adult
Laryngoscope handle, standard size
Straight laryngoscope blades, Miller, sizes No. 0 to 3
MacIntosh laryngoscope blades, size No. 3
Extra bulbs and batteries
Endotracheal tubes, sizes 2.5 to 6.0
Endotracheal tubes with cuff, sizes 6.0 to 7.0
Benzoin swabs
0.9% sodium chloride solution

Miscellaneous

Syringes, TB, 3, 10, 20 ml (4 each)
Needles, 25 to 18 gauge (5 each)
Cardiac needles, 3", 20 gauge (2)
Intraosseous needles, 18-gauge spinal or bone marrow needles
Blood tubes
Cotton balls
2" × 2" gauze
Medication labels
Isolation supplies (gloves, goggles, gowns, masks)
Cardiac arrest board

ORGANIZATIONAL ASPECTS OF CARDIOPULMONARY RESUSCITATION

Communication

A communication system for notifying personnel of an arrest is important, and the shortest amount of time possible should elapse between the discovery of the arrest situation and the arrival of the code team and resuscitation equipment. A standardized code recognized as a priority signal (Dr. Heart, Code Blue, Stat Page, Code 99, etc.) must be established in each hospital. This code can be communicated through overhead paging systems, hospital beeper systems, and direct lines to acute care areas (PICU, emergency department, operating room, etc.) to mobilize personnel and resuscitation equipment.

CPR Team

A key element to an effectively run code is an organized team response. Such a response might be by a "code team" assigned to respond to any location or by team members spontaneously formed during the crisis moment. The ideal members of the team would include (1) a charge physician knowledgeable in acute emergency care; (2) three to four nurses trained in advanced life support procedures who manage the areas of equipment, medication preparation, and recording; and (3) one to two respiratory therapists skilled in managing ventilatory support and external chest compressions. Additional assistance may be needed by an anesthesiologist, cardiologist, surgeon, or pharmacist. Support from social work and chaplains may be helpful to the team members and the patient's family. The effectiveness of the team depends on clearly delineated roles and responsibilities for each team member to avoid confusion and duplication of efforts.

Equipment

Resuscitation equipment must be readily available in all areas of a hospital and quickly mobilized to the arrest area. Pediatric resuscitation equipment needs to include (1) an emergency cart stocked with drugs and supplies, (2) defibrillator with strip recorder and pediatric paddles, (3) portable O_2 cylinder, and (4) portable suction machine. An upright rolling cart is often used to house the equipment. The defibrillator often can be placed on top of the cart with the O_2 cylinder taped or bracketed to the side of the cart so the equipment can be moved as one unit.

Supplies stocked on the emergency cart need to be limited to those needed during the initial phase of resuscitation. Standardizing all carts so that the number, type, and location of supplies are the same greatly aids in the efficiency of a code, especially if personnel are unfamiliar with the setting. Supplies can be categorized in drawers and the drawers labeled based on function (drugs, IV, suction/NG, airway, etc.). Supplies needed for monitoring and defibrillation (electrodes, paste or gel, extra ECG paper) must be readily accessible to the defibrillator.

To ensure that the resuscitative equipment is ready for use and functioning properly, daily checks must be made. Expiration dates of drugs and IV fluids need to be noted and a system established for replacing these drugs once expired. The defibrillator must be checked daily based on manufacturer recommendations.

Record of Resuscitation

The resuscitation record is an essential component of the resuscitation process. Its purpose is to account for the events that occur during a code. It is important therefore that a form be developed so that documentation can be quick, efficient, and accurate. The record is often referred to by team members responding to a code to verify when procedures were last performed. The resuscitation record must capture the following (Fig. 23-6):

1. Demographic patient data (including weight)
2. Time of arrest
3. Drug administration
4. IV therapy
5. Vital signs
6. Defibrillation or cardioversion
7. Laboratory values
8. Sequence of procedures
9. Effectiveness of treatments
10. Final disposition of the child
11. Notation of team members
12. Signature of recording nurse and physician

ECG strips can be affixed to the back of the resuscitation record to provide further documentation. The resuscitation record can be a valuable tool in evaluating the appropriateness of care and the effects of training. Making the form a carbon record allows the original form to be used in the patient's record and the carbon to be used for evaluation.

Training

The performance demonstrated in response to a code reflects the education and training of personnel. Physicians, nurses, respiratory therapists, and other

CHILDREN'S MEDICAL CENTER OF DALLAS
1935 Motor Street
Dallas, Texas 75235

CARDIOPULMONARY RESUSCITATION REPORT

DATE _____

NAME _____

AGE _____ WEIGHT _____ Kg

TIME STARTED _____   TIME ENDED _____

DRUGS

Note if route other than IV is used.

ET = ENDOTRACHEAL   IO = INTRAOSSEOUS   IC = INTRACARDIAC

EPINEPHRINE 0.1 mg/ml	TIME								
	AMOUNT								
ATROPINE 0.1 mg/ml	TIME								
	AMOUNT								
Na BICARBONATE 1 mEq/ml	TIME								
	AMOUNT								
NORMAL SALINE	TIME								
	AMOUNT								
	TIME								
	AMOUNT								
	TIME								
	AMOUNT								
	TIME								
	AMOUNT								

VITAL SIGNS

Note if other than spontaneous
C = COMPRESSIONS
B = BAGGING

TIME	B/P	HR	RESP

IV SOLUTIONS AND BLOOD PRODUCTS

LINE 1

TIME	RATE	MS	PT

LINE 2

TIME	RATE	MS	PT

LINE 3

TIME	RATE	MS	PT

LINE 4

TIME	RATE	MS	PT

DEFIBRILLATION

TIME	WATT-SECS.	RHYTHM RESPONSE

LAB VALUES

TIME	TEST	RESULT	TIME	TEST	RESULT

BLOOD GASES

TIME	PaO$_2$	PaCO$_2$	pH	△B

Fig. 23-6   Resuscitation record. (Courtesy Children's Medical Center of Dallas.)

ATTENDING PHYSICIAN NOTIFIED (Name) _____

TIME_____ BY _____

FAMILY NOTIFIED _____ RELATION_____

TIME_____ BY_____ DOB_____ MR_____

TIME	NURSING OBSERVATIONS	TIME	NURSING OBSERVATIONS
	INITIAL ASSESSMENT:		
		RECORDER SIGNATURE:	
		PHYSICIAN SIGNATURE:	
		STAFF (List by name, title, function)	
		ER Cart Used Yes ☐ No ☐	

Continued.

EMERGENCY DRUG DOSAGES

DRUG	DOSAGE	CONCENTRATION	ROUTE
ATROPINE	0.02 mg/kg (not less than 0.1 mg/dose) q 5 minutes	0.1 mg/ml	IV, IM, ET, IC*
CALCIUM CHLORIDE (10%)	20 mg/kg q 10 minutes	100 mg/ml	IV, IC*
DEXTROSE (50%)	Dilute to D25% 500 mg/kg	(50%) 500 mg/ml	IV
DIAZEPAM (Valium)	0.3 mg/kg/dose	5 mg/ml	IV
EPINEPHRINE (Adrenalin)	0.01 mg/kg q 5 minutes	1:10,000 = 0.1 mg/ml	IV, ET, IC*
		1:1,000 = 1 mg/ml Dilute for IV Admin.	IV
LIDOCAINE (Xylocaine)	1 mg/kg	20 mg/ml	IV, ET
NALOXONE (Narcan)	5-10 mcg/kg/dose	0.4 mg/ml	IV, IM, SQ
PHENOBARBITAL	10-15 mg/kg (Loading Dose)	65 mg/ml	IV, IM
SODIUM BICARBONATE	Based on ABG's only. 1mEq/kg/dose or 0.3 x kg x base deficit Repeat q 10 mins.	1 mEq/ml	IV, IC*

* IC only as a last resort

DEFIBRILLATION DOSAGE - 1-2 watt/seconds/kg.

AGE		ET TUBE SIZE (mm)
	PREMIE	2.0 - 3.0
0 - 6	MONTHS	3.0 - 3.5
6 - 12	MONTHS	3.5 - 4.0
12 - 18	MONTHS	4.0 - 4.5
2 - 4	YEARS	4.5 - 5.5
4 - 6	YEARS	5.5 - 6.5
> 6	YEARS	6.5 - 7.5

Length of insertion of ET tube
(in older children)

$$\frac{age}{2} + 12 \text{ mm (for oral)}$$

add 4 mm for nasal

CATECHOLAMINE INFUSION GUIDELINES

DOPAMINE
DOBUTAMINE   6 mg x body weight (kg) added to diluent to make 100 ml   then 1 ml/hr = 1 mcg/kg/min.

DOSE RANGE

DOPAMINE   2.0 - 20.0 mcg/kg/min.
DOBUTAMINE   5.0 - 15.0 mcg/kg/min.

ISOPROTERENOL
EPINEPHRINE   0.6 mg x body weight (kg) added to diluent to make 100 ml   then 1 ml/hr = 0.1 mcg/kg/min.

DOSE RANGE

ISOPROTERENOL   0.1 - 1.0 mcg/kg/min.
EPINEPHRINE   0.1 - 1.0 mcg/kg/min.

TIME TIME TIME TIME

CARDIOPULMONARY RESUSCITATION REPORT

CMC 26016

Fig. 23-6, cont'd   Resuscitation record.

health care professionals must maintain proficiency at all times in the skills of CPR. Basic life support can be required for all health care professionals who are involved in direct patient care. Both basic and advanced life support can be a component of orientation programs. An annual review of advanced life support standards and guidelines and hospital policies and procedures related to codes can be required of all personnel who might participate in resuscitation measures. Simulated mock codes can be a useful teaching method to allow personnel the practical experience in the procedures of an arrest.

Administrative Coordination

A successful CPR program requires close observation and evaluation. A committee composed of multidisciplinary members can provide the expertise for evaluation and critique. Disciplines most commonly included in such committees are critical care medicine, anesthesiology, cardiology, nursing, hospital administration, respiratory therapy, pharmacy, central supply, and nursing and medical education. The function of such a committee would be to:

1. Provide ongoing monitoring and evaluation of resuscitations
2. Develop policies and protocols for resuscitation (i.e., communication system for announcing arrests, function of arrest team members, documentation on CPR record, staff training requirements, do not resuscitate orders)
3. Standardize resuscitation equipment
4. Design, implement, and evaluate educational programs in basic and advanced life support

ADDITIONAL READING

American Heart Association. Instructor's Manual for Basic Life Support. Dallas: The Association, 1987.

• American Heart Association. Textbook of Advanced Pediatric Life Support. Dallas: The Association, 1987.

• American Heart Association. Standards and guidelines for cardiopulmonary resuscitation (CPR) and emergency cardiac care (ECC). JAMA 255:2972, 1986.

American Heart Association. Standards and guidelines for cardiopulmonary resuscitation (CPR) and emergency cardiac care (ECC). JAMA 244:435, 1980.

Brill JE. Cardiopulmonary resuscitation. Pediatr Ann 15:1, 1986.

Eisenberg M, Bergner L, Hallstrom A. Epidemiology of cardiac arrest and resuscitation in children. Ann Emerg Med 23:672, 1983.

Gillis J, Dickson D, Rieer M, et al. Results of inpatient pediatric resuscitation. Crit Care Med 14:469, 1986.

Ludwig S, Kettrick R, Parker M. Pediatric cardiopulmonary resuscitation. Clin Pediatr 23:2, 1984.

Moloney-Harmon P. Managing Pediatric Emergencies: Cardiopulmonary Arrest. Baltimore: Resource Applications, 1984.

Orlowski JP. Optimal position for external cardiac massage in infants and children. Crit Care Med 12:224, 1984.

Torphy D, Miner M, Thompson B. Cardiorespiratory arrest and resuscitation of children. Am J Dis Child 138:1099, 1984.

Zaritsky A. Cardiopulmonary resuscitation in children. Clin Chest Med 8:561, 1987.

Zaritsky A. Advanced pediatric life support: State of the art. Circulation 74(Suppl IV):124, 1986.

24 Brain Death

Mary M. Farrell · Gary R. Turner

BACKGROUND

Brain death is the irreversible cessation of the function of the entire brain, including the cerebral cortex and brain stem. Since the original publication of criteria for the diagnosis of brain death by the Ad Hoc Committee of the Harvard Medical School in 1968, over 30 different criteria for the diagnosis of brain death have been published. Until recently no criteria specifically addressed the particular problems associated with making a diagnosis of brain death in young children. In 1981 The Report of the Medical Consultants on the Diagnosis of Death to the President's Commission for the Study of Ethical Problems in Medicine and Biomedical and Behavioral Research stated, "The brains of infants and young children have increased resistance to damage and may recover substantial functions even after exhibiting unresponsiveness on neurological examination for longer periods compared with adults. Physicians should be particularly cautious in applying neurological criteria to determine death in children younger than 5 years." Problems in applying adult criteria to young children have included ascertaining the period of observation necessary to ensure irreversibility of the patient's condition and determining the appropriateness of applying ancillary tests such as EEG and radionuclide angiography to confirm the clinical diagnosis of brain death. Recently these issues were addressed by a national task force in published guidelines for the determination of brain death in children.

These guidelines emphasize determination of the cause of the patient's condition, physical examination criteria, observation periods according to the patient's age and etiology of the coma, and ancillary laboratory studies.

ETIOLOGY OF COMA

A thorough history of events preceding the patient's lapse into the comatose state must be obtained to exclude the presence of remedial conditions that mimic coma. Obtaining a toxicology screen can be helpful in ruling out coma from drug overdoses (e.g., barbiturates, sedatives) and in many institutions is required to confirm the diagnosis of brain death. It must be determined that the patient is in reasonable metaboblic balance by the absence of significant hypernatremia, hyponatremia, or hypoglycemia. Diabetes insipidus often occurs in brain-dead patients; however, its presence is not a prerequisite for the diagnosis of brain death. The presence of neuromuscular blockade may be excluded by the use of a nerve stimulator (see Chapter 130). Drug levels of sedative or hypnotic drugs must be below the toxic range.

PHYSICAL EXAMINATION

Before neurologic evaluation can be performed the patient's systemic arterial blood pressure must be within the range of normal for age, and body temperature must be normothermic; temperature <35° C is considered hypothermic. The patient can exhibit no response to pain, including decorticate and decerebrate posturing, in the area of the cranial nerve distribution. Brain stem reflexes must be absent (Fig. 24-1). Neurologic evaluation encompasses assessment of the following:

Pupils: The pupils may be fully dilated or in midposition but must not respond to light. Topical mydriatics, anticholinergic drugs, or preexisting ocular disease may impair testing. Glutethimide and scopolamine intoxication can cause dilated pupils that do not react to light stimulation.

Corneal reflexes: Absence of the corneal reflexes must be demonstrated as the inability of the orbicularis oculi to constrict following corneal stimulation.

Oculovestibular reflexes: The ear canals must be

CHECKLIST FOR DOCUMENTATION OF BRAIN DEATH

I. Diagnosis: _____
    Etiology of coma: _____

II. Laboratory information
    1. Electrolytes _____ Date/time _____
    2. Glucose _____ Date/time _____
    3. CNS depressant drugs and toxins
       a. Most recent blood level _____ Date/time _____
       b. Date/time of last dose _____
    4. Toxicology screen _____

III. Clinical examinations   *Exam #1*   *Exam #2*
     Date   _____   _____
     Time   _____   _____
     Temperature   _____   _____
     Blood pressure   _____   _____
     Response to nerve stimulator   _____   _____
     A. No spontaneous movements, including no decorticate or decerebrate postur-   _____   _____
        ing and no shivering
     B. Cranial nerves
        1. Pupils dilated and fixed to light   _____   _____
           a. Pupil diameter (mm)   _____   _____
        2. No corneal reflexes   _____   _____
        3. No eye movement in response to head turning   _____   _____
        4. No eye movement with irrigation of auditory canal with ice water (20 ml)   _____   _____
           after tympanic membranes visualized
        5. No gag or cough with suctioning of pharynx and endotracheal tube   _____   _____
        6. No motor response within the cranial nerve distribution with painful   _____   _____
           stimulation
     C. Apnea (after second examination)
        1. Pco_2 at end of apnea test   _____
        2. Po_2 at end of apnea test   _____
        3. pH at end of apnea test   _____
        4. Time in minutes off ventilator   _____

IV. Ancillary studies
    1. Study _____ Date/time _____ Results _____

Certification of Death

Having considered the above findings, we hereby certify as to the irreversible cessation of all spontaneous brain
function of, and the death of, _____
_____

Date _____ Time _____

_____ M.D.   _____ M.D.
Signature of physician   Signature of physician

Fig. 24-1 Brain death protocol. (Courtesy Children's Medical Center of Dallas.)

visualized before testing. Lack of eye movement after irrigation of each ear canal with 20 ml of ice-cold water indicates an absent response.

Oculocephalic reflexes: The "doll's eyes" maneuver is performed by observing the patient's eyes while rotating the head to one side and then 180 degrees in the opposite direction. In the brain-dead patient the head and eyes move together. This test must not be performed if a cervical fracture is suspected.

Other reflexes: Gag and cough reflexes must be absent; this can be ensured by suctioning of the posterior pharynx and endotracheal tube. Sucking and rooting reflexes must be absent when attempting to establish the diagnosis of brain death in the infant. Spinal reflexes may be present in up to 50% of brain-dead patients; for example, plantar withdrawal, muscle stretch reflexes, abdominal reflexes, and flexor-plantar response may be present.

Presence of apnea: The apnea test must be performed after the patient has fulfilled the other physical examination criteria and the findings of ancillary tests are consistent with the diagnosis of brain death. Test for apnea as follows:

1. Adjust the ventilator rate until the $PaCO_2$, $PetCO_2$, or $tcCO_2$ is approximately 45 mm Hg.
2. Preoxygenate the patient with 100% oxygen for 5 minutes before testing.
3. Disconnect the patient from ventilator for 5 minutes.
4. Deliver oxygen at 6 L/min to the endotracheal tube during testing.
5. Oxygen saturation and $PaCO_2$ may be followed by pulse oximetry and transcutaneous PCO_2 monitoring. Arterial blood gases and pH must be obtained at the end of the test.
6. To confirm the presence of apnea the arterial PCO_2 must reach 60 mm Hg during testing. The rate of rise of PCO_2 in brain-dead children is approximately 4 mm Hg/min.
7. The test must be discontinued if spontaneous respirations resume, cyanosis sets in, or there is a change in systemic arterial blood pressure >10% of baseline values.

OBSERVATION PERIODS

The special task force has recommended an observation period according to the age of the child. Obviously the physical examination must be unchanged during this observation period. For children from 7 days to 2 months of age two examinations and EEGs separated by at least 48 hours are necessary. Children from 2 months to 1 year of age must receive two examinations and EEGs separated by at least 24 hours. If the absence of flow is demonstrated on a radionuclide study the second examination and EEG may be omitted. For children over 1 year of age an observation period of at least 12 hours in the presence of an irreversible cause is necessary. A longer period of 24 hours may be required in certain instances such as hypoxic-ischemic encephalopathy. However, if the EEG is isoelectric or interpretation of the radionuclide study indicates no flow, the observation period may be shortened.

ANCILLARY STUDIES

Ancillary studies include EEG, cerebral arteriography, and radionuclide brain scan. The EEG must be performed over 30 minutes using standardized techniques. The pitfalls of EEG testing include the following: (1) electrocerebral silence may be difficult to record in the PICU setting because of the additional monitoring equipment; (2) many EEGs show multiple artifacts that may be bizarre and difficult to identify and locate; (3) extreme prematurity or asphyxia of the newborn, hypothermia, barbiturates, and other drugs may in and of themselves cause an isoelectric EEG; and (4) the incidence of discordance between clinicians interpreting the records is 3%.

The determination of the absence of cerebral blood flow on four-vessel cerebral arteriography is the sine qua non of brain death. In the presence of barbiturate coma this is the only method available to diagnose brain death.

Radionuclide cerebral imaging consists of IV injection of technetium-99m pertechnetate, which passes through the cervical circulation into the intracranial vault. A tourniquet is placed around the patient's forehead to prevent detection of scalp circulation, and images are obtained utilizing a portable y-scintillation camera. Demonstration of absence of intracranial circulation is confirmatory evidence of brain death. The presence of sagittal sinus activity in the absence of intracranial arterial circulation does not militate against the diagnosis of brain death. The advantages of this technique are that it is noninvasive; it can be performed at the bedside, which obviates the necessity of transporting unstable children or children attached to a great deal of equipment; and it is less expensive than cerebral arteriography. However, it has not been proved effective in the premature infant and young child less than 2 months of age.

Xenon CT, digital subtraction angiography, Doppler determination of cerebral blood flow, brain stem auditory-evoked and visual-evoked potentials, and visualization of cerebral arterial pulsations by real-time cranial ultrasonography are additional ancillary studies that may be helpful in the diagnosis of brain death; however, further experience with these methods is needed.

MEDICOLEGAL

Currently in the United States brain death legislation has been enacted in over 38 states. Legislation regarding the responsibilities of the examining physician and supporting ancillary studies may vary from state to state.

ADDITIONAL READING

Ad Hoc Committee on Brain Death, The Children's Hospital, Boston: Determination of brain death. J Pediatr 110:15-19, 1987.

Ad Hoc Committee of the Harvard Medical School. A definition of irreversible coma. JAMA 205:337-340, 1968.

Ashwal S, Smith A, Torres F, et al. Radionuclide bolus angiography: A technique for verification of brain death in infants and children. J Pediatr 91:722-728, 1977.

Black P McL. Brain death. N Engl J Med 299:338-344, 393-401, 1978.

Coulter D. Neurologic uncertainty in newborn intensive care. N Engl J Med 316:840-844, 1987.

Drake B, Ashwal S, Schneider S. Determination of cerebral death in the pediatric intensive care unit. Pediatrics 78:107-112, 1986.

Fiser D, Jimenez J, Wrape V, Woody R. Diabetes insipidus in children with brain death. Crit Care Med 15:551-553, 1987.

Freeman J, Ferry P. New brain death guidelines in children: Further confusion. Pediatrics 81:301-303, 1988.

Holzman B, Curless R, Sfakianakis G, et al. Radionuclide cerebral perfusion scintigraphy in determination of brain death in children. Neurology 33:1027-1031, 1983.

Outwater K, Rockoff M. Apnea testing to confirm brain death in children. Crit Care Med 12:357-358, 1984.

President's Commission for the Study of Ethical Problems in Medicine and Biomedical and Behavioral Research: Guidelines for the determination of death. JAMA 246:2184-2186, 1981.

Rowland T, Donnelly J, Jackson A. Apnea documentation for determination of brain death in children. Pediatrics 74:505-508, 1984.

Schaffer J, Caronna J. Duration of apnea needed to confirm brain death. Neurology 28:661-666, 1978.

Schwartz JA, Baxter J, Brill D. Diagnosis of brain death in children by radionuclide cerebral imaging. Pediatrics 73:14-18, 1984.

Steinhart C, Weiss I. Use of brain stem auditory evoked potentials in pediatric brain death. Crit Care Med 13:560-562, 1985.

• Task Force on Brain Death in Children: Guidelines for the determination of brain death in children. Pediatrics 80:298-300, 1987.

• Volpe JJ. Brain death determination in the newborn. Pediatrics 80:293-297, 1987.

25 Identification and Medical Management of the Pediatric Organ Donor

Alison B. Ballew · *Stephen D. Haid*

BACKGROUND

Organ transplantation in the late 1980s has proved to be a successful therapeutic modality for the treatment of end-stage organ failure. Development and refinement of posttransplant immunosuppressive regimens have resulted in 1-year graft survival rates >80% for kidney and heart transplantation, with 1-year success rates for liver transplants in the 70% range. Because organ transplantation is now recognized as a successful treatment and indeed is the preferred treatment in most cases, the number of new transplant centers has increased dramatically each year.

Although the supply of available cadaveric organs for transplantation has increased annually, the demand continues to increase at an even more accelerated rate. Further exacerbating the problem is the qualification that liver, heart, and heart-lung transplants must be matched for size (within 10% to 20%) plus blood group compatibility. This is particularly a problem for children awaiting transplants because organs from pediatric donors are so scarce. Fortunately there is more flexibility in the implantation of kidneys and pancreas because size is generally not a factor. However, transplantation of an extremely large kidney into a very small child or an infant's kidney into a large adult is not preferred. In fact, both kidneys from pediatric donors are frequently used en bloc in adult recipients. Because kidney transplantation in small infants is limited by the availability of pediatric kidneys, many centers will not transplant pediatric kidneys en bloc into an adult unless no suitable pediatric recipient is available. The absolute number of available organ donors in many cases is not as critical as the timeliness of the availability of donors of appropriate size for those recipients on the waiting list.

Although the importance of appropriate organ preservation in these situations cannot be overstated, one cannot even get to that point without acknowledging the gift from the parents of a child who has suddenly died. Giving consent to donate the organs of a loved one is, at best, an emotional decision that must be made over a short period of time by the immediate next of kin. When that loved one is a child, the decision to donate can be even more emotionally charged. A Gallup poll performed in 1987 showed that 82% of individuals would be willing to donate the organs of a loved adult, but only 61% would donate their own child's organs. Another public attitude survey of residents from North Carolina similarly showed that population less willing to donate a child's organs than those of self or spouse.

One may postulate that obtaining consent from the parents of a deceased child may be more difficult than from the family of an adult. However, in our experience we have found that many parents in this situation find comfort in knowing that others can benefit from this otherwise tragic situation and in some cases are not only willing to donate but actually initiate the conversation. Unfortunately there are times when the discussion never takes place and the opportunity to donate is lost. Many states have passed "Required Request" or "Routine Inquiry" laws mandating hospitals to offer the option of organ donation to the next of kin at the time of death. Additionally, federal legislation (P.L. 99-509) requires hospitals to have organ recovery policies in place, including procedures for approaching families about the issue of organ donation, in order to receive Medicare reimbursement. The Joint Commission on Accreditation of Health Associations has also issued new regulations along those same lines. Compliance is required for hospitals to receive accreditation. It is anticipated that, over time, the process of approaching families to offer the option of organ donation will become routine in all hospitals. Subsequently the incidence of organ donation should increase.

As the number of organ transplant centers increases, the demands on procurement organizations and organ recovery coordinators become greater. These individuals must be concerned not only about organ availability, but they are also faced with an expanding range of duties. One important function of the organ recovery coordinator is to ensure that the retrieved organs are in optimal condition, which is accomplished through appropriate medical management of the organ donor. Although much has been written about medical management of the adult organ donor, similar information for the pediatric organ donor is not widely available, and adult management principles cannot always be applied to the pediatric situation.

IDENTIFICATION AND CRITERIA

Several variables must be considered when evaluating the medical acceptability of potential pediatric donors. For the purpose of definition the upper age limit of a pediatric donor is generally considered to be 14 to 16 years with weight being the critical determinant. The information provided in this chapter describes pediatric donor criteria up to the point at which normal limits coincide with adult criteria. In most instances the pediatric donor is a previously healthy child who has sustained a head injury that ultimately results in brain death. In-depth evaluation must include (1) cause of death, (2) past medical history, (3) current hospital history, and (4) specific organ function.

Cause of Death

The initial evaluation of a brain-dead child considered as a potential organ donor begins with ascertaining the documented cause of death. A death of unknown cause may ultimately preclude donation; however, the referral of such cases should still be made to the local organ procurement organization for thorough evaluation.

Past Medical History

In all potential donor situations reviewing past medical history is important. It is important to note any congenital abnormalities and corresponding treatment (e.g., hydrocephalus and subsequent placement of a ventriculoperitoneal shunt). Inquiries about prior surgeries, chronic diseases such as diabetes, recurrent disease such as streptococcus infections or frequent urinary tract infections, and, finally, blood transfusion history must also be made. Whether either parent has a history of IV drug abuse or a communicable disease such as hepatitis B must also be determined.

Current Hospital History

The current hospital history must be a precise and detailed account of the donor's hospital course. Some widely accepted contraindications to donation include current sepsis, any history of malignancy other than primary CNS tumors, and a positive result on testing for human immunodeficiency virus. Additionally, a donor who tests positive for hepatitis B surface antigen or syphilis will be excluded from donation in most cases. All donors are screened for the above-mentioned conditions.

Evaluation of the potential donor begins with ascertaining the circumstances surrounding the preadmission and admission period, noting all injuries, chest or abdominal trauma, plus cardiac or respiratory arrests, including the duration and interventions used in attempting stabilization. Any surgery during the hospitalization must be documented, with findings of the primary surgeon relayed to the organ procurement organization.

A donor's hemodynamic status must also be carefully reviewed. Fluid balance must be determined early because variations in systemic arterial blood pressure, cardiopulmonary status, and interpretation of laboratory results are all affected by the state of hydration. All episodes of hypotension must be analyzed closely, assessing the degree, duration, type of therapy and response to therapy. For example, the use of vasopressors vs. simple fluid restoration can affect the suitability for transplantation of certain organs.

Infection is another area that demands close attention. Infection can occur through multiple avenues. All potential organ donors need mechanical ventilation, thereby subjecting them to the risk of pulmonary infection. Maximal support of the patient, and later the donor, involves multiple invasive procedures such as central venous, arterial, and bladder catheters. All of this, in conjunction with steroid therapy commonly used to treat cerebral edema, renders the potential donor a prime target for almost any type of infection. Any rise in temperature above normal must be investigated fully. In the brain-injured or brain-dead child determining the cause of an elevation in temperature can be difficult because of damage that commonly occurs to the hypothalamus. An abrupt temperature elevation may be totally unrelated to an infectious process; it may result from

Table 25-1   Standard Criteria for Organ Donation

	Heart	Heart/Lung	Lung	Liver	Kidney	Pancreas
Age range (yr)	Male 0-35 Female 0-40	Male 0-35 Female 0-40	Male 0-35 Female 0-40	0-50	0-60	1-60
ABO required	Yes	Yes	Yes	Yes	Yes	Yes
Accurate weight	Yes	Yes	Yes	Yes	No	No
Chest circumference	Yes	Yes	Yes	Yes	No	No
Presence of active systemic infections	Rule out	Rule out	Rule out	Rule out	Rule out	Rule out
Recent history of communicable disease	Rule out	Rule out	Rule out	Rule out	Rule out	Rule out
Disease of specific organ	Rule out	Rule out	Rule out	Rule out	Rule out	Rule out
Accepted level of vasopressor	Minimal	Minimal	Minimal-moderate	Minimal-moderate	Moderate	Minimal-moderate
Presence of abdominal trauma	Usually acceptable	Usually acceptable	Usually acceptable	May rule out	May rule out	May rule out
Incidence of cardiac arrest or extended hypotension	Cardiac arrest or hypotension does not preclude donation unless specific organ function is impaired as a result of those events					
Presence of chest trauma	May rule out	May rule out	May rule out	Acceptable	Acceptable	Acceptable
Additional physician consult	Cardiologist	Cardiologist and pulmonologist	Pulmonologist	None needed	None needed	None needed
Organ-specific laboratory workup required	ECG, CXR, echo, cardiac consult, cardiac enzymes	ECG, CXR, ABG, echo, cardiac consult, cardiac enzymes	ABGs, CXR	PT, PTT, direct and total bilirubin, AST, ALT, H/H	BUN, creatinine, electrolytes, U/A	Serum glucose amylase

H/H = hemoglobin and hematocrit; echo = echocardiogram; U/A = urinalysis; CXR = chest roentgenogram.

the inability of the patient to maintain normothermia. Conversely, one must be cautious not to overlook an infection-related temperature spike on the premise that the elevation is central in origin. Hence any elevation must be correlated specifically with the white blood cell and differential counts. An increase in neutrophils may indicate a bacterial infection, whereas an increase in lymphocytes may indicate a viral infection. Obtaining blood and urine cultures and a chest roentgenogram is routine with all organ donors. Other cultures such as CSF and sputum may be useful to rule out or identify any suspected infectious process. Open drains are a cause for concern because of the potential for contamination; therefore their presence must be noted.

Specific Organ Function

The result of specific laboratory tests must be obtained as part of the evaluation process. Some tests are necessary in all cases, and others are needed to evaluate specific organ function. Table 25-1 gives the criteria assessed in evaluating each organ for suitability. Normal laboratory values for various age ranges are listed in Table 25-2.

Donor Monitoring

To manage the pediatric donor adequately, frequent monitoring (every 4 hours) of electrolytes, complete blood count, arterial blood gases, and pH is essential. In those donors who are unstable a laboratory workup every 2 hours is necessary for effective donor management.

Management Challenges

Once brain death has been determined a change in philosophy takes place, shifting focus from caring for the patient to maintaining the viability of organs for transplantation. Various management problems are inherent in the care of an organ donor. The most frequently encountered is hemodynamic instability, which can result from fluctuations in (1) intravascular volume, (2) vascular resistance, and (3) cardiac function.

Intravascular volume

Because most children considered as donors have been involved in a traumatic situation, hemorrhage can be a primary cause of decreased intravascular volume. In the organ donor an increase in capillary permeability is frequently considered a physiologic response to the traumatic injury. This response further diminishes the volume of circulating blood by allowing easy passage of intravascular fluid into the extravascular space.

Another factor that influences intravascular volume is therapeutic dehydration. Most brain-injured patients are placed on fluid restriction and are treated with diuretics and steroids to reduce cerebral edema. The line between therapeutic dehydration and clinical hypovolemia is fine, and the situation must be

Table 25-2 Laboratory Values

Test	Unit	Newborn	Infant	Child	Adult
Albumin	g/dl	3.0-5.4	3.5-5.3	4.0-5.8	3.5-5
Alkaline phosphatase	IU	30-205	*	*	25-80
BUN	mg/dl	5-15	5-15	10-20	8-20
Bilirubin, total	mg/dl	<12	<1.0	<1.0	<1.0
Calcium, total	mg/dl	7.4-14	11-13	9-11	9-11
Chloride	mEq/L	100-105	100-105	100-105	100-105
Serum creatinine	mg/dl	0.5-1.3	0.5-1.3	0.5-1.3	0.5-1.3
GGT	IU/L	0-200	5-110	0-23	0.50
Potassium	mEq/L	4.0-5.5	4.0-5.5	4.0-5.5	4.0-5.5
Sodium	mEq/L	135-144	135-144	135-144	135-144
Protein	g/dl	4.6-7.0	5.4-7.5	6.2-8.1	5.5-7.8
AST	IU/L	Up to 120	8-50	8-30	8-40
ALT	IU/L	0-25	16-50	3-30	3-36

GGT = gamma glutamyl transferase; AST = aspartate transaminase; ALT = alanine transaminase.
*Higher than adult; very high in adolescence.

frequently assessed to prevent hemodynamic instability as a result of inadequate vascular volume. Untreated volume depletion can result in oliguria (urinary output <1 ml/kg/hr) or anuria and ultimately impaired renal function.

Diabetes insipidus may be the most significant factor affecting a child's volume status. In the presence of a pituitary injury the neurohypophysis (posterior pituitary) ceases its activation and release of antidiuretic hormone. Without this hormonal influence the body loses its ability to maintain normovolemia. This phenomenon can occur even in the presence of hypovolemia (see Chapter 58).

Vascular resistance

The second factor affecting hemodynamic status is vascular resistance. The loss of brain stem function dictates that the brain-dead individual no longer has control over autonomically regulated responses. The brain can no longer elicit a vasoconstrictive response to counteract the decreased intravascular volume, and profound vasodilatation often occurs at the time brain stem function is lost. This response, coupled with the difficulties encountered maintaining normovolemia, can severely impact cardiovascular function, which notably is the final factor influencing a donor's hemodynamic stability.

Cardiac function

Cardiac output is determined primarily by volume status and resistance. Hypovolemia and vascular dilatation combine to cause a decreased return of blood to the right heart, resulting in a tachycardia mediated by baroreceptors of the atrium and aorta. Through spinal pathways that may still be intact even in the brain-dead child, these baroreceptors stimulate the heart to beat faster. In addition low atrial filling pressures can trigger the release of endogenous catecholamines, which will also potentiate the tachycardia. Tachycardia untreated for prolonged periods can result in myocardial damage and also add to the difficulties encountered in maintaining donor stability.

TREATMENT
Fluid Management

The first step in stabilization of the organ donor is aggressive fluid replacement. An adequate initial fluid bolus of lactated Ringer's solution or 0.9% sodium chloride solution at a maximal rate of 20 to 30 ml/kg over a period of 20 minutes is administered. This therapy may be repeated a second time if needed. In the presence of severe depletion a colloid solution is often used to supplement fluid replacement and volume expansion. Administering a 5% albumin solution, 20 ml/kg, is usually an effective adjunct to crystalloid therapy. It is, however, generally not necessary to use blood products for restoration of fluid volume. Their use is restricted to treatment of an unacceptably low hematocrit (<20%).

Once adequate volume has been restored, maintenance fluids can be given in an amount equal to hourly urinary output plus an additional 3 ml/kg/hr of a solution similar to 5% dextrose in 0.25% sodium chloride solution. Minimal acceptable urinary output in the organ donor is 2 to 5 ml/kg/hr. If necessary, diuresis can be induced with the use of an osmotic diuretic such as mannitol at a dosage of 0.25 to 0.5 g/kg administered intravenously. However, diuretics must not be used to increase urinary output unless hemodynamic monitoring indicates adequate hydration has been achieved. Conversely, to restore and maintain normal volume status in the presence of diabetes insipidus, an infusion of aqueous pitressin is often used. The IV route is preferred over intramuscular and subcutaneous administration because the immediate response allows for easier titration of dosage to maintain an adequate urinary output. The method used in preparing a pitressin infusion varies widely; however, the most important consideration is the response (see Chapter 58).

Use of Vasopressors

Frequently vasopressors are used to maintain an acceptable systemic arterial blood pressure (Table 25-3). Aggressive use of vasopressors in conjunction with volume depletion can lead to significant ischemic damage to transplantable organs; therefore they must be used cautiously. In organ donor situations dopamine is the drug of choice when a vasopressor is needed. Supplementing dopamine with dobutamine is also an acceptable therapy that can aid in maintaining normotension. Although the optimal dose of dopamine is <10 μg/kg/min, the use of higher dosages does not preclude donation. However, in doses >20 μg/kg/min dopamine can cause ischemic damage to the heart and liver and may preclude donation of those organs. Other vasopressors such as norepinephrine (Levophed), metaraminol (Aramine), and phenylephrine (Neo-Synephrine) are potent vasoconstrictors, and their use must be

Table 25-3 Normal Systolic Blood Pressures

Age (yr)	Mean Systolic Pressure Range (mm Hg)
<1	80-89
1-7	94-100
7-10	102-107
10-14	111-118

avoided since they may render vascular organs unsuitable for transplantation.

Ventilator Management

Once the diagnosis of brain death is established, treatments for atelectasis that may have been contraindicated when attempting to reduce cerebral edema may be used. These therapies include (1) increasing the tidal volume and positive end-respiratory pressure to expand alveoli, enhance oxygen exchange, and decrease perfusion-ventilation mismatch and (2) instituting chest percussion therapy to aid in the mobilization of pulmonary secretions and mucous plugs. Ventilator therapy must be directed toward optimizing gas exchange, particularly oxygenation. Although a PaO_2 >100 mm Hg is optimal, organ oxygenation is not compromised until SaO_2 is <90% or PaO_2 is <70 mm Hg. Ventilator therapy must be monitored through frequent chest roentgenograms and arterial blood gas and pH determinations in addition to the usual noninvasive monitors of pulmonary gas exchange function.

Should pulmonary edema develop that compromises oxygenation, diuretics may be used cautiously.

ADDITIONAL READING

Ascher NL, Evans RW. Designation of liver transplant centers in the United States. Transplant Proc 19:2405, 1987.

Blaine EM, Tallman RD Jr, Frolicher D, et al. Vasopressin supplementation in a porcine model of brain-dead potential organ donors. Transplantation 38:459-464, 1984.

Bolman RM III, Olivari MT, Saffitz J, et al. Current results with triple therapy for heart transplantation. Transplant Proc 19:2490-2491, 1987.

Brown AM. Cardiac reflexes. In Geiger SR, Sperelakis N, Berne RM, eds. The Handbook of Physiology. Bethesda, Md.: American Physiological Society, 1979, pp 677-689.

Delerhoi MH, Sollinger HW, Kalayoglu M, et al. Quadruple therapy for cadaver renal transplantation. Transplant Proc 19:1917-1919, 1987.

1987 Dow Chemical Survey conducted by the Gallop Organization. The U.S. public's attitudes toward organ transplants/organ donation. Princeton: The Gallop Organization, 1979.

Ettner BJ, Youngstein KP, Ames JE. Professional attitudes toward organ donation and transplantation. Dialysis Transplant 17:72-73, 1988.

Evans RW, Manninen DL. Public opinion concerning organ donation, procurement and distribution: Results of a national probability sample survey. Seattle: Battelle Human Affairs Research Centers, 1987.

Evans RW, Manninen DL, Maier AM. Selected characteristics of 444 heart donors. Transplant Proc 19:2501-2502, 1987.

Finberg L. Severe dehydration secondary to diarrhea. In Dickerman JD, Lucey JF, eds. Smith's the Critically Ill Child, ed 3. Philadelphia: WB Saunders, 1985, pp 74-76.

Ford RD, ed. Diagnostic Tests Handbook. Springhouse, Pa.: Intermed Communications, 1987, pp 676-679.

Gordon RN, Starzi TE. Long-term survival after liver transplantation. Transplant Immunol Lett 4:2-4, 1988.

Hamilton HK, ed. Diagnostics. Springhouse, Pa.: Intermed Communications, 1983, pp 103-118.

Harris F. Paediatric Fluid Therapy. Oxford: Blackwell, 1972, pp 31-38, 55-64.

Iwatsuki S, Starzl TE, Gordon RD, et al. Late mortality and morbidity after liver transplantation. Transplant Proc 19:2373-2377, 1987.

Jamieson NV, Caine RYU, Rolles K, et al. Results and problems in pediatric liver transplantation in the Cambridge/Kings College Hospital series: 1968 to July 1986. Transplant Proc 19:2447-2448, 1987.

Jones RS, Owen-Thomas JB. Care of the Critically Ill Child. London: Edward Arnold, 1971, pp 15, 300-304.

Jordan CA, Snyder JV. Intensive care and intraoperative management of the brain dead organ donor. Transplant Proc 19:22-25, 1987.

Kaye MP. The Registry of the International Society for Heart Transplantation: Fourth Official Report. J Heart Transplant 6:63-67, 1987.

Lane SM, Haid SD, Jankiewicz T, et al. Multiple Organ and Tissue Recovery—A Hospital Manual. 1987. Dallas: Southwest Organ Bank, Inc., 1987, pp 22-27

Levy MN, Martin PG. Neural control of the heart. In Geiger SR, Sperelakis N, Berne RM, eds. The Handbook of Physiology. Bethesda, Md.: American Physiological Society, 1979, pp 581-619.

Lynn AM, Morray JP. Shock syndromes. In Morray JP, ed. Pediatric Intensive Care. Norwalk, Conn.: Appleton Lange, 1987, pp 60-69.

Miles MS, Frauman AC. Public attitudes toward organ donation. Dialysis Transplant 17:74-76, 1986.

Nadel SM. Adequate oxygenation. In Kinney MR, Dear CB, Packa DR, et al, eds. AACN's Clinical Reference for Critical Care. New York: McGraw-Hill, 1981, pp 363-387.

Otte JB, Yandza T, Tan KC, et al. Recent development in pediatric liver transplantation. Transplant Proc 19:4361-4364, 1987.

Rappaport FT. Living donor kidney transplantation. Transplant Proc 19:169-173, 1987.

Schmidt K, Burdelski M, Bernasau U, et al. Analysis of current results of liver transplantation in children. Transplant Proc 19:2449-2450, 1987.

Sleight P. Reflex control of the heart. Am J Cardiol 44:889-893, 1979.

Squifflet JP, Carlier M, Gribomont B, et al. The preoperative management in multiple organ donors: A crucial phase in organ transplantation. Acta Anaesthesiol Belg 37:71-76, 1986.

Tilkian SM, Conover MB, Tilkian AG. Clinical Implications of Laboratory Tests, 2nd ed. St. Louis: CV Mosby, 1979, pp 44-58.

Tiwari J, Terasaki PI, Mickey MR. Factors influencing kidney graft survival in the cyclosporine era: A multivariate analysis. Transplant Proc 19:1839-1841, 1987.

Wasserman E, Gromisch DS. Survey of Clinical Pediatrics, 7th ed. New York: McGraw-Hill, 1981, pp 9-10.

Whaley LF, Wong DL. Nursing Care of Infants and Children. St. Louis: CV Mosby, 1979, p 1601.

Yacoub M, Festenstein H, Doyle P, et al. The influence of HLA matching in cardiac allograft recipients receiving cyclosporine and azathioprine. Transplant Proc 19:2487-2489, 1987.

PART

III

Specific Diseases and Problems

26 Neurologic Complications of Hypoxia

Roy D. Elterman

BACKGROUND AND PHYSIOLOGY

The demand of the nervous system for oxygen is large and continuous. Since the capacity of neural tissue to store oxygen is negligible, a constant supply must be provided. Under normal conditions the brain derives its energy from aerobic metabolism. With glucose as a substrate, 38 molecules of ATP are produced per molecule of glucose consumed. For this metabolic process to take place a constant supply of oxygen is needed at a rate of 3.3 ml/100 g tissue/min. In an effort to ensure an adequate nutrient supply, cerebral blood flow is tightly controlled by the mechanism of autoregulation. This provides a buffering effect by which cerebral blood flow remains constant despite changes in systemic arterial blood pressure.

Interruption of the cerebral energy supply occurs when there is oxygen deprivation (hypoxia) and/or interruption of cerebral blood flow (ischemia). In the actual clinical situation both hypoxia and ischemia play a role in the insult suffered. Frequently it is difficult to determine in the clinical setting which of the two factors is the major contributor to the insult, leading to the concept of hypoxic-ischemic encephalopathy.

During periods of diminished oxygen supply the brain no longer can aerobically metabolize glucose or even utilize ketones, which can act as an energy source in the immature brain. Consequently energy must be obtained from anaerobic glycolysis, which yields only two ATP molecules per molecule of glucose consumed and produces lactic acid as its byproduct.

The impact of oxygen deprivation has systemic implications as well. Although autoregulation in the brain tends to increase cerebral blood flow to provide additional glucose for metabolism, the heart is often unable to respond with increased cardiac output since it has also been injured by lack of oxygen. Rather than receiving additional blood, the brain may actually experience a decrease in cerebral blood flow. Cerebral blood flow is further impaired by local cerebral acidosis, resulting from lactic acid production.

The effects of hypoxia are decreased energy production and increased local acidosis, which further impair cerebral circulation, resulting in a more rapid depletion of stored glycogen. As indicated earlier, rarely does hypoxia occur alone. Frequently it is combined with ischemia, and ischemia only serves to further exacerbate the metabolic derangement already present. Not only is the supply of oxygen and glucose further reduced by ischemia, but correction of local tissue acidosis is impeded. The metabolic waste products, lactic acid and carbon dioxide, are not removed.

Although the severity of hypoxic-ischemic injury varies with age, there are certain aspects that are always affected to some degree.

Cerebral Blood Flow

A variety of control mechanisms exists that attempt to keep cerebral oxygenation at an optimal level (3.3 ml/100 g/min). Cerebrovascular dilation results from lowered oxygen tensions, increased carbon dioxide tensions, and local accumulation of acid metabolites. Autoregulatory mechanisms in cerebral vasculature allow for the maintenance of a constant blood flow (50 to 60 ml/100 g/min) over a fairly wide range of systemic arterial blood pressures. As a result, cerebral blood flow in the adult does not drop until systemic mean arterial blood pressures drop below 60 to 70 mm Hg. Similarly, normal delivery of oxygen is maintained until arterial PO_2 tensions drop below 30 mm Hg. One mechanism by which the body does this is the redistribution of cardiac output when the organism is confronted with an asphyxial insult.

There comes a point, however, especially in the preterm and term infant, when asphyxia does impair cerebrovascular autoregulation. A "pressure-passive" relationship takes over. Increased cerebrovascular resistance, possibly secondary to edema, and decreased cardiac output by the injured or hypoxic myocardium result in decreased cerebral blood flow, exacerbating the hypoxic-ischemic condition. Studies of asphyxiated neonatal animals demonstrate major differences in regional blood flow and metabolic activity in different areas of the brain.

Cerebral Edema

The role of cerebral edema in hypoxic-ischemic injury is unclear. Although brain swelling is an inevitable occurrence after hypoxic-ischemic insult, it is unknown if the swelling is simply a result of the injury or may actually play a role in the pathogenesis of the injury. In adults swelling apparently is the result of intracellular or cytoxic edema. Whether this is true for the newborn or immature brain is unknown.

Only recently has electron microscopy been used to study changes in brain exposed to hypoxia. Early neuronal changes involve swelling of the mitochondria with loss of their inner membranes. Swelling of the endoplasmic reticulum and rarefaction (clumping) of the ribose-nucleoprotein granules are also seen. How much time must elapse between the insult and the onset of the above-mentioned changes remains unclear.

The use of light microscopy revealed significant cell changes 30 to 60 minutes after decapitation of rats. More sophisticated techniques showed mitochondrial swelling occurs within 1 hour of the hypoxic insult. More important, it was noted that all oxidative enzymes ceased to function and protein turnover was depressed at the time of the severe insult. Other workers have added support to the concept that brain edema is a consequence rather than a major cause of the ischemic injury in the immature animal. A better understanding of the precise nature of cerebral edema has major implications in the management of the asphyxiated newborn.

Role of Glucose in Hypoxic-Ischemic Encephalopathy

Several investigators have demonstrated a relationship between glucose levels and neuronal injury. The data suggest a direct relationship between the extent of brain injury and the accumulation in brain of lactic acid. The proposed mechanism for the deleterious effect of high blood glucose before the asphyxial insult is that the increased quantities of glucose allow for increased anaerobic glycolysis, resulting in increased formation of lactic acid. It has been suggested that lactic acid accumulation is actually far more damaging than oxygen deprivation per se. Some authors have hypothesized that lactic acid accumulation in the mature brain produces severe extracellular edema by damage to astrocytes. Injury to these cells produces endothelial leaks and disruption of the blood-brain barrier. The resulting cerebral edema may in part be responsible for the regional necrosis observed. Although this hypothesis may be valid in some situations, it clearly is not true in all cases. In immature brain, glycogen stores available for lactic acid production are small. In fact, at least in the mouse model, it has been demonstrated that lactic acid production after anoxia did not reach levels assumed necessary for tissue destruction.

To confuse the issue further, an experiment performed in 1952 using a cat model demonstrated that cerebral electrical activity and survival could be maintained for more than 1 hour if adequate cerebral profusion and oxygen supply were maintained, even with a solution devoid of glucose. In addition carbohydrate reserves in brain were exhausted 10 to 15 minutes after the initiation of the experiment. What was learned was that brain was able to maintain energy production by using its own structural components such as nucleic acid, proteins, and lipids as long as oxygen was also present. Support for these in vivo findings in the cat is found in a common clinical situation. During a seizure oxidation of noncarbohydrate substances is used to provide energy for the brain. After the seizure, when glucose is again available, the consumed components are then resynthesized.

Although experimental reports on the effect of hyperglycemia on hypoxic-ischemic encephalopathy appear contradictory, these different findings are in all likelihood the result of using different species at different levels of maturity. In addition experimental design may play a key role in the differing results. Consequently at present the precise effect of blood glucose levels on the extent of injury seen with hypoxic-ischemic insult during the perinatal period cannot be determined.

Ion Homeostasis

Ion homeostasis is also disrupted by hypoxic-ischemic injury. Increases in extracellular potassium occur and may accentuate cellular injury. Also there is a fall of extracellular sodium and calcium, with accumulations of calcium in the cell, which may have several deleterious consequences. The cell will use its already limited supply of ATP in an effort to correct the accumulation of cytosolic calcium. The increased intracellular calcium may also activate phospholipases, resulting in hydrolysis of membrane phospholipids and liberation of free fatty acids, some of which seem to have deleterious effects on brain structure and function. In some situations brain prostaglandins may also be increased. These agents may contribute to further constriction of cerebral arteries, thereby exacerbating the already impaired cerebral blood flow.

Some investigators have even suggested that hypoxic neuronal injury may be mediated in part through synaptic activity, whereby increased synaptic activity makes a cell more vulnerable to anoxic insult. In one study synaptic activity was blocked by magnesium before the hypoxic insult, and this blockade seemed to prevent cellular injury.

MONITORING AND LABORATORY TESTS

The clinical presentation of hypoxic-ischemic encephalopathy depends on several factors, including the age of the patient, the severity of the insult, and the acuteness of the insult.

In the newborn three clinical stages have been defined. They vary from stage I, which represents a mild encephalopathy, to stage III, which occurs in a severely asphyxiated infant.

In the older child who has suffered a severe asphyxial event, the patient is generally stuporous or comatose on admission. Seizures, both focal and generalized, are common. Posturing (decorticate or decerebrate), hyperreflexia, and extensor-plantar responses occur. Corneal and pupillary reflexes are frequently absent. Findings are usually bilaterally symmetric, although unilteral findings may occasionally be seen. Of key importance is that there is often significant involvement of other organ systems: cardiac, pulmonary, and renal.

It is critically important that a good baseline general and neurologic examination be performed on admission. Vital signs need continuous monitoring. One must constantly look for evidence of increased ICP. Repetitive neurologic evaluation remains the most effective tool in assessing the status of the patient.

The role of ICP monitoring is controversial; it has not been shown useful in the management of hypoxic-ischemic encephalopathy. Risks associated with ICP monitoring (particularly infection and bleeding) are greater than the benefit derived (see Chapters 7 and 118).

Laboratory studies that should be performed initially include sodium, potassium, chloride, glucose, calcium (preferably ionized calcium), magnesium, phosphorus, pH, Pao_2, $Paco_2$, and base excess. Since other organ systems are frequently involved in hypoxic-ischemic injury, assessment of liver function (aspartate aminotransferase [AST], alanine aminotransferase [ALT], total bilirubin), renal function (BUN, creatinine), and cardiac function (echocardiography) is indicated. The use of electroencephalography becomes very important if there is a question about whether or not seizure activity is present.

TREATMENT
Metabolic and Cardiorespiratory

Treatment is directed toward correction of derangements produced by the asphyxial event. Immediate attention must be directed toward ensuring adequate ventilation, good systemic perfusion, and metabolic homeostasis. Common metabolic abnormalities include hypoglycemia and hypocalcemia. Hypoglycemia can be corrected by the administration of 0.2 to 0.5 g glucose/kg, preferably as a 25% solution, followed by a constant infusion of 8 mg glucose/kg/min of a 10% solution. The blood glucose level is determined after the initial administration and periodically after that (see below). A glucose level of 40 to 60 mg/dl is adequate. Hypocalcemia is corrected by the slow IV administration of calcium chloride (5 to 10 mg/kg dose followed by 300 mg/kg/

day) or calcium gluconate (20 to 200 mg/kg dose followed by 200 to 700 mg/kg/day by infusion). Electrolytes, glucose, calcium, and phosphorus are measured and evaluated frequently (every 12 hours).

Volume expansion will be needed if the patient is hypotensive. However, fluid should be administered carefully to avoid exacerbating cerebral edema. Once systemic metabolic and cardiorespiratory problems are corrected, the issues of seizures and cerebral edema should be addressed.

Seizures (see also Chapter 9)

Seizures need aggressive treatment since they can cause systemic hypertension, which, in the presence of dysfunctional cerebrovascular autoregulation, produces increased cerebral blood flow and causes hemorrhage, especially in areas of previous infarction. Seizures further deplete already diminished stores of glucose and ATP. In general, seizures are treated initially with phenobarbital. A loading dose of 20 mg/kg is given intravenously. If seizures persist, a phenobarbital level must be obtained even though additional therapeutic measures may be needed before the results are available. If the patient's clinical condition permits waiting until the results are known before initiating additional treatment, the decision can then be made whether the use of additional phenobarbital is indicated or the addition of a second drug is needed. Clearly, if the phenobarbital level is low (<20 μg/ml), additional phenobarbital is indicated. If an adequate level is obtained (>40 μg/ml), a second anticonvulsant must be added. Generally phenytoin is the recommended agent. A loading dose of 18 to 20 mg/kg is given by slow IV push. The rate of administration cannot exceed 1 mg/kg/min. Pulse rate and systemic arterial blood pressure should be carefully monitored during IV administration of phenytoin. Phenytoin can also be used as the initial anticonvulsant since it has the advantage of not sedating the patient.

If seizures persist, intermittent doses of lorazepam (0.1 mg/kg dose) may be given every 3 to 4 hours. Diazepam in a dose of 0.1 to 0.2 mg/kg has also been used effectively. Very careful observation is necessary when this agent is used in conjunction with phenobarbital since respiratory suppression can occur and usually does occur during the treatment of a significant seizure disorder. At my institution lorazepam has become the preferred benzodiazepine for the

control of persistent seizures because its duration of action is 2 to 4 hours. The anticonvulsant action of diazepam lasts only approximately 30 minutes. Paraldehyde, which is very effective in stopping status epilepticus, is no longer available since production in the United States has ceased.

Once seizure control is established, maintenance anticonvulsant therapy is needed. Phenobarbital is given in a dose of 3 to 5 mg/kg/day to maintain therapeutic levels. Maintenance doses of phenytoin are in the range of 5 to 10 mg/kg/day. Phenytoin must be administered intravenously since gastrointestinal absorption in the neonate and intramuscular absorption in any age person are extremely poor. Hypoxia is almost always a generalized insult; thus there may be liver damage, which will alter the metabolism of these drugs. Generally the rate of metabolism is decreased, necessitating the use of lower doses to obtain the same therapeutic blood drug levels (see Chapter 6).

Cerebral Edema

The role of brain swelling remains unresolved. As previously mentioned, it is unclear if cerebral edema is simply the end result of neuronal injury or impaired blood flow, thus adding to the existing hypoxic-ischemic insult. To date there have been no controlled studies indicating the treatment of cerebral edema has immediate or long-term benefits in the neonate who has suffered a hypoxic-ischemic insult.

If an infant is deteriorating clinically and imaging studies demonstrate cerebral edema (see Chapter 7), it is appropriate to initiate steps to reduce the swelling. Simple measures such as raising the head of the bed 30 degrees and keeping the head in the neutral position to prevent "kinking" of the jugular veins have been shown to be helpful. Although free-water restriction may play a role in decreasing cerebral edema, care must be taken to prevent hypovolemia and to maintain adequate urinary output (1 ml/kg/hr) (see Chapter 7). Fluid restriction may also help treat the syndrome of inappropriate antidiuretic hormone secretion (SIADH) since it may be a sequela of hypoxic-ischemic encephalopathy (see Chapter 57).

Controlled hyperventilation is another effective means of decreasing ICP. Hypocarbia causes cerebral vasoconstriction, resulting in decreased cerebral blood flow, although the decrease in cerebral blood flow may further compromise an already insulted brain. If hyperventilation is to be used, it is suggested that the $Paco_2$ be kept in the range of 25 mm Hg (see Chapter 7). A pattern of ventilation must be chosen that allows adequate venous return to the thoracic cavity; high levels of positive end-expiratory pressure (PEEP) and large tidal volumes may increase intrathoracic pressure, impeding venous return and enhancing cerebral venous congestion.

The use of steroids has not been shown to be effective and in most situations should be avoided. Diuretics such as acetazolamide and furosemide may be helpful. Acetazolamide is given in a dose of 10 to 30 mg/kg/day, administered twice or three times daily. Furosemide is used in a dose of 0.5 to 1 mg/kg every 4 to 6 hours, not to exceed 6 mg/kg/day.

In a critical situation (i.e., impending herniation) osmotic diuretics such as mannitol can be used as a temporary measure to reduce cerebral blood volume and to dehydrate the brain. The suggested starting dose is 0.25 g/kg given every 4 to 6 hours, which may be increased up to 1 g/kg administered every 4 to 6 hours if necessary. After administration of mannitol, serum electrolyte values, osmolality, and urinary output must be monitored closely. Use of mannitol typically mandates placement of a urinary bladder catheter.

ADDITIONAL READING

Brann AW, Dykes FD. The effects of intrauterine asphyxia on the full-term neonate. Clin Perinatol 4:149, 1977.

Fenichel GM. Asphyxia. Neonatal Neurology. New York: Churchill Livingstone, 1985, pp 99-137.

Geiger A. Correlation of the brain metabolism and function by the use of a brain perfusion method in situ. Physiol Rev 38:1, 1958.

Hill A, Volpe JJ. Pathogenesis and management of hypoxic-ischemic encephalopathy in the term newborn. Neurol Clin 3:31, 1985.

Holowach-Thurston J, Hauhart RE, Jones EM. Anoxia in mice: Reduced glucose in brain with normal or elevated glucose in plasma and increased survival after glucose treatment. Pediatr Res 8:238, 1974.

Holowach-Thurston J, Hauhart RE, Jones EM, et al. Decrease in brain glucose in anoxia in spite of elevated plasma glucose levels. Pediatr Res 7:691, 1973.

Lindenberg R. Morphotrophic and morphostatic necrobiosis: Investigations on nerve cells of the brain. Am J Path 32:1147, 1956.

Lindenberg R. Patterns of CNC vulnerability in acute hypoxaemia, including anesthesia accidents. In Shade JP, McMenemey WH, eds. Selective Vulnerability of the Brain in Hypoxaemia. Oxford: Blackwell, 1963, pp 189-209.

Menkes JH. Anoxia and Hypoglycemia. Textbook of Child Neurology. Philadelphia: Lea & Febiger, 1980, pp 458-460.

Rothman SM. Synaptic activity mediates death of hypoxic neurons. Science 220:536, 1983.

Schneck SA. Cerebral anoxia. In Baker AB, Joynt RJ, eds. Clinical Neurology. Philadelphia: Harper & Row, 1987, chap 17.

Voorhies TM, Vannucci RC. Perinatal cerebral hypoxia-ischemia: Diagnosis and management. In Sarnat HB, ed. Topics in Neonatal Neurology. Orlando: Grune & Stratton, 1984, pp 61-82.

27 Reye's Syndrome

David B. Owen · Daniel L. Levin

BACKGROUND AND PHYSIOLOGY
Definition

In 1963 Reye and associates first published a series of 21 cases of encephalopathy and fatty degeneration of the viscera. The cause of Reye's syndrome remains unknown. The Communicable Disease Center provides the following case definition:

1. An acute noninflammatory encephalopathy documented clinically by an alteration of consciousness and, if available, a record of CSF containing 8 leukocytes/mm^3 or fewer or by histologic specimen demonstrating cerebral edema without perivascular meningeal inflammation
2. Hepatopathy documented either by a liver biopsy or autopsy considered to be diagnostic of Reye's syndrome or by a threefold or greater rise in the levels of either the AST, ALT, or serum ammonia
3. No more reasonable explanation for the cerebral or hepatic abnormalities

Although generally considered a disorder of pediatric age groups, a few cases suggestive of Reye's syndrome have been described in adults.

Clinical Presentation and Course

Usually there are two phases: First, an acute illness, usually a viral prodrome, is often caused by influenza B or varicella, but many other infectious agents have also been identified during the prodrome. The incidence of Reye's syndrome is 0.3 to 0.6 cases/100,000 influenza B infections, 2.5 to 4.3 cases/100,000 influenza A infections, and 0.3 to 0.4 cases/100,000 varicella infections. Second, after a period of time during which the patient seems to be improving (usually days to weeks later), an acute deterioration phase occurs that consists of recurrent vomiting followed by or concurrent with changes in mental status, which may progress rapidly. The second phase may also be associated with fever, seizures, and hyperpnea. Increased ICP may be present in the absence of papilledema since papilledema usually takes days of increased ICP to develop and therefore may not be seen initially. Young infants (<6 months) may not have these classic symptoms; they may present with irritability, coma, and convulsions, which are often hypoglycemic or apneic spells. Since these signs may be associated with many other diseases, careful investigation to exclude genetic disorders of metabolism must be done. The Lovejoy scale is well accepted as a means of staging the progression of the encephalopathy (Table 27-1). The second phase of the illness usually lasts 2 to 4 days but may persist for a week or more.

Pathophysiology

Multiple organ systems are involved in Reye's syndrome, including liver, brain, heart, kidneys, pancreas, and skeletal muscle. The liver is usually swollen and yellow. Panlobular accumulation of neutral lipids (oil red O positive) in microvesicles in the cytoplasm of the hepatocytes is noted on light microscopy, with little or no sign of inflammation or zonal necrosis. Ultrastructural examination of liver tissue reveals mitochondrial alterations, including pleomorphism, swelling, sometimes outer membrane rupture, matrix expansion, disorganization, and loss of dense bodies. If the patient survives the CNS insult, the liver usually returns to normal.

Analysis of CNS tissue (either biopsy or autopsy material) reveals multifocal infarction and astrocytosis of the cerebral cortex, periaqueductal gray matter, basal ganglia, and brain stem. Cerebral edema, with or without evidence of herniation, is also often seen. The edema is cytotoxic rather than vasogenic pathologically and therefore is probably not respon-

Table 27-1   Lovejoy Staging of Encephalopathy of Reye's Syndrome

Stage	Mental Status	Response to Pain	Other CNS Findings
I	Lethargic, follows verbal commands	Purposeful	Normal
II	Stuporous, combative, disoriented, delirious	Purposeful	Hyperventilates, hyperreflexic
III	Obtunded, comatose	Decorticate	Pupils dilated and react to light, normal to sluggish mentation
IV	Comatose	Decerebrate	Loss of oculocephalic reflex, dilated pupils with or without hippus, caloric reflex, dysconjugate
V	Comatose	Unresponsive	Flaccid with or without seizures, loss of brain stem reflex, Cheyne-Stokes respirations—apnea

sive to steroids. Mitochondria also may be dilated; inflammation is absent, and Alzheimer type II astrocytes are usually not seen.

The kidneys are pale and have a slightly yellow tinge. Pathologic evaluation of the kidneys can demonstrate fatty degeneration of the loops of Henle and proximal convoluted tubules. Cardiac involvement includes epicardial petechiae, oil red O–positive material in the ventricles and atria, and mitochondrial swelling.

The elevated catabolic state found in Reye's syndrome leads to an increase in ammonia production. In addition, intramitochondrial urea cycle enzymes have decreased activity, and therefore ammonia clearance via urea synthesis is decreased. All mitochondrial enzymes measured except for carnitine palmitoyl transferase are decreased, including ornithine carbamoyl transferase, carbamoyl-phosphate synthetase, the pyruvate dehydrogenase complex, pyruvate carboxylase, succinate dehydrogenase, cytochrome oxidase, glutamate dehydrogenase, isocitrate dehydrogenase, and monoamine oxidase. The encephalopathy of Reye's syndrome differs from other causes of hepatic encephalopathy with hyperammonemia in that the EEG changes usually differ and no Alzheimer type II astrocytes are usually seen in the brain. Increased lipolysis and impaired hepatic metabolism of fatty acids can lead to the microvesicular accumulation of lipids in hepatic, renal, and cardiac cells as well as increased serum fatty acids. Serum lactate is usually elevated, which may be caused by increased production from the brain and muscle, de-creased clearance by the liver and kidneys, and tissue hypoperfusion and hypoxia.

Pathologic and biochemical evidence of hepatic mitochondrial damage has led to speculation that Reye's syndrome is the metabolic response or result of a universal mitochondrial insult. There is also some evidence of mitochondrial damage in skeletal and cardiac muscle and in the pancreas, although there is less clear-cut evidence of CNS mitochondrial damage.

Possible Etiology

As stated before, the etiology of Reye's syndrome is currently unknown. Epidemiologic associations do not prove causation; however, in the United States several studies in the late 1970s and the early 1980s demonstrated a strong correlation of Reye's syndrome cases with aspirin use. Salicylates may be an added metabolic insult to an organism already burdened by a mitochondrial injury, whether the mitochondrial injury is caused by a virus, a genetic defect, or some combination of these factors. The additional metabolic insult might result from salicylate-induced dysfunction of the mitochondrial enzyme monoamine oxidase (MAO). When salicylate was added to the platelets of patients with Reye's syndrome, MAO activity was significantly inhibited when platelets were taken at the onset of illness, and the inhibiting effect was maintained throughout the illness. By comparison, salicylate had no inhibitory effect on platelet MAO activity when platelets were taken from recovered Reye's syndrome patients, healthy controls, and non-Reye's syndrome hospitalized patients. Since the ultrastructural, histochemical, and biochemical abnormalities in Reye's syndrome are fully recoverable, the mitochondrial lesion is probably acquired and transient.

An alternative explanation of the pathogenesis of Reye's syndrome involves the effect of aspirin on macrophages. Macrophages activated by viral infection, endotoxin, and phagocytosis release tumor necrosis factor (TNF) and interleukin-1 (IL-1). TNF and IL-1 have been shown to be mediators of the toxic and metabolic effects of endotoxemia, which are similar to those seen in Reye's syndrome. Therefore the salicylate stimulation of macrophages activated by viral infection may release TNF and IL-1, resulting in the metabolic abnormalities seen in Reye's syndrome, including hyperammonemia, lactic acidosis, and hyperfattyacidemia. These abnormalities result in encephalopathy, abnormal amino acid metabolism, and abnormal free fatty acids, with deposition of microvesicular fat in the liver as well as other organs.

In 1982 the Committee on Infectious Disease of the American Academy of Pediatrics issued a statement warning against the use of salicylates in children with possible varicella or influenza, and a public education program was initiated. In addition the CDC and the surgeon general have issued similar warnings. In the United States the number of cases reported to the CDC has dropped steadily since 1980. In 1985 the incidence was 0.15/100,000 population under 18 years of age, and the case fatality ratio was 32%. However, reporting bias probably underestimates the incidence and overestimates the case fatality ratio. Some authors have used the decrease in aspirin and the decrease in occurrence of Reye's syndrome as an additional argument to support the aspirin–Reye syndrome association. Other authors dispute these conclusions, pointing out that even the prospective controlled epidemiologic study by the U.S. Public Health Service showed that in only 15 patients (27%) was there histologic support for the diagnosis of Reye's syndrome, and no electron microscopic evidence of the diagnosis was presented. Also, they indicate it is not clear what steps were taken to exclude confounding genetic metabolic diseases.

In favor of the salicylate–Reye syndrome association are the reports of the occurrence of the syndrome in several patients with connective tissue diseases who were receiving chronic salicylate therapy. Other factors such as the predominant influenza strain type that year may have played some role in the decrease in the incidence of Reye's syndrome, although this later argument is contested by evidence that the same strain of influenza B was present in one community during times of both high and low incidences of Reye's syndrome. The difference was attributed to high vs. low rates of use of salicylates. Although there is much debate about the exact relationship of salicylates and Reye's syndrome, it is probably prudent to withhold salicylates from children with flulike syndromes and chickenpox.

Differential Diagnosis

The differential diagnosis includes infectious causes of altered mental status such as meningitis, encephalitis, intracranial abscess (bacterial, fungal, viral, microbacterial), and fulminating hepatitis. Metabolic and toxic syndromes must also be differentiated, including hypoxic-ischemic encephalopathy, errors of metabolism (acyl-CoA dehydrogenase deficiency, urea cycle defect, glutaric acidemia, orotic acidemia, carnitine deficiency, fructose intolerance), lead encephalopathy or other toxins such as aflatoxin and drug overdoses (e.g., aspirin), and diabetic ketoacidosis. In addition vascular syndromes such as occlusive or hemorrhagic events, hypertensive encephalopathy, and generalized shock can be confused with Reye's syndrome, as can CNS mass lesions such as traumatic hemorrhage, tumors, and other causes of hydrocephalus.

Prognosis

Morbidity and mortality figures vary greatly from study to study, but some general patterns are consistent. Early recognition and treatment with IV glucose of stage I Reye's syndrome may prevent some of these cases from progressing. Dr. Partin stated that "prompt treatment with IV glucose appears to reduce mortality and morbidity by at least ten-fold. Reye's syndrome is very much a front line office practice problem."

Several studies have pointed out that the more advanced the stage of Reye's syndrome on admission, the worse the patient's prognosis. Admission ammonia concentrations in patients with stage I Reye's syndrome ≥ 100 μg/dl and a prothrombin time ≥ 3 seconds longer than control correlate with progression of the illness to more advanced stages; therefore that patient must be observed in a PICU. Peak ammonia levels >5 times normal are associated with a severe course and a high mortality rate. Significantly more elevated plasma norepinephrine levels have also been reported in patients who did not survive as compared to survivors.

The neuropsychiatric prognosis is guarded. Some significantly neurologically damaged patients survive; however, some series report an optimistic picture, with little obvious lowering of the IQ in patients who were more than 7 years old when they developed Reye's syndrome and who did not have a severe case. Psychiatric problems, including attention-focusing problems, anxiety disorders, and depression, are common in survivors, and their families often suffer from depression and anxiety and demonstrate overprotective behavior.

MONITORING AND LABORATORY TESTS

AST and ALT values are elevated at least one and one-half times normal, but the bilirubin level is usually normal. The initial ammonia level very early on may be normal, leading to the misdiagnosis of other causes of encephalopathy, but usually within the first few hours of mental status change, it has risen to two times normal or more. The ammonia level may return to normal after 48 hours. The sample for ammonia analysis must be collected from free-flowing arterial blood and immediately placed on ice to give an accurate reading. Arterial ammonia levels will be higher than venous levels because of deposition of ammonia in the tissues. Prothrombin time (PT) and partial thromboplastin time (PTT) may be elevated. Hypoglycemia is more severe in younger patients and can cause hypoglycemic seizures early in the course of the illness. Electrolyte and mineral abnormalities can occur because of vomiting and poor intake.

The CSF may demonstrate an elevated opening pressure; usually the number of cells is normal, and the protein level is normal as well. The CSF glucose level reflects the serum glucose level. Some reports indicate that lumbar puncture in patients with stage II or greater Reye's syndrome increases the danger of herniation; however, it is difficult to know whether the deterioration of these patients is caused by the lumbar puncture or by the progression of the disease state. In cases in which the diagnosis of Reye's syndrome is unclear, meningitis must be strongly considered and excluded. CSF must be examined as soon as possible either by a lumbar puncture if the patient appears to have stage I or II Reye's syndrome or by a subarachnoid or intraventricular pressure monitor if the patient appears to have stage II Reye's syndrome or worse (see Chapter 118). Urinary and serum toxin screens must be performed, including a salicylate reading. A CT scan is most useful in ruling out structural lesions or intracranial hemorrhage as the cause of the encephalopathy. A CT scan may show evidence of cerebral edema, although a scan is not a substitute for direct ICP monitoring.

Since the background pattern of the EEG correlates with the stage of the disease, obtaining an EEG may be useful in situations in which the physical examination is altered by therapeutic measures (i.e., paralyzing agents). The EEG can assist in predicting survival; the typical EEG findings are listed in Table 27-2. The EEG does not usually demonstrate triphasic waves, which occur in patients with hepatic encephalopathies.

A higher level (>700 μg/L) of ammonia at the onset of the disease seems to correlate with a worse prognosis. In addition somatosensory-evoked potential abnormalities and their recovery to normal can be correlated with a good outcome. A cerebral perfusion pressure (CPP) of <40 mm Hg is better correlated with a poor outcome than the absolute level

Table 27-2 EEG Findings in Reye's Syndrome

Lovejoy Stage of Encephalopathy	EEG Grade	EEG Characteristic
I	I	Slowing for age
II	II	Marked slowing for age
III	III	Diffuse high-voltage delta activity (may become rhythmic)
IV	III and IV	Diffuse high-voltage delta activity
		Diffuse low-voltage delta activity (<50 μV)
		Burst suppression
		Epileptiform activity
V	IV	Diffuse low-voltage delta activity
		Burst suppression
		Epileptiform activity

of measured ICP. Liver biopsy is not as necessary to the diagnosis of Reye's syndrome as it may have been before clinical criteria for the diagnosis were as well established. In unusual cases, especially in an infant, a biopsy may be useful in ruling out other causes of encephalopathy and hepatopathy. It may also be indicated in research protocols to eliminate any doubt of the diagnosis.

TREATMENT

Treatment is supportive since an exact etiology(ies) is not known. A patient with stage I Reye's syndrome must be admitted to a hospital for close observation, optimally in a PICU or intermediate care unit, because the patient may deteriorate rapidly. IV hydration (maintenance and correction volume and electrolytes) using $D_{10}W$ or $D_{15}W$ to keep the serum glucose level normal to high normal is needed. The glucose level must be checked every 2 to 4 hours. Patients with stages II to V Reye's syndrome need aggressive therapy in a PICU. ICP monitoring must be instituted to calculate CPP, which is the systemic arterial mean blood pressure minus the mean intracranial pressure (see Chapter 7). Elevation of the ICP is usually the most life-threatening factor in Reye's syndrome. However, patients whose ICP was apparently not elevated have died. Generally accepted measures for treating intracranial hypertension include elevation of the head in a neutral position, some degree of volume restriction (keeping the serum osmolality between 290 and 310 mOsm), sedatives and paralyzing agents (never give neuromuscular blocking agents without sedation), intubation and hyperventilation to keep Pco_2 at 25 to 30 mm Hg, control of body temperature within normal range with a cooling blanket, and osmotic diuretics as needed (see Chapter 7).

Other General Measures for Treating Stage II to V Reye's Syndrome

Electrolytes and minerals: Perform serial measurements of serum Na, K, Ca, P, creatinine, glucose, and BUN every 4 hours. Make corrections if SIADH or diabetes insipidus is a possible complication.

Clotting disorders: Measure the PT and PTT initially and every 8 hours thereafter. Correct with fresh frozen plasma at approximately 10 ml/kg if bleeding is a problem or if liver biopsy, placement of an ICP measuring device, or other invasive procedures is needed. Also give vitamin K, 1 mg IV, every 2 to 3 days.

Metabolic dysfunction: Perform liver function tests daily until normal. Pancreatic involvement must be evaluated by obtaining a serum amylase level. If the course of the disease is prolonged more than 1 week and/or is complicated by pancreatitis, total parenteral nutrition will be needed (see Chapter 149).

Infections: Obtain daily blood cultures, a culture of removed vascular catheter tips, daily Gram's stains of tracheal secretions, and daily urinary cultures to help demonstrate early evidence of an infection.

Cardiovascular: Maintain normal systemic arterial blood pressure, central venous blood pressure, and urinary output using colloid to support volume needs. If needed, maintain a normal CPP with vasopressers and a normal oxygen-carrying capacity with transfusions; thus oxygen delivery to the brain will be assured. A complete ECG early in the course may reveal dysrhythmias; the patient must be on continuous ECG display.

Pulmonary: Perform good pulmonary toilet and chest physiotherapy (see Chapter 132).

Gastrointestinal: Consider nasogastric suction, gastric fluid pH determination, antacids, and neomycin (100 mg/kg orally) to decrease ammonia production.

Less well-proven therapies that have been tried at some centers include exchange transfusion, peritoneal dialysis, steroids, carnitine and/or citrulline supplements, insulin given with the IV fluids, barbiturates, and decompressive craniotomies. There is no evidence for the efficacy of any of these therapies, and they may be harmful. For example, exchange transfusion increases the risk of acquired infectious disease, and both barbiturate coma and cold therapy dramatically increase the incidence of serious nosocomial infections due to interference with white blood cell function.

ADDITIONAL READING

Arcinue EL. The metabolic course of Reye's syndrome: Distinction between survivors and nonsurvivors. Neurology 36:435-438, 1986.

Arrowsmith JB, Dennedy DL, Kuritsky JN, et al. National patterns of aspirin use and Reye syndrome reporting, United States, 1980 to 1985. Pediatrics 79:858-863, 1987.

Barrett MJ, Hurwitz ES, Schonberger LB, et al. Changing epidemiology of Reye syndrome in the United States. Pediatrics 77:598-602, 1986.

Benjamin PY. Intellectual and emotional sequelae of Reye's syndrome. Crit Care Med 10:583-587, 1982.

Clardy CW, Edwards KM, Gay JC. Increased susceptibility to infection in hypothermic children: Possible role of acquired neutrophil dysfunction. Pediatr Infect Dis 4:379-382, 1985.

DeLong GR. Encephalopathy of Reye's syndrome: A review of pathogenetic hypotheses. Pediatrics 69:53-63, 1982.

DeVivo DC. Reye syndrome. Neurol Clin 3:95-115, 1985.

• Dezateux CA. Recognition and early management of Reye's syndrome. Arch Dis Child 61:647-651, 1986.

Faraj BA, Caplan D, Lolies P, et al. Salicylate and mitochondrial monoamine oxidase function in Reye's syndrome. J Pharm Sci 76:423-426, 1987.

Frewen TC, Kissoon N. Cerebral blood flow and brain oxygen extraction in Reye syndrome. J Pediatr 110:903-905, 1987.

Fulginiti VA. Aspirin and Reye's syndrome. Pediatrics 69:810-812, 1982.

Glasgow JFT. Clinical features and prognosis of Reye's syndrome. Arch Dis Child 59:230-235, 1984.

Goff WR, Shaywitz GD, Goff MA, et al. Somatic evoked potential evaluation of cerebral status in Reye syndrome. Electroencephalogr Clin Neurophysiol 55:388-398, 1983.

Heubi JE, Daugherty CC, Partin JS, et al. Grade I Reye's syndrome—outcome and predictors of progression to deeper coma grades. N Engl J Med 311:1539-1542, 1984.

Hurwitz ES, Barrett MJ, Bregman D, et al. Public health service study on Reye's syndrome and medications. N Engl J Med 313:849-857, 1985.

Jenkins JG, Glasgow JFT, Black GW, et al. Reye's syndrome: Assessment of intracranial monitoring. Br Med J 294:337-338, 1987.

Larrick JW, Kunkel SL. Is Reye's syndrome caused by augmented release of tumour necrosis factor? Lancet 2:132-133, 1986.

• Lichtenstein PK. Grade I Reye's syndrome. Pediatr Ann 14:511-515, 1984.

Pellock JM. Neurologic Emergencies in Infancy and Childhood. Philadelphia: Harper & Row, 1984, pp 145-151.

Pribble C, Osborn L. Reye syndrome and aspirin therapy. Lancet 2:966-967, 1986.

Remington PL, Rowley D, McGee H, et al. Decreasing trends in Reye syndrome and aspirin use in Michigan, 1979 to 1984. Pediatrics 77:93-98, 1986.

Rennebohm RM, Heubi JE, Daugherty CC, et al. Reye syndrome in children receiving salicylate therapy for connective tissue disease. J Pediatr 107:877-880, 1985.

Reye's syndrome and aspirin: Epidemiological associations and inborn errors of metabolism. Lancet 1:429-434, 1987.

Reye's syndrome—Epidemiological considerations. Lancet 1:941-944, 1982.

Rogers MF, Schonberger LB, Hurwitz ES, et al. National Reye syndrome surveillance, 1982. Pediatrics 75:260-264, 1985.

Shaymitz BA. What is the best treatment for Reye's syndrome? Arch Neurol 43:730-737, 1986.

Shaymitz SE. Long term consequences of Reye's syndrome. J Pediatr 100:41-46, 1982.

Tarlow M. Reye's syndrome and aspirin. Br Med J 292:1543, 1986.

Trauner DA. What is the best treatment for Reye's syndrome? Arch Neurol 43:729-731, 1986.

White JM. Reye's syndrome and salicylates. N Engl J Med 314:920-921, 1986.

28 Guillain-Barré Syndrome

Jay D. Cook

BACKGROUND AND PHYSIOLOGY

Guillain-Barré syndrome (GBS) is a monophasic disease that presents with weakness. Its progression is unpredictable; but once recovery of function occurs, it is almost complete, and rarely is there a return of symptoms. The natural history of GBS can be divided into three main phases: (1) progressive loss of function, (2) plateau or nonprogression of symptoms, and (3) recovery of strength and function. The duration of each phase varies. The first phase can be as short as hours to as long as 4 weeks. The length of the second phase depends on the extent of lost function (i.e., the greater the loss of strength, the longer the second phase). The recovery phase is usually the longest of the three, being weeks to months. In general the rate of recovery seems to correspond to the extent of recovery. The faster the recovery, the more complete it is; thus the time can be from days to years.

The presentation often can be very subtle but is followed by rapid loss of neuromuscular power, leading to acute respiratory crisis resulting from weakness of the muscles of ventilation or aspiration pneumonia. Without mechanical ventilatory support, 20% of patients would die. Even in the best situations the mortality rate is 1% to 3%. Since the swine influenza vaccination program of 1973 to 1976 and the presumed association with GBS, much better epidemiologic data exist concerning the incidence of GBS, both for age and seasonal incidence. For children the incidence increases with age and follows the seasonal variation of viral syndromes, peaking in the late fall, winter, and early spring.

GBS is an acute autoimmune reaction directed primarily toward the myelin encasing the peripheral motor nerves. Pathologic features are predominantly macrophage infiltration and segmental demyelination of the peripheral nervous system. This reaction causes a delay or block in nerve conduction. Although progressive motor weakness is the hallmark of GBS, sensory, cranial nerve, and autonomic nerve dysfunction are usually present to some degree and may rarely constitute the primary neurologic dysfunction.

Diagnosis

As with many neurologic syndromes, there is no one laboratory test to establish the diagnosis of GBS, since the various syndromes cannot be separated by any pathophysiologic mechanism or test. Thus the diagnosis can be made only after a careful history, physical examination, and appropriate laboratory studies. In 70% of the cases a significant event occurs 1 to 4 weeks before the onset of motor symptoms (e.g., a viral, mycoplasmal, or bacterial infection, surgery, insect bite, medical treatment, vaccination). The features required for diagnosis are progressive weakness and areflexia, whereas the features strongly supportive of the diagnosis are quite variable. Thus the diagnosis of GBS is based on a history of a preceding event (e.g., viral syndrome), history of loss of motor function, neurologic examination showing areflexia and weakness, abnormal laboratory studies of CSF, albumino-cytologic disassociation, slow or blocked nerve conduction, and decreased motor action potentials with or without changes of acute denervation on electromyography (EMG).

History

Rarely does the child present with a complaint of ascending paralysis. Parents will note that "his play activity has decreased," "he hasn't felt well," "he has been lazy," or "he has been tired a lot." There may be sensory complaints; the parents often note that the child complains of "funny feelings" or "tingling," or in the case of the very perceptive child, "the floor isn't as cold as it used to be." If the disease process is affecting the brain stem (i.e., the Miller-Fisher syn-

FEATURES OF GBS*

Features required

Progressive motor weakness
Areflexia

Features strongly supportive of diagnosis

Typical clinical findings	*Acceptable variants*
Zenith by 4 wk	Beyond 4 wk
Symmetric involvement	
Mild sensory symptoms or signs	Severe sensory loss/pain
Cranial nerve dysfunction	
Recovery begins in 2-4 wk	
Autonomic dysfunction	Sphincter dysfunction at onset
Absence of fever at onset	Fever at onset
	CNS involvement

Typical laboratory findings	*Acceptable variants*
CSF Protein elevated	No rise in 1 to 10 wk
Less than 10 WBCs	10-50 WBCs
EMG Slow/blocked nerve conduction	Normal nerve conduction
	Active denervation

Features casting doubt on the diagnosis

Persistent asymmetric weakness
Persistent bladder and bowel dysfunction
Bladder and bowel dysfunction at onset
Greater than 50 CSF WBCs
Polymorphonuclear leukocytes in CSF
Sharp sensory level

Features that rule out the diagnosis

History of hexacarbon abuse (e.g., airplane glue)
Abnormal porphyrin metabolism
History or presence of diphtheritic infection
Findings consistent with lead intoxication
Pure sensory dysfunction
Definite diagnosis of a specific condition

*Modified from Asbury AK. Diagnostic considerations in Guillain-Barré syndrome. Ann Neurol 9 (Suppl): 1-6, 1980.

drome), complaints of "lazy eyes" (ptosis), "staggers" or "walks like a drunk" (gait ataxia), "weak voice" (dysphonia, involvement of cranial nerves IX and X), or "trouble with chewing food" (cranial nerve V) are common.

In addition to the chief complaints the parents will usually give a recent history of febrile illness with either upper respiratory infections or GI symptoms; however, other antecedent events have been linked to GBS, such as viral infection, *Mycoplasma* infection, surgery, treatment of elevated temperature, malignant disease (especially lymphoma), vaccination, and insect bites. Although the parents may connect this event with the child's present illness, often they do not; thus if a careful review of symptoms is not done, this antecedent event can be missed.

Physical Examination

Early, the physical examination may be completely normal except for areflexia and mild muscle weakness. However, the following abnormalities may be found (the order corresponds to the recording of the physical examination, not necessarily the order of disease symptom presentation).

Vital signs. Although abnormalities are not common early in the course of the disease, all abnormalities are of concern. Tachypnea occurs with respiratory failure. Tachycardia may be a reflection of respiratory failure or secondary to autonomic dysfunction. There may be an irregular pulse caused by autonomic dysfunction, presumably at the brain stem level. Hypertension rarely occurs early in the course of the disease; however, I have seen one such patient.

Fundoscopic examination. Rarely papilledema can be found. The exact mechanism is not known, but a low-grade obstructive hydrocephalus caused by the elevated protein level has been postulated and supported by CSF infusion studies.

Oral and pharyngeal examination. The breath may be foul or sour because of incomplete swallowing, resulting in trapped food in the pharyngeal clefts or in the oral saliva.

Chest examination. Nasal flaring, use of accessory muscles, tachypnea, monosyllabic speech, and cyanosis may all be present in severely weakened patients in respiratory failure. Single-breath counting can often be used in the older child to assess respiratory reserve; counts less than 10 suggest significant compromise. However, formal pulmonary studies are critical to the management of the GBS patient, and single-breath counting cannot be considered an adequate substitute but merely a supplementary bedside procedure. Rales and rhonchi can be present in the child who is aspirating secondary to dysphagia and who has developed pneumonia.

Abdominal examination. GBS can occur in patients with mononucleosis or hepatitis; thus hepatomegaly and/or splenomegaly may be found.

Skeletal examination. If muscle weakening has been gradual, heel cord contractures may be found by 2 weeks.

Neurologic examination: mental status. The literature regarding adult patients suggests that as many as 25% will present with some mental status changes (i.e., altered states of consciousness and/or confusional states secondary to respiratory failure). In addition I have been impressed by the high percentage of children who develop alterations in mood; whining, sadness, and emotional lability are the most frequent. These symptoms may lead some clinicians to consider a psychiatric illness and miss the true diagnosis.

Cranial nerve examination. Abnormalities of the third, fourth, and sixth cranial nerves are not that uncommon; ptosis, dysconjugate gaze, and rarely pupillary abnormalities are found. Involvement of the motor portion of the fifth cranial nerve may be missed, but if looked for, it will often be found. Jaw opening and closing are weak, the extreme case presenting with oral ptosis. The seventh cranial nerve is the most commonly involved cranial nerve; the child's abilities to blow out his cheeks, to smile, or

to close his eyes may all be affected. Involvement of the ninth and tenth cranial nerves may be life threatening. The child with involvement of cranial nerves IX and X will have decreased voice volume, decreased ability to cough, decreased ability to swallow, and depressed gag reflex. The first three can be tested easily and can be used to follow the patient's clinical course. Testing the gag reflex is not necessary if the other three findings are adequately evaluated. In addition the child often becomes fearful of the examiner because of gag reflex testing and thus less cooperative during subsequent examinations. Voice volume can be assessed by listening to the voice and asking the child to scream. The ability of the child to cough can be assessed by asking him to cough. The ability to swallow can be assessed by asking the child to drink some water; in fact, this latter activity can be made an objective test by simply measuring the quantity of water and timing the interval needed to drink the liquid (Table 28-1). Involvement of the eleventh cranial nerve is reflected in weak neck muscles, which may result in poor head control in the young child. Twelfth nerve involvement is reflected in poor tongue movement and dysarthric speech.

Motor examination. The muscle tone is decreased, but bulk is normal. Strength is decreased; legs are usually more involved than the arms and the distal motor groups more than proximal motor groups. Because neurologists are notoriously poor at examining muscle strength and I suspect pediatricians are no better, formal muscle grades are best assessed by a physical therapist. For the clinician, functional strength assessment is of more practical value. One

Table 28-1 Monitoring Respiratory and Swallowing Function in a Patient With GBS*

Day of Illness	Forced Vital Capacity (ml)	Time to Drink 4 oz. of Water (sec)
1	2500	11
8	2190	16
15	2240	20
21	2420	15
58	2940	6

*The course of a 15-year-old girl with areflexia, CSF protein of 78 mg/dl, and nerve conduction of 23 m/sec. Respiratory and swallowing function deteriorated for the first 15 days but then started to improve and became normal by 58 days.

needs to document whether or not the child can get to a sitting position, is able to crawl, is able to get up off the floor (if so, does he use Gowers' maneuver or does he need to pull himself using a chair), is able to walk, or is able to run. Does the child have enough strength to walk on his arms with his legs supported (i.e., wheelbarrow), to hold himself straight out "like Superman" if suspended at the waist, and to raise his arms over his head? These are all simple tasks that a child any age can understand and are much better assessments of muscle strength than "guesstimates" of formal muscle strength using the Kendall system.

Sensory system. Sensory dysfunction is less prominent on objective testing, often with only a slight stocking/glove dysfunction of touch, vibration, and/or position. A sensory level dysfunction is not associated with GBS and if found points to a spinal cord problem.

Reflexes. The hallmark of GBS is areflexia, which precedes the weakness in more than 95% of the patients. If it is not found, another diagnosis must be entertained.

Coordination. Early in the disease incoordination may be caused by weakness or sensory loss, but cerebellar ataxia (i.e., not being made worse by closing the eyes and movement in the plane of gravity) can be seen. Truncal instability is the hallmark of the Miller-Fisher variant. Later in the course of the disease all patients seem to go through a phase of significant incoordination.

Autonomic system. Dysfunction of the autonomic system is one of three causes of death (respiratory failure and dysphagia being the other two). Several abnormalities have already been discussed under "Vital Signs." Dysfunction can be assessed by measuring systemic arterial blood pressure in both the erect and lying positions and by measuring changes in heart rate with changes in body position, with the Valsalva maneuver, and with activity.

DIFFERENTIAL DIAGNOSIS

At least nine conditions have presentations similar to GBS: botulism, viral anterior horn cell diseases (e.g., poliomyelitis), posterior fossa tumors, transverse myelitis, organophosphate poisoning, tick paralysis, periodic paralysis, myasthenia gravis, and dermatopolymyositis complex. Table 28-2 lists the clinical and laboratory studies that help differentiate these conditions.

In addition to the usual malaise and GI symptoms, pupillary changes are very rare in GBS but are common for botulism; the dead-mouse test as well as blood *Clostridium botulinum* toxin levels can establish botulism as the diagnosis.

Anterior horn cell syndromes secondary to viruses (e.g., polioviruses, coxsackieviruses A and B) are characterized by a significant asymmetry in strength, painful cramps, and weakness associated with fever.

Alteration of the mental status along with long-tract signs can help differentiate posterior fossa tumors from GBS. The association of a sensory level and bowel/bladder dysfunction helps to differentiate transverse myelitis from GBS.

Tick paralysis will not be recognized unless a tick is sought. A thorough search will be rewarded since the complete removal of the tick will restore strength within hours.

Although ascending paralysis is common for both GBS and the periodic paralyses, laboratory studies easily differentiate the two; hypo- or hyperkalemia will suggest the diagnosis of either hypo- or hyperkalemic periodic paralysis. The EMG is silent with the periodic paralyses, and muscle contraction cannot be elicited by either nerve or muscle stimulation; however, response to muscle stimulation is always present in patients with GBS. Finally, the paralysis is not long lasting in periodic paralyses.

Children with organophosphate poisoning have a number of systemic symptoms, including vomiting, tachycardia, and no detectable cholinesterase activity in a blood sample.

A patient with myasthenia gravis (see Chapter 29) may have complete muscle paralysis, including respiratory paralysis, but the history usually reveals previous symptoms of weakness, and deep tendon reflexes are always present, no matter how weak.

Acute myositis can sometimes give the impression of an ascending paralysis, but reflexes are usually commensurate with weakness. Significant muscle pain, heliotropic rash (if present) and elevation of serum CK, aldolase, LDH, AST, and/or ALT all suggest an acute myositis.

MONITORING AND LABORATORY TESTS

Seven physiologic functions must be monitored to prevent serious complications. Monitoring the first two, respiratory function and swallowing function, is of paramount importance to prevent death. The third function, strength, must be followed to determine if the patient is in the worsening, zenith, or recovery phase of the disease. The fourth, assessing the autonomic system, is helpful in patients considered for therapeutic plasmapheresis or those who have a history of cardiac or renal dysfunction. The fifth, inattention to nutrition, will leave the child with a sig-

nificantly reduced muscle mass on which to depend during the rehabilitation stage. The sixth function, attention to good nursing care, will prevent occurrence of sources of infection (e.g., bed sores or nosocomial infections) and also prevent corneal scarring and residual bladder dysfunction. Seventh, the psychological status of the patient, parents, and staff

Table 28-2   Differential Diagnoses of GBS

Anatomic Site	Disorder	Deep Tendon Reflexes	CSF Protein	Clinical Points	Laboratory Studies
Upper motor neuron	Brain stem tumor	+ + +	NL/INC	Altered mental status, upgoing toes	MRI or CT scan
	Transverse myelitis	0/ + + +	NL/SL INC	Sensory level bowel/ bladder dysfunction	Myelogram
	Spinal cord tumor	+ + +	NL/S INC	Sensory level bowel/ bladder dysfunction	Myelogram
Anterior horn cell	Poliomyelitis	Absent	INC	Fever Pain Weakness, asymmetry	Culture of virus CSF cells
Neuromuscular junction	Botulism	Absent	NL	Pupillary abnormalities Systemic signs History of exposure	Serum toxins Dead-mouse test
	Tick paralysis	NL	NL	Tick found	
	Organophosphate poisoning	NL	NL	Vomiting Bradycardia Increased sweating Increased salivation History of exposure	Absence of cholinesterase
	Myasthenia gravis	NL	NL	Preservation of deep tendon reflexes History of weakness Prominent eye weakness Positive Tensilon test	Antiacetylcholine receptor antibody
Muscle	Periodic paralysis	NL	NL	Previous attacks Rapid onset and reversal	Hypo/hyperkalemia EMG silent
	Acute myositis	ETS	NL	Severe muscle pain Heliotropic rash	Elevated CK, aldolase, LDH, AST, ALT Electromyography—myopathy

NL = normal; INC = increased; SL = slightly; S = significantly; ETS = equal to strength.

must be constantly assessed to ensure all recognize that near-full, if not full, recovery is expected and every effort must be made to ensure that it occurs. Table 28-3 lists each of these areas, possible deleterious effects, and the suggested means for monitoring.

Initial orders need to include assessment of vital signs, appropriate monitoring (e.g., ECG, continuous systemic arterial blood pressure, transcutaneous oxygen saturation, carbon dioxide), nutritional intake, bowel and bladder assessments, and weight as fre-

quently as every other day. The physical therapist needs to assess the patient's strength, and for paralyzed patients the physical therapist needs to monitor the range of motion exercises and splinting of ankles and knees to prevent contractures.

Obviously respiratory function must be monitored closely. See Chapter 10 for more detailed discussion of respiratory failure.

The frequency of physician monitoring is dictated by the patient's clinical state. If the patient's condition is rapidly worsening, constant monitoring is advisa-

Table 28-3   Monitoring to Prevent Deleterious Effects of GBS

Area	Complications	Monitor
Respiratory dysfunction	Atelectasis, pneumonia	Auscultation Temperature q 6 hr Chest x-ray study
	Death	Po_2 Pco_2 ECG Respiratory rate Pulmonary function tests
Swallowing dysfunction	Aspiration pneumonia	Timed drinking Calorie count Body weight every other day
	Death by aspiration	As above
Strength	Loss of all motor skills (stage of disease)	Strength bid Functional test bid Patient evaluation
	Contractures	Check range of motion every day
Autonomic dysfunction	Hypertension Hypotension Cardiac dysrhythmia SIADH	Systemic arterial blood pressure ECG Input and output Urine/blood Osmolality Serum electrolytes
Nutrition	Loss of muscle mass	Body weight every other day Caloric intake
	Decubitus ulcers	Check skin daily
Nursing care	Corneal ulcers	Check ability to close eyes Check corneas daily
	Nosocomial infection	Good hand washing Isolation from other sick patients
Psychological status	Child anxiety Parent decompensation Health care team attitude	Mental status daily Mental status daily Mental status daily

ble; however, if stable, routine monitoring of the clinical state by the nursing staff is adequate.

Laboratory Studies

CSF. The hallmark of GBS is albumino-cytologic dissociation, which is found as early as the third day into the illness but may occur as late as the second or third week. In addition other findings are present: oligoclonal bands on CSF protein electrophoresis, elevated IgG or IgM, an elevated CSF IgG synthesis rate, and possibly an elevated opening pressure.

EMG. Electrophysiologic studies are the only other laboratory procedures helpful in establishing the diagnosis. The findings, however, are not uniform. Nerve conduction, which is a reflection of the myelination of the large fiber, may be normal, slow, or nonexistent (complete block). The motor potential amplitude (i.e., the number of muscle fibers fired by the electrical stimulus) is almost always reduced. The needle study can be normal or show signs of acute denervation with fibrillations and sharp waves. In general a poor prognosis is associated with an abnormal needle study (i.e., fibrillations, sharp waves).

Others. Other laboratory studies must be obtained early and followed because of differential diagnostic considerations or potential abnormalities during the course of the illness. CBC should be normal. If an elevated WBC is found, it may reflect a concurrent infection from aspiration pneumonia or an incorrect diagnosis. Serum electrolyte studies are needed to rule out hypokalemic or hyperkalemic periodic paralysis; patients in whom the autonomic system is involved need to have follow up studies because of potential SIADH. Muscle and liver enzymes should be normal; their elevation may suggest dermatopolymyositis complex or significant liver disease, which will also be associated with weakness. Immunologic studies have been unrewarding in general. ECG and chest roentgenograms are needed as early baseline studies. Although ECG abnormalities and aspiration pneumonia appear late in the disease, they are more easily identified when a previous ECG and/or chest roentgenogram is available for comparison.

TREATMENT
Preventive Treatment

After GBS has been diagnosed, the first decision is whether the child needs to be admitted to the hospital. The child with GBS can be safely followed up at home only if the respiratory and swallowing functions are normal, the family is well known to the physician and reliable (or the child is very verbal), the child is ambulatory, or the zenith of the disease has been reached (i.e., recovery has begun). All other children must be admitted for at least 24 hours for observation.

Special nursing care: Although bladder dysfunction is not an early symptom of GBS, it occurs quite frequently in those patients with respiratory failure and/or autonomic dysfunction. When the bladder's innervation is lost, it can be overstretched and become a flaccid bag. Early signs of dysfunction include difficulty with initiating urination, decreased force of stream, small volumes, fullness after voiding, decrease in frequency with large-volume voiding, and finally dribbling. Use of intermittent or continuous catheterization in selected patients will prevent any residual bladder dysfunction. Because the seventh cranial nerve is so frequently involved, careful attention to the corneas is a must to prevent exposure keratitis resulting from an inability to close the eyes. Finally, when the patient is severely weak and cannot move, a constant vigil for pressure sores must be kept. Following good nursing care plans (i.e., repositioning the patient every 2 hours and using a sheepskin blanket along with heel and elbow pads) will prevent skin ulcerations. If a decubitus ulcer develops, aggressive care must be initiated to prevent a secondary infection. Good handwashing and enforcement of visiting restrictions regarding sick relatives are paramount in preventing nosocomial infections. All infections must be treated aggressively.

Active Treatment

Nosocomial infections. The patient does not have the usual residual body strength to cough, to ward off secondary spread of an infection, or to prevent secondary opportunistic bacterial infections. Using aggressive bronchial toilet, increasing fluids, preventing contact with others with any illness, and using aggressive antibiotic therapy when appropriate will prevent significant problems.

Dysphagia. A child who frequently chokes during eating, refuses to eat, or cannot swallow water needs to have a nasogastric tube passed to ensure adequate nutrition (see Chapter 150).

Respiratory support. Management guidelines can be found in Chapters 10 and 128.

Reversing the disease process. Since GBS is presumed to be an immunologically mediated disease, the use of corticosteroids has been proposed to treat it. To date, studies show only that the use of corticosteroids is at best of no value and may even be harmful.

Recently therapeutic plasmapheresis (see Chapter 142) has been shown to be beneficial. In an adult cooperative study it was shown to halve the time patients were ventilator dependent and halved the time to ambulation. However, plasmapheresis is expensive and not without significant risks for the patient. The criteria for plasma exchange, in my opinion, are age dependent. Because of venous access problems, most children 5 years old and younger will need a central venous double-lumen catheter. Thus in these children plasma exchange should be reserved only for life-threatening situations (i.e., impending respiratory failure and/or significant feeding difficulties). For children more than 14 years of age loss of ambulation is a reason for plasma exchange since there is no question that plasma exchange reduces the recovery period by half. For children between the ages of 5 and 14 years the choice may be a balance between the adequacy of peripheral venous access and the rapidity of the progression of symptoms (i.e., the potential complications associated with a central catheter vs. a longer stay in the hospital). The recommended protocol is a total of five 1 to 1½ plasma volume exchanges done every other day over 8 days. Replacement fluids are purified plasma protein and 0.9% sodium chloride solution (see Chapter 142).

Autonomic dysfunction. Autonomic symptoms are possibly the result of dysfunction of the sympathetic nervous system. Hypertension has been correlated with elevated circulating levels of norepinephrine and increased muscle and nerve sympathetic activity. The symptoms result from an imbalance of the sympathetic and parasympathetic systems with end-organ denervation hypersensitivity. Stress will release catecholamines acting on the sympathetic terminals; however, because the usual parasympathetic balancing of this transient endogenous release of catecholamines is reduced, the patient will be tachycardic and/or hypertensive. As a result, any pharmacologic manipulation must be weighed against very probable adverse effects. A review of the literature revealed only one death ascribed to hypertension, but there are many documentations of

death caused by the use of vasopressors. In most instances conservative measures of fluid restriction or enhancement and posture in bed have been adequate to control either hypertensive or hypotensive crises. Propranolol (0.05 to 0.1 mg/kg bid to qid PO) is one agent well documented to control the hypertensive crises without resulting in significant hypotension in between episodes producing any significant cardiac dysrhythmias. Cardiac dysrhythmias are best controlled by careful monitoring and judicious use of propranolol or cardiac pacing in selected patients. Antidiuretic hormone dysfunction is best controlled by careful monitoring of fluids and serum electrolytes and not with hormone supplementation.

The dysesthesias that some patients experience are not unlike causalgia. They do respond to membrane stabilizers (i.e., carbamazepine, diphenylhydantoin, lorezapam, and desipramine); however, all of these drugs may affect the cardiovascular system, and the decision to use any must be weighed against possible deleterious effects of the drugs.

Psychological dysfunction. Sometimes at the beginning, but almost always during the recovery phase of GBS, the child demonstrates significant behavioral dysfunction. There is marked lability of mood, and because of the acuteness of onset and reversal, this mood dysfunction is most likely organic in nature. However, no matter the origin, behavioral dysfunction must be dealt with in a compassionate, consistent manner by all involved. In the acute care setting coordination is best handled by the nursing staff on advice of a clinical psychologist and the physician. Since most psychotropic drugs affect the autonomic system, it is best to avoid using them.

Special consideration must be given to the patient, parents, and the health care team when a child is on a ventilator. Nothing is more frightening to a child than being isolated from his family in an unfamiliar and frightening environment and being unable to move. Unless a special effort is made, the patient cannot make his wants known or call for his family. A system of eye blinking, hand signals, or letter spelling must be started early. This is also a tense time for the parents. The reality of their child's frailty, the economic burden, and the lack of "information on what is going on" even in the best of situations, create untold stresses for the parents. It is the task of the leader of the health care team to ensure that the child and parents get the special attention they need: regular parental visits; video-taped movies, television, and radio as much as possible for the child; and for the parents at least bidaily updates about the clinical situation and plan for care. The spokesman to the parents must be limited to one or two individuals; parents do not need a variety of messages. Finally, everyone must be apprised frequently of the general plan and be reassured of the realistic prognosis.

• • •

In general, the faster the loss of function the faster is the recovery; however, if the plateau stage is long, the recovery phase is always prolonged. Studies vary, but complete recovery is found in at least 70% to 90% of the patients. Electrophysiologic studies are helpful in making a prognosis for recovery; only 30% to 50% of the children with active denervation on EMG will have complete recovery.

ADDITIONAL READING

Arnason BGW. Acute inflammatory demyelinating polyradiculoneuropathies. In Dyck PJ, Thomas PK, Lambert EH, Bunge R, eds. Peripheral Neuropathy. Philadelphia: WB Saunders, 1984, pp 2050-2100.

Bos AP, van der Meche FGA, Witsenburg M, van der Voort E. Experience with Guillain-Barré syndrome in a pediatric intensive care unit. Intensive Care Med 13:328-331, 1987.

Cole GF, Matthew DJ. Prognosis in severe Guillain-Barré syndrome. Arch Dis Child 62:228-291, 1987.

Cook JD, Glass DS. Strength evaluation in neuromuscular disease. Neurol Clin 5:101-123, 1987.

Gruener G, Bosh EP, Strauss RG, Klugman M, Kimura J. Prediction of early beneficial response to plasma exchange in Guillain-Barré syndrome. Arch Neurol 44:295-298, 1987.

Mills N, Plasterer HH. Guillain-Barré syndrome: A framework for nursing care. Nurs Clin North Am 15:257-264, 1980.

Rossi LN, Mumenthaler M, Lutshg J, Ludin HP. Guillain-Barré syndrome in children with special reference to the natural history of 38 personal cases. Neuropadiatrie 7:42-51, 1976.

Singh NK, Jaiswal AK, Misra S, Srivastava PK. Assessment of autonomic dysfunction in Guillain-Barré syndrome and its prognostic implications. Acta Neurol Scand 75:101-105, 1987.

29 Myasthenia Gravis

Dwight Lee Lindholm · Jay D. Cook

BACKGROUND AND PHYSIOLOGY

Myasthenia (Greek for weakness) gravis (Latin for grave) is defined as an illness in which there is muscular weakness and fatigability due to dysfunction at the neuromuscular junction. The three main categories of childhood myasthenia gravis are (1) neonatal, (2) juvenile, and (3) congenital (Table 29-1). Neonatal and juvenile myasthenia gravis are autoimmune diseases, whereas the congenital form is an inherent structural or biochemical defect.

In the transient neonatal form the mother has myasthenia gravis. Recent studies have demonstrated a transient production of acetylcholine receptor antibody by the infant; thus neonatal myasthenia gravis is not merely the result of passively transferred antibodies from the mother.

In the juvenile form of myasthenia gravis there is an autoimmune reaction against the neuromuscular junction. IgG directed against the acetylcholine receptor has been shown to mediate this reaction by increasing the degradation and inhibiting the synthesis of acetylcholine receptors at the neuromuscular junction.

All three of these childhood myasthenia syndromes are treatable, but unexpected reversals in clinical status make doing so difficult. Without any treatment 30% of myasthenia gravis patients would die of their disease within a few years of onset. Treatment with only anticholinesterases and thymectomy still results in a mortality rate of up to 30% of patients with the autoimmune form of myasthenia gravis. With introduction of immunosuppression, plasma exchange, and improved ventilator support, the survival rate should be greater than 90%. Thus it is crucial to understand the newer methods of treatment fully so that after a myasthenia gravis patient is in crisis, proper treatment can be given.

The neuromuscular junction is a specialized area at the cleft between the motor axon and the muscle fiber. At the neuromuscular junction the motor axon's action potential is amplified by the release of acetylcholine, which binds to receptors, causing the opening of sodium and potassium ion channels. Five times the number of receptors needed for depolarization of the muscle are activated. Therefore the margin of safety for neuromuscular transmission is a factor of 5. Alteration of sodium and potassium permeability causes a depolarization of the muscle through the T-tubule system. Depolarization induces the release of calcium from the sarcoplasmic reticulum, activating the contractile apparatus of the actin-myosin complex. The reuptake of calcium induces the relaxation of the contractile apparatus.

Pathogenesis

Both transient neonatal myasthenia gravis and juvenile myasthenia gravis are mediated by autoimmune mechanisms. An antibody directed against the acetylcholine receptor is found in more than 90% of patients with adult-onset myasthenia gravis. An antibody has been found in the neonatal forms, but for the juvenile form the titers are often very low or undetectable. This acetylcholine receptor antibody leads to increased acetylcholine receptor destruction and a decreased acetylcholine receptor synthesis rate, resulting in significant loss of acetylcholine receptors. When this loss exceeds approximately 60% to 80% of normal acetylcholine receptors, the motor axon action potential does not result in muscle depolarization.

There are at least three different etiologies of congenital myasthenia gravis: (1) structural abnormalities that include small nerve terminals and decreased postsynaptic end-plate length; (2) an acetylcholine resynthesis or mobilization defect; and (3) decreased acetylcholine esterase.

241

Table 29-1   Childhood Myasthenic Syndromes and Their Treatment

Disorder Pathogenesis	Long-Term Therapy	Crisis Settings	Treatment of Crises
Neonatal			
Passive transfer and transient production of anti-acetylcholine receptor antibody	Respiratory and pharyngeal support Anticholinesterase drugs Anticholinergic drugs Blood exchange	Within the first week of life	Same as long term
Congenital			
Congenital dysfunction of neuromuscular junction	Respiratory and pharyngeal support Anticholinesterase drugs Ephedrine Anticholinergic drugs	Birth Aspiration Infection Improper medication (see p. 244)	Same as long term
Juvenile			
Autoimmune disease directed against neuromuscular junction	*Ocular* Anticholinesterase drugs Ephedrine Immunosuppressive drugs Thymectomy (rare) *Generalized* Immunosuppressive drugs Thymectomy Anticholinesterase drugs Ephedrine Anticholinergic drugs	Infection Aspiration Improper medication (see p. 244) Surgery Stress, emotional and/or physical Menses	*Ocular* Pulse methylprednisolone Pulse gamma globulin Plasma exchange *Generalized* Respiratory and pharyngeal support Pulse methylprednisolone Pulse gamma globulin Plasma exchange

Diagnosis: History and Physical Findings
Neonatal myasthenia gravis

Approximately 12% of infants born to mothers with myasthenia gravis will have neonatal myasthenia gravis. In transient neonatal myasthenia gravis the first symptoms usually occur within a few hours to 72 hours of birth. The duration of symptoms may be from 5 to 47 days, with a mean duration of 18 days. Feeding difficulties are the most common problem in these infants. Although initially they may suck vigorously, they quickly fatigue. The next most common manifestations are generalized weakness and hypotonia, which in some patients progress to respiratory failure. Approximately one half will have a weak cry and weak facial expression. Only 15% have limitation of eye movement and ptosis.

Crisis in myasthenia gravis is a condition in which there is marked decrease in strength and respiratory function. An infant with neonatal myasthenia gravis who is in crisis would have an increased respiratory rate, cyanosis, nasal flaring, and weak cry. The other two forms of myasthenia gravis have a somewhat different presentation.

Congenital myasthenia gravis

The first symptoms of congenital myasthenia gravis are usually present at birth and include ptosis, extraocular palsies, facial weakness, and swallowing problems. Because of the swallowing problem the child may tilt his head back to aid in swallowing or stick his hand into his mouth to self-gag. There are also limb weakness and delayed motor development.

Frequently the first symptoms are not noticed until approximately 6 months of age. The infant may have no known symptoms or only minor symptoms and then worsen at that time. The patient may present in crisis.

A patient with congenital myasthenia gravis will usually first be seen on an emergency basis with respiratory failure, associated inhalation of gastric or oral secretions, and/or pneumonia.

Juvenile myasthenia gravis

The onset of juvenile myasthenia gravis nearly always occurs after 1 year of age. The first symptoms most often involve the extraocular muscles (ptosis and diplopia). Other initial symptoms in decreasing order of frequency of occurrence are leg weakness, generalized fatigue, difficulty in swallowing, slurred speech, difficulty chewing, weakness of arms, neck, or face, and finally the most uncommon initial symptoms, which are weakness of trunk and shortness of breath. In the first month after symptoms are documented, the signs and symptoms remain ocular only in 40%, are generalized in 40%, are confined to extremities in 10%, and are bulbar only in 10%. All the symptoms of myasthenia gravis improve after the patient rests and are exacerbated by exercise, therefore being more prevalent by the end of a day.

Myasthenic crises are caused by acute pharyngeal or respiratory muscle failure. The following conditions often cause dysfunction.

Infection. Children with juvenile myasthenia gravis usually have a worsening of symptoms with any infection, although pneumonia is the infection most likely to cause a crisis. However, even a mild viral syndrome may cause a myasthenic crisis in a child who had only minor symptoms before the infection.

Medication problems. Medication problems usually are caused by (1) simultaneous use of anticholinesterases and steroids, which can be antagonistic to each other at the neuromuscular junction and cause weakness; (2) use of ancillary drugs (see p. 244); (3) lack of response to anticholinesterase medication; and (4) too rapid withdrawal of immunosuppressive therapy. If a patient has been receiving anticholinesterase medication, he may be in a myasthenic crisis because of unresponsiveness to the medication or in a cholinergic crisis, becoming weaker from too much anticholinesterase medication. Signs may be seen that will help distinguish these diagnoses. In a myasthenic crisis there is an adrenaline response to stress, which results in pupil dilatation and tachycardia. Muscle cramps and fasciculation are usually absent. In a cholinergic crisis the patient usually has small pupils, excessive sweating, lacrimation, increased salivation, bradycardia, diarrhea, muscle cramps, and muscle fasciculation.

Surgery. Stable symptomatic patients on anticholinesterase medications may go into a myasthenic crisis within 72 hours of surgery, possibly as a result of an adrenocorticosteroid surge with the stress of surgery. Corticosteroids have an antagonistic action at the neuromuscular junction when anticholinesterase medications are given.

Emotional stress. The worsening of myasthenia gravis with emotional stress may be caused by the increased adrenocorticosteroid surge (already explained as the mechanism of weakness postoperatively), but the exact mechanism is unknown.

DIAGNOSTIC TESTS AND MONITORING
Physical Examination

To test for myasthenia gravis by physical examination check for easy fatigue. This can be done by repetitive exercising of one muscle group while looking for weakness or by having the patient maintain upward gaze while looking for ptosis. A healthy person should be able to hold his arms horizontal or his legs off the bed for longer than 1 minute. Normally a child is able to move his wrist or ankle the full range of motion in 1 minute 45 times or more. After a myasthenic patient has rested, he may perform these tasks much better.

Edrophonium Test

The edrophonium (Tensilon) test is the principal test used to confirm the diagnosis of myasthenia gravis. Edrophonium is an acetylcholine esterase inhibitor with very short action that results in a decreased rate of acetylcholine breakdown; therefore more and more acetylcholine is available to bind to the acetylcholine receptors and the patient becomes stronger. When an acetycholine esterase deficiency is present, the patient does not have a positive response to edrophonium.

Resuscitation equipment must be available and a nurse present before starting the test should any respiratory, pharyngeal, or cardiac complications occur. To perform this test decide what variables need to be followed in muscle testing, select the muscle

DRUGS THAT MAY EXACERBATE MYASTHENIA GRAVIS*

Analgesics (narcotics)

Codeine
Dilaudid
Meperidine
Morphine
Pantopon

Antibiotics

Aminoglycosides
  Neomycin
  Streptomycin
  Kanamycin
  Gentamicin
  Tobramycin
Dihydrostreptomycin
Amikacin
Ampicillin (2 cases)
Bacitracin
Clindamycin
Colistimethate
Colistin
Erythromycin
Lincomycin
Polymyxin A
Polymyxin B
Sulfonamides (usually no
  problem with use)
Viomycin

Anticonvulsants

Barbiturates
Dilantin
Ethosuximide
Magnesium sulfate
Paraldehyde
Trimethadione

Anti-inflammatory

Chloroquine
Colchicine
D-Penicillamine

Antimalarials

Chloroquine
Quinine

Cardiovascular

Beta blockers
Dilantin
Lidocaine
Procainamide
Quinidine
Trimethaphan

Endocrine

Thyroid replacement

Eye drops

Echothiophate
Timolol

IV fluids

Sodium lactate solution

Neuromuscular blocking agents

Decamethonium
Dimethyltubocurarine
Gallamine
Pancuronium
Succinylcholine
Tubocurarine

Others

Amantadine
Diphenhydramine
Diuretics
Emetine
Muscle relaxants

Psychotropics

Amitriptyline
Benzodiazepines
Chlorpromazine
Droperidol
Haloperidol
Imipramine
Lithium carbonate
Paraldehyde
Trichloroethanol

Steroids

ACTH
Steroids (probably all steroids can
  make patient weaker when patient also takes anticholinesterase medication but can also
  make drug-free patient weaker
  before he begins a steady improvement on steroids)

*Modified from Adams SL, Mathews J, Grammer LC. Drugs that may exacerbate myasthenia gravis. Ann Emerg Med 137:532-538, 1984.

groups that were weak on physical examination, and grade their strength during the course of the test. The results must be made as objective as possible; therefore hand dynamometers for measuring grip strength in pounds of pressure and times for running a certain distance with maximal effort up and down the hall or up the stairs are used. When testing children too young to cooperate, observe whether head lag improves with the edrophonium test, that is, from the patient's head flopping in the dependent position to being able to hold his head erect in the pulling-to-sitting from supine maneuver and the vertical suspension maneuver. These children may also have a louder cry, fight the examiner more vigorously, get to a sitting position with more ease, walk and run better, and have resolution of ptosis and extraocular and facial palsies. For the profoundly weak child on a ventilator, only improved forced vital capacity (FVC) may be seen after edrophonium is given.

As with any test, the record of the test must convey all the important information concisely to any reader. We have found the data in Table 29-2 work best. The doses of atropine (used to counteract the muscarinic side effects of the edrophonium) and edrophonium are based on the child's weight: atropine, 0.01 mg/kg (maximum single dose, 1 mg), edrophonium, 0.2 mg/kg (maximum single dose, 10 mg). The parameters of muscle strength must be selected before the test is started. An evaluation of breathing ability should always be included; FVC or single-breath counting will do. If the patient has significant pharyngeal dysfunction, timed drinking can be helpful. To ensure good cooperation assess the child's strength before and after the IV infusion is started, after administration of the atropine, after the test dose of edrophonium (20% of the total dose), and after the high dose of edrophonium (80% of the total dose). A test is positive if one or more muscle groups improve a grade or more or if a timed test is improved by more than 25%. Patients who are very sensitive to edrophonium may show an improvement with the small dose but may worsen after the larger dose. The duration of benefit is said to be only 10 minutes, but it may last 6 to 8 hours.

Curare Test

Another test to diagnose myasthenia gravis is the curare test. Curare is a nondepolarizing muscle relaxant. Myasthenia gravis patients become weak with a much smaller dose of curare than normal people do.

Table 29-2   Edrophonium Test

Test	Before IV	After IV	After Atropine (0.01 mg/kg)	Edrophonium (0.04 mg/kg)	Edrophonium (0.16 mg/kg)	Response
Time of medication	—	—	0:00	8:00	13:00	
Time of test	−5:00	−3:00	2:00	10:00	15:00	
Pulse	96	128	148	—	104	
BP	112/62	128/80	—	—	100/50	
Single-breath count	40	47	50	50	46	None
Deltoids	4− both	4− both	4+ both	4+ both	5+ both	Positive
Biceps	4+ both	4+ both	4+ both	5+ both	5+ both	Equivocal
Triceps	4− both	4− both	4− both	4+ both	5+ both	Positive
Hip flexion	4− both	4− both	4+ both	4+ both	4+ both	None
Hip extension	5+ both	5+ both	5+ both	5+ both	5+ both	None
Sit up	Unable	Unable	Unable	Unable	Able	Positive
Ptosis	2 mm	Same	Same	Same	Same	None
Neck flexion	4−	4−	4−	4+	4+	Equivocal
Neck extension	4−	4−	5+	5+	5+	Positive
Ran hall	17.5 sec	14.0 sec	13.9 sec	10.9 sec	9.6 sec	Positive

This test can only be performed with personnel and equipment available to support respiration quickly in a PICU or operating room. Because of the logistics and danger of the curare test, a regional curare test has been developed using regional strength or electrophysiologic parameters. One twentieth of the usual dose of curare is infused into a superficial vein of one arm after the blood flow has been occluded. Measurements of hand-grip dynamometry or repetitive nerve stimulation (see below) will not be significantly affected in healthy patients but will be reduced by more than 50% in myasthenic patients.

Electrophysiologic Tests

The two electrophysiologic tests useful for confirming myasthenia gravis are repetitive nerve stimulation and single-fiber EMG. Repetitive nerve stimulation will show significant decrement of response in 80% of generalized myasthenia patients. Increased jitter is the result seen when myasthenia gravis patients are evaluated by single-fiber EMG. However, patients with other diseases such as myopathies and myotonic dystrophy can also have increased jitter.

Acetylcholine Receptor Antibody Levels

Determining acetylcholine receptor antibody levels is another objective means of establishing the diagnosis of myasthenia gravis. In 87% of adult patients with autoimmune myasthenia gravis these levels are elevated. Neonatal myasthenia gravis patients also have increased levels. However, in the juvenile myasthenia gravis patient the acetylcholine receptor antibody titers are often low or absent. With analysis of the clinical course and ancillary tests the diagnosis of myasthenia gravis can usually be established, and more appropriate monitoring and treatment can be applied.

Respiratory Status

A crisis situation arises from respiratory failure and pharyngeal dysfunction. Respiratory status must therefore be carefully followed and supported as needed to prevent death. A patient going into respiratory failure may have the following signs and symptoms: (1) increased respiratory rate, followed by a decrease, (2) panic, (3) decreased voice volume, (4) cyanosis, (5) inability to handle secretions, (6) air hunger, (7) gasping, (8) cardiac rate initially increased and then decreased, and (9) decreased

breath sounds. Monitoring must continue even after the patient apparently has recovered because with myasthenia gravis there is not only weakness, but also fatigue. To diagnose, monitor, and support a patient with respiratory failure appropriately, refer to Chapter 10.

Autonomic System
Cholinergic

Observe patients on anticholinesterase medication for cholinergic side effects, including salivation, lacrimation, profuse sweating, bradycardia, small pupils, and diarrhea.

Anticholinergic

Monitor patients who have received atropine or similar acting drugs for control of secretions. Side effects of these medications include dry skin, dilated pupils, altered mental status, tachycardia, and hypertension.

Pharyngeal System

The purpose of monitoring pharyngeal function is to prevent aspiration. This function must be assessed hourly by clinical observations. Symptoms include difficulty handling secretions, a problem with drinking water, inability to close the mouth and purse the lips, and dysphonia or aphonia. Laboratory investigations of pharyngeal function include time required to swallow 1 ounce of water. Normal time for ages 4 years and older is less than 7 seconds. Other studies include a chest roentgenogram and swallowing cineradiography. The recovery of pharyngeal function is not necessarily correlated to the clinical course of other motor strengths, and separate assessment is needed.

TREATMENT OF CRISIS
General Considerations

Since crisis in myasthenia gravis may be life threatening, the standard principles of cardiopulmonary resuscitation apply: maintain an airway and provide mechanically supporting ventilation when indicated (see Chapters 127 and 128). The underlying event causing the crisis must be treated as well. If it is infection, treat with the appropriate antimicrobial agent; if it is inappropriate dosage of a medication, adjust the dosage; if it is postoperative crisis in an autoimmune myasthenic patient on an anticholinesterase, give life-supportive care, discontinue anticholinesterase medication, and start steroids (anticholinesterase medications and steroids used together can be antagonistic and may worsen the patient's condition). Any infection, regardless of site or agent (viral or bacterial), can precipitate a crisis. Pneumonia is a more serious infection in a patient with myasthenia gravis since ventilation-perfusion mismatches are present in addition to poor inspiratory force.

Crisis in Autoimmune Juvenile Myasthenia Gravis

Crisis in the autoimmune juvenile myasthenia gravis patient may be treated by plasmapheresis either on a daily or an alternate day schedule with a 1 to 1½ volume exchange for five treatments. Additional treatments can be given if the response is not adequate (e.g., administer methylprednisolone in a dose of 30 mg/kg IV, with a maximum of 1 g in the early morning or every other morning for five doses). More recently gamma globulin (0.4 g/kg IV dose daily for 5 days) has been used.

If the patient has been receiving anticholinesterase medication, it must first be determined whether this is a myasthenic or a cholinergic crisis. If there has been an increase in the usual cholinergic side effects, there is greater probability that the weakness is caused by too much anticholinesterase medicine. An IV edrophonium test would further help distinguish these two groups. However, in the patient with myasthenic crisis in respiratory failure, the trachea must first be intubated and ventilation supported before an edrophonium test is done. Otherwise the patient may aspirate or go into complete respiratory failure and die. The patient in a myasthenic crisis will usually improve after the edrophonium test, although improvement may be minimal. The patient in a cholinergic crisis will usually worsen after this test.

If an autoimmune juvenile myasthenic patient is critically weak and is on anticholinesterase medication, the patient must first be stabilized by providing all supportive measures necessary (i.e., feeding tube and tracheal intubation), after which our approach to such a patient has been to stop all anticholinesterase medication and start prednisone at a dose of 3 mg/kg every other early morning up to a maximum of 100 mg every other morning. To help reduce steroid complications a strict diet of low sugar, low salt, high protein, and appropriate calories must be maintained.

After the patient returns to a stable condition (approximately 30 days), thymectomy is performed. Patients undergoing thymectomy must receive methylprednisolone, 30 mg/kg divided as follows: 7.5 mg/kg administered in the staging area, 7.5 mg/kg during anesthesia induction, 7.5 mg/kg during surgery, and 7.5 mg/kg postoperatively. Other immunosuppressive antimetabolic and cytotoxic drugs may be used in a patient with myasthenia gravis, but because of their toxicities and risk of malignancies, they must be used only as a last resort. Cyclosporine has been found useful in treating myasthenia gravis in experimental studies but should not be used routinely because of possible renal toxicity. If the patient has only autoimmune ocular myasthenia gravis, he may be treated with anticholinesterase medications. The most widely used anticholinesterase is pyridostigmine, which works by inhibiting acetylcholine esterase; thus more acetylcholine is available to interact with the receptors. Pyridostigmine comes in a 12 mg/ml syrup, a 60 mg tablet, or an injectable form, which can be given at one thirtieth of the oral dose.

Crisis in Neonatal Myasthenia Gravis

Because of improved physician and patient education an unexpected diagnosis of neonatal myasthenia gravis is quite rare today. Thus careful planning by the obstetrician, neurologist, pediatrician, and neonatologist can be done long before the delivery date. Treatment plan issues that must be resolved by all treating physicians include (1) a means to observe the child in the intensive care nursery, (2) feeding plans, (3) criteria and plan for ventilatory support, (4) criteria for blood exchange, (5) medications and dosages to be used if the child is symptomatic, and (6) criteria for going home. The pediatrician or neurologist can then discuss the treatment plan with the family. Doing this early will ensure that all controversy concerning the treatment plan will be resolved before the baby is born. Additionally, the parents can discuss the plan and ask questions during a nonstressful period.

When it is obvious from monitoring that the infant is in respiratory failure and has pharyngeal dysfunction, the first step is to support ventilation and provide adequate nutrition. Either nasogastric tube or parenteral nutrition if the infant is not able to swallow is acceptable treatment. Pyridostigmine (an anticholinesterase) may be given orally, 60 mg/5 ml, or by nasogastric tube, 0.05 mg/kg/dose initially, increasing the dosage until it is effective without significant side effects. The probable range of the effective oral dose is from 0.25 to 2 mg/kg per 4 hours (preferably 30 minutes before feeding). If the infant cannot swallow, one thirtieth of the oral neostigmine methylsulfate dose (0.1 mg in a full-term newborn) may be given intramuscularly 30 minutes before feeding. Ephedrine sulfate, 1 to 2 mg/kg/day orally in divided doses every 4 to 6 hours, may be added to prolong the anticholinesterase effect. Although the disease is autoimmune, use of immunosuppressive therapy is not indicated since the disease is transient. Exchange transfusion, however, may help speed recovery. For patients receiving anticholinesterase medications, anticholinergic drugs are useful in controlling the cholinergic side effects. The recommended dosages for two anticholinergic drugs are 0.02 mg/kg atropine (up to a 1.0 mg maximum single dose) or 0.004 mg/kg glycopyrrolate (Robinul, up to a 0.1 mg maximum single dose). The parenteral solution can be given intravenously, intramuscularly, or orally (if swallowing is adequate).

Crisis in Congenital Myasthenia Gravis

In patients with congenital myasthenia gravis the same principles apply for respiratory support, pharyngeal precautions, and nutrition. Immunosuppressive treatment is not effective since this is not an autoimmune disease. The medical treatment is similar to that for neonatal myasthenia gravis. The initial dose of pyridostigmine in children is 0.05 mg/kg (gradually increasing until optimal results are achieved without side effects). The expected optimal dose of pyridostigmine is usually 0.25 to 2.0 mg/kg every 4 hours (30 minutes before feedings) or 1.5 to 12 mg/kg/day. The onset of action is 30 to 60 minutes and duration is 4 hours. In more severe cases pyridostigmine must be given around the clock (every 4 to 6 hours). To potentiate the action of the anticholinesterases, ephedrine sulfate can be added to the treatment at a dose of 1 to 2 mg/day in divided doses every 6 hours or every 4 hours during the usual waking hours. The muscarinic cholinergic side effects of the anticholinesterase medication (pyridostigmine or neostigmine) include increased salivation, increased bronchial secretions, nausea, diarrhea, abdominal cramps, increased peristalsis, miosis, and diaphoresis. The nicotinic cholinergic side effects include weakness, muscle cramps, and fasciculations.

ADDITIONAL READING

Adams SL, Mathews J, Grammer LC. Drugs that may exacerbate myasthenia gravis. Ann Emerg Med 137:532-538, 1984.

Argov Z, Brenner T, Abramsky O. Ampicillin may aggravate clinical and experimental myasthenia gravis. Arch Neurol 43:255-256, 1986.

Arsura E, Brunmner NG, Namba T, et al. High-dose intravenous methylprednisolone in myasthenia gravis. Arch Neurol 42:1149-1153, 1985.

Bennett AE, Cash PT. Myasthenia gravis and curare sensitivity. Dis Nerv Syst 4:299-301, 1943.

Engel AG, Lambert EH, Gomez MR. A new myasthenic syndrome with endplate acetylcholinesterase deficiency, small nerve terminals and reduced acetylcholine release. Ann Neurol 1:315-330, 1977.

Engel AG, Lambert EH, Moulder OM, et al. A newly recognized congenital myasthenic syndrome attributed to a prolonged open time of the acetylcholine induced ion channel. Ann Neurol 11:553-569, 1982.

Fambrough DM, Drachman DB, Satyamurti S. Neuromuscular junction in myasthenia gravis: Decreased acetylcholine receptors. Science 182:293-295, 1973.

• Fenichel G. Clinical syndromes of myasthenia in infancy and childhood. Arch Neurol 35:97-103, 1978.

Foldes FF, Klonymus DH, Maisel W, Osserman KE. A new curare test for the diagnosis of myasthenia gravis. JAMA 203:133-137, 1968.

Genkins G. Studies in myasthenia gravis: Early thymectomy. Am J Med 58:517-524, 1975.

• Grob D, Brunner NG, Namba T. The natural course of myasthenia gravis and effect of therapeutic measures. Ann NY Acad Sci 377:614-639, 1981.

Hart ZH, Sahashi K, Lambert EH, et al. Congenital familial myasthenic syndrome caused by a presynaptic defect of transmitter resynthesis or mobilization. Neurology 29:556-557, 1979.

Horowitz SH, Sivak M. The regional curare test and electrophysiologic diagnosis of myasthenia gravis: Further studies. Muscle Nerve 1:432-434, 1978.

Hoyle G. How is muscle turned on and off. Sci Am 222:85-93, 1970.

Kennedy FS, Moersch FP. A clinical review of 87 cases observed between 1915 and the early part of 1932. Can Med Assoc J 37:216-223, 1937.

Lefvert AK, Osterman PO. Newborn infants to myasthenic mothers: A clinical study and an investigation of acetylcholine receptor antibodies in 17 children. Neurology 33:133-138, 1983.

Lieberman AT. Myasthenia gravis with acute fulminating onset in a child 5 years old. JAMA 120:1209-1211, 1942.

• Lindstrom JM, Seybold, Marjorie E, et al. Antibody to acetylcholine receptor in myasthenia gravis. Neurology 26:1054-1059, 1976.

• Namba T, Brown SE, Grob D. Neonatal myasthenia gravis: Report of two cases and review of literature. Pediatrics 45:488-504, 1970.

• Papatestas AE, Genkins G, Kornfeld P, et al. Effects of thymectomy in myasthenia gravis. Ann Surg 206:79-88, 1987.

Pascuzzi RM, Coslett HB, Johns TR. Long-term corticosteroid treatment of myasthenia gravis: Report of 116 patients. Ann Neurol 15:291-298, 1984.

Sarnat H, McGarry JD, Lewis JE Jr. Effective treatment of infantile myasthenia gravis by combined prednisone and thymectomy. Neurology 27:550-553, 1977.

Stalberg E, Ekstedt J, Broman A. Neuromuscular transmission in myasthenia gravis studied with single fiber electromyography. J Neurol Neurosurg Psychiatry 37:540-547, 1974.

Tindall RSA, Rollins J, Phillips JT, et al. Preliminary results of a double blind, randomized, placebo-controlled trial of cyclosporine in myasthenia gravis. N Engl J Med 316:719-724, 1987.

• Tronconi B, Brigonzi A, Fumagalli M, et al. Antibody induced degradation of acetylcholine receptors in myasthenia gravis: Clinical correlates and pathogenetic significance. Neurology 3:1440-1444, 1981.

Wand Dr, Wand BE. In vitro measurement of margin of safety of neuromuscular transmission. Am J Physiol 229:1632-1634, 1975.

30 Neonatal Respiratory Disease
Hyaline Membrane Disease and Meconium Aspiration Syndrome

Steven R. Mayfield

BACKGROUND AND PHYSIOLOGY

The identification, diagnosis, surveillance, and management of acute respiratory disorders of the newborn require an understanding of the epidemiology and pathophysiology of the disease and the experience to relate those elements to the patient's clinical course. Moreover, the baby may not have "read the book"; in other words, each patient is unique in terms of the magnitude of symptoms, effect of complicating conditions (e.g., patent ductus arteriosus), and length of the clinical course. Thus it is best to identify and treat pathophysiologic conditions and to use one's knowledge of the natural history of the disorder to make anticipatory management decisions. The physiology, symptoms, diagnostic considerations, and management of respiratory distress in the newborn are summarized briefly on pp. 252 and 253. The remainder of this chapter more specifically addresses these considerations, with particular emphasis on hyaline membrane disease and meconium aspiration syndrome.

The goal of ventilatory work is to effect an alveolar ventilation adequate for sufficient respiratory gas exchange. The ventilation–gas exchange unit can be separated into a ventilatory work unit and a gas-exchange unit. The ventilatory work unit includes the actively moving bony thorax and its muscular attachments and the resistive and elastic forces exerted by the lung parenchyma. The gas-exchange unit consists of respiratory bronchioles and alveoli, the alveolar-capillary membrane, and pulmonary capillaries. Defects in either unit can result in the signs and symptoms of respiratory distress.

Ventilatory work unit. The static lung volumes are illustrated in Fig. 30-1. Newborn infants typically have tidal volumes of 4 to 6 ml/kg, with intermittent "sigh" breaths to prevent end-expiratory alveolar collapse. The ability to perform ventilatory work requires an adequate CNS ventilatory drive, a stable, normally configured thorax, and an adequate ventilatory muscle mass to expand the thoracic volume. Inspiratory effort lifts the thorax up and forward with inferior diaphragmatic movement. These movements produce a negative intrapulmonic pressure as the lung, through its pleural attachments to the thorax, is actively expanded. Air is passively exhaled on relaxation.

Gas-exchange unit. The movement of O_2 from alveolus to pulmonary capillary and of CO_2 from pulmonary capillary to alveolus depends on characteristics of the alveolar-capillary membrane (thickness, effectively perfused surface area) and the alveolar-arterial pressure gradients for O_2 and CO_2. These gradients depend, in part, on the effectiveness of ventilation. Atelectasis reduces the effective surface area, as does hyperinflation, by increasing alveolar dead space ventilation (ventilation without effective respiratory gas exchange).

Pulmonary compliance. Pulmonary compliance is defined as the change in ventilatory volume per unit change in airway pressure ($\Delta V_E/\Delta P$) (Fig. 30-2). In practical terms pulmonary compliance translates to the force necessary to maintain alveolar patency. This force is described by Laplace's law as:

$$P = \frac{2ST}{r}$$

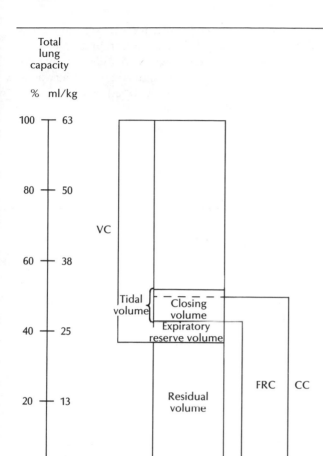

Fig. 30-1   Lung volumes in the infant. (VC = vital capacity; FRC = functional residual capacity; CC = closing capacity.) (Modified from Smith CA. Physiology of the Newborn, 4th ed. Springfield, Ill.: Charles C Thomas, 1976, pp 352, 356.)

Fig. 30-2   Extended compliance or lung expansion curve with "flattened" areas (*A* and *C*) at both ends. Area *A* represents the situation in diseases leading to atelectasis or lung collapse. Area *C* represents the situation in an over-expanded lung caused either by diseases in which there is significant air trapping (e.g., meconium aspiration) or by excessive application of distending pressure during assisted ventilation. (From Harris TR. Physiological principles. In Goldsmith JP, Karotkin EH, eds. Assisted Ventilation of the Neonate, 2nd ed. Philadelphia: WB Saunders, 1988, p 34.)

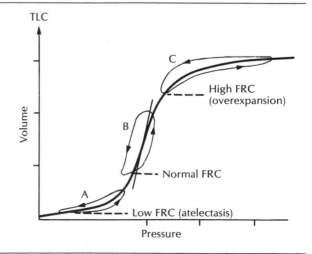

where P = distending pressure, ST = surface tension, and r = alveolar radius. Pulmonary compliance depends on the presence of surfactant, a phospholipoprotein produced by type II alveolar cells. Surfactant reduces surface tension at the alveolar liquid-air interface. Thus surfactant deficiency (such as occurs in hyaline membrane disease) results in decreased pulmonary compliance (i.e., "stiff" lungs).

Airway resistance. Airway resistance is defined as the change in airway pressure per unit change in airflow. In practical terms airway resistance translates to the force necessary to ventilate a small airway at a given airflow rate and is described by a rearrangement of Poiseulle's law as:

$$R = \frac{8n\ l}{r^4}$$

RESPIRATORY DISTRESS IN THE NEWBORN

Normal physiology

Fetus: Lungs are filled with fluid.

    Blood from the placenta enters the heart and bypasses the lungs by shunting right to left through the foramen ovale (FO) and ductus arteriosus (DA). Pulmonary vascular resistance (PVR) is high.

Newborn: The first breath expands the lungs and promotes clearing of lung fluid through the pulmonary lymphatics.

    PVR decreases.

    Left atrial pressure increases.

    Right atrial pressure decreases.

    FO closes.

    DA begins to close.

Pulmonary dynamics.

    Inspiration—negative airway pressure

    Expiration—positive airway pressure

    Lung volume = Airflow × Time

$$\text{Compliance} = \frac{\text{Change in lung volume}}{\text{Change in airway pressure}}$$

$$\text{Resistance} = \frac{\text{Change in airway pressure}}{\text{Change in airflow}}$$

    Ventilation-perfusion

        Perfusion decreases to poorly ventilated areas of lungs.

        Perfusion increases uniformly to lungs in response to diffuse atelectasis.

Symptoms

Tachypnea—respiratory rate ≥60/min

Retractions

    Suprasternal

    Substernal

    Intercostal

    Subcostal

Grunting

Nasal flaring

Cyanosis—≥3 to 5 g of desaturated hemoglobin/dl

    Peripheral—fingers and toes

    Central—lips and oral mucous membranes

Murmur of congenital heart disease

Diagnosis

History

Maternal

    Infection

    Prolonged rupture of membranes

    Elevated white blood count

    Vaginal discharge or bleeding

    Rh-negative blood type

    Meconium-stained fluid

Fetal

    Premature labor

    Intrauterine growth retardation

    Twin gestation

    Bradycardia or poor heart rate variability

    Ratio of lecithin to sphingomyelin in amniotic fluid ≤2:1

Newborn

    Cesarean section delivery

    Perinatal asphyxia

    Prematurity

    Meconium staining

    Foul odor

    Home delivery

where R = resistance, n = viscosity, l = length, and r = radius of the airway. Airway resistance is largely a function of the airway diameter at its narrowest point, which is the glottis in spontaneously breathing infants and the endotracheal tube in intubated infants.

Time constant. The time constant is the product of resistance and compliance and is described as:

Time constant (sec) =
Airway resistance (cm H_2O/ml/sec) ×
Pulmonary compliance (ml/cm H_2O)

The time constant is an index of the distribution of air within a ventilated space at a given resistance and compliance. In practical terms it represents an idealized minimum time required for inspiration (T_I) or expiration (T_E). Typically, three time constants represent the minimum T_I or T_E.

Physical examination

See "Symptoms."

Laboratory values

Arterial blood gases and pH
White blood cell count with differential count
Hemoglobin and hematocrit
Chest radiograph
Blood and urinary cultures as indicated
ECG as indicated

Differential diagnosis (incomplete list)
Pulmonary

Decreased lung compliance
    Hyaline membrane disease
    Pneumonia
    Meconium aspiration pneumonitis
Increased airway resistance—meconium aspiration
Ventilation-perfusion abnormalities
    Atelectasis
    Transient tachypnea of the newborn
    Persistent pulmonary artery hypertension
Restrictive abnormalities
    Congenital small thorax
    Pneumothorax
    Pleural effusions
    Thoracic masses

Cyanotic congenital heart disease

Often it presents with cyanosis without respiratory distress. One exception is total anomalous pulmonary venous return with obstruction below the diaphragm.

Upper airway obstruction

Choanal atresia
Micrognathia
Laryngeal-tracheal abnormality

Others

Hyperviscosity syndrome
Diaphragmatic hernia
Pulmonary hypoplasia

Management

Treat specific causes (e.g., infection, hyaline membrane disease).
Maintain Sao_2 >85% to 90%; monitor continuously.
Maintain pH >7.25 to 7.30; measure at least every 3 to 4 hours.
Institute positive pressure support as indicated.
    CPAP
    IMV with PEEP
Maintain intravascular euvolemia; monitor systemic arterial blood pressure and heart rate continuously. Obtain accurate measurement of fluid and electrolyte input and urinary output.
Maintain normal body temperature; monitor at least every 3 to 4 hours.
Monitor blood glucose, serum electrolytes, and hematocrit every 6 to 8 hr for 24 hr, then every 8 to 12 hr until respiratory distress is resolved.
Minimize unnecessary stimulation.
Treat with a penicillin and aminoglycoside until infection is excluded as a cause of respiratory distress.

Hyaline Membrane Disease

PHYSIOLOGY

Hyaline membrane disease is related to surfactant deficiency and hence is a disorder characterized by decreased pulmonary compliance. Surfactant is detectable at 20 to 23 weeks of gestation but is not present in sufficient quantities to ensure alveolar patency until ≥35 weeks of gestation. Surfactant deficiency results in a higher alveolar liquid-air surface tension with decreased pulmonary compliance (Fig. 30-3). The premature infant has a compliant bony thorax, which, combined with the stiff lungs characteristic of hyaline membrane disease, results in a marked increase in ventilatory work. As the infant attempts to achieve an adequate negative intrapulmonic pressure for effective ventilation, the stiff lungs may represent a greater inertial force relative to the momentum of chest wall movement. This means that the chest wall will retract more prominently in soft, nonbony intercostal, subcostal, or suprasternal regions.

The physiologic responses of infants with respiratory distress caused by decreased pulmonary compliance include attempts to maintain alveolar patency and minimize airway resistance. As arterial O_2 tension (Pao_2) falls and arterial CO_2 tension ($Paco_2$) rises, the infant attempts to improve ventilation by increasing the rate of breathing (tachypnea). As pulmonary compliance decreases, the infant may attempt to maintain alveolar patency at end-expiration by expiring against a semiclosed glottis (grunting) and/or by minimizing airway resistance with nasal flaring. As respiratory distress worsens, significant hypoxemia, acidosis, or pulmonary ischemia may occur, exacerbating the problem. Increased pulmonary capillary permeability results in accumulation of pulmonary interstitial and/or alveolar fluid, further decreasing lung compliance and worsening the gas diffusion abnormality. Pulmonary edema secondary to left-to-right shunting through a patent ductus arteriosus may also complicate the patient's pulmonary condition.

Ventilatory work performance may be affected by several factors. Central ventilatory drive and the hypercapnic and hypoxic ventilatory responses are blunted in premature infants. Moreover, many premature infants are in negative caloric balance in the first several days of life and, because body fat stores are low, must depend on body protein stores to compensate for the caloric deficit. The protein fuel reserve comes mainly from skeletal muscle, possibly reducing the ability to perform ventilatory work.

Hyaline membrane disease typically evolves during the first 24 hours of life, and infants who appear to be in little or no distress at birth may need intubation and mechanical ventilation by 6 to 24 hours of age (Fig. 30-4). Generally infants worsen to a plateau by 18 to 36 hours of age, although improvement in pulmonary compliance can be anticipated as early as 48 to 60 hours of age. Diuresis, which precedes improvement in pulmonary compliance by 12 to 36 hours, may be observed at 36 to 60 hours of age. Infants without hyaline membrane disease also have an increase in urinary output at approximately the same age. Thus, although diuresis may herald improvement in pulmonary function, the two events are probably not related.

The diagnosis of hyaline membrane disease in a premature infant depends on demonstration of decreased pulmonary compliance and a typical clinical course. The chest radiograph may demonstrate a diffuse reticulogranular pattern. The differential diagnosis must include pneumonia, which may be clinically and radiographically identical to hyaline membrane disease.

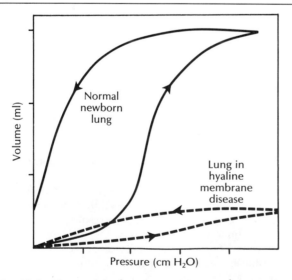

Fig. 30-3 Comparison between pressure-volume curves of normal infant and newborn with respiratory distress syndrome. (From Harris TR. Physiological principles. In Goldsmith JP, Karotkin EH, eds. Assisted Ventilation of the Neonate, 2nd ed. Philadelphia: WB Saunders, 1988, p 34.)

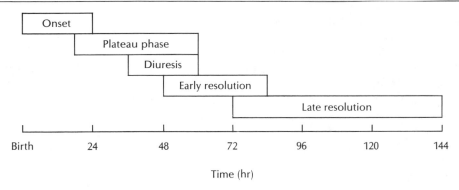

Fig. 30-4 Natural history of hyaline membrane disease. The early resolution phase reflects a 20% to 50% improvement. Late resolution results in extubation unless significant apnea is present.

MONITORING AND LABORATORY TESTS*

The physical examination should include the following:

1. Counting respiratory rate
2. Assessment of work of breathing, including retractions and grunting
3. Assessment of skin color, relating it to hemoglobin concentration (Cyanosis reflects 3 to 5 g of desaturated hemoglobin/dl.)
4. Auscultation and assessment of air movement and presence of adventitious airway sounds in all lung fields

Arterial blood gas tensions and pH must be measured at least every 2 hours until the patient is stable or improved, and the results must be related to changes in the work of breathing or the inspired O_2 requirement. *Remember, if the respiratory rate increases and the* $Paco_2$ *and pH do not change, the overall respiratory condition has worsened;* that is, increased ventilatory work is necessary to accomplish the same respiratory gas exchange. After the patient is stabilized, blood gas and pH measurements are obtained every 3 to 8 hours as indicated by the severity of illness.

Assessment of arterial O_2 saturation (pulse oximetry) may be used with the following caveats:

Arterial O_2 saturation (Sao_2) reflects the percent of hemoglobin bound to O_2 and hence the O_2 content

of the blood. Each gram of hemoglobin can carry 1.34 ml of O_2. The following example illustrates the relation of the Sao_2 to tissue O_2 availability:

1. If the hemoglobin is 20 g/dl and Sao_2 is 90%, the O_2 content and O_2 available to the tissues will be:

$$20 \text{ g/dl} \times 1.34 \text{ ml/g} \times 0.9 = 24 \text{ ml/dl}$$

2. At the typical rate of O_2 consumption the usual extraction of O_2 by the tissues is 20% to 30% of the total O_2 content, whereas maximum O_2 extraction is approximately 60% to 75%. Under typical conditions the O_2 released to tissues will be:

$$24 \text{ ml/dl} \times 0.25 = 6 \text{ ml/dl}$$

3. If the hemoglobin concentration falls to 10 g/dl, but the Sao_2 increases to 95%, the O_2 content will be:

$$10 \text{ g/dl} \times 1.34 \text{ ml/g} \times 0.95 = 12.7 \text{ ml/dl}$$

4. To extract 6 ml/dl of O_2:

$$6 \text{ ml/dl} \div 12.7 \text{ ml/dl} \times 100 =$$
$$47\% \text{ } O_2 \text{ extraction rate}$$

In the latter case, despite an increase in the Sao_2, there is less O_2 reserve in the event of an increased metabolic O_2 demand.

The maximum Sao_2 is 97.4% because of internally generated carbon monoxide. Thus the Sao_2 is 97% when the Pao_2 is ≥70 mm Hg, and a hyperoxic stress

*For electronic monitoring see Chapters 107, 108, 111, 120-122, and 125.

may occur that is not reflected by the Sao_2 value. Hyperoxia has been associated with retinopathy of prematurity and bronchopulmonary dysplasia.

A chest radiograph must be obtained daily or more often as indicated to assess the progression of the disease and the efficacy of therapy.

The hematocrit value must be determined every 8 hours, with transfusion of blood provided to maintain the hematocrit above 40%.

An umbilical or radial artery catheter for blood sampling and systemic arterial pressure monitoring must be placed in all infants needing 40% to 50% O_2.

TREATMENT

A multisystem approach to intensive care of the premature newborn is beyond the scope of this chapter, and the reader is referred to standard textbooks on neonatology for guidance. However, it is worthwhile to mention the problems associated with prematurity that may complicate the clinical course of an infant with hyaline membrane disease. These problems include fluid and electrolyte imbalance, thermal imbalance, patent ductus arteriosus, hypoglycemia, hyperglycemia, hyperbilirubinemia, hypocalcemia, intraventricular hemorrhage, apnea and/or bradycardia, and necrotizing enterocolitis.

The goal of intensive care medical practice is anticipatory management as opposed to crisis intervention. Thus the clinician must use all the tools and skills at his or her command and incorporate all findings into a coherent picture. The principles of management of hyaline membrane disease include:

1. Establish proper surveillance.
2. Relate signs, symptoms, and laboratory results to the natural history of the disease.
3. Maintain close follow-up after clinical interventions to assess efficacy.
4. When using positive pressure ventilatory support, try to make the ventilator fit the baby instead of making the baby fit the ventilator.

Supplemental Oxygen

Previous authors have recommended using supplemental O_2 to maintain a Pao_2 of 50 to 70 mm Hg. With the availability of continuous monitoring of Sao_2 using pulse oximetry, provision of supplemental O_2 sufficient to maintain an Sao_2 >85% to 90% when the hemoglobin concentration is ≥13 to 15 g/dl is

a reasonable goal and should provide adequate O_2 to meet the metabolic O_2 demands of the tissues. The maximum allowable Sao_2 as measured by pulse oximetry (generally ± 2%) depends on the variability of the oximeter. Since the theoretic maximum Sao_2 ($Sao_{2\ MAX}$) is 97.4%, any value measured by pulse oximetry from 93% to 101% (97% ± 2 SD) must be considered as representative of the $Sao_{2\ MAX}$. Thus values for Sao_2 by pulse oximetry that are consistently >93% may be associated with hyperoxia, and thus a blood sample for determination of Pao_2 must be obtained.

The decision to use continuous positive airway pressure (CPAP) depends on the diagnosis, the supplemental O_2 requirement, and the time point in the patient's clinical disease course. When using CPAP, the goal is to prevent end-expiratory atelectasis and to maintain the patient on the steep portion of the compliance curve. As shown in Fig. 30-2, the pressure necessary to accomplish this goal is greater if atelectasis has already occurred. Therefore CPAP must be instituted as a preventive therapy rather than as a means of rescue. CPAP may be provided through nasal prongs or a nasopharyngeal or endotracheal tube. The typical range of effective pressures is 4 to 8 cm H_2O. Infants needing >8 cm H_2O will probably benefit from intermittent mandatory ventilation (IMV) with positive end-expiratory pressure (PEEP). Most infants less than 24 hours old who need supplemental O_2 ≥50% to 60% will benefit from added CPAP. For infants older than 24 to 48 hours of age with a stable clinical course supported by acceptable blood gas and pH values, O_2 supplementation of up to 80% by hood may be acceptable. Infants needing O_2 supplementation >80%, regardless of the clinical course or postnatal age, usually benefit from either CPAP or IMV with PEEP.

IMV with PEEP

Indications for the institution of IMV with PEEP include:

1. O_2 requirement of ≥0.5 in the first 12 hours of life or ≥0.8 at any postnatal age
2. Respiratory acidosis with a pH of <7.25 in the first 12 hours of life or <7.20 at any postnatal age
3. Apnea while on CPAP

The goals of IMV with PEEP must relate to the pathophysiology of the pulmonary disorder. Hyaline membrane disease is characterized by decreased pulmonary compliance; thus the time constant is decreased, and the minimum inspiratory and expiratory times *at an adequate peak inspiratory pressure* are shortened. The goals are to support the patient with the following.

1. *Peak inspiratory pressure (PIP) sufficient to ventilate an adequate alveolar surface area without producing hyperinflation:* The minimum PIP can be assessed by adjusting the pressure on the ventilator while observing chest wall movement, auscultating for bilateral, basilar breath sounds, assessing changes in the work of breathing, and observing color and pulse oximetric values for the SaO_2. The initial, minimum PIP varies but is typically in the range of 15 to 30 cm H_2O for infants with hyaline membrane disease. Atelectasis is associated with a higher pressure requirement per unit change in ventilatory volume. Thus, if the patient has atelectasis at the onset of IMV with PEEP, considerable pressure may be necessary to open the airways. However, once the airways are open, the lungs are described by the steep portion of the compliance curve (Fig. 30-2). Thus the pressure needed to ventilate the patient initially may be higher than the pressure necessary to maintain adequate ventilation after overcoming atelectasis. This difference may vary from 0 to 10 cm H_2O. Only continued surveillance and appropriate follow-up of laboratory values can determine the patient's clinical condition. If no breath sounds are auscultated initially, increase the PIP until adequate basilar air movement is heard bilaterally and chest wall excursion is observed. After 2 to 5 minutes reduce the pressure while listening for breath sounds and observing chest wall movement. Note the PIP on the ventilator at the point at which breath sounds were no longer easily heard. Increase the PIP until breath sounds and chest wall movement are acceptable; note this "opening" pressure. As an allowance for the vagaries of physical assessments and with the knowledge that hyaline membrane disease continues to worsen during the first 24 hours of life, a margin of 1 to 2 cm H_2O above the opening pressure can be provided. Similar assessments must be made every 30 to 60 minutes during the first 6 to 12 hours of life until the patient is stable and blood gas and pH values are acceptable. An initial chest radiograph will confirm endotracheal tube placement, aid in diagnosis, and identify atelectasis, hyperinflation, or air leak.

2. *PEEP sufficient to prevent end-expiratory atelectasis:* PEEP is generally set initially at 3 to 5 cm H_2O.

3. *Inspiratory time adequate for sufficient gas exchange:* The inspiratory time must be related to the time constant. Typically infants with hyaline membrane disease have time constants of 0.02 to 0.05 second. Thus the expected minimum TI would be 0.06 to 0.15 second. However, a TI on the lower end of that range would not allow sufficient time for effective gas exchange. Therefore the usual starting range is 0.35 to 0.75 second, with 0.5 second as a reasonable starting point. The TI and TE must always be related to the IMV rate, and a respiratory rate change must never be ordered without indicating whether or not an associated change in TI and/or TE is desired. Never exceed a TI of 1.0 second.

4. *Expiratory time adequate to prevent air trapping:* The expiratory time, in the absence of hyperinflation and air trapping, does not need to exceed 3 time constants. Thus 0.15 second is probably adequate in most cases of hyaline membrane disease. If the IMV rate is set at 20 to 50 breaths/min and the TI at 0.5 second, the TE will necessarily be 0.7 to 2.5 seconds, more than enough time for expiration. Increasing the TI to as much as 1.0 second at IMV rates of 20 to 50 breaths/min will result in a range of values for TE of 0.2 to 2.0 seconds, which is probably adequate although a TE of ≥ 0.3 second is safer. Remember that the inspiratory to expiratory time I:E ratio is relevant only when the TI and TE are adequate. Calculate the I:E ratio as follows:

$$\frac{60 \text{ sec}}{\text{Minute}} \div \frac{\text{IMV rate (breaths)}}{\text{Minute}} = \text{Breath cycle (sec)}$$

$$\text{Breath cycle} - \text{TI} = \text{TE}$$

$$\text{TI:TE} = \text{I:E ratio}$$

5. *IMV rate initially set at 20 to 50 breaths/min depending on the ability of the infant to perform the work of breathing:* Some larger infants with mild hyaline membrane disease may need only 5 to 15 breaths/min. Infants ≤ 1250 g birthweight typically need at least 30 to 40 breaths/min. The decision to exceed 50 breaths/min should be made only after consultation with a neonatologist or pediatric intensivist since a high IMV rate, high PIP, high PEEP, and/or a long TI are all associated with air trapping. This may produce paradoxical CO_2 retention, hyperinflation, epithelial barotrauma, pulmonary interstitial

emphysema, and/or air leak into the pleural space, pericardium, or peritoneum.

Withdrawal of IMV with PEEP

During ventilator withdrawal the goals are consistent:

1. Maintain SaO_2 ≥85% to 90% without lability at a hemoglobin concentration of 13 to 15 g/dl.
2. Prevent respiratory acidosis in which the pH is ≤7.25 to 7.30 (measure blood gases and pH 20 to 30 minutes after each ventilator change).
3. Prevent increases in the clinical work of breathing.
4. Prevent radiographic and clinical evidence of atelectasis or hyperinflation/air leak.

Continued assessment of the minimum PIP should occur at least every 4 hours after the patient has reached the plateau phase of the disease. Clinical diuresis is defined as (1) the point at which the ratio of fluid input to urinary output is ≤0.8 or (2) an increase in urinary output of 3-fold to 5-fold in any 8- to 12-hour period after the first 24 hours of life. As previously noted, diuresis may be observed at 36 to 60 hours of age, preceding improvement in pulmonary function by 12 to 24 hours (Fig. 30-4). Therefore one can expect an increase in pulmonary compliance and a longer time constant at 48 to 72 hours of age. As compliance increases, the PIP will produce a larger change in ventilatory volume (see Fig. 30-2). The risk for hyperinflation and/or air leak is increased if the PIP remains high as pulmonary compliance improves. Thus with the onset of diuresis the clinician can begin looking for the following signs:

1. Greater chest wall excursion
2. Improved air movement on auscultation
3. Lower spontaneous work of breathing
4. Higher PaO_2 or SaO_2 with no change in FiO_2 or the maintenance of PaO_2 or SaO_2 on a lower FiO_2
5. Respiratory alkalosis
6. Respiratory acidosis with a paradoxical decrease in the O_2 requirement (indicative of hyperinflation and air trapping)

The PIP should be lowered using clinical criteria and prompt laboratory follow-up. If close attention is paid, individual reductions of the PIP will generally not exceed 2 to 4 cm H_2O. However, if air trapping has occurred, the need for greater reductions may be indicated. When the PIP is 12 to 16 cm H_2O, changes in IMV rate take priority over further pressure reductions.

Reductions of PEEP below 3 to 4 cm H_2O are rarely helpful, may unnecessarily delay extubation, and are potentially deleterious for infants on CPAP with high spontaneous inspiratory flow. In the latter case high inspiratory flow may create air turbulence in the endotracheal tube and increase airway resistance. As the infant attempts to inspire against the higher airway resistance, more negative intrapulmonic pressure may be generated, possibly resulting in atelectasis. For this reason some authors have advocated extubating infants while they are on a low IMV rate of 3 to 8 breaths/minute.

Reduction of the IMV rate should relate to the patient's efficiency in performing ventilatory work. Individual reductions of 3 to 5 breaths/min every 1 to 2 hours are reasonable, although more rapid reductions are warranted in some infants. Remember, make the ventilator fit the baby rather than making the baby fit the ventilator. Close monitoring of arterial blood gas and pH values must be done to assess the response to withdrawal of ventilator support.

The Ti can be maintained at 0.35 to 0.5 second. Remember to indicate the desired Ti with each change in IMV rate. As the IMV rate is decreased at a constant Ti, Te will necessarily increase, and the I:E ratio will decrease. Remember, the baby breathes spontaneously, and the ventilator I:E ratio only governs the *ventilator* breaths, not the infant's *spontaneous* breaths.

Typically infants with uncomplicated hyaline membrane disease demonstrate an improvement in pulmonary compliance within 24 hours of diuresis to the extent that the PIP, IMV rate, and FiO_2 can be reduced by 20% to 50% (Fig. 30-4). A new plateau is then established with further significant improvement occurring after another 12 to 36 hours. This latter improvement typically results in extubation unless significant apnea occurs.

Other Treatments

The use of chest physiotherapy with endotracheal suction is necessary in most cases to aid in removal of pulmonary secretions and to prevent atelectasis. Typically chest physiotherapy is needed every 3 to 6 hours.

An adequate O_2-carrying capacity must be maintained by keeping the hematocrit ≥40% during the acute phase of the disease.

An adequate vascular volume is ensured by continuously monitoring heart rate (normal range equals

120 to 160 bpm) and systemic arterial blood pressure. High heart rates with normal or low systemic arterial blood pressure or wide pulse pressures may reflect decreased vascular volume. O_2 delivery to tissues is the product of O_2 content (hemoglobin saturation) and blood flow (cardiac output and vascular volume).

Alkali may be used to maintain the arterial pH >7.25 with the following caveats:

1. Rapid IV administration of sodium bicarbonate to premature infants is associated with an increased incidence of intraventricular hemorrhage. Sodium bicarbonate must be administered over a minimum of 20 to 60 minutes.

2. Acid-base balance is related to the rate of CO_2 elimination:

$$pH = pK_a + \log \frac{Base}{Acid}$$

$$H^+ + HCO_3^- = H_2CO_3 = CO_2 + H_2O$$

As shown, if CO_2 is not eliminated (respiratory distress), the reaction is driven backward, resulting in acid accumulation. Therefore when providing bicarbonate, one must ensure that respiratory gas exchange is adequate to eliminate the CO_2 load. Otherwise adding bicarbonate will *worsen* the acidosis.

Occasionally, infants with hyaline membrane disease may struggle while receiving ventilatory support, potentially compromising lung ventilation and respiratory gas exchange. Judicious use of chloral hydrate (30 to 40 mg/kg/dose) may be helpful. Although the use of paralytic agents such as pancuronium is occasionally necessary, their use almost invariably leads to a higher level of positive pressure support. Thus any alternative therapies must be exhausted before using pancuronium (0.04 to 0.08 mg/kg/dose).

Meconium Aspiration Syndrome
BACKGROUND AND PHYSIOLOGY

Meconium is a viscous, green material that is formed in the fetal GI tract. It is composed of amniotic fluid, fetal hair, epithelial cells, and GI secretions. In 8% to 20% of all pregnancies meconium is passed by the fetus into the amniotic fluid. Meconium-stained amniotic fluid ranges in quality from green-tinged to a pea soup consistency. Although the trigger that evokes intrauterine defecation is unclear, fetal anoxic stress appears to be a common antecedent event.

Thus small-for-gestational-age and postmature infants or infants from a pregnancy complicated by uteroplacental insufficiency are at greatest risk. Meconium passage from the fetus into the amniotic fluid is rarely, if ever, seen before 34 weeks' gestational age.

In utero the net movement of lung fluid is usually from fetus to uterine cavity. Fetal distress and delivery of the neonate both result in gasping, with movement of amniotic fluid into the bronchial tree. Respiratory distress due to meconium aspiration is characterized by tachypnea, airway obstruction, and increased airway resistance from meconium plugs in the airways. These plugs may create a "ball-valve" effect in which inspiratory airflow is less impeded than expiratory airflow, resulting in overexpansion of distal airways. Adjacent airways may collapse because of meconium plugging. Thus the disease is heterogeneous, with areas of atelectasis adjacent to areas of overexpansion. The functional residual capacity (Fig. 30-1) may be increased, resulting in hypoxemia and/or hypercarbia.

Affected infants may demonstrate yellow-green staining of the skin and umbilical cord. Neurologic depression may be evident at birth, with cord blood gas and pH values indicating a nonrespiratory acidosis. Streaky pulmonary infiltrates may be seen on a chest radiograph, with an extrapulmonary air leak evident in up to 50% of affected infants. The arterial blood gas and pH values may reveal a respiratory acidosis, but significant hypoxemia is more common, often reflecting pulmonary arterial hypertension, which is commonly associated with the meconium aspiration syndrome. Other problems to consider relate to asphyxial injury and include hypocalcemia, hypoglycemia, hypoxic encephalopathy, seizures, renal tubular necrosis, DIC, and SIADH.

The natural history of meconium aspiration syndrome is variable. Most infants have resolved the respiratory distress by 24 to 48 hours of age. However, if pulmonary arterial hypertension is associated, the infant may be critically ill for 3 to 7 days followed by a further 3 to 21 days of convalescence (see Chapter 39).

MONITORING AND LABORATORY TESTS

Electronic monitoring, physical assessment, blood gas and pH determinations, and other laboratory and radiographic assessments are obtained as previously outlined for the management of hyaline membrane disease. If pulmonary arterial hypertension develops, both systemic arterial and central venous blood pressure monitoring are indicated. Hypotension must be avoided since pulmonary perfusion depends on the systemic arterial blood pressure/pulmonary arterial blood pressure ratio (SAP:PAP). Volume expanders and/or pressor agents must be used as indicated to maintain a positive SAP:PAP.

TREATMENT

The best management for the meconium aspiration syndrome is prevention, including careful prenatal surveillance with expeditious delivery in the event of fetal distress. During delivery the obstetrician needs to suction the hypopharynx while the head is on the perineum before the infant takes the first breath. After delivery the pediatrician must visually inspect the hypopharynx for the presence of meconium and promptly suction the trachea before providing positive pressure ventilatory support. This step will significantly reduce the mechanical component of the meconium aspiration syndrome by preventing migration of meconium-stained amniotic fluid into the distal airways. Hypopharyngeal or endotracheal suction has little or no impact on the incidence of pulmonary arterial hypertension. There is some controversy regarding the selection of infants who may benefit from endotracheal suction in the delivery room. However, the consensus is that all infants with moderately thick meconium will benefit from aggressive delivery room management. Endotracheal suction must be performed quickly along with continuous monitoring of the infant's color and heart rate. Many infants with meconium staining are depressed at birth and may be bradycardic. Prolonging the process of endotracheal suction will further promote anoxic stress. Therefore an experienced clinician must perform or directly supervise the delivery room management of meconium-stained infants.

Expectant management of the infant's respiratory distress due to meconium aspiration is indicated after stabilization in the delivery room. Endotracheal suction and chest physiotherapy are done every 2 hours. Use of saline lavage is of unproven benefit and may be deleterious. Meconium is sterile but can cause a chemical pneumonitis and can enhance bacterial growth. Moreover, bacterial sepsis may be the antecedent event in meconium staining of amniotic fluid. Therefore the administration of antibiotics is indicated while awaiting culture results (see Chapter 42).

Supplemental Oxygen

The use of supplemental O_2 is indicated to maintain the SaO_2 at 90% to 94% when the blood hemoglobin concentration is 13 to 15 g/dl. Infants with pulmonary arterial hypertension may have labile pulmonary perfusion with rapid swings in PaO_2 and SaO_2 values from hypoxic to hyperoxic levels. In infants with meconium aspiration and pulmonary arterial hypertension it is wise to maintain the PaO_2 and SaO_2 higher than is necessary for infants with hyaline membrane disease, in whom such extreme lability is less common.

IMV with PEEP

The indications for CPAP or IMV with PEEP are the same as for hyaline membrane disease with the following caveats:

1. Vasoactive changes in the pulmonary artery blood pressure may occur in response to changes in blood pH. Acidosis causes vasoconstriction, whereas alkalosis evokes vasodilation. Thus infants at risk for pulmonary arterial hypertension might benefit from earlier intervention, with IMV directed at maintaining the arterial pH ≥7.30 or, preferably, 7.40 to 7.50.

2. Although the meconium aspiration syndrome may be associated with decreased pulmonary compliance, the major pathophysiologic abnormality is an increase in airway resistance. This results in a lengthened time constant, necessitating a longer T_I to overcome airway resistance and a longer T_E to prevent pulmonary overexpansion. This paradoxical condition makes the severe case of meconium aspiration syndrome one of the most difficult ventilatory management problems.

3. When positive pressure ventilation is used, the incidence of pneumothorax is high among even the most fastidiously managed infants. While preparations take place for insertion of a chest tube (see Chapter 134), pleural air can be promptly evacuated using a 25-gauge butterfly needle attached to a stopcock and 60 ml syringe. To evacuate pleural air the needle should be clamped with a hemostat approximately 3 to 5 mm above the tip (Fig. 30-5). The needle is inserted into the chest wall lateral to the midclavicular or anterior axillary line in the second intercostal space. The needle must be inserted along the superior margin of the third rib to avoid the intercostal artery running along the inferior margin of the second rib. Air is *slowly* withdrawn into the 60 ml syringe. If more than 60 ml of air is present

or if the pneumothorax is under tension, the air in the syringe is evacuated into the atmosphere and air withdrawal resumed.

4. Infants with pulmonary arterial hypertension may struggle while on the ventilator. This movement can increase transthoracic pressure and pulmonary arterial blood pressure, increasing right-to-left shunting through a patent ductus arteriosus or a patent foramen ovale. Thus it is wise to minimize the activity of such infants by avoiding unnecessary stimulation and making judicious use of sedatives (chloral hydrate, 30 to 40 mg/kg) or, in severe cases, paralytic drugs (pancuronium, 0.04 to 0.08 mg/kg) (see Chapters 129 and 130).

The ventilator management of the meconium aspiration syndrome subsumes all of the principles and philosophies previously described for the management of hyaline membrane disease. Initial management depends on the ability of the infant to perform the work of breathing, the presence and severity of associated pulmonary arterial hypertension, and the extent of ventilation-perfusion mismatching caused by combined atelectasis and overexpansion. Guidelines for initial support include:

1. Peak inspiratory pressure of 15 to 35 cm H_2O
2. PEEP of 3 to 6 cm H_2O
3. IMV rate of 10 to 60 breaths/min
4. TI of 0.4 to 0.6 second
5. TE of 0.5 to 0.7 second

Withdrawal of IMV with PEEP is accomplished using the same approach outlined in the management of hyaline membrane disease. Respiratory distress caused by meconium aspiration syndrome is a disease characterized by increased airway resistance. Although pulmonary compliance may be decreased in areas of atelectasis, many infants may demonstrate little or no compliance abnormality. Thus the risk of hyperinflation and barotrauma is significant. Moreover, the clinical course of pulmonary arterial hypertension, if present, often dictates the need for ventilator support. As the pulmonary arterial hypertension resolves, ventilatory requirements may decline rapidly, and IMV with PEEP can be expeditiously withdrawn.

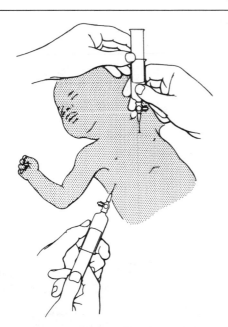

Fig. 30-5 Technique for needle pleuracentesis of intra- and extrapleural air. (From Brady JP, Lewis K. Quick Reference to Pediatric Emergencies, 3rd ed. Philadelphia: JB Lippincott, 1984, p 465.)

ADDITIONAL READING

• Brady JP, Gregory GA. Assisted ventilation. In Klaus MH, Fanaroff AA, eds. Care of the High Risk Neonate. Philadelphia: WB Saunders, 1986, pp 202-219.

• Carlo WA, Martin RJ. Principles of neonatal assisted ventilation. Pediatr Clin North Am 33:221-237, 1986.

Fanaroff AA, Martin RJ, Miller MJ. Meconium aspiration syndrome. In Martin RJ, Fanaroff AA, eds. Neonatal-Perinatal Medicine. St. Louis: CV Mosby, 1987, pp 604-606.

• Harris TR. Physiological principles. In Goldsmith JP, Karotkin EH, eds. Assisted Ventilation of the Neonate. Philadelphia: WB Saunders, 1981, pp 18-48.

Martin RJ, Fanaroff AA. The respiratory distress syndrome and its management. In Martin RJ, Fanaroff AA, eds. Neonatal-Perinatal Medicine. St. Louis: CV Mosby, 1987, pp 580-589.

Martin RJ, Klaus MH, Fanaroff AA. Respiratory problems. In Klaus MH, Fanaroff AA, eds. Care of the High Risk Neonate. Philadelphia: WB Saunders, 1986, pp 171-201.

Oh W, Stern L. Respiratory diseases of the newborn. In Stern L, Vert P, eds. Neonatal Medicine. Paris: Masson, 1987, pp 389-408.

Ting P, Brady J. Tracheal suction in meconium aspiration. Am J Obstet Gynecol 122:767-771, 1975.

31 Sudden Infant Death Syndrome and Apparent Life-Threatening Events

John G. Brooks

Sudden Infant Death Syndrome

BACKGROUND AND PHYSIOLOGY

Sudden infant death syndrome (SIDS) is defined as "The sudden death of any infant or young child which is unexpected by history, and in which a thorough postmortem examination fails to demonstrate an adequate cause for death." Without an autopsy this diagnosis cannot be established since this is the only definitive way to rule out other causes of sudden unexpected death in infants, such as meningitis, intracranial hemorrhage, myocarditis, aspiration pneumonia, or some other overwhelming infections.

SIDS is the leading cause of postneonatal infant mortality and results in approximately 7500 infant deaths each year in the United States. The incidence of SIDS in the general population is 1.5 to 2.0/1000 live births, but there are several subgroups of the population who are at varying degrees of increased risk of SIDS (Table 31-1, Fig. 31-1). SIDS is unusual in the first 2 weeks of life and has a peak incidence between 2 and 4 months of age; 70% to 90% of SIDS cases occur in the first 6 months of life. Rare cases occur in the second year of life. A variety of factors have been identified that are associated with an increased risk of SIDS. SIDS occurs more frequently during the winter months, in lower income families, in males, in subsequent siblings of previous SIDS victims, in infants of mothers who smoke, in infants who have experienced severe apparent life-threatening events, in infants of drug-addicted mothers, and in low birthweight infants. The risk for low birthweight infants is inversely proportional to the birthweight; newborn infants who weigh 1 kg have a SIDS risk of approximately 1%, or 10/1000 live births. The risk for subsequent siblings of SIDS victims is approximately 8/1000 live births, approximately four to five times the risk in the general population. It is likely that, as a group, these families were at increased risk for their first infant with SIDS because of their demographic characteristics and are at similar high risk with their next infant because these risk factors persist.

Although much is known about the circumstances of typical SIDS deaths, the cause of SIDS remains unknown. It is likely that several different mechanisms can produce the same clinical scenario. The

Table 31-1 Incidence of SIDS

Population	No./1000 Live Births
All infants	1.5-2.0
Infants having apparent life-threatening events (ALTE)	20-70
Low birthweight infants	5-10
SIDS siblings	7-8
Infants of addicts	10-15

death occurs when the infant is thought to be sleeping or silent, and it is often associated with a mild respiratory infection, although histologic findings at the postmortem examination do not implicate the respiratory infection as a cause of death. Two leading hypotheses of causation are the apnea hypothesis and the cardiac hypothesis. The former proposes that the primary cause of death is failure of respiration perhaps caused by failure of normal arousal mechanisms, neural reflex–mediated central apnea, or obstructive apnea. The cardiac hypothesis proposes a dysrhythmia leading to cardiac arrest as the primary cause of death, perhaps from abnormal dynamic regulation of cardiac repolarization caused by an imbalance in the autonomic innervation of the developing heart. A variety of other mechanisms such as botulism or rare genetic metabolic disorders may explain a very small proportion of SIDS deaths.

MANAGEMENT

An autopsy must be performed to establish the diagnosis of SIDS, and in most states there is a legal requirement that the coroner be notified of such a death. It is within the coroner's jurisdiction to insist on an autopsy.

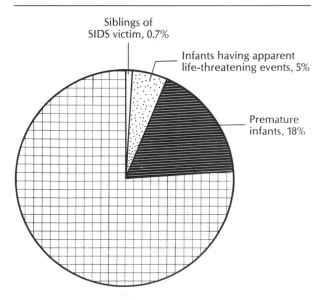

Siblings of
SIDS victim, 0.7%

Infants having apparent
life-threatening events, 5%

Premature
infants, 18%

Fig. 31-1 Sources of SIDS, showing percentage of total SIDS victims who are from each of these high-risk groups.

The therapeutic interventions must be directed toward the families of SIDS infants because the unexpected death of a previously healthy infant is a most devastating event for parents and other caretakers and is associated with a predictable grief reaction consisting of denial, guilt, anger, and depression. Initial interactions with the family in cases of probable SIDS must emphasize that SIDS is currently unpredictable and unpreventable. Professional and/or peer support can be offered to the family immediately and again after several days or weeks. It is important that the family be notified of the preliminary results of the autopsy within 24 hours and, with supportive individuals, have the opportunity to discuss the results of the final autopsy several months after the death. Feelings of guilt and anger as well as behavior problems are likely to occur in surviving siblings. Parents need to be advised how to discuss the infant's death with older siblings at an age-appropriate level.

Education of the public and first responders (e.g., emergency medical technicians, police, and firemen) about SIDS will minimize the risk of inappropriate accusations and insensitive interactions with the family at the time of the infant's death. Many communities have local chapters of the National Sudden Infant Death Syndrome Foundation or other appropriate support groups that can assist with both the individual parental support and the community education efforts.*

Apparent Life-Threatening Events
BACKGROUND AND PHYSIOLOGY

Infants who have experienced episodes of apnea and/ or color change (who, on some occasions, observers have thought to be dead) have attracted increased attention in the medical and lay communities over the past two decades. The 1986 National Institutes of Health (NIH) Consensus Development Conference on Infantile Apnea and Home Monitoring recommended that these infants be classified as undergoing apparent life-threatening events (ALTE) to describe the circumstances that bring them to medical atten-

---

*Locations and contacts for local SIDS Foundation chapters as well as other information about SIDS can be obtained by calling the National Sudden Infant Death Syndrome Foundation at 1-800-221-SIDS.

tion. These frightening episodes can occur during sleep, quiet or active wakefulness, or feeding. They are usually described as some combination of central or obstructive apnea, change of color (e.g., pallid, cyanotic, mottled) and muscle tone (hypertonic, hypotonic, seizing), and choking or gagging. In some such infants appropriate evaluation will demonstrate a specific diagnosis that is likely to explain the frightening episode (e.g., ALTE caused by seizure or gastroesophageal reflux), but in approximately 50% of cases no specific cause is identified.

Relationship of ALTE to SIDS

As a basis for management decisions and for counseling of families of affected infants, the relationship between ALTE and SIDS must be considered from two perspectives. First, only approximately 5% of SIDS victims have been noted to experience ALTE before their demise, so most SIDS victims do not come from the ALTE population (Fig. 31-1). Stated differently, the incidence of ALTE among the SIDS population of infants is approximately 5% as compared to a 2% to 3% incidence of ALTE in the non-SIDS infant population. Second, the incidence of SIDS among the heterogeneous group of ALTE infants is approximately 1% to 2%, but subgroups with significantly higher SIDS risk have been identified. Those whose frightening episode occurred during sleep and was perceived to require cardiopulmonary resuscitation have a 10% to 13% risk of subsequent sudden unexpected death, even with the prescription of home monitoring devices. The very rare infant who experiences two such severe episodes has a 28% risk of subsequent sudden and unexpected death. In most cases the second episode occurs within 3½ weeks of the first. These data about high-risk ALTE subgroups apply to infants in whom evaluation revealed no specific cause of the frightening episodes. The precise risk for infants who experience less severe ALTE events has not been determined, but in many cases it may be no greater than the general population. Identification of a specific cause of ALTE (e.g., infection, seizures) does not necessarily eliminate the increased risk of sudden and unexpected death.

Etiology

Specific causes of apparent life-threatening events are:

Chalasia with laryngeal chemoreceptor-mediated apnea
Seizure disorder
Infection (e.g., respiratory syncytial virus, pertussis, sepsis)
Upper airway obstruction
Cardiac disease
Breath holding
Severe anemia
Central hypoventilation syndromes
CNS tumors
Idiopathic apnea of infancy

Three general categories can be identified: "normal" infants, infants with acute infection, and infants with chronic conditions. No specific causative mechanism is identified in approximately 50% of ALTE infants. Of those in whom a specific diagnosis is established or highly likely, seizure disorder, laryngeal chemoreceptor-mediated apnea related to dysfunction of the upper GI tract (e.g., pharyngeal incoordination, gastroesophageal reflux), and infection (especially respiratory syncytial virus) are most common.

MONITORING AND LABORATORY TESTS

All infants who are hospitalized because of ALTE must be continuously monitored with an electronic cardiorespiratory impedance monitor for the duration of hospitalization. For infants <3 months of age the alarms in the hospital must be set to sound for a heart rate <80 bpm or a respiratory pause of 15 seconds or longer. Any respiratory pause >20 seconds or a shorter pause associated with bradycardia or hypoxemia is abnormal at any age. Most ALTE infants are stable at the time of admission and do not have subsequent frightening episodes during hospitalization. Some, however, will have repeat episodes, and occasional infants, particularly those who have experienced significant asphyxial episodes, may need much more extensive intensive care monitoring and intervention.

After a careful history and physical examination are performed, appropriate laboratory testing can be selected, depending on the most likely identifiable disease processes. Minimal laboratory evaluation for all ALTE infants consists of:

Continuous cardiorespiratory monitoring
Complete and differential blood count (especially for lymphocytosis of pertussis)
Serum bicarbonate

The bicarbonate value must be obtained as soon as possible after the infant is seen in the medical facility since persistent lactic acidosis may be objective evidence to support the parental report of a significant episode even though the infant may no longer be clinically symptomatic. An ECG, echocardiogram, chest roentgenogram, lateral neck roentgenogram, EEG, oximetry, arterial blood gases and pH, barium esophagram, esophageal pH probe, serum electrolytes, CT scan, laryngoscopy, or bronchoscopy are indicated in some infants. The history about the ALTE must be taken directly from the individual who observed it rather than as a secondhand report.

Polysomnography, which is the continuous recording of multiple physiologic variables (e.g., oximetry, end-tidal CO_2, EEG, EMG), is only occasionally necessary. Limited versions of polysomnography (e.g., continuous oximetry recording during sleep) may be appropriate more frequently. Polysomnography is essential for the diagnosis of central hypoventilation syndromes. "Pneumograms," which are hard-copy recordings of the cardiorespiratory pattern over 12 to 24 hours, have only a very limited role. As currently analyzed, such recordings do not identify infants who are at increased risk for sudden and unexpected death and therefore should not serve as a basis for therapeutic decisions. Intermittent ("event recordings") or continuous pneumogram recordings may be helpful in distinguishing artifactual from real monitor alarms in the hospital or at home.

MANAGEMENT

The issue of first concern for an ALTE infant is whether the baby's life is in immediate danger. If it is, appropriate supportive or resuscitative efforts are undertaken immediately. Second, one must decide whether it is likely that some abnormal event occurred or whether the observer's fright was an overreaction to a normal event. Unless one is quite certain that it was a normal event or unless there has been an interval of several days or weeks since the episode, the infant must be hospitalized for monitoring and evaluation. The goals of the hospitalization are (1) to watch for a repeat episode, (2) to look for direct or indirect signs of hypoxemia or hypoventilation, and (3) to identify treatable disease.

The two major categories of long-term intervention for ALTE infants are pharmacologic intervention and electronic home monitoring systems. If a specific disease process that is likely to respond to pharmacologic intervention is identified, appropriate drug therapy can be initiated (e.g., anticonvulsants for seizure disorders). Some centers advocate the use of methylxanthines as respiratory stimulants for some ALTE infants, but the merits of this practice are unproved.

The NIH Consensus Conference on Infantile Apnea and Home Monitoring addressed the issue of indications for home monitoring by identifying three groups of infants: one for whom it was inappropriate to use home monitors, one for whom it was inappropriate not to use home monitors, and one for whom decisions should be individualized through consultation between the family and the health care team. Infants for whom home monitoring is indicated include those who have experienced at least one severe ALTE perceived to require resuscitation, siblings of multiple SIDS victims, prematurely born infants whose apnea of prematurity persists when they are otherwise ready for hospital discharge, and infants with central hypoventilation syndrome. Home monitors should not be used for normal infants or for asymptomatic premature infants. Definite criteria cannot be provided for infants with less severe ALTE episodes, the subsequent siblings of one SIDS victim, or infants of drug-addicted mothers. In this intermediate risk group for whom specific guidelines are not possible, families should not be pressured to use home monitors against their wishes. Although not a specific recommendation of the consensus panel, two other categories that are widely monitored include infants with tracheostomies and infants requiring home oxygen therapy for bronchopulmonary dysplasia.

Combined cardiorespiratory impedance-type monitors are generally recommended. Those prescribing home monitors need to understand the reliability of the particular monitor types used and must provide a system for continuous, easy availability of technical and medical help for the families who are using these monitors in the home. Before the infant is discharged from the hospital, the parents and other key caretakers must be effectively taught about infant resuscitation, monitor use, and troubleshooting. A plan for duration of home monitoring and for regular follow-up by the health care team must be clearly established and conveyed to the family.

Although use of electronic home monitors makes

intuitive sense for many of these infants, there is only anecdotal evidence that they are effective in helping to save lives. There are multiple reported cases of infants dying despite the prescription of home monitors. Many of the monitors themselves are quite effective but the overall program of home monitoring is less so. In only approximately one third of the infants who have reportedly died despite the use of home monitors was the monitor use and response to monitor alarms apparently fully appropriate. This emphasizes the need for effective ongoing training of and communication with the parents.

Home monitoring should be continued until the infant has been free of significant episodes for at least 2 to 3 months and has successfully demonstrated the ability to tolerate stress such as an infection without real alarms. Decisions about monitor discontinuation cannot be based on pneumogram results. The potential adverse effects of home monitoring—false alarms, sleep disruption for the infant and the parents, and decreased mobility of the caretaking parent—must be presented to the family before a final decision about home monitoring is made.

It is appropriate to be quite optimistic about long-term prognosis to the families of most ALTE infants. The majority of infants do not experience recurrent severe ALTEs, and most appear to develop normally without any significant residual deficit.

ADDITIONAL READING

American Academy of Pediatrics Task Force on Prolonged Apnea. Prolonged infantile apnea: 1985. Pediatrics 76:129-131, 1985.

Davidson Ward SL, Keens TG, Chan LS, et al. Sudden infant death syndrome in infants evaluated by apnea programs in California. Pediatrics 77:451-455, 1986.

Guntheroth WG. Crib Death: The Sudden Infant Death Syndrome. Mt Kisco, N.Y.: Futura, 1982.

• Harper RM, Hoffman HJ, eds. Sudden Infant Death Syndrome: Risk Factors and Basic Mechanisms. New York: Pergamon, 1987.

Hoffman HJ, Hunter JC, Damus K, et al. Diphtheria-tetanus-pertussis immunization and sudden infant death: Results of the National Institute of Child Health and Human Development Cooperative Epidemiological Study of Sudden Infant Death Syndrome Risk Factors. Pediatrics 79:598-610, 1987.

• National Institutes of Health Consensus Development Conference on Infantile Apnea and Home Monitoring, Sept 29 to Oct 1, 1986: Consensus statement. Pediatrics 79:292-299, 1987.

Oren J, Kelly DH, Shannon DC. Identification of a high risk group for sudden infant death syndrome among infants who were resuscitated for sleep apnea. Pediatrics 77:495-499, 1986.

Peterson DR. Infant mortality among subsequent siblings of infants who died of sudden infant death syndrome. J Pediatr 108:911-914, 1986.

32 Croup

Nick G. Anas · Gary Goodman

BACKGROUND AND PHYSIOLOGY

Subglottic croup (laryngotracheobronchitis) is a fall and winter disease of viral etiology characterized by inspiratory stridor, hoarseness, and a barking or "seal-like" cough. Croup, a syndrome that begins gradually with a low-grade fever and upper respiratory infection and progresses to airway obstruction and respiratory distress, is most common in children aged 6 months to 3 years. Viral croup primarily involves the subglottis and trachea.

The propensity for symptomatic upper airway obstruction developing in young children is a function of several factors:

1. The viruses most commonly implicated (i.e., *parainfluenzae* 1, 2, 3; *influenzae* a, b; respiratory syncytial viruses) are capable of inducing inflammation, increased mucous production, and loss of ciliary activity all along the respiratory tract.
2. The diameter of the child's airway is small so that obstruction due to mucus and inflammation is greatly exaggerated; resistance to airflow is inversely related to the fourth power of the radius (Poiseuille's law).
3. The subglottis includes the complete, rigid ring of the cricoid cartilage; inflammation and swelling in this area can occur only at the expense of the internal airway diameter.
4. Dynamic collapse (i.e., upper airway narrowing during the inspiratory phase of the respiratory cycle) tends to occur more often in young children in whom the supporting cartilaginous structure of the trachea may be incompletely developed.
5. The infant and the young child are prone to respiratory muscle fatigue and failure from increased respiratory work (see Chapter 10).

Adverse physiologic effects occur as the result of the initial fever and upper airway obstruction associated with croup. Dehydration secondary to reduced intake and increased fluid losses (fever, insensible losses for increased respiratory work) is commonly documented. Demands for greater cardiac output are increased because of fever, hypermetabolism, and increased respiratory muscle output. Gas exchange is impaired by several mechanisms. Upper airway obstruction results in hypercapnia and in hypoxemia with a normal alveolar-arterial (A-a) oxygen difference (see Chapter 10). Upper airway obstruction is a cause of pulmonary edema; the mechanisms that explain this phenomenon are outlined in Fig. 33-2. The viruses responsible for upper airway disease may also involve the small airways, leading to atelectasis, gas trapping, or pneumonitis, and all of these processes interfere with normal ventilation-perfusion matching. If the respiratory muscles fatigue, hypoventilation or apnea and ultimately hypercapnia may ensue (Fig. 32-1).

Estimation of the degree of upper airway obstruction and resulting gas-exchange impairment determines management of the child with croup. This approach differs from the management of the child with epiglottitis in whom artificial airway support (i.e., nasotracheal intubation, tracheostomy) is always instituted. Table 32-1 compares the clinical presentations of the child with croup vs. the child with epiglottitis.

The severity and constancy of airway obstruction in the child with croup is best determined by observation at the bedside and by chest auscultation.

1. Respiratory rate and effort (i.e., use of accessory muscles of respiration) and color are the most important indicators of the adequacy of air exchange; a labored respiratory pattern or evidence of fatigue (e.g., paradoxical chest wall–abdominal motion, intermittent apnea) suggests respiratory failure. The intensity of stridor is not as helpful in gauging the degree of upper

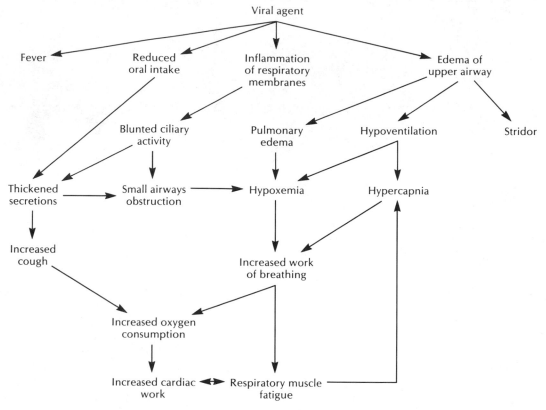

Fig. 32-1 Pathophysiology of croup leading to acute respiratory failure.

Table 32-1 Clinical Presentation: Croup and Epiglottitis

	Croup	Epiglottitis
Age	6 mo to 3 yr	1 to 5 yr
Seasonal occurrence	Fall/winter	None
Etiology	Parainfluenza viruses	*Haemophilus influenzae* type b
	Respiratory syncytial viruses	*Streptococcus*
	Influenza viruses	*Staphylococcus aureus*
Clinical findings		
Onset	Gradual after upper respiratory infection	Sudden
Fever	Variable	Marked
Voice	Hoarse	Muffled
Sore throat	Variable	Marked
Postural preference	None	Upright
Drooling	Absent	Present
Dysphagia	Variable	Present
Cough	Seal-like	Weak
Airway obstruction	Intermittent to constant	Constant
Laboratory findings		
Roentgenogram	Subglottic narrowing	Thumblike epiglottis
White blood cell count	Normal	Elevated
Blood culture	Negative	Positive

airway obstruction, although the absence of stridor along with evidence of excessive respiratory work indicates significant airflow obstruction.

2. Chest auscultation by an experienced practitioner is useful in determining the adequacy of air entry; because croup is a disease of varying airway obstruction, the same person must assess breath sounds to follow the course of the disease process.

3. The child's mental status is an important indicator of the adequacy of gas exchange. Anxiety is commonly seen in children with air hunger and associated hypoxemia (i.e., Pao_2 <50 mm Hg). Lethargy, obtundation, or coma may be seen with severe hypercapnia (i.e., $Paco_2$ >70 mm Hg).

Table 32-2 provides a clinical scoring system designed to quantitate the significance of upper airway obstruction in a child with croup; severity is determined by total points in all five categories.

The differential diagnosis of acute upper airway obstruction includes:

1. Croup
2. Epiglottitis
3. Bacterial tracheitis
4. Retropharyngeal/peritonsillar/cervical abscess
5. Foreign body inhalation
6. Trauma to larynx/trachea
7. Thermal and chemical burns
8. Angioneurotic edema
9. Cervical/mediastinal tumor
10. Postextubation swelling
11. Increased intracranial pressure
12. Narcotic or sedative overdose
13. Status epilepticus
14. Trauma to recurrent laryngeal nerve (accidental, postoperative)

Because each entity is managed in a different manner, proper diagnosis may be lifesaving. The diagnosis of subglottic croup (laryngotracheobronchitis) is made by eliciting the history and documenting the physical findings outlined in Table 32-1. Chest and lateral neck roentgenograms (Fig. 32-2) that demonstrate subglottic swelling but normal supraglottic structures confirm the diagnosis. A favorable response to either cool mist or nebulized racemic epinephrine (see "Treatment") is diagnostic although not pathognomonic for croup. Epiglottitis may be confused with croup in the very young infant (e.g., <18 months of

Table 32-2 Clinical Scoring System for Croup*

Clinical Finding	No. of Points
Color	
Normal	0
Dusky	1
Cyanotic in room air	2
Cyanotic in 40% oxygen	3
Air entry	
Normal	0
Mildly diminished	1
Moderately diminished	2
Severely diminished	3
Stridor	
None	0
Mild	1
Moderate	2
Severe	3
Intercostal or suprasternal retractions	
None	0
Mild	1
Moderate	2
Severe	3
Level of consciousness	
Normal	0
Agitated	1
Lethargic or obtunded	2
Mild disease	0-3
Moderate disease	4-8
Severe disease	9-14

*Modified from Taussig LM, Castro O, Beaudry PH, et al. Treatment of laryngotracheobronchitis (croup): Use of intermittent positive pressure breathing and racemic epinephrine. Am J Dis Child 129:790-793, 1975. Copyright 1975, American Medical Association.

age) since the severe sore throat, drooling, and toxicity typical of epiglottitis may not be obvious. Bacterial tracheitis generally is first seen as a *Staphylococcus aureus* superinfection of a primary viral upper airway process; the clinical findings often are consistent with either croup or epiglottitis, and therefore performing a laryngoscopy and obtaining a positive culture of tracheal secretions from the patient are necessary to confirm the diagnosis of bacterial tracheitis. Infections or malignant masses may develop suddenly, and careful physical and roentgenographic examinations are needed to rule them out. Disorders characterized by chronic stridor (e.g., congenital or acquired subglottic stenosis, laryngotracheomalacia, vascular rings) along with sudden deterioration of

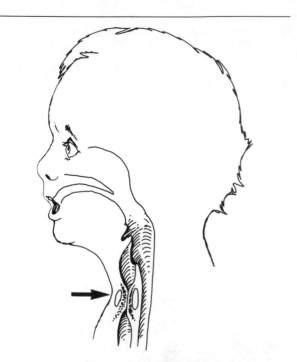

Fig. 32-2 Diagrammatic representation of lateral neck roentgenogram showing subglottic narrowing of croup (arrow).

upper airway function may be associated with an upper respiratory infection. Severe or intractable croup should suggest the presence of an underlying anatomic abnormality that predisposes to upper airway obstruction.

MONITORING AND LABORATORY TESTS

The goal in monitoring the child with croup is to assess the severity of airway obstruction and to follow the response to therapy. Every effort must be made to minimize agitation of the child; thus evaluation must be noninvasive as much as possible, and the parents must be allowed to remain with the child to provide comfort and security.

Once the diagnosis of croup is suspected, begin continuous observation of the child. Place equipment necessary for bag and mask ventilation, endotracheal intubation, tracheostomy, and cardiopulmonary resuscitation at the bedside. Contact the physician team previously assigned the responsibility of airway support in the acutely ill child (see Chapter 33 for the

protocol); these team members are to remain on standby call in the event that airway intervention is necessary.

Begin frequent assessment of the child using the clinical scoring system outlined in Table 32-2.

Begin continuous cardiac (ECG) and respiratory monitoring and continuous pulse oximetry if available. **Do not** obtain percutaneous arterial blood gas and pH samples routinely. The procedure is painful and likely to worsen the child's upper airway obstruction and will not provide any useful steady-state data. If the child's airway obstruction is judged severe and/or the decision for airway intervention is to be based on the results of arterial blood gas tension and pH analysis, an indwelling arterial catheter must be placed to obtain meaningful results.

Obtain chest and lateral neck roentgenograms to confirm the diagnosis of croup and to rule out other diagnostic considerations. Check the lung fields for the presence of atelectasis, pneumonitis, or pulmonary edema.

TREATMENT

The goals in the management of the child with croup are (1) to relieve the upper airway obstruction, (2) to treat hypoxemia, (3) to provide adequate hydration (in terms of previous losses and ongoing requirements), and (4) to determine the need for artificial airway support.

The first point of therapy is to give the child cool mist to breathe, which may be delivered either by face mask or within a transparent tent. Cool mist is effective in reducing upper airway swelling, presumably by inducing topical vasoconstriction. Care must be taken not to use mist to the extent that close observation of the child is not possible. The parents must remain at the bedside. Provide supplemental oxygen at a rate sufficient to maintain oxygen saturation (Sao_2) >90%.

Provide intravenous hydration with D_5 0.25% sodium chloride solution at a rate 1¼ to 1½ times maintenance requirements to compensate for insensible losses because of increased respiratory work, although these losses may be minimized by breathing the humidified cool mist. Do not allow the patient to drink or eat if the respiratory work is excessive or if the likelihood of using artificial airway support is high.

Control fever (temperature >38.4° C) with rectal antipyretics (e.g., acetaminophen at 10 mg/kg every

Table 32-3 Dose of Racemic Epinephrine
for Aerosol Administration

Weight (kg)	Dose (ml in 2 ml normal saline solution [0.9% sodium chloride solution])
20	0.25
20-40	0.50
>40 kg	0.75

4 hours). Neither antibiotics nor steroids are indicated for uncomplicated croup. The efficacy of antiviral agents (e.g., ribavirin) in the management of croup is unproved.

Administer nebulized racemic epinephrine (2.25%) for symptomatic upper airway obstruction (e.g., stridor, retractions, cyanosis). Raccmic epinephrine is effective in reducing edema by inducing local vasoconstriction. Most children prefer delivery by a nebulizer rather than by positive pressure (e.g., intermittent positive pressure breathing). Racemic epinephrine may be given safely every 2 to 4 hours; it may be given more often if its effectiveness continues and if the severity of the airway obstruction warrants this frequency. However, if racemic epinephrine must be administered more often than every 15 minutes, airway support is indicated as a rule. Table 32-3 gives the dosage recommendations for racemic epinephrine based on body weight.

Indications for airway support are based on the findings that gas exchange is significantly impaired and/or that the upper airway obstruction has not been relieved by the standard therapy outlined previously. The specific indications for airway support are outlined above.

Which type of artificial airway to use for the child with croup is a controversial topic. Unlike the management of epiglottitis, it has not been proved that nasotracheal intubation is safe for the management of croup. That is, it may be that a nasotracheal tube is a cause of further inflammation and edema formation at the level of the cricoid cartilage. Furthermore, the subglottic swelling may be of sufficient severity that an endotracheal tube large enough to provide adequate ventilation and pulmonary function cannot be placed. For these reasons many physicians prefer tracheotomy to nasotracheal intubation in children with croup. In either event the protocol for

---

TREATMENT OF THE CHILD WITH CROUP

Continuous close observation and noninvasive monitoring

Minimal agitation; parents at bedside

Cool mist by face mask or within tent

Supplemental oxygen sufficient to maintain oxygen saturation >90%

Racemic epinephrine (2.25%) by aerosol delivery system

No need for antibiotics or steroids routinely

Airway support for:

    Marked progressive anxiety or air hunger

    Hypoxemia (Pao_2 <50 mm Hg) despite supplemental oxygen at 50%

    Hypercapnia ($Paco_2$ >55 mm Hg)

    Requirement for frequent racemic epinephrine treatments (e.g., every 15 minutes)

    Clinical evidence of respiratory muscle fatigue

    Positive end-expiratory pressure

---

airway support and PICU management is outlined in Chapter 33. It includes the use of inhalation agents for induction of anesthesia in the operating room and sedation and restraint of the child in the PICU.

If the child has developed pulmonary edema as the result of upper airway obstruction and needs endotracheal intubation or tracheotomy, positive end-expiratory pressure may be used if the oxygen requirement exceeds 50%.

Administering helium-oxygen (80%/20%) mixtures to a patient with upper airway obstruction may provide temporary relief, particularly while he is prepared for nasotracheal intubation or tracheotomy. A helium-oxygen mixture improves gas flow in the upper airway because it is a less dense gas mixture than room air and results in reduced airflow turbulence.

Unlike epiglottitis, the subglottis cannot be visualized before extubation; therefore the decision to extubate the child is based on clinical findings of reduced swelling and the ability to maintain an adequate spontaneous minute ventilation. A change in the pressure at which an air leak is occurring will indicate reduced subglottic swelling (e.g., if a leak was first noted when 25 cm H_2O positive pressure was applied and now is noted at 20 cm H_2O). As a rule the endotracheal tube is removed as soon as possible. Administration of dexamethasone (Decadron) at 0.1 to 0.2 mg/kg for four doses may reduce edema that has occurred as the result of intubation of the airway, although this has not yet been shown effective in a prospective randomized trial. After extubation, fiberoptic bronchoscopy may be useful in providing more direct information about the structure and function of the upper airway, particularly at the level of the cricoid cartilage.

ADDITIONAL READING

Davis HW, Gartner JC, Galvis AG, et al. Acute upper airway obstruction: Croup and epiglottitis. Pediatr Clin North Am 28:859-979, 1981.

Denny FW, Murphy JF, Clyde WA, et al. Croup: An 11-year study in pediatric practice. Pediatrics 71:871-876, 1983.

Duncan PG. Efficacy of helium-oxygen mixtures in the management of severe viral and post-intubation croup. Can Anaesth Soc J 26:206-208, 1979.

Jones R, Santos J, Overall J. Bacterial tracheitis. JAMA 242:721-726, 1979.

• Newth CJL, Levinson H, Bryan AC. The respiratory status of children with croup. J Pediatr 81:1068-1072, 1975.

• Taussig LM, Castro O, Beaudry PH, et al. Treatment of laryngotracheobronchitis (croup): Use of intermittent positive pressure breathing and racemic epinephrine. Am J Dis Child 129:790-793, 1975.

• Tunnessen WW, Feinstein AR. The steroid-croup controversy: An analytic review of methodologic problems. J Pediatr 96:751-756, 1980.

Westley CR, Cotton EK, Brooks JE. Nebulized racemic epinephrine by IPPB for the treatment of croup. Am J Dis Child 132:484-487, 1978.

33   Epiglottitis

Gary Goodman · Nick G. Anas · Jane D. Siegel

BACKGROUND AND PHYSIOLOGY

Epiglottitis is an infectious disease of the supraglottic airway that is seen after a short prodrome (6 to 10 hours) of high fever (≥39° C) and sore throat and usually progresses to symptomatic upper airway obstruction. Children aged 2 to 7 years are affected most commonly, although infants less than 1 year of age represent 10% to 20% of the population in some studies. Rarely older children or adults have epiglottitis. All physicians and medical facilities responsible for the management of acutely ill children must have a protocol designed to confirm the diagnosis rapidly and safely and to achieve airway support in children with epiglottitis as well as other life-threatening disorders such as croup, foreign body aspiration, angioneurotic edema, and tracheal injury. Failure to do so will result in unnecessary morbidity and mortality.

Epiglottitis is an inflammatory reaction of the epiglottis and supraglottic soft tissues, including the aryepiglottic folds and arytenoids (Fig. 33-1). *Haemophilus influenzae* type b is by far the most common etiologic agent, accounting for approximately 75% of cases. Even though the patient has received the *H. influenzae* b (Hib) vaccine, the diagnosis of epiglottitis is not precluded since the vaccine does not provide 100% protection. Sporadic cases may be associated with *Staphylococcus aureus* and *H. parainfluenzae*. These organisms reach the supraglottic structures either by direct extension from the nasopharynx or as a result of bacteremia. Inspection of the larynx demonstrates a swollen, cherry-red epiglottis; the vocal cords and subglottis are spared. The severity of airway obstruction is a function of many factors, including the degree of enlargement of these supraglottic structures relative to the diameter of the glottic opening, the propensity for vocal cord spasm (laryngospasm) to occur as a result of the aspiration of oropharyngeal secretions, and the extent of dynamic airway collapse secondary to vigorous breathing by an anxious child.

Although 50% to 90% of all children with epiglottitis will have positive blood cultures for *H. influenzae* type b, it is unusual to document secondary sites of infection. Pneumonia, cervical adenitis, suppurative arthritis, and meningitis have been reported; meningitis occurs in <1% of cases.

The diagnosis of epiglottitis must be made within minutes of obtaining the history and observing the child. Important diagnoses to exclude that are also initially seen with acute respiratory distress are foreign body inhalation, spasmodic croup, and angioneurotic edema (see Chapter 32, p. 269). Epiglottitis is heralded by sudden onset of fever and followed by signs of difficulty in swallowing, vocalizing, and breathing. The child complains of a severe sore throat, and the parents report drooling, a muffled voice, and a labored respiratory effort. Hoarseness, cough, and inspiratory stridor are uncommon, being more characteristic of laryngotracheobronchitis or subglottic croup (see Chapter 32, Table 32-1). Examination generally reveals an apprehensive, toxic-appearing child who assumes a sitting position with head forward, neck extended, and mouth open, a position often referred to as "tripoding" or "flower-sniffing." The face appears pale or ashen gray. The severity of airway obstruction is determined most accurately by observation for the level of consciousness, color, respiratory rate and effort (including use of accessory muscles of respiration), the presence of audible breath sounds, and the quality of the voice. Cyanosis and/or a depressed level of consciousness are late signs indicating severe hypoxia. Respiratory compromise may be aggravated by disturbing the child, particularly by examining the pharynx or placing him in a supine position.

The most significant, although uncommon, complication of acute upper airway obstruction is pul-

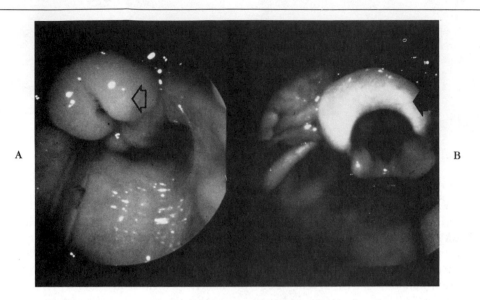

Fig. 33-1   A, Swollen epiglottis (open arrow). **B,** Diminished swelling 72 hours later (solid arrow). (Courtesy Max Klein, M.D.)

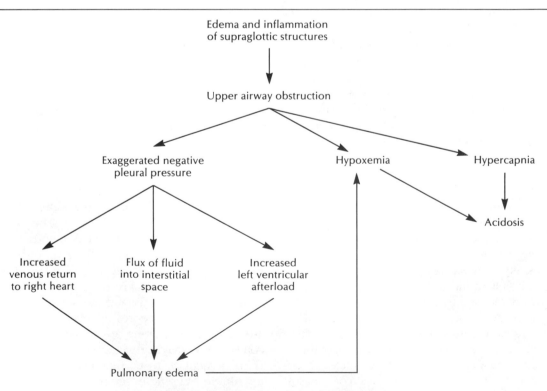

Fig. 33-2   Pathophysiology of epiglottitis.

monary edema resulting in hypoxemia. It most typically occurs after relief of the obstruction. The mechanisms responsible for pulmonary edema in this circumstance include (1) increased left ventricular afterload and elevated end-diastolic and pulmonary venous blood pressures, (2) increased negative pleural pressure favoring the flux of fluid from the capillary bed into the pulmonary interstitium, (3) damage to the alveolar-capillary membrane, leading to permeability pulmonary edema (adult respiratory distress syndrome), and (4) increased hydrostatic pressure in the pulmonary arterial vasculature, resulting from augmented peripheral venous return to the central circulation (Fig. 33-2).

MONITORING AND LABORATORY TESTS

Once the diagnosis of epiglottitis is suspected, the child must never be left unattended until the airway is secured. If the initial evaluation was in the physician's office or in an outlying emergency department, the child must be accompanied by the physician during transport to the referral facility or the physician must remain in attendance until the critical care transport team has arrived.

The importance of minimizing disturbance and avoiding attempts at visualization of the epiglottis in the absence of the intubation team cannot be overemphasized. The child must be maintained in the sitting position, preferably with the parents at the bedside. Do not place the patient supine until ready to intubate him. Inhalation induction is performed with the patient sitting up.

The medical personnel designated to secure the airway in children with life-threatening disorders such as epiglottitis must be notified even if the diagnosis is uncertain. The responsible persons vary depending on the institution but must include a physician skilled in endotracheal intubation and a physician able to perform emergency tracheostomy or cricothyrotomy. The operating room and/or the PICU must be notified that a child with suspected epiglottitis will be arriving.

Equipment and medications necessary for bag and mask ventilation, intubation, tracheostomy, and cardiopulmonary resuscitation, including oxygen and suction, must be immediately available at the patient's bedside. The use of bag and face mask ventilation can be effective in patients with epiglottitis; therefore, when necessary, ventilation usually can be maintained by this technique until the patient reaches the operating room or PICU.

Continuous ECG and respiratory monitoring must be instituted, as must pulse oximetry if available. The child's respiratory rate and effort, color, and level of consciousness must be ascertained without agitating the child. Arterial or venous blood samples are delayed until the airway is secured. An IV catheter can be placed at the time of anesthesia for endotracheal intubation.

If the child is clinically stable and the diagnosis is uncertain, a lateral roentgenogram of soft tissues of the neck will confirm the diagnosis of epiglottitis; a thickened epiglottic shadow that resembles an adult thumb in size and shape is pathognomonic of this condition (Fig. 33-3).

TREATMENT

All children with epiglottitis and evidence of airway obstruction must have an artificial airway securely placed. Rarely epiglottitis is confirmed and yet the child's respiration is not compromised; in such a case the child can be managed without immediate airway intervention, but provision must be made for continuous observation in the PICU and for immediate intubation or tracheostomy should evidence of obstruction appear.

Examination of the epiglottis must be performed when airway intervention is established. Until then the child must remain in a sitting position while being given oxygen at 1 to 2 L/min or at a rate sufficient to maintain oxygen saturation (Sao_2) >90%. If the child is agitated by the oxygen face mask or nasal cannula, it is preferable to have a parent hold the apparatus as close to the child as possible. Racemic epinephrine (2.25%) can be administered by nebulizer (0.2 ml in 2 ml 0.9% sodium chloride solution) to provide temporary improvement in airway obstruction; however, this will probably not be helpful if the child is struggling. If complete airway obstruction ensues before intubation, the prompt use of bag ventilation and tightly applied face mask ventilation with good head and jaw positioning is necessary. Steroids are not beneficial.

The type of airway support chosen depends on the personnel available to the institution. Orotracheal intubation followed by elective replacement of the tube nasally is safe and effective when performed by an experienced practitioner; tracheostomy is an ac-

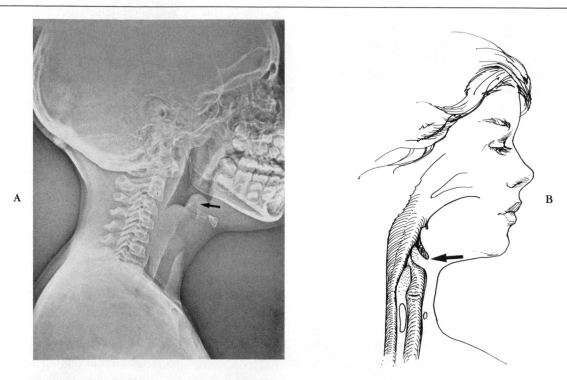

Fig. 33-3 **A,** A lateral neck xeroradiograph of patient with epiglottitis. Arrow indicates "thumblike" appearance of swollen epiglottis. **B,** Diagrammatic representation of lateral neck roentgenogram showing swollen, thumblike epiglottis (arrow).

ceptable alternative, but it has the added possible complications of bleeding, pneumomediastinum, pneumothorax, and scar formation. Because the duration of intubation is short (generally 48 hours) and because performing a tracheostomy is technically more difficult in young children, most protocols recommend endotracheal intubation as the mode of airway support in children with epiglottitis.

Once epiglottitis is confirmed by laryngoscopy, intubation should be performed with the patient under general anesthesia. Induction is instituted with the patient in a sitting position using an inhalation agent (e.g., halothane), helium if available, and oxygen. Another approach is endotracheal intubation over a flexible fiberoptic bronchoscope; this mode may be the least well tolerated by the child since the device must be passed through the nose while the patient is awake. Although use of paralytic agents to

facilitate intubation is recommended by some authors, it is a potentially dangerous practice. Patients with an obstructed airway must not be paralyzed unless the operator is absolutely certain he can provide ventilation before successful intubation. Failure to do so may cause the patient to go into arrest and suffer hypoxic injury or death. In addition, even if ventilation can be provided before intubation, the only clue to the location of the glottic opening in a patient with severely distorted anatomy may be some air bubbling seen at the time of laryngoscopy (see Chapter 127). Regardless of the method chosen for endotracheal intubation, a physician skilled in rigid bronchoscopy and tracheostomy must be in attendance should the endotracheal intubation attempt fail. The trachea initially should be intubated by the oral route using an endotracheal tube one size smaller than recommended for that age patient to allow for airway narrowing caused by edema and to allow breathing around the endotracheal tube. Once the oral tube is secured and the patient is adequately oxygenated (approximately 2 minutes of hand ventilation with oxygen), a nasotracheal tube can be placed before transport to the PICU. The tube must be checked for a leak at <20 cm H_2O inflating pressure and the chest auscultated for breath sounds.

After the airway is secured, all blood samples (including cultures) may be obtained and IV catheters placed. Tracheal secretions and the epiglottis must be cultured. If meningitis is suspected clinically when the patient is assessed following intubation, a lumbar puncture must be performed and CSF obtained for culture, Gram's stain, cell count, glucose, protein, and *H. influenzae* type b antigen detection by latex particle agglutination test. *H. influenzae* type b antigen may be detected in the urine of patients with uncomplicated epiglottitis. Antibiotics appropriate to treat *H. influenzae* type b, *Streptococcus pneumoniae*, group A *Streptococcus*, and *S. aureus* must be administered parenterally (Table 33-1). Cefuroxime is preferred in the absence of meningitis because of its activity against staphylococci, streptococci, and β-lactamase–producing *Haemophilus* sepsis. Chloramphenicol may not be suitable in geographic areas

where strains of *Haemophilus* sp resistant to chloramphenicol have been isolated. A chest roentgenogram must be obtained to confirm abnormalities. The patient needs to be in respiratory isolation for 24 hours after initiation of effective therapy.

Artificial airway support will be needed for 48 hours in most cases. Care in the PICU is directed at preventing inadvertent extubation; sedation (see Chapter 129) and No-No arm restraints will help to control the child, who usually feels tired, but much better after intubation. Usually the patient will sleep quietly for a few hours. Neuromuscular paralysis and assisted ventilation usually are not necessary if adequate sedation of the child is achieved. Maintaining patency of the endotracheal tube and optimizing pulmonary function are important; humidified gas must be administered by face mask or blow-by connector through the endotracheal tube until the time of extubation. Chest percussion therapy and suctioning three or four times a day may limit or prevent atelectasis. Continuous positive airway pressure, used as a method for optimizing end-expiratory lung volume, may be instituted to treat pulmonary edema. Rarely diuretics will be necessary to decrease interstitial or alveolar water. Continuous oximetry or intermittent arterial blood gas tension analysis must be done to

Table 33-1 Antimicrobial Agents Recommended for Treatment of Epiglottitis

Agent	Dosage (mg/kg/day)	Interval
*Parenteral**		
Cefuroxime†	150	q8h
Ceftriaxone	80	q12h x 2, then q24h
Cefotaxime	200	q4h
Chloramphenicol†	75	q6h
Oral‡		
Amoxicillin	50	q8h
Amoxicillin plus clavulanate potassium (Augmentin)	50 (amoxicillin component)	q8h
Cefaclor	80	q8h
Penicillin§	100	q6h
Cephalexin‖	50	q6h

*Only cefuroxime is active against *Staphylococcus aureus*; if *S. aureus* is suspected, nafcillin, 150 mg/kg/day q6h, should be added to agents other than cefuroxime.

†Dosages are increased in the presence of meningitis—cefuroxime, 300 mg/kg/day; chloramphenicol, 100 mg/kg/day.

‡Choice of agent is guided by identification and susceptibility of pathogen; if pathogen is unknown, cefaclor or Augmentin is preferred.

§Effective against streptococci only.

‖Effective against streptococci and staphylococci only.

ensure adequate oxygenation (i.e., Sao_2 >90%); if necessary, supplemental oxygen can be administered to maintain this minimum level.

Supportive care includes the use of IV fluids (D_5 0.25% sodium chloride solution) at a maintenance rate until the patient can swallow clear liquids. Antipyretics (e.g., acetaminophen suppository at 10 mg/kg) can be used to maintain normal body temperature.

Most children with epiglottitis can be extubated within 48 hours of the institution of airway support and antibiotic therapy. The criteria for extubation include (1) resolution of fever and other signs of sepsis and (2) evidence of a reduction of epiglottic swelling, as indicated by the presence of an air leak around the endotracheal tube and confirmed by direct visualization of the epiglottis using either a laryngoscope or bronchoscope. An appropriate short acting agent should be used to sedate the patient for this procedure.

After extubation the child must receive nothing by mouth and needs to remain in the PICU for 8 to 24 hours to be certain that reintubation will not be necessary. Postextubation sequelae such as stridor or a

---

PROTOCOL FOR MANAGEMENT OF EPIGLOTTITIS

I. *Once the diagnosis of epiglottitis is suspected,* the following steps are to be followed without exception:
   A. Begin continuous observation of the patient. Allow the parents to remain with the patient. Do not place the child in a supine position.
   B. Contact the team designated to secure the airway—anesthesiologist, intensivist, otolaryngologist.
   C. Place equipment for bag/face mask ventilation, intubation, oxygen, suction, tracheostomy, and cardiopulmonary resuscitation at bedside.
   D. Do not agitate the child with noxious procedures such as oral examination, blood drawing, or IV catheter placement.
   E. Begin continuous ECG, respiratory, and pulse oximetry monitoring.
   F. Obtain lateral neck roentgenogram only if the child is stable and the diagnosis is uncertain. A physician capable of intubation must accompany the child to the radiology department.
   G. Administer oxygen at 1 to 2 L/min or at a rate sufficient to maintain oxygen saturation >90% by pulse oximetry.
   H. Consider administering nebulized racemic epinephrine (2.25%) at 0.2 ml in 2 ml 0.9% sodium chloride solution for worsening airway obstruction.
   I. If *complete* airway obstruction occurs before the arrival of the airway team, begin assisted ventilation with bag and face mask.

II. *Once the airway team has arrived,* perform the following:
   A. Transport the child to the operating room or PICU.
   B. Ask the otolaryngologist to be prepared for fiberoptic examination, rigid bronchoscopy, or tracheostomy and to remain in the room.
   C. Induce anesthesia with the patient in a sitting position using an inhalation agent and oxygen. Confirm the diagnosis of epiglottitis. Intubate the child through the oral route with an endotracheal tube one size smaller than recommended for that age patient.
   D. Hyperoxygenate the child for 2 minutes. Replace the oral endotracheal tube with a nasotracheal tube.
   E. Obtain a chest roentgenogram to ensure proper placement of the endotracheal tube and to evaluate for pulmonary abnormalities.
   F. Place an IV catheter; obtain blood and pharyngeal cultures.
   G. Begin antibiotic therapy.
   H. Transfer to the PICU after administering a sedative (e.g., midazolam) and placing arm restraints.

crouplike cough may be treated with either cool mist or nebulized racemic epinephrine.

The duration of antibiotic treatment for uncomplicated epiglottitis is 5 to 7 days. Treatment duration is prolonged in the presence of infection at another site. Once the repeat blood cultures taken at 24 to 48 hours are sterile, the patient's fever has subsided, and he has been extubated and is tolerating oral fluids, oral antibiotics may be used to complete the course of therapy (Table 33-1). When *H. influenzae* type b is confirmed as the etiologic agent and there is a household contact less than 4 years of age, a 4-day course of prophylactic rifampin should be administered to all household members as soon as possible as recommended by the Academy of Pediatrics, regardless of immunization status of the one at risk.

ADDITIONAL READING

• Battaglia JD, Lockhart CH. Management of acute epiglottitis by nasotracheal intubation. Am J Dis Child 129:334-336, 1975.

• Blackshock D, Adderley RJ, Stewart DJ. Epiglottitis in young infants. Anesthesiology 67:97-100, 1987.

Butt W, Shann F, Walker C, et al. Acute epiglottitis: A different approach to management. Crit Care Med 16:43-47, 1988.

Glicklich M, Cohen RD, Jona JZ. Steroids and bag and mask ventilation in the treatment of acute epiglottitis. J Pediatr Surg 14:247-251, 1979.

Kanter RK, Watchdo JF. Pulmonary edema associated with upper airway obstruction. Am J Dis Child 138:356-359, 1984.

Kimmons HC, Peterson BM. Management of acute epiglottitis in pediatric patients. Crit Care Med 14:278-279, 1986.

Kinnefors A, Olofsson J. Acute epiglottitis in children: Experiences with tracheostomy and intubation. Clin Otolaryngol 8:25-29, 1983.

• Lewis JK, Gardner JC, Galvis AG, et al. A protocol for management of acute epiglottitis. Clin Pediatr 17:494-498, 1978.

Report of the Committee on Infectious Diseases, 21st ed. Chicago: American Academy of Pediatrics, 1988, p 208.

Travis KW, Todres ID, Shannon DC. Pulmonary edema associated with croup and epiglottitis. Pediatrics 59:695-698, 1977.

Vernon DD, Sarnaik AP. Acute epiglottitis in children: A conservative approach to diagnosis and management. Crit Care Med 14:23-27, 1986.

34 Acute Severe Asthma

Paul Lubinsky · Nick G. Anas · Stan L. Davis

BACKGROUND AND PHYSIOLOGY

Asthma, the most common chronic disease of childhood, affects 5% to 10% of children and results in approximately 400,000 hospital admissions and 4000 deaths a year in the United States. Asthma is defined as airways obstruction that reverses with time or treatment. Acute severe asthma is a disorder in which intensive therapy by skilled nurses, respiratory therapists, and physicians is needed. Acute severe asthma (also known as status asthmaticus) is an episode of airways obstruction that does not reverse after three bronchodilator treatments (subcutaneous epinephrine or aerosolized β-sympathomimetic agent) and further inpatient therapy is necessary. Not all children with asthma wheeze; some may present with cough, dyspnea, or emesis. Alternatively wheezing may be a sign of a variety of diseases.

The pathophysiologic triad of asthma comprises bronchial smooth muscle contraction, inflammation and edema of the bronchial mucosa, and production and retention of tenacious secretions. These factors produce increased airways resistance and prolongation of time constants (see Chapters 125 and 128), resulting in (1) decreased expiratory volume and flow rates and (2) premature closure of the airways, leading to air trapping in some regions and atelectasis in others. The reduction in ventilation-perfusion ($\dot{V}/\dot{Q}$) matching results in hypoxemia (Pao_2 <50 mm Hg). Hypoxemia stimulates respiratory drive, and the patient may present with hypocapnic alkalosis ($Paco_2$ <35 mm Hg) (see Chapter 10). As the degree of airway obstruction increases, hyperinflation and decreased lung compliance ensue, resulting in excessive work of breathing and impaired function of the respiratory muscles. Fatigue occurs, minute ventilation is reduced, and hypercapnic acidosis ($Paco_2$ >55 mm Hg) develops. Fig. 34-1 outlines the pathophysiology of acute severe asthma.

DIFFERENTIAL DIAGNOSIS OF WHEEZING

Asthma
Foreign body inhalation
Epiglottitis
Tracheitis
Laryngotracheomalacia
Bronchiolitis
Bronchopulmonary dysplasia
Pertussis
Inhalation pneumonia
Kussmaul's respirations
Cystic fibrosis
Anomalies of great vessels
Pulmonary arterial hypertension
Pulmonary edema

The severity of acute severe asthma in infants and young children is related to a number of anatomic and physiologic features, including smaller airways in which a reduction in radius has a greater effect on airways resistance since resistance is inversely related to the fourth power of the radius; limited elastic lung recoil, resulting in early airway closure; deficient collateral channels of ventilation, promoting atelectasis; an unstable rib cage, which limits the generation of tidal volume; and the propensity for respiratory muscles to fatigue (see Chapter 10).

MONITORING AND LABORATORY TESTS

The goals of monitoring are (1) to ascertain the cause, course, and outcome of previous episodes of acute severe asthma in the child, (2) to assess the severity of airways obstruction and gas exchange impairment,

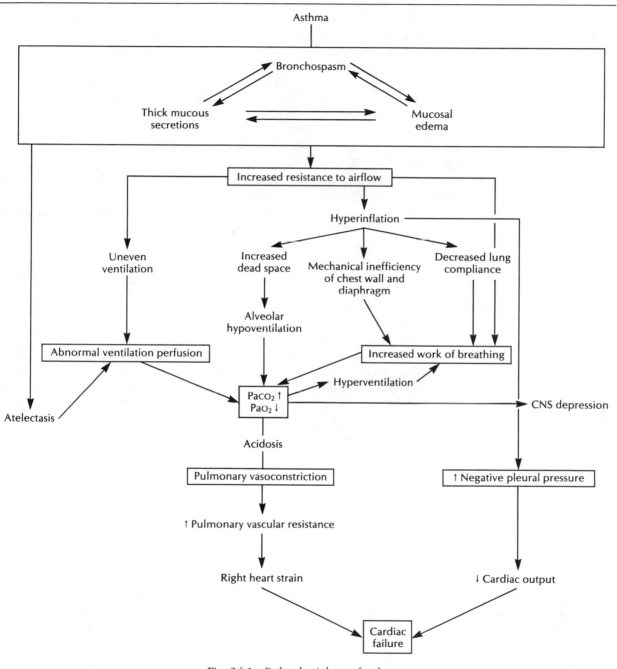

Fig. 34-1   Pathophysiology of asthma.

and (3) to follow the patient's neurologic and hemodynamic status.

Obtain historical information pertinent to the immediate management of the patient. Important factors include maintenance medications and compliance and the outcome of previous episodes of acute severe asthma, including frequency, duration, and use of continuous IV infusion, steroids, or assisted ventilation.

Document the severity of the attack by physical examination and laboratory investigation. Begin continuous respiratory and ECG monitoring. In addition to respiratory rate the degree of respiratory effort is an important indication of the severity of airways obstruction. Tachypnea, grunting respirations, and the use of the accessory muscles of respiration (i.e., intercostal, abdominal, and supraclavicular muscles) are signs of increased work of breathing. Alternating use of the diaphragm and the intercostal muscles, paradoxical movement of the diaphragm on inspiration, and intermittent apnea are signs of respiratory muscle fatigue. Restlessness, agitation, and confusion are nonspecific but important signs of hypoxemia, whereas lethargy or obtundation suggests hypercapnia. Cyanosis indicates severe gas exchange impairment.

Perform frequent assessment of air exchange by chest auscultation. To most effectively follow the course of the disease the same person should examine the patient during the acute phase. Wheezing signifies obstruction to airflow; prolongation of the expiratory phase of the respiratory cycle (e.g., >3 seconds) occurs with physiologically significant obstruction. Decreased breath sounds or the absence of wheezing in the presence of a labored respiratory effort indicates severe disease. Asymmetry of breath sounds suggests atelectasis, tension pneumothorax, or the presence of a foreign body.

Determine the hemodynamic status of the patient. Severe airways obstruction impairs cardiac output because of the development of very large negative intrapleural pressures during inspiration (e.g., < -100 mm Hg), which increases systemic afterload (i.e., left ventricular wall tension at end-systole). At the bedside this effect is best evaluated by the measurement of pulsus paradoxus. A reduction in systemic systolic arterial blood pressure of >15 mm Hg during inspiration (i.e., when intrapleural pressure is negative) is abnormal. Pulsus paradoxus >20 mm Hg correlates well with the presence of severe airways obstruction (i.e., forced expiratory volume in 1 second [FEV_1] <60% predicted).

Assess the state of hydration and monitor urinary output. These children may be dehydrated because of events before hospitalization, such as decreased oral intake, increased insensible losses, and the diuretic effect of theophylline.

Determine the adequacy of gas exchange. Obtain arterial blood gas and pH values at the time of admission to assess alveolar ventilation. Alveolar ventilation is inversely proportional to the arterial CO_2 tension (i.e., $Paco_2$). A capillary blood gas (CBG) analysis is an acceptable alternative, may be less traumatic to the frightened child, and requires less technical expertise. An arteriolized CBG sample is obtained by prewarming an extremity to produce vasodilation (usually accomplished by wrapping the hand or foot in a diaper or cloth warmed with warm water) and then puncturing the skin of a digit or the heel in infants with a lancet to produce free-flowing drops of blood. The sample is collected in a heparinized capillary tube for analysis. The pH and Pco_2 of samples obtained in this manner closely approximate those of arterial samples, whereas the O_2 tension value (i.e., Po_2) does not. Assess systemic oxygenation via continuous pulse oximetry if available or obtain arterial blood gas samples to measure the Pao_2. In most instances pulse oximetry provides the most useful data since it continuously monitors O_2 saturation during therapeutic maneuvers. Place an indwelling arterial catheter for monitoring of arterial blood gases in the following situations: (1) pulse oximetry is unavailable, (2) respiratory failure has been documented, (3) the patient is treated with a continuous IV infusion of isoproterenol, or (4) the patient is placed on mechanical ventilation. See Chapter 10 for a more detailed discussion of arterial blood gas and pH interpretation.

Obtain a chest roentgenogram to assess the degree of hyperinflation and mucous plugging. Check for the presence of pneumonia, pneumothorax or pneumomediastinum, cardiomegaly, pulmonary edema, or findings consistent with foreign body inhalation (see Chapter 93).

Do not perform forced expiratory pulmonary function tests in children with acute severe asthma. The results are not reproducible, and the maneuver may aggravate bronchospasm.

Check the serum theophylline level if a patient previously has been taking theophylline preparations. Obtain a complete and differential blood count and serum electrolyte and glucose values. Clinical and laboratory findings useful in determining the severity of an episode of acute severe asthma are as follows:

History of previous hospitalizations
Recurrent episodes in a 24-hour period
Tachycardia (heart rate >120 bpm)
Tachypnea (respiratory rate >30/min)
Pulsus paradoxus >15 mm Hg (spontaneous breathing)
Diaphoresis
Agitation progressing to lethargy and coma
Use of accessory respiratory muscles (e.g., sternocleidomastoid and scalene)
Cyanosis
Wheezing throughout the expiratory phase of the respiratory cycle
Decreased inspiratory breath sounds
Metabolic or respiratory acidosis (pH <7.30)
$Paco_2$ >45 mm Hg
Pao_2 <70 mm Hg
Pneumothorax
Pneumomediastinum
Associated pneumonia

TREATMENT

The goals of therapy are to correct hypoxemia, assure adequate alveolar ventilation, and reverse airways obstruction. The initial management with oxygen, β-sympathomimetic agents, and aminophylline will usually have been initiated before arrival in the PICU and must not be interrupted.

General Measures
Oxygen

Patients with acute severe asthma always are hypoxemic because of $\dot{V}/\dot{Q}$ imbalance. Furthermore, therapy with β-sympathomimetic agents and methylxanthines produces pulmonary vasodilation and increased cardiac output, further aggravating the $\dot{V}/\dot{Q}$ mismatch. Administer O_2 to all patients with acute severe asthma at a concentration sufficient to maintain Sao_2 >90% or Pao_2 >70 mm Hg. Initiate O_2 administration at a rate of 2 L/min by nasal cannula or at a concentration of 40% O_2 by face mask. Some patients may need a higher O_2 concentration, which can be achieved using various masks (see Chapter

126). Mist tents are not recommended since the mist may aggravate bronchospasm and impair close observation of the patient. Continue administering O_2 until the patient is well enough to receive oral bronchodilator therapy and the Sao_2 value exceeds 90% in room air.

Fluids

Begin fluid therapy to maintain hydration and replace fluid deficits that occur because of reduced intake and increased insensible losses. A total daily fluid intake of 1800 to 2000 ml/m²/day (120 ml/kg/day if <10 kg body weight) generally is adequate using a maintenance IV solution of D_5 0.45% sodium chloride with 30 mEq/L potassium chloride. The maintenance IV rate must be adjusted to allow other infusions and oral intake. The value of using overhydration to enhance mobilization of secretions is not scientifically proved and may lead to pulmonary edema formation.

Percussion, vibration, and postural drainage

Percussion, vibration, and postural drainage are important measures designed to mobilize secretions and to minimize the development of mucous plugging. They must be carried out in a way that will not create further stress for the child and at a frequency of every 3 or 4 hours (i.e., the child needs to be informed and the parents permitted to remain in attendance during the therapy).

Pharmacologic sedation

Sedatives may be useful in an extremely agitated child. However, sedative use is contraindicated unless the adequacy of oxygenation and ventilation can be constantly assessed. Chloral hydrate at 30 to 50 mg/kg per rectum every 4 to 6 hours as needed is a sedative that affects respiratory drive minimally.

Specific Therapy

The aim of drug therapy is to promote bronchodilation by increasing cyclic AMP, the active metabolite responsible for bronchial smooth muscle relaxation. This is achieved by stimulating synthesis of cyclic AMP with β-sympathomimetic agents (e.g., isoproterenol, albuterol) or by blocking its degradation by phosphodiesterases with methylxanthines (e.g., theophylline). In addition the bronchoconstrictor effect of cyclic guanosine monophosphate can be blocked using anticholinergic agents (e.g., atropine). Steroids have an anti-inflammatory effect due to modulation of synthesis, release, and activity of lipid mediators of inflammation. Steroids also increase the sensitivity and number of β-receptors, thereby decreasing the tachyphylaxis that develops in response to β-sympathomimetic agents.

Nebulized bronchodilators

Begin aerosol nebulization of β-sympathomimetic drugs since they are safely and effectively administered with minimal patient cooperation. In addition to promoting bronchodilation these agents improve mucociliary clearance. They must not be administered by positive pressure to avoid the risk of pneumothorax or pneumomediastinum. For patients with acute severe asthma β-sympathomimetic agents to be administered by aerosol include isoproterenol (0.5%) at 0.01 ml/kg, albuterol (0.5%) at 0.01 ml/kg, or metaproterenol (5%) at 0.01 ml/kg. All must be diluted in 2 ml 0.9% sodium chloride solution and are delivered over a period of 10 to 15 minutes every 30 minutes to 3 hours. Atropine (0.01%) at 0.05 ml/kg can be added to these treatments every 4 hours (see Chapter 133).

Aminophylline

Administer aminophylline intravenously to all patients with acute severe asthma. If more than two routine oral theophylline doses have been missed, a loading dose of 6 mg/kg must be administered over 20 to 30 minutes (a 1 mg/kg bolus will elevate the serum level by 2 μg/ml). Always inquire about sustained-release preparations and extra doses; if an adequate level is suspected, administer 3 mg/kg aminophylline IV over 20 to 30 minutes unless the clinical assessment suggests toxicity or the serum level is greater than that recommended as therapeutic (10 to 20 mg/dl). Manifestations and management of theophylline toxicity are discussed in Chapter 79. After administering the aminophylline bolus begin a maintenance infusion at the rates recommended in Table 34-1. Differences in infusion rates are based on the volume of distribution and clearance rate of aminophylline as a function of age. Since serum levels vary widely with the same dose, past history and theophylline clearance rates are essential in guiding therapy. The theophylline level must be checked 1 hour following a bolus to determine that a therapeutic level was achieved, again at 12 hours to check for steady-state level, and then every 12 to 24 hours.

Table 34-1 Aminophylline Infusion Rate*

Age	Infusion Rate (mg/kg/hr)†
Neonate	0.16
2-6 mo	0.5
6-11 mo	0.85
1-9 yr	1.0
9 yr	0.8

*Modified from Weinberger M, Hendeles L, Ahrens R, et al. Clinical pharmacology of drugs used for asthma. Pediatr Clin North Am 28:47, 1981.
†Add 250 mg aminophylline to 250 ml D₅ so that 1 ml/kg/hr equals 1 mg/kg/hr.

Check the theophylline level any time there is an inadequate clinical response or toxicity is suspected. A number of drugs decrease theophylline clearance (i.e., result in an increase in serum levels); most important are erythromycin, cimetidine, and oral contraceptives. In addition liver disease prolongs the half-life of theophylline. After resolution of the acute attack, begin administration of a sustained-release preparation at 80% of the total daily dose of aminophylline needed to achieve a therapeutic level (i.e., infusion drip rate in mg/hr × 24 hr × 0.8 = total daily dose of theophylline). Continue the theophylline infusion for 3 hours after the oral sustained-release preparation is given to allow absorption and maintenance of the serum theophylline level. A steady-state level must be checked while the patient is receiving an oral preparation. In addition to monitoring theophylline levels monitor the patient for clinical evidence of side effects.

Steroids

Begin administration of IV steroids in all patients admitted to the hospital with acute severe asthma. They improve the response to β-sympathomimetic agents and have anti-inflammatory properties. A 5- to 7-day course of steroids does not result in pituitary-adrenal axis suppression. Administer methylprednisolone (Solu-Medrol) at 125 mg/m² or 5 mg/kg/day in four divided doses. When changing from intravenous to oral medication, use prednisone at doses equivalent to IV methylprednisolone. The concurrent administration of antacids or an H₁-receptor agonist is recommended, as is monitoring of gastric pH in the intubated patient.

Isoproterenol infusion

If the previous measures fail to improve or maintain oxygenation and ventilation at an acceptable level (i.e., PaO_2 >70 mm Hg, $PaCO_2$ <55 mm Hg, SaO_2 >90%) or if a nebulized β-sympathomimetic agent is needed more frequently than every 30 minutes, begin a continuous IV isoproterenol infusion. It must be administered through a separate secure IV line that cannot be interrupted or flushed. An arterial catheter must also be placed for frequent monitoring of arterial blood gases, pH, and systemic arterial blood pressure.

The infusion is started at 0.1 μg/kg/min and increased by 0.1 μg/kg/min approximately every 15 minutes until clinical, arterial blood gas, and pH improvement occurs or until the heart rate exceeds 200 bpm or ventricular ectopy develops. Administration of nebulized β-sympathomimetic agents is discontinued during the isoproterenol infusion. The calculation (weight in kilograms × 0.6) will give the amount of isoproterenol in milligrams to add to 100 ml D_5 so that 1 ml/hr provides 0.1 μg/kg/min (e.g., for a 10 kg child, 6 mg of isoproterenol in 100 ml D_5W infused at 1 ml/hr will provide 0.1 μg/kg/min). The aminophylline infusion must be continued and may need to be increased (based on serum levels) since the isoproterenol will increase its clearance.

Isoproterenol has serious side effects, including myocardial ischemia and cardiac dysrhythmia but is generally well tolerated in children. It may also induce hyperglycemia, but this is rarely clinically significant. When arterial blood gas values have normalized, (i.e., PaO_2 >70 mm Hg, $PaCO_2$ <40 mm Hg) and the patient demonstrates clinical improvement for 6 to 12 hours, the isoproterenol infusion is weaned by 0.1 μg/kg/hr every 2 hours. If the clinical condition deteriorates, as seen by increased work of breathing, recurrence of wheezing, decreased PaO_2, or increased $PaCO_2$, the infusion rate will need to be increased. Once the infusion is discontinued, nebulized β-sympathomimetics may be needed. Aminophylline levels must be monitored since its clearance will decrease.

An alternative to continuous IV isoproterenol is continuous aerosol delivery of albuterol in patients with severe asthma. It is usually given as 1 ml albuterol/10 ml 0.9% sodium chloride solution (using a 250 ml bag)/hr through a nebulizer, noting patient improvement by clinical assessment to decrease the rate of administration.

Mechanical ventilation

If deterioration continues, begin assisted ventilation. Airways obstruction results in increased time constants (i.e., prolonged time for emptying of lung units); therefore the mechanical ventilation must be instituted in a fashion that allows a prolonged expiratory phase of the respiratory cycle and yet sustains normal or increased minute ventilation. A volume-limited ventilator can be used, with tidal volume set at 15 ml/kg, respiratory rate at 15 to 20/min, and an expiratory time of at least 1 to 1½ seconds. The inspired O_2 concentration must be sufficient to maintain an SaO_2 >90%. Begin with FiO_2 = 1.0 and wean FiO_2 as tolerated to maintain SaO_2 >90% (see Chapter 128).

The use of PEEP is controversial; in general it is contraindicated since the patient's functional residual capacity is already increased because of early airway closure and subsequent gas trapping. However, a few studies have shown it to be effective in treating severe asthma, perhaps by maintaining airway patency during the expiratory phase of the respiratory cycle and thereby enhancing the emptying of lung units.

Analysis of arterial blood gas tensions and pH must be instituted immediately after beginning mechanical ventilation and at a frequency of every 30 to 60 minutes until patient stability is achieved.

Intubation of the acute asthmatic patient

The decision to institute mechanical ventilation of the acute asthmatic patient ideally is made early enough to allow a semielective intubation to be performed by the most experienced available personnel. The goal is to secure an endotracheal airway while preserving oxygenation and preventing worsening of bronchospasm caused by either a struggling, agitated patient or stimulation of tracheal reflexes in the inadequately anesthetized patient. While preparations for intubation are being made (see Chapter 127), a history of the most recent oral intake must be obtained and the patient provided with 100% O_2 by face mask.

There is no consensus on the ideal technique for the induction and intubation of the acute asthmatic patient; however, certain drugs should be avoided because of their potential to induce bronchospasm. The administration of morphine, meperidine, *d*-tubocurarine, and atracurium is associated with histamine release, and all have been reported to induce bronchospasm. The use of thiopental (Pentothal) is more controversial, but it too causes histamine release and has the greatest potential of all the IV anesthetics to evoke bronchospasm.

Traditionally the potent halogenated inhalational agents (i.e., halothane) have been used for the induction of asthmatic patients in the operating room but have little application to the asthmatic patient with acute respiratory failure in the PICU. Occasionally inhalational therapy with halothane is indicated for severe cases of asthma refractory to standard therapy and mechanical ventilation. Halothane, however, possesses several adverse side effects, including myocardial depression and vasodilation, leading to systemic hypotension; inhibition of hypoxic pulmonary vasoconstriction, resulting in increased $\dot{V}/\dot{Q}$ mismatch; and sensitization of the myocardium to catecholamine and β-adrenergic agonist, inducing dysrhythmias. In addition it may increase the toxic cardiac effects of aminophylline. Therefore halothane must only be used in the presence of a person experienced with its administration and familiar with the potential complications.

The IV induction agent of choice for the acute asthmatic patient is ketamine (1 to 2 mg/kg IV). Ketamine acts as a bronchodilator through stimulation of the sympathetic nervous system and a direct effect on bronchial smooth muscle. Pretreatment with an antisialagogue such as glycopyrrolate (0.005 mg/kg IV) or atropine (0.01 mg/kg/IV) is effective in reducing ketamine-induced salivary secretions. The addition of lidocaine (1.5 mg/kg IV) to the induction agent is effective in blunting unwanted tracheal reflexes in response to laryngoscopy and intubation. Emergence delirium associated with ketamine (5% to 30% incidence) can be prevented by the inclusion of a benzodiazepine, midazolam (0.1 to 0.2 mg/kg IV) or diazepam (0.2 mg/kg IV). Ketamine is contraindicated in patients with increased ICP or severe systemic arterial hypertension.

Technically the asthmatic patient should be treated as a "full-stomach" case, thus necessitating a rapid-sequence induction, including succinylcholine (see Chapter 127). However, most asthmatic patients who need intubation have inadequate O$_2$ reserve to tolerate the 45 to 60 seconds of apnea required for rapid-sequence intubation and rarely have eaten in the preceding 6 to 8 hours. The stomach may be emptied with an orally placed gastric tube and the patient given a nonparticulate antacid (sodium citrate and citric acid, 15 ml by nasogastric tube) to neu-

---

INTUBATION SEQUENCE FOR THE ACUTE ASTHMATIC

Premedication

Glycopyrrolate (0.005 mg/kg) or atropine (0.01 mg/kg) IV

Oxygen

Induction

Lidocaine (1.5 mg/kg) IV

Ketamine (1-2 mg/kg) IV

Midazolam (0.1-0.2 mg/kg) or diazepam (0.2 mg/kg) IV

Muscle relaxant

Vecuronium (0.1-0.5 mg/kg) or pancuronium (0.1 mg/kg)

Bag and mask ventilation with cricoid pressure

---

tralize stomach pH if intake has occurred within 4 hours. The use of bag and mask ventilation with cricoid pressure after induction and administration of a nondepolarizing muscle relaxant such as vecuronium (0.15 to 0.2 mg/kg) is the preferred technique. This dose is somewhat greater than the usual recommended dose of 0.08 to 0.1 mg/kg; however, in this situation the period until onset of paralysis will be reduced by several minutes, allowing a shorter period of bag and mask ventilation. As always with an emergency intubation, the initial intubation should be via the oral-tracheal route, and the tube can be changed to a nasal-tracheal position once the airway is secured and ventilation maintained.

Patients on mechanical ventilation must be sedated (midazolam or diazepam at 0.1 to 0.2 mg/kg every 2 hours) (see Chapter 129); in addition, pharmacologic paralysis can be instituted to enhance the efficiency and decrease the risks of mechanical ventilation (e.g., vecuronium at a 0.075 mg/kg bolus followed by 0.075 mg/kg/hr with the IV infusion rate adjusted by monitoring twitch responses; see Chapter 130). Ketamine and halothane anesthesia have been used for the mechanically ventilated patient with acute severe asthma since they are bronchodilators; they must be administered only by experienced phy-

———————————————————— INITIAL EVALUATION IN THE ICU ————————————————————

1. *History*
2. *Physical examination*
3. *Laboratory values*
   Arterial blood gas and pH
   Chest roentgenogram
   Theophylline level
   Serum electrolytes and complete blood count

———————————————————————— INITIAL MANAGEMENT ————————————————————————

1. *General measures*   2. *Nebulized medications*   3. *Aminophylline*   4. *Minimum laboratory*
   Oxygen   Albuterol every 3 hrs   No recent use   Recent use   *values*
   Fluids   Atropine every 3 hrs   6 mg/kg bolus   3 mg/kg bolus   Every 12 hr theophyl-
   Drainage and percussion   Inadequate response   line level
   Solu-Medrol 2 mg/kg IV q6h   Maintenance infusion   Blood gas and pH if
                                                                                                        deteriorating
                                  Change to isoproterenol   Chest roentgenogram
                                  every 1 hr   if sudden deterioration

Check theophylline level 1 hour after bolus

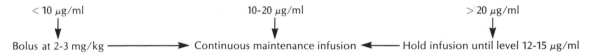

< 10 μg/ml   10-20 μg/ml   > 20 μg/ml

Bolus at 2-3 mg/kg ─────────────▶ Continuous maintenance infusion ◀───────── Hold infusion until level 12-15 μg/ml

———————————————————— DETERIORATION OR NO IMPROVEMENT ————————————————————

Increase fraction of inspired oxygen (FiO₂)
Increase frequency of aerosols
Continuous albuterol aerosol
Recheck theophylline level

< 10 μg/ml   10-20 μg/ml   > 20 μg/ml

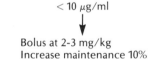   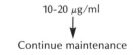   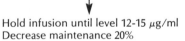

Bolus at 2-3 mg/kg   Continue maintenance   Hold infusion until level 12-15 μg/ml
Increase maintenance 10%   Decrease maintenance 20%

———————————————————————— CONTINUED DETERIORATION ————————————————————————

1. *Isoproterenol infusion*
   Arterial catheter
   Secure separate IV
   Start infusion and increase as tolerated or until improvement
   Check theophylline level (increased clearance)
   Hold isoproterenol aerosol

   Further deterioration
         ↓

2. *Assisted ventilation*
   Sedation and paralysis or ketamine anesthesia
   Volume ventilator
      Large tidal volumes
      Slow rate
      Prolonged expiratory phase
      Monitor for pneumothorax

Fig. 34-2   Management protocol for acute severe asthma.

sicians who are knowledgeable about their side effects. (For a full discussion on mechanical ventilation, see Chapter 128.)

Pneumothorax

If there is a sudden deterioration in a patient's arterial blood gas values and pH at any time, but particularly in a patient on positive pressure mechanical ventilation, the possibility of tension pneumothorax must be considered. Hypotension may be caused by either pneumothorax or pneumopericardium (see Chapter 134). Physical examination and a chest roentgenogram will confirm this diagnosis; tube thoracostomy placement and continuous suction will be needed for treating pneumothorax in a patient with acute severe asthma.

Fig. 34-2 summarizes the management protocol for acute severe asthma.

ADDITIONAL READING

Boushey HA, Holtzman MJ, Sheller JR, et al. Bronchial hyperactivity. Am Rev Respir Dis 121:389, 1980.

Dolan LM, Keshrwala MH, Holroyde JL, et al. Short-term, high-dose, systemic steroids in children with asthma: The effect on the hypothalamic-pituitary-adrenal axis. J Allergy Clin Immunol 80:81, 1987.

Fanta CH, Rossing TH, McFadden R Jr. Treatment of acute asthma. Is combination therapy with sympathomimetics and methylxanthines indicated? Am J Med 80:5, 1986.

Herman JJ, Noah ZL, Moody RR. Use of intravenous isoproterenol for status asthmaticus in children. Crit Care Med 11:716, 1983.

• L'Hommedieu CS, Arens JJ. The use of ketamine for the emergency intubation of patients with status asthmaticus. Ann Emerg Med 16:87, 1987.

McGuire JF, Geha RS, Umetsu DT. Myocardial specific creatinine phosphokinase isoenzyme elevation in children with asthma treated with intravenous isoproterenol. J Allergy Clin Immunol 78:631, 1986.

Skoner DR, Fischer TJ, Gormley C, et al. Pediatric predictive index for hospitalization in acute asthma. Ann Emerg Med 16:25, 1987.

• Weinberger M, Hendels L. Theophylline use: An overview. J Allergy Clin Immunol 76:277, 1985.

• Weiss EB, Siegel MS, Stern M, eds. Bronchial Asthma. Mechanisms and Therapeutic, 2nd ed. Boston: Little Brown, 1980.

Wood DW, Downes JJ, Scheinkopf H, et al. Intravenous isoproterenol in the management of respiratory failure in childhood status asthmaticus. J Allergy Clin Immunol 50:75, 1972.

35 Adult Respiratory Distress Syndrome

James A. Royall

BACKGROUND AND PHYSIOLOGY

Adult respiratory distress syndrome (ARDS) is a clinical syndrome of acute respiratory failure following almost any severe physiologic insult that may or may not have injured the lungs primarily. The hallmark of the syndrome is increased permeability of the alveolar-capillary membrane, resulting in pulmonary edema. Common precipitating insults include shock of any etiology, sepsis, viral or bacterial pneumonia, near-drowning, aspiration pneumonia, ingestions, and trauma. It was first described as a distinct entity in 1967; the pathologic appearance of the lungs was similar to that of neonatal respiratory distress syndrome and the term "adult respiratory distress syndrome" became accepted. The word "adult" is therefore of historical origin only, and ARDS can occur in patients of any age. The clinical course, pathophysiologic alterations, and pathologic findings are well described, as summarized in Table 35-1.

The diagnosis of ARDS is made on the basis of the clinical course and exclusion of other potential causes of pulmonary edema such as hydrostatic edema from cardiac failure. The clinical course can be divided into four stages: acute injury, latent period, acute respiratory failure, and severe physiologic abnormalities. With the acute injury there may be no signs related to the lungs unless they are injured primarily. Some patients will hyperventilate, developing hypocarbia and respiratory alkalosis despite adequate oxygenation. A latent period of approximately 6 to 48 hours follows, during which the patient appears to be recovering and the cardiovascular and pulmonary status is stable. Hyperventilation will persist, and the chest roentgenogram may show a fine reticular pattern due to interstitial pulmonary fluid. Acute respiratory failure is often of sudden onset, with hypoxemia that responds poorly to O_2 therapy because of a large intrapulmonary shunt; the $Paco_2$ is often low because of secondary hyperventilation. Diffuse crackles are heard on chest auscultation, and the chest roentgenogram has diffuse, hazy, bilateral infiltrates (Fig. 35-1). Most patients will need intubation for respiratory support, and decreased pulmonary compliance will be noted. Development of these signs after the initial insult is sufficient to make the diagnosis of ARDS. Not all patients will progress to the fourth phase of severe physiologic abnormalities. Some will recover and some will die from causes other than respiratory failure. There is no clear point of transition into the phase of severe physiologic abnormalities, but development of CO_2 retention indicates severe pulmonary disease, primarily from progressive pulmonary fibrosis. Intractable respiratory failure may eventually develop, or the patient may need prolonged respiratory support while the chronic lung changes slowly resolve.

Mortality rates vary with the population evaluated but are generally greater than 50% in both pediatric and adult patients. Early mortality, within the first 3 days, is most often related to the severity of the precipitating insult. Later mortality is due primarily to secondary infection and multiple organ system failure. Intractable respiratory failure causes only approximately 16% of the deaths. Therefore ARDS should be viewed as a multiple organ system insult, and rather than concentrating on the lungs as an isolated system, a more global approach to therapy, including attention to tissue oxygenation, nutritional support, and aggressive management of potential secondary infections, must be taken.

The pathophysiologic mechanisms in ARDS include abnormalities of both arterial oxygenation and

289

Table 35-1   Sequential Clinical, Pathophysiologic, and Pathologic Changes in ARDS*

Change	Acute Injury	Latent Period	Acute Respiratory Failure	Severe Physiologic Abnormalities
Clinical		Chest x-ray Possibly fine reticular markings →	Bilateral, diffuse, hazy infiltrates	→ Chronic lung changes with fibrosis
		Possible hyperventilation →	Tachypnea, dyspnea, rales on auscultation	Intractable respiratory failure
			Hypocarbia or normocarbia ↗ → Hypercarbia	Metabolic and respiratory acidosis
		Possible hypocarbia ↘		Eventual death
				or
			Hypoxemia with poor response to increased F_{IO_2} → Worsening hypoxemia	Chronic lung disease requiring prolonged respiratory support
Pathophysiology	Primary or secondary injury to the alveolar-capillary membrane with increased permeability	Possible increased pulmonary vascular resistance	Usually increased pulmonary vascular resistance and pulmonary hypertension Ventilation/perfusion mismatching and increased intrapulmonary shunt Decreased functional residual capacity, decreased pulmonary compliance, and increased dead space	
Pathology		Possible increased interstitial fluid	*Early exudative phase (24-96 hr)* Interstitial and intra-alveolar fluid Epithelial degeneration Microemboli (polymorphonuclear leukocytes, fibrin, platelets) *Cellular proliferative phase (3-10 days)* Proliferation of type II pneumocytes Interstitial cellular infiltrates *Fibrotic proliferative phase (>7 days)* Disruption of acinar architecture of lung Alveolar fibrosis Alveolar duct fibrosis	

*Modified from Royall JA, Levin DL. Adult respiratory distress syndrome in pediatric patients. J Pediatr 112:335, 1988.

cardiac function. This disorder is primarily one in which tissue O_2 delivery and consumption are inadequate to meet the metabolic demands of the vital organ systems.

$$O_2 \text{ delivery (ml } O_2/\text{min}/\text{m}^2) = \quad (1)$$
$$\text{Arterial } O_2 \text{ content (ml } O_2/\text{dl}) \times$$
$$\text{Cardiac index (L/min/m}^2) \times 10 \text{ (dl/L)}$$

Pulmonary interstitial fluid and alveolar fluid lead to abnormalities in pulmonary mechanics, with decreased functional residual capacity, decreased compliance, and increased dead space ventilation. Gas exchange is altered with ventilation/perfusion mismatching (primarily lung units with very low or no ventilation), resulting in severe hypoxemia from large venous admixture. The cardiac dysfunction is not manifest as clinical cardiac failure but rather as an inability to increase cardiac function appropriately. Pulmonary hypertension with increased right ventricular afterload and the adverse effects of positive end-expiratory pressure (PEEP) reduce cardiac output.

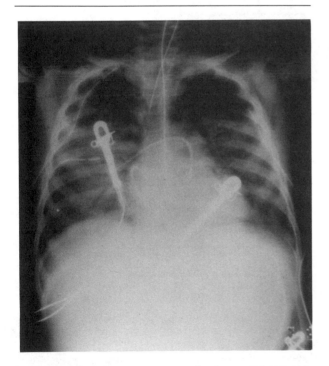

Fig. 35-1 Chest roentgenogram of a 2-year-old girl with ARDS subsequent to kerosene ingestion/inhalation.

Additionally, there is an alteration in the normal relationship of O_2 consumption to delivery (Fig. 35-2). Normally O_2 consumption is independent of O_2 delivery except when O_2 delivery is reduced to very low levels. In patients with ARDS O_2 consumption is linearly related to O_2 delivery even when O_2 delivery is well above the range that would usually be adequate. Allowing O_2 delivery to remain in the range in which this linear relationship exists potentially maintains the patient in a constant state of O_2 debt. Because of abnormalities of peripheral O_2 use, mixed venous O_2 is an unreliable indicator of tissue oxygenation; lactic acidosis, although reflecting inadequate tissue oxygenation, is a late indicator. Therefore one goal of therapy is to maintain tissue O_2 delivery at a high normal or supranormal level.

The underlying pathogenic mechanisms causing ARDS are not clearly delineated; however, a variety of mechanisms and mediators have been proposed. ARDS is a syndrome resulting from diverse initiating insults; this clinical event is the result of different sets of pathologic events, with the common end point being injury to the alveolar-capillary barrier. Therefore it is not surprising that one mechanism or mediator cannot explain every case of ARDS. A given pathologic event will be occurring to a greater or lesser degree, depending on the initiating insult and the stage of ARDS. Additionally, one mediator may exert its pathologic effect via another mediator. Fig. 35-3 is a schematic representation of potential mechanisms by which a distant event (sepsis) leads to ARDS. These mechanisms can be placed into four categories, mainly for the sake of clarity. As is evident from the discussion to follow, this categorization is somewhat arbitrary, considering the overlap and feedback involving the various processes.

First are the processes that can initiate ARDS, causing endothelial injury; inflammatory cell activation is of central importance in sepsis-induced ARDS. Approximately 10 years ago there was considerable enthusiasm for the hypothesis that complement-mediated polymorphonuclear leukocyte activation was a necessary event. Although it may be important in many cases of ARDS, it is not a necessary process, and ARDS can occur in the setting of profound neutropenia. This does not detract, however, from the central role of inflammatory cells. Evidence is mounting for an important role for mononuclear phagocytes (monocytes and macrophages) in sepsis and ARDS. Even with neutropenia the tissue and alveolar

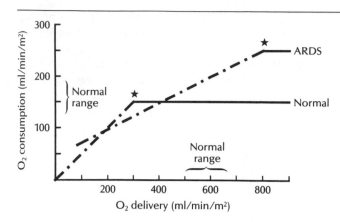

Fig. 35-2   Relationship of O₂ consumption to O₂ delivery in normal person and patient with ARDS. O₂ supply dependency is represented by broken lines in each curve. The points at which O₂ consumption becomes independent of O₂ delivery are noted by stars. The slope of the line in the O₂ supply dependency region indicates how efficiently the available O₂ is used. In patients with ARDS the slope is less, indicating a reduced ability of the tissues to extract O₂.

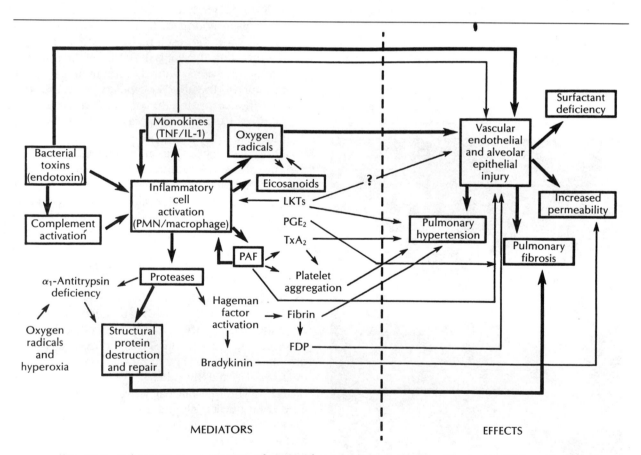

Fig. 35-3   Schematic representation of potential mechanisms in ARDS with sepsis. (FDP = fibrin degradation products, IL-1 = interleukin-1, LKTs = leukotrienes; PAF = platelet-activating factor; PGE₂ = prostaglandin E₂; PMN = polymorphonuclear leukocyte; TNF = tumor necrosis factor; TxA₂ = thromboxane A₂.)

macrophages represent a resident population of inflammatory cells within the lung capable of causing injury. However, isolated inflammatory cell activation probably is not sufficient to cause ARDS, and a concomitant direct injury to the endothelial cell may be required. Endotoxin itself, as well as the macrophage products, tumor necrosis factor and interleukin-1, causes direct endothelial cell injury and activates inflammatory cells. With activation these inflammatory cells release O_2 radicals, proteases, eicosanoid, and other substances such as platelet-activating factor, which are the mediators of the injury. The ability of O_2 radicals to produce vascular endothelial cell injury is well established, but the role of the other substances is less certain. The generation of fibrin microthrombi and fibrin degradation products can cause alveolar-capillary injury. Although this may occur in patients with sepsis via proteolytic enzyme activation of Hageman factor, resulting in fibrin formation and fibrinolysis, this process may have a more central role in ARDS associated with other insults such as trauma than in ARDS associated with sepsis.

The second category includes processes that may not independently cause alveolar-capillary injury but, once ARDS occurs, result in pathophysiologic disturbances and additional amplification of the injury. Proteolytic enzymes and platelet aggregation would be in this category. Although still controversial, proteolytic enzymes probably do not independently result in increased vascular endothelial permeability but may act synergistically with O_2 radicals. They can activate Hageman factor, as described previously, and can activate complement, thereby amplifying the injury. Proteolytic enzymes disrupt lung structural protein, and during its repair fewer elastic collagen types are deposited. Additionally, proteolytic enzymes (as well as hyperoxia and O_2 radicals) can inactivate α-antitrypsin, which is the endogenous protection against proteolytic enzymes. Endotoxin, macrophages, PGE_2, and lymphocytes also have modulating effects on fibroblasts. These processes are of particular importance in the patient who progresses to a later stage of ARDS in which severe pulmonary fibrosis develops. Platelet aggregation, through thromboxane A_2 release, is one factor in the pulmonary hypertension that occurs with ARDS. Thromboxane A_2 itself induces further platelet aggregation and increases PMN adherence to endothelial cells, which are processes that would amplify injury.

The third category comprises processes that are

PROPOSED PATHOGENIC MECHANISMS IN ARDS

Cellular mediators

Polymorphonuclear leukocytes
Mononuclear phagocytes (monocytes, macrophages)
Platelets
Fibroblasts
Lymphocytes

Secondary effects of lung injury

Surfactant deficiency
Pulmonary fibrosis
α_1-Antitrypsin deficiency

Iatrogenic factors

O_2 toxicity
Malnutrition
Barotrauma

Secretory/circulating mediators

Bacterial toxins (endotoxin)
Activated complement
Oxygen radicals
Eicosanoids (thromboxane, prostaglandins, leukotrienes)
Proteases
Platelet-activating factor
Monokines (tumor necrosis factor, interleukin-1)
Free fatty acids
Fibrin platelet microthrombi
Fibrin degradation products
Fat emboli
Tissue thromboplastin (tissue factor)
Hageman factor (factor XII)
Serotonin
Bradykinin
Histamine

MONITORING AND LABORATORY STUDIES

Cardiorespiratory system

Hemoglobin or hematocrit (O_2-carrying capacity) every 12 hr
Systemic arterial catheter
Pulse oximeter
Pulmonary arterial catheter often needed; indications for use include:
1. Therapeutic maneuvers that are likely to inhibit cardiac function (PEEP $\geq$15 cm H_2O)
2. Precipitating disease process that is likely to cause myocardial dysfunction
3. Clinical status, based on urinary output, peripheral perfusion, heart rate, and systemic arterial blood pressure, that indicates a low cardiac output responding poorly to volume infusion
4. Etiology of pulmonary edema is unclear

Potential for multiple organ system failure

Renal: BUN and creatinine (initial screen; repeat as needed); clinical signs of renal insufficiency (weight gain, decreased urinary output, positive fluid balance, hyponatremia, decreased hematocrit, abnormal fractional excretion of sodium)
Gastrointestinal: Gastric aspirate pH every 2 hr (must be >4.0 to ensure adequate prophylaxis against GI bleeds)
Disseminated intravascular coagulation: PT/PTT and platelet count (initial screen; repeat as needed)
Thrombocytopenia: Platelet count (initial screen; repeat as needed)
Hepatic: AST, ALT, bilirubin (initial screen; repeat as needed)

---

the result of the lung injury and result in a specific pathophysiologic disturbance. Surfactant deficiency from damage to type II alveolar epithelial cells, resulting in alveolar collapse, would be in this category. Some recent evidence suggests that surfactant has antioxidant properties; therefore surfactant depletion may eventually prove to be in the second category.

The fourth category is for iatrogenic processes such as O_2 toxicity and poor nutrition. Although sometimes necessary for therapy, these processes can also have adverse effects. O_2 toxicity can increase lung injury and delay healing. Poor nutrition can also delay healing and, if sufficiently severe, can leave the patient more susceptible to secondary infection.

MONITORING AND LABORATORY TESTS

The routine monitoring needed for a critically ill child is discussed in Chapters 10 and 12. The child with ARDS will need cardiorespiratory monitoring, including the measurements obtained using a systemic arterial catheter, pulse oximeter, and often a pulmonary arterial catheter for sequential measurement of O_2 delivery and consumption (see Chapter 10). Dysfunction of any organ system can be associated with ARDS. Renal dysfunction, gastrointestinal bleeding, disseminated intravascular coagulation, and thrombocytopenia are commonly encountered. Reviewing clinical signs and laboratory studies will be necessary to screen for and monitor the progression of these problems. Secondary infection, most commonly bacterial bronchopneumonia often caused by gram-negative organisms, is an important cause of poor outcome, but the definitive diagnosis of bronchopneumonia is difficult to make. The usual signs that suggest pneumonia, including new infiltrates on chest roentgenogram, fever, abnormal white blood cell count, purulent secretions, and apparent response to antibiotics, are unfortunately neither specific nor sensitive in the patient with ARDS.

THERAPY

Therapy is primarily supportive but is directed by an understanding of the pathophysiologic alterations associated with ARDS. Attempts at specific treatment after the onset of ARDS, including the use of steroids, PGE_1, and extracorporeal membrane oxygenation, have been disappointing. Tissue oxygen delivery must be maintained in a high normal or supranormal range (ideally an O_2 delivery >600 ml/min/m²). This is accomplished by maintaining the primary deter-

---

GENERAL GUIDELINES FOR MANAGEMENT

Provide therapy for the precipitating insult.

Perform appropriate monitoring (see p. 294).

Maintain adequate tissue oxygenation with minimal supplemental O_2.

Hematocrit, 40%-49%

Arterial O_2 saturation ≥90%

Cardiac index ≥4.5 L/min/m²

O_2 delivery >600 ml O_2/min/m²

PEEP as needed to maintain Fio₂ ≤0.50-0.60

See text for end points of PEEP therapy and criteria for weaning PEEP.

Support cardiac function with fluids and inotropic agents.

Provide fluids initially at 70% maintenance.

Provide additional fluids for cardiac and nutritional support.

Provide early and aggressive nutritional support.

See text for goals of early and late nutritional support.

React early to evidence of secondary infection.

Prescribe broad-spectrum antibiotic coverage for *Pseudomonas* and *Staphylococcus.*

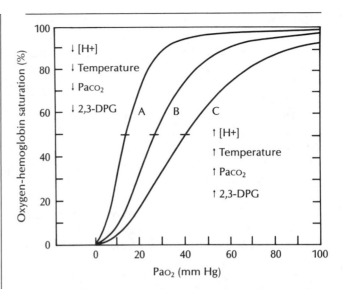

Fig. 35-4 Oxygen-hemoglobin dissociation curve. Curve *B* is the normal curve. Curve *A* represents a left shift and curve *C* a right shift. ([H⁺] = hydrogen ion concentration, DPG = diphosphoglycerate.) (Reproduced by permission from Levin DL, Morris FC, Moore GC, eds. A Practical Guide to Pediatric Intensive Care, 2nd ed. St. Louis: CV Mosby, 1984.)

---

minants of tissue O_2 delivery, that is, hemoglobin, arterial O_2 saturation, and cardiac index, within defined ranges. O_2 delivery is determined by the product of arterial O_2 content and cardiac index (see equation 1). Equation 2 is used to determine arterial O_2 content.

$$\text{Arterial } O_2 \text{ content (ml } O_2/dl) = \quad (2)$$
$$[\text{Hb (g/dl)} \times 1.36 \text{ (ml } O_2/\text{g Hb)} \times$$
$$O_2 \text{ saturation of Hb (\%)] +}$$
$$[\text{Pao}_2 \text{ (mm Hg)} \times 0.003 \text{ (ml } O_2/dl/\text{mm Hg)}]$$

The first half of the equation (within first brackets) describes the contribution of hemoglobin-bound O_2, which is the majority of O_2 in the blood. The second half of the equation describes the dissolved O_2, which is only a small fraction of the total O_2 content. Therefore, when considering arterial O_2 content, the important determinants are the hemoglobin level and percent saturation. The relationship of Pao₂ to O_2 saturation is described by the oxygen-hemoglobin dissociation curve (Fig. 35-4). Note that the curve is **S** shaped and can be shifted to the left or right. Above a saturation of approximately 90% the curve is rel-

atively flat so that large changes in Pao₂ yield little change in saturation and total O_2 content. Below 90% saturation small changes in Pao₂ can result in significant decreases in saturation. Therefore the arterial saturation is maintained at approximately 90% and can be monitored continuously by the pulse oximeter. O_2-carrying capacity is maintained with a hematocrit level of 40% to 49% (hemoglobin value of approximately 13 to 15 g/dl). Above this range hyperviscosity may be detrimental to tissue perfusion. The cardiac index is maintained at 4.5 L/min/m² or greater. If these values are attained, that is, a hemoglobin of 13 to 15 g/dl, O_2 saturation of 90%, and cardiac index of 4.5 L/min/m², tissue O_2 delivery will be in the desired range of >600 ml O_2/min/m².

These goals of O_2 delivery must be achieved at an Fio₂ of <0.50 to 0.60, which will cause minimal additional damage to the lungs. The use of PEEP increases oxygenation at lower levels of Fio₂. When the patient is initially intubated, 100% O_2 and a low level of PEEP (2 to 4 cm H_2O) are used. If the arterial saturation is >90%, the Fio₂ is decreased in decrements of 3% to 5% until the saturation is close to

90%. If the FiO_2 is still in the potentially toxic range (>0.50), the PEEP is increased in increments of 2 to 3 cm H_2O; the effect on oxygenation and cardiac function is evaluated approximately 30 minutes after the PEEP is increased, and the FiO_2 is decreased as tolerated. If the increase in PEEP causes a decreased cardiac index, cardiac function is supported with fluids, inotropic agents, or both as guided by the hemodynamic measurements (see Chapter 12). The end points of PEEP therapy are (1) the goals for tissue O_2 delivery are achieved; (2) increases in PEEP actually result in a decreased arterial O_2 saturation, indicating that PEEP has been increased beyond the beneficial range; and (3) increases in PEEP result in cardiac depression that is not reversible with fluids and inotropy.

There is no absolute upper limit for PEEP. To interpret the effects of an increase in PEEP it is important to make sequential hemodynamic observations before and after each change. Small incremental changes are also made when decreasing the level of PEEP. A common occurrence is hypoxemia after decreasing PEEP that necessitates a higher than baseline level of PEEP to correct. To prevent this occurrence PEEP must be decreased slowly (no more often than every 6 hours) and in small decrements (2 to 3 cm H_2O). The patient must be stable, the FiO_2 0.40 or less, the arterial saturation 95% (PaO_2 of approximately 80 mm Hg) and stable for 12 hours, and the pulmonary compliance stable or improving for 12 hours.

The routine use of diuretics, hemodialysis, or hemofiltration in an effort to reduce lung water is not beneficial in the patient with an appropriate intravascular volume. This is not surprising since the pathophysiologic alteration causing pulmonary edema is increased permeability, not increased hydrostatic pressure. However, if intravascular volume is inappropriately elevated, there will be worsening of edema and potentially decreased cardiac function. Therefore the goal of fluid therapy is to maintain cardiac function with the lowest effective intravascular volume. Although a reasonable initial approach is to maintain moderate fluid restriction, there should be no hesitation in giving additional fluid as needed to support cardiac function. Also, additional fluids will be needed to supply adequate nutritional support. Some patients may be unable to tolerate the increased fluids; measures to decrease intravascular volume (diuretics, dialysis, hemofiltration) must be used rather than decreasing nutritional support.

Malnutrition is a common problem among hospitalized pediatric patients (see Chapter 74). Adverse effects of malnutrition include poor tissue repair, respiratory muscle weakness, multiple organ system failure, and immunodeficiency. Patients with ARDS have increased caloric requirements due to hypercatabolism. This need is met by mobilization of endogenous energy stores, including protein. Early nutritional support is aimed at preventing the depletion of endogenous energy stores and requires approximately 50 to 60 kcal/kg/day in infants, 35 to 40 kcal/kg/day in children, and 20 to 40 kcal/kg/day in adults. Protein intake must be approximately 1 to 3 g/kg/day, and 20% to 30% of the caloric intake must be fat. After the acute phase of illness, caloric requirements will be 25% to 50% above the usual age requirements for repletion of losses, tissue repair, resting energy requirements, and growth. Although the main concern is prevention of malnutrition, there are also potential problems with the use of aggressive nutritional support. Increased carbohydrate loads may result in elevated CO_2 production, which can cause hypercarbia and respiratory acidosis or can hinder weaning the patient from ventilatory support.

Despite the problems in establishing the definitive diagnosis of secondary infection, the clinician must institute aggressive therapy once infection is suspected because of the associated poor outcome. Appropriate cultures must be obtained and empiric therapy with broad-spectrum antibiotics started for both gram-negative bacteria, including *Pseudomonas,* and gram-positive bacteria, primarily *Staphylococcus.* An aminoglycoside, antipseudomonal penicillin, and antistaphylococcal penicillin will offer this coverage. Another option is a combination of an antistaphylococcal penicillin and a third-generation cephalosporin with antipseudomonal activity such as ceftazidime, although the effectiveness of these as single agents for *Pseudomonas* infections is still being evaluated.

The approach outlined above provides general guidelines. Because of the diversity of initial insults associated with ARDS and the myriad of considerations in adjusting therapy for individual patients, it would be impossible to deal with all the possibilities. One must make a risk/benefit analysis for each intervention, whether it be a monitoring technique such as the use of a pulmonary arterial catheter or a therapeutic maneuver such as an increase in the level of PEEP, and decide that the risks associated with the maneuver are justified by the potential benefits.

ADDITIONAL READING

Alberts WM, Priest GR, Moser KM. The outlook of survivors of ARDS. Chest 84:272-274, 1983.

Ashbaugh DG, Bigelow DB, Petty TL, Levine BE. Acute respiratory distress in adults. Lancet 2:319-323, 1967.

Bachofen M, Weibel ER. Structural alterations of the lung parenchyma in the adult respiratory distress syndrome. Clin Chest Med 3:35-56, 1982.

Bell RC, Coalson JJ, Smith JD, Johanson WG. Multiple organ system failure and infection in adult respiratory distress syndrome. Ann Intern Med 99:293-298, 1983.

Bernard GR, Luce JM, Sprung CL, et al. High-dose corticosteroids in patients with the adult respiratory distress syndrome. N Engl J Med 317:1565-1570, 1987.

Bihari D, Smithies M, Gimson A, Tinker J. The effects of vasodilation with prostacyclin on oxygen delivery and uptake in critically ill patients. N Engl J Med 317:397-403, 1987.

Czer LS, Appel P, Shoemaker WC. Pathogenesis of respiratory failure (ARDS) after hemorrhage and trauma. II. Cardiorespiratory patterns after development of ARDS. Crit Care Med 8:513-518, 1980.

Dantzker DR. Gas exchange in the adult respiratory distress syndrome. Clin Chest Med 3:57-67, 1982.

• Demling RH. The role of mediators in human ARDS. J Crit Care 3:56-72, 1988.

Katz R, Pollack M, Spady D. Cardiopulmonary abnormalities in severe acute respiratory failure. J Pediatr 104:357-364, 1984.

Montgomery AB, Stager MA, Carrico J, Hudson LD. Causes of mortality in patients with the adult respiratory distress syndrome. Am Rev Respir Dis 132:485 489, 1985.

Pingleton SK. Complications associated with the adult respiratory distress syndrome. Clin Chest Med 3:143-155, 1982.

Pingleton SK, Harmon GS. Nutritional management in acute respiratory failure. JAMA 2157:3094-3099, 1987.

• Rinaldo JE, Rogers RM. Adult respiratory-distress syndrome: Changing concepts of lung injury and repair. N Engl J Med 306:900-909, 1982.

Royall JA, Levin DL. Adult respiratory distress syndrome in children. In Nussbaum E, ed. Pediatric Intensive Care. New York: Futura (in press).

Royall JA, Levin DL. Adult respiratory distress syndrome in pediatric patients. Part I. Clinical aspects, pathophysiology, pathology, and mechanisms of lung injury. J Pediatr 112:169-180, 1988.

Royall JA, Levin DL. Adult respiratory distress syndrome in pediatric patients. Part II: Management. J Pediatr 112:335-350, 1988.

Shapiro BA, Cane RD, Harrison RA. Positive end-expiratory pressure therapy in adults with special reference to acute lung injury: A review of literature and suggested clinical correlations. Crit Care Med 12:127-141, 1984.

Sibbald WJ, Driedger AA, Myers ML, Short AIK, Wells GA. Biventricular function in the adult respiratory distress syndrome: Hemodynamic and radionuclide assessment, with special emphasis on right ventricular function. Chest 84:126-134, 1983.

Zapol WM, Snider MT, Hill JD, et al. Extracorporeal membrane oxygenation in severe acute respiratory failure. JAMA 242:2193-2196, 1979.

36 Sequelae of Intubation

Scott C. Manning · Orval E. Brown

BACKGROUND AND PHYSIOLOGY

The development of a relatively safe means of endotracheal intubation for infants and young children in the mid-1960s constituted a much needed technologic solution to the problem of assisted ventilation. In the United States 45% of neonatal intensive care patients will need endotracheal intubation for >7 days. Unfortunately endotracheal intubation has created its own set of problems in the upper airway. Dental and pharyngeal injuries during the act of intubation, fortunately rare, are related to the skill of the intubator. Sinusitis and otitis media secondary to intubation are related to bypass and disturbance of the normal upper airway mucociliary protective mechanism as well as to direct obstruction of sinus and eustachian tube openings in patients intubated nasally. Direct mechanical trauma from the tube is the principal etiologic factor in the remainder of significant complications (Table 36-1).

Supraglottic and Glottic Laryngeal Sequelae

The relatively wide and flexible supraglottic airway is able to accommodate endotracheal tubes easily, and significant complications at this level are rare. Tissue injuries secondary to traumatic or prolonged intubation can lead eventually to webs and stenosis between false cords, aryepiglottic folds, and epiglottis. However, these sequelae do not usually result in symptomatic airway obstruction, and they can be managed with endoscopic surgery.

Because of its relatively small size and because of the continuous rubbing and shearing from vocal cord motion, the glottic larynx is at much greater risk for tissue injury. Traumatic intubations can result in vocal cord contusions and lacerations and even in complete subluxation of arytenoid cartilages with subsequent vocal cord fixation. The indwelling tube inevitably causes some degree of epithelial injury and subepithelial edema related to the length and num-

Table 36-1 Sequelae of Intubation

Nose	Stenosis secondary to columellar/ alar necrosis
	Choanal stenosis
	Sinusitis
Ear	Otitis media
Mouth	Dental trauma
	Lip lacerations
Pharynx	Sore throat
	Lacerations
Supraglottic larynx	Laryngitis
	Webs and stenosis
Glottic larynx	Vocal cord laceration
	Vocal cord paralysis
	Vocal cord ulceration, granulation, edema
	Anterior web
	Arytenoid subluxation
	Posterior glottic stenosis
Subglottic larynx	Edema
	Ulceration, granulation
	Firm stenosis
	Cysts, webs
Trachea	Necrotizing tracheobronchitis
	Granulation
	Firm stenosis
Bronchus	Granulation
	Stenosis
	Bronchitis
Lung	Pneumonia

ber of intubations, the size of the tube, and the relative motion between tube and vocal cords. The greatest degree of injury is usually seen in the posterior glottis because the tube is forced back by (1) the front-to-rear pushing effect of vocal cord closure in the triangular-shaped glottis and (2) the angulation between the relatively high anterior infant larynx and the posteriorly sloping cervical trachea. Severe injury can lead to sufficient edema, granulation tissue, and fibrosis to result in significant obstruction after extubation.

Acquired Subglottic Stenosis

With the development of soft, inert, siliconized polyvinyl chloride endotracheal tubes the incidence of severe obstructive airway complications in intubated pediatric patients has decreased from 12% to 20% in the late 1960s to 1% to 8% at present. Overall, endotracheal intubation is safer in children than in adults to the degree that tracheotomy based solely on prolonged ventilatory support is now rarely recommended for infants. However, clinicians are still faced with the problem of obstructing lesions developing in a small percentage of intubated patients. The most common and the most difficult to treat of the lesions is acquired subglottic stenosis.

The subglottic larynx extends from the vocal cords to the inferior border of the cricoid cartilage. It is more prone to injury than other portions of the intubated pediatric airway because (1) it is the narrowest part of the airway, (2) the cricoid constitutes the only complete circumferential cartilaginous ring in the upper airway and is therefore less yielding to expansile forces, and (3) the subglottic mucosa is especially fragile and prone to edema. Autopsy studies have documented subglottic injury in 75% to 100% of intubated infants, and the pathophysiology of acquired subglottic stenosis has been fairly well outlined (Table 36-2). Shearing and pressure forces of the endotracheal tube lead to mucosal erosions and ulcerations and submucosal edema within a few hours of intubation. As with glottic injuries, these changes are most pronounced in the posterior subglottis. A longer duration of intubation is associated with necrosis of the subepithelial stroma and in the presence of bacteria leads to perichondritis and chondritis of the arytenoid and cricoid cartilages. Wound healing, as evidenced by granulation tissue and epithelial migration, is usually seen a few days after intubation, and in the majority of patients subglottic injury resolves without sequelae. However, in a small minority, subepithelial fibrosis, cricoid collapse, and organizing scar will lead to symptomatic subglottic stenosis.

Factors involved in the development of subglottic stenosis can be divided into those relating to tube

Table 36-2   Pathogenesis of Acquired Subglottic Stenosis

Mechanical Factors	Events	Systemic Factors
Duration of intubation Number of intubations Tube size Tube motion Mucosal drying	Shearing and pressure forces of tube Disruption of mucociliary clearance Mucosal erosion	 Vitamin A deficiency
	Edema	Fluid and electrolyte imbalance Congestive heart failure Hepatic failure GE reflux
	Perichondritis Ischemic necrosis	GE reflux Local and systemic infection
	Wound healing (granulation and reepithelialization)	Anemia Hypotension Hypoxia
Tracheotomy?	Fibrosis, mature stenosis	

trauma and those that influence edema formation and wound healing. Regarding tube trauma, well-designed prospective studies have consistently determined that intubation for longer than 7 to 10 days is the most significant factor. Frequent reintubations, spontaneous head motion in poorly sedated patients, and passive head motion during nursing care are factors that have been implicated in the development of acquired subglottic stenosis in retrospective studies. In addition more recent studies have described a higher risk of trauma in patients with hyaline membrane disease, presumably because of the need for larger tubes to sustain high ventilatory pressures and the pistonlike motion of the tube in response to mechanical ventilation. In older infants a presenting diagnosis of laryngotracheobronchitis has been associated with an increased risk for acquired subglottic stenosis, presumably because the already greatly narrowed and infected subglottis is more susceptible to tube trauma.

Factors that can influence edema formation in the injured glottic and subglottic larynx include liver failure, kidney disease, congestive heart failure, and fluid and electrolyte imbalance. Wound-healing influences include the presence of local or systemic infection, vitamin A deficiency, and poor tissue oxygenation secondary to systemic hypotension, hypoxia, or anemia.

Tracheal and Bronchial Sequelae

Tracheal stenosis can occur in much the same manner as acquired subglottic stenosis, although its incidence is far lower because of the larger relative size and increased pliability of the tracheal airway. Recently the phenomenon of acute airway obstruction secondary to massive desquamation of tracheal epithelium has been described. The entity of so-called necrotizing tracheobronchitis is more common with high-frequency jet ventilation, but it can also occur in intubated patients and can be seen as unexpected hypercarbia and poor chest motion with increasing ventilatory pressure and increasing air leak. Potential contributors to development of necrotizing tracheobronchitis include shock, local and systemic infection, high oxygen concentrations, and mucosal drying from too little humidity or from use of anesthetic gases. In addition tracheal and bronchial obstruction can occur as a result of epithelial injury from overzealous suctioning with catheters extending beyond the distal tip of the endotracheal tube.

The most common presentation is persistent right upper lobe or total right lung atelectasis secondary to granulation tissue in the proximal right mainstem bronchus.

MONITORING AND LABORATORY TESTS

After extubation all patients must be monitored closely for respiratory failure in an area in which intubation equipment and physicians skilled in intubation are immediately available. Extubated patients who develop progressive stridor, retractions, aphonia, or cyanosis must be carefully evaluated via blood gas analyses or noninvasive oxygen saturation and carbon dioxide determinations. Should an immediate or progressive deterioration in respiratory status necessitate reintubation, quick resolution of the distress by insertion of the tube is a strong indicator of upper airway obstructive pathology.

Flexible Laryngoscopy

Flexible laryngoscopy is an invaluable tool in the assessment of symptomatic patients after extubation. It allows detailed examination of the supraglottic and glottic larynx, and it often yields a strong impression about subglottic pathology. Prospective studies using flexible laryngoscopy have demonstrated significant airway disease in 40% to 50% of neonatal ICU patients at the time of extubation. Up to 8% of patients have been found to have severe obstructing lesions, including acquired subglottic stenoses, laryngeal webs, and true vocal cord paralysis.

Newborn and premature infants must be watched especially carefully for progressive development of upper airway obstruction hours after extubation. The initial laryngoscopic findings may be normal because of the stenting effect of the endotracheal tube, but subsequent laryngoscopy will show development of glottic and subglottic edema. These same infants are also more prone to acute upper airway obstruction secondary to the formation of firm subglottic scar or cysts weeks or months after extubation. Late obstruction usually manifests itself during an upper respiratory illness, and the clinician must always consider subglottic pathology in the differential diagnosis of any previously intubated child undergoing evaluation for recurrent or refractory airway disease. If flexible laryngoscopy is nondiagnostic in the patient with signs and symptoms of upper airway obstruction, the use of rigid bronchoscopy is indicated to evaluate the subglottic larynx and trachea.

TREATMENT

The treatment of postextubation sequelae is a team effort involving pediatricians, anesthesiologists, nurses, respiratory therapists, and airway surgeons. Close communication and cooperation between team members are essential for early diagnosis and appropriate successful treatment.

Medical Treatment of Postextubation Distress with Croupy Cough and Stridor

For treatment of postextubation distress withhold oral feedings and deep suctioning. Administer humidified cool mist with oxygen as needed for hypoxia. Monitor oxygen saturation and transcutaneous carbon dioxide if possible. For patients with inspiratory stridor administer racemic epinephrine by aerosol as follows:

1. For patients <20 kg, 0.25 ml in 3 to 5 ml saline solution
2. For patients 20 to 40 kg, 0.5 ml in 3 to 5 ml saline solution
3. For patients >40 kg, 0.75 ml in 3 to 5 ml saline solution

Racemic epinephrine treatments can be repeated as needed, usually every 2 to 4 hours. Monitor heart rate and ECG closely during the treatment to identify excess sympathetic stimulation (e.g., heart rate >200 bpm) and dysrhythmias. Recurrence of symptoms within 30 to 60 minutes of a treatment should alert the physician to the possible need for reintubation. Reintubation is preferably carried out in the operating room, with a surgical team ready to perform a tracheotomy if necessary. The efficacy of steroids for postextubation croup has not been proved in clinical studies to date.

Medical Management of Second and Subsequent Extubation Attempts

Administer dexamethasone (Decadron), 0.5 mg/kg up to a maximum of 4 mg, 6 hours before extubation, at the time of extubation, and at 6 and 12 hours after extubation. Although this is a standard recommendation, studies to prove the efficacy of the recommendation are currently being performed. Withhold feedings and administer aerosolized racemic epinephrine to the patient's nose and mouth immediately after extubation. The use of nasal continuous positive airway pressure may be attempted in young infants for a period of time to allow resolution of glottic and subglottic edema. Flexible laryngoscopy may be used to define the specific type and location of airway pathology. Always remember to monitor respiratory and cardiovascular variables as suggested previously.

Surgical Treatment

The key to successful surgical treatment of postintubation sequelae is the appropriate diagnosis of specific airway lesions with the use of flexible laryngoscopy and rigid bronchoscopy. Advances in surgical techniques, including the development of fiberoptic telescopes and the carbon dioxide laser, have allowed endoscopic treatment of many airway problems, including webs, granulations, and subglottic cysts. Tracheotomy is still the "gold standard" for relieving upper airway obstruction, and indications for its use are outlined in Chapter 136. Specifically, firm cicatricial subglottic stenosis resulting in obstruction is managed initially with a tracheotomy. If the stenosis fails to show signs of resolution with growth and development in the first year of life, surgical procedures designed to augment the circumference of the subglottis such as rib grafting can be undertaken.

Cricoid split

The cricoid splitting procedure, first described by Cotton and Seid in 1980, is designed to allow decannulation and avoid tracheotomy. Its use is indicated primarily for newborn and premature infants with extubation failure on the basis of soft, edematous subglottic stenosis that has not yet progressed to mature, firm fibrosis. The criteria for cricoid splitting are strict and include infants with the following:

1. At least two failed extubations
2. Weight ≥1500 g
3. Laryngeal pathology as stated above demonstrated by endoscopy
4. No need for assisted ventilation for at least 1 week
5. Need for <35% supplemental oxygen
6. No evidence of congestive heart failure for 1 month
7. No evidence of local or systemic infection

After surgery these patients are kept intubated and are given systemic broad-spectrum antibiotics for 10 days before extubation is attempted. Although many centers report good results in properly selected patients, the procedure is still new and must be used with caution.

ADDITIONAL READING

Abbott TR. Complications of prolonged nasotracheal intubation in children. Br J Anaesth 40:347-352, 1968.

Blanc VF, Tremblay NAG. The complications of tracheal intubation: A new classification with a review of the literature. Anesth Analg 53:202-212, 1974.

Brodsky L, Reidy M, Stanievich JF. The effects of suctioning techniques of the distal tracheal mucosa in intubated low birth weight infants. Int J Pediatr Otorhinolaryngol 14:1-14, 1987.

Cotton RT, Seid AB. Management of the extubation problem in the premature child: Anterior cricoid split as an alternative to tracheotomy. Ann Otol Rhinol Laryngol 89:508-511, 1980.

Dankle SK, Schuller DE, McClead RE. Prolonged intubation of neonates. Arch Otolaryngol 113:841-843, 1987.

• Donnelly WH. Histopathology of endotracheal intubation. Arch Pathol 88:511-520, 1969.

Drew JH. Immediate intubation at birth of the very-low-birth-weight infant. Am J Dis Child 136:207-210, 1982.

Fan LL, Flynn JW, Pathak DR. Risk factors in predicting laryngeal injury in intubated neonates. Crit Care Med 11:431-433, 1983.

Fan LL, Flynn JW, Pathak DR, Madden WA. Predictive value of stridor in detecting laryngeal injury in extubated neonates. Crit Care Med 10:453-455, 1982.

Gould SJ, Grahm JM. Acquired subglottic stenosis in neonates. Clin Otolaryngol 10:299-302, 1985.

Hilding AC. Laryngotracheal damage during intratracheal anesthesia. Ann Otol Rhinol Laryngol 80:565-581, 1971.

Jones R, Bodnar A, Roan Y, Johnson D. Subglottic stenosis in newborn intensive care unit graduates. Am J Dis Child 135:367-368, 1981.

Jordan WS, Graves CL, Elwyn RA. New therapy for postintubation laryngeal edema and tracheitis in children. JAMA 212:585-588, 1970.

Kiripalami H, Higa T, Perlman M, Friedberg J, Cutz E. Diagnosis and therapy of necrotizing tracheobronchitis in ventilated neonates. Crit Care Med 13:792-797, 1985.

Marshak G, Grundfast KM. Subglottic stenosis. Pediatr Clin North Am 28:941-946, 1981.

Orlowski JP, Ellis NG, Amin NP, Crumrine RS. Complications of airway intrusion in 100 consecutive cases in a pediatric ICU. Crit Care Med 8:324-331, 1980.

Othersen HB. Intubation injuries of the trachea in children. Ann Surg 189:601-606, 1979.

Postma DS, Prosma J, Woods CI, Sidman J, Pisslbury C. Use of steroids and a long-acting vasoconstrictor in the treatment of postintubation croup—a ferret model. Arch Otolaryngol 113:844-849, 1987.

• Pransky SM, Grundfast KM. Differentiating upper from lower airway compromise in neonates. Ann Otol Rhinol Laryngol 94:509-515, 1985.

Quiney RE, Gold SJ. Subglottic stenosis: A clinicopathological study. Clin Otolaryngol 10:315-327, 1985.

Stetson JB, Guess WL. Causes of damage to tissues by polymers and elastomers used in fabrication of tracheal devices. Anesthesiology 33:635-652, 1970.

Strong RM, Passy V. Endotracheal intubation. Arch Otolaryngol 103:329-335, 1977.

Zulliger JJ, Schuller DE, Beach TP, Garvin JP, Birck HG, Frank JE. Assessment of intubation in croup and epiglottitis. Ann Otol Rhinol Laryngol 91:403-406, 1982.

37 Bronchopulmonary Dysplasia

Ronald M. Perkin

BACKGROUND AND PHYSIOLOGY

Bronchopulmonary dysplasia (BPD) is a chronic respiratory disease of infants manifested by tachypnea, dyspnea, hypoxemia, and hypercapnia. Chest radiographic features are characteristic and include overinflation, with multiple cystic areas interspersed with linear densities due to collapse, fibrosis, or both. The disorder commonly follows the treatment of hyaline membrane disease with O_2 and positive pressure ventilation but also may follow pneumonia, meconium aspiration syndrome, tracheoesophageal fistula, and congenital heart disease. Thus it is likely that this form of chronic lung disease represents a nonspecific reaction of the lung to slowly resolving acute injury.

Although this disorder is characterized by profound lung damage during the neonatal period, the potential for improvement during early childhood exists. The underlying pathologic conditions are potentially treatable or reversible or produce secondary complications that are amenable to therapy. Most infants with BPD need rehospitalization during the first 2 to 3 years of life, frequently for respiratory tract symptoms, which often necessitate intensive care, support, and observation.

Pathologic involvement of the airways, parenchyma, and pulmonary vascular bed is extensive. Marked airway changes are found, including squamous metaplasia or necrosis of large and small airways, increased amounts of peribronchial smooth muscle and fibrosis, edematous submucosal glands, inflammatory cell infiltrates, and occasionally granulomatous obstructive lesions. Lung volume loss from atelectasis and fibrosis alternates with regions of hyperinflation of emphysema. Interstitial spaces are thickened with edema fluid, inflammatory cell infiltrates, and connective tissue proliferation.

Pulmonary function in patients with BPD can be characterized generally by rapid, shallow breathing patterns, increased dead space ventilation, decreased dynamic compliance, maldistribution of ventilation, and abnormal ventilation-perfusion matching. Infants with BPD characteristically have a marked increase in airways resistance. Many mechanisms can be responsible for this elevated airways resistance, including marked metaplasia of the bronchial epithelium with partial luminal obstruction; increased mucous production; inflammation or infection; decreased mucociliary clearance; mucosal edema; reactive bronchoconstriction; small airways closure at low lung volumes; and pulmonary vascular engorgement or edema.

Although airways obstruction in patients with BPD is often related to bronchial hyperactivity and small airways dysfunction, large airway injury can also contribute to acute respiratory exacerbations. If an infant's respiratory distress is atypical or unresponsive to the usual therapeutic maneuvers, airway lesions of the trachea and bronchial tree must be considered. The use of flexible bronchoscopy has documented a wide spectrum of laryngeal, tracheal, and bronchial lesions in infants with BPD. Demonstrated lesions include tracheomalacia, bronchomalacia, polyps, granulomas, and inspissated secretions. Early diagnosis of these abnormalities is useful because the therapies instituted in the treatment of such lesions may not be a usual part of the therapeutic regimen.

Patients with BPD have respiratory failure with varying degrees of hypoxemia, hypercapnia, and compensatory metabolic alkalosis. They often need supplemental O_2 to maintain a PaO_2 >55 mm Hg. The amount and duration of O_2 therapy vary with the severity of pulmonary damage. The O_2 requirement decreases gradually as the disease process improves but increases during feedings, physical activity, sleep states, or episodes of pulmonary infection or edema.

Pulmonary hypertension apparently contributes significantly to the morbidity and mortality of infants with BPD. The pulmonary circulation is characterized by elevation of vascular resistance and abnormal vasoreactivity, reflecting both structural and functional abnormalities. Structural abnormalities include intimal proliferation, medial muscle thickening, peripheral extension of smooth muscle to intra-acinar vessels, adventitial edema and fibrosis, and occasional thrombo-obliterative vascular changes. The bronchial circulation is often dilated and tortuous. Infants with BPD have an exaggerated pulmonary vasoconstrictor response to acute hypoxia. Elevated right ventricular afterload leads to cor pulmonale or perhaps left ventricular dysfunction, which adversely affects ventilation-perfusion matching, promotes pulmonary edema, and further decreases oxygenation.

There is a high incidence of left ventricular hypertrophy in many of the older or sick infants with BPD. Chronic hypoxia, systemic hypertension, chronic adrenergic stimulation from stress or drug therapy, cor pulmonale, or metabolic and nutritional factors are suggested mechanisms for the development of left ventricular hypertrophy.

Infants with BPD admitted to the intensive care unit with acute respiratory symptoms present a difficult diagnostic and therapeutic problem because of the severity and complexity of their cardiorespiratory disease. The usual presenting symptoms of increased respiratory distress with cyanosis and wheezing may result from a multitude of factors, many of which are interrelated. Diagnosis, monitoring, and therapy

must be instituted promptly to interrupt potentially lethal cycles and prevent intubation and mechanical ventilation of a child with underlying severe lung disease. Although initiation of mechanical ventilation is inevitable in some infants, the focus of this discussion is the spontaneously breathing infant with BPD and acute respiratory symptoms.

MONITORING AND LABORATORY TESTS
Respiratory System

Continuous observation for retractions, flaring, fatigue, and apnea is necessary. The quality of air movement and the presence of wheezing and rales must be recorded. Any acute change must be reported and investigated.

Measure and record inspired O_2 concentration every 2 to 3 hours and initiate continuous pulse oximetry. Record circumstances of any decrease in O_2 saturation. Obtain capillary or arterial blood samples on admission and then as indicated for measurement of gas tension and pH. An acceptable limit for $Paco_2$ is up to 60 mm Hg. In some cases higher $Paco_2$ levels must be accepted, depending on each infant's degree of illness, history, and previous blood gas values.

Obtain a chest roentgenogram on admission and as needed to evaluate hyperinflation, atelectasis, edema, and heart size. If possible, prior chest roentgenograms should be obtained for comparison. Perform pulmonary function testing if possible. Observe the patient closely for an increase in secretions obtained when suctioning and obtain cultures as indicated.

Institute a "minimal touch" policy, organizing care and monitoring (nursing, respiratory, laboratory) so the infant is disturbed as little as possible.

Cardiovascular System

Obtain an ECG and echocardiogram to assess cardiac function and estimate pulmonary arterial blood pressure. Observe the patient for signs of right heart failure, including such signs as edema, weight gain, oliguria, tachycardia, tachypnea, and increased O_2 requirements. Cardiac catheterization may be indicated to accurately measure pulmonary arterial blood pressures, identify anatomy, and assess response to O_2 and other vasodilators.

Renal-Metabolic Status

Obtain serum electrolyte samples initially and as needed, especially in infants receiving long-term di-

---

> POSSIBLE CONTRIBUTIONS
> TO ACUTE RESPIRATORY DISTRESS
> IN INFANTS WITH BPD
>
> Bronchospasm
> Airway abnormalities
>   Mucous plugging
>   Bronchomalacia
>   Granuloma
>   Stenosis
> Infection and inflammation
> Aspiration pneumonia
> Pulmonary edema
> Pulmonary hypertensive crisis
> Agitation
> Heart failure

uretics. Assess the nutritional status and liver and renal function. Weigh the infant at least daily and investigate excessive weight gains (i.e., >30 g/day in infants <12 months of age).

TREATMENT
Respiratory System

Oxygen. O_2 is the most essential medication; proper O_2 therapy can decrease the work of breathing, improve weight gain, and reduce pulmonary vascular resistance. Supplemental O_2 therapy is indicated in infants when the Pao_2 is <55 mm Hg or the O_2 saturation is <90% at rest. O_2 therapy does not produce respiratory depression in infants with chronic lung damage. It can be administered via a hood, tent, face mask, or nasal catheter. Requirements may vary, depending on illness, agitation, feeding, or sleeping. The state of oxygenation must be continuously or frequently monitored and Fio_2 adjusted to maintain O_2 saturation >90%. Unrecognized and untreated hypoxemia has been proposed as one mechanism by which chronic pulmonary hypertension develops in patients with advanced lung disease. O_2 therapy will probably be indicated for several months or even years; therefore arrangements to provide O_2 for home use must be part of discharge planning.

Methylxanthines. Infants with BPD have bronchiolar smooth muscle hypertrophy and hyperactive airways, and bronchodilators improve pulmonary function in these infants. Methylxanthines may improve the function of respiratory muscles and central ventilatory drive in addition to relaxing bronchial smooth muscle and stimulating ciliary motility. Worrisome side effects include gastrointestinal irritation, reduced esophageal sphincter pressure, irritability, vomiting, and alteration in sleep patterns. These complications may contribute to nutritional and respiratory problems. Careful dosing must be done and adjusted according to blood levels of theophylline.

Inhaled medications (see also Chapter 133). Aerosolized β-adrenergic agents may prove beneficial and in general should be used before other bronchodilators because of their effectiveness and relative safety. Recent data show that inhaled atropine may improve small airways function in some infants with BPD. Inflammation may play an important role in mediating pulmonary edema formation and in altering bronchial vascular reactivity. Preliminary data indicate that cromolyn therapy may prove useful in reducing the effects of inflammation.

Corticosteroids. Corticosteroids suppress inflammation and the release of chemical mediators that may trigger bronchospasm. These drugs also increase responsiveness to β-adrenergic agonists. Benefits of steroid therapy in nonventilator-dependent infants with BPD have not been assessed. Short-term steroid use during acute episodes of wheezing and bronchospasm may be useful, just as it is in older children with asthma. Long-term steroid use is discouraged.

Percussion and postural drainage. In general infants with BPD have difficulty clearing secretions, and during acute illness when secretions are more copious, they need frequent percussion, postural drainage, and suctioning to prevent mucous plugging and atelectasis.

Antimicrobial therapy. Infants with BPD are at risk for developing respiratory failure with viral or bacterial infections. If pneumonia or bronchitis is suspected, cultures must be obtained and appropriate antibiotics started. During the peak respiratory syncytial virus season, nasal washings must be sent for serologic diagnostic testing and ribavirin therapy initiated when respiratory syncytial virus preparations are positive.

Cardiovascular System

Fluid management. Infants with BPD tolerate excessive or even normal amounts of fluid intake poorly and tend to accumulate fluid in the interstitium of the lung.

Fluid administration must be limited to the minimum needed to provide necessary calories for the infants' metabolic needs and growth. It is important to provide patients in respiratory distress (for whatever reason) with an adequate O_2-carrying capacity. The hematocrit level is maintained at approximately 40%. Blood transfusions are administered over 2 to 3 hours; bolus IV infusions (>10 ml/kg/hr) are avoided.

Diuretics. When increased lung water persists despite fluid restriction, diuretic therapy can be used. The use of furosemide (1 to 2 mg/kg/dose IV) is associated with improvement in lung compliance and a decrease in airways resistance, but gas exchange is usually unaffected. The beneficial effects of furosemide on lung function appear to be in part nondiuretic in nature and due to nonrenal effects either in the lung or in the systemic circulation.

Long-term furosemide use is associated with many complications. Electrolyte imbalance, alteration in calcium and phosphate homeostasis, renal stone formation, and undesirable effects on bone growth have been described. In addition furosemide-induced hypochloremia will promote bicarbonate retention, which is an undesirable effect in patients with chronic hypercarbic respiratory failure. Oral therapy with chlorothiazide (15 to 40 mg/kg/day) or a combination of chlorothiazide and spironolactone (2 to 4 mg/kg/day) results in a diuresis equivalent to that from furosemide therapy but may not provide equal improvement in lung function. Overzealous use of diuretics resulting in volume contraction may decrease cardiac output and stimulate neurohormonal systems much like antidiuretic hormone or catecholamines, which may be detrimental.

Vasodilators. Despite O_2 administration, pulmonary hypertension often persists and prevents acceptable cardiac function and interferes with gas exchange. Although vasodilator therapy may be beneficial in decreasing pulmonary arterial blood pressure in selected patients, if cardiac output falls or ventilation-perfusion ratios become more abnormal, the net effect on O_2 delivery may be detrimental. Vasodilators such as hydralazine are not selective for the pulmonary circulation and can potentially worsen hypoxemia, increase pulmonary edema, and cause systemic hypotension.

Cardiac catheterization is useful in determining the hemodynamic response to vasodilator therapy, and it can rule out congenital heart disease and assess whether significant shunting through collateral vessels is present. In the presence of elevated systemic arterial blood pressure and decreased cardiac output, vasodilator therapy may lead to an overall improvement in cardiac output and hence pulmonary blood flow.

Digitalis. The use of digitalis preparations in patients with chronic pulmonary diseases is controversial and lacks firm experimental support. Although digitalis increases myocardial contractility, the inotrope may also increase pulmonary vascular resistance and right ventricular afterload.

Nutritional Support

Poor nutritional status can adversely affect cardiopulmonary function by impairing respiratory muscle function, ventilatory drive, and pulmonary defense mechanisms. These adverse effects are additive in patients with respiratory failure and increase morbidity and mortality. Patients with BPD often suffer from inadequate caloric intake. Frequent episodes of pneumonia, sepsis, and bronchospasm often necessitate discontinuing oral feeding for days to weeks. Giving constant attention to provision of adequate calories for growth is critical. In addition patients with BPD have increased caloric requirements and O_2 consumption. The requirement of 100 to 120 cal/kg/day for growth in normal infants is inadequate for these patients, many of whom need 130 to 150 cal/kg/day or more. If severe fluid restriction limits caloric intake, judicious use of diuretics can be instituted to permit larger volumes of feeding. Food supplements such as Polycose can be used to increase the caloric density of the feeds. However, the increased osmotic load may result in diarrhea or insufficient free water to maintain normal renal function. Attention must also be given to requirements for iron, vitamins, and mineral supplementation.

Total parenteral nutrition delivered by means of a central venous catheter can be initiated early and at any time oral intake is compromised. Hyperalimentation with high carbohydrate load must be given cautiously to patients whose impaired pulmonary function limits their ability to handle increased CO_2 production.

Infants with BPD commonly have feeding difficulties, which are often exacerbated by acute respiratory symptoms. These difficulties may be caused by gastroesophageal reflux, prolonged gastric emptying time, rumination, or bulbar dysfunction, causing food inhalation on swallowing. Recognition of recurrent inhalations can sometimes lead to a dramatic improvement after institution of appropriate medical or surgical therapy. Infants with inhalation because of bulbar dysfunction may benefit from bypassing the swallowing mechanism temporarily through nasogastric or gastrostomy feedings. Infants with recurrent inhalation caused by gastroesophageal reflux may also benefit from bypassing the swallowing mechanism temporarily through nasogastric or gastrostomy feedings and from therapy with metoclopramide (0.1 to 0.2 mg/kg/dose), with the exact dosage titrated by pH probe. Fundoplication occasionally is necessary. The condition of infants with rumination often improves when the same caretaker is allowed to participate consistently in feedings.

Abnormalities resulting from complications arising during the neonatal period may seriously affect the overall nutritional management of infants with BPD. Examples include IV hyperalimentation–induced damage to liver and gallbladder and the residual effects of necrotizing enterocolitis with or without bowel resection.

Behavioral and Developmental Support

Many behavioral, physiologic, and autonomic effects are apparent in infants with BPD. Common characteristics include excessive drops in O_2 saturation secondary to external stimuli, skin mottling, difficulty in temperature regulation, and poor tolerance to any nursing procedure. In the absence of hypoxemia administering doses of sedative medications may facilitate management (chloral hydrate, 25 to 50 mg/kg/dose). All care must be organized so that the infant is disturbed as little as possible, and the infant needs to be involved in an infant-developmental intervention program.

ADDITIONAL READING

Abman SH. The Aspen conference on bronchopulmonary dysplasia. Pediatr Pulmonol 3:185-196, 1987.

Abman SH, Wolfe RR, Accurso FJ, et al. Pulmonary vascular response to oxygen in infants with severe bronchopulmonary dysplasia. Pediatrics 75:80-84, 1985.

Bancalari E, Gerhardt T. Bronchopulmonary dysplasia. Pediatr Clin North Am 33:1-23, 1986.

Berman W, Katz R, Yabek SM, et al. Long-term follow-up of bronchopulmonary dysplasia. J Pediatr 109:45-50, 1986.

Engelhardt B, Elliot S, Hazinski T. Short and long term effects of furosemide on lung function in infants with bronchopulmonary dysplasia. J Pediatr 109:1034-1039, 1986.

• Farrell PM, Taussig LM, eds. Bronchopulmonary dysplasia and related chronic respiratory disorders. Columbus, Ohio: Ross Laboratories, 1986.

Goodman G, Perkin RM, Anas NG, et al. Pulmonary hypertension in infants with bronchopulmonary dysplasia. J Pediatr 112:67-71, 1988.

Groothius JR, Rosenberg AA. Home oxygen promotes weight gain in infants with bronchopulmonary dysplasia. Am J Dis Child 141:992-995, 1987.

Guiftre RM, Rubin S, Mitchell I. Antireflux surgery in infants with bronchopulmonary dysplasia. Am J Dis Child 141:648-651, 1987.

Hazinski TA. Furosemide decreases ventilation in young rabbits. J Pediatr 106:81-85, 1985.

Kao LL, Warburton D, Sargent CW, et al. Furosemide acutely decreases airways resistance in chronic bronchopulmonary dysplasia. J Pediatr 103:624-629, 1983.

• Koops BL, Abman SH, Accurso FJ. Outpatient management and follow-up of bronchopulmonary dysplasia. Clin Perinatol 11:101-122, 1984.

Miller RW, Woo P, Kellman RK, et al. Tracheobronchial abnormalities in infants with bronchopulmonary dysplasia. J Pediatr 111:779-782, 1987.

• Nickerson BG. Bronchopulmonary dysplasia: Chronic pulmonary disease following neonatal respiratory failure. Chest 87:528-535, 1985.

• O'Brodovich HM, Mellins RB. Bronchopulmonary dysplasia: Unresolved neonatal acute lung injury. Am Rev Respir Dis 132:694-709, 1985.

Perkin RM, Anas NG. Pulmonary hypertension in pediatric patients. J Pediatr 105:511-522, 1984.

Pingleton SK, Harmon GS. Nutritional management in acute respiratory failure. JAMA 257:3094-3099, 1987.

Roberts RJ. Pharmacologic approaches to the prevention and treatment of bronchopulmonary dysplasia. Respir Care 31:581-590, 1986.

Sauve RS, Singhal N. Long-term morbidity of infants with bronchopulmonary dysplasia. Pediatrics 76:725-733, 1985.

Sibbald WJ, Driedger AA, Cunningham DG, et al. Right and left ventricular performance in acute hypoxemic respiratory failure. Crit Care Med 14:852-857, 1986.

Vandenplus Y, DeWolf D, Sacre L. Influence of xanthines on gastroesophageal reflux in infants at risk for sudden infant death syndrome. Pediatrics 77:807-810, 1986.

Weinstein MR, Oh W. Oxygen consumption in infants with bronchopulmonary dysplasia. J Pediatr 99:958-961, 1981.

38 Cyanotic Congenital Heart Disease and Neonatal Polycythemia

Edgar A. Newfeld

Cyanotic Congenital Heart Disease

BACKGROUND AND PHYSIOLOGY

A patient with cyanotic congenital heart disease is usually initially seen in the PICU as a newborn; therefore this chapter is directed toward the diagnosis and management of the cyanotic newborn. These infants have central cyanosis noted at birth or soon thereafter. Central cyanosis results from cardiac right-to-left shunts or from a ventilatory insufficiency and intrapulmonary right-to-left shunt secondary to pulmonary parenchymal disease. When pulmonary disease is the cause, usually the $PaCO_2$ is elevated, and the chest roentgenogram often reveals pulmonary parenchymal abnormalities. The infant with cyanotic heart disease usually has a normal $PaCO_2$ and clear lungs (unless congestive heart failure is present), and the PaO_2 can range from 20 to 50 mm Hg, with no significant improvement produced by increasing the FiO_2. Other seriously ill neonates can have cyanosis secondary to hypoventilation or apnea produced by hypocalcemia, hypoglycemia, and sepsis and low cardiac output and/or shock.

Use of new techniques, with optimization of oxygenation and cardiac output, can help to stabilize satisfactorily a cyanotic infant born in a primary or secondary care medical facility and can help in transferring him safely to a tertiary care facility for further diagnosis and management.

Mild degrees of arterial unsaturation (PaO_2 of 40 to 60 mm Hg) are usually well tolerated by the newborn, but PaO_2 in the 20 to 30 mm Hg range can result in tissue hypoxia and metabolic acidosis. In the latter case the patient represents an emergency

and needs prompt diagnosis and treatment to prevent clinical deterioration and death.

MONITORING AND LABORATORY TESTS

Noncardiac causes of cyanosis can be excluded by appropriate laboratory tests. Ruling out methemoglobinemia is necessary (see Chapter 49). Routinely obtaining serum glucose and calcium levels, complete blood count, and temperature determinations on all neonates admitted to the PICU is necessary. Sepsis must be considered in all ill neonates, and cultures must be drawn before beginning antibiotic treatment. A complete physical examination with an emphasis on the cardiovascular system should be performed after taking the patient's history and obtaining baseline laboratory tests essential to adequate diagnosis. Cardiac monitoring with display of the ECG heart rate is mandatory.

Chest Roentgenogram

A chest roentgenogram can help exclude pulmonary disease and congenital anomalies of the respiratory tract. It also demonstrates the heart size and shape and whether the pulmonary vascularity is increased, normal, or decreased.

Electrocardiogram

An ECG can show cardiac chamber enlargement and suggest certain specific defects. In addition it can rule out dysrhythmias.

Echocardiogram

State-of-the-art improvement in imaging quality and the use of Doppler flow studies have made echocardiography the diagnostic technique of choice for the cyanotic newborn; in many cases it can even replace the need for cardiac catheterization before surgical treatment. Exact anatomic and hemodynamic diagnosis is usually possible if probes designed for the small infant or neonate are used.

Arterial Blood Gas Tensions and pH

Blood gas studies can indicate the presence of pulmonary disease (elevated $PaCO_2$), metabolic acidosis, and the degree of hypoxemia. Increasing the FIO_2 usually will not increase the PaO_2 by more than 10 to 15 mm Hg in a patient with cyanotic heart disease, but with pulmonary disease the PaO_2 may increase more than 100 mm Hg.

Hemoglobin and Hematocrit

The hemoglobin and hematocrit determinations can rule out neonatal polycythemia (see below), which can clinically mimic cyanotic heart disease. Cardiorespiratory symptoms such as tachypnea and congestive heart failure can be seen when the hemoglobin is 20 to 25 g/dl and the hematocrit is 65% to 70% or greater.

Cardiac Catheterization

Before the modern improvements in echocardiography, cardiac catheterization was considered the definitive diagnostic test for cyanotic congenital heart disease. It is still needed in certain neonates, often when intracardiac repair is contemplated, and in some infants needing systemic-pulmonary shunts (see below).

DIAGNOSIS AND MANAGEMENT OF SPECIFIC CARDIAC DEFECTS

In general patients with various forms of obstruction of pulmonary blood flow are not in congestive heart failure and usually do not need digoxin or diuretics. Often an immediate increase in pulmonary blood flow can be lifesaving in a severely hypoxemic infant and can be accomplished by a prostaglandin E_1 (PGE_1) infusion at a dose of 0.05 μg/kg/min to maintain or increase patency of the ductus arteriosus. PGE_1 is a potent vasodilator, and ductal tissue is extremely sensitive to its action. If this infusion is begun at a referring center, careful observation and maintenance of ventilation during transport are essential since PGE_1 can produce apnea.

Patients with increased pulmonary blood flow may

be in congestive heart failure and may benefit from receiving diuretics and from beginning digitalization before transport to the tertiary center for definitive diagnosis and treatment.

Lesions With Diminished Pulmonary Blood Flow
Tetralogy of Fallot

Pathophysiology. Pulmonary blood flow in patients with tetralogy of Fallot is reduced by pulmonary stenosis, both infundibular and valvar, and a right-to-left shunt occurs through a large, high ventricular septal defect (VSD). Aortic overriding of the VSD is common.

History. These patients usually are not severely cyanotic at birth and may be first seen in the PICU at several months of age, perhaps because of a hypercyanotic "Tet spell," characterized by a marked increase in cyanosis, irritability, and tachypnea, often followed by limpness and/or sleep or loss of consciousness. A severe spell can produce brain damage because of the dramatic fall in PaO_2 values.

Physical examination. Cyanosis, a systolic ejection murmur at the middle left sternal border, and an accentuated right ventricular (RV) impulse are typical. The second heart sound (S_2) may be single or may split with a diminished pulmonic component.

Laboratory tests. A boot-shaped heart and decreased pulmonary vascular markings are common features of the chest roentgenogram, and a right aortic arch is seen in 20% to 40% of patients. The ECG reveals right axis deviation (RAD) and right ventricular hypertrophy (RVH). The echocardiogram will show the large VSD with aortic overriding and the pulmonic stenosis (Doppler study).

Cardiac catheterization. The angiocardiogram is characteristic and is usually only performed in early infancy if a shunt operation (systemic-pulmonary artery shunt) is needed to visualize the pulmonary artery anatomy so that the surgeon can select the best surgical approach.

Management. Administering morphine sulfate (0.1 mg IM), providing oxygen by face mask, and placing the infant in a prone knee-chest position are used to treat the Tet spell. Propranolol (1 to 4 mg/kg/day in three or four divided doses by mouth) is used to reduce the frequency of the spells and may eliminate them in some patients. Physicians at some centers use this treatment as palliation until the infant reaches a size for intracardiac repair, although physicians at other centers suggest performing a shunt operation as palliation. Intracardiac repair is usually delayed until the patient is 2 or 3 years old or until he weighs 10 kg since intracardiac repair in early infancy has a higher surgical mortality rate.

Pulmonary atresia with VSD (pseudotruncus)

Pathophysiology. In this lesion there is complete atresia of the RV outflow tract and/or pulmonary valve. Pulmonary blood flow is supplied by the patent ductus arteriosus (PDA) or bronchial collateral vessel, and there is a right-to-left shunt through a large VSD. This is considered to be an extreme form of tetralogy of Fallot.

History. Cyanosis is present usually from birth and can be marked except for patients with large collateral vessels.

Physical examination. Cyanosis, an RV impulse, an ejection click caused by a dilated aorta, a soft continuous murmur at the base or in the back, and a single S_2 are typical findings.

Laboratory tests. Analysis of the chest roentgenogram usually reveals a boot-shaped heart with decreased pulmonary vascular markings and possibly a right aortic arch. The ECG shows RVH. The echocardiogram will demonstrate the large VSD and aortic overriding, and the Doppler study will show absence of antegrade flow from RV outflow into the main pulmonary artery or even an atretic pulmonary valve.

Cardiac catheterization. Aortic root angiography will show the collateral vessels or a PDA supplying the pulmonary arteries (which may or may not be confluent). The RV angiogram shows a right-to-left shunt through the VSD and the pulmonary atresia.

Management. PGE_1 infusion is often used to maintain ductal patency until surgery can be done. A systemic-pulmonary shunt operation is performed to establish more reliable pulmonary blood flow, and this is often an emergency procedure. Corrective surgery using a pulmonary homograft or Dacron tube and VSD closure is deferred until the patient is older.

Pulmonary atresia without VSD

Pathophysiology. The pulmonary valve is atretic, the right ventricle is usually quite hypoplastic, and a right-to-left atrial shunt is present. The pulmonary blood flow is via a PDA.

History. Patients are markedly cyanotic at birth, and rapid deterioration is common when the PDA shunt diminishes.

Physical examination. Marked cyanosis, no murmur or a soft continuous murmur, and a single S_2 are found.

Laboratory tests. Arterial blood gas studies reveal Pao_2 in the 20 to 30 mm Hg range. The chest roentgenogram demonstrates a normal-sized heart and oligemic lung fields. The ECG reveals normal or left axis deviation (RAD is normal for a newborn) and relative left ventricular hypertrophy (LVH) for age without the usual RV potential expected for a newborn. The echocardiogram reveals an atretic pulmonary valve and small RV cavity. An atrial septal defect (ASD) with right-to-left shunt is always present on a Doppler study.

Cardiac catheterization. The RV angiogram is diagnostic, showing the small RV cavity and the atretic pulmonary valve. A balloon atrial septostomy is done to ensure unobstructed interatrial communication.

Management. A PGE_1 infusion is used until a systemic-pulmonary shunt operation can be performed. RV outflow reconstruction or pulmonary valvotomy can restore flow through the pulmonary artery and promote RV cavity growth in some cases, ultimately leading to corrective surgery.

Critical pulmonary valve stenosis

Pathophysiology. This condition is similar to pulmonary atresia without VSD with only a small amount of flow across the severely stenotic pulmonary valve. The RV cavity may be hypoplastic or may be dilated if congestive heart failure is present. A PDA is often present, and a right-to-left shunt through a patent foramen ovale or ASD produces cyanosis. Tricuspid regurgitation may be present.

History. Cyanosis and a heart murmur are noted from birth.

Physical examination. Findings include cyanosis of a variable degree, a systolic ejection murmur at the base, and possibly a blowing systolic murmur at the lower left sternal border if tricuspid regurgitation is present. A single S_2 or split heart sound with a very soft pulmonic component is typical. Hepatomegaly and peripheral edema can result from RV failure.

Laboratory tests. A chest roentgenogram reveals oligemic lung fields and either a normal-sized heart or globular cardiomegaly. The ECG reveals RAD, right atrial hypertrophy (RAH), and severe RVH or absent RV potential if the right ventricle is hypoplastic as in pulmonary atresia. The echocardiogram reveals a relatively immobile pulmonary valve, a hypertrophied right ventricle, and an ASD or patent foramen ovale. Doppler studies reveal high-frequency flow through the stenotic valve and a right-to-left atrial shunt.

Cardiac catheterization. The RV pressure can be suprasystemic, and the angiogram demonstrates a thickened dome-shaped pulmonic valve with a small jet of dye passing through it.

Management. If the RV cavity is of adequate size, a systemic-pulmonary shunt is performed; a systemic-pulmonary shunt is done in addition to the valvotomy if the right ventricle is hypoplastic. The ASD may need closure at a later date. Recent reports have indicated successful emergency treatment with balloon pulmonary valvuloplasty during the cardiac catheterization. This procedure carries substantial risk in inexperienced hands, especially when performed on very young infants.

Tricuspid atresia

Pathophysiology. In a patient with tricuspid atresia there is no tricuspid orifice, and the systemic venous blood passes from the right to the left atrium through an ASD. A VSD (small, moderate, or rarely large in size) shunts blood into the hypoplastic right ventricle and into the pulmonary artery. Pulmonary blood flow is usually diminished except when the VSD is large. A PDA may be present.

History. Cyanosis is usually noted at birth or soon thereafter. PDA closure will often result in significant clinical deterioration.

Physical examination. A VSD or PDA murmur and cyanosis are typical findings.

Laboratory tests. The chest roentgenogram will usually show decreased pulmonary vascularity without significant cardiomegaly. The ECG will reveal left axis deviation (LAD), LVH for age, and an absence of the expected RV forces. An echocardiogram can establish the anatomic diagnosis, and a two-dimensional Doppler study will reveal a right-to-left atrial shunt and other details. The tricuspid valve will be absent.

Cardiac catheterization. Angiograms are helpful in demonstrating the VSD and the pulmonary artery anatomy. Balloon atrial septostomy will ensure unobstructed atrial shunting.

Management. A systemic-pulmonary arterial shunt operation will improve the pulmonary blood flow and is often needed as an emergency procedure, although the use of PGE_1 can maintain ductal patency in the younger infant.

Ebstein's malformation of the tricuspid valve

Pathophysiology. The tricuspid valve annulus is displaced downward into the right ventricular cavity, and the valve tissue often adheres to the ventricular wall, producing tricuspid insufficiency of a significant degree. The increased pressure and flow in the right atrium produces a right-to-left atrial shunt through the foramen ovale, and therefore pulmonary blood flow is diminished. Occasionally pulmonic stenosis can be present as well, but this is uncommon. Severe tricuspid regurgitation can produce congestive heart failure in some neonates.

History. Cyanosis can be present at birth or soon thereafter, and some neonates are initially seen with marked cyanosis and congestive heart failure.

Physical examination. Cyanosis, a gallop rhythm (triple or quadruple sounds), a blowing regurgitant systolic murmur, and occasionally a diastolic murmur are found. Peripheral edema and hepatomegaly are present when congestive heart failure is marked.

Laboratory tests. Marked cardiomegaly and diminished pulmonary markings are found on the chest roentgenogram. The ECG shows RAD, RAH, and right bundle-branch block pattern in some patients. The echocardiogram will reveal the downward displacement of the tricuspid valve and large right atrium. Doppler study demonstrates tricuspid regurgitation, right-to-left atrial shunt, antegrade flow through the pulmonary valve (ruling out pulmonary atresia), and a PDA when present.

Cardiac catheterization. Cardiac catheterization is usually not needed after an adequate two-dimensional echocardiogram and a Doppler flow study, but angiograms of the right atrium and left ventricle are occasionally needed to rule out other anomalies.

Management. Digitalization and diuretic therapy may be useful in treating the neonate with congestive heart failure. Surgical treatment is usually not indicated in the neonate as long as pulmonary atresia has been excluded.

Other lesions

Pulmonary stenosis or atresia can be associated with complex single ventricle or other complex lesions, and complete discussions of these conditions can be found in standard textbooks of pediatric cardiology. Treatment usually consists of a systemic-pulmonary shunt operation in the very cyanotic neonate, and PGE_1 infusion will promote ductal patency until surgery can be performed.

Lesions With Increased Pulmonary Blood Flow

Complete transposition of the great vessels

Pathophysiology. The origins of both great arteries are reversed (i.e., the aorta arises from the right ventricle and the pulmonary artery from the left ventricle). Intracardiac mixing of oxygenated and unoxygenated blood occurs at either the atrial level (patent foramen ovale), the ventricular level (ventricular septal defect present in approximately 50% of cases), or the great vessel level (PDA) to sustain life. If mixing is inadequate, severe cyanosis leads to metabolic acidosis, deterioration, and death within the first few days or weeks of life. A large PDA or VSD will improve oxygenation but usually causes markedly increased pulmonary blood flow, pulmonary hypertension, and congestive heart failure.

History. Cyanosis, usually marked, is present from birth and is unaffected by the administration of oxygen or assisted ventilation in the case of inadequate intracardiac mixing. The birth history is usually normal.

Physical examination. Marked cyanosis, an accentuated right ventricular impulse, often no cardiac murmur, and generally a lack of respiratory distress are found. A single loud S_2 is common. Mild tachypnea is occasionally present, but except for this and the cyanosis some infants can appear quite comfortable and normal for the first few days of life.

Laboratory tests. Classically (approximately 40% to 50% of cases), the chest roentgenogram reveals an egg-shaped heart with increased pulmonary blood flow, but it can be normal in many neonates. Pao_2 is usually <35 mm Hg unless a VSD or PDA is present and can be in the 20 to 30 mm Hg range in some infants. Rarely patients with D-transposition of the great vessels and concurrent persistent pulmonary hypertension of the newborn will shunt large volumes of highly oxygenated blood from the pulmonary artery via the PDA to the aorta (anatomic right-to-left), resulting in much higher aortic Pao_2 values. The descending aortic Pao_2 may be as high as 200 mm Hg in these patients. The ECG, revealing RAD and RVH, is usually within normal limits for a newborn. The two-dimensional echocardiogram shows the anterior aorta arising from the right ventricle and any other associated defects.

Cardiac catheterization. Angiograms of each ventricle reveal the anatomy and associated defects. Balloon atrial septostomy is performed during catheterization to create an adequate-sized ASD to allow favorable intracardiac mixing unless the infant is scheduled for prompt intracardiac repair (arterial switch operation).

Management. Balloon atrial septostomy provides palliation and will usually increase Pao_2 into the 30 to 40 mm Hg range. Metabolic acidosis must be corrected. A PGE_1 infusion can be used before balloon atrial septostomy if severe cyanosis and metabolic acidosis threaten life; however, if the infant is comfortable and in no immediate difficulty, it should not be used routinely, since hypotension and apnea are its side effects. The PGE_1 increases pulmonary blood flow and dilates the ductus arteriosus, both of which can increase systemic oxygenation by an interatrial shunt and ductus shunt, respectively. If inadequate palliation follows balloon atrial septostomy because of an inadequate size of interatrial communication (echocardiogram can define the size of the ASD and the presence of bidirectional shunting), repeat septostomy or emergency surgery to increase the size of the atrial defect (i.e., atrial septectomy) is indicated. If inadequate pulmonary blood flow is the reason for a decreased bidirectional atrial shunt, intracardiac repair can be done, including a venous redirection procedure (Mustard or Senning operation) or an arterial switch procedure. Physicians at some centers routinely perform arterial switch (Jatene operation) procedures during the neonatal period; this procedure involves transecting both the aorta and main pulmonary artery and anastomosing the aorta to the left ventricle and the pulmonary artery to the right ventricle.

Total anomalous pulmonary venous drainage

Pathophysiology. In this lesion the pulmonary veins do not connect directly to the left atrium and instead join together to form a common vein that drains to one of several sites carrying the pulmonary venous blood into the right side of the heart. The common forms of drainage are supracardiac, including a vertical vein that empties into the innominate vein; cardiac, with the veins draining to the coronary sinus or draining directly into the right atrium; combinations of these forms; and infracardiac, usually draining into the portal venous system via a common pulmonary vein passing down through the diaphragm. The pulmonary venous drainage can be obstructed to some degree anywhere along its pathway back to the heart in any type of drainage. The oxygenated and nonoxygenated blood mix completely in the right atrium, and the systemic blood flow depends on a right-to-left atrial shunt. In the case of significant pulmonary venous obstruction (all cases of infradiaphragmatic drainage) there is severe pulmonary venous congestion in the lungs, with pulmonary venous and pulmonary arterial hypertension often to suprasystemic levels. In the absence of venous obstruction there is markedly increased pulmonary blood flow, and congestive heart failure is common.

History. This lesion is often confused with respiratory distress (e.g., hyaline membrane disease) of a pulmonary origin because of tachypnea and cyanosis noted soon after birth. This mistaken impression often leads to intubation and management with assisted mechanical ventilation, and clinical improvement to some degree is common. The cardiac origin of the problem often does not become evident until attempts are made to wean the infant from ventilatory support.

Physical examination. Dyspnea, tachypnea, cyanosis, a gallop rhythm, an accentuated RV impulse, a loud S_2 (may be single), and occasionally systolic and diastolic murmurs are found. If pulmonary venous obstruction is present, hepatomegaly and pulmonary rales may be present.

Laboratory tests. The ECG usually shows RAD, RAH, and severe RVH. The chest roentgenogram is characteristic when there is obstruction to the pulmonary venous drainage, showing marked pulmonary venous congestion but with a heart often normal in size. The neonate is often misdiagnosed as having hyaline membrane disease because of the similarity in appearance of the diffuse reticular congestion that occurs in both conditions. An echocardiogram shows absence of connection of the left pulmonary veins to the left atrium, right-to-left atrial shunt, and the common pulmonary vein posterior to the left atrium, and with infradiaphragmatic drainage the vertical vein may be seen descending through the diaphragm. Arterial blood gas and pH values usually reveal decreased PaO_2, possibly some elevation of $PaCO_2$, and metabolic acidosis in cases of obstructed venous drainage.

Cardiac catheterization. Pulmonary hypertension is present with obstructed venous drainage, and pulmonary angiography reveals the anomalous pulmonary venous drainage pathway as the dye returns from the lungs. The presence of a PDA must be doc-

umented since its ligation is necessary at the time of surgical repair.

Management. With obstructed venous drainage, assisted ventilation may be necessary, and the use of digitalization and diuretics is beneficial when congestive heart failure secondary to a large pulmonary blood flow is present. Surgical correction consists of anastomosis of the common pulmonary vein to the left atrium and ligation of the anomalous vein. Total circulatory arrest under deep hypothermia with cardiopulmonary bypass is required for repair in the neonate.

Hypoplastic left heart syndrome

Pathophysiology. There is underdevelopment of the entire left side of the heart, and anomalies include combinations of mitral and aortic atresia or severe stenosis and hypoplasia of the left ventricle, often to a marked degree in the typical case. Pulmonary venous return must pass from left to right through the foramen ovale to the right side of the heart when the mitral valve is atretic, and systemic circulation depends entirely on a right-to-left shunt through a PDA. Because the PDA closes within the first few hours (or occasionally days) of life, systemic circulation decreases, resulting in metabolic acidosis, shock, and death, which often occurs within the first few days of life if the neonate does not receive treatment.

History. Infants often appear healthy at birth, but tachypnea and cyanosis usually appear within the first 24 hours after birth. Clinical deterioration and progressive heart failure can be very rapid.

Physical examination. In the typical patient there are tachypnea, slight cyanosis, a markedly hyperdynamic precordial impulse, usually without a palpable thrill, and decreased peripheral pulses. A systolic murmur at the left sternal border, a single accentuated S_2, gallop rhythm (commonly), and marked hepatomegaly are common findings. There is often a characteristic ashen and mottled appearance of the skin.

Laboratory tests. Arterial blood gas and pH values reveal mild hypoxemia, with PaO_2 usually from 40 to 50 mm Hg, $PaCO_2$ usually normal, but pH often low because of metabolic acidosis. The chest roentgenogram shows cardiomegaly and both active and passive congestion of the lungs. The ECG reveals RAD, RAH, and severe RVH, with little if any left-sided forces. The echocardiogram is usually diagnostic and can clearly show the atretic aortic and mitral valves and the marked hypoplasia of the left ventricle and aorta.

Cardiac catheterization. Cardiac catheterization is usually not necessary for diagnosis except in those cases in which the echocardiogram is inconclusive. An angiogram through an umbilical artery catheter placed near the PDA will reveal the markedly hypoplastic aorta and atretic aortic valve.

Management. The Norwood operation, performed in two stages, results in a single-ventricle heart that is amenable to a modified Fontan operation as the second stage. This procedure is still considered experimental by physicians at many centers, and state and federal programs have been unwilling to pay for the surgery. The first stage must be done soon after birth, and PGE_1 infusion is begun immediately after the diagnosis is made to maintain ductal patency and thereby sustain systemic circulation and prevent progressive acidosis before surgery. The use of assisted mechanical ventilation, digitalization, and diuretics to treat heart failure is only indicated if surgical palliation is planned; otherwise their use may simply delay the inevitable death for these infants. Some patients are doing well after the second-stage Norwood operation. The alternate treatment is heart transplantation, which has been very effective in some centers.

Persistent common truncus arteriosus

Pathophysiology. In a patient with persistent common truncus arteriosus both the pulmonary artery and the aorta arise from the heart as a common vessel as a result of a failure of septation and division during fetal development. In the most common type the vessel appears as an aorta, from which the pulmonary arteries arise in several different anatomic configurations. Systemic pressure is transmitted directly to the lungs, and there is markedly increased pulmonary blood flow and congestive heart failure. A large VSD allows both ventricles to eject directly into the common truncal vessel.

History. Congestive heart failure develops within the first few weeks of life, and cyanosis is usually not severe.

Physical examination. Mild cyanosis, a systolic murmur at the base, a diastolic murmur at the apex, a markedly hyperdynamic precordial impulse, and bounding peripheral pulses are common features. A single S_2, an ejection systolic click, and a gallop rhythm are also frequently present.

Laboratory tests. Pao_2 is often in the 40 to 50 mm Hg range. An ECG reveals combined ventricular hypertrophy, with prominent midprecordial voltages, RAD, and occasionally LAH. The chest roentgenogram shows cardiac enlargement and markedly increased pulmonary vascular markings, and a right aortic arch is often associated. An echocardiogram will show a single large vessel overriding a high VSD, with no separate pulmonic valve. The truncal valve can be quadricuspid or stenotic, and these features can often be well visualized on an echocardiogram.

Cardiac catheterization. Angiography with injection in the truncal root will define the anatomy and the manner in which the pulmonary arteries arise. Pulmonary hypertension and increased pulmonary blood flow are common, and a ventricular-truncal vessel pressure difference will be demonstrated in the presence of truncal valve stenosis. Left ventricular angiography will define the VSD and show the truncus overriding the septum.

Management. Digitalization and diuresis are used for congestive heart failure. Corrective surgery is necessary and is usually performed in early infancy since these infants fail to thrive. A conduit is used to connect the right ventricle to the pulmonary arteries, which are separated from the truncus vessel, and the VSD is patched. Primary repair is considered the procedure of choice, replacing the previous two-stage repair of pulmonary artery banding in early infancy and intracardiac repair at a later age.

Neonatal Polycythemia
BACKGROUND AND PHYSIOLOGY

The neonate has a normal hematocrit value that ranges from 44% to 65%; values >65% should prompt consideration of polycythemia. Hemoglobin levels of 14 to 24 g/dl are considered within normal range, although levels >20 to 22 g/dl have also been considered abnormal. Elevated hematocrit can cause an increase in the blood viscosity, leading to decreased rates of blood flow, especially in the smaller blood vessels, with the possibility of clumping of red cells and microthrombosis. Elevations of hematocrit to >65% occur in 3% to 5% of newborns. Polycythemia has a deleterious effect on various organ systems, with increased viscosity causing an increase in systemic and pulmonary vascular resistances and a decrease in tissue perfusion. Increased pulmonary vascular resistance leads to right-to-left shunting across the foramen ovale and ductus arteriosus. Increased systemic vascular resistance reduces cardiac output, leading to decreased tissue perfusion and hypoxia in many organs, including the heart, brain, liver, kidney, and bowel.

Chronic intrauterine hypoxia can lead to polycythemia and occurs in small-for-gestational-age infants, infants with twin-twin, maternal-twin, and placental-fetal transfusions, infants of diabetic mothers, infants of toxemic mothers, and infants with various genetic abnormalities such as trisomy 21, trisomy D, α-chain hemoglobinopathies, and adrenal hyperplasia.

Polycythemic infants can exhibit respiratory distress, cyanosis, and congestive heart failure, and these neonates can be confused with patients with congenital cardiac disease or respiratory disease. CNS findings such as tremulousness, agitation or depression, abnormal cry, convulsions, and poor feeding are common. Residual brain damage may occur in some infants. Enlarged kidneys, oligemia, hematuria, renal vein thrombosis, and anuria reflect renal abnormalities. Hypocalcemia and hypoglycemia, seen often in infants of diabetic mothers, may also be present in polycythemic neonates, causing further decrease in cardiac function. With destruction of the excess red blood cells hyperbilirubinemia may occur. Necrotizing enterocolitis can occur, probably related to decreased blood flow to the intestines because of the increased blood viscosity.

MONITORING AND LABORATORY TESTS

Patients must be on a cardiac and respiratory monitor and must be closely observed for seizures, apnea, poor feeding, and decreased urinary output. Blood for laboratory tests (see below) must be drawn regularly to monitor progress and to help detect signs of organ system failure. Stools must be checked for signs of blood, and abdominal girth must be measured.

All newborns must have a capillary hematocrit determination at 2 to 4 hours of age, and if it is >65% a free-flowing venous sample should be obtained. Platelet counts must be checked, since they may fall if sludging of blood occurs and if renal vein thrombosis occurs. Arterial blood gas and pH values must be obtained before and after partial exchange transfusion (see below), and if cyanosis is present, both a pre- and a postductal sample will help determine the site of the right-to-left shunt. A chest roentgenogram will help determine cardiac size and rule out pulmonary disease. A complete ECG must be obtained, and an echocardiogram will help rule out cardiac defects and assess cardiac function. Serum bilirubin levels must be followed closely (late rise at 2 to 4 days) and urine samples checked for blood.

TREATMENT

There is no general agreement on the preferred management of these infants with polycythemia, especially the asymptomatic neonate with a hematocrit >65%. Studies have shown an increased incidence of necrotizing enterocolitis in patients treated by partial exchange transfusion. However, the major risk of not lowering the hematocrit may be permanent CNS damage. In a symptomatic infant less controversy exists about whether to treat; treatment involves several methods of lowering the hematocrit (i.e., partial exchange transfusion or simple phlebotomy), and the choice depends on the clinical situation.

Congestive Heart Failure With Hypervolemia

This condition may rarely be seen within the first few hours of life. Phlebotomy should be performed by slowly removing 10 ml/kg blood. Hematocrit levels must be rechecked since polycythemia may be seen after 2 to 6 hours.

Hypervolemia and Polycythemia (Without Congestive Heart Failure)

A partial exchange transfusion must be performed, using 4 g/dl albumin (16 ml of 25% albumin and 84 ml of 0.9% sodium chloride solution) to decrease the red blood cell mass isovolumically. Fresh frozen plasma may be used instead of albumin, but it is associated with an increased risk of infection. The hematocrit must be decreased to 50% to 55%, using this formula:

$$V = \frac{Hct_i - Hct_f \times \text{Body weight (kg)} \times 90 \text{ ml/kg}}{Hct_i}$$

where V = volume to be exchanged; Hct_i = initial hematocrit; Hct_f = final hematocrit; and 90 ml/kg =

blood volume per kilogram of body weight. Use the routes suggested in Chapter 141 for exchange.

Albumin can be infused and whole blood withdrawn in 5 ml aliquots. After the partial exchange is completed, the blood volume should be lowered by phlebotomy of 10 ml/kg body weight. If the neonate is not hypervolemic, the blood volume is not to be reduced by phlebotomy, but the partial exchange should be performed as outlined.

Management of Organ Systems

Cardiorespiratory. Supplemental oxygen should be administered when indicated for hypoxemia. Symptoms are usually relieved after partial exchange transfusions.

Central nervous system. Seizures must be treated with calcium, glucose, or oxygen as needed. Phenobarbital, 10 mg/kg IV loading dose followed by 5 mg/kg/day in three divided doses if above measures do not prevent the seizures, should be administered.

Renal metabolic. Hypocalcemia can be treated with calcium gluconate, 100 mg/kg IV slow push for a calcium level <7.5 mg/dl. Dextrostix readings must be maintained at 45 to 90 mg/dl with IV glucose. When hematuria is present and renal vein thrombosis suspected, BUN and creatinine levels must be monitored, and sonography may document an enlarged kidney and even delineate the clot. Blood detected in the stools should prompt a search for necrotizing enterocolitis with serial abdominal roentgenograms. Serum bilirubin levels must be monitored until safe levels are assured.

These infants need careful follow-up evaluation to detect the presence of any permanent sequelae (especially of the CNS).

ADDITIONAL READING
Cyanotic Congenital Heart Disease

Byrum CJ, Bove EL, Sondheimer HM, Kavey REW, Blackman MS. Hemodynamic and electrophysiologic results of the Senning procedure for transposition of the great arteries. Am J Cardiol 58:138-142, 1986.

Cumming GR, Carr W. Hemodynamic effects of propranolol in patients with Fallot's tetralogy. Am Heart J 74:29-36, 1967.

• Daskalopoulos DA, Edwards WD, Driscoll DL, Seward JB, Tajik AJ, Hagler DL. Correlation of two-dimensional echocardiographic and autopsy findings in complete transposition of the great arteries. J Am Coll Cardiol 2:1151-1157, 1983.

Fellows KE, Radtke W, Keane JF, Lock JE. Acute complications of catheter therapy for congenital heart disease. Am J Cardiol 60:679-683, 1987.

• Foker JE, Braunlin EA, St Cyr JA, Hunter D, Molina JE, Moller JE, Ring WS. Management of pulmonary atresia with intact ventricular septum. J Thorac Cardiovasc Surg 92:706-715, 1986.

• Freed MD, Heymann MA, Lewis AB, Roehl SL, Kensey RC. Prostaglandin E₁ in infants with ductus arteriosus dependent congenital heart disease. Circulation 64:899-905, 1981.

Hammerman C, Aramburo MJ, Bui K. Endogenous dilator prostaglandins in congenital heart disease. Pediatr Cardiol 8:155-159, 1987.

Kveselis DA, Rocchini AP, Snider R, Rosenthal A, Crowley DC, Dick M II. Results of balloon valvuloplasty in the treatment of congenital valvar pulmonary stenosis in children. Am J Cardiol 56:527-532, 1985.

Lang P, Norwood WI. Hemodynamic assessment after palliative surgery for hypoplastic left heart syndrome. Circulation 68:104-108, 1983.

Levin DL, Paul MH, Muster AJ, Newfeld EA, Waldman JD. D-transposition of the great vessels in the neonate. Arch Intern Med 137:1421-1425, 1977.

Lewis AB, Wells W, Lindesmith GG. Right ventricular growth potential in neonates with pulmonary atresia and intact ventricular septum. J Thorac Cardiovasc Surg 91:835-840, 1986.

• Lewis AB, Wells W, Lindesmith GG. Evaluation and surgical treatment of pulmonary atresia and intact ventricular septum in infancy. Circulation 67:1318-1323, 1983.

• Lewis AB, Freed MD, Heymann MA, Roehl SL, Kensey RC. Side effects of the therapy with prostaglandin E₁ in infants with critical congenital heart disease. Circulation 64:893-898, 1981.

Main DD, Ritter DG. Truncus arteriosus. In Moss AJ, Adams FH, Emmanuolides GC, eds. Heart Disease in Infants, Children and Adolescents, 2nd ed. Baltimore: Williams & Wilkins, 1977.

McFaul RG, Main DD, Feldt RH, Ritter DG, McGoon DC. Truncus arteriosus and previous pulmonary arterial banding: Clinical and hemodynamic assessment. Am J Cardiol 38:626-632, 1976.

Newfeld EA, Cole RB, Paul MH. Ebstein's malformation of the tricuspid valve in the neonate. Am J Cardiol 19:727-731, 1967.

Olley PM, Coceani F, Bodach E. E-type prostaglandins: A new emergency therapy for certain cyanotic congenital heart malformations. Circulation 53:728-731, 1976.

• Sharma AK, Brawn WJ, Mee RBB. Truncus arteriosus: Surgical approach. J Thorac Cardiovasc Surg 90:45-49, 1985.

Shiina A, Seward JB, Edwards WD, Hagler DJ, Tajik AJ. Two-dimensional echocardiographic spectrum of Ebstein's anomaly: Detailed anatomic assessment. J Am Coll Cardiol 3:356-370, 1984.

• Sidi D, Planche C, Kachaner J, Bruniaux J, Villain E, Bidois J, Prichard JF, Lacour-Gayet F. Anatomic correction of simple transposition of the great arteries in 50 neonates. Circulation 75:429-435, 1987.

• Smallhorn JF, Freedom RM. Pulsed Doppler echocardiography in the preoperative evaluation of total anomalous pulmonary venous connection. J Am Coll Cardiol 8:1413-1420, 1986.

Teixeira OHP, Carpenter B, MacMurray SB, Vlad P. Long-term prostaglandin E_1 therapy in congenital heart defects. J Am Coll Cardiol 3:838-843, 1984.

• Trusler GA, Castaneda AR, Rosenthal A, Blackstone EH, Kirklin JW, Congenital Heart Surgeons Society. Current results of management in transposition of the great arteries, with special emphasis on patients with associated ventricular septal defect. J Am Coll Cardiol 10:1061-1071, 1987.

Van Praagh R, Ando M, Dungan WT. Anatomic types of tricuspid atresia: Clinical and developmental implications. Circulation 44:111-115, 1971.

• Zhao HX, Miller DC, Reitz BA, Shumway NE. Surgical repair of tetralogy of Fallot. Long-term follow-up with particular emphasis on late death and reoperation. J Thorac Cardiovasc Surg 89:204-220, 1985.

Neonatal Polycythemia

• Black VD, Rumack CM, Lubchenco LO, Koops BL. Gastrointestinal injury in polycythemic term infants. Pediatrics 76:225-231, 1985.

• Black VD, Lubchenco LO, Koops BL, Poland RL, Powell DP. Neonatal hyperviscosity: Randomized study of effect of partial plasma exchange transfusion on long-term outcome. Pediatrics 75:1048-1053, 1985.

Gatti RA, Muster AJ, Cole RB, Paul MH: Neonatal polycythemia with transient cyanosis and cardiorespiratory abnormalities. J Pediatr 69:1063-1072, 1966.

Geierman C, Young G, Pyk W. Echocardiographic study of pulmonary vascular resistance (PVR) in polycythemia in neonates. Pediatr Res 12:381, 1978.

Hakanson DO, Oh W. Necrotizing enterocolitis and hyperviscosity in the newborn infant. J Pediatr 90:458-461, 1977.

Herson VC, Raye JR, Rowe JC, Phillips AF. Acute renal failure associated with polycythemia in a neonate. J Pediatr 100:137-139, 1982.

Murphy DJ Jr, Reller MD, Meyer RA, Kaplan S. Left ventricular function in normal newborn infants and asymptomatic infants with neonatal polycythemia. Am Heart J 112:542-547, 1986.

• Murphy DJ Jr, Reller MD, Meyer RA, Kaplan S. Effects of neonatal polycythemia and partial exchange transfusion on cardiac function: An echocardiographic study. Pediatrics 76:909-913, 1985.

Ramamurthy RS, Brans YW. Neonatal polycythemia. I. Criteria for diagnosis and treatment. Pediatrics 68:168-174, 1981.

Stevens K, Wirth FH. Incidence of neonatal hyperviscosity at sea level. J Pediatr 97:118-119, 1980.

• Swetnam SM, Yabek SM, Alverson DC. Hemodynamic consequences of neonatal polycythemia. J Pediatr 110:443-447, 1987.

39 Persistent Pulmonary Hypertension of the Newborn

Daniel L. Levin

BACKGROUND AND PHYSIOLOGY
Definition

Persistent pulmonary hypertension of the newborn (PPHN) is defined as a physiologic syndrome in which pulmonary vascular resistance in the newborn infant remains elevated at the fetal level rather than rapidly falling as it normally does in the newborn's transitional circulation. The effects of the prolonged elevation in pulmonary vascular resistance are elevated pulmonary arterial blood pressure, decreased pulmonary blood flow, right-to-left shunting through the patent foramen ovale at the atrial level, and, if it is patent, right-to-left shunting through the ductus arteriosus.

Etiology

Since there are many physiologic and physical factors that control the pulmonary vascular resistance and its normal fall during the transitional circulation after birth, many alterations in or failures of these several mechanisms acting on the pulmonary vascular bed are possible. PPHN is, therefore, a syndrome with many etiologies, which can be thought of as either primary (i.e., caused by abnormalities altering the muscularity, numbers, and/or degree of constriction of pulmonary vessels) or secondary (i.e, associated with conditions that increase pulmonary vascular resistance and pulmonary vascular blood pressure).

It is difficult in many cases to know whether an association is primary or secondary. For example, an otherwise normal infant who has a sudden intrapartum obstetric mishap (e.g., prolapsed cord) may be acutely stressed, pass meconium, aspirate, and de-velop secondary PPHN due to vasospasm of otherwise normal pulmonary vessels. Alternatively, a fetus who is chronically stressed in utero may have fetal pulmonary arterial hypertension and a remodeling of the pulmonary vessels with increased muscularity. This, in turn, may cause abnormal transitional circulation, resulting in intrapartum distress and passage of meconium with aspiration. This infant would have primary PPHN associated secondarily with meconium aspiration.

In another example, thromboxane A_2 (TxA_2) may be abnormally elevated because of some intrapartum stimulus to the fetus. The elevated TXA_2 can cause pulmonary vasospasm in an otherwise normal pulmonary vascular bed, intrapartum distress, and an abnormal transitional circulation with passage of meconium and aspiration. Either TxA_2 or meconium can cause clumping of platelets in the pulmonary vasculature, which can cause PPHN both by a further release of TxA_2 from platelets and a physical decrease in the cross-sectional area of the pulmonary vascular bed. In this case elevated TxA_2 is a cause of primary PPHN. Alternatively, in newborn infants with group B β-hemolytic streptococcal pneumonia and/or sepsis, TxA_2 may be released from blood vessels or platelets and cause pulmonary vasospasm and secondary PPHN.

Some mediators of pulmonary vasoconstriction may have other effects on the lungs that further alter lung mechanics and enhance pulmonary hypertension due to vasoconstriction. For example, leukotriene C_4 (LTC_4) and leukotriene D_4 (LTD_4) may also increase lung vascular permeability, leading to pul-

POSSIBLE ETIOLOGIES OF PERSISTENT PULMONARY HYPERTENSION OF THE NEWBORN

Primary: Physical or physiologic pulmonary vessel disease

1. Intrauterine increase in pulmonary arterial smooth muscle because wall thickening and/or degree of peripheral extension into vessels not normally muscularized
   a. Genetic differences
   b. Secondary to chronic intrauterine stress resulting from hypoxemia and/or fetal pulmonary arterial hypertension
   c. Intrauterine constriction of the ductus arteriosus (anatomic, physiologic, pharmacologic)
2. Decrease in total number of pulmonary arterial resistance vessels (decreased cross-sectional area of pulmonary vascular bed) either because of reduction in actual number of vessels or because of intraluminal occlusion of vessels by, for example, thrombi or emboli
3. Alteration in levels of vasoactive agents either naturally occurring or exogenously introduced prenatally and/or in newborn period
   a. Increase in availability of pulmonary vasoconstrictors before or after birth (e.g., angiotensin II, thromboxane A_2 [TxA_2], prostaglandin $F_{2\alpha}$ [$PGF_{2\alpha}$], leukotrienes C_4, D_4, and E_4 [LTC_4, LTD_4, LTE_4], platelet activating factor [PAF])
   b. Decrease in availability of vasodilators before or after birth (e.g., bradykinins, prostaglandin E_1, E_2, and D_2 [PGE_1, PGE_2, PGD_2], prostacyclin [PGI_2], and oxygen)
4. Pulmonary vessel misalignment
5. Main pulmonary artery distention
6. Abnormal endothelial-myocardial cell interactions

Secondary: Diseases with anatomic and/or physiologic abnormalities associated with persistent pulmonary hypertension in the newborn

1. CNS disorders (e.g., hypoventilation)
2. Infection (e.g., group B β-hemolytic streptococcal pneumonia, ureaplasmal pneumonia)
3. Polycythemia/hyperviscosity syndrome
4. Upper airway obstruction (e.g., Pierre Robin syndrome)
5. Pulmonary parenchymal disorders
   a. Retained fetal lung fluid
   b. Hyaline membrane disease
   c. Meconium aspiration syndrome
6. Congenital lung disorders
   a. Diaphragmatic hernia and hypoplastic lung
   b. Primary pulmonary hypoplasia
7. Congenital heart disease
   a. Obstructed pulmonary venous return (e.g., total anomalous pulmonary venous return)
   b. Myopathic left ventricular disease (e.g., myocardial ischemia)
   c. Obstruction to left ventricular outflow (e.g., aortic stenosis, coarctation of aorta)
   d. Obligatory left-to-right shunt (e.g., atrioventricular canal, arteriovenous malformation)
   e. Miscellaneous (e.g., Ebstein's anomaly)

monary edema and increased lung water, thereby decreasing lung compliance.

Whether or not exposure of the fetal ductus arteriosus to exogenously introduced pharmacologic agents (via the maternal circulation and transplacental passage) causes PPHN is a subject of much debate. An abundance of data indicates that prostaglandin synthetase inhibitors such as naproxen, salicylates, and indomethacin cross from the maternal circulation into the fetus via the placenta and cause constriction of the fetal ductus arteriosus in a variety of experimental animal conditions (Fig. 39-1). This has been demonstrated also in human fetuses by using fetal echocardiography and Doppler techniques. These agents have a direct vasoconstrictive effect on the pulmonary vasculature and possibly result in a decreased number of vessels in the newborn. These mechanisms have been associated with an increase in pulmonary vascular smooth muscle in fetal and newborn lungs fixed by the perfusion technique. In some experimental models ischemia of the tricuspid papillary muscle and right ventricular myocardial

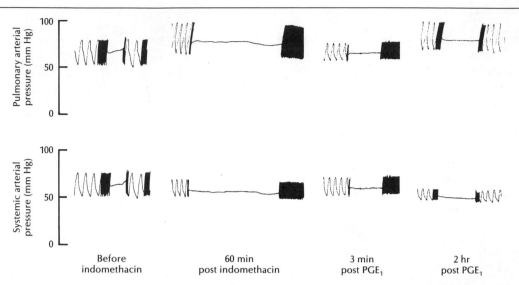

Fig. 39-1   Fetal pulmonary and systemic arterial blood pressures (minus intra-amniotic pressure) obtained from continuous, simultaneous recordings in one fetus before and 60 minutes after maternal administration of indomethacin, 3 minutes after one dose of 5 μg of PGE_1 into the fetal inferior vena cava, and 2 hours later. Note the pulmonary-systemic arterial blood pressure differences, which are due to pulmonary arterial hypertension. (From Levin DL, Mills LJ, Weinberg AG, et al. Constriction of the fetal ductus arteriosus after administration of indomethacin to the pregnant ewe. J Pediatr 94:647-650, 1979.)

wall has resulted in tricuspid insufficiency. Whether or not these events following exposure of the fetus to these agents result in newborn animals or infants with PPHN is the subject of debate. Some, but not all, infants of mothers receiving these agents during pregnancy have PPHN. The effects of these agents on constriction of the fetal ductus arteriosus and fetal pulmonary vasculature may vary, depending on the amount and timing of the exposure. Certainly in clinical trials in which these prostaglandin synthetase inhibitors are studied for their potential beneficial effects such as inhibition of premature labor, it is necessary for the investigators to examine the fetus and newborn carefully for possible alterations such as PPHN that may be caused by the experimental agent.

Common Names

In such a complex and evolving area it should not be surprising that the syndrome is known by many different names, including persistent fetal circulation, persistent pulmonary vascular obstruction, progressive pulmonary hypertension, persistent fetal cardiopulmonary circulatory pathway, and persistent transitional circulation.

Clinical Presentation

These infants usually are full- or postterm newborns with, in many cases, identifiable prenatal and perinatal risk factors such as passage of meconium, maternal fever, maternal anemia (abruptio placentae, placenta previa), maternal pulmonary distress (asthma, pneumonia), cesarean section, abnormal presentation, fetal distress, and vaginal bleeding. Shortly after birth these infants are cyanotic, tachypneic, or in some cases apneic and may have a systolic murmur. Hypoxemia, hypercarbia, acidemia, hypocalcemia, and hypoglycemia are characteristic. Occasionally the syndrome is seen in preterm infants as well.

Diagnosis

Simultaneous Pao_2 measurements from preductus arteriosus (temporal or right radial artery) and postductus arteriosus (abdominal aorta, posterior tibial artery) sites are helpful in making the diagnosis if there is a large right-to-left shunt through the ductus arteriosus. In this case the Pao_2 will be ≥ 10 mm Hg lower in the descending aorta than in the ascending aorta. This information may also be ellicited by proper placement of either tco_2 or Sao_2 (pulse oximeter) electrodes in preductus and postductus arteriosus sites. In some patients right-to-left shunting at the level of the atrial septum is so great that the well-oxygenated blood returning to the left atrium from the pulmonary veins is rapidly diluted with poorly oxygenated blood so that ascending aortic blood is also unsaturated. In other infants the ductus arteriosus may be prematurely closed in utero. In both of these cases, a significant difference (>10 mm Hg oxygen tension) between preductus and postductus arteriosus blood samples would not be expected. Use of contrast M-mode and Doppler echocardiography is helpful in documenting the right-to-left atrial shunt and right-to-left ductus shunt (see Chapter 119). Use of two-dimensional echocardiography can also demonstrate dilatation of the right ventricle and pulmonary artery and abnormal prolonged right ventricular systolic time intervals. When tricuspid or pulmonic valve regurgitation is detected by Doppler signals, the right ventricular pressure can be estimated. The combination of history, physical examination, chest roentgenogram, oxygen saturation data, ECG, echocardiogram, and Doppler studies can be used to diagnose PPHN. Differentiating PPHN from total anomalous pulmonary venous return is especially challenging and may take color-flow Doppler studies to localize entry of the pulmonary veins or cardiac catheterization and angiography.

Chest roentgenograms in patients with primary PPHN usually show normal lung fields and a normal or mildly enlarged heart. In patients with secondary PPHN the chest roentgenogram will show evidence of the associated condition (e.g., meconium aspiration, hyaline membrane disease). The ECG is helpful in diagnosing some primary cardiac defects and myocardial ischemia.

Course

Infants with a transient imbalance of circulating vasoactive agents would be expected to have a short course, whereas those with remodeling of the pulmonary vasculature by excessive pulmonary arterial smooth muscle may be ill for several days until the muscle mass regresses. Some infants with extensive remodeling of the pulmonary vasculature may not be able to overcome the limitations of pulmonary blood flow because of the severity of the morphologic abnormalities. Infants with a small pulmonary vascular bed or intraluminal obstruction may not improve. Infants with secondary PPHN usually improve with treatment of the primary disease process. In all cases the course may be prolonged by the superimposition of chronic lung disease due to oxygen toxicity and barotrauma resulting from the treatment.

Outcome

Although some centers report a fatality rate of 50% to 90% for infants with severe PPHN, other centers report a 10% to 15% mortality rate for infants who receive conventional medical management. Despite the concerns about chronic lung disease from treatment, hypoxic-ischemic encephalopathy, and hearing loss, most follow-up studies performed thus far indicate no greater risk of poor outcome for these infants than for comparable groups of sick infants without PPHN.

MONITORING AND LABORATORY TESTS

In addition to the standard monitoring of a sick infant with cardiorespiratory disease (see Chapter 4), careful attention must be given to the adequacy of systemic oxygenation and possible right-to-left ductus shunting. An initial determination of arterial blood gas tensions and pH must be done on any infant with respiratory abnormality or cyanosis. Both the inspired oxygen concentration and the sampling site must be carefully noted (e.g., $Fio_2 = 0.4$, right radial artery). All such infants will need a continuous noninvasive means of assessing oxygenation either by tco_2 or Sao_2 techniques; I prefer Sao_2. The results of the initial determination can be used in conjunction with the clinical picture to assess the need for further intra-arterial sampling.

In most cases infants with PPHN are unstable and can deteriorate rapidly. Therefore in addition to noninvasive monitoring they will need repetitive arterial blood gas tension and pH determinations during the acute phase of the illness (usually 2 to 4 days). If at all possible the arterial catheter should be placed in the right radial artery to sample blood from a preductus arteriosus site. The intra-arterial catheter is also needed for continuous systemic arterial blood pressure monitoring, especially in infants who receive tolazoline. Noninvasive monitors are placed in both the upper right quadrant (preductus) and lower extremity (postductus) sites for continuous monitoring.

Initially arterial blood gas and pH sampling must be done every hour as well as 10 minutes after every respiratory support change until some degree of stability at a satisfactory level of oxygenation, carbon dioxide elimination, and pH is achieved. Once these levels are achieved, the rate of arterial blood gas and pH sampling can be decreased to every 4 hours if the noninvasive monitoring is providing accurate and sufficient information.

When patients are in the recovery phase, evaluation by arterial blood sampling and noninvasive monitors must continue at a frequent rate since these infants may deteriorate rapidly during the recovery process, especially when respiratory support is withdrawn. Only after they are clearly recovered is the arterial catheter removed.

In addition to continuous noninvasive oxygen monitoring it is helpful to use continuous noninvasive carbon dioxide monitoring either by transcutaneous ($tcco_2$) (see Chapter 121) or end-tidal ($etco_2$) (see Chapter 123) methods.

TREATMENT

The overall goals in treating PPHN are to maintain oxygenation and oxygen delivery until the process resolves, to treat any associated condition (e.g., group B β-hemolytic streptococcal pneumonia), and to avoid significant insults to organs (e.g., lung, brain) during the treatment phase.

The specific goals for arterial blood gas and pH levels are to maintain the preductus arteriosus blood samples at a Pao_2 of 100 to 125 mm Hg (in full-term infants) or an Sao_2 of 96% to 100% to provide a margin of safety for the sudden and unexpected dips (or "flips") seen in these patients.

The optimal $Paco_2$ level is controversial. Although most clinical protocols advocate the use of hyperventilation ($Paco_2$ of 20 to 25 mm Hg or even lower) to establish respiratory alkalosis (pH ≥7.5), some authors debate the necessity of its use, choosing to provide just enough alveolar ventilation to maintain a normal level ($Paco_2$ of 35 to 45 mm Hg). Other evidence indicates it may be more a matter of met-

abolic alkalosis rather than respiratory alkalosis that causes an apparent increase in systemic oxygenation, presumably because of relaxation of pulmonary vasospasm. Other authors advocate the use of high-frequency jet ventilation or high-frequency oscillatory ventilation in these patients and have had some success, which in part may be the result of less barotrauma to the lungs than with conventional mechanical ventilation.

The optimal arterial blood pH is controversial, as indicated previously, and may be normal or elevated by either hyperventilation or continuous sodium bicarbonate (1 mEq/kg/day) infusion to a pHa ≥7.5. In patients who are also receiving tolazoline, which can cause gastric hypersecretion and HCl loss, the pH may become dangerously alkalotic, and these patients may need HCl replacement if the base excess is greater than 10 to 15 mEq/L or if blood pH exceeds 7.6.

To achieve the above goals it is necessary to follow a series of successive maneuvers initiated by increasing the Fio_2 to as high as 1.0 and intubating the patient if the Pao_2 is <100 mm Hg with an Fio_2 of 1.0. Alveolar oxygen (Pao_2) is a potent regulator of pulmonary vascular tone, with more relaxation of the pulmonary resistance vessels the higher the Pao_2. This effect is probably modulated by oxygen diffusing through the alveolar epithelium and influencing local production of vasodilatory prostaglandins. Once the patient is intubated, continuous positive airway pressure (CPAP) is used, starting at 2 cm H_2O and increasing by 2 cm H_2O successively to 10 cm H_2O if the Pao_2 does not increase to 100 mm Hg. This procedure may be helpful in treating patients with lung disease and decreased functional residual capacity (FRC). In patients with healthy lung parenchyma or with lung disease not associated with a decreased FRC, the CPAP must be kept at 2 cm H_2O.

If oxygenation is not improved with an increased Fio_2 and CPAP, mechanical ventilation must be initiated using peak inspiratory pressures (PIP) starting at approximately 20 cm H_2O and maintaining PIP as low as possible to provide adequate alveolar ventilation as assessed by good breath sounds, chest wall movement, and carbon dioxide elimination. Use of sedation (see Chapter 129) and paralytic agents (see Chapter 130) may be helpful in maintaining low PIP and decreasing the risk of barotrauma. The PIP and respiratory rate used to provide minute ventilation will depend on the desired $Paco_2$. In my unit the PIP is increased as indicated above, and the rate is increased to as high as 80 to 100 breaths per minute to achieve a $Paco_2$ of 20 to 25 mm Hg. An inspiratory to expiratory (I:E) time ratio of 1:1 is generally used.

In some patients with extremely low total lung compliance (CL) who need excessively high PIP and whose CL may vary frequently, there may be an advantage in switching from a pressure-limited to a volume-limited mechanical ventilator (e.g., Siemens 900C; see Chapter 128). The pressure provided by the volume ventilator will be appropriate to deliver the preset tidal volume and can vary from breath to breath as CL changes. Under these conditions, although the risk of barotrauma still exists, a stable $Paco_2$ may be easier to achieve.

If oxygenation and oxygen delivery are still not adequate, the use of pulmonary vasodilators may be tried. There is no generally accepted agent that can be used with reasonable certainty of success. All the agents used, including tolazoline, prostaglandins (PGI_2, PGE_1, PGD_2), acetylcholine, nitroprusside, isoproterenol, bradykinin, chlorpromazine, methylprednisolone sodium succinate, morphine sulfate, and amrinone, have met with variable or no success. In the future specific blockers of the possible mediators of hypoxic, septic, and platelet-induced PPHN such as LTC_4, leukotriene D_4 (LTD_4), TxA_2, and platelet activating factor may be available for human trials. These blockers have shown some success in animal studies.

For now tolazoline (an alpha-adrenergic blocker with histamine receptor stimulating properties) is the only commonly used agent. If one chooses to use tolazoline (Priscoline), a test dose is used of 1 mg/kg (total dose) in four divided doses of 0.25 mg/kg/dose over several (5 to 10) minutes. This is administered into any vein or into the umbilical or pulmonary artery catheter. Tolazoline has a long (3.3 to 33 hours) half-life and will eventually reach the pulmonary circulation after being given by any route. One must continuously display and watch systemic arterial blood pressure when giving tolazoline since it is also a systemic vasodilator.

If a positive response to tolazoline is documented with an increase in upper body Pao_2 of ≥ 15 mm Hg, a continuous infusion may be started. The dose, as determined by pharmacokinetic studies, is 0.16 mg/kg/hr for every 1.0 mg/kg loading dose used. Because of the long half-life higher doses may give elevated and toxic plasma levels. Tolazoline may cause systemic hypotension and hemorrhage, and all secretions (endotracheal, nasogastric, stool) and urine must be checked for blood. The effect of tolazoline on H_1 and H_2 receptors is to increase GI secretions, including HCl, which predispose to GI hemorrhage. The use of cimetidine to counteract this effect is not indicated because some of the pulmonary vasodilation by tolazoline may be due to stimulation of pulmonary vascular H_1 receptors as well as alpha blockade. Use of tolazoline is also associated with a decrease in platelet counts, although it is not known if this is a cause and effect or just an association. Providing volume expansion with use of a continuous infusion may be necessary to maintain adequate organ perfusion, especially renal.

Although the use of tolazoline is controversial, it apparently is a direct pulmonary vasodilator under hypoxic conditions and an indirect pulmonary vasodilator under normoxic conditions and with its use the effects of hyperventilation and respiratory alkalosis are enhanced. It is also a systemic vasodilator, and systemic hypotension may occur and need treatment with volume expansion and/or a vasotonic agent such as dopamine (4 to 5 $\mu g/kg/min$). There is a possibility that some of the benefit of tolazoline may result from systemic vasodilation in asphyxiated patients, with an elevated systemic vascular resistance (SVR) and poor left ventricular function exacerbating pulmonary vascular hypertension. A lowering of SVR toward normal by vasodilation may improve left ventricular function, decrease pulmonary venous and arterial hypertension, improve pulmonary blood flow, decrease right-to-left shunting, and improve systemic oxygenation and oxygen delivery.

Tolazoline may be administered for at least 24 hours while the Fio_2, PIP, and respiratory rates (see below) are decreased as tolerated, as determined by assessment of oxygenation and oxygen delivery. If patient stability is maintained, tolazoline may be decreased by one fourth of the dose every 6 to 8 hours, closely watching for signs of decreased oxygenation. Remember tolazoline can have a very long half-life. After administration of tolazoline is discontinued and progress has been made in weaning the patient from the high Fio_2, PIP, and respiratory rates, the muscle relaxant may be discontinued. If this is successful, the dose of sedative/narcotic may be decreased slowly.

The Fio_2 must be decreased slowly. Pao_2 is a primary determinant of pulmonary vascular tone since oxygen is a potent vasodilator. Small decrements in Pa_{O_2} may not only decrease the diffusion gradient for oxygen-lowering Pa_{O_2} but also cause pulmonary vasoconstriction and increased right-to-left shunting via the patent foramen ovale and ductus arteriosus, resulting in dramatic drops in Pa_{O_2}. PIP should be decreased sequentially by 2 cm H_2O decrements until 20 cm H_2O is reached. If elevated positive end-expiratory pressure (PEEP) has been used, decrease it by 2 cm H_2O until 2 cm H_2O is reached, and, finally, decrease the respiratory rate by 2 breaths/min until the patient is ready for extubation (see Chapter 135).

Many patients who fail vasodilator therapy are ultimately discovered to have some lesion such as congenital heart disease or pulmonary vascular thrombi that would explain the failure of therapy. Some do not have these lesions.

There has been a great deal of interest lately in using extracorporeal membrane oxygenation (ECMO) for patients who fail or are anticipated to fail conventional medical management with mechanical ventilation and vasodilator therapy. Patients treated with ECMO (see Chapter 137) do quite well, with a reasonable rate of complications attributable to this invasive therapy. Some investigators note that the therapy ECMO attempts to supplement (i.e., mechanical ventilation) is invasive and harmful with its own set of complications as well. The major problem thus far has been to identify convincingly the patient at high risk for a poor outcome with conventional treatment so that ECMO can be started on that infant before irreversible deterioration occurs.

As far as the cardiovascular system is concerned, adequate circulating blood volume and systemic arterial blood pressure must be ensured; special attention to this system is needed when vasodilator therapy is used. Administer 0.9% sodium chloride solution in pushes of 10 ml/kg IV as the initial volume expander. If total serum protein levels are less than 5 mg/dl, administer 5% albumin (10 ml/kg IV) or 25% albumin (1 g/kg IV) or fresh frozen plasma (10 ml/kg IV) if clotting factors need replacement. If the patient needs an improved oxygen-carrying capacity (Hct <35%), give packed RBCs (10 ml/kg IV).

Maintain the serum glucose at approximately 90 mg/dl. These patients are frequently hypoglycemic, a condition that may, among other things, decrease myocardial function. Maintain normal body temperature (36.5° to 37.2° C). Cooling the blood may increase pulmonary vascular resistance. These patients are frequently hypocalcemic and hypomagnesemic. Administer calcium gluconate at 200 mg/kg/24 hrs IV as a maintenance dose and administer more if necessary to correct deficits (ionized <3.5 mEq/L). Give magnesium sulfate (0.8 mEq/kg/24 hr) in three divided doses IV during 1 hour if the serum magnesium is <1.2 mg/dl. Patients receiving antacids with magnesium and patients with poor renal function may have high levels of magnesium, which can cause systemic hypotension. Use enough volume to ensure a urinary output of at least 0.5 ml/kg/hr.

ADDITIONAL READING

Abman SH, Shanley PF, Accurso FJ. Chronic intrauterine pulmonary hypertension alters perinatal pulmonary vasoreactivity and structure. Pediatr Res 23:561A, 1988.

Adams JM, Hyde WH, Proceanoy RS, et al. Hypochloremic metabolic alkalosis following tolazoline-induced gastric hypersecretion. Pediatrics 66:298-300, 1980.

Andrews AF, Roloff DW, Bartlett RH. Use of extracorporeal membrane oxygenators in persistent pulmonary hypertension of the newborn. Clin Perinatol 11:729-735, 1984.

Arnold J, O'Brodovich H, Whyte R, et al. Pulmonary thromboemboli after neonatal asphyxia. J Pediatr 106:806-809, 1985.

Ballard RA, Leonard CH. Developmental follow-up of infants with persistent pulmonary hypertension of the newborn. Clin Perinatol 11:737-744, 1984.

Bartlett RH, Roloff DW, Cornell RG, et al. Extracorporeal circulation in neonatal respiratory failure: A prospective randomized study. Pediatrics 76:479-487, 1985.

Baylen GB, Emmanouildes GC, Jusatsch CE, et al. Main pulmonary artery distention: A potential mechanism for acute pulmonary hypertension in the human newborn infant. J Pediatr 96:540-544, 1980.

Beachy P, Powers LK. Nursing care of the infant with persistent pulmonary hypertension of the newborn. Clin Perinatol 11:681-693, 1984.

Beck R. Chronic lung disease following hypocapnic alkalosis for persistent pulmonary hypertension. J Pediatr 106:527-528, 1985.

Beck R, Anderson KD, Pearson GD, et al. Criteria for extracorporeal membrane oxygenation in a population of infants with persistent pulmonary hypertension of the newborn. J Pediatr Surg 21:297-302, 1986.

Benitz WE, Malachowski N, Cohen RS, et al. Use of sodium nitroprusside in neonates: Efficacy and safety. J Pediatr 106:102-110, 1985.

Boros SJ, Mammel MC, Coleman JM, et al. Neonatal high-frequency jet ventilation: 4 years' experience. Pediatrics 75:657-663, 1985.

Boyle RJ, Oh W. Transcutaneous Po₂ monitoring in infants with persistent fetal circulation who are receiving tolazoline therapy. Pediatrics 62:605-607, 1978.

Bradley LM, Goldstein RE, Feuerstein G. Influence of thromboxane A₂ receptor antagonism on pulmonary vasoconstrictor responses in the newborn. Pediatr Res 23:431A, 1988.

Bradley LM, Goldstein RE, Feuerstein G, et al. Leukotriene D₄ and the pathogenesis of hypoxic pulmonary constriction in the newborn. Pediatr Res 23:432A, 1988.

Brett C, Dekle M, Leonard CH, et al. Developmental follow-up of hyperventilated neonates: Preliminary observations. Pediatrics 68:588-591, 1981.

Bruce DA. Effects of hyperventilation on cerebral blood flow and metabolism. Clin Perinatol 11:673-680, 1984.

Bucciarelli RL, Egan EA, Gessner IH, et al. Persistence of fetal cardiopulmonary circulation: One manifestation of transient tachypnea of the newborn. Pediatrics 58:192-197, 1976.

Cohen RS, Stevenson DK, Malachowski N, et al. Late morbidity among survivors of respiratory failure treated with tolazoline. J Pediatr 97:644-647, 1980.

Cole CH, Jillson E, Kessler D. ECMO selection criteria: Evaluation of two populations. Pediatr Res 23:502A, 1988.

Davidson D. Hemodynamic adjustments to acute alveolar hypoxia during the transition after birth in lambs: Effect of leukotriene antagonism. Pediatr Res 23:503A, 1988.

Demello De, Murphy JD, Aronovitz MJ, et al. Effects of indomethacin in utero on the pulmonary vasculature of the newborn guinea pig. Pediatr Res 22:693-697, 1987.

Donnelly WH, Bucciarelli RL, Nelson RM. Ischemic papillary muscle necrosis in stressed newborn infants. J Pediatr 96:295-300, 1980.

Drummond WH. Use of cardiotonic therapy in the management of infants with PPHN. Clin Perinatol 11:715-729, 1984.

Drummond WH, Gregory GA, Heymann MA, et al. The independent effects of hyperventilation, tolazoline, and dopamine on infants with persistent pulmonary hypertension. J Pediatr 98:606-611, 1981.

Dworetz AR, Moya FR, Sabo B, et al. Survival in infants with persistent pulmonary hypertension (PPHN) without extracorporeal membrane oxygenation (ECMO). Pediatr Res 21:360A, 1987.

• Fox WW, Duara S. Persistent pulmonary hypertension in the neonate: Diagnosis and management. J Pediatr 103:505-514, 1983.

Fox WW, Gewitz MH, Dinwiddie R, et al. Pulmonary hypertension in the perinatal aspiration syndromes. Pediatrics 59:205-211, 1977.

Frantz EG, Soifer SJ, Heymann MA. Bradykinin-induced pulmonary vasodilation in fetal lambs is independent of cyclooxygenase metabolism. Pediatr Res 23:506A, 1988.

Frattallone JM, Fuhrman BP, Kochanek PM, et al. Management of pulmonary barotrauma by extracorporeal membrane oxygenation, apnea, and lung rest. J Pediatr 112:787-789, 1988.

Geggel RL, Reid LM. The structural basis of PPHN. Clin Perinatol 11:525-549, 1984.

• Gersony WM. Neonatal pulmonary hypertension: Pathophysiology, classification, and etiology. Clin Perinatol 11:517-524, 1984.

Gersony WM, Duc GV, Sinclair JC. "PFC" syndrome (persistence of the fetal circulation). Circulation 40(Suppl III):111, 1969.

Glass P, Short B. ECMO: Developmental outcome at age 2. Pediatr Res 23:447A, 1988.

Hageman JR, Dusik J, Keuler H, et al. Outcome of persistent pulmonary hypertension in relation to severity of presentation. Am J Dis Child 142:293-296, 1988.

Hammerman C, Komar K, Abbu-Khudair H. Hypoxic vs septic pulmonary hypertension. Am J Dis Child 142:319-325, 1988.

Hammerman C, Lass N, Strates E, et al. Prostanoids in neonates with persistent pulmonary hypertension. J Pediatr 110:470-472, 1987.

Hansen TN, Gest AL. Oxygen toxicity and other ventilatory complications of treatment of infants with persistent pulmonary hypertension. Clin Perinatol 11:653-672, 1984.

Harker LC, Kirkpatrick SE, Friedman WF, et al. Effects of indomethacin on fetal rat lungs: A possible cause of persistent fetal circulation (PFC). Pediatr Res 15:147-151, 1981.

Haworth SG. Normal structural and functional adaptation to extrauterine life. J Pediatr 98:915-918, 1981.

Hendricks-Munoz KD, Walton JP. Hearing loss in infants with persistent fetal circulation. Pediatrics 81:650-656, 1988.

Henry GW. Noninvasive assessment of cardiac function and pulmonary hypertension in persistent pulmonary hypertension of the newborn. Clin Perinatol 11:627-640, 1984.

• Heymann MA, Hoffman JIE. Persistent pulmonary hypertension syndromes in the newborn. In Weir EK, Reeves JT, eds. Pulmonary Hypertension. Mount Kisco, N.Y.: Futura, 1984, pp 45-71.

Hofkosh D, Trento A, Thompson AE, et al. Outcome among infants treated with extracorporeal membrane oxygenation (ECMO): Children's Hospital of Pittsburgh (CHP) 1979-1986. Pediatr Res 23:449A, 1988.

Huhta JC, Moise KJ. Human fetal ductus arteriosus constriction from nonsteroidal anti-inflammatory drugs. Am J Cardiol 60:643, 1987.

Huhta JC, Moise KJ, Fisher DJ, et al. Detection and quantitation of constriction of the fetal ductus arteriosus by Doppler echocardiography. Circulation 75:406-412, 1987.

Kaapa P. Platelet thromboxane B₂ production in neonatal pulmonary hypertension. Arch Dis Child 62:195-196, 1987.

Kaapa P, Koivisto M, Ylikorkala O, et al. Prostacyclin in the treatment of neonatal pulmonary hypertension. J Pediatr 107:951-953, 1985.

Klesh KW, Murphy TF, Scher MS, et al. Cerebral infarction in persistent pulmonary hypertension of the newborn. Am J Dis Child 141:852-857, 1987.

Kulik TJ, Lock JE. Pulmonary vasodilator therapy in persistent pulmonary hypertension of the newborn. Clin Perinatol 11:693-701, 1984.

Levin DL. Effects of inhibition of prostaglandin synthesis on fetal development, oxygenation, and the fetal circulation. Semin Perinatol 4:35-44, 1980.

Levin DL. Primary pulmonary hypoplasia. J Pediatr 95:550-551, 1979.

Levin DL. Morphologic analysis of the pulmonary vascular bed in congenital left-sided diaphragmatic hernia. J Pediatr 92:805-809, 1978.

Levin DL. Idiopathic persistent pulmonary hypertension of the newborn. In Rudolph AM, ed. Pediatrics, 20th ed. New York: Appleton-Century-Crofts (in press).

Levin DL, Gregory GA. The effect of tolazoline on right-to-left shunting via a patent ductus arteriosus in meconium aspiration syndrome. Crit Care Med 4:304-307, 1976.

Levin DL, Weinberg AG, Perkin RM. Pulmonary microthrombi syndrome in newborn infants with unresponsive persistent pulmonary hypertension. J Pediatr 102:299-303, 1983.

Levin DL, Mills LJ, Parkey M, et al. Constriction of the fetal ductus arteriosus after administration of indomethacin to the pregnant ewe. J Pediatr 94:647-650, 1979.

Levin DL, Mills LJ, Weinberg AG, et al. Hemodynamic, pulmonary vascular, and myocardial abnormalities secondary to pharmacologic constriction of the fetal ductus arteriosus: A possible mechanism for persistent pulmonary hypertension and transient tricuspid insufficiency in the newborn infant. Circulation 60:360-364, 1979.

Levin DL, Fixler DE, Morriss FC, et al. Morphologic analysis of the pulmonary vascular bed in infants exposed in utero to prostaglandin synthetase inhibitors. J Pediatr 92:478-483, 1978.

Levin DL, Hyman AI, Heymann MA, et al. Fetal hypertension and the development of increased pulmonary vascular smooth muscle: A possible mechanism for persistent pulmonary hypertension of the newborn infant. J Pediatr 92:265-269, 1978.

Levin DL, Heymann MA, Kitterman JA, et al. Persistent pulmonary hypertension of the newborn infant. J Pediatr 89:626-630, 1976.

Levin DL, Cates L, Newfeld EA, et al. Persistence of the fetal cardiopulmonary circulatory pathway: Survival of an infant after a prolonged course. Pediatrics 56:56-64, 1975.

Lock JE, Coceani F, Olley PM. Direct and indirect pulmonary vascular effects of tolazoline in the newborn lamb. J Pediatr 95:600-605, 1979.

Lock JE, Olley PM, Coceani F, et al. Use of prostacyclin in persistent fetal circulation. Lancet 1:1343, 1979.

Long WA. Structural cardiovascular abnormalities presenting as persistent pulmonary hypertension of the newborn. Clin Perinatol 11:601-626, 1984.

Mammel M, Einzig S, Kulik TJ, et al. Pulmonary dilation from amrinone in unsedated lamb. Pediatr Res 16:1264, 1982.

McIntosh N, Walters RO. Effect of tolazoline in severe hyaline membrane disease. Arch Dis Child 54:105-110, 1979.

Meadow W, Benn A, Giardini N, et al. Clinical correlates do not predict Pao_2 response after tolazoline administration in hypoxic newborns. Crit Care Med 14:548-551, 1986.

Moise KJ, Huhta JC, Sharif DS, et al. Indomethacin in the treatment of premature labor: Effects on the fetal ductus arteriosus. N Engl J Med 319:327-331, 1988.

Momma K, Takao A. In vivo constriction of the ductus arteriosus by nonsteroidal antiinflammatory drugs in near-term and preterm fetal rats. Pediatr Res 22:567-572, 1987.

Morray JP, Lynn AM, Mansfield PB. Effect of pH and Pco_2 on pulmonary and systemic hemodynamics after surgery in children with congenital heart disease and pulmonary hypertension. J Pediatr 113:474-479, 1988.

Murphy JD, Rabinowitch M, Goldstein JD, et al. The structural basis of persistent pulmonary hypertension of the newborn infant. J Pediatr 98:962-967, 1981.

Phillips JB III, Lyrene RK. Prostaglandins, related compounds, and the perinatal pulmonary circulation. Clin Perinatol 11:565-579, 1984.

Philips JB, Westfall M, Oliver J, et al. Effects of prostaglandins in two types of pulmonary hypertension. Pediatr Res 23:519A, 1988.

Pinheiro JMB, Pitt BR. Roles of thromboxane (TxA_2) and platelet-activating factor (PAF) in group B streptococcus induced pulmonary hypertension in piglets. Pediatr Res 23:520A, 1988.

Reece EA, Moya F, Yazigi R, et al. Persistent pulmonary hypertension: Assessment of perinatal risk factors. Obstet Gynecol 70:696-700, 1987.

Reid LM. Structure and function in pulmonary hypertension: New perceptions. Chest 89:279-288, 1986.

Riggs T, Hirschfeld S, Bormuth C, et al. Neonatal circulatory changes: An echocardiographic study. Pediatrics 59:338-344, 1977.

Riggs T, Hirshfeld S, Fanaroff A, et al. Persistence of fetal circulation syndrome: An echocardiographic study. J Pediatr 91:626-631, 1977.

Rowe RD. Abnormal pulmonary vasconstriction in the newborn. Pediatrics 59:318-321, 1977.

• Rudolph AM. High pulmonary vascular resistance after birth. I. Pathophysiologic considerations and etiologic classification. Clin Pediatr 19:585-590, 1980.

Rudolph AM, Yuan S. Response of the pulmonary vasculature to hypoxia and H^+ ion concentration changes. J Clin Invest 45:399-411, 1966.

Scanlon JW. Persistent pulmonary hypertension: Possible pathogenesis. Perinatal Press 2:97, 1978.

Schapira D, Solimano A. Is extracorporeal membrane oxygenation (ECMO) necessary to reduce mortality and morbidity in patients with meconium aspiration syndrome (MAS)? Pediatr Res 23:474A, 1988.

Schreiber MD, Heymann MA, Soifer SJ. Increased arterial pH, not decreased $Paco_2$, attenuates hypoxia-induced pulmonary vasoconstriction in newborn lambs. Pediatr Res 20:113-117, 1986.

Setzer E, Ermocilla R, Tonkin I, et al. Papillary muscle necrosis in a neonatal autopsy population: Incidence and associated clinical manifestations. J Pediatr 96:289-294, 1980.

Shaffer TH, Douglas PR, Sivieri EM, et al. Liquid ventilation (LV): Improved oxygenation in meconium stained lambs with persistent fetal circulation. Pediatr Res 16:361A, 1982.

Soifer SJ, Schreiber MD. Arachidonic acid metabolites mediate pulmonary hypertension caused by platelet activating factor in newborn lambs. Pediatr Res 23:525A, 1988.

Soifer SJ, Clyman RI, Heymann MA. Effects of prostaglandin D_2 on pulmonary arterial pressure and oxygenation in newborn infants with persistent pulmonary hypertension. J Pediatr 112:774-777, 1988.

Soifer SJ, Morin FC, Heymann MA. Developmental changes in the effect of prostaglandin D_2 on the pulmonary circulation in the newborn lamb. J Pediatr 100:458-463, 1982.

Spitz B, Magness RR, Cox SM, et al. I. Effect on angiotensin II pressor responses and blood prostaglandin concentrations in pregnant women sensitive to angiotensin II. Am J Obstet Gynecol 159:1035-1043, 1988.

Stenmark KR, James SL, Voelkel NF, et al. Leukotriene C_4 and D_4 in neonates with hypoxemia and pulmonary hypertension. N Engl J Med 309:77-80, 1983.

Tarpey MN, Graybar GB, Lyrene RK, et al. Thromboxane synthesis inhibition reverses group B streptococcus-induced pulmonary hypertension. Crit Care Med 15:644-647, 1987.

Taylor BJ. Leukotriene antagonist FPL 55712 reverses hypoxic pulmonary vasoconstriction in piglets. Pediatr Res 23:527A, 1988.

Tiefenbrunn LJ, Riemenschneider TA. Persistent pulmonary hypertension of the newborn. Am Heart J 111:564-572, 1986.

Truog WE, Feusner JF, Baker DL. Association of hemorrhagic disease and the syndrome of persistent fetal circulation with the fetal hydantoin syndrome. J Pediatr 96:112-114, 1980.

Turner GR, Levin DL. Prostaglandin synthesis inhibition in persistent pulmonary hypertension of the newborn. Clin Perinatol 11:581-589, 1984.

Valdes-Cruz LM, Dudell GG, Ferrara A. Utility of M-mode echocardiography for early identification of infants with persistent pulmonary hypertension of the newborn. Pediatrics 68:515-525, 1981.

Wagenvoort CA. Misalignment of lung vessels: A syndrome causing persistent neonatal pulmonary hypertension. Hum Pathol 17:727-730, 1986.

Wagenvoort CA, Dingemans KP. Pulmonary vascular smooth muscle and its interaction with endothelium. Chest 88:200S-202S, 1985.

Waites KB, Crouse DT, Philips JB III, et al. Ureaplasmal pneumonia and sepsis associated with persistent pulmonary hypertension of the newborn. Pediatrics 83:79-85, 1989.

Ward RM. Pharmacology of tolazoline. Clin Perinatol 11:703-713, 1984.

Ward RM, Daniel CH, Kendig JW, et al. Oliguria and tolazoline pharmacokinetics in the newborn. Pediatrics 77:307-315, 1986.

Wecsner KM, Bucher JR, Roberts RJ. Hypoxia alters lung vascular development. Pediatr Res 16:107A, 1982.

Wilkinson AR, Aynsley-Green A, Mitchell MD. Persistent pulmonary hypertension and abnormal prostaglandin E levels in preterm infants after maternal treatment with naproxen. Arch Dis Child 54:942-945, 1979.

Wung JT, James LS, Kilchevsky E, et al. Management of infants with severe respiratory failure and persistence of the fetal circulation, without hyperventilation. Pediatrics 76:488-494, 1985.

Yeh TF, Lilien LD. Altered lung mechanics in neonates with persistent fetal circulation syndrome. Crit Care Med 9:83-84, 1981.

40 Cardiac Tamponade

Timothy F. Feltes

BACKGROUND AND PHYSIOLOGY

Accumulation of fluid in the pericardial space may lead to compression of the heart with impairment of diastolic filling, resulting in a decrease in cardiac output, a condition known as cardiac tamponade. Early detection and swift management of this condition are necessary to prevent a clinical catastrophe.

Venous return to the heart occurs primarily during two phases of the cardiac cycle and is reflected by changes that occur in the central venous blood pressure. During ventricular ejection the total cardiac volume decreases, allowing venous spillage to the atria, and corresponds to the systolic x-descent of the systemic venous blood pressure tracing (Fig. 40-1, *A*). During early diastole venous return again increases as the tricuspid valve opens and is marked by a y-descent of the central venous pressure (Fig. 40-1, *A*).

Normally the intrapericardial pressure closely parallels pleural pressure and is significantly less than the diastolic pressures inside of the heart. The transmural pressure difference allows the various cardiac chambers to remain distended throughout the cardiac cycle and offers no significant resistance to venous return to the heart. With the accumulation of fluid in the pericardial space the intrapericardial pressure gradually increases and reduces the transmural pressure difference. When the intrapericardial pressure equals that of the right heart's diastolic pressure, collapse of the right atrium and ventricle occurs. Despite opening of the tricuspid valve, ventricular filling is impaired by the equilibration of the diastolic right atrial, ventricular, and pericardial pressures. This diastolic dysfunction results in an elevation in central venous blood pressure and attenuation or loss of the y-descent (Fig. 40-1, *B*). Because the left heart normally has a slightly higher diastolic pressure than the right, collapse of the left atrium and left ventricle generally does not occur until the intrapericardial

pressure increases further. However, left ventricular end-diastolic volume is reduced, resulting in a decrease in stroke volume and cardiac output. The body attempts to compensate for this reduction in output by increasing systemic vascular resistance (increasing systemic arterial blood pressure), heart rate, and myocardial contractility. When these compensatory mechanisms fail, cardiovascular collapse ensues.

The development of cardiac tamponade depends greatly on the compliance of the pericardial sac. Slowly developing pericardial effusions generally allow time for the pericardium to distend gradually without a significant change in intrapericardial pressure so that sizable accumulations may occur without evidence of tamponade. In contrast a small volume of intrapericardial fluid may lead to tamponade if accumulation occurs rapidly before a change in pericardial compliance can occur.

Clinical Setting and Recognition

Cardiac tamponade in the pediatric age group may be encountered in a variety of clinical settings. Pericardial fluid accumulation leading to tamponade may consist of blood (e.g., acute postoperative hemorrhage), a transudate (e.g., postpericardiotomy syndrome), an exudate (e.g., purulent pericarditis), crystalloid solution (e.g., erosion of a central venous catheter tip through a vessel wall), or even air (pneumopericardium in patients on positive pressure ventilation) and may accumulate slowly or rapidly.

Physical Examination

Cardiac tamponade is a cause of shock but does not necessarily initially appear as cardiovascular collapse. Therefore this diagnosis must always be considered in the patient presenting with early signs of a low cardiac output state of unknown etiology.

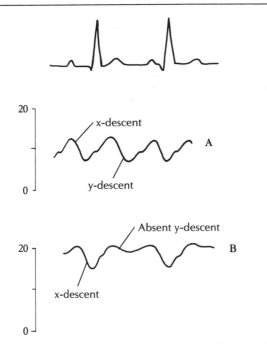

Fig. 40-1 Central venous pressure tracings in the normal patient, **A**, and in patient with cardiac tamponade, **B**. Note the elevation of pressure and loss of the y-descent in the patient with tamponade.

Typically the patient with cardiac tamponade is distressed, dyspneic, and tachycardic and may lose consciousness. The extremities are cold and clammy. By mechanisms outlined previously the systemic arterial blood pressure is maintained early in the course of tamponade, but the pulse pressure becomes progressively narrow as a result of decreased cardiac filling with eventual loss of systemic blood pressure. Reduced urinary output may precede declines in the systemic blood pressure. The central venous blood pressure is increased as reflected by jugular venous distention, and the y-descent is characteristically lost in the pressure tracing (Fig. 40-1, *B*). Kussmaul's sign, distention of the jugular vein during inspiration, has been described in patients with cardiac tamponade. Cardiac tones become muffled on auscultation. In addition other signs of venous hypertension such as hepatosplenomegaly may be present.

Pulsus Paradoxus

Pulsus paradoxus is a regular finding in patients with cardiac tamponade but may also occur in other low cardiac output states. The term "pulsus paradoxus" in the setting of cardiac tamponade is actually a misnomer since the change in the pulses represents only an exaggeration of a normal physiologic response. Normally systolic arterial blood pressure falls a slight amount during inspiration, but the change does not exceed 10 mm Hg. Decreases in excess of this amount represent pulsus paradoxus (Fig. 40-2). Testing for pulsus paradoxus may be conducted using either an indwelling arterial pressure tracing or a cuff sphygmomanometer reading. In the latter the cuff must be inflated to a level approximately 20 mm Hg above systolic arterial pressure. As the cuff is deflated, the pressure at which intermittent Korotkoff sounds become audible (associated with expiration) is recorded. As the cuff is further deflated, the pressure at which the Korotkoff sounds become constant throughout the respiratory cycle can be noted. A difference between these two systolic pressures of 10 mm Hg or more constitutes pulsus paradoxus. Since these findings occur only during normal respiratory activity, mechanically ventilated patients will not demonstrate this type response and may, in fact, reverse the order of the paradox.

The mechanisms of pulsus paradoxus are complex and not fully understood. Considerable evidence suggests that at least three mechanisms that occur during inspiration contribute to this condition: (1) increased venous return to the right heart causes a leftward shift of the interventricular septum and reduces left ventricular volume; (2) increased transit time for pulmonary blood flow in the lung reduces left ventricular venous return; and (3) decreased intrathoracic pressure transiently reduces systolic arterial pressure. All of these mechanisms are enhanced in the tamponade state.

MONITORING AND LABORATORY TESTS
Chest Roentgenogram

The chest roentgenogram in cardiac tamponade is nonspecific and may appear completely normal. In tamponade secondary to chronic effusions the cardiac silhouette is likely to appear enlarged, taking on a globular or water-bottle shape. The pulmonary vascular markings may be reduced and the mediastinum widened. Serial chest roentgenograms using an iden-

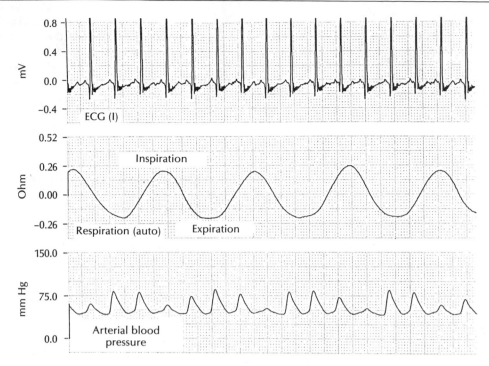

Fig. 40-2   Pulsus paradoxus in patient with cardiac tamponade. Note the decrease in systolic blood pressure with inspiration.

tical technique each time may be helpful in confirming the suspicion of pericardial effusions, particularly in the postoperative patient.

Electrocardiogram

It is not unusual for the ECG of the patient with cardiac tamponade to demonstrate reduced QRS voltages and ST segment elevation consistent with changes seen in pericarditis. Electrical alternans has also been described in patients with tamponade. This phenomenon is characterized by a phasic change in the QRS amplitude and is thought to be related to a "swinging" effect of the heart within the pericardial space (Fig. 40-3).

Echocardiogram

The echocardiogram is a reliable tool in the diagnosis of pericardial effusions and identification of signs of cardiac tamponade. In experienced hands two-dimensional and Doppler echocardiography assists

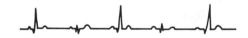

Fig. 40-3   Electrical alternans in cardiac tamponade.

in localizing and characterizing the pericardial effusion (e.g., anterior/posterior, fibrous), potentially identifying the source of the effusion (e.g., dehiscent suture line) and identifying signs of impending cardiovascular collapse (e.g., diastolic collapse of atria and ventricles).

Other

Compulsive monitoring of chest tube output in postoperative patients must always be exercised. A sudden decrease of output from a previously briskly draining mediastinal chest tube may indicate blockage of the tube either by a clot or kink. "Milking" or suctioning of the tube is indicated.

Because intravascular catheter tips can erode vascular walls, confirmation of catheter location by chest roentgenograms must be obtained intermittently. If there is a question of extravascular erosion, the IV fluid container and line can be removed from the mechanical pump, then lowered to a level below the heart. A solid blood return in the line usually indicates an intravascular location.

TREATMENT

As with all patients in a low cardiac output state, a reliable IV catheter, preferably with central venous blood pressure monitoring capacity, must be established in patients with cardiac tamponade. IV fluids must be initiated and administered liberally. However, caution must be used in employing central venous catheters that were in place at the time of tamponade since erosion of a vessel by these catheters may represent the source of the problem. Positive inotropic agents may be necessary to maintain systemic arterial blood pressure, but digoxin, which may cause an undesirable slowing of the heart rate, must be avoided. Because tachycardia may temporarily delay the cardiovascular collapse that occurs in tamponade, isoproterenol infusion is the inotropic agent of choice in these patients. Although some investigators have advocated the use of afterload-reducing agents in patients with cardiac tamponade as a means of increasing cardiac output, this treatment plan remains controversial. Because of potential ill effects of afterload-reducing agents on systemic arterial blood pressure in patients with cardiac tamponade and depleted intravascular volume, liberal use of IV fluids in conjunction with these agents is recommended. If respiratory arrest ensues, intubation and ventilation are necessary. However, positive pressure ventilation reduces pulmonary blood flow in the presence of cardiac tamponade and must, therefore, be used cautiously.

One thing is certain about the management of cardiac tamponade: the pericardial effusion must be evacuated. But who is to perform the procedure? Is a pericardiocentesis safe to perform, or should the patient be surgically explored? If cardiac tamponade is a suspected cause of low cardiac output in a patient, an echocardiogram must be obtained promptly. This study is not only confirmatory, but also provides ad-

ditional information that helps determine the most effective course of action in relieving the pericardial effusion. A variety of conditions may exist that either increase the potential risks of pericardiocentesis or reduce the success of adequate evacuation of the effusion by this technique: (1) small pericardial effusion, (2) lack of anterior extension of the effusion (i.e., posterior pericardial effusion that is difficult to reach), (3) loculated effusions, (4) effusion caused by active bleeding (posttraumatic, postoperative), and (5) formed clot that is difficult to aspirate. If any of these conditions is encountered, the patient needs referral for surgical evacuation.

The anesthetic agent selected must be one that does not result in significant vasodilatation and drop in systemic blood pressure or myocardial depression. Recommendations include induction with ketamine (1 mg/kg) and pancuronium (0.1 mg/kg) and maintenance with fentanyl and nitrous oxide in oxygen. Inhalation agents may not be well tolerated. Again, positive pressure ventilation must be used cautiously in these patients.

If the pericardial effusion appears reasonably large and nonloculated and extends anteriorly in the pericardial space, uncomplicated pericardiocentesis can be anticipated. For acute relief of the tamponade and/or for diagnostic purposes, pericardiocentesis may be performed by, or supervised by, someone experienced with the procedure in the intensive care setting; the procedure is greatly facilitated by the use of echocardiographic or portable fluoroscopic guidance of needle placement.

The patient's chest and head are tilted up approximately 20 to 30 degrees to displace the pericardial fluid anteriorly and inferiorly. An aseptic preparation of the chest and upper abdomen is performed with an iodine solution, and a local anesthetic (1% lidocaine) is infiltrated in the left subxiphoid region. Depending on the patient's age, a small nick using a No. 11 scalpel blade may facilitate entry of the piercing needle. A long 18-guage thin-walled needle is attached to the end of a syringe containing a small amount of nonbacteriostatic 0.9% sodium chloride solution. Use of lumbar puncture needles should be avoided since they tend to have long bevels and may injure the epicardium. The size of the syringe used depends, in part, on the size of the patient. Five or 10 ml syringes may be adequate for the newborn, whereas 60 ml syringes are more appropriate for the teenaged patient. Remember the larger the syringe the greater the negative pressure generated at the needle tip with aspiration. Overzealous aspiration may cause local tissue to be sucked into the bevel, making it difficult to confirm placement of the needle in the pericardial space. A metal alligator clamp may be attached to the hub of this needle, and connected to a precordial lead (V), and a continuous ECG may be recorded during the procedure (Fig. 40-4). If the equipment being used does not have equipotential grounding, the inserted needle could function as a current conductor and induce ventricular fibrillation during the procedure. If there is any question about what setup is available, the electrode method should not be used.

The puncture site is just to the left of the xiphoid process at its junction with the costal margin. The tip of the needle is directed posteriorly just deep enough to clear the bony structures. The hub of the needle is then tilted posteriorly by approximately 15 degrees and the tip of the needle directed toward the left shoulder. The needle should not be advanced during

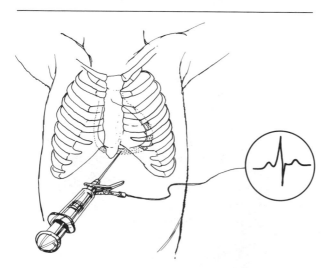

Fig. 40-4 Subxiphoid approach to pericardiocentesis. The hub of the needle is angled 15 degrees caudally, and the needle tip is directed toward the left shoulder while being advanced from a puncture site just to the left of the xiphoid process. An alligator clip is attached to the hub of the needle and is connected to a precordial lead to monitor for a myocardial injury current.

this directing process. Once aimed, the needle tip is then advanced by steady, deliberate moves, and aspiration with the syringe is attempted after every few millimeters. Trying to maintain a constant negative pressure with the syringe is cumbersome and gives the operator less fine motor control. The ECG, either by surface or needle electrography, must be constantly observed, preferably by an assistant. Acute ST-T wave changes (Fig. 40-4) or the presence of ectopic beats suggests that the needle tip has come in contact with the epicardium. If this occurs, avoid any unsteady movements and slowly withdraw the needle, attempting to aspirate pericardial fluid once the ECG changes have disappeared.

If blood is aspirated and it is uncertain where the needle tip is located, a small amount of contrast material may be injected into the space and visualized under fluoroscopy. A small amount of agitated sterile 0.9% sodium chloride solution injected under echocardiographic visualization will also confirm needle tip location. If the procedure is performed blindly and blood is aspirated but there is no hemodynamic improvement, the tip of the needle can be assumed to be in the heart, and the needle must be withdrawn in the manner described previously.

Complete evacuation of the pericardial effusion through a blindly placed needle may be dangerous. It is preferable to relieve the tamponade by this technique and then place an indwelling catheter into the pericardial space for complete relief of the effusion. This can be performed effectively by introducing the soft end of a spring guidewire through the needle and advancing the wire into the desired location of the catheter (anterior vs. posterior). The needle is then removed, and a catheter such as a No. 4 pigtail is advanced into the pericardial space over the guidewire. The wire is then removed, and gentle aspiration pressure is placed on the catheter. It is commonly necessary to reposition the catheter intermittently for complete evacuation of the effusion. Because this latter technique requires the ability to distinguish anterior and posterior placement in the pericardial sac, this procedure is best performed in a catheterization laboratory if available.

Fluid obtained from a pericardiocentesis must be submitted for several laboratory tests, including Gram's stain, white and red blood cell counts, and glucose, protein, and amylase levels. If the cause of the effusion is uncertain, consider obtaining specimens for cytologic studies (in heparinized tubes) and aerobic, anaerobic, and fungal cultures.

Remember, what has collected once may collect again, and treatment of the primary cause of the pericardial effusion needs further consideration.

RISKS AND COMPLICATIONS

The principal risks of pericardiocentesis are perforation of the myocardium, coronary artery injury, and pneumothorax.

ADDITIONAL READING

• Darsee JR, Braunwald E. Diseases of the pericardium. In Braunwald E, ed. Heart Disease: A Textbook of Cardiovascular Medicine. Philadelphia: WB Saunders, 1984.

Fowler NO. Physiology of cardiac tamponade and pulsus paradoxus. I. Mechanisms of pulsus paradoxus in cardiac tamponade. Mod Concepts Cardiovasc Dis 47:109, 1978.

• Fowler NO. Physiology of cardiac tamponade and pulsus paradoxus. II. Physiologic, circulatory, and pharmacological responses in cardiac tamponade. Mod Concepts Cardiovasc Dis 47:115, 1978.

Hudson RB. Diseases of the pericardium. In Hurst JW, Logue RB, Schlant RC, Wenger NK, eds. The Heart, Arteries and Veins. New York: McGraw-Hill, 1978.

Lell WA, Reves JG, Samuelson PN. Anesthesia for cardiovascular surgery. In Kirklin JW, Barratt-Boyes BG, eds. Cardiac Surgery. New York: John Wiley, 1986.

41 Nosocomial Infection

Jane D. Siegel · Patti Duer

BACKGROUND AND PHYSIOLOGY

A nosocomial infection is a localized or systemic condition acquired after admission to the hospital as an adverse reaction to the presence of an infectious agent(s) or its toxin(s). Onset of symptoms must appear at least 48 to 72 hours after admission. The highest priority for infection control resources is assigned to surveillance of patients in ICUs. Studies in general hospitals have reported a 3- to 20-fold increase in the incidence of hospital-acquired infection in the ICU as compared with other inpatient areas. Although beds in ICUs account for only 6% of all hospital beds in the United States, 25% of all nosocomial infections and 35% to 50% of hospital-acquired bacteremias and pneumonias occur in ICU patients. ICU patients constitute a large proportion of patients infected with multiply resistant organisms, outbreaks occur more frequently in ICUs, and there is a significant increase in morbidity and mortality in infected vs. noninfected ICU patients.

The PICU is the only area of the pediatric hospital in which patients are not segregated by age or diagnosis. Neonates, older children, and surgical and medical patients are cared for in the same closed environment. Recent studies of PICUs and neonatal intensive care units (NICUs) have found a similar increase in the incidence of nosocomial infection as compared with other areas of the hospital. In a review of the epidemiology of nosocomial infection in pediatric patients from 1970 to 1986 the overall rate of hospital-acquired infection in pediatric hospitals was found to be 4.1%, with the highest rates occurring in the NICU (22.5%) and the PICU (13.5%) (Table 41-1). The higher rates of infection were reported in prospective studies that included viral cultures of symptomatic patients. In pediatric patients more than 50% of nosocomial infections are attributable to bacteremias and infections of the respiratory and gastrointestinal tracts, and infections of the urinary tract

and surgical wounds each account for less than 10% of infections. In contrast more than 40% of hospital-acquired infections in adults are urinary tract infections, and 20% are surgical wound infections. Cutaneous infections occur frequently in the neonate but are rare in older patients.

During the past decade gram-positive bacteria and viruses have accounted for more nosocomial infections than gram-negative bacteria. *Staphylococcus aureus* is the most frequently reported pathogen from pediatric services, and coagulase-negative staphylococci have assumed a major role in catheter-related sepsis in both the NICU and PICU. Methicillin-resistant *S. aureus* is now endemic to many large (≥200 beds) pediatric hospitals in the United States. In studies in which viral infections are detected, rotavirus and respiratory syncytial virus (RSV) may be the most important hospital-aquired pathogens during the winter season. Outbreaks of RSV within a PICU or NICU cause significant morbidity and mortality among infants with chronic bronchopulmonary dis-

Table 41-1 Incidence of Nosocomial Infection in Children*

Site	Incidence (%) and Range
Neonatal ICU (NICU)	22.5 (5.9-30.4)
Normal newborn nursery	0.9 (0.6-2.0)
Pediatric ICU (PICU)	13.5 (6.2-24.1)
Pediatric hospitals, overall	4.1 (2.8-10.3)
Pediatric services in general hospitals	1.2 (1.2-5.5)
Adult medical-surgical ICUs	5-24

*Modified from Jarvis WR. Epidemiology of nosocomial infections in pediatric patients. Pediatr Infect Dis 6:344, 1987. Copyright by William & Wilkins.

ease, congenital heart disease, and immunodeficiency syndromes. Fungi, mainly *Candida* sp and *Aspergillus,* may account for only 3% to 15% of nosocomial infections in the PICU but are difficult to treat and are associated with substantial morbidity and mortality in low birthweight infants and immunocompromised patients. The most frequently encountered nosocomial pathogens and their associated clinical manifestations are presented in Table 41-2.

Risk Factors

Host factors. PICU patients have compromised host defenses by virtue of the complexity of their primary disease, the associated immunosuppressive therapy, and their poor nutritional state. The underlying disease is the most important factor in predicting mortality as a result of nosocomial infection. All components of the neonate's host defense system are deficient as compared with older infants and adults, and these deficiencies are more severe in the premature infant.

Device and procedure-related factors. The intensive monitoring and life support procedures needed by PICU patients violate the natural barriers to infection and facilitate invasion by pathogens. Contaminated equipment and fluids that have been associated with outbreaks of infection in ICUs and nurseries are as follows:

Scalp electrodes	Resuscitation equipment
Eye or umbilical cord wash	Bulb syringes
	Rectal thermometers
Disinfectants	Catheters
Topical ointment	Pressure transducers
Hand lotion	IV fluids, TPN, heparin
Scrub brushes	Blood products
Laundry	Banked breast milk
Elastoplast	

Respiratory support equipment has the potential for contamination with "water bugs" such as *Pseudomonas* sp. Additionally, endotracheal and nasotracheal intubation are associated with an increased risk of purulent otitis media and sinusitis due to obstruction of the normal drainage of the eustachian tubes and the maxillary and ethmoid sinuses. Purulent otitis media has been identified as a "silent" source of sepsis in the PICU. *P. aeruginosa* inoculated into the eye at the time of endotracheal suctioning has been responsible for outbreaks of bacterial conjunctivitis in both adult and pediatric ICUs.

Invasive vascular access lines, especially central venous catheters (CVCs) and arterial catheters, contribute substantially to the risk of bacteremia and, in rare instances, endocarditis. Reported rates of infections from indwelling CVCs (e.g., Broviac, Hickman) are 0.2 to 0.5/1000 catheter days, with the highest rates occurring in neonates, immunosuppressed patients, and patients receiving hyperalimentation fluids. Cannula colonization with skin pathogens re-

---

RISK FACTORS ASSOCIATED WITH NOSOCOMIAL INFECTION IN THE PICU PATIENT

Heterogeneity of patients
Crowding, understaffing
Duration of stay
Compromised host defenses
   Neonates
   Immunodeficiency syndromes: congenital, acquired
   Immunosuppressive therapy: oncology, organ or bone marrow transplant
Device- and procedure-related risk factors
   Respiratory therapy equipment
   Intravascular catheters: central venous, multiple use, arterial
   Pressure-monitoring transducers
   Intracranial pressure monitors
   Peritoneal dialysis catheters
   Urinary catheters
   Nasogastric and nasotracheal intubation
Acquisition of hospital flora
   Multiply resistant gram-negative bacilli
   Methicillin-resistant staphylococci: methicillin-resistant *S. aureus* (MRSA), coagulase-negative staphylococci (e.g., *S. epidermidis, S. haemolyticus*)
   Seasonal viruses: respiratory syncytial virus, rotavirus, enteroviruses
Transfused blood products
   Hepatitis (hepatitis B; non-A, non-B), human immunodeficiency virus (HIV), cytomegalovirus (CMV)
Contaminated air
   Construction-associated aspergillosis
   Varicella
   Tuberculosis

Table 41-2 Etiology and Clinical Manifestations of Hospital-Acquired Infections

Pathogen	Septicemia	Central Venous Catheter	Endocarditis	Meningitis/Ventriculo-peritoneal Shunt	Bone/Joint	Pneumonia	Diarrhea*	Urinary Tract Infection	Hepatitis	Skin/Soft Tissue
Gram-positive bacteria										
S. aureus†	+	+	+		+	+				+
Coagulase-negative staphylococci	+	+	+	+						
Streptococci										
Group A†	+									+
Group B	+			+	+					+
Group D (enterococcus)	+	+	+					+		
Gram-negative bacteria										
E. coli, Klebsiella, Enterobacter, Serratia, Pseudomonas	+	+	+	+	+	+		+		+
Salmonella sp	+				+					
Citrobacter diversus	+			+				+		
Anaerobes										
Clostridium difficile							+			
Fungus										
Candida sp	+	+	+	+	+	+				+
Aspergillus	+			+	+	+				
Malassezia furfur	+	+				+				
Virus										
Respiratory syncytial (RSV)	+					+				
Rotavirus							+			
Herpes simplex	+			+					+	+
Cytomegalovirus	+			+		+			+	
Enteroviruses (Coxsackie, ECHO)	+		+‡	+					+	

*May be associated with necrotizing enterocolitis in neonates.
†May be associated with toxic shock syndrome.
‡Myocarditis.

sults in invasion and occasionally dissemination of infection. Each port of a multilumen catheter must be considered a potential entry site for microorganisms. Disease rather than colonization in a symptomatic patient is likely when a microorganism is isolated simultaneously from peripheral and central venous blood cultures or when a semiquantitative catheter tip culture yields ≥15 colonies/ml. Specific guidelines for insertion and care of catheters have been developed by the CDC. The decreased rate of complications associated with team care of CVCs used for administration of TPN fluids reflects the efficacy of consistent protocol-guided care. Additionally, pressure-monitoring transducers used with intravascular catheters have been reported as sources of nosocomial infection. Therefore disposable transducers or domes should not be reused, and reusable equipment must be adequately cleansed and sterilized after each patient use.

Iodophor solutions used for routine CVC care may be intrinsically contaminated during the manufacturing process. Both true infection and pseudoinfection (positive culture of normally sterile body fluid in the absence of clinical disease) may result from such contamination. Pseudobacteremia and pseudomeningitis may also occur in ICU patients as a result of contamination of commercial culture media or of blood culture analyzers. Pathogens that commonly cause disease as well as unusual pathogens (e.g., *P. cepacia, P. putida, Bacillus* sp) are recovered from patients with pseudoinfections.

Acquisition of hospital flora. PICU patients may develop mucosal and skin colonization with hospital flora (gram-negative bacilli, staphylococci, fungi) soon after admission. Increased pharyngeal colonization with gram-negative bacilli correlates best with the clinical severity of illness. Oropharyngeal colonization may be enhanced by retrograde spread of organisms in the stomach. The stomach becomes a more favorable environment for bacterial growth when the gastric pH is elevated by agents administered for the prevention of stress gastritis and gastric ulceration. The risk of stool colonization with *Klebsiella, Enterobacter,* and *Citrobacter* species is increased with the duration of hospitalization. Selective pressure exerted by liberal use of broad-spectrum antimicrobial agents within a closed environment facilitates the emergence of multiply resistant strains of bacteria. Plasmid-mediated resistance results in several different species with a similar pattern of resistance. Resistance of hospital-acquired gram-negative bacilli to third-generation cephalosporins (e.g., cefotaxime, ceftriaxone, ceftazidime) may develop within weeks of introduction of these agents as first-line agents for empiric treatment of all patients with suspected sepsis. A PICU that is located within a teaching hospital complex and accepts transfers from other institutions is at increased risk of acquiring methicillin-resistant *S. aureus* as part of the endemic flora.

Transfused blood products. Routine screening of blood donors for hepatitis B surface antigen (HBsAg) and antihuman immunodeficiency virus and heat treatment of factor concentrates have nearly eliminated the transmission of hepatitis B (HBV) and human immunodeficiency virus (HIV). The risk of transmission of HIV by transfusion is estimated at present to be <1 in 40,000. More than 90% of posttransfusion hepatitis is attributed to non-A, non-B hepatitis agents. The risk of transmitting non-A, non-B hepatitis is approximately 10 to 15 cases/1000 units of transfused blood derived from volunteer donors. The frequency of posttransfusion hepatitis is expected to be reduced by 30% to 40% since universal screening for non-A, non-B hepatitis surrogate markers, ALT and anti-HBc, became a requirement in 1987. Approximately 2.5% to 12% of blood donors may transmit CMV. The likelihood of acquiring symptomatic disease is greatest in immunosuppressed recipients who are CMV seronegative, and it is significantly correlated with the volume of transfused blood. CMV-seronegative blood is required for transfusion of infants who weigh <1500 g at birth. CMV-seronegative organ and blood donors are preferred whenever possible for seronegative organ or bone marrow transplant recipients.

Mode of transmission. Hand carriage of pathogens is by far the single most important mode of transmission of infective agents and is most likely to occur in overcrowded conditions and during understaffed periods. The fecal-oral route plays a major role in the spread of enteric pathogens (e.g., rotavirus, hepatitis A virus, *Salmonella* sp, *Shigella* sp, *Clostridium difficile*), several of which have been associated with outbreaks of necrotizing enterocolitis among neonates. Airborne transmission of varicella and tuberculosis in the hospital setting has been observed. Patients with varicella can harbor the virus in the nasopharynx for 24 hours before the eruption of skin lesions and therefore are considered infectious from this time until all lesions are completely crusted, even if being treated wth acyclovir. Similarly, immuno-compromised patients with herpes zoster (shingles) are at risk for dissemination and may transmit the virus by the respiratory route. Only patients with cavitary lesions of pulmonary tuberculosis are able to transmit infection by aerosolization of tubercle bacilli in sputum. However, visiting family members with previously undiagnosed cavitary tuberculosis may be unsuspected disseminators of infection within a unit. Nosocomial outbreaks of aspergillosis in immuno-compromised hosts have been associated with airborne spread from hospital construction sites or a poorly functioning air-filtering system.

Direct infusion or ingestion of fluids contaminated with bacteria is infrequent.

Infectious Risks for Personnel

Hospital personnel with direct patient care responsibilities are at increased risk of acquiring blood-borne infections after percutaneous (e.g., needle-stick) or mucous membrane (splash onto conjunctivae, nose, mouth, nonintact skin) exposure. The risk of acquiring hepatitis B viral infection after percutaneous or mucous membrane exposure is approximately 20%. Although 75% of these cases are not clinically recognizable, 5% of those infected are hospitalized, and 1.7% die from acute and chronic effects of the HBV infection. In contrast the risk of an HIV infection after percutaneous or mucous membrane exposure is, at most, 0.4% to 0.9%. However, recognition that HIV-infected individuals will eventually develop clinical symptoms of AIDS that is associated with ≥70% case fatality rate, combined with the fact that patients with HIV infection are not identified reliably by history or physical examination, has led most U.S. hospitals to adopt the universal precautions policy recommended by the CDC in 1987.

Several agents such as RSV, rotavirus, and *Bordetella pertussis* readily infect and produce clinical disease in health care workers. Similar infection rates for RSV and rotavirus infection have been reported in both personnel and patients during outbreaks. Although the adult caregiver develops only minor symptoms, he will transmit infection to other patients if proper precautions are not observed.

Some infections transmitted by blood and respiratory secretions have special implications for pregnant health care workers because of the potentially adverse effect on the fetus. The risk of their acquiring

---

INFECTIONS THAT MAY BE ACQUIRED BY HOSPITAL PERSONNEL FROM PATIENTS

Blood, body fluids

HIV,* hepatitis B,* non-A, non-B hepatitis, CMV,* meningococcal infection,* syphilis,* adenoviral conjunctivitis

Respiratory tract

RSV, influenza, varicella,* rubella,* rubeola* (measles), pertussis, meningococcal infection, tuberculosis

Enteric source

Rotavirus, hepatitis A, salmonellosis,* shigellosis, *Campylobacter* infection

Skin

Herpes simplex, herpes zoster, staphylococcal dermatitis (MRSA), scabies

*Serious implications for the fetus of a pregnant employee.

CMV infection has been questioned most frequently. However, clinical studies have not demonstrated an increased risk of acquisition of CMV infection by health care workers. In fact, the greater risk occurs during household exposure to toddlers enrolled in day care centers. Having the antibody to CMV before pregnancy is protective against the clinical manifestations of intrauterine infection.

MONITORING AND LABORATORY TESTS

An effective infection surveillance and control program in the PICU has the following components:

1. Development and updating of policies for invasive procedures and for disinfection and sterilization of devices and equipment with which patients come in contact
2. *Prospective* surveillance of infection rates and etiologic agents
3. Periodic review of antibiotic susceptibility patterns of pathogens acquired during the PICU stay
4. Regularly scheduled communication of surveillance results with the PICU staff

5. Focused educational programs
6. Prompt investigation and implementation of appropriate intervention programs when clusters of infections occur

Although the hospital infection control officer is responsible for the PICU, it is advantageous to designate one full-time PICU staff member as the infection control liaison. A hospital epidemiology computer program permits timely analysis and reporting of infection rates. Use of a case-mix adjuster scoring system (e.g., Acute Physiology and Chronic Health Evaluation [APACHE], Therapeutic Intervention Scoring System [TISS]) has been suggested by some hospital epidemiologists to account for the wide variation in severity of underlying disease. Overall infection rates are maintained optimally at ≤10%. Routine environmental and body surface cultures are not useful. However, colonization cultures will facilitate proper cohorting during an outbreak of disease or in the presence of colonization and/or disease caused by a multiply resistant organism such as MRSA or a gram-negative bacillus. The following sites are recommended for survey cultures: anterior nares (staphylococci), nasopharynx, rectum, axilla, umbilicus (neonate), endotracheal secretions, and purulent wound drainage. Swabs obtained from two separate sites may be incubated in one broth tube since identification of the specific site of colonization is not important in most unit surveys. The frequency of surveillance may vary from every 2 to 8 weeks, depending on how rapidly the results become available, conditions are changing, and transmission of infection is continuing. It is prudent to obtain body-surface cultures from new admissions who have been hospitalized for more than 5 days in another health care facility, especially if it is known that multiply resistant organisms are endemic to the referring institution. Colonized or infected patients are cohorted and cared for by personnel different from those for newly admitted or noncolonized patients.

When an outbreak of infection is suspected, appropriate investigations are performed cooperatively by the PICU staff, hospital infection control officer, and microbiology laboratory personnel to determine the source and to establish the identity of the pathogens isolated from the affected patients. Rapid diagnostic antigen detection tests are especially useful for RSV, rotavirus, and *Clostridium difficile*. More specific techniques such as phage typing, plasmid analysis, and restriction endonuclease enzyme analysis may be performed in a reference laboratory if necessary.

PREVENTION
Handwashing

Handwashing before and after each patient contact is the single most important method of interrupting transmission of hospital-acquired pathogens. Sinks for handwashing must be located at all entrances and exits to the PICU as well as among the patient beds. Ideally, one sink is located between each two beds. Separate sinks for cleaning equipment away from bed spaces must be available. The content of the antiseptic agent used for handwashing is of secondary importance under routine conditions. However, during outbreaks agents containing an iodophor for increased activity against gram-negative enteric bacilli or chlorhexidine for increased activity against staphylococci should be used, depending on the cause of the outbreak. Agents must be nonirritating to ensure compliance and to prevent dermatitis that may increase the likelihood of colonization of personnel with pathogens. Handwashing procedures must last long enough for all surfaces of fingers and hands to be cleansed. Alcohol-containing foams have bactericidal and virucidal activity against the commonly encountered pathogens. If used in sufficient quantity, these foams are a useful adjunct as the "quick handwash" between patients when substantial contamination with body fluids has not occurred. They cannot be substituted for the initial and final handwashes or for handwashing after extensive contamination with body fluids.

Space

Adequate floor space must be available so that each patient's equipment and supplies can be contained without overflow into adjacent patient care areas. Ideal allocations are 80 to 100 square feet per patient in the NICU and 300 to 400 square feet per patient in the PICU, with additional space for storage and utility and ancillary services. Physically separate clean and dirty storage areas must be designated.

Isolation

The CDC guidelines published in 1983 designated seven categories of isolation: strict, contact, respiratory, acid-fast bacillus for tuberculosis (AFB), enteric, drainage/secretion, and blood/body fluids. A private room is always required for strict, AFB, and respiratory isolation, although patients infected with the same organism may be cohorted together in one room. A room with negative pressure ventilation is required for all patients with cavitary tuberculosis, all patients with varicella or disseminated herpes zoster, and immunocompromised patients with localized herpes zoster. Negative pressure ventilation is preferred for patients with measles. The patient's hygiene and ability to contain infective body fluids will determine the need for a private room for enteric, blood/body fluid, and drainage/secretion precautions. Wearing masks is required for all persons entering a room in strict isolation, with the exception of individuals known to be immune to varicella when they are in the room of a patient with varicella or disseminated herpes zoster. Wearing masks is also required for only those individuals coming into close contact with patients in contact and respiratory isolation or when splatter of blood or secretions is likely to occur. The use of gowns and gloves is indicated whenever contact with infective material is likely to occur. The CDC guidelines for isolation and the biannual report of the Academy of Pediatrics Committee on Infectious Diseases, the *Redbook,* must be consulted for specific information concerning the appropriate isolation of PICU patients with infections at the time of bed assignment.

Routine use of gowns on entrance into the PICU has been traditional in many units. In a study of four crossover periods of 3 months of gown and no-gown use in a six-bed PICU, it was found that wearing gowns had no effect on the nosocomial infection rate, vascular catheter colonization rate, or compliance with handwashing between patient or support equipment contacts. The occurrence of visits per patient per hour and total visits per hour were, however, significantly decreased during the gown periods. Thus, when direct handling of patients and their secretions is unlikely to occur, gowning is not necessary. However, when patients are likely to be handled for examination, observation, feeding, or procedures, proper gowning may limit horizontal spread of infection. Less costly methods to decrease unnecessary traffic through the PICU are preferred.

Universal Precautions

Recognition that patients infected with HIV cannot be identified reliably by history and physical examination led the CDC to recommend in 1987 the ex-

> **APPLICATION OF UNIVERSAL PRECAUTIONS TO BODY FLUIDS AND PROCEDURES**
>
> *Apply*
> Body fluids: Blood, any fluid containing visible blood, semen, vaginal secretions, breast milk, amniotic fluid; normally sterile body fluids—CSF, synovial, pleural, pericardial, peritoneal
> Procedures: Endoscopy, intubation, endotracheal suctioning, rinsing of used instruments, lumbar puncture, puncture of normally sterile body cavities
>
> *Do not apply**
> Body fluids: Feces, nasal secretions, saliva, sputum, sweat, tears, urine, vomitus
> Procedures: Diaper change

*Unless these body fluids contain visible blood.

tension of blood and body fluid precautions to all patients (i.e., universal precautions). The goal of universal precautions is to prevent parenteral, mucous membrane, and nonintact skin exposures of health care workers to blood-borne pathogens. Other isolation categories such as enteric, AFB, and respiratory are applied in addition to universal blood and body fluid precautions when specific infectious agents are suspected or confirmed. It is prudent for every PICU to institute a policy of universal precautions even in areas with low HIV seroprevalence ($\leq 1:1000$) because of the increased exposure of blood. According to the revised recommendations published in 1988, universal precautions apply to contact with blood, tissues, normally sterile body fluids, and any body fluid containing visible blood. Since the risk of occupational transmission of HIV or HBV from patient to health care worker through certain body fluids such as saliva, urine, or feces is minimal or nonexistent, universal precautions do not apply routinely for such contacts. Specifically, gloves are not required for all diaper changes of infants without diarrhea.

The basic principles of universal precautions are as follows:

1. Prevent penetrating injuries when needles and other sharp instruments are handled. Do not recap

needles by hand but use a flat surface, hemostats, or other commercially available devices when recapping is necessary (e.g., inoculation of blood culture tubes). Locate puncture-resistant containers as close to the patient use area as is practical.

2. Use appropriate barriers to protect nonintact skin and mucous membranes from contact with the patient's blood or high-risk body fluids, mucous membranes, or nonintact skin. The use of nonsterile examination gloves made of vinyl or latex is appropriate for procedures that do not involve contact with normally sterile areas of the body. Gloves should be changed after contact with each patient and should not be washed or disinfected for reuse. Masks, goggles, gowns, or aprons should be worn during procedures that are likely to generate splattering of blood or high-risk body fluids.

3. Hands or skin surfaces should be washed after glove removal and immediately after accidental contamination with blood and high-risk body fluids. Contaminated surfaces or equipment are cleaned with a 1:10 diluted bleach solution.

4. The need for mouth-to-mouth resuscitation should be minimized by increasing the availability of appropriately sized bag and mask.

5. All laboratory specimens are considered contaminated and should be transported in plastic bags.

Catheters and Respiratory Therapy Equipment

Important features of established guidelines for use of catheters and respiratory therapy equipment are as follows:

1. IV catheters are changed every 72 hours or are inspected daily if left in place beyond that time.
2. Intravascular administration sets and extension tubing are changed every 24 hours for hyperalimentation fluids and every 72 hours for routine fluids.
3. Intravascular infusion fluid is changed every 12 hours if it contains lipid; otherwise it is changed every 24 hours.
4. Dressing changes and entries into CVCs are performed under aseptic conditions while wearing gloves and mask. Dressing changes are performed every 48 to 72 hours unless a transparent occlusive dressing is used, in which case daily inspection is recommended.
5. Infusion of blood products must be completed within 4 hours.

6. Mechanical ventilator tubing is changed every 48 to 72 hours.
7. In and out straight catheterization of the bladder is preferred over indwelling urinary catheterization whenever possible. When the use of indwelling urinary catheters is medically indicated, a sterile closed drainage system is used, and antibiotics are not added.

Housekeeping

The risk of disease transmission from soiled linen or most infective waste is negligible. Soiled linen is handled as little as possible and is bagged at the location at which it was used. Linens soiled with blood or body fluids are transported in bags that prevent leakage. All sharp instruments are placed in puncture-proof containers at the location of use and are autoclaved before disposal. Bulk blood and fluid-filled suction cannisters are disposed of according to state regulations for infective wastes. Excretions and secretions are disposed into a sanitary sewer.

Staff

Observation of appropriate precautions will protect against transmission of infection from patients to staff. These include:

1. Determine susceptibility of the health care worker to frequently encountered infections (varicella, rubella, measles) by history or serologic testing.
2. Comply with prophylaxis regimens.
   Before exposure: Immunization against hepatitis B, rubella, measles, influenza
   After exposure: Immunoglobulin for varicella, hepatitis B, non-A, non-B hepatitis; antibiotics for meningococcal infection, syphilis, pertussis
3. Know mode of transmission and recommended isolation techniques for specific infections of patients cared for.
4. Adhere meticulously to *universal* precautions.
5. Request factual counseling if exposure or potential exposure to an infectious agent has caused concern.

For infections such as hepatitis B, rubella, and measles, preexposure immunizations are recommended for individuals who are susceptible by history or by serologic testing. In the absence of a history of varicella, serologic testing is performed on the staff member to determine susceptibility. A susceptible health care worker must be removed from patient care from day 10 to 21 after exposure to a patient with varicella-zoster infection to prevent transmission to patients during the 24-hour period before eruption of the skin rash. Administration of varicella zoster immunoglobulin within 96 hours of exposure may be considered. Use of antibiotics is recommended after blood or mucous membrane exposure to the untreated patient with meningococcal disease or syphilis or after respiratory exposure to a patient with pertussis. Contact of the patient's respiratory secretions with the caregiver's mucous membranes or nonintact skin or a needlestick constitutes a significant exposure to *Neisseria meningitidis,* warranting antimicrobial prophylaxis. Presence in the room without direct blood or mucous membrane contact does not increase the risk of meningococcal infection for hospital personnel. Skin testing with purified protein derivative (PPD) is performed at 10 weeks after exposure to a patient with cavitary tuberculosis, and treatment with isoniazid is recommended if skin test conversion occurs and the individual is less than 35 years old.

A well-defined protocol for evaluation of percutaneous and mucous membrane exposures will facilitate appropriate testing of the source patient and the health care worker. Administration of immune serum globulin is recommended for significant mucous membrane or percutaneous exposures to non-A, non-B hepatitis and hepatitis B immune globulin, and administration of hepatitis B vaccine is recommended after exposure of the nonimmune employee to hepatitis B. The decision to perform serial determinations of antibody to HIV is based on the HIV seroprevalence of the geographic area, presence of risk factors, clinical suspicion in the source patient, and employee anxiety. It is prudent for members of the PICU staff who become pregnant to review with the employee health nurse the guidelines for pre-

vention of infections that may present special risks for her. Prepregnancy immunizations and adherence to universal precautions are protective against most infections likely to be encountered in the PICU.

Health care workers with direct patient contact must be aware that they can transmit to their patients respiratory and gastrointestinal tract infections as well as pathogens from weeping skin lesions *(herpes simplex, S. aureus)*. Individuals with these infections or lesions are best removed from direct patient contact until no longer infective. Employees with HIV infection should be restricted from direct patient care responsibilities only in the presence of weeping skin lesions or a transmissible secondary infection. In the presence of clinically significant immunocompromise, the employee with AIDS should avoid exposure to infectious agents that would jeopardize his health. Ongoing evaluation with the employee's private physician is advised.

ADDITIONAL READING

Centers for Disease Control recommendations for prevention of HIV transmission in health-care settings. MMWR 36(Suppl 25):3S-18S, 1987.

• Centers for Disease Control update: Universal precautions for prevention of transmission of human immunodeficiency virus, hepatitis B virus, and other bloodborne pathogens in health care settings. MMWR 37:377-387, 1988.

Donowitz LG. Failure of the overgown to prevent nosocomial infection in a pediatric intensive care unit. Pediatrics 77:35-38, 1986.

Garner JS, Simmons BP. Guidelines for isolation precautions in hospital. Infect Control 4(Suppl):245-348, 1983.

• Jarvis WR. Epidemiology of nosocomial infections in pediatric patients. Pediatr Infect Dis 6:344-351, 1987.

• Plotkin SA. Cytomegalovirus in hospitals. Pediatr Infect Dis 5:177-178, 1986.

• Report of the Committee on Infectious Diseases. Elk Grove Village, Ill.: American Academy of Pediatrics, 1988.

42 Sepsis

Octavio Ramilo · Jane D. Siegel

BACKGROUND AND PHYSIOLOGY

Sepsis is a clinical condition defined by the presence of microorganisms or their toxic products in the bloodstream. Approximately 15% to 20% of children admitted to the PICU have an infectious disease as the primary indication for intensive monitoring and treatment. Another 5% of PICU patients may have an episode of sepsis during their stay after admision for treatment of another condition (see Chaper 41).

Bacteria are the most common etiologic agents of clinical sepsis, but fungi, viruses, and rickettsiae are associated with similar clinical findings. These infectious agents or their toxins are capable of activating a cascade of mediators of inflammation that results in a characteristic host response. The actions of cachectin, interleukin-1 (IL-1), prostaglandins, complement, platelet-activating factor (PAF), and kinins are responsible for the complex pathophysiologic changes and clinical manifestations of septicemia. The lipid A moiety of the lipopolysaccharide of gram-negative organisms and the cell wall components of pneumococci have been identified as specific triggers of the host inflammatory response. Once these deleterious mechanisms are set in motion, the patient will progress to a stage of circulatory insufficiency, shock, or purpura fulminans in the most severe cases unless promptly and effectively managed.

The clinical manifestations and etiologic organisms associated with sepsis vary in different age groups.

The Neonate

In the neonate the presentation of sepsis is often subtle and difficult to distinguish from noninfectious disorders. Respiratory distress, temperature instability, and gastrointestinal signs such as abdominal distention and diarrhea are frequent clinical findings. The infection usually involves the bloodstream, without evidence of a primary focus. However, there is spread to the meninges in 25% of cases.

The most common pathogens are those frequently isolated from the maternal gastrointestinal and genital tracts, and group B streptococcus is currently the predominant etiologic agent of neonatal sepsis in most geographic areas of the United States. Two distinct forms of streptococcal disease have been described. The early-onset syndrome usually occurs during the first 3 days of life and is characterized by respiratory distress, pulmonary arterial hypertension, hypoxemia, severe shock, and disseminated intravascular coagulation (DIC). The late-onset form is more insidious and is associated with meningitis, osteomyelitis, or other soft tissue foci of infection. *Escherichia coli,* enterococcus, *Listeria monocytogenes,* nongroup D α-hemolytic streptococcus, and nontypable *Haemophilus influenzae* are other microorganisms responsible for sepsis neonatorum. Less frequently isolated pathogens that are important in late-onset infections, especially those acquired in the hospital, include coagulase-negative staphylococci, *Staphylococcus aureus,* gram-negative enteric rods, *Pseudomonas* sp, and *Candida* sp. *H. influenzae* type b and *Salmonella* species may be either maternally or community acquired.

Herpes simplex, enteroviruses (coxsackie and ECHO), and adenovirus must be considered in the differential diagnosis of a septic neonate if no improvement is observed after initiation of antibiotic therapy and bacterial cultures are sterile. Hepatic and CNS involvement are frequently observed in patients with these viruses. Enteroviruses are associated with myocarditis, and adenovirus has a characteristic biphasic clinical course.

Children 3 Months to 5 Years of Age

Children from 3 months to 5 years of age typically present with high fever, tachycardia, tachypnea, and poor perfusion. Petechial rash, altered consciousness, and seizures may also be encountered. *H. influenzae* type b (Hib), *Streptococcus pneumoniae*, and *Neisseria meningitidis* are the most common pathogens. The risk of concomitant meningitis is greatest with *N. meningitidis* and Hib and least with *Str. pneumoniae*. Clinical signs specific for meningitis are not always present; therefore a lumbar puncture is needed to rule out meningitis in children under 2 years of age who are septic. Hib bacteremia may occur without a localized site, but more commonly meningitis, pneumonia, cellulitis, arthritis, or epiglottitis is present. A petechial or purpuric skin rash is most often associated with *N. meningitidis* infection, but petechiae and DIC may be associated with other pathogenic organisms.

Organisms associated with sepsis and petechial rash

N. meningitidis (all ages; severe purpura and shock)
H. influenzae type b
Str. pneumoniae
Enteroviruses
Herpes simplex
Rickettsia rickettsii (Rocky Mountain spotted fever)
S. aureus
N. gonorrhoeae (teenagers)
Branhamella catarrhalis (young children, uncommon)

Meningococcemia is an extremely severe disease that frequently results in DIC and shock, which can be worsened by endotoxin released from rapid killing of microorganisms during the first few hours after the first dose of antibiotics.

The presence of diarrhea in a toxic-appearing child suggests the possibility of infection with *Shigella* sp, *Salmonella* sp, *Campylobacter* sp, or *E. coli* 0157. *Shigella* and *E. coli* 0157 may be associated with the hemolytic-uremic syndrome. Children with invasive amebiasis may present with the clinical finding of overwhelming septicemia without specific gastrointestinal signs or symptoms. A urinary tract focus must always be ruled out in any child with possible gram-negative sepsis.

Children Over 5 Years of Age

Sepsis not associated with an obvious site of infection is less common in patients without underlying disorders who are older than 5 years of age. Meningococcemia can occur in this age group, and acute disseminated staphylococcal syndrome has been described in otherwise healthy children 8 to 15 years of age without any other risk factors. Such patients usually have *S. aureus* bacteremia with two or more foci of infection in lung, bone, joint, heart, or brain. This syndrome has a male predominance and has

---

CLINICAL MANIFESTATIONS OF SEPSIS

Cardiopulmonary

Tachypnea
Tachycardia
Systemic arterial blood pressure instability
Congestive heart failure
Poor peripheral perfusion
Increased capillary permeability, edema
Decreased urinary flow

Neurologic

Altered level of consciousness
Temperature instability
Seizures

Gastrointestinal

Ileus
Diarrhea
Poor feeding
Vomiting

Hematologic

Anemia
Neutrophilia and neutropenia
Thrombocytopenia
Disseminated intravascular coagulation (DIC)

Metabolic

Hypoglycemia
Hypocalcemia

Dermatologic (skin rashes)

Petechial
Ecchymotic
Pustular
Ecthymatous
Scarlatiniform

been associated with a case fatality rate of 25%. Disseminated gonococcal infection in sexually active adolescents rarely progresses to a fulminant septic shock that mimics meningococcemia. Rocky Mountain spotted fever is another important diagnosis to consider in a septic child with a maculopapular and petechial rash involving the palms and soles. The presence of conjunctivitis, a petechial rash involving the palms and soles with centripetal spread, peripheral edema, hyponatremia, and a history of tick exposure are valuable clues.

Coagulase-negative staphylococci, *S. aureus,* gram-negative bacilli, and *Pseudomonas* species are likely bacterial pathogens associated with sepsis in immunocompromised hosts. Children with hypogammaglobulinemia or agammaglobulinemia, splenic dysfunction, and AIDS are at increased risk for developing overwhelming sepsis associated with the usual encapsulated bacteria (e.g., *Str. pneumoniae, H. influenzae* type b, *N. meningitidis, E. coli*). Young infants with immunodeficiency syndromes, either acquired or congenital, may present with serious bacterial infection as their first clinical manifestation of disease. Historical and laboratory evidence for such underlying disorders must be pursued as indicated in each case. Sepsis may also be the initial presentation of ketoacidosis in patients with newly developed diabetes.

CMV infection must be considered in the immunocompromised host who presents with a clinical sepsis syndrome. The manifestations of disseminated CMV may vary from fever and thrombocytopenia to overwhelming shock and DIC.

Diagnosis

The clinical diagnosis of sepsis can be confirmed by the following laboratory studies:

Indirect indicators

Complete and differential blood cell count, platelet count; calculation of immature-to-total neutrophil (I:T) ratio in newborn
Erythrocyte sedimentation rate (ESR)
C-reactive protein (CRP)

Microbiologic indicators

Bacterial cultures: blood, CSF, urine, soft tissue site, abscess, empyema, CVC tips
Latex particle agglutination tests (LPA) for detection of bacterial antigens (group B streptococcus, Hib, meningococcus, pneumococcus, *E. coli* K₁)

Gram and acridine orange stains of buffy coat preparations, CSF, urine, infected body fluids
Fungal cultures: blood, urine, CSF, tissue biopsy, infected body fluids, CVC tips
Viral cultures: buffy coat preparations, CSF, urine, nasopharynx, conjunctiva, stool, infected skin/tissue sites; Tzanck smear of vesicles
Immunofluorescent or enzyme-linked immunosorbent assay (ELISA) tests for detection of viral antigen in nasopharyngeal secretions or stool (e.g., RSV, rotavirus, adenovirus, parainfluenza viruses)
Acute, convalescent serologic titers: viral, rickettsial

The most useful indirect indicators are the white blood cell (WBC) and differential count, the ESR, and the CRP. Neutrophilia ($\geq$20,000 WBC/mm^3) and neutropenia ($<$5000 WBC/mm^3) with a shift to the left are more likely to be associated with infection. In newborns the immature/total neutrophil ratio $\geq$0.2 is the most useful indirect indicator of sepsis. Other noninfectious conditions of the neonate that may be associated with neutrophilia or neutropenia do not have an elevated immature-to-total neutrophil ratio. Both ESR and CRP tend to increase in association with acute bacterial infections. The CRP rises significantly within a few hours after the onset of infection. The CRP concentration decreases more rapidly than the ESR if there is a response to therapy, and it is persistently elevated if the patient does not improve.

Identification of the specific etiologic agent necessitates appropriate microbiologic cultures and/or serologic studies. Cultures of blood (at least 0.5 to 1 ml), CSF, urine (obtained by suprapubic bladder aspiration or bladder catheterization), and needle aspirate of any infected body fluid or soft tissue site of infection must be obtained before antimicrobial therapy is initiated. Patients with intravascular catheters, especially long-term catheters (e.g., TPN line), must have blood cultures taken from the catheters as well as from another site (see Chapter 41). An antibiotic removal device may be used for obtaining blood cultures in selected high-risk patients, but the increased rate of contamination of the cultures makes this method less desirable for routine use. Patients with suspected infective endocarditis who have been treated with antimicrobial agents before admission are most likely to benefit from the use of blood cultures obtained with the antibiotic removal device.

Detection of bacterial antigens in body fluids (concentrated urine, CSF) permits a rapid diagnosis even after antimicrobial treatment has been initiated. Commercially available LPA tests are easy to perform and have high sensitivity and specificity. They are most useful in the diagnosis of infection caused by *H. influenzae* type b and group B streptococcus. The antigen detection tests for *Str. pneumoniae* and *N. meningitidis* are somewhat less sensitive and specific. It is preferable to perform antigen detection tests on urine obtained through suprapubic bladder aspiration or catheterization since bag specimen urine samples may be contaminated with perineal organisms that may be detected by the LPA test. The choice of antimicrobial agents cannot be determined by the results of antigen detection tests. Acridine orange stain can detect bacteria in the CSF of children who received previous antibiotics or in buffy coat preparations from septicemic neonates.

Fungal as well as viral cultures must be considered in selected clinical cases. Biopsy of skin lesions or aspirates from solid organ abscesses are particularly useful in confirming the diagnosis of disseminated fungal infection. Buffy coat preparations for viral culture may be particularly helpful for the diagnosis of disseminated herpes simplex infection or disseminated CMV in the neonate. A Tzanck preparation of scrapings from the base of cutaneous vesicles will correctly identify herpes simplex or varicella zoster virus in approximately 70% to 80% of cases. The serologic tests for *Rickettsia* are not helpful in the management of the acutely ill patient but are useful for retrospective confirmation of the diagnosis.

Sonography, technetium bone scan, CT, and MRI are helpful for the identification of localized foci of infection. Echocardiography is especially useful for identification of vegetations in the heart and pericardial effusion. In recent years CT scans and MRI studies have identified an increased number of cases of focal hepatic, splenic, and renal candidiasis in immunocompromised hosts. Additionally, these scans are used to guide the percutaneous aspiration of localized abscesses. Purulent material from such sites may be the only means of identifying the pathogen. Gallium scans are less frequently used because of the exposure to large doses of radiation.

MONITORING AND LABORATORY TESTS
Supportive Care

All infants and children with sepsis must be monitored as described in Chapter 4. Cardiovascular status must be meticulously monitored during the first 4 to 12 hours after initiation of antimicrobial therapy since this is the period of greatest risk for developing endotoxin-mediated shock. Because the patient's fluid needs are often underestimated, a CVC or a Swan-Ganz catheter must be placed. A widening pulse pressure and persistent tachycardia may indicate ongoing vasodilation resulting from endotoxin release, but measurement of a low systemic vascular resistance is more specific. Large volumes of colloid or crystalloid solutions or blood may be needed to maintain a urinary output of 1 to 2 ml/kg/hr and adequate tissue perfusion. Narrowed pulse pressure or pulsus paradoxus may be associated with significant pericardial effusion. Large volumes of fluid must be administered to such patients to increase their cardiac output before pericardiocentesis (see Chapters 40 and 143). Oxygenation and acid-base balance must be assessed every 2 to 4 hours during the acute phases of sepsis.

Infection

Specific recommendations for monitoring the efficacy of treatment of infection are presented on p. 347. Overall clinical improvement should be evident within 24 to 48 hours after the initiation of appropriate antimicrobial therapy. Although complete defervescence may not occur for several days, the maximum daily temperature should be decreasing each day. Specific soft tissue sites such as septic joints, pyomyositis, and abscesses may need drainage for complete resolution of the infectious process. Certain bacteria may need determination of minimum bactericidal concentrations (MBC) of penicillin (group B streptococcus, *Str. viridans*) or nafcillin *(S. aureus)* when associated with serious infections such as endocarditis and a delayed clinical response. MBC:MIC ratios ≥ 32 for penicillin or nafcillin indicate the need for the addition of an aminoglycoside for complete killing.

Serum creatinine and peak and trough serum levels of several antimicrobial agents must be determined after the first 24 hours of therapy to assure safe and therapeutic levels. If adjustment of dosages or dosage intervals is needed in the presence of hepatic or renal dysfunction, repeated measurements of serum antibiotic levels must be performed. If a constant dosage regimen is followed, weekly determinations of trough levels only are needed to prevent toxicity. Serum bacteriostatic and bactericidal titers provide indirect evidence of drug levels. This test is performed when the clinical response is poor or when patients with serious infection complete their course of treatment with high-dose oral antibiotics. Serum is obtained 1 hour after the patient receives a dose of antibiotics, and serial twofold dilutions are made against the infecting pathogen. Titers ≥1:8 are generally needed for efficacy. Serum levels of amphotericin B are not routinely determined since this drug is so highly bound to tissue that drug activity at the site of infection is not reflected in serum levels.

RECOMMENDATIONS FOR MONITORING THE EFFICACY OF TREATMENT OF INFECTION

1. Repeat blood and CSF cultures after 24-36 hours of effective therapy to document sterilization.
2. Obtain CBC, differential, platelet count, PT, PTT every 12-24 hours until normal.
3. Perform daily evaluation of soft tissue sites of bacterial infection for possible needle aspiration or surgical drainage.
4. Determine minimum inhibitory concentration (MIC) and minimum bactericidal concentration (MBC) of penicillin for group B streptococcus and *Str. viridans* and of nafcillin for *S. aureus* in patients with serious infections (e.g., endocarditis) who have delayed clinical response.
5. Obtain serum bacteriostatic and bactericidal titers 1 hour after antibiotic dose if efficacy of antimicrobial agent is uncertain.*
6. Measure peak and trough levels of the following antimicrobial agents:

Agent	Peak (μg/ml)	Trough (μg/ml)
Vancomycin, amikacin, chloramphenicol	20-30	<10
Gentamicin, tobramycin	6-8	<2

*For peak serum antibiotic concentrations or bactericidal titers, blood samples are obtained 30 minutes after IV infusion or 60 minutes after IM injection or oral administration of the antimicrobial agent. Blood samples for trough serum concentrations are obtained less than 30 minutes before administration of the next dose.

ANTIBIOTIC TREATMENT

Once the appropriate diagnostic workup has been completed, empiric antimicrobial treatment is initiated as soon as possible. The choice of antimicrobial agents is determined by several factors: the likely etiologic agent, susceptibility patterns within a specific institution, CNS penetration, toxicity, and the patient's hepatic and renal function. Third-generation cephalosporins such as cefotaxime, ceftriaxone, and ceftazidime must not be used routinely for empiric therapy of suspected sepsis because of the rapid emergence of resistance associated with heavy usage in a closed unit. Specific indications for usage of these newer drugs include prevalence of multiply resistant gram-negative rods, persistent gram-negative bacteremia, poor clinical response to aminoglycosides, extensive deep tissue infection or abscess, and gram-negative meningitis. The decreased activity of aminoglycosides under acidotic and anaerobic conditions characteristic of abscesses and deep tissue infections makes this class of drugs less desirable for treatment of such clinical conditions. The use of chloramphenicol must be avoided in patients with cardiovascular instability since poor liver perfusion is associated with decreased clearance, resulting in elevated levels and thus toxicity (gray baby syndrome). Recommended treatment regimens are presented in Table 42-1.

Neonates

The rapidly changing metabolic and physiologic processes as well as hepatic and renal immaturity of the neonate demand special considerations. For example, dosage schedules of antibiotics vary according to age and birthweight because of the improved renal function and clearance of drugs associated with increasing gestational and chronologic age. The half-life of vancomycin and the aminoglycosides is usually prolonged in low birthweight infants; therefore serum levels of these drugs as well as serum creatinine must be monitored routinely for determination of the appropriate dosing interval in an individual patient. Aminoglycosides are frequently administered at 18- to 24-hour intervals in the very low birthweight infant.

Sulfonamides and ceftriaxone should not be administered to the newborn because of their displacement of bilirubin from albumin and the resulting increased risk of kernicterus. Nafcillin must be used with caution because it is metabolized primarily by the liver. Chloramphenicol is no longer recommended for treatment of neonatal infections for the following reasons: (1) its action against most gram-negative enteric pathogens is bacteriostatic rather than bactericidal; (2) in vitro antagonism with ampicillin against enteric gram-negative rods and group B streptococci has been demonstrated and may be associated with clinical failure; and (3) wide individual variations in pharmacokinetics in neonates in-

crease the risk of toxicity and necessitate frequent determinations of serum drug levels. Recommended dosage schedules for the most frequently used antimicrobial agents are presented in Table 42-2.

The regimen favored for empiric therapy of early-onset sepsis within the first 5 days of life is administration of ampicillin and aminoglycoside. Ampicillin is preferred over penicillin for its activity against *L. monocytogenes* and enterococci. The aminoglyco-

Table 42-1 Recommended Antimicrobial Therapy for the Most Common Etiologic Agents of Sepsis

Organism	Antibiotics	Organism	Antibiotics
Bacteria		**Bacteria—cont'd**	
Enterobacter sp	Aminoglycoside, third-generation cephalosporin*	*Serratia marcescens*	Aminoglycoside, third-generation cephalosporin
Escherichia coli	Aminoglycoside, third-generation cephalosporin	Streptococcus	
		Enterococcus	Ampicillin plus aminoglycoside, vancomycin
Haemophilus influenzae	Ampicillin if susceptible, cefotaxime, ceftriaxone, cefuroxime	Streptococcus group B	Ampicillin, penicillin,‡ cefotaxime if tolerant to penicillin
Klebsiella sp	Aminoglycoside, third-generation cephalosporin	*Str. pneumoniae*	Penicillin if susceptible, cefuroxime, cefotaxime, ceftriaxone, vancomycin if relatively resistant to penicillin
Listeria monocytogenes	Ampicillin†		
Neisseria meningitidis	Penicillin		
Pseudomonas aeruginosa	Ceftazidime plus aminoglycoside, mezlocillin plus aminoglycoside, imipenem-cilastatin, aztreonam if resistant	*Str. viridans*	Penicillin§
		Staphylococcus aureus	Nafcillin, methicillin, vancomycin if resistant (MRSA)‖
Pseudomonas cepacia	Trimethoprim-sulfamethoxazole, ceftazidime	Staphylococcus coagulase negative	Vancomycin,‖ nafcillin, methicillin if susceptible
Xanthomonas maltophilia	Aminoglycoside, trimethoprim-sulfamethoxazole	**Others**	
Salmonella sp	Trimethoprim-sulfamethoxazole, ceftriaxone, ampicillin, chloramphenicol	*Candida* sp	Amphotericin B¶
		Herpes simplex	Acyclovir, vidarabine
		Rickettsia rickettsii (Rocky Mountain spotted fever)	Chloramphenicol, tetracycline

*Increased resistance to third-generation cephalosporins.
†Synergy of ampicillin plus aminoglycoside may be beneficial.
‡Add aminoglycoside to ampicillin if tolerant to penicillin.
§Add aminoglycoside if endocarditis or poor response present.
‖Addition of rifampin may be beneficial in serious disease or with poor response.
¶Flucytosine synergy beneficial in serious infections.

side provides synergistic activity with ampicillin against group B streptococcus, enterococcus, and *L. monocytogenes* in addition to broad gram-negative coverage. If a third-generation cephalosporin is administered before identification of the infecting pathogen, ampicillin must be administered additionally because cephalosporins are inactive against *L. monocytogenes* and enterococci. The second-generation cephalosporin, cefuroxime, is inappropriate for empiric treatment of neonatal infections because of its limited spectrum of activity against the gram-negative enteric organisms and the lack of experience with treatment of group B streptococcal infections. Staphylococci become more likely pathogens in infants over 5 days of age, necessitating substitution of methicillin or vancomycin for ampicillin. Vancomycin is preferred if methicillin-resistant staphylococci are prevalent within an institution or if the patient has been hospitalized previously and treated with antibiotics. Antistaphylococcal coverage is indicated when a CVC or ventricular shunt is in place.

Infants 1 to 3 Months of Age

Community-acquired infection in patients who are 1 to 3 months old may be caused by organisms characteristic of the newborn period (group B streptococcus, *E. coli, Listeria,* enterococcus) or those commonly isolated in older infants and children (*H. influenzae* type b, *Str. pneumoniae, N. meningitidis*). Combined ampicillin and cefotaxime is therefore recommended, especially if meningitis has not been ruled out.

Children 3 Months to 5 Years of Age

Two important changes in the susceptibility pattern of the principal pathogens, *H. influenzae* type b (Hib) and *Str. pneumoniae,* have been observed in recent years: (1) 10% to 35% of Hib strains may be resistant to ampicillin as a result of β-lactamase production, and less than 1% of strains may be resistant to both ampicillin and chloramphenicol; and (2) up to 10% to 15% of strains of *Str. pneumoniae* are relatively resistant to penicillin (MIC, 0.1 to 1.0 µg/ml). The relatively resistant pneumococci are also susceptible to vancomycin. These organisms are, however, susceptible to cefuroxime, cefotaxime, or ceftriaxone. Cefuroxime is preferred for patients 3 months to 5 years of age in the absence of meningitis because of its activity against the major community-acquired pathogens—Hib, *Str. pneumoniae, N. men-*

ingitidis, and *S. aureus.* Cefotaxime or ceftriaxone need the addition of an antistaphylococcal agent such as nafcillin. If enteric pathogens such as *Salmonella* sp or *Shigella* sp are suspected, a third-generation cephalosporin (cefotaxime, ceftriaxone) or trimethoprim-sulfamethoxazole must be administered. When urinary tract infection is suspected, the combination of ampicillin and an aminoglycoside or a third-generation cephalosporin is recommended. Children with presumed Rocky Mountain spotted fever need treatment with either chloramphenicol or, if older than 7 years of age, tetracycline.

Children Over 5 Years of Age

Cefuroxime provides optimal coverage in a normal host with community-acquired infection. In the presence of diarrhea or urinary tract infections the choices are modified as above.

Special Considerations

The use of nafcillin or vancomycin in combination with an aminoglycoside or ceftazidime is indicated for empiric treatment of febrile neutropenic patients or of PICU patients with hospital-acquired sepsis. Patients with an intra-abdominal focus of infection need treatment with a combination of antibiotics that includes antianaerobic activity as discussed in Chapter 45. Empiric antifungal therapy with amphotericin B must be considered after 7 days of empiric antibacterial therapy without response in febrile neutropenic patients. Flucytosine may be combined with amphotericin B for synergism when disseminated fungal infection is documented.

Two new antimicrobial agents, aztreonam and imipenem-cilastatin, are highly active against multiply resistant gram-negative bacilli but as of this writing are not yet approved for use in children younger than 12 years of age. Aztreonam is a monobactam antibiotic that is active against aerobic gram-negative bacilli only and must therefore be combined with an agent active against gram-positive pathogens. Aztreonam offers two advantages: (1) spectrum of activity comparable to amikacin without the associated renal toxicity and (2) safety in penicillin-sensitive patients because of its absence of cross-sensitivity with β-lactam agents. Imipenem-cilastatin is a unique broad-spectrum β-lactam antibiotic that is active against nearly all anaerobes and aerobic gram-positive and aerobic gram-negative microorganisms and can therefore be used as a single-drug regimen. Caution

Table 42-2 Recommended Dosage Schedule for Antimicrobial Agents Frequently Used for Treatment of Sepsis*

Antimicrobial Agent	Body Weight <2000 g		Body Weight >2000 g		Older Infants and Children	Maximum Daily Dose
	Age 0-7 Days	>7 Days	Age 0-7 Days	>7 Days		
Acyclovir	—	—	—	—	20-50 mg/kg/day div q 8 hr† or 750-1500 mg/m²/day div q 8 hr	—
Amikacin	15 div q 12 hr	22.5 div q 8 hr	20 div q 12 hr	30 div q 8 hr	30 div q 8 hr	1-2 g
Ampicillin	50-100 div q 12 hr	75-150 div q 8 hr	75-150 div q 8 hr	100-300 div q 6 hr	100-200 div q 6 hr	8-10 g
Amphotericin B‡	1 once daily	1 once daily	1 once daily	1 once daily	1-1.5 once daily	—
Aztreonam	60 div q 12 hr	90 div q 8 hr	90 div q 8 hr	120 div q 6 hr	75-150 div q 6 hr	6-8 g
Cefotaxime	100 div q 12 hr	150 div q 8 hr	100 div q 12 hr	150 div q 8 hr	150-200 div q 6-8 hr	8-10 g
Ceftazidime	100 div q 12 hr	150 div q 8 hr	100 div q 8 hr	150 div q 8 hr	100-150 div q 8 hr	4-6 g
Ceftriaxone	50 once daily	50 once daily	50 once daily	75 once daily	50-100 div q 12-24 hr	1-2 g
Cefuroxime	—	—	—	—	75-300 div q 6-8 hr	4-6 g
Chloramphenicol	—	—	—	—	75-100 div q 6 hr	2-4 g
Clindamycin	10 div q 12 hr	15 div q 8 hr	15 div q 8 hr	20 div q 6 hr	30-40 div q 6-8 hr	2-4 g
Flucytosine§	100-150 div q 8 hr	100-150 div q 6 hr	100-150 div q 6 hr	100-150 div q 6 hr	100-150 div q 6 hr	300 mg
Gentamicin	5 div q 12 hr	7.5 div q 8 hr	5 div q 12 hr	7.5 div q 8 hr	3-7.5 div q 8 hr	300 mg
Imipenem-cilastatin	—	—	—	—	60-100 div q 8 hr	2-4 g
Methicillin	50-100 div q 12 hr	75-150 div q 8 hr	75-150 div q 8 hr	100-200 div q 6 hr	150-200 div q 6 hr	8-10 g
Metronidazole	15 div q 12 hr	15 div q 12 hr	15 div q 12 hr	30 div q 12 hr	30 div q 6 hr	2-4 g
Mezlocillin	150 div q 12 hr	225 div q 8 hr	150 div q 12 hr	225 div q 8 hr	200-300 div q 4-6 hr	18-24 g
Nafcillin	50 div q 12 hr	75 div q 8 hr	50 div q 8 hr	75 div q 6 hr	150 div q 6 hr	8-10 g
Penicillin G	50-100,000 U	75-150,000 U	50-150,000 U	100-200,000 U	100-250,000 U div q 4 hr	20 million U
Tetracycline	—	—	—	—	20-30 div q 8-12 hr	1-2 g
Ticarcillin‖	150 div q 12 hr	225 div q 8 hr	225 div q 8 hr	300 div q 6 hr	200-300 div q 4-6 hr	18-24 g

Drug					
Tobramycin	4 div q 12 hr	6 div q 8 hr	4 div q 12 hr	6 div q 8 hr	3-7.5 div q 8 hr	300 mg
Trimethoprim-sulfamethoxazole	—	—	—	—	8-12 trimethoprim div q 12 hr	1 g
Vancomycin	30 div q 12 hr	45 div q 8 hr	30 div q 12 hr	45 div q 8 hr	40-60 div q 6 hr	2-4 g

*Modified from Nelson JD, ed. 1989-1990 Pocketbook of Pediatric Antimicrobial Therapy, 8th ed. Baltimore: Williams & Wilkins, 1989. For detailed information about antibiotics in newborns, see McCracken HG, Nelson JD. Antimicrobial Therapy for Newborns, 2nd ed. New York: Grune & Stratton, 1983.

†The same dosage schedule is used for all ages; the lower range is recommended for treatment of herpes simplex infections, but the higher range is required for treatment of varicella-zoster infections.

‡Initial dose, 0.25 mg/kg/day × 2; then 0.5 mg/kg/day × 2; then 0.75 mg/kg/day × 2; then 1.0 mg/kg/day. Dose may be increased daily with severe disease. Maintenance dose, 0.75-1.0 mg/kg/day. Every other day dosing may be considered after good clinical response. IV infusions, over 4-6 hr.

§Routinely administered PO, but IV formulation available by special request for use when PO not tolerated.

‖Clavulanate potassium (Timentin) dosage is the same as for ticarcillin, but clavulanate potassium is not yet approved for use in children.

is advised in the use of this drug because of the CNS and renal toxicity that have been observed, especially in the neonate. These agents may prove particularly useful for treatment of infections associated with multiply resistant pathogens.

Acyclovir is indicated for treatment of disseminated herpes simplex or varicella zoster infections. The combination of ganciclovir and IV immunoglobulin is the only therapeutic regimen that may be effective against invasive cytomegalovirus infection in compromised hosts. The presence of retinitis or identification of the virus in lung or liver tissue is required to obtain this drug under a compassionate-use protocol.

Adjunctive measures such as steroids, IV immunoglobulin infusions, and WBC transfusions have been proposed for treatment of overwhelming sepsis. Sufficient evidence now supports the use of dexamethasone for the treatment of bacterial meningitis (Chapter 44). Results of studies of the use of steroids for gram-negative sepsis are more variable, and at present steroids are not routinely recommended for treatment of sepsis without meningitis. Indications for replacement of deficient components of the host defense are discussed in Chapter 20. To date there is insufficient evidence to support routine use of these products. However, individual patients who are particularly compromised hosts may benefit from such adjunctive therapy.

The duration of therapy is determined by the clinical course and the results of diagnostic microbiologic studies. A 7- to 10-day course of antibiotics active against the infecting organism is recommended for treating uncomplicated bacterial infection or clinical sepsis without documentation of the pathogenic agent. Suppurative complications such as empyema, endocarditis, or osteomyelitis necessitate prolonged therapy for at least 3 to 6 weeks. Antimicrobial therapy is frequently initiated for suspected sepsis that remains unproved. If after 72 hours of therapy the clinical course and the laboratory data do not support the diagnosis of bacterial infection, it is appropriate to discontinue antibiotics, to observe the patient, and to reevaluate therapy. Initiation of antiviral or antifungal therapy is guided by evidence supportive of a viral or fungal cause of sepsis. Nelson's book (see Additional Reading) provides complete and updated recommendations for therapy of specific conditions.

For other supportive measures that aid in treating a patient with sepsis see Chapters 10-12, 14-16, 19, and 22.

ADDITIONAL READING

Beutler B, Cerami A. Cachectin: More than a tumor necrosis factor. N Engl J Med 316:379-85, 1987.

Manroe BL, Rosenfeld CR, Weinberg AG, et al. The differential leukocyte count in the assessment and outcome of early onset group B streptococcal disease. J Pediatr 91:632, 1977.

• McCracken GH, Freij BJ. Infectious diseases of the fetus and newborn. In Feigin RD, Cherry JD, eds. Textbook of Pediatric Infectious Disease. Philadelphia: WB Saunders, 1987, pp 940-966.

• Nelson JD. Antibiotic therapy for newborns. In Nelson JD, ed. 1989-1990 Pocketbook of Pediatric Antimicrobial Therapy, 8th ed. Baltimore: Williams & Wilkins, 1989, pp 12-21.

Weinstein MP, Stratton CW, Achley A, et al. Multicenter collaborative evaluation of a standardized serum bactericidal test as a diagnostic indicator in infective endocarditis. Am J Med 78:262-269, 1985.

43 Toxic Shock Syndrome

Jane D. Siegel

BACKGROUND AND PHYSIOLOGY
Epidemiology

Toxic shock syndrome (TSS) was first described in children and teenagers ages 8 to 17 years in 1978. During the next 18 months there was a dramatic increase in the number of TSS cases reported to the CDC, with nearly 900 cases in 1980. More than 3000 cases meeting the case definition have been reported to the CDC to date. Since 1980 the yearly number of cases has declined, but the incidence of TSS is still many times higher than it was before 1979. Based on retrospective analysis, the earliest cases to meet the strict definition of TSS occurred in 1972. A literature review suggests that severe cases of staphylococcal scarlet fever reported in 1927 may have been, in reality, the first cases of TSS. Because most cases are associated with a unique toxin produced by some strains of *Staphylococcus aureus,* this condition is generally referred to as "staphylococcal" TSS. However, similar clinical manifestations have been associated with a pyrogenic exotoxin A produced by group A streptococcus. As a result of intensive surveillance and investigation of affected patients identified during the past decade, the epidemiology, pathogenesis, and clinical manifestations of TSS have been well described.

Approximately 70% of TSS cases occur in women 16 to 30 years of age, with a peak time of onset on the fourth day of menstruation. Menstrual-related TSS is more common in women who use high-absorbency tampons and are sexually inactive. There has been no definite seasonal or regional distribution of cases. Apparent increases most likely reflect the presence of active surveillance programs, although some regional differences in the degree of immunity to TSS-associated toxins and in the distribution of toxin-producing organisms have been suggested. Nonmenstrual *S. aureus* infections account for 20% to 30% of reported cases of TSS, only 5% of which occur

in males. Sources of toxin-producing staphylococci in nonmenstrual cases are as follows: nonsurgical cutaneous and subcutaneous infections, 30%; childbirth/abortion, 27%; surgical procedures (e.g., otolaryngologic, mammoplasty), 18%; vaginal infections unrelated to menstruation, 5%; and unknown sources, 20%. The age of these patients has varied from the neonatal period to the seventh decade. TSS associated with surgical procedures usually develops 2 to 5 days after surgery. TSS after an influenza viral illness complicated by a secondary focal *S. aureus* infection of the respiratory tract was reported in 10 patients in 1987.

Pathogenesis

Within 2 years of the recognition of TSS an association with menstruation, use of tampons, and *S. aureus* was established. Two putative toxins—pyrogenic exotoxin C and staphylococcal enterotoxin F—identified in 1981 by two independent groups of investigators have proved identical and are referred to as toxic shock syndrome toxin-1 (TSST-1). Distinct immunologically and biologically active fragments of the TSST-1 molecule have been described. In vitro TSST-1 is a potent T-cell mitogen, a suppressor of antibody production, and a more potent inducer of interleukin-1 (IL-1) production by peripheral blood mononuclear cells than bacterial lipopolysaccharide (LPS). TSST-1 stimulation of both IL-1 and tumor necrosis factor (TNF) production by mononuclear cells explains many of the clinical features of TSS and provides a mechanism through which corticosteroids may be beneficial when administered early in the course. The pathogenetic role of IL-1 in bacterial meningitis and the therapeutic effect of early dexamethasone treatment are discussed in Chapter 44. A small number of cases of TSS have been associated with the production of staphylococcal enterotoxin B (SEB) rather than TSST-1, but only one case has been associated with the production of both toxins. Interestingly an amino acid homology of nearly 50% between the streptococcal pyrogenic exotoxin type A and the SEB have been associated with TSS cases; furthermore, SEB shares many biologic properties with TSST-1 and the streptococcal pyrogenic exotoxin.

Evidence to support the pathogenetic role of TSST-1 is as follows: (1) TSST-1 is produced by 93% of strains of *S. aureus* isolated from vaginal cultures of women with menstrual-related TSS and by 62% of strains of *S. aureus* isolated from normally sterile body fluids in patients with nonmenstrual-related TSS as compared with 1% to 5% of *S. aureus* strains isolated from vaginal cultures of healthy women. (2) Similar pathophysiologic changes may be produced after injection of purified TSST-1 into rabbits and baboons. (3) Antibody to TSST-1 is present in 70% to 80% of normal teens and young adults and in 90% to 95% of individuals in the fourth decade, but there is no measurable antibody in TSS patients at the time of presentation. There is an increase in antibody during recovery in nonmenstrual cases of TSS, and failure of antibody formation in patients with menstrual TSS has been associated with recurrent disease. (4) IL-1 stimulation and other in vivo responses to TSST-1 are neutralized by antibody to TSST-1.

The epidemiologic association with high-absorbency tampons led to the elucidation of an important pathogenetic mechanism. The production and release of TSST-1 as well as other exoproteins from replicating *S. aureus* strains are significantly increased under conditions of magnesium deficiency. Of note, the polyester foam and polyacrylate rayon in high-absorbency tampons readily combine with magnesium ions and are associated with an increased amount of TSST-1 production in vitro. No other trace metals have been shown to have an effect on the production of staphylococcal exoproteins. The decreased risk of TSS during the first 3 days of menstruation and in sexually active women may be explained by the increase in magnesium concentration in blood associated with heavier flow in the early phase of menstruation and in semen. This effect on magnesium concentration is the most likely explanation of the association of tampons with TSS. Additionally, many surgical packing materials that have been associated with nonmenstrual cases are composed of similar materials that bind magnesium.

Clinical Manifestations and Diagnosis

The case definition of TSS that has been adopted by the CDC is presented on p. 355. These patients are initially seen with a 1- to 2-day history of fever >38.5° C, sore throat, myalgias, vomiting, and watery diarrhea. They typically develop a diffuse, blanching rash that has a characteristic "sunburn" appearance and is mainly truncal in distribution, with accentuation in the inguinal and axillary folds as well as in areas of pressure. Indurative edema of the palms and soles may develop. Desquamation of the involved skin and of the palms and soles occurs during the second week of illness. Examination of the mucous membranes reveals hyperemia of the conjunctivae, pharynx, and genital mucosa. A vaginal discharge may be observed. Micro ulcerations of the vaginal mucosa may develop as a result of the disease process, even in the absence of tampon usage. Exquisite muscle tenderness is characteristic of patients with TSS. Hypotension occurs during the first 48 to 72 hours of illness and may be severe and prolonged because of massive vasodilation and rapid movement of serum proteins and fluid from the intravascular to the extravascular compartment. The multisystem involvement may be a reflection of the rapid onset of hypotension and decreased organ perfusion or the result of the action of a toxin with multiple target organs. Diffuse vasculitis has been observed in skin biopsies and autopsy specimens. Acute renal failure results from both prerenal impairment and intrinsic renal disease. The acute course may be further complicated by the development of adult respiratory distress syndrome and toxic cardiomyopathy. Late sequelae include reversible hair and nail loss, vocal cord paralysis, and peripheral neuropathy.

Initial laboratory findings reveal leukocytosis with a high proportion of immature neutrophils in most patients. Other findings include thrombocytopenia, hyponatremia, hypocalcemia, evidence of hepatic and renal dysfunction, elevated CPK, and myoglobinuria. CSF is usually normal but may rarely show a pleocytosis <100 cells/mm³ with normal glucose and protein levels. Blood cultures are sterile in 95% of TSS patients. Toxin-producing *S. aureus* may be recovered from focal sites of infection or from mucosal surfaces. The clinical diagnosis is confirmed by identification TSST-1–producing strains of *S. aureus*. Suspect isolates should be referred to the state laboratory or CDC for appropriate studies.

The recurrence rate of TSS is approximately 30% in menstruating females. These women usually experience recurrences within 1 or 2 months of the initial episode, but an interval of ≥1 year has been documented. The recurrences are most often milder than the initial episode but have on occasion been more severe, with individual patients needing multiple ICU admissions. The maximum number of reported recurrences is five. Failure to eradicate the toxin-producing staphylococci and to produce antibody to the toxin during convalescence increases the risk of recurrence. The overall case fatality rate for TSS is 3% to 8%. The differential diagnosis of staphylococcal TSS includes bacterial septicemia, Kawasaki disease, staphylococcal scalded skin syndrome, scarlet fever, Rocky Mountain spotted fever, leptospirosis, rubeola, Stevens-Johnson syndrome, viral hepatitis, Legionnaires' disease, and hemolytic-uremic syndrome.

CASE DEFINITION OF TOXIC SHOCK SYNDROME*

Fever: Temperature ≥38.9° C

Rash: Diffuse macular erythroderma ("sunburn" appearance)

Desquamation of palms and soles 1 to 2 weeks after onset of illness

Hypotension: Systolic arterial blood pressure ≤90 mm Hg for adults or below fifth percentile by age for children <16 years of age; orthostatic drop in diastolic arterial blood pressure ≥15 mm Hg from lying to sitting; or orthostatic syncope

Multisystem involvement—three or more of the following:

Gastrointestinal: Vomiting or diarrhea at onset of illness

Muscular: Severe myalgia or CPK level at least twice the upper limit of normal laboratory values

Mucous membrane: Vaginal, oropharyngeal, or conjunctival hyperemia

Renal: BUN or creatinine at least twice the upper limit of normal laboratory values or urinary sediment with ≥5 white cells per high-power field in the absence of urinary tract infection

Hepatic: Total bilirubin, AST, or ALT at least twice the upper limit of normal for laboratory values

Hematologic: Platelets ≤100,000/mm³

Central nervous system: Disorientation or alterations in consciousness without focal neurologic signs when fever and hypotension are absent

Negative results for other pathogens on the following tests (if obtained):

Blood, throat, CSF cultures

Rise in titer to Rocky Mountain spotted fever, leptospirosis, or rubeola

*Modified from Perkin RM. Toxic shock syndrome. In Nelson J, ed. Current Therapy in Pediatric Infectious Disease. Toronto: BC Decker, 1988; modified from information appearing in Shands KN, Schmid GP, Dan DB, et al. Toxic shock syndrome in menstruating women. N Engl J Med 303:1436-1442, 1980.

MONITORING AND LABORATORY TESTS

All infants and children with TSS must be monitored as described in Chapter 4. Cardiovascular status must be meticulously monitored. Vomiting, diarrhea, vasodilation, and greatly increased vascular permeability account for the massive amounts of fluid needed to stabilize systemic arterial blood pressure and to maintain organ perfusion. A CVC or a Swan-Ganz catheter is therefore usually needed to assess volume status accurately, and urinary ouput is determined hourly. Cardiopulmonary status is further assessed through a chest roentgenogram and arterial blood gas and pH values. Echocardiography is indicated in the presence of cardiac enlargement or dysfunction. Hematologic monitoring includes a complete blood cell and differential count and platelet count. If DIC is suspected clinically, prothrombin time, partial thromboplastin time, and fibrin split products are measured. Assessment of the renal-metabolic systems includes determination of electrolytes, calcium, phosphorus, total serum protein, albumin, BUN, creatinine, bilirubin, AST, ALT, and CPK and examination of the urinary sediment. Oxygenation and acid-base balance are reassessed every 2 to 4 hours until the patient has stabilized.

Before the initiation of antimicrobial therapy, cultures of blood, soft tissue sites of infection, and all mucosal surfaces (nasopharynx, conjunctivae, trachea if intubation is performed, rectum, vagina) are obtained. Lumbar puncture is performed only in the presence of clinical signs of CNS involvement or in the young infant. It is advisable to forewarn the microbiology laboratory that *S. aureus* isolates from any site are significant and must be saved for toxin determination. Appropriate cultures and serologic studies are obtained to rule out other diagnostic possibilities as indicated for individual patients.

TREATMENT

The recommendations in Chapter 12 for management of shock must be followed aggressively for patients with TSS. A successful outcome is determined by the adequacy of supportive care, the elimination of the source of staphylococcal infection, and eradication of the toxin-producing organism. Large volumes of colloid or crystalloid solutions or blood are needed to maintain a urinary output of 1 to 2 ml/kg/hr, and adequate tissue perfusion and vasopressors are indicated in the most severe cases. Inotropic support may be needed for treatment of the toxic cardiomyopathy. Tampons or surgical packings must be removed immediately. Any soft tissue abscess or empyema is drained promptly, and infected wounds are debrided and irrigated generously with sterile saline solution. Vaginal irrigation with sterile saline solution is performed when clots and purulent material are present. However, there is a theoretic consideration that vaginal irrigation may enhance absorption of toxin or result in bacteremia.

A β-lactamase–resistant antistaphylococcal agent such as nafcillin (150 mg/kg/day, divided q6h) or vancomycin (40 mg/kg/day, divided q6h) must be administered intravenously as soon as TSS is suspected clinically to decrease toxin production. Although the effect of antimicrobial therapy on the acute phase of TSS is uncertain, using effective antimicrobials has reduced dramatically the recurrence rate of menstrual-related TSS. The administration of antibiotics is continued for a minimum of 7 days. An appropriate oral agent such as cephalexin or dicloxacillin may be substituted for the last few days of therapy if permitted by the clinical condition. Experience from only one retrospective study demonstrates an association between administration of a short course of methylprednisolone or dexamethasone and a decrease in the duration of fever and severity of disease. Based on the pathogenetic functions of TSST-1, it is reasonable to consider the administration of dexamethasone (0.6 mg/kg/day, divided q6h) for 2 to 4 days in severely affected patients. This therapy must be initiated early in the course to have a beneficial effect. Although there is no evidence for person-to-person transmission of TSS, the use of drainage/secretion isolation precautions for the duration of the patient's hospitalization is recommended.

ADDITIONAL READING

• Cone LA, Woodard DR, Schlievert PM, et al. Clinical and bacteriologic observations of a toxic shock-like syndrome due to *Streptococcus pyogenes*. N Engl J Med 317:146-149, 1987.

• International Symposium on Toxic Shock Syndrome Proceedings. Rev Infect Dis II (Suppl):S1:S333, 1989.

• Kass EH, Parsonnet J. On the pathogenesis of toxic shock syndrome. Rev Infect Dis 9(Suppl):S482-S489, 1987.

McDonald CL, Osterhold MT, Hedberg CW, et al. Toxic shock syndrome: A newly recognized complication of influenza and influenza-like illness. JAMA 257:2053-1058, 1987.

Shands KN, Schmid GP, Dan DB, et al. Toxic shock syndrome in menstruating women. N Engl J Med 303:1436-1442, 1980.

Smith CB, Jacobson JA. Toxic shock syndrome. DM 31:77-118, 1986.

• Todd JK, Ressman M, Caston SA, et al. Corticosteroid therapy for patients with toxic shock syndrome. JAMA 252:3399-3404, 1984.

44 Meningitis/Encephalitis

David C. Waagner · George H. McCracken, Jr.

BACKGROUND AND PHYSIOLOGY

Meningitis is an inflammation of the meningeal covering of the CNS, as reflected by an increased number of WBCs in CSF. *Encephalitis* refers to inflammation of the brain. *Meningoencephalitis* indicates an inflammation of both the meninges and brain. *Aseptic meningitis* describes inflammation of the meninges in the absence of microorganisms on a Gram-stained smear and routine bacteriologic culture of CSF. Approximately 15,000 cases of bacterial meningitis occur annually, with the highest attack rates occurring in neonates and in infants younger than 1 year of age. Prompt diagnosis and appropriate medical management are paramount to reducing the incidence of sequelae of CNS infection.

Pathogenesis

Invasion of the CNS by pathogenic organisms can occur by three routes. The primary route involves hematogenous spread from a distant focus of infection. Accordingly, the most common organisms causing bacterial sepsis for a given pediatric age range are the most common causes of bacterial meningitis. Direct invasion can occur through a communication between the CSF and the environment, an example of which is a fracture through a sinus or the cribriform plate. Pathogens can also spread from contiguous structures such as the mastoid or paranasal sinuses to the CNS.

Most often, CNS bacterial or viral infections result from an initial focus in the respiratory tract. After establishing an infection or colonization in the respiratory tract, organisms invade the bloodstream and eventually seed the brain and meninges. In newborn infants organisms from the intrauterine environment or maternal genital tract gain access to the bloodstream through the respiratory or gastrointestinal tract or through the umbilical cord. The site of entry into the CSF from blood-borne organisms ap-

pears to be the highly vascularized choroid plexus. Minimal clearance of organisms from the CSF space occurs through the subarachnoid villi and lymphatic channels and by phagocytes.

The host inflammatory response results in marked CSF pleocytosis. The inflammation disrupts the selective permeability of the cerebral capillary cells, altering the structure and function of the capillary endothelium and permitting serum protein to "leak" into the CSF. Inflammation of the arachnoid villi can alter CSF flow, which, coupled with loss of autoregulation of cerebral blood flow, can result in increased ICP. The release of cytotoxic agents from granulocytes in the CSF contributes to the cerebral edema. Anaerobic glycolysis by poorly perfused cerebral tissues results in hypoglycorrhachia, which further potentiates swelling of glial and neuronal cells through failure of the ATP-dependent sodium pump, resulting in accumulation of intracellular sodium. The syndrome of inappropriate secretion of antidiuretic hormone (SIADH), resulting acutely in serum hyposmolality, can also contribute to cerebral edema. Edema of vascular endothelial cells and increased ICP contribute to reduced blood flow to vital areas of the brain and possibly to cerebral infarction. The inflammatory exudate around the brain can produce scarring, with damage to cranial nerves, especially the eighth cranial nerve. Hydrocephalus results from either aqueductal obstruction by fibrinous debris or reduced CSF outflow caused by inflammation of the arachnoid villi.

Etiology

Bacterial meningitis. In the newborn infant the most common cause of bacterial meningitis is group B streptococcus, followed by *Escherichia coli* and *Listeria monocytogenes*. In low birthweight premature infants nosocomial pathogens such as *Staphylococcus* species, gram-negative enteric organisms, and *Can-*

357

dida species can cause meningitis during the period of intensive care management. Rarely, *Haemophilus influenzae* type b and *Streptococcus pneumoniae* meningitis occur in newborn infants. From 3 months to 5 years of age, the period with the highest incidence of meningitis, the most common pathogen is *H. influenzae* type b, followed by *Neisseria meningitidis,* and *Str. pneumoniae.* After 5 years of age, *N. meningitidis* and *Str. pneumoniae* are the most common causes of bacterial meningitis. *L. monocytogenes* may cause meningitis in an immunocompromised patient of any age. *Mycobacterium tuberculosis* is an uncommon but frequently overlooked cause of childhood meningitis. Primary amebic meningoencephalitis caused by *Naegleria* species is an uncommon but usually fatal condition that is often misdiagnosed as bacterial meningitis with sterile cultures.

Encephalitis. Approximately three fourths of the cases of encephalitis are of undetermined etiology. Frequent outbreaks occur during warm, wet seasons of the year, depending on arthropod vectors. Table 44-1 lists the most commonly identified causes of encephalitis in the United States. The herpesvirus family comprises only 7% of the total causes of encephalitis but is associated with the highest mortality rate (44%).

Aseptic meningitis. Both infectious and noninfectious causes can produce CNS inflammation in children with aseptic meningitis or meningoencephalitis. Enteroviruses are estimated to cause 85% to 90% of all cases of aseptic meningitis.

*Causes of aseptic meningitis**

Bacterial: Partially treated meningitis, leptospirosis, *Borrelia burgdorferi, Mycobacterium tuberculosis, Rickettsiae, Mycoplasma,* syphilis, bacterial endocarditis, brain abscess

Viral: Enteroviruses, mumps, herpes simplex type II, adenoviruses, Epstein-Barr virus, cytomegalovirus, influenza viruses, rubella, rubeola, lymphocytic choriomeningitis virus

Fungal: *Cryptococcus, Candida, Aspergillus, Coccidioides*

Parasites: *Toxoplasma, Naegleria* species, *Taenia solium* (cysticercosis)

Immune disorders: Systemic lupus erythematosus, Guillain-Barré syndrome

---

*Modified from Klein JO, Feigin RD, McCracken GH. Report of the task force on diagnosis and management of meningitis. Pediatrics 78(Suppl):959-982, 1986. Reproduced by permission.

Malignancy: Leukemia, lymphoma, Hodgkin's disease, medulloblastoma

Miscellaneous: Intrathecal injections, heavy metal poisoning, Kawasaki disease, multiple sclerosis, neurosurgery

Clinical Manifestations

The symptoms of bacterial meningitis in infants are subtle, requiring a detailed history and a high index of suspicion to identify the patient at high risk. Meningitis can appear abruptly, progressing rapidly in a few hours, or can develop insidiously over several days. Nonspecific findings include fever, irritability, lethargy, apnea, poor feeding, vomiting, jaundice, skin lesions, respiratory distress, and change in mental status. Older children may complain of headache, nausea, and photophobia.

There are no pathognomonic signs of meningitis. The characteristic stiff neck and positive Kernig's and Brudzinski's signs are often found late in the course of illness and are seen infrequently in children younger than 15 months. The absence of nuchal rigidity should never be used to exclude the diagnosis of meningitis, particularly in the young infant. A bulging or tense fontanelle can be present. Focal neurologic findings may appear at the onset of illness. Seizures occur in 20% to 30% of patients before admission to the hospital. A petechial rash may be present and may be associated with *N. meningitidis, H. influenzae* type b, or *Str. pneumoniae.* Purpuric lesions indicate a rapid and fulminant onset and are associated with a high mortality rate. The risk of meningitis is increased in the presence of focal infections such as buccal or periorbital cellulitis, pneumonia, or septic arthritis.

Manifestations of encephalitis in children are variable. Headache, fever, photophobia, vomiting, alterations in consciousness and personality, and loss of bowel and bladder control can occur. Seizures occur frequently and are often focal in nature. Neurologic findings can fluctuate or progress rapidly. Nuchal rigidity is uncommon. Clinical improvement after lumbar puncture is frequently observed.

MONITORING AND LABORATORY TESTS
Lumbar Puncture

Diagnosis of bacterial meningitis depends on examination of the CSF. A lumbar puncture must be performed in all patients in whom meningitis is sus-

Table 44-1   Etiology and Deaths From Encephalitis in the United States, 1978*

Etiology	Percent of Total	Death: Case Ratio (%)
Herpesviruses (herpes simplex, Ebstein-Barr, cytomegalovirus, herpes zoster)	7	44
Arboviruses (St. Louis, eastern equine, western equine, California)	10	3.5
Postchildhood infections (measles, mumps, rubella, chickenpox)	5	7.5
Enteroviruses	3	2.5
Indeterminate	75	8.5

*Modified from the Centers for Disease Control. Encephalitis surveillance, Annual Summary 1978. Atlanta: CDC, May 1981.

pected. In patients with significant cardiorespiratory instability, evidence of increased ICP, or localized infection at the site of the puncture, the lumbar puncture can be delayed.

Once obtained the CSF must be evaluated for cell count and differential count, protein and glucose concentrations, latex agglutination and culture, and presence of organisms on a Gram-stained smear. Serum glucose concentration must be measured simultaneously to determine the CSF/blood glucose ratio. Children at risk for tuberculosis or opportunistic infections must have appropriately stained smears and cultures performed. Latex agglutination to identify bacterial antigen in body fluids is a rapid, sensitive, and specific technique to detect *H. influenzae* type b and group B streptococcus but is less reliable for other pathogens. Healthy preterm and newborn infants have significantly different normal CSF values than do healthy infants and children (Table 44-2). Characteristic findings in patients with a CNS infection are described in Table 44-3.

The presence of blood from a traumatic lumbar puncture can cause confusion in interpreting the CSF findings. If the ratio of WBCs to RBCs in the CSF is greater than that in the peripheral blood, CSF pleocytosis is likely. To correct the CSF protein level in a traumatic tap, 1 to 1.5 mg/dl of protein may be subtracted from the total CSF protein for every 1000 RBCs/ml. The CSF findings associated with subarachnoid bleeding may be indistinguishable from bacterial infection.

In a patient with encephalitis the CSF can be clear but usually shows pleocytosis, ranging from 10 to 500 cells and rarely exceeding 1000 cells/mm³. Early in the course of the illness, neutrophils can predomi-

Table 44-2   Normal CSF Values*

	Newborn Infants		Infants and Children
	Preterm	Term	
WBC count (cells/mm³)			
Mean	9.0	8.2	0
± 2 SD	0-25.4	0-22.4	0-7
PMN (%)	57.2	61.3	0
Glucose (mg/dl)			
Mean	50	52	>40
Range	24-63	34-119	40-80
CSF/blood glucose (%)			
Mean	74	81	50
Range	55-105	44-248	40-60
Protein (mg/dl)			
Mean	115	90	<40
Range	65-150	20-170	5-40

PMN = polymorphonuclear leukocytes.
*Modified from Sarf LD, Platt LH, McCracken GH. Cerebrospinal fluid evaluation in neonates: Comparison of high-risk infants with and without meningitis. J Pediatr 88:473-477, 1976.

nate, later shifting to a lymphocytic predominance. CSF protein concentration can be slightly elevated, but the CSF/blood glucose ratio is usually normal. Viral cultures of the CSF must be obtained if encephalitis is suspected. In encephalitis caused by arboviruses or enteroviruses the CSF viral culture is frequently positive, whereas in herpes simplex encephalitis the culture is usually negative. In amebic meningoencephalitis the CSF is grossly purulent and hemorrhagic, and there is elevation of the protein concentration. Amebas are not commonly observed on a Gram-stained smear but are best detected on a wet mount of the CSF.

Treating the patient with an oral antibiotic before lumbar puncture does not significantly alter CSF characteristics other than the Gram-stained smear in bacterial meningitis. Rarely CSF cultures can be sterile if prior oral therapy was given, in which case latex agglutination for bacterial antigen may identify the pathogen.

Additional Diagnostic Studies

In addition to examination of the CSF other diagnostic tests can be useful. Blood cultures must be obtained on all patients suspected of meningitis because bacteria often reenter the bloodstream from the arachnoid villi. All strains of *H. influenzae* must be checked for β-lactamase production and for susceptibility to the antimicrobial agents used for therapy. If *Str. pneumoniae* is the pathogen, susceptibility to penicillin must be determined because 5% to 10% of strains are relatively penicillin resistant. Urine cul-

Table 44-3　CSF Findings in Patients With CNS Infection

Condition	Leukocytes/ mm³	Cell Differential	Protein (mg/dl)	Glucose (mg/dl)	Comment
Acute bacterial meningitis	Several hundred to >30,000 (may have <100 in early disease)	PMN predominance (may see monocytosis in *Listeria* infection)	Increased, >100	Decreased, <40	Cultures may be negative in partially treated disease; latex agglutination of CSF may be helpful
Enteroviral meningoencephalitis	Usually <500	Lymphocytic predominance (PMN predominance early in infection)	Normal to slightly elevated	Normal	Viral cultures of CSF may be positive
Herpes simplex encephalitis	50-2000	Lymphocytic predominance (PMN predominance early in infection); red blood cells present in most cases, indicating hemorrhagic necrosis	Normal to slightly elevated	Normal to slightly decreased	CSF cultures are seldom positive; rare cases may have normal CSF characteristics
Brain abscess	10-200	Lymphocytic or PMN predominance	Increased, >100	Normal	Gram's stain and cultures of CSF seldom reveal pathogen
Tuberculous meningitis	50-500 (rarely, up to 1000)	Lymphocytic predominance (PMN predominance early in infection)	Increased, >100	Decreased, <40	Stains and cultures for acid-fast bacilli may be positive
Amebic meningoencephalitis	Several hundred to >20,000	PMN predominance (many red blood cells usually present)	Increased, >100	Decreased, <40	Organisms can be seen on a wet mount of CSF

ture and latex agglutination are useful in diagnosing the neonate and young infant but are less helpful in older children. Leukocytosis with a shift to the left and elevation of the erythrocyte sedimentation rate are usually present but are nonspecific. A very low peripheral WBC count with thrombocytopenia can be indicative of severe disease. CT or MRI should be performed in all infants with *Citrobacter diversus* meningitis because of the association with brain abscess in 75% of cases.

Other studies can provide helpful information in the evaluation of a patient with encephalitis. The EEG can show the characteristic paroxysmal lateral epileptiform discharges suggestive of infection with herpes simplex. MRI is very sensitive in detecting edema or hemorrhage in the temporal lobes, a finding suggestive of herpes simplex encephalitis. If en-

cephalitis caused by herpes simplex is suspected, a brain biopsy and culture can be considered for diagnosis.

TREATMENT
Antimicrobial Therapy for Bacterial Meningitis

The selection of antimicrobial therapy for bacterial meningitis is based on providing CSF bactericidal activity against the most likely pathogens for a given age. Empiric broad-spectrum antibiotic therapy must be used in all patients suspected of meningitis until culture results are available. With the advent of the newer cephalosporins many effective regimens exist. Table 44-4 lists the most frequently used antimicrobials for bacterial meningitis, with the dosage and frequency adjusted for age.

Table 44-4   Antimicrobials and Daily Dosages for Treating Bacterial Meningitis*

Drug	Neonates <7 days old	Neonates 8 days to 1 month old	Infants and Children
Amikacin†	15-20 divided q 12 hr	20-30 divided q 8 hr	20-30 divided q 8 hr
Ampicillin	100-150 divided q 12 hr	150-200 divided q 8 or 6 hr	200-300 divided q 6 hr
Cefotaxime	100 divided q 12 hr	150-200 divided q 8 or 6 hr	200 divided q 6 hr
Ceftriaxone	—	—	75-100 divided q 24 or 12 hr
Ceftazidime	60 divided q 12 hr	90 divided q 8 hr	125-150 divided q 8 hr
Cefuroxime	—	—	240 divided q 8 hr
Chloramphenicol†	25 divided q 24 hr	50 divided q 12 hr	75-100 divided q 6 hr
Gentamicin†	5 divided q 12 hr	7.5 divided q 8 hr	7.5 divided q 8 hr
Isoniazid (oral)‡	—	—	15-20 divided q 24 or 12 hr
Penicillin G	100,000-150,000 divided q 12 hr	150,000-200,000 divided q 8 or 6 hr	250,000 divided q 6 hr
Pyrazinamide (oral)‡	—	—	30 divided q 24 or 12 hr
Rifampin (oral)‡	—	—	15-20 divided q 24 or 12 hr
Streptomycin (IM)‡	—	—	30 divided q 12 hr
Ticarcillin	150-225 divided q 12 or 8 hr	225-300 divided q 8 or 6 hr	300 divided q 6 hr
Tobramycin†	4 divided q 12	6 divided q 12 hr	6 divided q 8 hr
Vancomycin†	20 divided q 12 hr	30 divided q 8 hr	40-60 divided q 6 hr

*Dosages in milligrams per kilogram per day divided into every (q) 4, 6, 8, 12, or 24 hours. Penicillin G is listed as units per kilogram per day.
†Serum concentrations should be determined to ensure safe and therapeutic values.
‡Denotes antimicrobials for treating tuberculous meningitis.

Newborn infants

The combination of ampicillin and an aminoglycoside has been shown to be a safe and effective regimen for initial empirical therapy of neonatal meningitis. Ampicillin can be used alone in patients with meningitis caused by *L. monocytogenes* or group B streptococcus, although many authorities continue therapy with an aminoglycoside. Synergism between ampicillin and aminoglycosides has been demonstrated in in vitro studies and in an experimental meningitis model. Most gram-negative enteric pathogens are effectively treated with ampicillin and an aminoglycoside or with cefotaxime. Adjustment of the aminoglycoside dosage or substitution with a cephalosporin such as cefotaxime or ceftazidime are necessary in infants with renal compromise. These latter agents are effective therapy for meningitis caused by group B streptococcus and most gram-negative enterics. Cefotaxime is preferred for therapy in neonates because of greater experience in this age group, less inhibition of bilirubin binding to albumin, and less suppression of the bacterial intestinal flora. The newer cephalosporins do not provide adequate coverage for *L. monocytogenes* and enterococci and cannot be used alone for initial empiric treatment of neonatal meningitis. The routine use of cephalosporins in neonates, especially those in ICUs, is discouraged because of the likelihood of rapid development of resistant organisms, especially *Enterobacter* and *Serratia* species.

Uncomplicated meningitis caused by group B streptococcus and *L. monocytogenes* is treated for 10 to 14 days, whereas infants with gram-negative enteric meningitis must receive a minimum of 3 weeks of therapy (at least 2 weeks of therapy after sterilization of the CSF culture). Some patients need therapy for 4 to 6 weeks.

Infants 1 to 3 months old

Infants 1 to 3 months of age are considered separately because the pathogens in this age group include those of both the newborn and of early childhood. The combination of cefotaxime and ampicillin provides broad coverage for the pathogens common in those patients. The use of ampicillin combined with chloramphenicol is effective in most cases but may result in antagonism for group B streptococcal and *Listeria* infections. Cefotaxime would be effective alone for most patients, with the exception of the rare patient with *Listeria* or enterococcal infection. The duration of therapy is usually 10 to 14 days, except for disease caused by gram-negative enteric organisms or *Pseudomonas* species, in which case a minimum of 3 weeks is necessary.

Children over 3 months of age

There is no unanimity regarding the optimal antimicrobial regimen in older children and infants. The combination of ampicillin and chloramphenicol has been effectively used for many years. The new cephalosporins, cefotaxime and ceftriaxone, provide equally effective therapy, with the potential benefit of greater safety. Cefuroxime is somewhat less active in vitro against the common pathogens of meningitis. Cephalosporins have not been proved more efficacious than conventional therapy with ampicillin and chloramphenicol despite the fact that the former drugs are considerably more active in CSF. The variable metabolism of chloramphenicol in young infants, in those with hypotension and hepatic dysfunction, and in patients receiving anticonvulsants or rifampin therapy necessitates monitoring serum chloramphenicol concentrations to ensure safe and therapeutic values. The prolonged half-life and extraordinary CSF bactericidal titers achieved with ceftriaxone permit single daily dosing. With the increasing frequency of β-lactamase–producing *H. influenzae* strains and the emergence of penicillin-resistant *Str. pneumoniae,* the newer cephalosporins offer an advantage over conventional therapy for meningitis.

The child with tuberculous meningitis must be treated empirically with isoniazid, rifampin, and pyrazinamide or streptomycin until susceptibilities are available. In areas with isoniazid-resistant tuberculosis, streptomycin must be added routinely as a fourth drug.

The duration of therapy has traditionally been 10 to 14 days; however, recent studies indicate that uncomplicated meningitis caused by *H. influenzae* or *N. meningitidis* can be treated for 7 to 10 days. A 10- to 14-day regimen is needed for meningitis caused by *Str. pneumoniae.* Patients with tuberculous meningitis need therapy for the first 4 to 8 weeks with isoniazid, rifampin, pyrazinamide, and/or streptomycin, after which streptomycin may be discontinued.

Immunocompromised children

Neonates and children with primary or acquired immunodeficiency or those receiving intensive care management are susceptible to a wide array of pathogens that may not be adequately treated with conventional therapy. Empiric treatment with ceftazidime and vancomycin provides coverage against the most common pathogens as well as against most *Pseudomonas* species, gram-negative enterics, and *Staphylococcus* species. Once the pathogen has been identified, results of susceptibility testing can be used to guide therapy. Another suitable alternative is the combination of ticarcillin, nafcillin, and an aminoglycoside.

Antimicrobial Therapy for Encephalitis

Only a few agents are effective for the treatment of encephalitis. Encephalitis caused by herpes simplex has been successfully treated with acyclovir or vidarabine. Acyclovir is preferred in children because of its superior outcome in comparison to vidarabine and is preferred in newborn infants because it can be administered in a smaller infusion volume. Recurrence of symptoms may be secondary to relapse or may be caused by postinfectious encephalopathy. MRI may help demonstrate demyelination in the latter condition. Varicella-zoster encephalitis may respond to treatment with acyclovir, but a larger dosage (50 mg/kg/day) than that prescribed for herpes simplex infection (30 mg/kg/day) is needed. For treating meningoencephalitis caused by *Naegleria* species a combination of amphotericin B, miconazole, and rifampin has been proposed, but effectiveness of the regimen has not been established.

Supportive Therapy

Supportive therapy is based on correcting the pathologic alterations of the CNS. Immediate attention must be given to support of the cardiovascular system and reduction of increased ICP and cerebral edema. Increased ICP reduces cerebral perfusion pressure (CPP). If systemic hypotension is present, decreased cerebral blood flow can result, predisposing the patient to cerebral ischemia. Noninvasive ICP monitoring and appropriate cardiovascular support in an intensive care surrounding are paramount in treating the hypotensive child with meningitis. Based on studies in experimental meningitis, dexamethasone should be useful for therapy to decrease ICP and brain edema. The management of ICP is described in detail in Chapter 7.

Management of fluid and electrolyte balance is of great importance. SIADH has been noted in almost 90% of children with meningitis on admission to the hospital, and intravenously administered fluids are traditionally restricted to 800 to 1000 ml/m²/24 hr (approximately 50% to 75% of normal maintenance requirements). Fluid composition must consist of an electrolyte solution containing 0.25% to 0.45% sodium chloride solution (depending on the patient's serum sodium concentration) and 5% dextrose. Potassium must be added to the electrolyte solution, based on the serum potassium concentration and renal status. Hyponatremia will usually resolve within 24 to 48 hours with fluid restriction. The duration of hyponatremia correlates with neurologic sequelae.

Fluids should not be restricted in the patient with hypotension because of the importance of maintaining systemic arterial blood pressure. In addition the patient needs a sufficient glucose infusion to maintain the blood glucose in the normal range. The use of vasopressors such as dopamine and dobutamine can improve systemic arterial blood pressure and perfusion sufficiently to permit the infusion of a lesser fluid volume to maintain circulation. Placement of a central catheter to monitor central venous blood pressure is useful in assessing fluid status in patients in shock. Serum sodium and urinary specific gravity must be followed closely to avoid fluid overload. Oral intake must be prohibited until mental status is sufficiently recovered to minimize the risk of aspiration.

Once serum sodium concentrations are approximately 135 mEq/L, fluids may be slowly increased during the ensuing 24 to 48 hours to 1500 to 1700 ml/m²/day (100% of maintenance requirements). Vasopressors must be decreased slowly as the cardiovascular status improves to avoid any rapid fluctuations in systemic arterial blood pressure. Once the patient is well enough to take fluids orally, IV fluids must be tapered accordingly.

Seizures occur in as many as one third of patients hospitalized with meningitis. If seizure activity is present, an artificial airway must be maintained and anticonvulsant medication initiated. Diazepam or lorazepam can be given intravenously to stop convulsions until a loading dose of phenytoin can be given, followed by daily maintenance dosages. Phenytoin is preferred to phenobarbitol because it produces less sedation and respiratory depression. Both phenobarbitol and phenytoin substantially alter the metabolism of chloramphenicol; when these drugs are administered concomitantly, chloramphenicol serum concentrations must be monitored.

Regular neurologic examinations must be performed to evaluate any change in neurologic status. Daily measurements of head circumference and head transillumination provide early information about the development of hydrocephalus or effusions in neonates. CT or MRI is indicated in any patient with meningitis who has persistent obtundation, a rapidly enlarging head circumference, persistent or prolonged fever, focal seizure activity, focal neurologic abnormalities, or evidence of increased ICP. The use of IV contrast media helps differentiate subdural effusion from empyema.

Although controversial, a repeat lumbar puncture 24 to 36 hours after initiation of therapy can document bacteriologic cure. Delayed sterilization of CSF cultures correlates significantly with poor outcome. In children in whom no organisms are seen on a Gram-stained smear and CSF findings are not indicative of bacterial meningitis, a repeat lumbar puncture 6 to 8 hours after admission usually demonstrates a shift of the cell type predominance to lymphocytes in the CSF and continued normal glucose and protein concentrations; these findings usually indicate a nonbacterial cause of meningitis.

In addition to antimicrobial therapy and supportive care the patient with bacterial meningitis must be kept in respiratory isolation for 24 hours after initiation of appropriate antimicrobial therapy. Persons who have been in contact with patients who have *H. influenzae* type b and *N. meningitidis* meningitis should undergo prophylaxis with orally administered rifampin. The patients also need to receive rifampin prophylaxis near or directly after completion of parenteral antibiotic therapy. Rifampin produces sufficient concentrations in nasopharyngeal secretions to eliminate colonization, thereby reducing the risk of transmission or invasion of the pathogen. Table 44-5 lists the dosage of rifampin and indications for its administration to contacts.

Recent evidence indicates that the use of dexamethasone in a dose of 0.15 mg/kg (given intravenously) every 6 hours for the first 4 days of therapy significantly reduces the incidence of severe to profound hearing loss. Based on further investigation, dexamethasone is expected to become routine adjunctive therapy in patients with bacterial meningitis.

Most patients with bacterial meningitis have normal body temperatures by 5 to 7 days after initiation of antimicrobial therapy. Persistent fever for 5 to 9 days and prolonged fever for 10 days or longer occur in approximately 13% of all patients; those with *Haemophilus* meningitis have a greater incidence of persistent fever. Secondary fever (i.e., fever occurring after at least one afebrile 24-hour period) occurs in 16%. Patients with prolonged or persistent fever must be evaluated for subdural collection of fluid, concomitant arthritis or pneumonia, and drug fever. In addition patients with secondary fever must also be evaluated for nosocomially acquired infections.

Table 44-5   Rifampin Prophylaxis Recommendations*

Pathogen	Rifampin Dosage	Indications
N. meningitidis	Infants ≤1 mo of age: 5 mg/kg q 12 hr for four doses Children: 10 mg/kg q 12 hr for four doses Adults: 600 mg q 12 hr for four doses	All household, day care, and school contacts
H. influenzae	Infants ≤1 mo of age: 10 mg/kg in one dose q 24 hr for four doses Children: 20 mg/kg in one dose q 24 hr for four doses Adults: 600 mg in one dose q 24 hr for four doses	All contacts, including adults, within a household with at least one household contact younger than 48 mo not immunized with Hib vaccine

HIB = *H. influenzae* type b vaccine.
NOTE: Day care and nursery school contact prophylaxis should be individualized. In most situations prophylaxis is not initiated until two or more cases of documented *H. influenzae* invasive disease occur.
*Modified from Committee on Infectious Disease, American Academy of Pediatrics. *Haemophilus Influenzae* Infections. Report of the Committee on Infectious Diseases. Evanston, Ill.: American Academy of Pediatrics, 1986, pp 169-174. Reproduced by permission.

PROGNOSIS

The case fatality rate in patients with bacterial meningitis is influenced by age, the specific pathogen, length of illness before hospitalization, and the competency of the immune system. Neonates have a fatality rate of 15% to 20%, whereas infants and older children have a rate of approximately 5%.

Neurologic, developmental, and behavioral sequelae occur in 30% to 50% of patients after meningitis. Approximately 30% of postmeningitic patients demonstrate a mean IQ that is 1 SD below that of their siblings. Mental retardation and learning disorders can occur in 10% and 15%, respectively. Hearing impairment, ranging from mild and unilateral to profound and bilateral, occurs in as many as 30% to 40% of patients after meningitis. Visual impairment can be noted in 2% to 4%. Permanent seizure disorders occur in 2% to 8%.

Relapse of bacterial meningitis occurs in fewer than 1% of patients and is most often associated with group B streptococcus, gram-negative enteric organisms, or *H. influenzae* type b and in some patients can be associated with resistant strains, inadequate dosage of antimicrobials, or insufficient duration of therapy. Recurrent meningitis can occur in those with inherent defects in the immune system. Recurrent pneumococcal meningitis is often associated with a communication of CSF to mucosal surfaces.

ADDITIONAL READING

Feigin RD, Shackleford PG. Sequential lumbar puncture as a diagnostic aid in aseptic meningitis. N Engl J Med 289:571-574, 1973.

• Kaplan SL, Fishman MA. Supportive therapy for bacterial meningitis. Pediatr Infect Dis 6:679-667, 1987.

Klein JO, Feigin RD, McCracken GH. Report of the task force on diagnosis and management of meningitis. Pediatrics 78(Suppl):959-982, 1986.

• Lebel MH, Freij BJ, Syrogiannopouos GA, et al. Dexamethasone therapy for bacterial meningitis. Results of two double-blind, placebo-controlled trials. N Engl J Med 319:964-977, 1988.

Lebel MH, McCracken GH. Delayed cerebrospinal fluid sterilization and adverse outcome of bacterial meningitis in infants and children. Pediatrics 83:161-167, 1989.

• Sande MA, Scheld WM, McCracken GH, and the Meningitis Study Group. Report of a workshop: Pathophysiology of bacterial meningitis—implications for new management strategies. Pediatr Infect Dis 6:1145-1171, 1987.

• Whitley RJ, Alford CA, Hirsch MS, et al. Vidarabine vs. acyclovir therapy in herpes simplex encephalitis. N Engl J Med 314:144-149, 1986.

45 Peritonitis

Mahmoud M. Mustafa · Jane D. Siegel

BACKGROUND AND PHYSIOLOGY

Peritonitis, inflammation of the serous lining of the peritoneal cavity, is classified as primary or secondary. Primary peritonitis is caused by bacterial invasion from an inapparent site outside of the abdominal cavity in the absence of an intra-abdominal source. Secondary peritonitis results from contamination of the peritoneal cavity with microorganisms and/or chemical substances that have leaked from the bowel, hepatobiliary tract, or genitourinary tract. Despite the differences in pathogenesis, both primary and secondary peritonitis are considered medical emergencies that require frequent monitoring, intensive supportive measures, antimicrobial therapy, and appropriate diagnostic studies to determine if there is a need for surgical intervention.

Primary Peritonitis

Primary or spontaneous bacterial peritonitis (SBP) accounts for approximately 2% to 3% of all pediatric intra-abdominal emergencies for which surgical exploration is done. A bimodal age distribution has been recognized with infants in the first 2 months of life and children 5 to 9 years of age. SBP may occur in previously healthy infants and children, but it is more frequent in those with the following underlying conditions: nephrotic syndrome, chronic liver disease, and systemic lupus erythematosus. Preexisting ascites is noted as a risk factor in most clinical reviews. An incidence of 17.3% for SBP in children with nephrotic syndrome and 8% to 10% in children with chronic liver disease was recently reported. A single microorganism is recovered from the peritoneal fluid in 65% to 75% of cases of SBP, the remainder being sterile. The same organism may be isolated from blood cultures in 75% of cases, but isolates from other body fluids or mucosal surfaces do not correlate well with isolates from peritoneal fluid cultures. The most frequently isolated pathogen is *Strep-*

tococcus pneumoniae. Other pathogens encountered include *Streptococcus pyogenes, Haemophilus influenzae* type b, *Neisseria meningitidis, Staphylococcus aureus, Escherichia coli,* and other gram-negative rods. Some centers have observed an increase in the incidence of gram-negative rods during the past 20 years. Anaerobes are rarely recovered from peritoneal fluid of patients with SBP.

Secondary Peritonitis

Secondary peritonitis results from direct extension of intra-abdominal or external infection and accounts for the majority of cases of peritonitis. Secondary peritonitis may be bacterial, chemical, or both. Chemical peritonitis develops after the introduction of blood, bile, pancreatic or gastric juices, or meconium into the peritoneal cavity. Meconium peritonitis occurs most often as a complication of meconium ileus in infants with cystic fibrosis and perforation of the gut in utero or shortly after birth. Most cases of secondary peritonitis are bacterial and are caused by contamination of the peritoneum from a perforated hollow viscus before surgery or during intra-abdominal surgery or by extension from an abscess of one of the solid organs within the abdominal cavity. The most frequently encountered underlying processes include acute appendicitis, volvulus, incarcerated hernia, intussusception, ruptured Meckel's diverticulum, and inflammatory bowel disease. In neonates secondary peritonitis is usually due to direct extension from umbilical infection or to perforation of the bowel associated with necrotizing enterocolitis.

Secondary bacterial peritonitis is a polymicrobial infection with a mean of 1.8 aerobic species and 2.4 anaerobic species per patient. An increase in the proportion of anaerobes isolated occurs in association with colonic or rectal perforation as compared with perforation of the stomach or small intestine. The major aerobes isolated include *E. coli, Klebsiella-En-*

terobacter species, enterococcus, and *Proteus* species. *Pseudomonas aeruginosa* has been isolated from peritoneal fluid in approximately 20% of healthy children with acute perforated appendicitis, and *S. epidermidis* may be isolated in pure culture from infants with necrotizing enterocolitis. *Bacteroides fragilis* is the most commonly encountered anaerobe and is associated with an increased risk of intra-abdominal abscess. Other anaerobes include clostridia, anaerobic cocci, eubacteria, and fusobacteria. Fungi, most commonly *Candida* species, may also be associated with secondary peritonitis. Contamination of the peritoneal cavity with *Candida* species at the time of construction of the Roux-en-Y limb during liver transplantation has been identified as the primary focus from which early disseminated candidiasis develops in such patients. Other adjuvants such as chemical irritants, blood, or foreign bodies may act to increase the virulence of intraperitoneal microorganisms.

Whatever the initiating cause of peritonitis, a similar series of local and systemic reactions occur. Initially there is a local peritoneal inflammation with exudation of fluid rich in antibodies, complement, neutrophils, and macrophages. These elements of the defense system are essential to enhance bacterial phagocytosis and killing. The sealing action of the greater omentum, coupled with formation of fibrinous adhesions in the peritoneal cavity, further limit the inflammatory process. The actions of the host defense system may lead to resolution of the inflammatory process or localized abscess formation. If not contained, there is diffuse spread of infection, resulting in a generalized peritonitis. Bacteria and toxins are absorbed by the peritoneum, resulting in bacteremia and endotoxemia. Infected fluid may diffuse into the subhepatic, subphrenic, or pelvic spaces and result in abscess formation.

Massive shifts of fluids and electrolytes into the bowel lumen and peritoneal cavity result in decreased circulating blood volume, which is further compounded by fluid loss associated with fever, vomiting, diarrhea, and nasogastric suction. In addition endotoxin release increases capillary permeability and extravasation of fluids into peripheral tissues. Respiratory function may be compromised by the mechanical effect of the fluid interfering with diaphragmatic movement. Limitation of movement leads to hypoventilation and loss of functional residual capacity and eventually ventilation/perfusion mis-

match. In addition low-pressure pulmonary edema develops and decreases lung complicance. The ultimate effects of uncontrolled infection may be septic shock, with hypotension, hypoxemia, a hypermetabolic state, metabolic acidosis, renal failure, DIC, and death.

Clinical Manifestations and Diagnosis

The characteristic clinical findings on presentation include fever, abdominal pain and distention, shallow breathing not associated with movement of abdominal muscles, decreased or absent bowel sounds, rigidity of the abdominal wall, rebound tenderness, shifting dullness to percussion, tenderness on rectal examinatin, and diarrhea. Signs of shock may be present in the most severely affected patients. Very young infants and children receiving immunosuppressive therapy may have an atypical presentation, with poor feeding, lethargy, normal tempcrature, or hypothermia. Also, abdominal muscle spasm may be absent. In such cases peritonitis must be considered in the presence of a completely silent abdomen with a rapid pulse or decrease in systemic arterial blood pressure.

Other conditions that may have a clinical presentation similar to that of peritonitis include pneumonia, acute rheumatic fever, diabetic ketoacidosis, and porphyria. A cardiopulmonary process as the cause of abdominal distress must be excluded by chest roentgenogram. Children with acute rheumatic fever may present with an aseptic peritonitis as one component of their immunologically mediated polyserositis; therefore a careful cardiac evaluation, including an ECG and echocardiogram, may be helpful in diagnosing patients without any risk factors for SBP or evidence for an intra-abdominal source of peritonitis.

MONITORING AND LABORATORY TESTS

All infants and children with peritonitis must be monitored as described in Chapter 4. Until the patient becomes stable, the abdominal examination must be repeated every 2 to 4 hours to assess the following: distention, abdominal girth, anterior abdominal wall cellulitis, bowel sounds, tenderness, and involuntary spasm of abdominal musculature. As long as bowel perforation is a possibility, a cross-table lateral abdominal roentgenogram is repeated at 8- to 12-hour intervals to look for free air. Another sample of peritoneal fluid must be obtained for a Gram stain, culture, and cell count if the patient has not responded within 24 to 48 hours to appropriate antibiotic therapy. In patients with compromised cardiorespiratory function or moderate to severe dehydration, a CVC or a Swan-Ganz catheter should be used (see Chapter 12). In addition arterial cannulation is advantageous for accurate systemic blood pressure measurements plus is a convenient source of blood for serial determination of blood gas and pH determinations and other laboratory tests.

The usual laboratory findings include a peripheral leukocytosis more than 15,000 to 20,000 WBCs/mm³ with a moderate to marked left shift and an elevated hematocrit, BUN, and urine specific gravity reflecting dehydration and hemoconcentration. Serum amylase levels may be increased in patients with peritonitis from almost any cause, but very high levels are observed only in children with acute pancreatitis. Metabolic and/or respiratory acidosis is present in patients with severe and late peritonitis. Supine upright and cross-table lateral roentgenograms of the abdomen may reveal distention of both small and large intestines or free air in the peritoneal cavity if there is a ruptured viscus. Ultrasonography, CT, or MRI of the abdomen may be helpful in identifying the underlying cause of the peritonitis.

Cultures of blood and urine must always be obtained. When predisposing factors are present and there is no evidence to suggest an acute surgical emergency, abdominal paracentesis with or without peritoneal lavage may be performed to confirm the diagnosis (see Chapters 89 and 144). Relative contraindications to peritoneal tap include previous abdominal surgery or the possibility of meconium peritonitis in neonates from bowel adhering to the anterior abdominal wall and the risk of puncture associated with the procedure. Ascitic fluid must be cultured both aerobically and anaerobically. An ascitic fluid leukocyte count >300 WBCs/mm³ with more than 30% neutrophils is diagnostic of intraperitoneal bacterial infection. The presence of only gram-positive organisms on the stained smear is highly suggestive of primary peritonitis. If a Gram stain of the sediment of peritoneal fluid shows no organisms, gram-negative bacteria, or mixed organisms, an exploratory laparatomy may be indicated to rule out a ruptured viscus. Although organisms may reach the peritoneal cavity via the genital tract in females, vaginal cultures have not proved helpful.

Specific laboratory tests to be repeated will be determined by the initial results. An evaluation of the immune system should be undertaken after the patient's recovery from primary peritonitis, especially in the absence of an associated chronic disease state. Studies to consider include serum immunoglobulins, measurement of acute and convalescent antibody to the specific pathogen in the case of *Str. pneumoniae* or *H. influenzae* type b, intradermal test with a control antigen, C3, C4, CH₅₀, human immunodeficiency virus antibody and/or antigen, plus liver spleen scan to rule out functional or anatomic asplenia. In appropriate cases a sickle cell preparation is indicated.

TREATMENT

Appropriate treatment of children with bacterial peritonitis includes general supportive measures, use of appropriate antimicrobial agents, and surgical repair of gangrenous or perforated bowel or drainage of an intra-abdominal abscess.

Supportive Care

Hypovolemia is a frequent complication of peritonitis, and volume must be replaced with crystalloid or colloid solutions or blood to maintain a urinary output of 1 to 2 ml/kg/hr and adequate tissue perfusion. Oxygen administration and elevation of the head are indicated for patients who are hypoxemic, and mechanical ventilation is indicated for those with respiratory failure (see Chapter 10). Oral feedings are contraindicated during the early phases of treatment of peritonitis, and the stomach must be decompressed by placement of a nasogastric tube and suction. Patients with peritonitis who have serious underlying disease and/or a perforated viscus may be unable to tolerate oral feedings for a prolonged period of time. Hyperalimentation fluid infusions via a CVC may be necessary to provide sufficient calories for replacement of losses incurred during the acute illness plus for ongoing maintenance in patients who are unlikely to recover promptly.

Antimicrobial Therapy

Antimicrobial therapy is initiated intravenously as soon as the clinical diagnosis of peritonitis is made and appropriate microbiologic cultures are obtained. Antimicrobial agents active against the infecting pathogens are necessary for prompt resolution of the local infection and bacteremia as well as for prevention of abscess formation and seeding of distal sites. Recommended regimens are presented in Table 45-1. Traditionally, primary peritonitis has been treated

Table 45-1   Recommended Antimicrobial Agents for Treatment of Peritonitis

Clinical Condition	Empiric Choice	Alternatives
Primary peritonitis	Cefotaxime	Penicillin G
Secondary peritonitis		
Community acquired	Clindamycin plus gentamicin	Clindamycin plus ceftazidime
Previous hospitalization or treatment with antibiotics	Ampicillin, clindamycin, amikacin	Ampicillin, clindamycin, ceftazidime
Neonate	Ticarcillin, gentamicin	Clindamycin, gentamicin; consider vancomycin, ceftazidime, metronidazole as discussed in text

successfully with penicillin G alone. A third-generation cephalosporin such as cefotaxime or ceftriaxone is currently preferred because of the increased incidence of *H. influenzae* type b and gram-negative enteric bacilli reported by some centers in recent years. In some geographic areas 8% to 15% of pneumonococci are relatively insensitive to penicillin (MIC >0.125 μg/ml, <2 μg/ml) and may not be eradicated by penicillin alone, but they are completely killed by cefotaxime or ceftriaxone. Ceftazidime as a single drug is less desirable in this setting because of its relatively decreased activity against *Str. pneumoniae*.

The initial choice of antibiotics for treatment of secondary peritonitis is based on the knowledge of the source of infection and the microorganisms that are potentially responsible for peritoneal contamination. Since secondary peritonitis is most often associated with bowel perforation, the combination of clindamycin and an aminoglycoside remains the preferred treatment regimen. The choice of aminoglycoside is determined primarily by the antibiotic susceptibility pattern within an institution and secondarily by the cost of the agent. In patients who have had prolonged hospitalization and/or a previous course of antibiotics, amikacin is preferred over gentamicin or tobramycin because of the likelihood of previous colonization with resistant gram-negative enteric bacilli. Such patients may also benefit from the addition of ampicillin for its activity against enterococci.

Alternative regimens warrant discussion. Metronidazole is preferred over clindamycin combined with an aminoglycoside for treatment of clindamycin-resistant strains of *B. fragilis* or very extensive persistent infection associated with *B. fragilis*. Cefoxitin is not used frequently because of its poor activity against clostridial species, resistance of *Bacteroides* species in some geographic areas, and its narrow spectrum of activity against aerobes. Ceftazidime, a third-generation cephalosporin that is active against *Pseudomonas* species and multiply resistant aerobic gram-negative rods, is a suitable alternative to an aminoglycoside for treatment of secondary peritonitis, especially in patients with renal dysfunction. Ceftazidime should be combined with either clindamycin or metronidazole because of its poor activity against *Bacteroides* species plus many other anaerobes. Like other third-generation cephalosporins, ceftazidime is more effective than aminoglycosides in the treatment of deep tissue infection or an abscess because of its relatively increased activity under anaerobic conditions and at an acidic pH. In patients who develop peritonitis as a postoperative complication in a hospital in which methicillin-resistant *S. aureus* (MRSA) is prevalent, vancomycin is included as part of a two- or three-drug regimen.

Two new antimicrobial agents, aztreonam and imipenem-cilastatin, as of this writing are not yet approved for use in children younger than 12 years of age. Aztreonam is a monobactam antibiotic that is active against aerobic gram-negative bacilli only and must therefore be combined with clindamycin. Aztreonam may be used in penicillin-allergic patients since there is no cross-sensitivity with β-lactam agents. Imipenem-cilastatin is a unique broad-spectrum β-lactam antibiotic that is active against nearly all anaerobes plus aerobic gram-positive and gram-negative microorganisms and therefore can be used as a single-drug regimen. Caution is advised in the use of this drug because of the CNS and renal toxicity that have been observed. These two regimens have exhibited efficacy equivalent to the standard clindamycin-aminoglycoside combination in clinical trials in adults. These agents may prove particularly useful for treatment of infections associated with multiply resistant pathogens.

The choice of an appropriate combination of antimicrobial agents for use in neonates is more difficult. Metabolism of clindamycin by the neonate is highly variable, and no high-pressure liquid chromatography methods are available for rapid and easy measurement of serum clindamycin concentrations. Metabolism of metronidazole by the liver and the potential mutagenicity of this drug make it undesirable as a first-line drug in neonates. Therefore clindamycin in combination with an aminoglycoside is recommended only if there is definite evidence for serious anaerobic infection (e.g., gross fecal contamination of the peritoneal cavity, putrid peritoneal fluid, abscess contents with Gram-stain evidence of

Bacteroides or clostridial species). In most other cases either ticarcillin or mezlocillin in combination with an aminoglycoside is preferred.

Infants with CVCs in place before peritonitis developed are at increased risk of endocarditis as a result of *S. epidermidis* bacteremia; therefore vancomycin is included in the antimicrobial regimen of such patients.

Recommended dosage schedules for frequently used antimicrobial agents are presented in Table 45-2.

Although a minimum course of 10 to 14 days is recommended, duration of therapy must be individualized. Patients who have normal function of the gastrointestinal tract plus uncomplicated primary peritonitis caused by a single highly susceptible pathogen may complete the course of therapy with an appropriate oral antibiotic in high dosages (two to three times the routine dosage). Such management requires very close physician monitoring of the adequacy of oral therapy. Patients with secondary peri-

Table 45-2 Antimicrobial Agents Frequently Used for Treatment of Intra-abdominal Sepsis

Drug	Dosage (mg/kg/day)	Comments
Clindamycin*	30 divided q 8 hr	Resistant *Bacteroides* species in some areas of country
Metronidazole*	30 divided q 6 hr	Excellent activity against anaerobes; inactive against aerobes
Cefoxitin	160 divided q 6 hr	Poor activity against clostridial species
Chloramphenicol*	75 divided q 6 hr	Inactivated by anaerobic bacteria; bacteriostatic against aerobic gram-negative rods
Ceftazidime	150 divided q 8 hr	Variable activity against anaerobes; very active against aerobic gram-negative rods; little experience
Moxalactam	150 divided q 8 hr	Associated bleeding tendency makes this drug less desirable in surgical patients; variable activity against anaerobes; inactive against *Pseudomonas* species
Cefotaxime	150 divided q 6 hr	Variable activity against anaerobes; inactive against *Pseudomonas* species
Ceftriaxone	50-75 divided q 12 hr	Variable activity against anaerobes; inactive against *Pseudomonas* species; little experience
Ampicillin	100 divided q 6 hr	Active against enterococcus
Ticarcillin	200-300 divided q 6 hr	Adequate activity against enterococcus when combined with an aminoglycoside; variable activity against anaerobes
Mezlocillin	200-300 divided q 4 to 6 hr	Active against enterococcus; variable activity against anaerobes
Gentamicin	5-7.5 divided q 8 hr	Reduced activity at acid pH and in anaerobic environment of abscesses and deep tissue infections
Tobramycin	5-7.5 divided q 8 hr	
Amikacin	22.5 divided q 8 hr	

*Oral route may be considered when gastrointestinal function is normal.

tonitis who have signs of persistent infection may need prolonged parenteral therapy. Such patients need a complete evaluation for possible abscess formation or development of metastatic foci of infection.

Surgical Management

Aggressive surgical management of secondary peritonitis is indicated for prompt resolution. An exploratory laparotomy is indicated for any patient with an acute abdomen in whom secondary peritonitis cannot be excluded. Removal of necrotic tissue, drainage of abscesses, and closure of perforations are the major surgical procedures in the management of this form of peritonitis. Surgical drainage of primary peritonitis is not indicated.

ADDITIONAL READING

• Bartlett JG. Recent developments in the management of anaerobic infection. Rev Infect Dis 5:235-245, 1983.

• Clark JH, Fitzgerald JF, Kleinman MB. Spontaneous bacterial peritonitis. J Pediatr 104:495-500, 1984.

Gorensek MJ, Lebel MH, Nelson JD. Peritonitis in children with nephrotic syndrome. Pediatrics 81:849-856, 1988.

Larcher VG, Manolaki N, Vegnente A, et al. Spontaneous bacterial peritonitis in children with chronic liver disease: Clinical features and etiologic factors. J Pediatr 106:907-912, 1985.

46 Pneumonia

John D. Nelson

BACKGROUND AND PHYSIOLOGY

Pneumonia is a common primary disease leading to admission to an intensive care unit, and it is also a common secondary event in those patients who are hospitalized for other reasons. This chapter focuses on identifying the etiologic agents and selecting antimicrobial therapy for pneumonias caused by infection. Inhalation (i.e., aspiration) pneumonia and general supportive care for pneumonia patients are discussed in other chapters.

Establishing the Diagnosis

The definitive diagnostic test for pneumonia is obtaining a sample of lung tissue by percutaneous needle aspiration or by open biopsy of an infected area, but these invasive procedures are reserved for special situations. Formerly it was standard practice to obtain lung tissue in all cases of suspected *Pneumocystis carinii* infection, but in recent years that practice has given way to an empiric course of trimethoprim-sulfamethoxazole (TMP/SMX) therapy. In general aspiration or biopsy is considered in two situations: (1) when there is doubt whether the disease is infection or another type of pulmonary pathology and (2) when the patient has failed to respond to a course of antimicrobial therapy. A practical problem in the latter course of action is that by the time the decision is made that direct examination of lung tissue is needed, the procedure is sometimes contraindicated because the patient is receiving high ventilation pressures or has a bleeding problem. Biopsy is important in patients with human immunodeficiency virus (HIV) infection to differentiate between infection and lymphoid interstitial pneumonia.

Blood cultures are positive in as many as 20% of cases of bacterial pneumonia. When pleural fluid is present, it must be obtained for direct microscopic examination and cultures. Antibody to adenovirus can be detected in pleural fluid. Antigen detection tests by latex agglutination, immunofluorescence, counterimmunoelectrophoresis, and enzyme-linked immunosorbent assay (ELISA) methods are available for several bacterial and viral agents. They can be used on specimens of tracheal secretions, pleural fluid, or concentrated urine.

Bronchoalveolar lavage for detection of *P. carinii* or bacteria has been used in adults, and there is limited experience with the technique in young children suggesting it is useful.

Microbiologic findings in tracheobronchial secretions obtained at the time a patient's airway is intubated or shortly thereafter correlate well with findings in lung tissue itself, but within an hour or so the trachea is colonized with the patient's oral flora and with organisms inhaled from the environment or inoculated during suctioning. At that time the culture results are difficult to interpret.

Cold agglutinins in the blood develop within several days in more than half the patients with viral or *Mycoplasma* infection; however, they are nonspecific, and their presence does not rule out the possibility of bacterial superinfection.

Acute and convalescent serologic tests for antibody are useful for retrospective diagnosis of certain infections.

Results of nasopharyngeal cultures for bacteria do not correlate well with cultures of lung tissue and in individual cases are more likely to be confounding than helpful because potential bacterial pathogens are commonly present in the nasopharynx of healthy children. However, finding viral antigen in nasopharyngeal mucosal cells is highly predictive that the same virus is present in the lung because prolonged, asymptomatic carriage of respiratory viruses is uncommon.

Etiologic Agents in Immunocompetent Patients

Infants and children who do not have an underlying immune or anatomic defect that predisposes them to unusual infections develop pneumonia from a limited number of infectious agents. Viruses are the most common causes in any age group, but in patients who are ill enough to need hospitalization the proportion of cases caused by bacteria increases. Age is an important factor in considering likely infectious agents (Table 46-1).

Newborn infants. Pneumonia as an isolated disease is uncommon in the newborn. It is generally part of sepsis or multisystem disease. Group B streptococcus is the most common bacterial agent. Coliform bacteria are rare causes except in cases of nosocomial infection in low birthweight babies or those in intensive care. Cytomegalovirus (CMV) acquired perinatally causes interstitial pneumonia at 2 or 3 weeks of age and is usually self-limited in otherwise healthy neonates. Syphilis and herpes simplex are rare causes of pneumonia, and other manifestations suggest the diagnosis.

Infants 1 to 3 months of age. Bacterial pneumonia is uncommon in this age group. The principal pathogens in the "afebrile" pneumonia syndrome of early infancy (many infants actually have low-grade fever) are respiratory syncytial virus (RSV), *Chlamydia trachomatis,* and to a lesser extent parainfluenza viruses. They characteristically cause a diffuse interstitial pneumonia, and the infants sometimes are initially seen with apnea as the initial event. Rapid antigen detection tests are very useful. The possible role of *P. carinii* and *Ureaplasma urealyticum* in this age group is uncertain. *Staphylococcus aureus* is uncommon and, when it does occur, usually complicates a primary viral infection. Pertussis is common in this age group, but the *Bordetella pertussis* organism itself does not invade tissue and cause pneumonia; however, secondary bacterial pneumonias can complicate pertussis.

Children 4 months to 2 years of age. Because of waning transplacentally acquired antibodies to encapsulated bacteria, the infant in this age group begins having serious infections caused by *Haemophilus influenzae* type b and *Streptococcus pneumoniae.* These infections can be manifest as either bronchopneumonia or lobar pneumonia with or without pleural effusion. They cannot be differentiated clinically. This is also the peak age for adenovirus infection, which is manifest as interstitial pneumonia or bronchopneumonia. In some severe cases there is multisystem infection with myocarditis, nephritis, hepatitis, or encephalitis.

Table 46-1 Etiologic Agents of Pneumonia in Immunocompetent Hospitalized Patients

Age	Common Pathogens	Less Common Pathogens
Newborn	Group B streptococcus Cytomegalovirus Nosocomial pathogens (infants in intensive care)	Coliform bacilli *Treponema pallidum* Herpes simplex
1-3 mo	*Chlamydia trachomatis* Respiratory syncytial virus Cytomegalovirus	Parainfluenza viruses *Staphylococcus aureus*
4 mo-2 yr	*Haemophilus influenzae* type b *Streptococcus pneumoniae* Adenoviruses Parainfluenza viruses	*Staphylococcus aureus* Respiratory syncytial virus Influenza viruses
2-5 yr	*Streptococcus pneumoniae* *Haemophilus influenzae* type b Adenovirus	Influenza viruses *Mycoplasma pneumoniae*
>5 yr	*Mycoplasma pneumoniae* *Streptococcus pneumoniae*	Respiratory viruses

Children 2 to 5 years of age. *Haemophilus* pneumonia becomes progressively less common during this period, but pneumococcal pneumonia persists. Adenovirus and influenza virus pneumonia still occur, but in general the overall incidence of pneumonia declines.

Children over 5 years of age. The peak age for *Mycoplasma pneumoniae* infection is 5 to 15 years. It is usually confined to one lobe and does not result in consolidation. Symptoms are typically worse than the radiographic appearance suggests. Sometimes infiltrate appears in a new area after approximately a week. Around 20% of cases are associated with pleural effusion that is small in quantity and may only be detected in decubitus roentgenograms. Pneumococcal and viral pneumonias occur.

Etiologic Agents in Compromised Hosts

A number of host factors or iatrogenic interventions result in either unusually severe disease with common pathogens or pneumonia caused by agents of low inherent virulence (Table 46-2).

Prematurity. The premature infant is deficient in virtually all elements of host defense mechanisms, and the many invasive procedures needed for management violate natural defense barriers. *Pseudomonas aeruginosa, S. aureus,* and coliform bacilli take advantage of the situation and are common causes of pneumonia in premature infants. The premature infant is probably no more susceptible to RSV infection than is the term newborn since maternally derived antibody is not protective, but the disease is more severe in the premature baby. The case fatality rate is approximately 20% and rises to as much as 80% in premature infants with underlying cardiopulmonary problems.

Intravascular catheters. Coagulase-negative staphylococci, which include *S. epidermidis* and other species, are the most common pathogens associated with indwelling vascular catheters. Most strains are resistant to β-lactam antibiotics and must be treated with vancomycin. *Candida* sp and multiply antibiotic-resistant *Enterobacter* and *Serratia* strains are other prominent pathogens. These infections are usually limited to septicemia, but on occasion pulmonary infection occurs, usually caused by *Candida*.

Sickle cell disease. Children with sickle cell disease have a sharply increased risk of pneumococcal infection, and the younger ones have an increased risk of *H. influenzae* type b infection. It can take the

form of a fulminating, rapidly fatal sepsis, especially in children younger than 5 years of age. When older children develop *M. pneumoniae* infection, they have an unusually severe form of the disease.

Previous broad-spectrum antibiotic therapy. Children with viral or bacterial respiratory infections who are treated with broad-spectrum antibiotics develop an alteration in their normal respiratory flora. An overgrowth of organisms such as *S. aureus, P. aeruginosa, Klebsiella pneumoniae,* and *Candida* sp occurs. Any of them is capable of serving as a secondary invader of the lower respiratory tract.

Immunosuppression and/or neutropenia. Any immunosuppressed patient is at risk for *Pneumocystis* pneumonia; the greatest risk is in patients with HIV infection or leukemia. Giant cell pneumonia can occur with measles, RSV, and parainfluenza virus infections. Patients with neutropenia are at risk for all types

---

Table 46-2   Likely Etiologic Agents in Compromising Situations

Situation	Pathogens
Prematurity	Respiratory syncytial virus *Staphylococcus aureus* Coliform bacilli *Pseudomonas aeruginosa*
Intravascular catheters	Coagulase-negative staphylococci *Candida* sp *Enterobacter cloacae* *Serratia marcescens*
Sickle cell disease	*Streptococcus pneumoniae* *Mycoplasma pneumoniae*
Previous broad-spectrum antibiotic therapy	*Staphylococcus aureus* *Pseudomonas aeruginosa* *Klebsiella pneumoniae* *Candida* sp
Immunosuppression and/or neutropenia*	*Pneumocystis carinii* *Pseudomonas aeruginosa* *Aspergillus* sp *Candida* sp Coliform bacilli Cytomegalovirus

*Such patients also are at increased risk of infection with the common respiratory pathogens.

of infection, but the most serious are those caused by *P. aeruginosa* and fungal infections.

TREATMENT
Initial Empiric Antimicrobial Therapy

In most seriously ill persons with pneumonia the cause is not known at the time therapy is initiated. After appropriate and available specimens for culture are obtained, the physician makes a judgment about therapy based on the considerations discussed previously in this chapter. Bacterial, fungal, or acid-fast stains of pleural fluid or freshly obtained tracheo-bronchial secretions and results of rapid antigen detection tests help guide the selection. Conditions commonly encountered in intensive care units are summarized in Table 46-3.

Interstitial pneumonia syndrome of early infancy

If the rapid test for RSV is positive, ribavirin aerosol therapy is considered. The drug is not used routinely because it is expensive and difficult to administer. Infants with bronchopulmonary dysplasia or any cardiac, pulmonary, or neuromuscular disorder that compromises pulmonary function are treated with ribavirin even if the illness is not severe. Postoperative patients with RSV infection probably need treatment as well. In any other situation ribavirin therapy is reserved for infants with severe infection. If the drug is aerosolized through tubing in a patient with an artificial airway, care must be taken to assure that precipitated drug does not clog the tubing. The drug must be aerosolized for at least 18 hours of every 24-hour period for 3 to 5 days.

If the rapid test for *C. trachomatis* is positive or if there are other reasons to suspect that pathogen, erythromycin is the drug of choice, but sulfonamides or ampicillin are also effective. If *P. carinii* infection is suspected, TMP/SMX would be appropriate therapy for that disease and also for chlamydial infection.

Community-acquired pneumonia in normal hosts

In a patient with RSV infection ribavirin therapy is considered as discussed above. Amantadine is indicated for pneumonia caused by influenza A virus, but treatment loses effectiveness if started more than 72 hours after onset of symptoms. Ribavirin is also effective, but this pneumonia is easier to treat with amantadine.

In cases of suspected bacterial pneumonia cefuroxime is appropriate for patients younger than 5 years of age in whom *Haemophilus* and gram-positive cocci are the major pathogens. In older children erythromycin is appropriate therapy for mycoplasmal or pneumococcal infection, but nafcillin or a related drug must be used if staphylococcal infection is suspected.

Table 46-3 Initial Empiric Antimicrobial Therapy in Selected Conditions

Condition	Preferred Therapy	Alternative Therapy
Interstitial pneumonia syndrome of early infancy	Erythromycin	Ampicillin, a sulfonamide
Pertussis	Erythromycin	Trimethoprim-sulfamethoxazole, ampicillin
Cystic fibrosis	An anti-*Pseudomonas* penicillin and an aminoglycoside*	Ceftazidime, piperacillin
Leukemia or immunocompromised		
Interstitial pneumonia (presumed *Pneumocystis*)	Trimethoprim-sulfamethoxazole	Pentamidine
Bronchopneumonia	Nafcillin (or vancomycin) and ceftazidime	Nafcillin, an anti-*Pseudomonas* penicillin and an aminoglycoside
Nosocomial pneumonia	(Same as for bronchopneumonia in immunocompromised patients)	

*Patients with cystic fibrosis usually require dosages of aminoglycosides two to three times those normally used in order to achieve therapeutic serum concentrations.

Acute pulmonary exacerbations in patients with cystic fibrosis

The role of bacteria in acute pulmonary exacerbations in patients with cystic fibrosis is uncertain. Traditionally, antibiotic therapy is directed against the organism that most commonly is isolated from the sputum, which is *P. aeruginosa*. The organisms persist in most patients after antibiotic therapy and clinical improvement. Although it has not been conclusively proved, most physicians who treat cystic fibrosis patients believe that antibiotics are beneficial. For many years an anti-*Pseudomonas* penicillin such as

ticarcillin has been given along with an aminoglycoside such as tobramycin, gentamicin, or amikacin. Cystic fibrosis patients have altered pharmacologic disposition of antibiotics that complicates the use of aminoglycosides. Larger dosages are needed to achieve therapeutic serum concentrations than in other patients. For example, in the case of tobramycin desired peak serum concentrations of 5 to 8 μg/ml are usually achieved with individual doses of 1.5 mg/kg every 8 hr (4.5 mg/kg/day). In cystic fibrosis patients an average dose of 3 mg/kg (9 mg/kg/day) is needed, and the range of daily dosage is wide (7.5

Table 46-4   Therapy for Specific Pathogens

Organism	Preferred Therapy	Alternative Therapy
Acinetobacter calcoaceticus	Imipenem-cilastatin	TMP/SMX; anti-*Pseudomonas* penicillin + amikacin
Actinomyces sp	Penicillin G	Tetracycline, ampicillin
Bacteroides sp	Clindamycin or chloramphenicol	Metronidazole, cefoxitin
Bordetella pertussis	Erythromycin	TMP/SMX, ampicillin
Chlamydia trachomatis, C. psittaci or TWAR strain	Erythromycin	Tetracycline
Coliform bacilli	A cephalosporin (e.g., cefotaxime)	An aminoglycoside
Cytomegalovirus	Ganciclovir (experimental)	—
Francisella tularensis	Gentamicin or streptomycin	Tetracycline
Haemophilus sp	Cefuroxime or chloramphenicol	Other cephalosporins; ampicillin (if β-lactamase negative)
Herpes simplex	Acyclovir	Vidarabine
Human immunodeficiency virus	Zidovudine	—
Influenza A	Amantadine	Ribavirin
Legionella sp	Erythromycin	Add rifampin
Listeria monocytogenes	Ampicillin + an aminoglycoside	TMP/SMX
Mycobacterium tuberculosis	Rifampin + isoniazid	Add pyrizinamide or aminoglycoside as third drug
Nocardia asteroides	A sulfonamide	Amikacin, TMP/SMX
Pseudomonas aeruginosa	Anti-*Pseudomonas* β-lactam + an aminoglycoside	Imipenem-cilastatin
Pseudomonas cepacia	Ceftazidime	TMP/SMX
Respiratory syncytial virus	Ribavirin	—
Rickettsia	Tetracycline (>7 yr of age)	Chloramphenicol
Staphylococcus sp	Nafcillin	A cephalosporin, vancomycin if nafcillin resistant
Streptococcus, groups A or B or pneumococcus	Penicillin G	Erythromycin, a cephalosporin, vancomycin for penicillin-resistant pneumococci
Treponema pallidum	Penicillin G	Erythromycin, tetracycline
Varicella-Zoster virus	Acyclovir	Vidarabine

TMP/SMX = trimethoprim-sulfamethoxazole.

to 15 mg/kg/day). Therefore it is essential to monitor serum concentrations in individual patients and to make adjustments in the dosage to stay in the safe and therapeutic range.

To avoid these problems with aminoglycosides β-lactam antibiotics alone have been used in clinical trials, and in the case of ceftazidime and piperacillin it appears that using either one is as effective as combination drug therapy.

Leukemic or other immunocompromised patients

When an immunocompromised patient develops interstitial pneumonia, the major probable causes are *P. carinii,* viruses, and fungi. Tuberculosis also must be considered. TMP/SMX therapy is usually initiated unless there are clinical conditions suggesting the likelihood of viral, fungal, or tuberculous infection. Lymphoid interstitial pneumonia is a condition of uncertain etiology in patients with HIV infection that appears to respond to corticosteroid therapy.

In the febrile, neutropenic patient it is customary to initiate therapy directed against a broad spectrum of gram-positive and gram-negative aerobic pathogens. The regimens listed in Table 46-3 are commonly used.

When a cause for the pneumonia has not been uncovered and empiric antibiotic therapy has failed to result in clinical improvement after 5 to 7 days, the possibility of fungal infection increases. It is common practice to initiate antifungal therapy with amphotericin B while continuing the antibiotic regimen.

Nosocomial pneumonia

In most instances of nosocomially acquired pneumonia in an intensive care environment the spectrum of anticipated pathogens is similar to that for neutropenic or immunosuppressed patients, and those treatment regimens would be appropriate initial, empiric therapy. Most important is the knowledge of the current nosocomial pathogens and their antimicrobial susceptibilities. For example, if methicillin-resistant staphylococci are a problem, vancomycin is used instead of nafcillin or a related β-lactam antibiotic. If aminoglycoside-resistant gram-negative pathogens are prevalent in the unit, a cephalosporin such as cefotaxime or ceftriaxone is used instead of an aminoglycoside.

Specific Antimicrobial Therapy

Table 46-4 lists pulmonary pathogens likely to be encountered in patients in an intensive care environment, along with antimicrobial regimens of choice and alternative drugs to use when a specific pathogen has been identified. Other regimens could be used since there are so many available antibiotics with similar spectra and activity. Selection of an appropriate drug or combination of drugs must always be based on antimicrobial susceptibility testing results and physiologic abnormalities in the patient (e.g., altered renal or hepatic function) that could affect the pharmacology, pharmacodynamics, or pharmacokinetics of a given antimicrobial drug.

ADDITIONAL READING

Chartrand SA, McCracken GH. Staphylococcal pneumonia in infants and children. Pediatr Infect Dis 1:10-23, 1982.

• Freij BJ, Kusmiesz H, Nelson JD, et al. Parapneumonic effusions and empyema in hospitalized children: A retrospective review of 227 cases. Pediatr Infect Dis 3:578-591, 1984.

• Golden SE, Shehab ZM, Bjelland JC, et al. Microbiology of endotracheal aspirates in intubated pediatric intensive care unit patients: Correlations with radiographic findings. Pediatr Infect Dis 6:665-669, 1987.

Nelson JD. Management of acute pulmonary exacerbations in cystic fibrosis: A critical appraisal. J Pediatr 106:1030-1034, 1985.

Ramsey BW, Marcuse EK, Foy HM, et al. Use of bacterial antigen detection in the diagnosis of pediatric lower respiratory tract infections. Pediatrics 78:1-9, 1986.

• Teele D. Pneumonia: Antimicrobial therapy for infants and children. Pediatr Infect Dis 4:330-335, 1985.

Thorpe JE, Baughman, RP, Frame PT, et al. Bronchoalveolar lavage for diagnosing acute bacterial pneumonia. J Infect Dis 155:855-861, 1987.

47 AIDS

Richard L. Wasserman

BACKGROUND AND PHYSIOLOGY

As of October 31, 1989, 112,241 cases of acquired immunodeficiency syndrome (AIDS) had been reported to the CDC: 1908 of these patients were children under 13 years of age. AIDS was first recognized in late 1979 simultaneously in Los Angeles, San Francisco, and New York with the occurrence of opportunistic infections and Kaposi's sarcoma in young, homosexual men, who as a group were not known to be at risk for these disorders. Within 2 years a syndrome similar to the inherited disorders severe combined immunodeficiency disease and Wiskott-Aldrich syndrome was recognized in infants and toddlers. Before 1983, when the human immunodeficiency virus type 1 (HIV 1; formerly called human T-cell leukemia virus type III [HTLV-III] or lymphadenopathy-associated virus [LAV]) was identified as the etiologic agent of AIDS, epidemiologic studies played a major role in understanding AIDS, and the apparent clusters of rare inherited immunodeficiencies led investigators to realize that these children had a disease similar to AIDS in adults. Case definitions for AIDS in children under 13 years of age were initially developed before the pathogenic role of HIV was known and before a test for HIV was available. The definition was revised in 1987 but is useful primarily as an epidemiologic tool since HIV-infected patients may not meet the diagnostic criteria for AIDS.

Risk factors for HIV infection include having a parent who has AIDS or who is a member of a high-risk group for AIDS or being exposed to blood or blood products. Most transfusion-associated HIV infections resulted from transfusions received during the 1979-1985 period. However, the inability of the present screening test to detect a recently infected donor who has not yet formed HIV antibody is associated with an estimated risk of transmission of 1 in 40,000. The primary risk groups for HIV infections are as follows:

IV drug abusers
Homosexual and bisexual males
Hemophiliacs
Blood transfusion recipients (before 1985)
Natives of countries where heterosexual HIV infection is prevalent
Sexual partners of risk-group members
Children of risk-group members or their sexual partners

Of HIV-infected children under 13 years of age who were identified by the CDC AIDS surveillance, 78% had a parent with AIDS or who was at risk for AIDS and acquired the infection perinatally, 13% received contaminated blood products, 6% were hemophiliacs, and 3% had undetermined risk factors. Perinatal transmission can, however, occur from asymptomatic women. Identifying and characterizing AIDS in children was much more difficult than in adults because many of the clinical and laboratory features of the syndrome as they appear in young children are similar to well-known pediatric entities such as failure to thrive, cystic fibrosis, and the inherited immunodeficiencies mentioned previously. Until the etiologic agent HIV-1 was found and a reliable, specific test for infection was developed, it was difficult or impossible to differentiate AIDS in children from other conditions.

HIV infection is becoming more common among pediatric patients in general as well as those admitted to the ICU. It is estimated that by 1991 1 in 10 pediatric beds in the United States will be occupied by HIV-infected patients. Often the diagnosis is not considered until after the critically ill child is admitted to the PICU. The most common presentations of HIV-infected patients in the PICU are (1) interstitial pneumonitis due to cytomegalovirus, *Pneumocystis carinii,* or lymphocytic interstitial pneumonia and (2) overwhelming sepsis due to common bacterial pathogens such as gram-positive cocci, *Salmonella, Escherichia coli,* or bacteria that are usually not considered invasive pathogens such as nontypable *Haemophilus* species or *Mycobacterium avium-intracellulare* (MAI). Unusually severe manifestations of common viral infections such as varicella and rubeola also suggest an underlying immunodeficiency.

SUMMARY OF SEPTEMBER 1987 REVISION OF SURVEILLANCE CASE DEFINITION FOR AIDS*

I. Without laboratory evidence of HIV infection (tests not done or inconclusive, infants of HIV infected mothers who are under 15 months of age and have no other evidence for immunodeficiency) a patient with AIDS:

  A. Does not have another cause of immunodeficiency (e.g., malignancy, chemotherapy, congenital syndrome)

and

  B. Has had one AIDS indicator disease definitively diagnosed

II. With laboratory evidence of HIV infection a patient with AIDS:

  A. Has had one AIDS indicator disease definitively diagnosed

or

  B. One of the following AIDS indicator diseases presumptively diagnosed: esophageal candidiasis, CMV retinitis with loss of vision, Kaposi's sarcoma, lymphoid interstitial pneumonia, mycobacterial infection disseminated to a site other than lungs, skin, or cervical or hilar lymph nodes, *Pneumocystis carinii* pneumonia, toxoplasmosis of brain at more than 1 month of age

III. With laboratory evidence against HIV infection (negative test results) a patient with AIDS:

  A. Does not have another cause of underlying immunodeficiency

and

  B. Has had *P. carinii* pneumonia definitively diagnosed

or

  C. Has had definitive diagnosis of one of the AIDS indicator diseases plus a T-helper lymphocyte count $<400/mm^3$

---

*From MMWR 36:1S-15S, 1987.

AIDS, the most severe expression of HIV infection, is a progressive combined immunodeficiency disease secondary to infection with HIV that may initially be seen as virtually any syndrome or unusual infection. HIV has been shown to infect hepatocytes, lymphocytes, monocytes, macrophages, brain, and bowel. Although there may be direct effects of viral infection of these tissues, the most important effect of HIV infection is the elimination of most or all T4 helper cells (CD4 cells), rendering the specific immune system essentially nonfunctional. The possible effects of HIV infection include the spectrum of infections mentioned in Chapter 20 and certain problems unique to AIDS. In addition to recurrent bacterial infections and infections with opportunistic organisms, neurologic deterioration manifested as developmental delay, seizures, or coma; cardiomyopathy; lymphoid interstitial pneumonitis; and autoimmune blood dyscrasias, particularly idiopathic thrombocytopenic purpura (ITP), are also part of the constellation of disorders seen in patients with AIDS. HIV infection must be considered in any risk-group member, regardless of the presenting complaint, and in any patient with an unusual infectious disease presentation, regardless of the stated risk-group history. Organ system disorders seen in children with AIDS are listed on p. 380.

There are virtually no useful data in children to determine the rate of progression from asymptomatic HIV infection to clinical AIDS or the rate of survival. Although estimates of the duration of latency have been revised several times, it is currently thought that most infected adults will demonstrate signs and symptoms of AIDS within 14 years of infection, with approximately 7% to 10% of infected patients becoming sick each year. Similar data in children are not available, but incubation periods as short as a few months and as long as 7 years have been reported for perinatally acquired HIV. The diagnosis of AIDS is made within the first year of life in 40% of children and by 5 years of age in 82%. Reported survival rates are influenced by the case definition of AIDS in children. HIV-infected children who did not meet the CDC case definition are not included in the calculations of survival rates. In addition the treatment of HIV-infected children is constantly changing. Improved diagnosis, supportive care, antimicrobial therapy, and antiviral drugs have invalidated the early prognostic data.

CLINICAL MANIFESTATIONS OF AIDS IN CHILDREN

Hematologic system

Immunodeficiency
ITP, anemia
Leukopenia
Lymphoma
Sepsis

Central nervous system

Encephalopathy, dementia
Developmental delay
Hypertonicity, hyperreflexia
Seizures, coma
Meningitis, encephalitis

Upper respiratory tract

Sinusitis
Otitis

Lower respiratory tract

Pneumonia—bacterial, viral, fungal, parasitic
Lymphoid interstitial pneumonitis

Cardiac system

Cardiomyopathy

Hepatic system

Hepatitis

Gastrointestinal tract

Oral candidiasis
Parotitis
Chronic diarrhea and wasting
Enteritis—fungal, parasitic, viral

Renal system

Nephrosis

MONITORING AND LABORATORY TESTS

Once suspected, the diagnosis of HIV infections must be confirmed by enzyme-linked immunosorbent assay (ELISA) and Western blot techniques. This two-step procedure, which is followed automatically by most laboratories, measures anti-HIV antibodies produced by the patient in response to HIV infection. ELISA is a screening test that measures antibody in the patient's serum that is reactive with any component of HIV. It is a rapid screening test that is quite sensitive but is subject to false positive reactions. Because of the potential for false positive reactions, the Western blot test is performed on all patients with positive ELISA reactions. It detects antibody against the individual protein antigens of HIV. For the Western blot to be positive the patient's serum must react with three viral proteins.

Virtually all patients infected with HIV postnatally produce antibody within 3 months of exposure to the virus. Biologic false negative reactions may occur if the patient is tested very early after infection before antibody is produced (<8 to 12 weeks) or very late in the course of AIDS when antibody is absorbed by high titers of virus. These two situations have minimal clinical relevance because the patients with early false negative antibody tests rarely present for evaluation of an HIV-related illness, and the patients with late false negative tests may be diagnosed on clinical criteria alone. Technical false negative reactions are rare. Tests looking for the presence of HIV by detecting the viral core protein p24 in serum (the HIV antigen test) or by detecting viral genes in leukocytes (the HIV polymerase chain reaction [PCP] test) are occasionally useful for monitoring or diagnosis.

The diagnosis of perinatal HIV infection is much more difficult. Most newborns of infected mothers will be ELISA and Western blot positive because of transplacentally acquired maternal antibody. Only 20% to 50% of infants born to infected mothers will be infected, but most will test positive at birth. Maternal antibody has persisted in infants for as long as 15 months. Consequently, it is often impossible to conclusively determine the infant's HIV status until after the first year of life. The HIV antigen test and an IgM anti-HIV antibody test have been used in an effort to differentiate passive antibody transfer from actual infection in the neonate. Although each test has successfully identified infected infants, false positive and false negative reactions occur commonly, and neither the HIV antigen test nor the IgM test is clinically useful. Some ELISA-positive newborns can be definitively diagnosed as infected by comparing simultaneous Western blot tests performed on the mother and the child. If the child's serum reacts with viral components different from the maternal sample, those antibodies must have been made by the infected child himself. The HIV PCR test is not subject to false positive results but may be falsely negative if the amount of virus in infected leukocytes is small. There is no way to eliminate completely the possibility of HIV infection until at least 15 months of age. Until the results of the HIV antibody test are known, blood and body fluid precautions are observed and the patient treated as though HIV infection were present. (See Chapter 41 for discussion of universal precautions and the risk of occupational transmission.)

Specific immunologic testing of cell-mediated immunity or antibody function has limited clinical use. Skin test anergy or the lack of in vitro responsiveness is a poor prognostic sign, but this information rarely alters clinical management. There is some evidence, derived from adult patients, that the absolute number of T4 (CD4) or T-helper cells correlates with disease progression. Some clinicians use the absolute T4 (CD4) count when considering the initiation of antiviral therapy. In the PICU setting the laboratory investigation is focused on the acute problem. Perhaps the most important point is that vigorous efforts, including early lung biopsy, must be made to establish the etiologic diagnosis of pulmonary disease. Treatment of acute infectious processes is considered in Chapters 42 to 46.

TREATMENT

At the time of this writing there is no curative treatment for AIDS. Studies in adults strongly support the use of zidovudine (AZT, Retrovir), which has been shown to decrease morbidity and prolong life. Preliminary studies in children suggest that similar effects will be seen. Several other drugs with less toxicity and different sites of action are also undergoing clinical trials in children. Efficacy of AZT in asymptomatic HIV-infected patients is presently under investigation.

Lymphoid interstitial pneumonitis is usually, but not always, responsive to steroids. In the absence of studies establishing an appropriate steroid regimen, the choice of a particular approach is somewhat arbitrary. Several regimens that have been used to treat lymphoid interstitial pneumonitis in patients with AIDS are as follows:

1. Administer methylprednisolone (30-50 mg/kg or 1.5 g/m²) every other day for three doses, followed by 2 mg/kg/day, with weaning as tolerated.
2. Administer prednisone (1-2 mg/kg/day) until a significant response is achieved; then wean as tolerated.
3. Bronchodilator therapy may be useful.
4. Provide supplemental oxygen.
5. Treat heart failure.
6. Pneumonitis may be incompletely responsive to steroids. Attempts should be made to wean the patient from steroids at clinical "plateaus," not just when the patient is completely asymptomatic. Because of the association of lymphoid interstitial pneumonitis and Epstein-Barr virus, acyclovir has been used in some patients. The efficacy of acyclovir for lymphoid interstitial pneumonitis has not been established.

Children with AIDS do not mount a normal antibody response to infection and therefore benefit from treatment with intravenous immunoglobulin during acute infections. Both clinical improvement with a decrease in the number of febrile episodes and sepsis episodes and improved laboratory tests of immune function have been reported in children given intravenous immune globulin prophylactically (200 to 400 mg/kg every 4 weeks). Therefore most investigators recommend this regimen for young children with AIDS. Antibiotic prophylaxis with trimethoprim/sulfamethoxazole (TMP/SMX) (5 mg/kg of trimethoprim) is effective in the prevention of PCP and apparently reduces the incidence of bacterial infections as well. Many patients become neutropenic when treated daily with TMP/SMX. Regimens using TMP/SMX only on Monday, Wednesday, and Friday or Monday, Tuesday, and Wednesday appear equally effective and cause less neutropenia. Administration of aerosolized pentamidine once a month is effective in preventing PCP in adults, but there is no experience in children. Similarly, aerosolized pentamidine has been used as an adjunctive therapeutic agent in selected adult patients who have not responded to the usual therapeutic modalities.

ADDITIONAL READING

• Falloon J, Eddy J, Wiener, et al. Human immunodeficiency virus infection in children. J Pediatr 114:1-30, 1989.

Fischel MA, Richman DD, Grieco MH, et al. The efficacy of azidothymidine (AZT) in the treatment of patients with AIDS and AIDS-related complex. N Engl J Med 317:185-191, 1987.

• Pizzo PA, Eddy J, Fallon J, et al. Effect of continuous infusion of zidovudine (AZT) in children with symptomatic HIV infection. N Engl J Med 319:889-896, 1988.

• Rubenstein A, Morechi R, Silverman B, et al. Pulmonary disease in children with acquired immune deficiency syndrome and AIDS related complex. J Pediatr 108:498-503, 1986.

Scott GB, Buck B, Letterman JG, et al. Acquired immunodeficiency syndrome in infants. N Engl J Med 310:76-81, 1984.

Ward JW, Holmberg SD, Allen JR, et al. Transmission of human immunodeficiency virus (HIV) by blood transfusions screened as negative for HIV antibody. N Engl J Med 318:473-478, 1988.

48 Life-Threatening Complications of Sickle Cell Disease

Joann M. Sanders

BACKGROUND AND PHYSIOLOGY

Sickle cell anemia and related hemoglobinopathies (sickle hemoglobin C disease and S-β thalassemia) are characterized by chronic hemolysis in the steady state, which can be interrupted by episodes of acute sickling. Irreversibly sickled cells can block capillary beds as well as the arterial blood supply to various organs, resulting in ischemia with subsequent infarction of bone, bone marrow, or other organs. A variety of events can trigger these episodes, which vary in severity from patient to patient. Children with sickle cell C disease and S-β thalassemia usually have fewer episodes than children with homozygous sickle cell disease. Most of the time the management of sickle cell disease does not necessitate admitting the patient to the PICU. However, acute crises can lead to life-threatening complications that demand intensive care.

Bacterial Septicemia

Patients with homozygous sickle cell disease have an increased susceptibility to septicemia and meningitis, with *Streptococcus pneumoniae, Haemophilus influenzae* type b, and enteric pathogens as the most common offending organisms. The pathologic basis for this complication involves impaired splenic function and defective opsonization. Children less than 5 years of age with homozygous sickle cell disease have the highest incidence of septicemia. The risk of infection is much less pronounced in the child with sickle cell C disease or S-β thalassemia.

Aplastic Crisis

Evidence suggests that aplastic crisis results from a primary erythropoietic failure associated with a parvovirus infection. These brief periods of decreased RBC production can result in a life-threatening anemia in a patient with a significantly decreased RBC life span. Presenting symptoms usually include increasing listlessness and pallor, sometimes associated with an upper respiratory infection. The hemoglobin values are markedly below steady-state values, and the reticulocyte count is very low. If the hemoglobin value is low enough, symptoms of congestive heart failure can occur.

Splenic Sequestration Crisis

Acute splenic sequestration can be the first major clinical manifestation of sickle cell disease and is an important cause of mortality. The spleen undergoes acute enlargement secondary to engorgement of the splenic sinuses with blood. A significant proportion of the red cell mass can become entrapped in the spleen, resulting in a precipitous fall in hemoglobin levels and sometimes death from peripheral circulatory failure. The etiology of this complication is unknown, and the severity of sequestration can vary from mild splenic enlargement with a minimal decrease in hemoglobin level to massive splenomegaly, life-threatening anemia, shock, and occasionally death. Splenic sequestration may recur and most commonly occurs in patients who already have some splenomegaly.

Organ-Related Sickling

Sickling can occur within the capillary bed of any organ, causing obstruction to normal blood flow. The arterial blood supply of these organs can also be occluded by irreversibly sickled cells, and the ensuing ischemia can lead to episodes of stroke, pulmonary infarction, jaundice and hepatic enlargement, gross hematuria, priapism, and bone infarction.

MONITORING AND LABORATORY TESTS

Close monitoring of several variables, including hemoglobin and hematocrit values daily and reticulocyte count and total and differential WBC count every other day, is imperative in the care of critically ill patients with sickle cell disease. At steady state children with sickle cell disease have a mild leukocytosis but a normal WBC differential count. Increases in the WBC count are common during crises; however, a left shift can be a warning of possible bacterial infection. Temperature and vital signs must be monitored and hydration status assessed every 2 hours. Frequent neurologic checks are important since neurologic abnormalities or altered states of consciousness can be early indications of stroke.

TREATMENT
Bacterial Sepsis

Bacterial sepsis in patients with sickle cell disease is managed the same way as in children without hemoglobinopathy (see Chapter 42). In addition to administering the appropriate IV antibiotic, it is important to try to prevent further sickling by maintaining temperature, hydration, pH, and oxygen tension in the normal range.

Aplastic Crisis

Peripheral oxygen delivery must be maintained through transfusions. Approximately 5 to 7 ml/kg of packed RBCs must be given over 3 to 4 hours and then repeated as necessary to increase the hematocrit to 18% to 20%. The hematocrit and reticulocyte counts must be monitored frequently during an aplastic crisis. Spontaneous recovery of active production of red cells usually occurs within 5 to 10 days.

Splenic Sequestration Crisis

Splenic sequestration crises can occur rapidly. Whole blood or volume expanders and packed RBCs are indicated if the patient is hypovolemic secondary to splenic sequestration of blood. Subsequent transfusions may be necessary to keep the hemoglobin level stable until the spleen is reduced in size. Systemic arterial blood pressure and vital signs must be closely observed and monitored until the patient is hemodynamically stable.

Vaso-Occlusive Crisis

Precipitating factors. The elimination of precipitating factors for vaso-occlusive crisis is necessary. Sickling can be exacerbated by episodes of infection, dehydration, acidosis, hypoxemia, and fever. Thus antibiotics, IV fluids, alkali, supplemental oxygen, and antipyretics must be administered as clinically indicated.

Hydration. Any fluid deficit must be corrected and the patient's hydration status monitored closely. Although increased IV fluids may dilute sickled cells, their use can result in pulmonary edema, especially in patients who are receiving continuous IV infusions of narcotics.

Analgesia. Analgesics usually can control and alleviate pain. Depending on the severity of the painful crisis, acetaminophen, aspirin, codeine, morphine, or meperidine may be administered. Repetitive or continuous IV infusions of morphine or meperidine may be necessary to control pain.

Transfusion. The use of exchange or modified exchange transfusion in a patient with vaso-occlusive crisis remains controversial. In patients with recurrent, incapacitating episodes of pain, transfusion can be of benefit. The two broad indications for blood transfusion in patients with sickle cell disease are maintaining oxygen-carrying capacity and decreasing or diluting the level of hemoglobin S–containing cells. Thus transfusions may be of benefit to patients with stroke, pulmonary infarction, or severe recurrent episodes of pain.

If a patient in crisis needs a surgical procedure (e.g., appendectomy), some physicians would perform an exchange transfusion before surgery to prevent intraoperative sickling. Whether or not to perform an exchange transfusion before elective surgery is a more controversial issue. No good data support routine use of preoperative blood transfusions.

ADDITIONAL READING

Charache S. The treatment of sickle cell anemia. Arch Intern Med 133:698-705, 1974.

• Davis JR, Vichinsky EP, Lubin BH. Current treatment of sickle cell disease. Curr Probl Pediatr 10(12):1-64, 1980.

Keeley K, Buchanan GR. Acute infarction of long bones in children with sickle cell anemia. J Pediatr 101:170-175, 1982.

• Pearson JA, Diamond IK. Sickle cell disease crises and their management. In Smith CA, ed. The Critically Ill Child: Diagnosis and Management, 2nd ed. Philadelphia: WB Saunders, 1977.

Schwartz E, ed. Hemoglobinopathies in Children. Littleton, Mass.: PSG Publishing, 1980.

Serjeant GR, ed. Sickle Cell Disease. Oxford: Oxford University Press, 1985.

49   Methemoglobinemia

James S. Roloff

BACKGROUND AND PHYSIOLOGY

The primary function of the red blood cell is the efficient movement of oxygen from lungs to tissue and of carbon dioxide and other products of metabolism from tissue to the lungs for disposal. Pivotal to the transport of oxygen is the respiratory pigment hemoglobin. Throughout phylogeny respiratory pigments have a stereotypic structure and function, predicated on the modulation of electron orbitals in coordination with a metal ion. Typically this is iron in the ferrous form in a metalloporphyrin complex, which, in turn, is enclosed in the "protected" environment of an amino acid cage, typically globin. Hemoglobin is tetrameric in structure, comprising four globin cages, each containing the prosthetic heme group tucked into the hydrophobic pocket. An essential feature of hemoglobin is referred to as "cooperativity," the sequential modification of components of a biocomplex resulting in a "changed" overall function of the complex. In hemoglobin the uptake of a single molecule of oxygen by one component of the tetramer results in a changed ability to pick up or release additional oxygen molecules. This is accomplished through multiple mechanisms, including the making and breaking of salt bridges, hydrogen ion uptake, and interaction of the organic phosphate molecule 2,3-diphosphoglycerate (2,3-DPG) with the tetramer. The result of these mechanisms is a subtle, albeit dramatic, intra- and intermonomeric shift that presents ("opens" the pocket) or withdraws ("closes" the pocket) the heme unit for coordination ("bonding") with an oxygen molecule. The release or uptake of oxygen is thus affected (Fig. 49-1).

At the atomic level the interaction between iron and oxygen is orchestrated by a constellation of local environmental changes in the exchange of electrons. The iron molecule is actually moved from the "deoxy" position slightly behind the plane of the porphyrin ring to the "oxy" position within the porphyrin ring. This movement is accomplished by a shift of the amino acids in the globin chain lining the heme pocket. The pocket "opens" ever so slightly, allowing improved access of the oxygen molecule (as well as other ligands such as carbon monoxide and sulfur). In the deoxy state the electrons in the iron are maintained in a "low-energy state" by the nitrogens of the porphyrin and the amino acid of the surrounding globin chain. In the latter the most significant amino acids are histidines, located at key points lining the pocket (Fig. 49-2).

Since oxygen is more electrophilic than iron, an electron is shifted reversibly from iron to the oxygen molecule, creating a superoxide molecule (O_2^-). The iron loses an electron, moving from a divalent ferrous (Fe^{+2}) state to a temporary trivalent ferric (Fe^{+3}) state. During the normal oxy to deoxy shift, release of the oxygen results in return of the electron shared between the iron and oxygen to the iron, reducing the iron to the ferrous state. Such opening and closing of the pocket and shifting of electrons back and forth to bind or release oxygen has been likened to the respiratory cycle itself.

This electron sharing may be contrasted with methemoglobin in which the iron's electron is completely lost (oxidized), creating a permanent ferric state (Fig. 49-3). Any factor(s) that disrupt(s) the environment surrounding the heme molecule may facilitate this removal of an electron, irreversibly impeding oxygen uptake and disturbing the cooperativity of the hemoglobin molecule itself. To return the methemoglobin to its reduced state, alternative chemical reactions must provide the "lost" electron.

Several reactions and various substrates can provide this electron replacement. Three of these reactions have been identified as having physiologic or pharmacologic significance in humans. Necessary components of the reduction include (1) a source of electrons, (2) an enzyme to carry out the reaction,

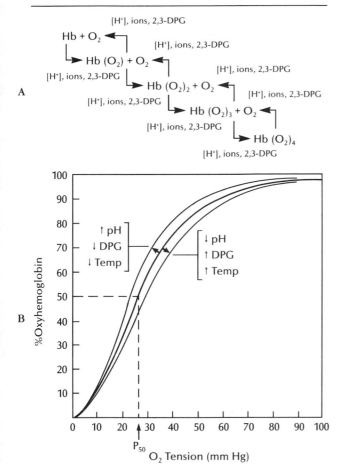

Fig. 49-1 Hemoglobin interaction with oxygen. **A**, Oxygen, variably and sequentially bound or released by hemoglobin, is influenced by the number of oxygen molecules already coordinated with subunits of the hemoglobin tetramer ("cooperativity") as well as hydrogen ion concentration ([H$^+$] or pH), various other ions, and the organic phosphate molecule 2,3-diphosphoglycerate (2,3-DPG or DPG). **B**, These influences result in the characteristic sigmoid oxyhemoglobin dissociation curve.

Fig. 49-2 Schematic diagram of a globin chain with the prosthetic heme group tucked in the hydrophobic pocket. A proximal histidine and a distal histidine in the pocket are indicated. They influence the Fe molecule within the heme unit. Substitutions for these histidines are seen in hemoglobin M diseases.

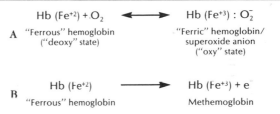

Fig. 49-3 **A**, Oxygen normally is coordinated with heme by reversibly shifting an electron from the ferrous iron (Fe^{+2}) to the oxygen, creating a superoxide anion (O^{-2}) and a temporary ferric (Fe^{+3}) iron in the heme. **B**, If an electron (e$^-$) is irreversibly lost (by interaction with "oxidant stress"), the iron is permanently left in the ferric form, resulting in methemoglobin formation.

and (3) (in most cases) a cofactor to provide the link for the electron transfer to methemoglobin. Consistently the electron source proves to be a pyridine nucleotide—either NADH or NADPH (Fig. 49-4). The former is supplied by the Embden-Meyerhof pathway in the oxidation of glyceraldehyde-3-phosphate and oxidation of lactate to pyruvate. NADPH is supplied by the hexose monophosphate shunt through the conversion of glucose-6-phosphate to ribulose-5-phosphate.

Enzymes responsible for the reduction of methemoglobin back to hemoglobin have been identified and are designated either NADH dependent or NADPH dependent. The NADH-dependent forms (and probably others) use flavin as a cofactor. The NADH-dependent enzymes (e.g., NAD-methemoglo-

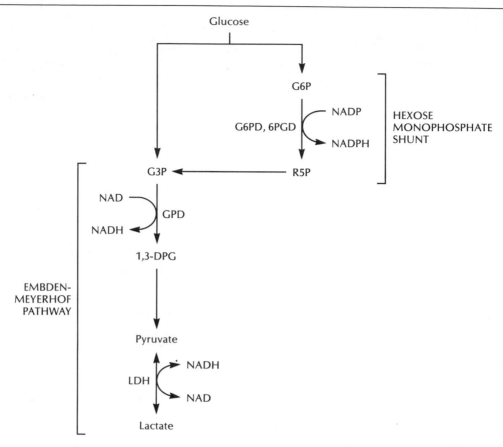

Fig. 49-4 Glucose metabolism in red blood cells is limited to glycolysis either by the Embden-Meyerhof pathway or the hexose monophosphate shunt. Important metabolic products (used in reducing methemoglobin) are reduced pyridine nucleotides—NADH and NADPH. (G3P = glyceraldehyde-3-phosphate; 1,3-DPG = 1,3-diphosphoglycerate; G6P = glucose-6-phosphate; R5P = ribulose-5-phosphate; NAD/NADH = oxidized/reduced nicotinamide adenine dinucleotide; NADP/NADPH = oxidized/reduced nicotinamide adenine dinucleotide phosphate; GPD = glyceraldehyde phosphate dehydrogenase; LDH = lactate dehydrogenase; G6PD = glucose-6-phosphate dehydrogenase; 6PGD = 6-phosphogluconate dehydrogenase.)

$$NADH + FAD \xrightarrow{R} NAD + FADH$$

$$FADH + Cyto\ b_5 \xrightarrow{R} FAD + R\text{---}Cyto\ b_5$$

$$R\text{---}Cyto\ b_5 + Hb\ (Fe^{+3}) \xrightarrow{sp} Cyto\ b_5 + Hb\ (Fe^{+2})$$

Fig. 49-5 Methemoglobin is reduced to hemoglobin under physiologic conditions by NADH-dependent methemoglobin reductase *(R)*. This enzyme is the same as cytochrome b_5 reductase. It uses flavin (FAD/FADH = oxidized/reduced flavin adenine dinucleotide) as an intermediate electron carrier as well as cytochrome b_5 (cyto b_5/R-cyto b_5 = oxidized/reduced cytochrome b_5) as the link to methemoglobin reduction. The last step is non-enzymatic (sp = spontaneous).

bin reductase) apparently are the same as cyto-chrome b_5 reductases (Fig. 49-5). Cytochrome b_5 serves as the link between the reductase and the methemoglobin, efficiently transferring the electron to the oxidized iron. Interestingly, this family of reductases does not use NADPH as an electron donor. Variations in this reductase have been found and may explain the familial methemoglobin reductase deficiency (see below).

In contrast, the enzyme dependent on NADPH as the primary electron donor (NADP-methemoglobin reductase) has little to no physiologic role under normal circumstances because of a lack of linking cofactor. Although not apparently important for normal physiology, pharmacologic manipulation of this system provides a therapeutic alternative for patients with excessive amounts of methemoglobin (Fig. 49-6).

At the cellular level the consequences of oxidation of hemoglobin to methemoglobin are the inability of oxidized hemoglobin to bind oxygen, subsequent impairment of oxygen transport to tissues, and increased affinity of oxyhemoglobin for oxygen, which interferes with its release. Characteristically, oxyhemoglobin demonstrates a bright red color, and deoxyhemoglobin appears deep purple (turning bright red when exposed to oxygen in the air). Methemoglobin is a mahogany-brown color, which does not change on exposure to oxygen.

Normally there is a homeostatic balance between the spontaneous production of methemoglobin (approximately 2% to 4% per day (0.15 to 0.45 g/dl/day) and its reduction by routine protective mechanisms. The normal steady-state concentration of methemoglobin in the adult is less than 0.6% (0.09 g/dl). In normal infants it is slightly higher. The physiologic tolerance of this loss of oxygen-transporting ability is usually quite good. A normal individual can have up to 10% methemoglobin (1.5 g/dl) without any clinical evidence of abnormality. Above this level the characteristic slate-gray cyanosis appears and is especially visible in the lips and nail beds. Concen-

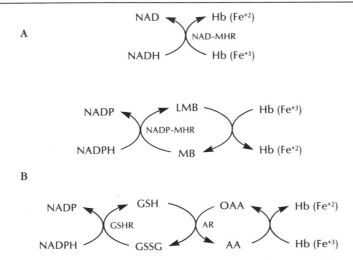

Fig. 49-6 A, Normal methemoglobin reduction. **B,** In contrast to physiologic reduction of methemoglobin to hemoglobin by NAD-methemoglobin reductase *(NAD-MHR),* pharmacologic agents are needed to supply the link for electron transport from NADPH supplied by the hexose monophosphate shunt. Methylene blue *(MB)* is rapidly converted to leukomethylene blue *(LMB),* which in turn nonenzymatically reduces methemoglobin. Ascorbic acid *(AA)* more slowly reduces methemoglobin directly. It is converted to an oxidized form *(OAA)* that must be reduced by ascorbate reductase *(AR).* The latter uses reduced glutathione *(GSH)* as the electron donor, which in turn is coupled to the hexose monophosphate shunt by glutathione reductase *(GSHR),* using the oxidized glutathione *(GSSG)* as an intermediary.

trations up to 25% to 30% (3.25 to 4.5 g/dl) of methemoglobin may occur without causing significant clinical problems. Above 30% to 35% methemoglobin a succession of clinical signs and symptoms appear, including mild fatigue and tachycardia, particularly on exertion. At 50% methemoglobin (7.5 g/dl), tachypnea, headache, and disorientation occur. Coma and death may occur at levels of methemoglobin >70% to 75% (10.5 to 11.25 g/dl). With chronic methemoglobinemia the patient may have mild erythrocytosis, which is probably a function of the persistent decrease of oxygen availability and subsequent marrow response.

The abnormality may be either congenital (familial) or acquired. The congenital form is noted at birth and is lifelong, although it is usually more apparent during the newborn period. It is inherited as an autosomal recessive phenomenon and may represent a heterogenous process, with different gene products accounting for the variability of the clinical picture. The gene responsible for methemoglobin reductase/cytochrome b_5 reductase is found on chromosome 22. Examination of the patient reveals noteworthy cyanosis and mild exercise intolerance but otherwise relatively few clinical problems. Patients usually have a normal life expectancy. Nevertheless, a subgroup of patients with accompanying mental retardation has been described and appears to have a foreshortened life expectancy. This group may represent an abnormality in levels of cytochrome b_5 reductase, not only in the red cell but other tissues as well, including the brain.

Acquired (toxic) methemoglobinemia is seen when the red cell is exposed to various oxidant drugs or chemicals that increase the production of methemoglobin, overwhelming the normal protective reductive mechanisms. The manifestations of clinically significant toxic methemoglobinemia result from the summation of factors, including the type of oxidizing agent, the dose, the duration of exposure, the clearance of the agent, and the relative amount and activity of reductive enzymes and cofactors. Toxic methemoglobinemia may be seen in all age groups, but the newborn and infant are particularly susceptible to the process, probably reflecting their naturally reduced amount of functional enzyme (approximately 60% of adult levels in neonatal red cells). This process may be exaggerated in those infants heterozygous for an abnormal NADH-dependent methemoglobin reductase. Probably the most readily

recognized condition in the pediatric population is toxic methemoglobinemia resulting from ingested nitrates (in well water), which are subsequently modified to nitrites by gut flora. Symptoms of an incompletely characterized syndrome in very young infants include severe diarrhea and acidosis with concomitant acquired methemoglobinemia (usually <40%). Etiology has not been determined, although gut flora, particularly enteropathogenic *Escherichia coli,* have been suggested as contributory. Therapy has been directed at correction of the acidosis and rehydration. Methylene blue therapy is needed on an individual basis, depending on symptoms.

Hemoglobin M disease comprises a rare group of hemoglobinopathies characterized by the presence of significant cyanosis, usually with minimal clinical symptoms. These abnormalities have the unique feature of abnormal substitutions of amino acids in the pocket of the globin chains. Specifically, the histidines are replaced by tyrosine (Fig. 49-2). As mentioned previously, these histidines play a role in maintaining the iron in a receptive state for oxygen binding. The substitution of an aberrant amino acid at these key sites in either the α-globin or β-globin chain alters the electron availability, although this does not significantly impair overall oxygen uptake. Characteristic cyanosis occurs in these individuals. Remarkably, patients with hemoglobin M disease have minimal clinical symptoms. Occasionally hemolytic anemia may be found. The process is inherited as an autosomal dominant trait, although spontaneous mutations account for a large fraction of reported cases. There are five recognized hemoglobin M diseases, two involving the α-globin chain and three the β-globin chain. The onset of the cyanosis is recognized at birth in those individuals whose abnormality involves the α chain. However, because β-chain synthesis is not maximal at birth, hemoglobin M diseases involving β-chain substitutions may not become apparent until the infant is 6 months of age or older as the γ-chain synthesis diminishes and β-chain synthesis becomes dominant. Diagnosis depends on excluding other causes of cyanosis (see above) and specific spectral determinations for hemoglobin M. Hemoglobin electrophoresis and spectrophotometry may be necessary to characterize the specific abnormality.

Sulfhemoglobinemia is an extremely rare abnormality that is a part of noncardiac/nonpulmonary cyanosis. In this entity sulfur replaces iron in the por-

---

CAUSATIVE AGENTS OF METHEMOGLOBIN

Nitrites/nitrates

Amyl nitrate, butyl nitrate
Bismuth subnitrite
Food—sausages, spinach, carrots
Isobutyl nitrate ingestion or sniffing
Nitroglycerin
Nitrous gases
Silver nitrate (for burns)
Well water contamination

Anilines

Disinfectants
Laundry dyes
Red crayons
Shoe dyes

Drugs

Benzocaine
Cetacaine
Chlorates
Chloroquine, primaquine
Dapsone
EDTA
Hydralazine
Lidocaine
Nitroprusside
Phenacetin
Phenazopyridine
Prilocaine
Propitocaine
Sulfonamides
Vitamin K analogs

Miscellaneous

Lysol
Naphthalene
Nitrobenzene

---

phyrin ring, rendering the respiratory pigment not only incapable of oxygen transport but also unstable. Various agents appear responsible for this substitution, but the particular mechanism(s) has (have) not been determined. Causative agents of sulfhemoglobinemia include phenacetin and acetanilide (rarely used) as well as acetaminophen; sulfur-containing compounds such as trimethoprim-sulfamethoxazole; hydrogen sulfide (in vitro); and constipation (rectal stricture) plus exposure to aniline dyes. Usually the patient is asymptomatic, so intervention is seldom indicated. A congenital form of this abnormality has been suggested in two kindreds, but the exact nature and validity of these observations has not been established. Sulfhemoglobinemia has been reported in patients with rectal strictures or severe constipation (often in association with use of aniline dyes). This problem is reversed by correcting the anatomic lesion. The only treatment is removal of the offending agent. Specific spectral analysis is necessary to establish the diagnosis.

DIAGNOSIS

Clinical observations. Patients with methemoglobinemia have a characteristic slate-gray cyanosis that is not responsive to increased Fio_2. Cardiac and/or pulmonary abnormalities are absent. Variable symptoms are a function of the percent methemoglobin present. A drop of the characteristically mahogany-brown blood placed on a filter paper fails to turn bright red on exposure to room air (or $Fio_2 = 1.0$).

Laboratory tests. The CBC is usually normal (occasionally erythrocytosis may be seen in patients with chronic methemoglobinemia). Characteristic spectrophotometric peaks of the methemoglobin appear at 500 and 631 nm; the latter peak rapidly disappears with the addition of a cyanide anion. (If the peak at 600 to 640 nm is abnormal or the 631 nm peak does not disappear with the addition of cyanide, one of the hemoglobin M abnormalities should be suspected.)

A confirmatory test is the direct assay of NADH-methemoglobin reductase, although it is rarely needed.

TREATMENT

For treating acquired (toxic) methemoglobinemia the toxic agent or stress should first be removed and methylene blue administered as indicated in Table 49-1. The dose of methylene blue (adult dose) is 100 to 300 mg/day PO (dose determined empirically) or 1 to 2 mg/kg IV (slowly) in 1% (1 mg/dl) solution in 0.9% sodium chloride solution. Ascorbic acid plays no role in acquired (toxic) methemoglobinemia.

The side effects of methylene blue administration are blue-green urine and blue-gray skin color. If it is administered in excess, methemoglobinemia and hemolysis (if patient is subject to oxidant hemolysis such as having an enzyme deficiency) may be induced.

Table 49-1   Treatment of Methemoglobinemia

Methemoglobin (%)	Symptoms	Therapy†
<40	−	No therapy needed
<40* or	+	Methylene blue PO
40-60	+	Methylene blue IV; (exchange)
>60	+	Exchange/hemodialysis; (hyperbaric oxygen)

*Rapidly rising level.
†If there is no response to therapy, suspect either a hyaline membrane disease abnormality (e.g., G6PD deficiency), sulfhemoglobinemia, or hemoglobin M disease. Treatments in parentheses are rarely needed.

For patients with congenital (familial) methemoglobinemia symptoms are usually mild, or there are cosmetic changes. Initially methylene blue IV should be administered, followed by ascorbic acid PO (chronically) and possibly riboflavin PO. The methylene blue IV dose is 1 to 2 mg/kg (slowly) as 1% (1 mg/dl) solution in 0.9% sodium chloride solution. The adult dose of ascorbic acid is 200 to 1000 mg/day PO (dose determined empirically), and the dose for riboflavin is 20 to 60 mg/day PO (dose determined empirically). The side effects of ascorbic acid are hypoxaluria, renal stones, and gastrointestinal upset.

ADDITIONAL READING

Feig SA. Methemoglobinemia. In Nathan DG, Oski FA, eds. Hematology of Infancy and Childhood. Philadelphia: WB Saunders, 1987, pp 641-654.

Jaffe ER. Methaemoglobinaemia. Clin Haematol 10:99-122, 1981.

50 Severe Anemia

Naomi J. Winick

BACKGROUND AND PHYSIOLOGY

Severe anemia is defined numerically as an Hb value of <4 g/dl or an Hct value of <12%. Anemia of this magnitude can lead to (1) fatigue, malaise, lethargy, and decreased exercise tolerance; (2) congestive heart failure with pulmonary edema and possible cardiac arrest; (3) hypovolemia if the anemia is secondary to acute blood loss; (4) tissue hypoxia with ischemia or infarction of vital organs; and/or (5) acute renal failure if the anemia is secondary to intravascular hemolysis. However, children with rapid blood loss or limited compensatory mechanisms caused by previously existing disease may have signs and symptoms of severe anemia at hemoglobin concentrations much greater than 4 g/dl.

The differential diagnosis of severe anemia in childhood commonly includes hemorrhage, leukemia, severe iron deficiency, transient erythroblastopenia of childhood, immune-mediated hemolysis, sickle cell disease with aplastic crisis or splenic sequestration, and microangiopathic hemolysis. These entities can be distinguished rapidly through a brief history, physical examination, complete blood count, reticulocyte count, and examination of the peripheral blood smear (Table 50-1). Confirmatory tests (e.g., a Coombs test and a haptoglobin test to diagnose suspected immune-mediated hemolysis, hemoglobin electrophoresis to diagnose sickle cell disease, a serum ferritin determination to establish the diagnosis of iron deficiency) may be useful adjuvants.

MONITORING AND LABORATORY TESTS

In addition to Hb and Hct determinations the cardiorespiratory effects of anemia, including heart rate, cardiac size, pulmonary edema, respiratory rate, and effort of breathing, must be monitored.

TREATMENT
Chronic Anemia

The treatment of severe chronic anemia can be difficult. Rapid correction and expansion of the child's intravascular volume can precipitate congestive heart failure and cardiovascular decompensation, whereas the severe anemia places continued stress on the cardiovascular system and diminished oxygen delivery jeopardizes vital organs. The key to treatment is to initiate the therapy rapidly but deliver it gently. A simple packed red blood cell transfusion can be given at a dose of 3 to 5 ml/kg over 3 to 4 hours. It will raise the child's Hb level 1 to 1½ g/dl. The transfusion can be repeated after a 6- to 8-hour interval, which will allow for equilibration and diuresis.

Should increasing tachycardia, tachypnea, or signs of worsening congestive heart failure develop, diuretic therapy can be considered, although an alternative approach is to perform a partial exchange transfusion (see Chapter 141). Once vascular access is achieved, 10 to 30 ml aliquots of the patient's blood can be exchanged with equivalent aliquots of packed red blood cells using the following equation to determine the exchange volume (Hb is in g/dl):

Exchange volume (ml) =
[Weight (kg) × 75 ml/kg × Desired rise in Hb] ÷
25 g/dl − [(Initial Hb + Desired Hb) ÷ 2]

The advantage to using a partial exchange vs. a simple packed red blood cell transfusion is that increasing the red blood cell volume can rapidly correct the severe anemia without making great changes in the total blood volume. The primary disadvantage is the need for obtaining vascular access, which can delay the onset of transfusion therapy. Regardless of which

Table 50-1 Differential Diagnosis of Severe Anemia in Childhood

Condition	History*	Physical Examination†	Mean Corpuscular Volume (ml)	Reticulocyte Count	Peripheral Blood Smear/Complete Blood Count‡
Hemorrhage	Hematemesis, hematochezia, trauma, child abuse	Evidence of trauma, acute abdomen	Normal	↑	—
Leukemia	Fever, malaise, bone pain	Adenopathy, hepatosplenomegaly, petechia	Normal or elevated	↓	Blast forms, nucleated RBCs, neutropenia, decreased platelets
Iron deficiency	Poor diet, pica, black stools	Poor dentition	Decreased	↓	Occasionally decreased platelets; usually increased platelets
Transient erythroblastopenia of childhood	Viral illness	—	Normal	↓	Occasionally neutropenia
Immune-mediated hemolysis	Viral illness, sudden pallor, dark urine	—	Normal or elevated	↑ (usually)	Spherocytosis
Sickle cell disease/aplastic crisis	Sudden pallor	—	Normal	↓	Sickled forms
Sickle cell disease/splenic sequestration	Sudden pallor	Splenomegaly	Normal or elevated	↑	Sickled forms
Microangiopathic hemolysis	Hematuria, oliguria, cough, coryza, vomiting, diarrhea	Petechia, bruises, acute abdomen, edema, hypertension, bloody stools	Normal	↑	Schistocytes, decreased platelets, leukocytosis

*Fatigue, malaise, lethargy, decreased exercise tolerance are common to all.
†Pallor, increased heart rate, increased respiratory rate are common to all.
‡Decreased hemoglobin and hematocrit are common to all.

Table 50-2 Therapy in Addition to
Transfusion in Severe Anemia in Childhood

Etiology of Anemia	Adjuvant Therapy
Hemorrhage	Stop bleeding
Leukemia	Chemotherapy
Severe iron deficiency anemia	Iron therapy
Immune-mediated he-molysis	Steroids
Microangiopathic he-molysis	Dialysis, fresh frozen plasma, platelet transfusion

approach is chosen, careful monitoring of the patient (heart rate, respiratory rate, systemic arterial blood pressure, capillary perfusion) and oxygen supplementation can safely and expeditiously correct severe anemia. Additional support may be needed as well, depending on the etiology of the severe anemia (Table 50-2).

Acute Anemia

Severe, acute anemia secondary to blood loss must be treated as rapidly as possible with fresh whole citrated blood (<72 hours old) or packed red blood cells resuspended in fresh frozen plasma or Plasmanate to achieve an Hct of approximately 35%. General risks and complications of transfusion therapy are discussed in Chapter 139; however, the following unique problems are associated with massive transfusion (i.e., >1 blood volume).

Dilutional thrombocytopenia. Frequently the patient's platelet count will fall below 150,000/mm³. Unless there is continued significant bleeding, a platelet transfusion is not indicated for a platelet count of ≥50,000/mm³. This thrombocytopenia may persist for 1 week, but intervention is rarely necessary once the bleeding has stopped.

Coagulation factors. These plasma proteins may be depleted by massive blood loss. Fresh frozen plasma can be used when a patient develops a prolonged PTT with continued bleeding.

Microaggregates. Transfused leukocyte and platelet remnants may aggregate in the pulmonary vasculature, leading to pulmonary compromise. The use of a microaggregate filter will prevent this complication.

Citrate toxicity. Whole blood prepared for transfusion contains 2.5 mg of citrate ion/ml. Citrate will lower the ionized calcium when given at a rate of ≥1 mg of citrate/kg/min or 0.4 ml/kg/min. This rate is well within the range that might be used to treat a hypovolemic, bleeding child. Accordingly, total serum calcium and ionized calcium levels must be monitored closely. Calcium replacement will circumvent both hypotension and decreased cardiac output.

Alkalosis and hypokalemia. When fresh citrated whole blood (<72 hours old) is used for massive transfusions, the citrate is metabolized to bicarbonate, and the recipient often becomes alkalotic and hypokalemic. Potassium moves into the cells as hydrogen ions leave in response to the increase in bicarbonate. The converse, hyperkalemia, rarely occurs and only when very old blood is used for transfusion support. Serum potassium concentrations must be monitored every 2 to 4 hours during massive transfusions.

Drug dilution. It may be necessary to repeat drug doses given before a massive transfusion, depending on the distribution and binding characteristics of the drug.

ADDITIONAL READING

Geha A. Coronary and cardiovascular dynamics and oxygen availability during acute normovolemic anemia. Surgery 80:47-53, 1976.
• Miller DR, Baehner RL, McMillan CW, eds. Blood Diseases of Infancy and Childhood. St. Louis: CV Mosby, 1984, pp 97-115.
• Nathan DG, Oski FA, eds. Hematology of Infancy and Children. Philadelphia: WB Saunders, 1987, pp 265-274.
Schwartz S, Frantz R, Shoemaker W. Sequential hemodynamic and oxygen transport responses in hypovolemia, anemia, and hypoxia. Am Physiol Soc 241:H868-H870, 1981.
Varat M, Adolph RJ, Fowler NO. Fundamentals of clinical cardiology. Am Heart J 83:415-424, 1972.

51 Oncology in the PICU

Steven Weitman · Barton A. Kamen

BACKGROUND

Pediatric oncology has made great strides as a subspecialty during the past two decades, partly because of the empiric, aggressive use of potent antineoplastic agents. Probably no other pediatric subspecialty faces such myriad problems secondary to the primary disease and its therapy. In fact, it is the ability to treat iatrogenic problems in the PICU setting that is at least in part responsible for the more aggressive, potentially curative chemotherapy that is now being tested.

Children with a malignant disease need PICU level care generally at predictable times: (1) at diagnosis when tumor bulk can cause both metabolic and anatomic life-threatening problems and (2) when they have chemotherapy-induced toxicity. This chapter is divided into sections designed to detail these special situations. The treatment of some problems (e.g., hyponatremia) is discussed in other chapters. Thus this chapter on oncology in the PICU is as much an aid to define a given problem as an outline of specific therapy. Potential iatrogenic complications caused by drugs are too numerous to elaborate completely; therefore this section should serve not only as a specific, but also as a general reminder for the PICU staff to refer to the patient's specific treatment protocol and consult with the attending oncologist about any unique pharmacologic toxicities associated with specific drugs.

METABOLIC PROBLEMS
Hyperuricemia

Increased uric acid production results from enhanced degradation of purines, possibly reflecting either increased turnover from rapidly proliferating cancer cells or lysis of tumors that are exquisitely sensitive to chemotherapeutic agents (tumor lysis syndrome). Burkitt's (B-cell) lymphoma and T-cell leukemias/lymphoma are prime examples of neoplasms likely to produce acute tumor lysis. Tumor lysis can produce sudden and often unexpected renal failure, especially with the institution of cytotoxic therapy. Therefore, before any intervention (pharmacologic or surgical), large-diameter central venous access must be obtained for both monitoring purposes and fluid administration.

Hyperuricemia results when renal transport or excretion of urate is impaired or overwhelmed. Factors adversely influencing transport of urate include dehydration or persistently low urinary pH. Urinary pH may also be decreased iatrogenically secondary to furosemide administration. Obstructive uropathy producing azotemia/oliguria results from precipitation of uric acid crystals in the distal renal tubules.

Clinical manifestations of hyperuricemia include lethargy, nausea, and vomiting, which result when serum levels exceed 10 to 15 mg/dl.

Management of hyperuricemia involves either inhibiting production or enhancing elimination of uric acid. Administration of allopurinol at doses of either 50 mg PO tid in patients under 6 years old or 100 mg PO tid in patients over 6 years old inhibits xanthine oxidase, thereby reducing production of urate. Higher doses may be used if tumor lysis syndrome is anticipated. However, allopurinol must be used cautiously if renal failure is present or imminent because allopurinol and its metabolites are excreted by the kidneys. If the creatinine clearance rate falls below 10 to 20 ml/min, the dose must be decreased by two thirds. Further decline would necessitate increasing the time interval between doses. Secondarily, enhanced elimination of uric acid results from hydration (150% to 200% of maintenance) and alkalinization with $NaHCO_3$ (150 to 200 mEq/m²/day). Inadequate aveolar ventilation is a contraindication for $NaHCO_3$ use.

Acetazolamide (5 mg/kg/dose repeated two to

three times over 24 hours) will also alkalinize urine. The pharmacology of acetazolamide suggests that its combined use with $NaHCO_3$ may be beneficial in maintaining an alkalinized urine. However, acetazolamide must be used with caution since it may competitively inhibit the tubular secretion of organic acids (e.g., uric acid). Ideally, a urinary specific gravity of ≤ 1.015 and pH of 7.5 will facilitate excretion, but caution must be exerted not to alkalinize excessively or hyperphosphotemia and hypokalemia may occur (see below).

Dialysis must be considered when uric acid levels exceed 10 mg/dl and/or renal failure and oliguria are present. Members of the nephrology service must be consulted at this point for determination of an appropriate method of dialysis. Peritoneal dialysis cannot be considered when a large abdominal mass is present. The combination of hemodialysis and continuous arteriovenous hemofiltration may be the best approach for managing these patients (see Chapters 146 and 148).

Hyperkalemia

Elevated levels of potassium in the pediatric age group with cancer can result from several mechanisms. Lysis of neoplastic cells (tumor lysis syndrome) releases large amounts of intracellular potassium, and acute renal failure secondary to hyperuricemia may accentuate hyperkalemia. Iatrogenically, hyperkalemia can result from the potassium salts of several drugs, including antibiotics, diuretics, and antihypertensives, and blood transfusions may further increase potassium concentrations. Caution must be exercised when interpreting blood potassium concentrations in this group of patients, since pseudohyperkalemia can result from lysis of white cells in vitro, especially when the WBCs exceed $50,000/mm^3$. In addition lysis of either platelets or erythrocytes can increase potassium concentrations in vitro. Comparison of serum and plasma potassium levels or ECG changes (peaked T waves, especially in precordial leads) may avoid using unnecessary therapeutic intervention (see Chapter 14).

Clinical effects of hyperkalemia include muscle weakness, paralysis, and gastrointestinal disturbances. Ultimately ECG changes occur in patients with hyperkalemia, and when they do, immediate intervention is needed. The initial management of acute hyperkalemia includes removing potassium-containing salts from fluids being given to the patient.

ONCOLOGY PROBLEMS IN THE PICU

Metabolic problems

Hyperuricemia
Hyperkalemia
Hyperphosphatemia
Hypocalcemia
Hyponatremia
Hypokalemia
Hypercalcemia
Hypomagnesemia
Hyperammonemia

Anatomic problems

Superior vena cava syndrome
Superior mediastinal syndrome
CNS:
    Increased intracranial pressure
    Spinal cord compression
Pleural effusions
Pericardial tamponade
Abdominal/retroperitoneal masses

Hematologic problems

Anemia
Leukopenia
Thrombocytopenia
Hyperleukocytosis
Thrombocytosis
DIC

Infection/immunocompromised host

Bacterial
Opportunistic
    Fungal
    Pneumocystis
Viral
    Varicella
    Cytomegalovirus

Chemotherapy-related problems

Marrow suppression
Mucositis
Pulmonary
Cardiac
Renal
Other (rare/unique)

Pain

Psychosocial problems

Pharmacologic treatment is aimed first at counteracting the actions of potassium, followed by a slower process to remove excess ions from the body. The most rapid effect is achieved by infusion of calcium gluconate (0.5 ml/kg of 10% solution) over 10 minutes since it directly antagonizes the toxic actions of potassium. The initial therapy may be followed by administration of 1 to 2 mEq/kg sodium bicarbonate intravenously over 10 minutes and, if necessary, 0.5 g/kg glucose, with 0.3 unit regular insulin/g glucose infused intravenously over 2 hours. Potassium may also be removed from the body (although this takes longer to accomplish than alteration of membrane potential by the methods just described) by administering sodium polystyrene sulfonate resin (Kayexalate), 1 to 2 g/kg/day qid given by mouth or by enema. Finally, dialysis can be considered if hyperkalemia appears imminently life threatening. See Chapter 14 for more details of therapeutic intervention.

Hyperphosphatemia

An elevated serum phosphate level results from tumor lysis syndrome and is especially prevalent in lymphoproliferative disorders. Hyperphosphatemia is potentially deleterious due to the interaction between calcium and phosphate, which may result in crystal formation and hypocalcemia. However, adverse reactions to hyperphosphatemia may not develop unless concurrent hypocalcemia is present. Acute renal failure may also contribute to hyperphosphatemia.

Clinical effects of hyperphosphatemia result from precipitation of calcium phosphate crystals, producing lesions involving skin, eyes, and joints and potentially causing acute renal failure. Overalkalinization of urine in an attempt to prevent uric acid nephropathy can exacerbate calcium phosphate crystal formation in the kidneys. Calcium phosphate formation also results in hypocalcemia, leading to disturbances in consciousness, photophobia, carpopedal spasms, and convulsions.

Initial management of hyperphosphatemia involves use of hydration and diuretics (see Chapter 15). Caution must be exercised when using most diuretics, including thiazides, mercurials, and furosemide, since they may contribute to hyperuricemia. Hyperphosphatemia may also be treated by preventing further phosphate absorption through use of aluminum hydroxide (50 to 150 mg/kg/day divided q 4 to 6 hr). However, phosphate binders may be of limited use since the majority of patients will be on an NPO regimen or on parenteral nutrition. Concurrent hypocalcemia can be treated with calcium supplements, including calcium gluconate.

Miscellaneous Electrolyte Abnormalities

Miscellaneous electrolyte abnormalities, including hyponatremia, hypercalcemia, hyperammonemia, and hypomagnesemia, occasionally occur in patients with cancer. They are either a direct result of tumor physiology/pharmacology or a consequence of chemotherapy.

Hyponatremia. Hyponatremia results from vomiting, diarrhea, and adrenal insufficiency. Low sodium concentration can also be iatrogenic from inappropriate secretion of antidiuretic hormone caused by chemotherapy (e.g., vincristine). In addition many antibiotics, including ampicillin or carbenicillin, depend on sodium for elimination and can contribute to hyponatremia. Treatment depends on either fluid restriction or hypertonic saline solution (3% sodium chloride solution) when serum sodium is <120 mEq/L.

Hypercalcemia. Hypercalcemia occurs rarely in children as a result of bone resorption (potentially occurring in patients with Burkitt's lymphoma or multiple myeloma) and of parathyroid-secreting tumors such as soft tissue sarcomas. Clinically, a patient with hypercalcemia can present with a life-threatening syndrome of profound weakness, abdominal pain, severe dehydration, dysrhythmias, and then coma. Treatment must be aimed at correcting dehydration, but careful cardiac monitoring is necessary. Specific therapy includes mithramycin, an antitumor agent that prevents osteoclastic bone resorption. The dose is 5 to 10 μg/kg q 8 to 12 hr. In addition, if oral administration is possible, phosphate can be tried at doses of 10 to 20 mg/kg bid or tid. It may take days for either mithramycin or phosphate to produce the desired response; therefore, in severe cases of hypercalcemia, calcitonin, a serum calcium-lowering hormone, must be administered immediately. Human or salmon calcitonin is administered twice daily either intramuscularly or subcutaneously in doses of 4 to 8 units/kg/dose. IV calcitonin has been used during life-threatening hypercalcemia; however, experience is limited. The risk of anaphylactic reaction to salmon calcitonin must be considered, especially with IV administration. If elevated serum calcium levels persist 36 to 48 hours after initiation of therapy or if acute life-threatening hypercalcemia is present, dialysis must be considered.

Hyperammonemia. Hyperammonemia can be seen in cases of severe liver failure secondary to tumor or drug toxicity. Almost 50% of patients who receive L-asparaginase will demonstrate biochemical evidence of hepatic injury, of which many have significant elevations of ammonia. Hyperammonemia has also been seen in patients with lymphoma receiving cytarabine and may in part be secondary to perturbation in pyrimidine biosynthesis and degradation. Treatment must be aimed at eliminating the cause and providing supportive measures as outlined in Chapter 16.

Hypomagnesemia. Hypomagnesemia often occurs after chemotherapy with cisplatin. Polystyrene sulfonate resin may also cause or exacerbate this condition. If hypomagnesemia occurs acutely, magnesium sulfate supplementation must be given intravenously (25 to 50 mg/kg/dose q 4 to 6 hr). If chronic hypomagnesemia is present and oral administration is feasible, magnesium gluconate can be given at a dose of 3 g/m²/day.

ANATOMIC PROBLEMS
Superior Vena Cava Syndrome

Superior vena cava syndrome (SVCS) is caused by obstruction of venous drainage of the superior vena cava in the right upper thorax. It is manifested by swelling of the face and upper trunk, dilation of the veins of the same distribution, and "wet brain" syndrome (stupor/seizures). Widening of the superior mediastinum is noted on a chest radiograph. If there is associated coughing, wheezing, or respiratory distress with deviation of the trachea or main bronchi, superior mediastinal syndrome may coexist, which is not uncommon.

In children 95% of cases of SVCS are due to malignant diseases, most commonly lymphomas because the superior vena cava is in the right antero-superior mediastinum, encircled by lymphatics. However, other mediastinal tumors (e.g., germ cell tumor) or metastatic diseases (e.g., neuroblastoma, Ewing's tumor) can also cause SVCS. Tumors that cause SVCS can also cause spinal cord compression; therefore, when a child presents with SVCS compli-

cations and also with low-back pain or neurologic abnormalities, appropriate diagnostic procedures (e.g., CT, MRI of the spine) must be undertaken quickly to avoid permanent spinal cord injury (see below).

Treatment of SVCS may be divided into supportive and specific modalities. Supportive therapy includes giving all IV fluids in the lower extremity veins and treating associated pleural effusions if necessary with a thoracentesis. Specific therapy includes radiation or chemotherapy. Since almost all children with SVCS have a T-cell lymphoma, steroids are the treatment of choice. We have observed complete disappearance of large mediastinal masses within 36 to 48 hours of initiation of 2 mg/kg/day of prednisone or its equivalent on a bid or tid dosing schedule. Rapid elimination of the tumor mass may result in metabolic problems characteristic of the acute tumor lysis syndrome described previously.

Pleural Effusions

Pleural effusions are generally due to obstruction of venous or lymphatic drainage or to direct involvement of the pleural surface by tumor or infection with associated inflammation. In children the most common malignancies associated with pleural effusions are Hodgkin's disease, non-Hodgkin's (especially T-cell) lymphoma, osteogenic sarcoma, neuroblastoma, and soft tissue sarcomas. Pleural effusions can be one component of SVCS.

Treatment is as for any effusion. First, if acute respiratory distress is present, therapeutic thoracentesis must be performed immediately using an 18- to 20-gauge angiocatheter. Fluid must be sent for routine diagnostic studies, including cytologic examination. If symptoms persist or fluid reaccumulates, chest tube placement (see Chapter 134) may be necessary. If the diagnosis cannot be made through thoracentesis, thoracostomy and biopsy may be needed or other procedures such as bone marrow aspirate may be done, depending on the patient's status. If an abnormal CBC (increased WBC with blasts) is present, the diagnosis of T-cell lymphoma is likely. Treatment, in this case steroids, can be started without performing thoracentesis if no respiratory distress is present and if tissue from another source (e.g., bone marrow) has been obtained. Tumor lysis syndrome must be anticipated when treating T-cell lymphoma, especially if rapid tumor shrinkage occurs.

Pericardial Tamponade

Pericardial tamponade (see Chapter 40) rarely occurs. When it does, it is usually in patients with mediastinal tumors or after extensive chemotherapy with cardiotoxic drugs such as the anthracyclines (doxorubicin and daunorubicin) or in patients in septic shock. Clinical manifestations include precordial pain, hypotension, diminished heart sounds, dyspnea, and pulsus paradoxus. Emergency treatment includes aspiration of fluid. If tamponade is directly due to malignancy, it will almost always recur; therefore instillation of sclerosing agents (e.g., tetracycline) or anticancer agents may be necessary. Surgically, formation of a pericardial window or pericardial stripping can be done.

Neurologic Space-Occupying Tumors

Space-occupying tumors impinging on the brain or spinal cord can be seen as acute emergencies at the time of diagnosis or at relapse. Spinal cord compression for as little as 24 hours can result in permanent sequelae; therefore it is important to do a complete and careful neurologic examination even when a child is admitted for another emergency such as pleural effusion or SVCS because tumors that cause these anatomic lesions (e.g., lymphomas, neuroblastoma) can also cause CNS disease.

Spinal cord involvement can be intramedullary, intradural, or epidural. Epidural masses are the most common finding. Intradural masses would most likely be secondary to cerebrospinal seeding by CNS tumors such as medulloblastoma. Intramedullary involvement is usually due to primary tumors such as astrocytomas and ependymomas. The neurologic findings depend on localization of the tumor. Neurologic deficits depend on the location of the lesion (vertebral space) and the portion of the cord that is under pressure. Spinal cord compression in the low back results in signs and symptoms similar to those of a ruptured disk. In particular, severe back pain is a frequent finding.

Diagnosis is through clinical examination and is confirmed by appropriate radiologic studies. For example, paraspinous neuroblastoma can often be seen on plain chest and abdominal roentgenograms. More involved or invasive procedures would include a CT-directed myelogram or, depending on time, an MRI for diagnosing soft tissue masses. At the time of myelography, CSF must be evaluated for the presence or absence of malignant cells.

Treatment includes relieving acute pressure, making a diagnosis, and initiating specific therapy for a particular disease. Major methods for relieving pressure include laminectomy, radiotherapy, and chemotherapy for treating neuroblastoma. In addition dexamethasone in "neurosurgical" doses (1 to 2 mg/kg/push, then 0.5 to 1 mg/kg q 6 to 8 hr) can be initiated. Choice of the modality to use depends on factors such as whether tissue is needed for diagnosis and whether chemotherapy can work fast enough (e.g., lymphoma, neuroblastoma).

Problems and treatment of intracranial lesions (i.e., increased intracranial pressure) are discussed in Chapter 7.

Abdominal and Retroperitoneal Masses

Abdominal and retroperitoneal masses are generally of primary origin; however, metastatic lesions do occur. Problems revolve around whether the mass is intrinsic to, impinging on, and/or disrupting normal organ function. For example, treatment for renal failure secondary to a tumor mass causing obstructive hydronephrosis is to treat the tumor via chemotherapy and possibly to relieve the obstruction surgically. The most common tumors in the abdominal/retroperitoneal space in children include Wilms' tumor, neuroblastoma, and lymphoma. Large abdominal Burkitt's lymphomas can cause all the problems noted in the metabolic section, bowel obstruction, and anatomic obstructive renal failure, further complicating treatment.

Once the child is older than 18 months to 2 years of age, the most common cause of an intussusception in the pediatric population is an abdominal lymphoma, often at the ileocecal junction.

HEMATOLOGIC PROBLEMS

Anemia. Anemia results from either hypoproduction of RBCs or from hemorrhage. Leukemia is the most common pediatric malignancy to produce anemia. Hypoproduction also occurs iatrogenically, secondary to chemotherapy or radiotherapy if the treatment volume is large enough (i.e., cranial-spinal axis). Although most antineoplastic agents cause anemia through a mechanism of hypoproduction, they also cause gastrointestinal bleeding (mucositis). Finally, anemia also results from hemorrhage and is most commonly associated with thrombocytopenia. See Chapter 50 for more details about the cause and treatment of anemias.

Hyperleukocytosis. Hyperleukocytosis (leukocyte count >100,000/mm^3) occurs in 5% to 20% of children with leukemia. Most patients with hyperleukocytosis have acute leukemia; however, a few have chronic myelocytic leukemia in "blast crisis." This condition is associated with increased blood viscosity, hemorrhage, or obstruction of vessels by leukemic aggregates or thrombi. It can especially affect brain and lung tissue and is associated with marked early mortality. These patients can initially be seen with dyspnea, hypoxemia, and right ventricular failure secondary to pulmonary involvement or with death because of intracerebral hemorrhage. Prompt evaluation is necessary, and treatment is aimed at decreasing blood viscosity. Initially, IV fluids and avoiding packed red blood cell transfusion and diuretics are essential. Further reduction in viscosity can be achieved through exchange transfusion or leukopheresis (Chapter 141). The former allows rapid correction of severe anemia and electrolyte abnormalities if they are superimposed. Cranial radiation has been suggested to prevent intracerebral hemorrhage and may be beneficial as emergency treatment, especially in acute nonlymphocytic leukemia. Alternatively, hydroxyurea or high-dose cytarabine can be given; consultation with the attending oncologist should provide specifics.

Thrombocytopenia. Thrombocytopenia results from hypoproduction or consumptive coagulopathy, and the patient can be asymptomatic or present with petechiae or frank bleeding. Although pediatric malignancies can involve thrombocytopenia because of marrow infiltration by tumor, most cases of thrombocytopenia result from chemotherapy and occur 10 to 14 days after treatment. Thrombocytopenia may also be a complication of disseminated intravascular coagulation (DIC). This syndrome is associated with consumption of coagulation factors, producing prolonged PT or PTT in addition to thrombocytopenia. DIC occurs secondary to sepsis, acidosis, hypoxia, or organ failure or by interaction with tissue factors released by tumors. Treatment of DIC involves removal of the underlying condition that triggers consumption of coagulation factors. Further management includes transfusion of platelets and fresh frozen plasma to replenish coagulation deficiencies. The use of heparin should be reserved for patients with significant thrombotic manifestations or for thromboplastin-like releasing tumors. See Chapter 19 for more detailed information.

Thrombocytosis is often seen in patients with hepatoblastoma and neuroblastoma. Platelet counts of 1,000,000/mm^3, unless associated with hyperleukocytosis (as in patients with chronic myelocytic leukemia), generally do not require emergency reduction. In the absence of obvious thrombotic events, thrombocytosis is generally not a significant clinical problem in pediatric patients.

Transfusion reaction. Pediatric patients may require transfusions of multiple blood components at various times during their course of treatment, and most cases of significant transfusion reactions occur because of clerical error. Management of transfusion reactions is discussed extensively in Chapter 139.

INFECTION IN THE IMMUNOCOMPROMISED HOST

Patients with cancer are often treated with very aggressive myelo- and immunosuppressive agents. In addition many will have chronic or prolonged central venous line access devices (e.g., Hickman catheter or a completely implantable system such as a Port-a-Cath). Cancer, chemotherapy, and a central venous line all predispose the patient to infections, including viral, bacterial, and more esoteric opportunistic organisms such as fungi and *Pneumocystis carinii*. Since chemotherapy also causes mucositis, the skin as the first major barrier against infection is often disrupted, thus increasing the risk of infection by *Staphylococcus* and gram-negative enteric organisms. Patients with cancer are generally infected at the time the marrow is most compromised such as at presentation for leukemia or along with other malignancies that demonstrate significant metastatic disease involving bone marrow. In addition 1 to 3 weeks after intensive chemotherapy when the marrow has not fully recovered, children will have an increased risk of infection.

Since patients are at great risk, appropriate cultures and antibiotic therapy are initiated early in a febrile, neutropenic patient. Usually a third-generation cephalosporin, which has good gram-negative coverage, including *Pseudomonas,* is started empirically. Additional gram-positive coverage is achieved using nafcillin or, when central venous catheters have been placed, vancomycin. It is important to consult the infectious disease service since local susceptibilities and occurrence of methicillin-resistant species may affect antibiotic selection and duration of therapy.

Based on the patient's response to antibiotics (e.g., persistently febrile) and the state of his marrow function and physical findings (e.g., esophagitis), initiation of amphotericin B for treating suspected fungal infection is used in patients who have no response after receiving 5 days of broad-spectrum antibiotics. Esophagitis can also occur in a patient with herpes; therefore a Tzanck test and cultures of oral lesions are needed.

Since opportunistic infection or even simple bacteremia can have a fatal outcome in severely immunocompromised patients, routine care must include the following: (1) scrupulous handwashing by the caretaker, (2) optimal skin care, especially in

Table 51-1   Toxicities of Some Commonly Used Antineoplastic Agents

Antineoplastic Agents	"Other" Names	Major Acute Toxicities*	Other Toxicity and Comments
Alkylating agents			
Mechlorethamine	HN₂, Mustargen, nitrogen mustard	N/V, BM, V	Phlebitis
Cyclophosphamide	Cytoxan	HL, BM	Hemorrhagic cystitis
Ifosfamide	IFX, Ifex	BM	Neurotoxicity
Cisplatin	Platinol, CDDP, DDP	N/V, BM	Hearing loss; renal dysfunction
Carboplatin	CBDCA, Paraplatin	N/V, BM	Renal dysfunction
Antimetabolites and enzyme inhibitors			
Azacitidine	5-Aza	BM, M, N/V	—
Cytarabine	Ara-C, Cytosar-U	BM, N/V	Neurotoxicity (high doses); rhabdomyolysis
Fluorouracil	5-FU, Adrucil	M, N/V, BM	Phlebitis
Hydroxyurea	Hydrea	BM	—
Mercaptopurine	6MP, Purinethol	BM	Hepatotoxicity
Methotrexate	MTX, Mexate	M, BM	Hepatotoxicity, neurotoxicity
Thioguanine	6TG, Tabloid	BM	Hepatotoxicity
Teniposide	VM-26	A, BM	Hypotension
Etoposide	VP-16-213, VePeSID	A, BM	Hypotension (less than VM-26)
Antibiotics			
Actinomycin D	Act D, Cosmegen, AMD	V, M, BM	Radiation recall
Bleomycin	Blenoxane	F/C, A	Chronic pulmonary fibrosis
Daunorubicin	Daunomycin, Rubidomycin	V, HL, M, N/V, BM	Cardiotoxic; radiation recall
Doxorubicin	Adriamycin, ADR	V, HL, M, N/V, BM	Cardiotoxic; radiation recall
Miscellaneous			
Vinblastine	Velban	V, BM, HL	Neurotoxicity—seizures, depressed reflexes, ileus
Vincristine	Oncovin	V, HL	Neurotoxicity—seizures, depressed reflexes, ileus; pain
L-Asparaginase	Elspar	A, N/V	Pancreatitis; bleeding or thrombosis

N/V = nausea, vomiting; BM = bone marrow; V = vesicant; F/C = fever, chills; HL = hair loss; M = mucositis; A = allergic reaction.
*In cases of unexplained signs or symptoms, consult oncologist and/or pharmacist for more complete information.

pressure points and perianal area, (3) special care with invasive procedures and placement of indwelling venous and arterial catheters, and (4) cultures of nares, throat, and endotracheal tube, when appropriate, for nosocomial pathogens. Some institutions and/or treatment protocols recommend use of trimethoprim-sulfamethoxazole prophylactically for *P. carinii* and to lower the incidence of infection by enteric organisms.

After identification of an organism specific therapy must be promptly initiated: acyclovir for varicella; trimethoprim-sulfamethoxazole, pentamidine, or trimetrexate with leucovorin rescue for *P. carinii;* amphotericin for fungal infections; and specific antibiotics for bacterial infections. Although there was initial excitement about the use of neutrophil transfusion in leukopenic, febrile patients, its benefit is controversial. Except for the newborn infant, and even this use is not fully accepted, there are little data proving superiority of results in treatment of gram-positive or gram-negative sepsis with addition of granulocyte transfusions (See Chapter 140). Since granulocytes for transfusion are time consuming to obtain, difficult to give, and not proved efficacious, we generally do not initiate them. Consultation with the division of infectious disease or hematology/oncology is advised since prospective studies may be in progress to evaluate more completely the effectiveness of granulocytic transfusions.

CHEMOTHERAPY-RELATED PROBLEMS

Probably no other pediatric subspecialty has as much iatrogenic disease as oncology. Since there is no real selectivity in cell kill (normal vs. malignant), chemotherapy is associated with toxicity of rapidly renewing organ systems, including mucosa and marrow (platelets, leukocytes, erythrocytes). In addition some drugs have hepatic, renal, cardiac, and/or pulmonary toxicity.

The acute toxicities are generally predictable, based on knowledge of cell growth in marrow and gut. Leukocytes and platelets renew every 10 to 14 days; therefore marrow-suppressive doses of chemotherapy will have a significant effect on these two cell lines, generally 10 to 14 days from initiation of therapy. Earlier problems suggest more rapid chemotherapy (i.e., DIC or sepsis) or less marrow reserve. Since chemotherapy can have cumulative effects, neutropenia and thrombocytopenia may occur

earlier as more treatment is given. Hemoglobin will decline more slowly than WBCs and platelets unless there is increased loss (gastrointestinal blood) or shortened red cell life span secondary to chemotherapy. Gut mucosa renews approximately weekly; therefore it is highly susceptible to toxic effects of chemotherapy. As noted in the section on the immunocompromised host, the skin is an important first barrier to infection. Mucositis can lead to bacteremia from bowel flora.

Some specific sites of toxicity of commonly used drugs in pediatric oncology are noted in Table 51-1. The caretaker in the PICU is encouraged to confer with the patient's oncologist regarding past therapy and potential complications of the patient's chemotherapy. These drugs are cytostatic and/or cytocidal with a very low therapeutic index.

PAIN

Metastatic bone disease, spinal cord compression, nerve root involvement, or simply mass effect on normal tissue can cause severe pain for which treatment with narcotic agents may be beneficial. Important guidelines in treatment of patients in pain follow.

1. Use enough drug to eliminate pain; the concept of "too much" based on a mg/kg recommended dose is incorrect. We have often exceeded by 10-fold to 100-fold the standard morphine requirements for children to treat severe pain. Children often metabolize morphine faster than adults.

2. Determine the dose that works acutely and how long it is effective to determine the time interval between doses. If the time is short, consider using a continuous infusion. A typical starting dose for a morphine drip is approximately 0.05 to 0.1 mg/kg/hr.

3. If morphine fails to relieve the pain, newer synthetic narcotics can be tried. Tricyclic antidepressants or benzodiazepines can be added for treating anxiety. We generally prefer to use as few drugs as possible (i.e., avoid "polypharmacy") because of drug interactions, either synergistic or antagonistic.

4. Very rarely and usually in terminally ill children who should not be in the PICU, simple pharmacologic therapy will not control pain. Injection of alcohol or lidocaine or use of dorsal rhizotomy (destruction of dorsal nerve root) or

even more complete procedures such as cordotomy can be performed by a neurosurgeon.

5. When decreased platelets are not a problem, it is important to use peripherally acting agents (i.e., nonsteroidal anti-inflammatory drugs) rather than centrally acting drugs because of decreased somnolence and other side effects.

SOCIAL/PSYCHOLOGICAL PROBLEMS

Being in the PICU is a frightening experience, and when a child and a family are exposed to these facilities at the time of diagnosis, they are also facing the reality of cancer as well as their immediate acute needs. At the time of drug toxicity or relapse they are also faced with long-term problems of morbidity and mortality. Therefore, without belaboring the issues, the PICU caretakers should collaborate with the oncologist about short-term and long-term goals for the patient. Most oncology divisions have social workers and chaplains to assist all physicians responsible for the patient's care, especially when the child is known to the division.

ADDITIONAL READING

• Allegretta GJ, Weisman SJ, Altman AJ. Oncologic emergencies I; Metabolic and space-occupying consequences of cancer and cancer treatment. Pediatr Clin North Am 32:601, 1985.

• Allegretta GJ, Weisman SJ, Altman AJ. Oncologic emergencies II; Hematologic and infectious complications of cancer and cancer treatment. Pediatr Clin North Am 32:613, 1985.

Halpern J, Chatten J, Meadows AJ, et al. Anterior mediastinal masses: Anesthesia hazards and other problems. J Pediatr 102:407, 1983.

Kamen BA, Summers CP, Peason HA. Exchange transfusion as a treatment for hyperleukocytosis, anemia, and metabolic abnormalities in a patient with leukemia. J Pediatr 96:1045, 1980.

Pizzo PA, Hathorn JW, Heimenz J, et al. A randomized trial comparing ceftazidime along with combination antibiotic therapy in cancer patients with fever and neutropenia. N Engl J Med 315:552, 1986.

EORTC International Antimicrobial Therapy Cooperative Group. Ceftazidime combined with a short or long course of amikacin for empirical therapy of gram-negative bacteremia in cancer patients with granulocytopenia. N Engl J Med 317:1692, 1987.

52 Hemolytic-Uremic Syndrome

Richard F. Salmon · *Michel Baum*

BACKGROUND AND PHYSIOLOGY

Hemolytic-uremic syndrome (HUS) comprises the triad of acute renal failure, Coombs'-negative hemolytic anemia, and thrombocytopenia. HUS most frequently occurs in children 1 to 5 years of age. White children are affected more often than black children, and there is no sex predilection. The syndrome is often preceded by a prodromal illness. Typically gastroenteritis with diarrhea that frequently is bloody occurs in a previously healthy infant. Severe abdominal pain and vomiting are common. Occasionally the infant presents with an acute abdomen necessitating evaluation for bowel obstruction. A barium enema may reveal nonspecific changes such as "thumbprinting" and "transverse ridging," which have been associated with HUS. The prodrome usually lasts 1 to 4 days but can extend to 10 days.

In some cases the infant will recover from the prodome only to become symptomatic from one or more facets of HUS. A fall in the hemoglobin level with accompanying acute renal insufficiency and thrombocytopenia follows. The infant at presentation is frequently pale, has purpura or petechiae, and is hypertensive and edematous. Hepatosplenomegaly is common. The anemia at presentation is multifactorial in origin. The erythrocytes have a decreased life span because of ongoing hemolysis. A small dilutional component secondary to volume overload contributes to the anemia. Thrombocytopenia is present and lasts 7 to 14 days. Occasionally some patients do not demonstrate thrombocytopenia as part of the disease process. The degree of renal insufficiency influences the severity of volume and electrolyte abnormalities; patients with mild renal involvement may have only mild oliguria without electrolyte abnormalities, hypertension, or volume overload.

HUS is not limited to renal and hematologic involvement. In 30% of patients neurologic involvement of some magnitude is seen. Initial presentation with either coma and/or seizures is frequently associated with hypertension and electrolyte abnormalities such as hyponatremia and hypocalcemia secondary to the renal involvement. Often transient, mild irritability and lethargy are the only neurologic symptoms manifested, which may be caused by uremia, electrolyte abnormalities, vasculitis, or other unknown factors. Approximately 40% of patients with neurologic involvement develop further neurologic impairment from HUS, including hemiparesis, cortical blindness, and a persistent state of altered consciousness. It is not uncommon for these children to have residual neurologic disease after the other manifestations of HUS have resolved.

Other organ systems are less frequently involved in patients with HUS. Pancreatic damage leading to pancreatic insufficiency has caused both transient and permanent insulin-dependent diabetes mellitus. Hepatic involvement secondary to vascular congestion has been described and is usually transient. Elevations in hepatic transaminases and bilirubin occur, but these values return to normal with resolution of the hemolytic process.

Pathophysiology

There is evidence that HUS is the result of an infectious agent. The frequent occurrence of an infectious prodrome with epidemic episodes suggests that an infectious mechanism is the initiating stimulus in many cases. In one subset of patients with HUS multiple children will contract HUS at the same time of the year, will occasionally be from the same family, and will have the same organism cultured from either blood, urine, or stool. Frequently cultured agents include *Escherichia coli, Shigella, Salmonella, Yersinia,* and enteroviruses. Some studies report an increased incidence of epidemics during specific seasons of the year. This seasonality may be secondary to a higher prevalence of an infectious agent at that specific time of year for that geographic area. Other organisms have been isolated from patients during the prodromal phase, including *Streptococcus pneumoniae,* Epstein-Barr virus, coxsackievirus, *Pseudomonas,* and *Rickettsia.* Endemic areas with isolation of specific infectious agents have been described. In Argentina an arbovirus has been isolated, in Bangladesh multiple cases of *Shigella* with an associated endotoxin have been described, and in the Pacific Northwest association with a specific serotype of *E. coli* has been described.

The complement system has been considered a contributing factor in the development of HUS. Decreased levels of C3 and CH_{50}, in association with elevated IgM and breakdown products of C3, have been described in patients with HUS. Also, C3 and IgM deposits have been found in glomerular capillaries and small renal vessels. Conclusive studies evaluating complement activity in patients with HUS have yet to be performed.

Endothelial damage like that seen in patients with HUS can be induced by experimental administration of an endotoxin. A report of a group of patients from Bangladesh has identified the presence of a *Shigella*-related endotoxin in this population, and this endotoxin is believed the inciting agent for the endothelial damage seen in this disease. The presence of an endotoxin has been identified only in the Bangladesh population, and further confirmatory evidence about its role in HUS is still needed.

The events leading from an initial infection to the development of HUS are unknown. In patients with HUS the vascular endothelium (glomerular capillaries, interlobular arteries, arterioles) is damaged by some unknown event and initiates a cascade of events, leading to the triad of symptoms that characterize HUS. After the onset of endothelial cell wall damage, fibrin strands are formed in the microvasculature. As the RBCs pass through these vessels, they are sheared by these strands and damaged. When returned to the systemic circulation, the damaged cells are sequestered by the reticuloendothelial system, as demonstrated by the localization of radioactively labeled RBCs over the liver and spleen. The sequestering of RBCs results in a decrease in the RBC count, with an associated decrease in the hemoglobin level.

The platelets are sequestered in a similar manner. The endothelial cell wall damage that is present also contributes to decreasing the number of circulating platelets via increased platelet aggregation around these damaged vessel walls. As platelets adhere to the damaged vessels and are subsequently destroyed, they liberate a potent vasoconstrictor (thromboxane A_2) and platelet aggregatory stimulating factor, which causes further depletion of the platelet number. The ongoing damage to the endothelial walls in the kidney with release of vasoconstrictors and the deposition of fibrin strands and platelets results in vascular congestion within the renal microvasculature, leading to decreased glomerular filtration, which results in renal insufficiency in these patients. Renal failure will continue until this series of events stops and the microvasculature is permitted to heal. Platelet consumption with fibrin deposition in the kidney suggests that an intravascular coagulopathic process may be central to this syndrome. However, the inability to demonstrate consistent evidence of a consumptive process and documentation of adequate replacement of fibrinogen do not support this theory.

The histopathologic changes in kidneys of patients with HUS are very characteristic for this syndrome. Glomerular capillary wall thickening and subendothelial electron-dense deposits of fibrin are common. Thrombi, seen on light microscopic examination, are found within the glomerular capillaries and arterioles. Immunoglobulin deposition in the glomeruli has been reported, but this is not universally described. Focal areas of cortical necrosis can be seen, and a generalized bilateral cortical necrosis has been described, demonstrating that HUS can cause irreversible lesions that lead to permanent damage. Biopsy specimens of other organ systems such as the brain and pancreas have demonstrated similar endothelial damage.

Many other factors have been evaluated as contributors to the abnormalities seen in HUS. Prostacyclin, produced by the endothelial cell wall, is a potent vasodilator and antiplatelet aggregatory agent. Serum from patients with HUS has been shown not to stimulate the production of prostacyclin to the same degree as that from control patients. Other studies have identified lower levels of prostacyclin precursors in patients with HUS. RBCs from patients with HUS are more fragile than normal RBCs. An association with lower levels of antioxidant factors such as tocopherol has been suggested.

There is evidence that some cases of HUS have a genetic link. Family groups have been described in which multiple children of the same family contract

HUS at the same age. These isolated cases usually have a poor outcome. No specific inheritance has been described at this time. Also, the expression of HUS is not limited to the pediatric population since there are multiple cases documenting its occurrence in adults. It has been seen in postpartum women as well as in women who use oral contraceptives. Thrombotic thrombocytopenic purpura, a clinical syndrome occurring predominantly in adults, is considered an expression of the same microangiopathic process seen in infants afflicted with HUS. The association of renal and neurologic dysfunction in the presence of thrombocytopenia and hemolytic anemia is highly suggestive of thrombotic thrombocytopenic purpura. As with HUS, coagulation studies are usually normal; but in contrast to HUS, therapy with exchange transfusion and plasmapheresis is beneficial in approximately 70% of cases. On biopsy patients with HUS and thrombotic thrombocytopenic purpura have been shown to have endothelial damage with formation of microthrombi.

MONITORING AND LABORATORY TESTS

The patient with HUS has multisystem involvement, and each system must be frequently monitored. Serial physical examinations, including daily weights and complete record of fluid intake and output, are essential. The presence of edema, hypertension, S_3 gallop, and rales reflects the total body fluid excess that often occurs during acute renal failure. The presence of pallor and petcchiae or purpura reflects the hematologic abnormality associated with this disease. Frequent neurologic assessment is necessary to determine the magnitude and progression of CNS involvement. Patients with generalized seizures or coma with thrombocytopenia and anemia must be evaluated for CNS hemorrhage. Patients with abdominal distention and persistent vomiting may need surgical evaluation for bowel obstruction.

Frequent evaluation of hematologic status, serum chemistries, and renal function is critical for appropriate management of these patients. Serum electrolytes, calcium, phosphate, creatinine, and BUN must be monitored initially as often as every 4 hours, depending on the abnormalities present. Hematologic evaluation via CBC, platelet count, evaluation of the peripheral smear by the physician managing the patient, reticulocyte count, and coagulation profile, including PT, PTT, fibrinogen, and fibrin split products with haptoglobin, must be performed. Since the he-matologic variables can change rapidly, they may need monitoring as often as every 4 hours. Stool, blood, and urinary cultures must be obtained since an infectious agent is frequently isolated from these patients.

Hyponatremia and hypocalcemia, with an elevated serum creatinine and BUN values in patients with significant renal involvement, are not uncommon. Frequently these electrolyte abnormalities predispose the patients to seizure activity in the presenting stage of HUS. Hemoglobin and platelet counts are low. The reticulocyte count is elevated, and the haptoglobin level is decreased, consistent with a hemolytic process. A direct and an indirect Coombs test will yield negative results. The coagulation profile should not demonstrate any abnormalities. If there is evidence of any coagulation defect, further studies to rule out the possibility of DIC must be performed since this defect does not typically occur in association with HUS. The peripheral blood smear will demonstrate normochromic normocytic anemia, with the presence of schistocytes and a paucity of platelets. The association of insulin-dependent diabetes mellitus in patients with HUS necessitates frequent evaluations of serum glucose, especially in those patients on peritoneal dialysis. Elevation of liver enzymes can occur in patients with HUS and need evaluation.

TREATMENT

Early institution of peritoneal dialysis has improved the outcome for patients with this syndrome. The indication for dialysis in any patient is correction of azotemia, fluid, and electrolyte abnormalities that are refractory to medical management. The patient with HUS may not initially have an absolute indication for dialysis, but with the early use of peritoneal dialysis, the risks associated with therapies commonly used early in the course of HUS are reduced. At presentation patients with HUS may be anemic and azotemic and frequently will have fluid and electrolyte abnormalities. These patients invariably need multiple blood transfusions that are tolerated poorly in the absence of dialysis because of the already increased intravascular volume. Electrolyte abnormalities such as hyperkalemia, hyperphosphatemia, hyponatremia, and hypocalcemia can be managed efficiently with peritoneal dialysis. Similarly, reducing BUN, creatinine, and unmeasured middle molecular weight toxins associated with renal insufficiency is virtually impossible in anuric or oliguric patients without adjuvant use of peritoneal dialysis. These patients are highly catabolic and have increased nutrition needs. Peritoneal dialysis allows delivery of a large caloric volume without further compromising the volume or electrolyte status of the patient, ensuring that the patient is able to receive the nutrition needed during a sometimes prolonged illness.

Although hemodialysis is an alternative for renal replacement therapy, peritoneal dialysis offers a continuous mode of treatment without the complications of hemodialyzing the smaller patient. Care must be taken to prevent development of iatrogenic electrolyte abnormalities such as hypokalemia and hypophosphatemia associated with frequent dialysate exchanges. Hyperglycemia secondary to the high concentrations of dextrose used in the dialysate to facilitate ultrafiltration must be prevented.

Generalized seizures are common in patients with HUS. Frequently electrolyte and pH abnormalities such as hyponatremia, hypocalcemia, and acidosis are seen in conjunction with seizure activity. Hypertension is also common in the presence of seizure activity. Electroencephalography may demonstrate generalized, nonfocal abnormalities in some infants or specific focal abnormalities in others. Treatment of the underlying electrolyte abnormalities and hypertension is necessary for control of seizure activity. When there are no metabolic abnormalities or hypertension and seizures are present, anticonvulsant therapy is required to stop the seizure.

Hypertension is common at presentation in patients with HUS. Multifactorial causes contribute to this problem. Many children receive fluid challenges to generate urine output; when given in the presence of acute renal failure, this leads to volume overload. The liberation of vasoconstrictors such as thromboxane A_2 from increased platelet destruction in the microvasculature and decreased production of prostacylin (PGI_2) also contribute to hypertension as do increased renin levels secondary to the underlying renal injury. Until adequate control of hypervolemia is achieved, hypertension will persist. Providing acute therapy with vasodilator agents is mandatory for initial control until euvolemia is achieved by either ultrafiltration via peritoneal dialysis or forced diuresis. Some patients may have persistent hypertension even when euvolemic and need continued antihypertensive therapy.

Blood products must be given to patients before hemodynamic compromise develops from anemia or thrombocytopenia. RBC transfusions are given when the hematocrit continues to fall below 20% and the hemolytic process has not ceased. Since the transfused RBCs will be subjected to the same hemolytic process that created the anemia initially, the cells will have a shorter survival time. Use of platelet infusions is avoided unless there is evidence of bleeding or the platelet count is consistently below $20,000/mm^3$. The complications caused by further platelet plugging of the microvasculature by the infused platelets justifies withholding therapy in these patients unless necessary. Again, as with the RBCs, the survival time of the platelets is shortened. Blood product tranfusions are not without risks, including volume overload, non-A, non-B hepatitis, acquired immunodeficiency syndrome, or cytomegaloviral infections; therefore judicious use of these products is recommended.

There is no conclusive evidence about the benefit of adjunctive therapies, including the use of fresh frozen plasma, antiplatelet therapies, anticoagulants, and antioxidant therapies. Infusion of fresh frozen plasma was thought to replace a deficiency of an unknown circulating factor contributing to the pathogenesis of HUS. Plasmaphoresis has been used in conjunction with fresh frozen plasma infusions with no demonstrable benefit over conservative management. Antiplatelet therapy with aspirin and dipyridamole has been used in an effort to decrease the increased aggregatory nature of the platelets causing microvasculature plugging, but this has not been demonstrated to be beneficial. Heparin and vitamin E were used to treat the presumed consumptive coagulopathy and decrease the instability of the red blood cells, respectively. No apparent benefit has resulted from either therapy, and fatal complications have occurred with the use of heparin.

Systemic Complications and Prognosis

HUS is usually a self-limited syndrome that resolves 1 to 3 months after presentation. Occasionally complete resolution may not occur for 12 months. The patients return to their previously healthy state and suffer no residual complications in 70% of the cases. Residual disease includes HUS nephropathy and CNS dysfunction. Patients who are at greater risk for morbidity and mortality are isolated, nonepidemic cases, have a prior family history of HUS, or have recurrent HUS. Patients who have a prodrome other than diarrhea, develop HUS outside of the summer months, and are more than 3.4 years of age at onset may have a worse prognosis. Complications occurring during the initial phase of the illness usually are due to fluid and electrolyte abnormalities secondary to renal insufficiency. In patients who recover completely the period of oliguria or anuria averages 7 to 14 days. One study showed children with HUS had a lower incidence of chronic renal failure (6%) when the mean period of oliguria was 9 days vs. a 43% incidence when the mean period was 26 days. In approximately 10% to 15% of patients renal function does not return to normal. The anemia in patients with HUS may persist for a few months, with RBC transfusions needed beyond the initial phase of the illness. In patients who have complete recovery of renal function, the prognosis for recovery from anemia is excellent.

The degree of CNS involvement affects morbidity and mortality. In one review of more than 600 patients, 41% experienced either stupor, coma, convulsions, or hemiparesis. Another study of 60 children reported 50% had major CNS involvement, including seizures, decerebrate posturing, and transient hemiparesis. All children in the latter series who died during the acute phase of HUS had CNS involvement. Patients who have prolonged neurologic impairment may be at a higher risk for residual disease such as cortical blindness or hemiparesis.

Overall mortality in HUS has decreased in recent years because of early use of dialysis. Approximately 10% of patients who develop HUS suffer some residual disease with either renal or neurologic involvement.

ADDITIONAL READING

Bale JF, Brasher C, Siegler RL. CNS manifestations of the hemolytic-uremic syndrome. Am J Dis Child 134:869-872, 1980.

Berry PL, Siegler RL, Hogg RJ. A multicenter study of the outcome of children with the hemolytic-uremic syndrome (HUS). Kidney Int 29:179, 1986.

Campos A, Sibley R, Kim Y, Miller K, Michael AF. The hemolytic uremic syndrome. Am J Kidney Dis 14:23-28, 1981.

Cooper RA, Bunn HF. Hemolytic anemias. In Braunwald E, ed. Harrison's Principles of Internal Medicine, 11th ed. New York: McGraw-Hill, 1987, pp 1511-1512.

Coulthard MG. An evaluation of treatment with heparin in the haemolytic-uremic syndrome successfully treated by peritoneal dialysis. Arch Dis Child 55:393-397, 1980.

Gaynor E, Bouvier C, Spaet TH. Vascular lesions: Possible pathogenetic basis of the generalized Schwartzman reaction. Science 170:986-988, 1970.

• Gianatonio CA, Vitacco M, Mendilaharzu F, Gallo GE, Sogo ET. The hemolytic-uremic syndrome. Nephron 11:174-192, 1973.

• Kaplan BS, Thomson PD, deChadarevian JP. The hemolytic uremic syndrome. Pediatr Clin North Am 23:761-777, 1976.

Kosler F, Levin J, Walker L, Tung KSK, Gilman RH, Rahaman MM, Majid A, Islam S, Williams RC. Hemolytic-uremic syndrome after shigellosis: Relation to endotoxemia and circulating immune complexes. N Engl J Med 298:927-933, 1978.

Neill MA, Tan PL, Calusen CR, Christie DL, Hickman RO. *Escherichia coli* 0157:H7 as the predominant pathogen associated with the hemolytic uremic syndrome: A prospective study in the Pacific Northwest. Pediatrics 80:37-40, 1987.

O'Regan S, Chesney RW, Kaplan BS, Drummond KN. Red cell membrane phospholipid abnormalities in the hemolytic uremic syndrome. Clin Nephrol 15:14-17, 1980.

Peterson RB, Meseroll WP, Shrago GG, Gooding CA. Radiographic features of colitis associated with the hemolytic-uremic syndrome. Radiology 118:667-671, 1976.

Powell HR, McCredie DA, Taylor CM, Burke JR, Walker RG. Vitamin E treatment of haemolytic uraemic syndrome. Arch Dis Child 59:401-404, 1984.

Rao SP, Sutton AL, Falter ML, Robinson MG. Chronic microangiopathic hemolytic anemia. NY State J Med 79:1763-1765, 1979.

Remuzzi G, Misiani R, Marchesi D, Livio M, Mecca G, de Gaetano G, Donati MB. Treatment of the hemolytic uremic syndrome with plasma. Clin Nephrol 12:279-284, 1979.

Rogers MF, Rutherford GW, Alexander SR, Diliberti JH, Foster L, Schonberger LB, Hurwitz ES. A population-based study of hemolytic-uremic syndrome in Oregon, 1979, 1982. Am J Epidemiol 123:137-142, 1986.

Schlegel N, Maclouf J, Loirat C, Cronet L, Marotte R, Scarabin PY, Mathieu H. Absence of plasma prostacylin stimulating activity deficiency in hemolytic uremic syndrome. J Pediatr 111:71-76, 1987.

Sheth KJ, Swick HM, Haworth N. Neurological involvement in hemolytic-uremic syndrome. Ann Neurol 19:90-93, 1986.

Trompeter RS, Schwartz R, Chantler C, Dillon MS, Haycock GB, Kay R, Barratt TM. Haemolytic-uraemic syndrome: An analysis of prognostic features. Arch Dis Child 58:101-105, 1983.

• Vitsky BH, Suzuki Y, Strauss L, Charg J. The hemolytic-uremic syndrome: A study of renal pathologic alterations. Am J Pathol 57:627-639, 1969.

53 Hypertensive Crisis

Mouin G. Seikaly

BACKGROUND AND PHYSIOLOGY

In children systemic arterial BP is a continuous variable dependent on age, sex, size, genetics, and environmental factors. Defining limits for normal BP in children is difficult; it is arbitrary, however, to consider any BP elevation above the 95th percentile for a matched population as hypertension (Table 53-1).

Table 53-1 Classification of Hypertension by Age Group*

Age Group	Significant Hypertension (mm Hg)*	Severe Hypertension (mm Hg)
Newborns		
7 days	SBP ≥96	SBP ≥106
8-30 days	SBP ≥104	SBP ≥110
Infants (≤2 yr)	SBP ≥112	SBP ≥118
	DBP ≥74	DBP ≥82
Children (3-5 yr)	SBP ≥116	SBP ≥118
	DBP ≥76	DBP ≥84
Children (6-9 yr)	SBP ≥122	SBP ≥130
	DBP ≥78	DBP ≥86
Children (10-12 yr)	SBP ≥126	SBP ≥134
	DBP ≥82	DBP ≥90
Adolescents (13-15 yr)	SBP ≥136	SBP ≥144
	DBP ≥86	DBP ≥92
Adolescents (16-18 yr)	SBP ≥142	SBP ≥150
	DBP ≥92	DBP ≥98

SBP = systolic blood pressure; DBP = diastolic blood pressure.
*Modified from Horan MK, et al. Task force on blood pressure control in children. Pediatrics 79:1, 1987. Reproduced by permission.

When BP values increase rapidly or exceed the upper limits of normal diastolic BP for age by 55%, an acute hypertensive emergency situation exists. Hypertensive emergencies can occur during the course of preexisting hypertension (accelerated) or can develop in children with previously unrecognized disease (de novo). When arteriolar pressure reaches critical levels, fibrinoid necrosis develops in the arterial wall. Vascular changes are manifested in several organ systems: in the retina as exudates and hemorrhage, in the CNS as papilledema, in the kidneys as proteinuria or hematuria, and in the vascular system as angiopathic changes causing thrombosis and hemolytic anemia.

Compared to adults, children are more prone to hypertensive encephalopathy than to malignant hypertension. Several theories attempt to explain the involvement of the CNS in patients with severe hypertension. Cerebral blood flow is maintained nearly constant over a wide range of blood pressure changes from 70 to 200 mm Hg (Fig. 53-1). The major mechanism through which the brain autoregulates its blood flow is altering its intracerebral vascular resistance; with acute hypertension "overregulation" of cerebral blood flow may occur, causing intense focal arteriolar spasm and resulting in ischemia, microinfarcts, and necrosis. Alternatively, the "breakthrough" theory hypothesizes that the cerebral arteriolar vessels may fail to constrict sufficiently during an abrupt rise in BP, resulting in an increase of transcapillary pressure and cerebral edema, and, in turn, encephalopathy.

Signs and Symptoms

Patients with severe hypertension may initially have a spectrum of clinical symptoms related to the CNS,

CAUSES OF HYPERTENSIVE CRISIS IN CHILDREN

Renal causes

Vascular
  Hemolytic-uremic syndrome
  Renal artery stenosis or thrombosis
  Polyarteritis nodosa
  Kawasaki disease
  Sickle cell nephropathy
Nephritides
  Henoch-Schönlein purpura
  Postinfectious glomerulonephritis
  Systemic lupus nephritis
  Membranoproliferative glomerulonephritis
  Rapidly progressive glomerulonephritis
Congenital malformation
  Polycystic kidney disease
  Tuberous sclerosis
  Hydronephrosis
Miscellaneous
  Iatrogenic fluid overload
  End-stage renal disease with volume overload
  Renal transplant
  Reflux nephropathy

Central nervous system

Meningoencephalitis
Tumor
Trauma/child abuse
Hydrocephalus

Drugs

Corticosteroids
Cyclosporin A
Clonidine and beta blockers—withdrawal
Reserpine, amphetamines, phenylephrine, pseudo-
  ephedrine
Licorice; phenylpropanolamine overdose
Selected "recreational" drugs

Tumors

Renin-secreting tumor
Pheochromocytoma
Wilms' tumor or neuroblastoma

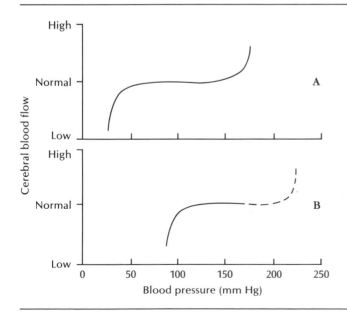

Fig. 53-1   Relationship between cerebral blood flow and mean arterial pressure in normotensive individuals, **A**, and in those with chronic hypertension, **B**. Arterial pressure has been altered rapidly by ganglionic blockers or pressors. The broken line indicates a hypothetical curve. (From Cuneo RA, Caronna JJ. The neurologic complications of hypertension. Med Clin North Am 61:568, 1977.)

kidneys, and heart. Hypertensive encephalopathy has characteristic clinical features:

1. Abrupt rise in BP to levels exceeding upper limits of normal by 55%
2. Severe headache and vomiting
3. Blurred vision with or without papilledema
4. Altered sensorium
5. Localized neurologic signs
6. Convulsions

It is mandatory to distinguish other clinical conditions that may be confused with hypertensive encephalopathy (e.g., stroke, subarachnoid hemorrhage). Stroke is usually associated with lateralizing neurologic signs and symptoms. Subarachnoid hemorrhage has been reported in hypertensive children undergoing hemodialysis and receiving heparin. Fortunately stroke and subarachnoid hemorrhage occur less frequently in children than in adults.

Sustained elevation in BP results in an increase in left ventricular afterload, which, if not corrected, will eventually lead to cardiac decompensation. Congestive heart failure is the presenting sign of coarctation of the aorta, aortic thrombosis, and renal artery stenosis. Patients with postinfectious acute glomerulonephritis may be seen with acute hypertension and congestive heart failure caused by volume overload.

MONITORING AND LABORATORY TESTS

A major factor determining the outcome of a hypertensive crisis is the speed of initiating an effective plan to lower BP. The initial plan of action should include the following:

1. Obtain a concise medical history, stressing cardiac, endocrine, renal, and neurologic systems, current medications or ingestions, and hydration.
2. Perform physical examination, emphasizing cardiovascular, genitourinary, and neurologic systems.
3. Gain vascular access for therapy.
4. Obtain baseline studies, including CBC, BUN, creatinine, serum electrolytes and glucose, plasma catecholamine, renin activity, and aldosterone. Urinalysis and urine culture should also be obtained.
5. Institute appropriate parenteral therapy based on initial assessment.
6. Request stat chest roentgenogram, renal ultrasound examination, and depending on neu-

rologic status, head CT, with or without contrast. An echocardiogram should be obtained.
7. Admit patient to intensive care unit and insert intra-arterial catheter for continuous blood pressure monitoring.
8. Reassess clinical course and therapeutic strategy based on physical examination, laboratory studies, and initial response to therapy.

TREATMENT

Internists are always concerned about too rapid normalization of severe hypertension. During longstanding hypertension cerebral blood flow is maintained at higher perfusion pressure (Fig. 53-1); too rapid normalization of BP can carry significant risks. In adults rapid reduction in BP, even to normal levels, may produce cerebral ischemia. Similarly, coronary artery blood flow and renal perfusion may be compromised if BP is too rapidly reduced. Thus gradual reduction of BP to normal values over 24 hours, if permitted by the patient's clinical condition, is indicated. In patients with long-standing hypertension good BP control with antihypertensive therapy will usually normalize the autoregulation curve (Fig. 53-1).

However, during hypertensive emergencies associated with encephalopathy or during an episode of severe malignant hypertension accompanied by acute left ventricular failure, stroke, or renal insufficiency, risks of rapid normalization of BP appear to outweigh the risks of continued vascular damage. The speed and the level to which to reduce BP remain strictly a clinical decision. An arbitrary, yet safe regimen is to decrease BP during the first 6 hours by one third of the total reduction planned, with another decrement of one third during the next 12 to 36 hours. Normalization should be achieved over 2 to 3 days. Other clinicians, however, are more aggressive in attempting BP reduction in children.

Therapeutic Approaches to the Treatment of Severe Hypertension

Regardless of the cause of hypertension, the progressive use of potent vasodilators, combined with salt restriction and diuresis, is the most common approach for managing hypertensive emergencies. It is usually advisable to start with one antihypertensive agent at a time and increase the dose either to its maximum recommended dose or until side effects are noted. The simultaneous introduction of multiple therapeutic agents may lead to unpredictable responses, and it is not unusual that this nonspecific approach may fail to reduce elevated BP. The patient's clinical progress and the therapeutic strategies used must be reassessed periodically and necessary adjustments made. Understanding the underlying pathophysiology of hypertension and using a combination of physiologic and pharmacologic therapeutic modalities often ensure better and smoother control of hypertension.

Nifedipine

Calcium channel blockers decrease BP by blocking calcium-mediated electromechanical contractile tissue and producing peripheral arteriolar vasodilation. However, calcium channel blockers vary in their ability to dilate different vascular beds. Nifedipine lowers both systolic and diastolic BP by 49 and 38 mm Hg, respectively, within 30 minutes after sublingual administration. Heart rate, cardiac output, and glomerular filtration rate increase after nifedipine is given; however, cerebral blood flow is unaffected in adult patients. In contradistinction to other vasodilators, calcium channel blockers cause no sodium retention; and their renal vasodilatory effect may even favor sodium excretion. Furthermore, calcium channel blockers stimulate the renin-angiotensin system minimally compared to other vasodilators.

In children the dose of nifedipine is 0.25 to 0.50 mg/kg, which can be repeated within 30 minutes if additional lowering of BP is desirable. The dose could again be repeated within 3 to 4 hours. Use of the sublingual route has been recently criticized and the "bite and swallow" approach advocated; however, this may be difficult to achieve in the young, uncooperative patient. Nifedipine is commercially available in 10 and 20 mg gelatinous capsules. For a young patient the content of the capsule can be aspirated into a tuberculin syringe, its volume measured (approximately 0.34 ml/10 mg capsule), and a graded dose squirted into the patient's sublingual area. Of the oral vasodilators, nifedipine has a more prompt onset of action and more reliable absorption, making it the oral drug of choice in the treatment of hypertensive crises; furthermore, its ease of administration makes it the first line of drug therapy to give even in a clinic setting.

Side effects are usually moderate and tolerated and include flushing, dysrhythmia, dizziness, nausea, and syncope.

Hydralazine

Hydralazine is another peripheral vasodilator, which mainly affects the arterial beds and can lower peripheral vascular resistance up to 73%. However, because of reflex tachycardia, increased stroke volume, and fluid retention, its antihypertensive properties are only modest when used alone. Hydralazine is administered as a bolus IV infusion at an initial dose of 0.1 to 0.5 mg/kg. If the patient's systemic arterial BP has not been lowered satisfactorily within 20 minutes, the dose can be repeated as needed. The onset of action is within 5 to 20 minutes, with a duration of action of up to 5 hours. Parenteral hydralazine is available in ampules of 20 mg in a 1 ml solution. Its major side effects include tachycardia, palpitation, chest pain, hypotension, headaches, nasal congestion, vomiting, and diarrhea.

Diazoxide

Diazoxide is a benzothiadiazine derivative related to a thiazide diuretic in structure. When administered intravenously, it relaxes the arterial smooth muscles, most likely by stimulating prostacyclin synthesis, with minimal effect on the capacitance vessels. In patients with acute hypertension diazoxide lowers systemic arterial BP rapidly but rarely below age-related normal values. Because of increased venous return and heart rate the cardiac output increases; cardiac work, however, is reduced because of lowering of afterload. The drug is most commonly used as a rapid IV bolus in single or multiple doses at 2 to 10 mg/kg/dose, which may be repeated in 30 minutes if the desired response is not achieved. The onset of action is 1 to 3 minutes and may last up to 18 hours. After a precipitous, excessive, and prolonged drop in BP with diazoxide administration, serious neurologic complications have been reported in chronically hypertensive adults but not in children. In addition, profound hypotension can occur in patients with myocardial dysfunction. Continuous IV infusion has been used in adults as an alternative method for the administration of diazoxide; a loading dose of 7.5 mg/kg is given at a rate of 7.5 mg/min until the systemic BP falls by 25%. If additional systemic BP reduction is desired, the drug is infused at a rate of 3.75 mg/min. A maintenance dose of 10% of the loading dose is given as a continuous infusion over 6 hours. Higher drug levels are usually needed when the drug is given as a continuous infusion to maintain the reduced BP, as compared to the drug levels needed for lowering BP by bolus administration. This is probably due to an induced renin-angiotensin system. Administration of furosemide is often recommended to prevent fluid retention. Diazoxide is available in ampules containing 300 mg in a 70 ml solution.

Hyperglycemia, hyperuricemia, hypertrichosis, hypotension, fluid retention, nausea, vomiting, headache, flushing, and an unusual metallic taste in the mouth are the most frequent side effects of diazoxide therapy. Hyperglycemia secondary to the direct effect of diazoxide on the pancreatic beta cells is its most common serious side effect. Nonketotic hyperglycemic coma has been reported with diazoxide therapy; serum glucose levels ought to be monitored and insulin therapy instituted when glucose levels exceed 300 mg/dl.

Nitroglycerin

Nitroglycerin is a vasodilator of both the arterial and venous beds. Because of its rapid degradation by the liver, nitroglycerin can be titrated quickly and effectively when given intravenously; although there is no established pediatric dose, a suggested starting IV dose is 0.5 to 5.0 μg/kg/min, which is increased by increments of 0.5 to 1.0 μg/kg/min every 3 to 5 minutes. The maximal rate of infusion is approximately 50 μg/min. Parentral nitroglycerin is available in 50 mg vials (5 mg/ml). Nitroglycerin is diluted with dextrose in water or 0.9% sodium chloride solution to yield a final concentration of 100 μg/ml. If fluid intake is limited, use of a more concentrated preparation is possible but should not exceed 400 μg/ml. Nitroglycerin cannot be used in plastic bags and must be mixed in a special glass bottle administration set to maintain potency. Although its reported use in pediatric patients is limited to perioperative and intraoperative control of systemic arterial BP during heart surgery, we have successfully used it to control hypertension in one patient with end-stage renal disease who developed nitroprusside toxicity and in another patient with neurofibromatosis after repair of bilateral renal artery stenosis. Its beneficial dilating effects on the pulmonary vascular

bed give it an added advantage. Nitroglycerin is also available as an ointment for transdermal slow release. The onset of action is approximately 30 minutes and lasts for up to 24 hours.

Its major side effects include hypotension, tachycardia, nausea, vomiting, apprehension, restlessness, dysrhythmia, and abdominal pain.

Sodium nitroprusside

Sodium nitroprusside is a direct vasodilator of both resistance and capacitance vessels, and its effects on cardiac output and heart rate are often minimal. The short-lived antihypertensive response is dose-dependent and ensues within seconds of infusion, with an average decrement in both systolic and diastolic BP of 40 to 50 mm Hg. The drug is administered by continuous infusion; the initial starting dose is 0.5 to 1.0 μg/kg/min, incremently increased as needed every 2 to 3 minutes up to a maximum of 8 μg/kg/min. Desired systemic BP control is often achieved within 20 minutes, whereas cardiac failure and hypertensive encephalopathy are often reversed within 24 to 48 hours. Nitroprusside is available in a 50 mg vial, which, when dissolved in 500 ml of 5% dextrose in water, gives a final concentration of 100 μg/ml. The drug is stable in solution for 4 hours, but it is heat and light sensitive, and both the reservoir and tubing must be completely protected by aluminum foil. Throughout nitroprusside infusion attentive systemic BP monitoring is warranted, preferably via an arterial catheter. Nitroprusside is considered by some clinicians as the first drug of choice in hypertensive emergency. Its efficacy lies in its rapid onset of action and its ability to make a smooth transition to normal BP levels attainable. In contradistinction to other antihypertensive drugs, nitroprusside does not alter the level of the sensorium, making its use in patients with hypertensive encephalopathy and stroke advantageous. An additional advantage for use in patients with congestive heart failure is its action on the capacitance vessels, decreasing ventricular preload by shifting blood volume to the periphery.

Side effects of sodium nitroprusside include muscle twitching, sweating, apprehension, and vomiting. Nitroprusside is nonenzymatically metabolized by the liver and red blood cells to cyanide and thiocyanate, which are cleared by the kidney at a rate of 2.2 ml/min. In vitro photodegraded nitroprusside releases nitric oxide, followed by production of cyanide; hence degraded nitroprusside is potentially more toxic than intact nitroprusside. Side effects of nitroprusside related to thiocyanate or cyanide include hypothyroidism, bone marrow suppression, fatigue, anorexia, decline in renal function, mental confusion, psychosis, and coma. The earliest signs of nitroprusside toxicity are unexplained metabolic acidosis and tachyphylaxis. In patients with normal renal and liver function, serum thiocyanate levels must be monitored if the drug is used for more than 48 hours. In patients with even moderate renal or hepatic impairment, cyanide poisoning has been observed within 6 to 12 hours of initiating therapy. Nitroprusside is also more toxic in patients with poor nutritional support because of depleted stores of thiosulfate, a substrate for subsequent metabolism of the drug. A thiocyanate-cyanide level exceeding 10 mg/dl is considered toxic. Thiocyanate toxicity is treated by discontinuing the drug, performing peritoneal dialysis or hemodialysis, and infusing hydroxocobalamin.

Labetalol

Labetalol is a nonspecific beta-adrenoceptor antagonist with some alpha-adrenergic blocking activity. When given intravenously the drug has been shown to be effective in acutely reducing high systemic arterial BP and heart rate, but not stroke volume. The drug is administered as a continuous infusion at a rate of 1 to 3 mg/kg/hr. The starting infusion rate is 1 mg/kg/hr; in the absence of the desired response the rate is increased every 30 minutes up to a maximum dose of 3 mg/kg/hr. The infusion is discontinued when the desired BP control is achieved. The duration of BP response varies among patients. In adults the drug has been given as an IV bolus of 1 to 2 mg/kg. The onset of action is within 5 minutes and lasts at least 6 hours, and diastolic BP is lowered by at least 30 mm Hg. A mini-bolus schedule is also effective, using repeated injections of 0.5 mg/kg every 15 minutes until the desired BP or a total cumulative dose of 3.5 mg/kg has been achieved. Once the desired BP is achieved, oral maintenance therapy is started. Labetalol is supplied in ampules containing 100 mg in a 20 ml solution and in multidose vials with 300 mg in a 60 ml solution. Labetalol has been reported effective in treating patients during emergencies when they are resistant to treatment with other vasodilators, and it has been shown to be advantageous over hydralazine and diazoxide in treating peripartal women. Labetalol is of special advantage in treating hypertension associated with thyrotoxicosis, pheochromocytoma in the perioperative periods, laryngotracheal manipulation, and neurosurgical procedures.

Side effects of IV labetalol administration are minimal and include nausea, epigastric burning, rhinorrhea, premature ventricular contractions, and hypotension. The use of beta blockers is contraindicated for patients with bronchial hypersensitivity or congestive heart failure.

Labetalol has only recently been used in children; more studies are needed to ascertain its safety and efficacy in pediatric patients.

Sedatives and analgesics

Pain and anxiety are known causes of acute hypertension. Most parenteral sedatives and analgesics lower systemic arterial BP, especially when combined with vasodilators. In hypertensive patients in whom pain is part of their clinical picture, special effort is needed to alleviate pain and agitation before advancing antihypertensive therapy.

Choosing Among Antihypertensive Agents

The choice of an antihypertensive agent as the first line of action remains a matter of professional preference (Table 53-2). Usually nifedipine is administered first in the emergency department before the initiation of parentral therapy. Hydralazine and diazoxide are often started as soon as a venous access is placed if there has not been a desirable response to nifedipine. Although sodium nitroprusside is considered by many as the primary agent for treating hypertensive emergencies, it is unpredictable and has serious side effects, mainly those of cyanide poisoning—especially when renal or hepatic function is compromised as it often is in critically ill patients with hypertensive emergencies. Therefore its use as a first-line drug has major limitations. In my experience IV nitroglycerin has proved a safe, effective antihypertensive agent, and it may be used in place of nitroprusside. As for the use of labetalol, further evaluation is needed.

Table 53-2   Antihypertensive Agents Available for Treatment of Hypertensive Emergencies

Agent	Route	Dose	Interval	Onset of Action	Duration of Action	Major Acute Problems
Nifedipine (Procardia) (10 or 20 mg capsule)	SL/PO	0.25-0.5 mg/kg	30 min × 1, then q 3-4 hr	30 min	1-4 hr	Hypotension, dysrhythmias
Hydralazine (Apresoline) (20 mg/ml)	IV or IM	0.1-0.5 mg/kg/dose; maximum dose, 20 mg; repeat q 20 min if no response	q 3-6 hr	5-20 min	4-6 hr	Tachycardia, headaches, flushing, nasal congestion, palpitations, vomiting, diarrhea, acute hypotension, myocardial ischemia
Diazoxide (Hyperstat) (300 mg/20 ml)	IV push (rapid)	2.5-10 mg/kg; may repeat in 30 min if no response	prn	1-3 min	1/2-24 hr	Hyperglycemia, hyperuricemia, acute hypotension, nausea, vomiting, flushing, dysrhythmia, sodium retention
	IV infusion	7.5 mg/kg at a rate of 7.5 mg/min/70 kg	10% loading dose as continuous infusion	Minutes	5-6 hr	
Nitroglycerin (Nitro-Bid) (5 mg/ml)	IV	0.5-1 μg/kg/min	Continuous infusion	Immediate	Only effective during infusion	Hypotension, abdominal pain, dizziness, headache
Sodium nitroprusside (Nipride) (50 mg)	IV infusion by pump	0.5-10 μg/kg/min; maximum dose, 20 mg	Continuous infusion	Immediate	Only effective during infusion	Thiocyanate intoxication (maintain thiocyanate levels <10 mg/dl); chest pain, abdominal pain, headaches, rigidity, GI upset, seizures
Labetalol (Normodyne) (100 mg/20 ml)	IV	1 mg/kg/hr, up to 3 mg/kg/hr	Continuous infusion	5 min	Only effective during infusion	Nausea, premature ventricular contractions, rhinorrhea, hypotension, bronchospasm

ADDITIONAL READING

Arnold WP, Longnecker DE, Epstein RM. Photo-degradation of sodium nitroprusside: Biologic activity and cyanide release. Anesthesiology 61:254-260, 1984.

Ashe RG, Moodley J, Richards AM, et al. Comparison of labetalol and dihydralazine in hypertensive emergencies of pregnancy. S Afr Med J 72:354-356, 1987.

Bailey RR. Labetalol in the treatment of patients with hypertension and renal functional impairment. Br J Clin Pharmacol 8:135S-140S, 1979.

Balfe VW, Ranu CP. Recognition and management of hypertensive crises in childhood. Pediatr Clin North Am 25:159-172, 1978.

Boerth RC, Long WR. Dose response relation of diazoxide in children with hypertension. Circulation 56:1062-1067, 1971.

Byron FB. The pathogenesis of hypertensive encephalopathy and its relation to malignant phase of hypertension—experimental evidence from the hypertensive rat. Lancet 2:201-211, 1954.

Charles MA, Danforth E. Non-ketotic hyperglycemia and coma during intravenous diazoxide therapy in uremia. Diabetes 20:501-507, 1971.

Chauvin M, Deriaz H, Viars P. Continuous I.V. infusion of labetalol for postoperative hypertension. Br J Anaesth 59:1250-1256, 1987.

Cohn JN, Burke LP. Nitroprusside. Ann Intern Med 91:752-757, 1979.

Danzig LE. Dynamics of thiocynate dialysis. N Engl J Med 252:49-57, 1955.

• Dillon MJ. Drug treatment of hypertension. In Holliday MA, et al, eds. Pediatric Nephrology. Baltimore: Williams & Wilkins, 1987, pp 758-765.

Dillon MJ. Hypertension. In Postlethwaite RH, ed. Clinica Pediatric Nephrology. Bristol: Wright, 1986, pp 1-25.

Dilmen V, Caglar MK, et al. Nifedipine in hypertensive emergencies in children. Am J Dis Child 137:1162-1165, 1983.

Ferguson RK, Vlasses PH. Hypertensive emergencies and urgencies. JAMA 225:1607-1612, 1986.

Freis ED, Rose JC, Higgins TF, et al. The hemodynamic effects of hypotensive drugs in man. Circulation 5:199-204, 1953.

Gifford RW, Westbrook E. Hypertensive encephalopathy. Mechanisms, clinical features, and treatment. Progr Cardiovasc Dis 17:115-124, 1974.

Gordillo-Paniagua G, Velasquez-Jones L, Martini R, et al. Sodium nitroprusside treatment for severe arterial hypertension in children. J Pediatr 87:799-804, 1975.

• Gruskin AB, Baluarte HJ, Polinsky MS, et al. Treatment of severe hypertension in children with renal disease. In Strauss J, ed. Acute Renal Disorders and Renal Emergencies. Amsterdam: Martinus Nijhoff, 1984, pp 143-178.

Herling IM. Intravenous nitroglycerin: Clinical pharmacology and therapeutic consideration. Am Heart J 108:141-149, 1984.

Hollenberg NK. Strategies in antihypertensive therapy: Implications of the kidney. JAMA 81:15-19, 1985.

Ilbawi MN, Idriss FS, DeLeon SY, et al. Hemodynamic effects of intravenous nitroglycerin in pediatric patient after heart surgery. Circulation 72(Suppl 2):101-107, 1985.

McAllister RG. Kinetic and dynamics of nifedipine after oral and sublingual doses. JAMA 81:2-5, 1986.

Maharaj RJ, Thompson M, Brock-Utne JG, et al. Treatment of hypertension following endotracheal intubation. S Afr Med J 63:691-694, 1983.

Merotoja OA, Laaksonen VO. Hemodynamic effects of preload and sodium nitroprusside in patients subjected to coronary bypass surgery. Circulation 58:815-825, 1978.

Ngole PM. Intravenous labetalol in the management of resistant hypertensive emergency. Drug Intell Clin Pharm 21:512-514, 1987.

Ogilvie RI, Nadeau JH, Sitar DS. Diazoxide concentration-response relation in hypertension. Hypertension 4:167-170, 1982.

Palmer RF, Lasseter KC. Sodium nitroprusside. N Engl J Med 292:294-301, 1975.

Posner MA, Rodkey FL, Tobey RE. Nitroprusside-induced cyanide poisoning: Antidotal effect of hydroxycobalamin. Anesthesiology 44:330-335, 1976.

Puschstein C, Van Aken H, Hidding J, et al. Treatment of hypertension with labetalol in neurosurgical practice. Acta Neurochir 67:283-290, 1983.

Resnick L. Calcium metabolism, renin activity, and the antihypertensive effects of calcium channel blocker. JAMA 81:6-14, 1986.

Russell RP. Side effects of calcium channel blockers. Hypertension 2:42-43, 1988.

Siegler RL, Brewer ED. Effect of sublingual or oral nifedipine in the treatment of hypertension. J Pediatr 112:811-813, 1988.

Smith WB, Clifton GG, O'Neill WM, et al. Antihypertensive labetalol in accelerated hypertension. Hypertension 5:579-583, 1983.

Standgaard S, Olesen J, Skinhoj E, et al. Autoregulation of brain circulation in severe arterial hypertension. Br Med J 1:507-510, 1973.

Vana Stratum M, Levarler M, Lambilliote JP, et al. Use of labetalol during anesthesia for pheochromocytoma removal. Acta Anaesthesiol Belg 34:233-240, 1984.

Vidt DG. Intravenous labetalol in emergency treatment of hypertension. J Clin Hypertens 1:179-186, 1985.

Vlachakis ND, Maronde RF, Maloy JW, et al. Pharmacodynamics of intravenous labetalol and follow-up therapy with oral labetalol. Clin Pharmacol Ther 38:503-508, 1985.

54 Diabetic Ketoacidosis

James F. Marks

BACKGROUND AND PHYSIOLOGY

Diabetic ketoacidosis (DKA), with its attendant cardiovascular and neurologic instability, is a late sign of a chain of related pathophysiologic events. The physician's ability to manage this catastrophic scenario successfully depends on an understanding of these events.

Although ketoacidosis results from a combination of a subtle interplay of both insulin deficiency and glucagon excess, the initiating event in the development of type I diabetes mellitus is an absolute or relative lack of insulin. The precise molecular and biochemical causes of the insulin and glucagon defects are under continuing study, but a number of known pathophysiologic phenomena occur in individuals with DKA, including an elevation of blood sugar, an increase in osmolality of the plasma, electrolyte imbalance and dehydration, and ketoacidosis and buffer depletion.

Decreased peripheral use of glucose, increased gluconeogenesis, and increased glycogen breakdown lead to hyperglycemia. In the absence of insulin glucose is unable to enter the cell in a normal fashion. Because glucose is not available as a primary substrate, metabolic pathways move in the direction of increased lipolysis, gluconeogenesis, and ketogenesis to cope with energy requirements. With the mobilization of lipids the serum may become lipemic, and with the accumulation of acetoacetic acid and beta-hydroxybutyric acid, acidosis worsens and ammonium ion production increases. Without the use of exogenous insulin, fluids, electrolytes, and glucose, a predictable deterioration ensues.

Both osmotic diuresis from hyperglycemia and vomiting related to the ketoacidosis cause dehydration. Significant amounts of sodium and potassium are lost because of the combination of an osmotic diuresis from the glucose and from excretion of ketones. Signs and symptoms of prerenal azotemia and shock appear because of the fall in glomerular filtration rate and worsening dehydration. The typical patient with severe DKA frequently loses 100 ml water, 8 mEq of sodium, 6 mEq of chloride, and 6 to 10 mEq of potassium per kilogram of body weight.

Several mechanisms are involved in compensating for metabolic acidosis. With CNS stimulation alveolar ventilation increases, resulting in respiratory alkalosis. As a result of action of the bicarbonate buffer system, there is a shift to remove excess hydrogen ions. This system is helpful until a pH of approximately 7.10 is reached. Below pH 7.10 increasing acidosis tends to produce CNS narcosis, with respiratory depression rather than stimulation. With even greater decreases in pH there is less respiratory compensation (alkalosis) to balance metabolic acidosis. A difference in carbon dioxide (faster) and bicarbonate (slower) diffusion across the blood-brain barrier occurs, with a consequent lag in the CNS respiratory drive in response to changes in pH. In the recovery phase the patient may become alkalotic because of continued increase in alveolar ventilation as a result of this delay. During treatment bicarbonate must be used judiciously to avoid accentuating these problems. If enough bicarbonate is used to bring the patient into the range of respiratory compensation (i.e., to approximately pH 7.15), there is little risk of complications due to alkalosis during the course of therapy.

A number of factors contribute to the development of diabetic coma, including hyperosmolality, acidosis, contracted vascular volume, and increased oxygen consumption. The cause of the coma may not always be clear at the beginning. In addition to ketoacidosis, hypoglycemia, nonketotic hyperosmolality, drug ingestion, and infection may cause the coma or complicate DKA, and these possibilities must be considered. In addition DKA may mimic other conditions. For example, a patient in DKA with abdominal pain may mistakenly be thought to have an acute condition of the abdomen instead of ketoacidosis, or a patient in DKA coma may mistakenly be thought to have meningitis or encephalitis. In addition these entities can coexist with diabetic ketoacidosis. However, in the new, previously undiagnosed diabetic the differential diagnosis may delay the final diagnosis and the initiation of appropriate treatment. Management is not simply a matter of making the diagnosis and allowing the events and the treatment to follow automatically. A successful treatment outcome depends on frequent monitoring and changes of management consistent with clinical and metabolic changes in the individual patient.

Possible complications of management include cerebral edema, hypokalemia, and inadequate insulin levels. Clinical evidence of cerebral edema is present in some patients with DKA who die in spite of improving biochemical values. A recent study found that virtually all patients with severe DKA had some degree of cerebral swelling. Why some of these patients will have a catastrophic outcome with severe neurologic residua or death and the majority will recover with similar therapy is not clear. The mechanism for cerebral edema is not known. Some animal studies have shown that a rapid fall in blood glucose from a hyperosmolar state will cause cerebral swelling. Other mechanisms, including rapid administration of fluid, rapid correction of acidosis with alkali, and hypophosphatemia, have been suggested but remain unproved. No clinical study has been done that clearly documents the benefits of aggressive phosphate replacement treatment for diabetic ketoacidosis. Because the contribution of each of these variables to cerebral edema is unknown, frequent observation of the patient's response to management is the only way to deal with these concerns.

The serum potassium level in a patient with severe DKA does not reflect the marked intracellular losses of potassium. With the correction of DKA a number of factors tend to lower the serum potassium, including the following:

1. Potassium moves with glucose across cell membranes intracellularly during the insulin-mediated restoration of carbohydrate metabolism.
2. Expanding extracellular volume decreases the extracellular potassium concentration through dilution.

3. Correction of the acidosis leads to a shift of sodium, potassium, and hydrogen ions, with potassium and hydrogen going into the cell and sodium coming out of the cell, further reducing the serum potassium concentration.

Potassium replacement must be performed aggressively but cautiously since hyperkalemia can develop in a patient who still has poor renal perfusion. The ECG and the serum potassium levels must be monitored closely.

MONITORING AND LABORATORY TESTS

The patient's vital signs, including systemic arterial blood pressure, pulse rate, and respiratory rate, must be monitored constantly during the initial phase of DKA (Table 54-1). Values for these variables must be recorded on the flow sheet every hour and more frequently if the patient is unstable. The neurologic status must be monitored continuously since the most common complication in these individuals (and the most common cause of death) is cerebral edema. The patient must be monitored for signs of increased ICP as would any patient with a cerebral injury (see Chapter 7), and the patient's volume status must be monitored on a continuous basis by observing pulse rate, systemic arterial blood pressure, peripheral perfusion, and urinary output. All fluids administered must be meticulously recorded.

TREATMENT (Table 54-2)
Insulin Therapy

Although many types of therapy have been proposed for managing ketoacidosis, I prefer the use of the low-dose constant infusion of insulin. The use of a bolus of regular insulin at the start of low-dose constant infusion therapy has not significantly decreased the length of time for correction of DKA.

The IV insulin infusion must be started immediately with regular insulin given initially at a dose of 0.1 unit/kg/hr, diluting 50 units of regular insulin in 250 ml of 0.9% sodium chloride solution, and administering via a calibrated, continuous infusion pump. This solution must be changed every 8 to 12 hours. Monitoring the blood glucose will reveal whether or not the insulin infusion needs to be increased. Ideally, the blood glucose should fall between 50 and 100 mg/dl/hr. Blood pH determination should also show a significant improvement. In the absence of these results the insulin infusion should be increased, first to 0.15 unit/kg/hr and then to 0.2

unit/kg/hr. Roughly 95% of patients will respond to an infusion of 0.1 unit/kg/hr. Once the plasma acetone becomes undetectable, subcutaneous regular insulin can be used. The first dose is given 30 minutes before the cessation of the infusion. The time of the day will indicate the precise strategy for this procedure. If the patient's serum acetone becomes negative between midnight and 7 A.M., it may be more convenient to maintain an infusion and to continue to monitor the glucose throughout that time period by continuing the infusion rate at approximately one half the previous rate (i.e., approximately 0.05 unit/kg/hr) and providing glucose at a rate of 3 to 4 g per unit of insulin given. If the infusion is discontinued close to mealtime, 0.2 unit/kg of regular insulin should be administered before the meal and 0.1 unit/kg before a snack. To that regimen should be added a sliding scale of 1 unit of regular insulin for every 30 to 50 mg/dl of blood glucose >180 mg/dl. In a previously diagnosed diabetic patient for whom a prior dosage of NPH and/or regular insulin is known,

the previous insulin doses may be given before breakfast and supper and the patient placed on his old insulin regimen.

Fluid Therapy

Fluid therapy has four different components: (1) correction of acute vascular depletion, (2) provision of fluids for correction of dehydration, (3) provision of maintenance fluids, and (4) fluids for replacing continuing losses.

A patient who presents with vascular instability needs to receive a minimum of 20 ml/kg of 0.9% sodium chloride solution as rapidly as it can be infused, and this infusion may be followed by an additional dose of the same volume if there is not an adequate vascular response to the primary infusion. An adequate response is judged by a decrease in heart rate, increase in systemic arterial blood pressure, increase in CVP, and improved perfusion. Colloid solution may be used (see Chapter 12) if some degree of vascular stability is not obtained with the rapid

Table 54-1   Monitoring Plan

	Bedside				
	Vital Signs*	Neurologic Signs	Urinary Output	Chemstrip	Urine Sugar/ Acetone
First 8 hr	Continuous or q 30 min	q 30 min	q 1 hr	q 1 hr	q 1 hr
Second 8 hr	q 1 hr	q 1 hr	q 1 hr	q 1 hr	
Third 8 hr	q 1 hr	q 1 hr	q 1 hr	q 1 hr	

	Chemistry Laboratory					
	A/VBG	Acetone or β-OHB	Blood Glucose	Electrolytes	C/Phos	BUN/Creatinine
If initial pH is <7.15						
First 8 hr	q 1 hr	q 1 hr	q 1 hr	q 2 hr	q 4 hr	q 4 hr
If initial pH is >7.15						
First 8 hr	q 2 hr	q 2 hr	q 2 hr	q 2 hr	q 4 hr	q 4 hr
Second 8 hr	q 2 hr	q 2 hr	q 2 hr	q 4 hr	q 4 hr	q 4 hr
Third 8 hr	q 4 hr	q 4 hr	q 2 hr	q 4 hr	q 4 hr	q 8 hr

A/VBG = arterial/venous blood gas; β-OHB = beta-hydroxybutyric acid; C/Phos = calcium/phosphorus.
*If vascular instability is present, place central venous catheter for constant monitoring until patient stabilizes.

LABORATORY STUDIES FOR PATIENTS WITH DKA

Initial tests

Blood glucose
Plasma acetone
Serum beta-hydroxybutyric acid
Blood gases and pH
Serum electrolytes
Serum calcium and phosphorus
BUN
Serum creatinine

If the patient's pH is <7.15

Hourly
    Blood glucose (in addition to Chemstrip or Accu-
        check at bedside)
    Plasma venous blood gases and pH
    Urinary glucose and acetone
Every 2 hr
    Serum electrolytes
Every 4 hr
    Serum calcium and phosphorus

If the patient's pH is >7.15

Every 2 hr
    Serum glucose
    Plasma ketoacids (acetone, beta-hydroxybutyric
        acid)
    Blood gases and pH
    Serum electrolytes
Every 4 hr
    Serum calcium and phosphorus
Once the patient's pH is >7.30 (twice)
    Discontinue blood gases and pH
Once the patient's plasma acetone is normal (twice)
    Discontinue plasma acetone measurements

Table 54-2   Treatment Plan

Fluids	Insulin, Glucose, Potassium	HCO_3

1. Correction of shock
  a. 10-20 ml/kg 0.9% NaCl push or
  b. Colloid solution, 5% albumin for hypotension
2. 10 ml/kg/hr 0.9% NaCl for next hour; calculate maintenance and replacement
3. 1.5 × normal maintenance + one half of replacement in first 8 hr
4. 1.5 × normal maintenance + one half of replacement in next 16 hr
	1. 0.1-0.25 U regular insulin/kg (optional)
	2. Infusion 0.1 U/kg/hr
	  a. Increase to 0.15 U/kg/hr if BS falls <50 mg/dl/hr or if pH fails to start to correct by 2-4 hr
	  b. Increase to 0.2 U/kg/hr if pH not responsive to above
	3. Add glucose at 3-4 g per unit of insulin if:
	  a. BS falls <300 mg/dl
	  b. BS falls 20 mOsm/L (360 mg/dl), even if BS still >300 mg/dl
	4. Add potassium to 2-4 mEq/dl fluids if:
	  a. K <5.5 mEq/L and patient is not anuric
	  b. When glucose is added
	  c. If PO_4 <3.0 mg/dl (all as potassium phosphate)
	  d. If PO_4 >3.0 mg/dl (one half as potassium phosphate, one half as potassium chloride)
		1. If initial pH >7.1—no HCO_3
		2. If initial pH <7.1, 1 mEq/kg over 20 min
		3. Repeat if pH not >7.10

BS = blood sugar.

infusion of 20 ml/kg of 0.9% sodium chloride solution. The 0.9% sodium chloride solution can be continued at a rate of 10 ml/kg/hr for the next hour.

Next, precise maintenance and replacement fluids must be calculated. The patient needs to receive at least one and one half times the normal maintenance fluids. The patient's percent of dehydration must be estimated (the usual patient in DKA is approximately 7% to 10% dehydrated on presentation), calculating the percent dehydration at 8%. To obtain the appropriate rate of delivery of fluids, one and one half of the maintenance fluids plus half of the planned correction for dehydration must be administered in the first 8 hours. In the following 16 hours one and one half of maintenance amount should be continued, plus the remaining half of correction for dehydration. Monitoring for vascular stability must be done continuously to assess the success of fluid replacement therapy.

Glucose and potassium must be started as indicated by measured laboratory values. If the patient's potassium level is low on admission, potassium must be added when this information is known. If the serum potassium level is <5.5 mEq/L on admission, potassium should be added approximately 2 hours after starting treatment. The patient needs to receive 2 to 4 mEq/dl of solution delivered. If the serum phosphate level is normal, this solution can be half potassium phosphate and half potassium chloride. If the serum phosphate level is low, the solution must initially be potassium phosphate only.

Glucose is started when the blood glucose drops to approximately 300 mg/dl. However, in patients who have extremely high blood glucose values, glucose administration may be started at a higher level. For example, a fall of 20 mOsm (or 360 mg/dl), even if the glucose level is well above 300 mg/dl, is an indication for starting a glucose-containing solution. Glucose is normally started approximately 2 to 4 hours after the onset of therapy. It is extremely unusual to wait more than 4 hours after the initiation of insulin therapy to start glucose.

The initial glucose/insulin ratio is usually 3 to 4 g of glucose for every unit of insulin administered. The glucose/insulin ratio must be titrated so that the rate of decrease in blood sugar is not too rapid and the patient does not become hypoglycemic during the course of therapy. If the serum glucose drops too rapidly with no improvement in the degree of ketoacidosis, then the amount of both glucose and insulin delivered must be increased. If the rate of glucose drops precipitously at a point when the serum pH and plasma acetone are significantly improving, the glucose infusion may be increased and the insulin infusion decreased. If the serum glucose level is increasing at a point at which the plasma acetone level is decreasing and the pH is increasing, the rate of glucose administration must be decreased.

In the latter stage of the recovery phase from DKA, it is sometimes forgotten that insulin has a short half-life of less than 5 minutes. Thus subcutaneous insulin therapy must be begun approximately 30 minutes before an insulin infusion is stopped. If this is not done, an increase in blood glucose and a recurrence of ketosis are common occurrences.

ADDITIONAL READING

Foster DW, McGarry JD. The metabolic derangements and treatment of diabetic ketoacidosis. N Engl J Med 309:159-169, 1983.

Lightner ES, Kappy MS, Revsin B. Low-dose intravenous insulin infusion in patients with diabetic ketoacidosis: Biochemical effects in children. Pediatric 60:681-688, 1977.

Perkin RM, Marks JF. Low-dose continuous intravenous insulin infusion in childhood diabetic ketoacidosis. Clin Pediatr 18:540-548, 1979.

55 Acute Adrenocortical Insufficiency

James F. Marks

BACKGROUND AND PHYSIOLOGY

Acute adrenocortical insufficiency is occasionally seen in pediatric patients. Two specific types are of interest. The first type, by far the most common in infants, is the salt-losing form of 21-hydroxylase congenital adrenal hyperplasia. The second type of insufficiency occurs in older children. Its most common cause is "idiopathic" Addison's disease, sometimes associated with other endocrinopathies and currently believed to occur most commonly in association with an autoimmune disorder. Less common causes are congenital adrenal hypoplasia, acute infection, hemorrhage into the adrenal glands, inadequate replacement of adrenal corticoid therapy after surgery for removal of adrenal neoplasms, and inappropriate tapering of corticosteroids in children who have received long-term adrenal steroid therapy.

The underlying cause for sodium depletion in patients with 21-hydroxylase deficiency is still a matter of debate. Several different mechanisms have been suggested: (1) a deficiency in the formation of both aldosterone and hydrocortisone; (2) competitive inhibition of the action of aldosterone at the distal tubular site in the kidney, believed to be due to the production of metabolites such as 17-hydroxyprogesterone; or (3) a concept elucidated by New is that the glomerulosa and fasiculata of the adrenal gland behave as separate organs, with those patients who have the non-salt-losing form defective in the fasciculi only and not in the glomerulosa. Although these hypotheses are still debated, the resulting hormonal abnormalities lead to hyperkalemia, hyponatremia, acidosis, and hypoglycemia. Approximately two thirds of children with 21-hydroxylase deficiency have the salt-losing form, which will be clinically most severe in the first 2 years of life. One uncommon syndrome that mimics salt-losing congenital adrenal hyperplasia is pseudohypoaldosteronism, in which there is a defect at the aldosterone receptor site.

For the usual infant with the salt-losing form of congenital adrenal hyperplasia, dehydration and signs of acute and chronic hypovolemia, with and without peripheral vascular collapse, will appear sometime between the third and twenty-eighth day of life. Uncommonly such signs may appear as late as 3 to 4 months of age. Although male infants with this condition have normal external genitalia, female infants with this condition have ambiguous external genitalia because of excessive androgen production resulting from the response to the pituitary feedback, which stimulates the adrenal cortex because of the 21-hydroxylase deficiency. Of the initial cases in a given family, 60% of the patients seen are female. In a disease with autosomal-recessive inheritance, this percentage suggests that a substantial proportion of male infants with congenital adrenal hyperplasia are being missed.

In the recent past data have been accumulated regarding the genetics of congenital adrenal hyperplasia. Analysis of the work of many groups around the world indicates that the classic form of congenital adrenal hyperplasia and a new, previously unrecognized cryptic form are associated with human lymphocyte antigen (specifically HLA-B and HLA-DR) abnormalities, thus locating the genetic locus for this disease on the sixth chromosome in the immune region. Subsequent work has resulted in the elucidation of the structure of the gene. Patients with the classic 21-hydroxylase deficiency, with and without salt loss, have the same genetic abnormality, whereas patients with the cryptic form have a separate genetic abnormality but at the same locus. This is analogous to patients with hemoglobin S and C diseases.

MONITORING AND LABORATORY TESTS
(Tables 55-1 and 55-2)

The patient's vital signs, including systemic arterial blood pressure, heart rate, respiratory rate, and temperature, must be monitored hourly until he is stable. Patients may be hypothermic and also in peripheral vascular collapse.

The ECG must be monitored continuously since hyperkalemia can cause severe ventricular dysrhythmias. In patients who do not respond to the first two fluid challenges with an increase in systemic arterial blood pressure, peripheral perfusion, and urinary output, a central venous catheter should be placed to monitor central venous blood pressure.

Serum and urinary electrolyte (Na, K, Cl, HCO_3) values must be obtained initially, followed by serum electrolyte values at 4-hour intervals for the first 24 hours of management. Blood must be obtained for 17-hydroxyprogesterone and plasma renin studies. Obtaining 24-hour urine specimens for determination of 17-ketosteroids is not practical in children with vascular instability. The 17-hydroxyprogesterone study has been shown to be a reliable diagnostic technique for use in infants acutely ill with congenital adrenal hyperplasia.

In older children who have primary Addison's disease the initial level of serum cortisol and ACTH should be determined. In patients with primary (adrenal glandular) adrenal insufficiency the cortisol level will be low and the ACTH level will be extremely high. Usually time is not available in these circumstances to do an ACTH stimulation test.

TREATMENT (Table 55-3)
Endocrine Therapy

The aim of endocrine treatment is to replace the missing adrenocorticosteroids. It is necessary to continue acute therapy until replacement is sufficient to maintain the patient's stability.

Glucocorticoid replacement. An initial dose of glucocorticoid, specifically hydrocortisone sodium succinate, is initially administered by IV push (60 to 80 mg/m²). The initial dose must be no less than 25 mg in an infant and no more than a 100 mg in an older child. This dose can be repeated if there is inadequate initial response as judged by systemic arterial blood pressure and urinary output.

Glucocorticoid Equivalency	
Cortisone	25 mg
Hydrocortisone	20 mg
Prednisone	5 mg
Prednisolone	5 mg
Methylprednisolone	4 mg
Triamcinolone	4 mg
Dexamethasone	0.7 mg

Cortisone acetate, 60 mg/m², is administered IM as a repository dose of glucocorticoid at the same time as the initial treatment. The half-life of cortisone acetate is approximately 24 hours, and its duration of action could be up to 2 to 3 days. One third to one half of the initial dose of hydrocortisone sodium succinate is given every 4 hours for three doses, by which time the cortisone acetate should be effectively absorbed. The half-life of hydrocortisone sodium succinate is approximately 60 to 90 minutes, and its duration of action is approximately 4 hours.

On the second day of treatment cortisone acetate, 30 mg/m² IM, can can be given. It is usual to continue this dosage for 2 additional days and then change to oral hydrocortisone, 16 mg/m² divided into two to three daily doses.

Mineralocorticoid replacement. Previously the recommendation was to give mineralocorticoid replacement as IM aqueous deoxycorticosterone acetate. Unfortunately this drug has been withdrawn from the market so it is no longer available. The current recommendation is to give fludrocortisone acetate (Florinef), 0.05 to 0.2 mg daily orally, starting as soon as the patient is no longer vomiting and is able to retain oral fluids. The mineralocorticoid effect of administered hydrocortisone and the administration of IV saline solution are needed to help control hyponatremia and hyperkalemia until the fludrocortisone acetate is working.

General Therapy

Body temperature must be maintained in a neutral thermal environment to minimize oxygen consumption and maintain blood sugar levels greater than 60 mg/dl (use hourly Accucheck monitoring). Hypovolemia, hyponatremia, and hyperkalemia are cor-

Table 55-1 Monitoring Child with Addison's Disease

	Clinical Vital Signs	ECG	Chemstrip	Hormonal		
				Glucose	Cortisol	ACTH
First 12 hr	q 1 hr*	Continuous	q 1 hr	q 4 hr	Onset of treatment	Onset of treatment
Second 12 hr	q 2 hr	Continuous	q 2 hr	q 8 hr		
Second 24 hr	q 4 hr		q 4 hr	q 12 hr		

*CVP may be needed while patient's condition is unstable.

Table 55-2 Monitoring Patient with 21-Hydroxylase Congenital Adrenal Hyperplasia

	Clinical Vital Signs	ECG	Laboratory Electrolytes	Hormonal		Plasma Renin
				Glucose	17-Hydroxy-progesterone	
First 12 hr	q 1 hr*	Continuous	q 4 hr	q 4 hr (laboratory) q 1 hr (Chemstrip)	Onset of treatment	Onset of treatment
Second 12 hr	q 2 hr	Continuous	q 4 hr	q 4 hr (laboratory) q 1 hr (Chemstrip)		
Second 24 hr	q 4 hr		q 12 hr	q 12 hr (laboratory) q 2 hr (Chemstrip)		

*CVP may be needed while patient's condition is acutely unstable.

Table 55-3 Treatment

Fluids	Corticosteroids	
Onset—NaCl, 20 ml/kg IV push	Hydrocortisone sodium succinate— 60-80 mg/m^2 IV push (not less than 25 mg), then one third of initial dose q 4 hr × 3	Cortisone acetate—60 mg/m^2 IM
First 8 hr—0.9% NaCl with 5% dextrose (one third maintenance rate plus one half replacement rate)		
8-24 hr—0.9 NaCl with 5% dextrose (two thirds maintenance rate plus one half replacement rate)*		
Second 24 hr—0.9% or 0.45 NaCl with 5% dextrose (maintenance rate)*		Cortisone acetate—30 mg/m^2 IM

*May be decreased to 0.45% NaCl plus D 5% when Na ≥135 mEq/L.

rected in the following manner. Administer 0.9% sodium chloride solution with 5% glucose, initially giving 20 ml/kg over the first 20 minutes to correct acute volume depletion. Continue with 0.9% sodium chloride solution with 5% dextrose solution; the necessary volume is one third of maintenance plus replacement of 10% of body weight during the first 8 hours. The patient should be assessed at 4-hour intervals to determine if 10% replacement will be adequate and to adjust fluid for ongoing needs (see Chapter 15). Continue administering 0.9% sodium chloride solution with 5% glucose until the serum sodium level is >135 mEq/L; then change to 0.45% sodium chloride solution with 5% glucose.

The IV fluid should be potassium free for the first 24 hours unless the serum potassium level drops below 3 mEq/L. When signs of hyperkalemic electrocardiographic toxicity exists, administer sodium polystyrene sulfonate (Kayexalate) as indicated in Chapter 14. Use sodium bicarbonate at a rate of 1 mEq/kg/min IV to correct signs of cardiotoxicity until the effect of the sodium polystyrene sulfonate is observed, and repeat as necessary for treating elevated serum potassium levels and signs of cardiotoxicity.

When acute episodes are controlled, usually on the second day of therapy, continue to administer 0.45% sodium chloride solution with dextrose. Usually the institution of oral fluids will allow adequate potassium intake without resorting to administration of IV potassium. Once oral feedings are instituted, the patient can be started on formula as tolerated. It may be necessary to add 1.5 to 3 g of sodium a day to the patient's feedings. In the older child who has adrenal insufficiency secondary to an acute episode of Addison's disease, oral feedings can be restarted as soon as tolerated. Supplementary sodium may be needed in the child's diet, depending on the size and age of the patient.

Perioperative Considerations

Monitoring. The patient's preoperative vital signs and serum electrolyte and blood sugar levels are obtained to establish a baseline for the postoperative period. The patient must have his vital signs monitored every hour postoperatively for the first 8 hours, every 2 hours for the second 8 hours, and every 4 hours thereafter. Serum electrolyte and blood sugar levels should be determined every 4 hours for the first 8 hours and every 8 hours for the remainder of the 24 hours. For those patients who are to have nothing by mouth for a prolonged time period, serum electrolyte levels should be determined every 12 hours until they are receiving oral feedings; similarly, their vital signs must be monitored every 2 to every 4 hours, depending on their other clinical needs.

Steroid therapy. Cortisone acetate, 60 mg/m², is administered IM 12 hours before surgery. At this dose a high steroid level will be provided just before and during the induction of anesthesia, which are the periods of maximal stress normally associated with high levels of circulating endogenous steroid. Cortisone acetate, 30 mg/m² IM, is given with the preoperative medications to produce a peak steroid level during the postoperative period. These dosages have been chosen because prior studies have shown that a surgical patient who is undergoing general anesthesia and a major surgical procedure and who has normal adrenal corticoid function will produce four to eight times his maintenance amount of daily steroids (or 12 mg/m² of cortisone). Serum electrolyte and fluid imbalances must be monitored and corrected vigorously, and 0.9% sodium chloride solution with 5% glucose must be administered during the procedure. During a prolonged procedure 50 mg of hydrocortisone sodium succinate is given continuously during every 3-hour interval. Postoperatively 5% glucose with 0.45% sodium chloride solution is given if serum electrolyte levels remain abnormal. In emergency surgery patients need to receive 60 mg/m² of hydrocortisone sodium succinate immediately before surgery and 50 mg of hydrocortisone sodium succinate in the intraoperative IV fluids given continuously for every 3-hour period of surgery. The minimal dose of preoperative hydrocortisone sodium succinate should never be less than 25 mg in an infant or 50 mg in a young child. In progressively more complicated cases higher doses of steroids may be needed. IM cortisone acetate must be continued until the infant or child is able to take oral steroids, with 30 mg/m² administered every 24 hours in the postoperative period. Because deoxycorticosterone acetate is no longer available, sodium balance must be maintained through the mineralocorticoid effect from cortisone and hydrocortisone and IV sodium solutions. Frequent reassessment of the patient for signs and symptoms of adrenal insufficiency is necessary, and replacement of steroids is to be increased if necessary. Perioperatively the patient must be monitored as indicated above.

ADDITIONAL READING

New MI, Dupont B, Grumbach K, Levine LS. Congenital adrenal hyperplasia and related conditions. In Stanbury JB, Wyngaarden JB, Fredrickson DS, Goldstein JL, Brown MS, eds. The Metabolic Basis of Inherited Disease. New York: McGraw-Hill, 1983.

56 Thyrotoxic Crisis and Sick Thyroid Syndrome

James F. Marks

BACKGROUND AND PHYSIOLOGY

Thyrotoxicosis is uncommon in children, and probably less than 2% of all cases of thyrotoxicosis are initially seen before the patient is 15 years of age. Although there are multiple causes of thyrotoxicosis, the most common cause in children is Graves' disease. Another cause is the thyrotoxic phase of Hashimoto's disease (autoimmune thyroiditis). Rarely seen in children are several types that occur more commonly in adults (e.g., toxic nodular goiter, pituitary TSH-secreting adenomas, hyperthyroidism secondary to hydatidiform mole or choriocarcinoma).

The symptoms of hyperthyroidism arise from the excess of circulating thyroid hormone and the physiologic effects related to such an excess. An acute exacerbation of the thyrotoxicosis (thyroid storm) represents a life-threatening exaggeration of signs and symptoms of hyperthyroidism, specifically cardiac and CNS involvement. Thyrotoxic crisis cannot be separated from hyperthyroidism on the basis of laboratory studies but is diagnosed by clinical manifestations that are quite variable. A sign that suggests a patient is exhibiting a thyroid storm is a hypermetabolic state of unknown cause with symptoms such as extreme tachycardia, tachypnea, cardiac failure associated with hypertension and wide pulse pressure, profound hyperthermia of 40° to 42° C, nausea, vomiting, and diarrhea with dehydration, delirium, acute psychotic behavior, and coma. Thyroid storm left untreated can be fatal. On some rare occasions one may see an apathetic thyroid crisis in which a patient may be extremely lethargic rather than obviously agitated. Among the inciting events for thyrotoxic storm that occurs in a patient who is either undiagnosed or incompletely diagnosed are inappropriately timed surgery, abrupt withdrawal of antithyroid medication, acute severe infection, acute trauma, and other organ dysfunction such as diabetic ketoacidosis.

MONITORING AND LABORATORY TESTS

Vital signs, including systemic arterial blood pressure, heart rate, respiratory rate, and temperature must be obtained hourly in the initial acute phase of disease. As a patient becomes less acutely ill over the first 24 hours, the frequency may be decreased.

Endocrine studies, including serum thyroxine, triiodothyronine, and thyroid-stimulating hormone, must be performed and repeated as often as needed until a steady state has been reached. Steady state is defined as levels of pulse, respiration, systemic arterial blood pressure, and temperature that are safe for the patient. The patient may leave the PICU when he is no longer in danger of cardiovascular decompensation.

TREATMENT

Several levels of therapy are available for the patient with hyperthyroidism, including destruction of the thyroid gland by surgery or radiation (^{131}I), pharmacologic suppression of synthesis or release of thyroid hormone, and counteraction of related autonomic nervous system problems.

Therapy is directed first at diagnosis and treatment of any underlying illness or precipitating factor. General organ systems support (e.g., airway, ventilation) must be provided and steps taken to reduce the production and secretion of thyroid hormone and to diminish its metabolic effects (e.g., decrease temperature, nausea, vomiting, dehydration). If any surgery has been scheduled, it is to be canceled. The medication history or noncompliance in a known patient with thyrotoxicosis must be determined, as must a history of exogenous administration of thyroxine with no known prior history of thyroid disease.

Fluid replacement must be through the IV route. The use of aspirin is contraindicated in control of fever, so physical means must be used (see Chapter 21). Appropriate cultures must be obtained and antibiotics started if infection is suspected. The production and release of thyroid hormone must be reduced. Propylthiouracil can be given in maximum doses up to 1.2 g/24 hr (15 mg/kg in three to four divided doses) orally or by nasogastric tube to block thyroid synthesis. It will also inhibit extrathyroidal or peripheral conversion of thyroxine to its most active form (triiodothyronine). One hour after giving propylthiouracil administer a form of sodium or potassium iodide that blocks release of preformed hormone. Lugol's iodine solution, 500 mg orally every 6 hours or by tube, would be preferable. IV forms of sodium or potassium iodide are no longer available. Treatment of the effects of the pathophysiologic results of increased thyroid hormone secretion include starting beta blockade with propranolol (Inderal). A loading dose of 1 to 3 mg IV in increments of 0.5 mg every 1 minute may be given. The IV injection should be stopped when either the heart rate is normal for age or the maximum dose has been given. Then an oral maintenance therapy regimen of 2 mg/kg/day, divided into three or four doses, is started. Propranolol is contraindicated in patients with limited cardiac reserve, heart block, atrial flutter, or bronchospasm. Because propranolol may mask the symptoms of hypoglycemia, diabetic patients must have serum glucose measurements monitored, which can be done effectively using bedside glucose monitoring. Symptomatic bradycardia can be reversed with the use of atropine, 0.01 mg/kg IV or SC.

Corticosteroids have been used since they may possibly block peripheral conversion of thyroxine, and increased survival has been reported with their use. Prednisone, 2 mg/kg/24 hr orally; prednisolone, 2 mg/kg/24 hr IM or IV; or hydrocortisone, 3 to 7 mg/kg IV, may be administered every 4 to 6 hours for 24 to 48 hours.

ADDITIONAL READING

Ingbar SH. The thyroid gland. In Wilson JD, Foster DW, eds. Williams Textbook of Endocrinology, 7th ed. Philadelphia: WB Saunders, 1985.

57 Syndrome of Inappropriate Antidiuretic Hormone Secretion

James F. Marks · Billy S. Arant, Jr.

BACKGROUND AND PHYSIOLOGY

Antidiuretic hormone (ADH), or arginine vasopressin, is a neurohypophysial peptide that alters the permeability of the urinary collecting system to water and allows water to move into the extracellular compartment, thus concentrating urine.

Either a decrease in effective arterial blood volume (EABV) or a rise in plasma osmolarity will evoke release of ADH in healthy individuals. When ADH is secreted in the perceived absence of any stimulus, the condition is referred to as the syndrome of inappropriate ADH secretion (SIADH). Patients who manifest this clinical condition recover water from the renal collection tubule in excess of that needed to maintain euvolemia or normal tonicity of body fluids. The first evidence of the problem is an unexplained decrease in urinary volume associated with a gain in body weight. With continued fluid intake that is not excreted into the urine, plasma osmolarity gradually decreases and the EABV increases; under normal circumstances either of these stimuli would inhibit the further release of ADH. The expanded EABV will inhibit hormonal and nonhormonal mechanisms of renal tubular reabsorption of sodium. The urinary sodium concentration increases as less filtered sodium is reabsorbed along the nephron and as more water is reabsorbed from tubular fluid reaching the ADH-sensitive portion of the distal nephron; the fractional excretion of sodium (FE_{Na}), if calculated, will be >1%. When no ADH is released from the hypothalamus (e.g., in patients with central diabetes insipidus), the urinary osmolarity is reduced to the kidney's maximal diluting capacity (i.e., <50 mOsm/L [specific gravity, 1.001]). Any osmolarity >50 mOsm/L when body fluids are hypotonic (osmolarity <270) is *inappropriate*.

The diagnosis of SIADH can be made earliest when a patient considered at clinical risk for the problem exhibits a fall in urinary volume associated with an acute gain in body weight and received fluid intake is no greater than a maintenance volume. SIADH can be differentiated from other causes of oliguria by the rise in urinary osmolarity (or specific gravity) and by a decrease in BUN and plasma sodium concentration that parallels the decrease in plasma osmolarity. If one waits for hyponatremia to develop before suspecting the diagnosis of SIADH, the risk to the patient is greater, and the clinical management must be more aggressive.

SIADH occurs more commonly in children as an acute and self-limited event that may last only hours or continue for days. Any disturbance of the CNS (e.g., infection, hemorrhage, neurosurgical procedure, increased ICP, head trauma) can be associated with SIADH. Moreover, any change in intrathoracic hemodynamics that reduces cardiac output or EABV (most often seen in patients treated by mechanical ventilation) can cause a baroreceptor-mediated release of ADH and a condition that cannot be distinguished from SIADH. In adults SIADH may be associated with tumors that secrete an ADH-like substance.

There are several conditions in which hyponatremic events may mimic SIADH, including Addison's disease, myxedema, and hypopituitarism. In patients with myxedema the most likely cause is reduced renal perfusion rather than an excess secretion of vasopressin. Other mimickers of SIADH include a postanesthetic, apparently inappropriate vasopressin response, cardiac failure, and hypoproteinemia of various types. However, it has not been proved that vasopressin is present in inappropriately large amounts in patients with these syndromes, and such children tend to conserve rather than lose sodium as do children with SIADH (see Chapter 15).

MONITORING AND LABORATORY TESTS

The vital signs, including systemic arterial blood pressure, heart rate, and respiratory rate, should be recorded every 4 hours. Intake and output must be monitored closely. Measurements of serum and urinary osmolarities and concentrations of sodium, potassium, plus chloride must be simultaneously obtained initially and every 4 to 6 hours. The patient must be weighed twice daily and observed frequently for mental status changes.

TREATMENT

Since the pathophysiologic consequence of SIADH is excess body water, the only treatment is reduction of total body water. Anticipatory treatment of patients at risk for developing SIADH can be done best by calculating fluid therapy based only on insensible water loss and previous urinary volume plus other losses (e.g., nasogastric tube, chest tube, wound) instead of some arbitrary predetermined volume based on healthy individuals who can excrete any excess water as a dilute urine. In patients with obvious SIADH at the time of the first examination, further fluid intake must be restricted to only the minimum volume needed for administering medications or nutrition. Insensible water losses will augment the reduction in body water excess. Thirst in conscious patients with SIADH is unusual because the increased EABV inhibits renin release, and angiotensin II is, perhaps, the most important stimulus to thirst in a patient with hypotonic body fluid. When plasma os-

molarity has increased to >270 mOsm/L, fluid therapy can be prescribed based on insensible water loss plus urinary volume plus other losses.

Clinical management is facilitated when any factor contributing to SIADH can be reduced or removed (e.g., increase cardiac output, lower positive pressure settings for assisted ventilation, reduce intracranial pressure).

Hyponatremia and hypochloremia do not represent a reduction of total body sodium chloride, just its dilution by excess water in the extracellular fluid compartment. Additional sodium chloride administration is not necessary unless fluid restriction sufficient to prevent further weight gain is associated with a continued decrease in plasma sodium concentration. When plasma sodium concentration is decreased to <120 mEq/L, the risk of seizure activity increases. In the event of seizure activity treatment with hypertonic sodium chloride solution must be given. Usually an amount calculated to raise the plasma sodium concentration to 120 mEq/L is adequate to control seizure activity, that is, plasma Na^+ 120 − plasma Na^+ actual times body weight in kilograms times 0.6 equals mEq Na^+ needed to raise plasma sodium concentration to 120 mEq/L; half this amount can be infused rapidly over 5 to 10 minutes and the remainder given over the next 2 hours (see Chapter 15).

Although lithium carbonate and demethoxytetracycline have been used for treating chronic SIADH in adults, they are not indicated for the acute, self-limited situations seen in the PICU.

Recovery from SIADH is heralded by diuresis, urinary dilution, fall in body weight, and an increase in plasma osmolarity and sodium concentrations.

ADDITIONAL READING

Culpepper RM, Hekect SC, Andreoli TE. The posterior pituitary and water metabolism. In Wilson JD, Foster DW, eds. Williams Textbook of Endocrinology, 7th ed. Philadelphia: WB Saunders, 1985.

58 Central Diabetes Insipidus

James F. Marks · Billy S. Arant, Jr.

BACKGROUND AND PHYSIOLOGY

The failure of synthesis and/or release of arginine vasopressin from the hypothalamus or the posterior pituitary gland results in diabetes insipidus. Since the kidney is unable to conserve water in the absence of vasopressin, polyuria and polydipsia ensue. In the nonstressed state most children with intact thirst mechanisms are able to maintain their water requirements by ingesting large volumes of fluids.

Factors such as altered consciousness or stress that prevent children from voluntarily meeting these needs will result in the children's admission to the PICU for care. There are two groups of children in whom diabetes insipidus is encountered in the PICU. In the first group are children who have undergone neurosurgical procedures. Some will have had diabetes insipidus before surgery; however, others will develop this condition postoperatively. The best-known surgical cause for central diabetes insipidus of children is the resection of a craniopharyngioma. The second group includes children who develop the condition after head trauma or CNS infection.

The postoperative clinical course of children whose urinary concentrating mechanism is normal preoperatively but who develop diabetes insipidus postoperatively follows a biphasic or triphasic pattern. The polyuria is first observed within hours after surgery, and it may last 2 to 3 days. A 2- or 3-day period follows during which there is a decrease in urinary output because of a release of residual vasopressin. This period is usually followed by the onset of permanent diabetes insipidus. It is not uncommon for children with diabetes insipidus with postoperative onset to void as much as 200 to 300 ml/hr and develop hypovolemic shock. Because the volume deficit is water alone and because sodium is conserved maximally by the kidney in response to a decreased effective arterial blood volume, the degree to which hypernatremia and hyperosmolality develop is related to the water deficit.

MONITORING AND LABORATORY TESTS

Vital signs must be monitored hourly and body weight recorded every 12 hours. Placement of a central venous catheter is useful in following central venous blood pressure to plan fluid therapy more accurately. Fluid intake and urinary output must be monitored hourly or more often when urinary volume is large and the patient is hemodynamically unstable. Serum osmolality or electrolyte values must be measured initially and every hour until the patient is stable. The urinary specific gravity must be recorded at the bedside every hour after desmopressin complex (DDAVP) treatment is initiated. Blood sugar determinations must be obtained every 4 hours. The neurologic status of the patient must be carefully monitored (see Chapter 4).

TREATMENT
Fluid Therapy

If the patient is hypovolemic, 0.45% sodium chloride solution in 2.5% dextrose, 20 ml/kg IV, is administered over 10 to 20 minutes initially to correct acute volume depletion. While a response to vasopressin is awaited, the volume of fluids administered must equal urinary volume. After shock is corrected, solutions in which sodium concentration is no greater than 15 mEq/L can be used. As the effect of desmopressin treatment is seen (decreased urinary volume and increased urinary specific gravity), the rate of the IV infusion must be decreased. Failure to do so will cause rapid volume overload plus symptomatic hyponatremia. IV glucose must be regulated so that excessive glycosuria does not occur, having no glycosuria is preferred.

Hormonal Therapy

Desmopressin must be administered and can be given either intranasally or intravenously. In patients who have not had transsphenoidal neurosurgery the use of intranasal vasopressin will suffice. For patients who need to receive IV desmopressin, 0.025 μg/kg can be given up to a maximum dose of 1 μg per dose. Approximately 10 to 15 times this dose may be given intranasally.

The response in urinary volume in 15-minute intervals should be noted over the first hour and in hourly intervals thereafter. There should be an obvious response to the administration of the IV preparation in the first 15 to 30 minutes and to the administration of the intranasal preparation within 1 to 2 hours. IV fluids administered must be carefully adjusted, based on the urinary output once it starts to decline. If an appropriate fall in urinary output does not occur within 1 hour in a patient who has received IV therapy or within 2 hours in a patient given intranasal therapy, a larger dose must be given then or at some later time.

The patient needs to be on an NPO regimen until a satisfactory response to the initial management has been observed. Once it is apparent that an antidiuretic effect has been achieved, the patient must be monitored until urinary output increases again, indicating escape from the antidiuretic effect, thus establishing the time interval and the frequency with which medication must be given. In patients receiving intranasal desmopressin, this interval may be anywhere from 6 to 24 hours. A timed, repetitive order for desmopressin is not written until the duration of action has been firmly established in a particular patient. The dose established in the postoperative period for patients receiving intranasal desmopressin will usually be the long-term dose needed by the patient. In those patients in whom IV desmopressin was needed a new intranasal dose for chronic therapy must be established as indicated above. In those patients who have a triphasic pattern (i.e., patients who, 2 to 4 days after surgery, apparently use the residual hypothalamic vasopressin), a second duration of action period must be reestablished for an antidiuretic medication after the triphasic phase is over.

ADDITIONAL READING

Culpepper RM, Hekect SC, Andreoli TE. The posterior pituitary and water metabolism. In Wilson JD, Foster DW, eds. Williams Textbook of Endocrinology, 7th ed. Philadelphia: WB Saunders, 1985.

59 Anesthesia: Perioperative Principles

Frances C. Morriss

BACKGROUND

Anesthesia is a necessary concomitant of surgery, making it possible for a patient to undergo painful and often traumatic physical invasion without disruption of physiologic homeostasis or the occurrence of harmful side effects. This is accomplished by administration of potent pharmacologic agents that act either centrally or locally to produce analgesia. The ideal anesthetic agent would provide pain relief, muscle relaxation, amnesia, and obtundation of potentially harmful physiologic reflexes; in addition it would be inexpensive, easy to administer, and without harmful side effects for both the patient and operating room personnel.

Safe and rational use of anesthetics has become the basis for a specialized branch of medicine. The American Society of Anesthesiologists (ASA) delineated the areas of activity for the anesthesiologist; many of these concerns overlap with those of intensivists. In particular, monitoring (specifically for potential and expected problems based on the patient's health status) and procedures essential to good patient care throughout the perioperative period in the operating room, postanesthesia recovery unit (PARU), and the PICU are similar.

During the procedure the anesthesiologist is the patient's watchdog; he must oversee all aspects of patient care in conjunction with the surgeon and the nursing personnel. The more complex the procedure, the more preliminary communication that needs to take place among all caregivers to ensure a smooth, uneventful operation. Specific areas of concern include proper functioning of all equipment, proper anatomic positioning of the patient to prevent nerve or joint damage, compatibility of all pharmacologic agents—anesthetic and nonanesthetic—

with one another, maintenance of sterility and universal body fluid precautions, proper use of blood and blood products, and communication with the surgeon, particularly about problems or unexplained physiologic changes, throughout the case.

TECHNIQUES

Preanesthetic care. A basic standard for preanesthetic care as approved in 1987 by the ASA states the following:

I: An anesthesiologist shall be responsible for determining the medical status of the patient, developing a plan of anesthesia care, and acquainting that patient or the responsible adult with the proposed plan.

The development of an appropriate plan of anesthesia care is based upon:
1. Reviewing the medical record
2. Interviewing and examining the patient to:
   a. Discuss the medical history, previous anesthetic experience, and drug therapy
   b. Assess those aspects of the physical condition that might affect decisions regarding perioperative risk and management
3. Obtaining and/or reviewing tests and consultations necessary to the conduct of anesthesia
4. Determining the appropriate prescription of preoperative medications as necessary to the conduct of anesthesia

The responsible anesthesiologist shall verify that the above has been properly performed and documented in the patient's record.

To plan safe and effective anesthesia the anesthesiologist must be thoroughly informed about the patient's health status from a personal interview, chart review including laboratory and other diagnostic data, and physical examination. All anesthetics must be compatible with any existing disease processes so that these conditions are not exacerbated during surgery. If information is insufficient to establish a safe care plan and it is not an emergency procedure, appropriate laboratory, diagnostic, and consultative tests and interviews must be arranged. Every effort must be made to have the patient in the best physical and emotional condition possible before surgery.

Anesthetic agents. All anesthetic agents have physiologic actions that may be harmful or undesirable (Table 59-1). Some of these actions occur only in specific circumstances (e.g., in the presence of renal or hepatic failure) that must be identified preoperatively. Specifically, cardiorespiratory function, which is usually depressed by both inhalation and IV anesthetics, must be evaluated thoroughly as well as those systems involved with drug detoxification and metabolism (hepatic, renal, plasma, pulmonary). The differences between pediatric and adult physiology must be kept in mind (see Chapter 2). These differences are of critical importance in premature and newborn infants who may have immature or transitional organ systems. Unique physiologic characteristics of neonates that must be considered are listed in Table 59-2. Table 59-3 lists some of the more common problems encountered and the adaptations the anesthesiologist must make for these conditions.

ANESTHETIC RISKS

The relative risk of the procedure may be estimated from the ASA's physical status classification*:

P1   Normal, healthy individual
P2   Patient with mild systemic disease
P3   Patient with severe systemic disease
P4   Patient with severe systemic disease that is a constant threat to life
P5   Moribund patient who is not expected to survive without the operation
P6   A declared brain-dead patient whose organs are being removed for donor purposes
E   Emergency procedure

The higher the physical status class, the greater the chance that significant morbidity and mortality exist. Numerous studies show that difficulties encountered in class 1 or 2 patients are often the result of inattention, carelessness, or mishap. Patients in the higher classifications encounter problems related to their disease processes and experience a greater number of cardiac arrests. Although many of these problems are predictable based on the patient's pathophysiology, the pharmacology of anesthetic

---

*Modified from Relative Value Guide 1988. American Society of Anesthesiologists, 1988.

AMERICAN BOARD OF ANESTHESIOLOGY: DEFINITION OF SCOPE OF PRACTICE*

The American Board of Anesthesiology defines anesthesiology as a practice of medicine dealing with:

A. The provision of insensibility to pain during surgical, obstetric, therapeutic, and diagnostic procedures and the management of patients so affected.
B. The monitoring and restoration of homeostasis during the perioperative period, as well as homeostasis in the critically ill, injured, or otherwise seriously ill patient.
C. The diagnosis and treatment of painful syndromes.
D. The clinical management and teaching of cardiac and pulmonary resuscitation.
E. The evaluation of respiratory function and application of respiratory therapy in all of its forms.
F. The supervision, teaching, and evaluation of performance of both medical and paramedical personnel involved in anesthesia, respiratory, and critical care.
G. The conduct of research at the clinical and basic science levels to explain and improve the care of patients insofar as physiologic function and response to drugs are concerned.
H. The administrative involvement in hospitals, medical schools, and outpatient facilities necessary to implement these responsibilities.

*Modified from Miller R, ed. Anesthesia, 2nd ed. New York: Churchill Livingstone, 1986.

Table 59-1   Side Effects of Anesthetic Agents

Agents	Cardiac	Respiratory	Metabolic	Miscellaneous
Inhalation agents				
Halothane	Myocardial depression (negative inotropy) Dose-related myocardial sensitization to action of catecholamines Bradycardia Vasodilation, particularly of CNS	Inhibition of Hering-Breuer reflex leading to decreased minute ventilation and hypercarbia Dose-related reduction in ventilatory response to CO_2 Blunted ventilatory response to hypoxemia	Trigger for malignant hyperpyrexia Decreased hepatic blood flow Idiopathic hepatic reactions Shivering	Marked increase in cerebral blood flow
Isoflurane	Peripheral vasodilation Reactive tachycardia	Dose-related reduction in ventilatory response to CO_2 Blunted ventilatory response to hypoxemia	Shivering Trigger for malignant hyperpyrexia	
Nitrous oxide	Mild myocardial depression Pulmonary arterial spasm			Equilibrates with nitrogen in air-containing spaces with expansion of volume
Intravenous induction agents				
Ketamine	Centrally mediated tachycardia Hypertension (systemic and pulmonary) Direct mild myocardial depression	Increased airway secretions Obtundation of protective reflexes and mild respiratory depression Increased coughing Bronchodilation	Increased cerebral metabolic rate	Increased intracranial and intraocular pressure Postoperative hallucinations Purposeless movement CNS excitation seizures
Thiopental	Direct myocardial depression Hypotension from histamine release	Bronchospasm from histamine release Respiratory depression Potentiation of narcotic respiratory depression	Histamine release	No analgesia Myoclonic muscle movements
Local anesthetic agents				
	Direct myocardial depression Peripheral vasodilation			CNS excitation seizures CNS depression Tinnitus

Table 59-1   Side Effects of Anesthetic Agents—cont'd

Agents	Cardiac	Respiratory	Metabolic	Miscellaneous
Intravenous muscle relaxants				
Succinyl-choline	Dysrhythmias		Trigger for malignant hyperpyrexia Massive potassium release under special conditions Larger volume of distribution	Paralysis Fasciculations Myoglobinuria Masseter spasm Increased intra-ocular pressure Increased intra-gastric pressure
d-Tubocurarine	Histamine-related hypotension	Histamine-related bronchospasm	Histamine release Prolonged neuro-muscular blockade with renal disease	Muscle paralysis
Pancuronium Vecuronium Atracurium	Tachycardia	 Histamine release related to dose and speed of injection		Muscle paralysis Muscle paralysis Muscle paralysis
Intravenous narcotics				
Morphine	Hypotension, especially with associated hypovolemia Peripheral vasodilation	Central respiratory depression and apnea Euphoria, dysphoria Decreased response to hypercarbia	Central nausea and vomiting Decreased GI motility and gastric emptying Histamine release Spasm of sphincter of Oddi	Itching
Meperidine	Hypertension Tachycardia	Central respiratory depression by decreased tidal volume Decreased response to hypercarbia	Nausea and vomiting Less effect on sphincter of Oddi	Itching Tremors, muscle twitching
Fentanyl	Dose-related bradycardia	Central respiratory depression Decreased response to hypercarbia Dose-related chest wall rigidity		Itching

Table 59-2   Physiologically Unique Characteristics of Neonates*

System	Potential Problem	System	Potential Problem
Cardiovascular	Relative pulmonary hypertension Decreased cardiac reserve Transitional circulation with potential bidirectional shunts Vasomotor instability Increased cardiac output	Renal	Decreased GFR Diminished capacity to excrete sodium Decreased concentrating capacity (increased free-water clearance secondary to decreased sensitivity to ADH) Distal renal tubule unresponsive to aldosterone (premature)
Respiratory	Airway anatomy predisposing to difficult management and intubation Decreased functional residual capacity Increased tendency for small airway collapse (premature airway closure) Airway diameter small relative to airway length Increased chest wall compliance	Hepatic	Decreased glucuronide conjugation Decreased P-450 enzyme activity, limited glycogen stores
		Hematologic	Presence of fetal hemoglobin (low P_{50}) Physiologic marrow arrest shortly after birth
CNS	Generalized immaturity Presence of immature reflexes Relative tonicity of parasympathetic nervous system Potential for abnormalities of control of breathing Increased susceptibility to CNS hemorrhage Increased retinal sensitivity to high concentrations of oxygen Relative blood-brain barrier incompetency	Metabolic	Increased requirements for calories and energy substrate Increased susceptibility to heat loss Large water content (large volumes of circulation) Decreased plasma cholinesterase Inability to shiver
		Neuromuscular	Increased joint laxity Relatively immature acetylcholine receptors

*Modified by permission from Morriss FC. Anesthesia: Perioperative principles. In Levin DL, Morriss FC, Moore GC, eds. A Practical Guide to Pediatric Intensive Care, 2nd ed. St. Louis: CV Mosby, 1984.

agents, and the nature of the surgery, they may not be completely preventable. In these instances the benefits of the surgery should make the risk of known complication acceptable to the patient. It is crucial that the patient or parent understand the intraoperative risks of anesthesia, particularly for ASA classifications of 3 or greater, and the proposed solutions for these known risks before he agrees to the procedure. The extremes of age (<1 year and >70 years) also present greater risk for perioperative problems. Emergency procedures for which the patient often cannot be prepared adequately have an increased risk as well.

An adequate anesthetic plan cannot be formulated without considering the surgery itself. Many proce-dures have their own requirements with respect to patient position, use of specialized techniques (e.g., cardiopulmonary bypass, intraoperative somatosensory evoked potentials), pharmacologic agents used by the surgeon (e.g., bone cement, locally injected vasoconstrictors, cavitary antibiotics), and patient discharge status (e.g., ambulatory vs. hospitalized). All such eventualities must be anticipated to provide the surgeon with the best possible conditions in which to operate and to make the procedure as short and successful as possible.

Finally, the patient's preferences for specific agents and techniques should be honored if not contraindicated by health problems or surgical requirements. Having the patient participate in decisions about his

Table 59-3   Factors Affecting Anesthetic Characteristics in Neonates and Infants*

Agent	Altered Anesthetic Characteristics	
	Neonate	Infant
Inhalation agents	High minimal alveolar concentration needed to achieve surgical anesthesia	Highest minimal alveolar concentration needed to achieve surgical anesthesia
	More rapid rise in anesthetic blood levels due to high cardiac output	More rapid rise than adults, less than neonates
	More rapid pulmonary excretion	Same as neonate
	Reduction of baroreceptor responses (halothane)	None
	Very rapid uptake	Same
Neuromuscular blocking agents		
Succinylcholine	Larger volume of distribution	Same as neonates
	Decreased levels of pseudocholinesterase	Normal levels
		2% of myoglobinuria after single dose
	Increased incidence of postinjection bradycardia	Same as neonates
d-Tubocurarine	Large variation in effective dose	Not significant
	Early depression of ventilation, large volume of distribution, longer elimination half-life	
Pancuronium	Tachycardia may predispose to CNS hemorrhage and increased ICP	None
	Wide individual variation	
Vecuronium	Somewhat increased half-life (decreased glucuronide conjugation)	Same as adult
Atracurium	Volume of distribution larger, elimination half-life shorter	Same
Narcotics	Increased sensitivity to respiratory depression and early onset of apnea, especially in premature infants (most potent is morphine)	Same
	Increased elimination, especially in premature infants	
	CNS accumulation of drug, greater depression of CO_2 response	
Barbiturates	Increased sensitivity to respiratory depression, early onset of apnea in premature infants	None
	Greater penetration of blood-brain barrier	More rapid degradation
Ketamine	Efficacy questionable, elimination half-life prolonged	Decreased incidence of hallucinations as compared to adults; more rapid degradation
Ester-type local anesthetics	Decreased ability to metabolize, greater potential for toxicity	None
Amide-type local anesthetics	Plasma levels needed to produce cardiovascular depression 50% of adult	
Benzodiazepines	Slower elimination half-life	None

*Modified by permission from Morriss FC. Anesthesia: Perioperative principles. In Levin DL, Morriss FC, Moore GC, eds. A Practical Guide to Pediatric Intensive Care, 2nd ed. St. Louis: CV Mosby, 1984.

anesthetic is especially important in helping to establish a cooperative, comfortable attitude toward an otherwise frightening experience. When the patient's preferences must be superceded, the reasons and the risks and benefits of the technique or agent in question must be carefully explained. The more familiar the patient is with what will be occurring, the more able he will be to handle the experience. Child life specialists, surgically oriented play therapy, tours, and visual aids help patients, even very young ones, gain familiarity with the surgical environment, including anesthesia equipment, IV lines, monitors, the PARU, and the PICU.

The anesthetic care plan must include specific recommendations for preoperative preparation, including a discussion of any risks; induction, maintenance, and termination of anesthesia; intraoperative fluid management; and airway management and maintenance. The first decision concerns the use of general vs. local techniques; traditionally, regional and local techniques have not been used in children because of their inability to cooperate and to comprehend such methods without fear. Minimal inhalational and IV techniques are currently used more often to supplement spinal, caudal, epidural, and local nerve block anesthetics. The largest number of cases, however, are still done with the patient under general anesthesia, and this discussion concentrates on that technique.

PREOPERATIVE TEACHING AND PREPARATION

Preoperative preparation of any patient must include a discussion of the anesthetic plan and its risks so that the family members may know their options with respect to the anesthetic and may have a clear understanding of what is going to happen. This helps to allay parental anxiety and gain cooperation in handling a young or anxious child, particularly when the patient's condition or discharge status may preclude sedation. All procedures, particularly frightening or painful ones, must be explained to the child in understandable terms so he can deal with the experience on his own terms. It is inappropriate to conceal from a child what is going to happen; fear and anxiety will be increased and the procedure becomes more traumatic. Preoperative medication is often indicated to provide sedation and amnesia, pain relief, dry secretions, or neutralize gastric acid. In addition anticonvulsants, cardiac medications, bronchodilators,

histamine blocking agents, and glucocorticoids that the patient routinely receives should be continued; the timing of routine doses may have to be rescheduled with respect to NPO orders. Finally, antibiotic prophylaxis for treating cardiac lesions or prosthetic devices such as ventriculoperitoneal shunts or artificial joints must be given to patients likely to experience intraoperatiave bacteremia. Table 59-4 delineates the American Heart Association's recommendations for cardiac prophylaxis and appropriate antibiotic coverage for patients with implanted devices. Serum antibiotic levels must be adequate at the time of the highest incidence of bacteremia (airway instrumentation); therefore most antibiotics must be administered in sufficient time preoperatively to assure uptake into the blood. Oral administration is usually better tolerated than IM injection since fear of needles is almost universal among children.

Nothing by mouth. For safe induction of anesthesia the patient must have an empty stomach, thereby decreasing the opportunity for passive reflux and aspiration of stomach contents at times when the protective airway reflexes are obtunded. Table 59-5 outlines routine NPO guidelines. Hypoglycemia and dehydration can be avoided by paying careful attention to the period of time young infants are without fluid and caloric intake. Gastric emptying occurs within 4 hours after a clear liquid meal and is prolonged by the presence of fats or protein. Thus the last feeding is a glucose-containing clear liquid or breast milk (which is digested in the same way as a clear liquid) timed to occur 4 hours before surgery. Exceptions are made for small volumes necessary to take oral medication. For infants with a history of hypoglycemia or on feeding schedules less than every 4 hours, an IV line may be started to supply maintenance glucose needs. Specific orders must be written to ensure young infants are awakened and fed at appropriate times.

INDUCTION OF ANESTHESIA

Anesthesia has traditionally been induced with an IV agent such as thiopental; however, most children are frightened by needles, and the use of other techniques is more appropriate. Many nontraumatic techniques, including oral and nasal narcotic induction, have been investigated, but at present induction by mask with a potent inhalation agent combined with nitrous oxide and oxygen is commonly used and well tolerated. Rectal agents (benzodiazepines, barbitu-

Table 59-4 Antibiotic Prophylaxis for Prevention of Bacterial Endocarditis

Antibiotic	Dosage
Dental procedures, tonsillectomy, adenoidectomy, and bronchoscopy	
Penicillin (V or G)	>60 lb: 2 g orally 1 hr before procedure and 1 g in 6 hr or 2 million units IM or IV 30 to 60 min before procedure and 1 million units in 6 hr <60 lb: 1 g orally 1 hr before procedure and 500 mg in 6 hr or 50,000 units/kg IM or IV 30-60 min before procedure and 25,000 units/kg in 6 hr
Erythromycin (for patient with penicillin allergy)	20 mg/kg orally 1 hr before procedure, 10 mg/kg in 6 hr
Vancomycin (for patient with penicillin allergy)	20 mg/IV slowly over 1 hr, starting 1 hr before surgery
GI and GU tract surgery and instrumentation	
Ampicillin plus	50 mg/kg IM or IV
Gentamicin	2 mg/kg IM or IV, both given ½ hr before procedure; repeat dose in 8 hr
For patients with artificial valves	
Ampicillin and	50 mg/kg IM or IV
Gentamicin	2 mg/kg IM or IV; follow with
Penicillin	1 g orally after 6 hr
For patients with other implanted foreign materials	
Methicillin or	50 mg/kg IV before intubation
Vancomycin (for patient with allergy or who has resistant colonization) plus	10 mg/kg IV slowly over 1 hr, beginning 1 hr before intubation
Gentamicin	2 mg/kg IV or IM 30 min before intubation; may repeat both doses in 8 hr

Table 59-5 Anesthesia NPO Guidelines

Age	Type Fluids	Amount	Time
<1 mo	Clear liquids: specify glucose-containing fluid such as Pedialyte or breast milk	Usual amount of feeding	Up to 3 hr before surgery
	Formula	Usual amount	Up to 4 hr before surgery
1-12 mo	Clear liquids	Volume not to exceed 8 ml/kg	Up to 4 hr before surgery
	Formula or solid food	Any	Up to 6 hr before surgery
>12 mo	Clear liquids	Any	Up to 6 hr before surgery
	Food or milk	Any	Up to 8 hr before surgery

Comments

1. Patients with specific problems such as hypoglycemia, failure to thrive, hepatic disease, or gastroesophageal reflux will need individualized NPO orders and/or IV fluid after being made NPO.
2. Clear liquids include juices, soda, Jell-O, broth, Popsicles, Pedialyte, water. Milk is not a clear liquid.
3. NPO orders for infants <6 months of age should specify that the patient be awakened and fed at a specific time and that the type, time, and amount of last feeding be recorded in the chart.

rates) work well for children who are experiencing acute separation anxiety and in instances in which parents cannot be in the operating room. Such agents can be administered in a holding area and the child allowed to go to sleep in the parent's arms before moving him to the operating room. A rapid IV technique must be used for any patient with a full stomach (see Chapter 127). Even if IV access is difficult to establish, the induction technique should not be changed because a cutdown can be done using local anesthesia. In most patients it is preferable to begin noninvasive monitoring along with the induction since this period is one of changing physiology and statistically is associated with many problems, particularly hypotension, loss of protective reflexes, and dysrhythmias.

Maintenance of Adequate Level of Anesthesia

IV or inhalational drugs are the major anesthetic agents used to maintain an adequate depth of anesthesia; these agents may be supplemented by local anesthetic agents or regional nerve blocks. An ideal anesthetic agent should provide amnesia, pain relief, obtundation of reflexes, and muscle relaxation. Inhalation agents satisfy these requirements in varying degrees; most often muscle relaxants and analgesics must be supplemented. Varying degrees of surgical stimulation can be more easily accommodated by inhalational drugs than by IV or local agents. As the inhaled concentration of the gas is changed, the alveolar concentration changes in direct proportion. Since the amount of gas in the vascular compartment is in equilibrium with the amount of gas in the alveoli, changes in the inhaled anesthetic concentration will be rapidly reflected by changes in the serum concentration of inhaled agent.

If no potent inhalational agents are used, each component of anesthesia must be supplied by a different drug (e.g., narcotics for analgesia, neuromuscular blocking agents for muscle relaxation, nitrous oxide or sedatives for amnesia). Stable vital signs at the time of surgical stimulation indicate that an adequate depth of anesthesia and obtundation of reflex changes in heart rate, respiratory rate, and blood pressure have been achieved. IV drugs must be metabolically altered by renal or hepatic mechanisms before they become chemically inactive and are excreted from the body. This process allows their pharmacologic actions to last longer and prevents rapid alteration of the depth of anesthesia. Use of continuous drips (narcotics, neuromuscular blocking agents, neuroleptics, sedatives) offer a convenient method to control depth of anesthesia more accurately, particularly if short-acting agents such as fentanyl and vecuronium are selected.

Airway management in children is particularly im-

Table 59-6   Anesthetic Indications for Intubation

Indication	Associated Condition
Protection of airway from possible aspiration	Full stomach (unprepared patient), abnormal gastric emptying (shock, gastroesophageal reflux, esophageal foreign body) Trendelenburg position Absence of protective airway reflexes (coma)
Possibility of airway obstruction	Infant <6 mo, prone or sitting positions, shared airway (tonsillectomy, excision laryngeal papillomas) Abnormal airway anatomy (cleft palate, macroglossia, micrognathia, airway mass)
Necessity to control ventilation	Intentional hyperventilation (neurosurgical procedures) Thoracotomy Muscle relaxation for abdominal procedures Underlying respiratory abnormalities
Provision of adequate surgical field	Ophthalmologic procedures Otologic procedures Surgery of head and neck Abdominal or other muscle relaxation

portant because the infantile anatomy predisposes to upper airway obstruction and difficult intubation (see Chapters 2 and 127). Table 59-6 lists indications for intubation; otherwise the airway may be maintained with a bag and mask technique designed to prevent airway obstruction (jaw thrust, oral or nasal airway, sniffing position). Usually the patient is breathing spontaneously since manual control of ventilation with a bag may cause gastric distention with air and unacceptably increase the anesthetic depth.

The decision to control ventilation implies the use of neuromuscular blocking agents and ventilation by hand or mechanical ventilator. Use of mechanical ventilators must be accompanied with sufficiently sensitive monitoring of both the patient and the equipment to detect circuit disconnections, hypoxic gas mixtures, tube obstruction or kinking, ventilator malfunction, and other disruptions of the artificial airway and oxygen supply system. Standard FDA-approved anesthesia equipment (machines and ventilators) possess disconnect, high- and low-pressure alarms, and fail-safe devices to shut off gas anesthetics should partial pressure of oxygen fall to levels indicative of a hypoxic gas mixture. In addition expired gases (carbon dioxide and inhalation anesthetics); peak, mean, and end-expiratory airway pressures; and expired tidal volumes can be monitored, even in very small infants.

Fluid Management

Fluid management depends on several variables—the length of time preoperatively that the patient had nothing by mouth, the type of procedure, expectations regarding blood loss, and the patient's underlying volume status. Hourly maintenance fluids are calculated as outlined in Chapter 15, and the fluid deficit present is calculated based on the time of last intake. This deficit must be replaced over several hours, particularly if the patient is being discharged home from the PARU; maintenance and deficit fluids should have a composition of approximately 0.2% sodium chloride solution. Extra fluid losses occurring preoperatively from fever, diarrhea, nasogastric output, or bowel preparation must be corrected in an anticipatory fashion with IV replacement before surgery.

In addition to hourly maintenance fluid needs and the accrued deficit, the intraoperative fluid losses should be estimated. This may be difficult because such volumes, known as third-space losses, cannot be measured directly. Radioactive-labeled ions have shown these third-space losses to occur as evaporation from exposed tissue surfaces, particularly in the GI tract, or as sequestration of fluid into tissue as a result of extensive surgical dissection. The magnitude of such losses have been estimated as follows: 8 to 10 ml/kg/hr for abdominal, pelvic, or retroperitoneal procedures; 6 to 8 ml/kg/hr for thoracic, neurosurgical, and orthopedic procedures; and a negligible amount for most endoscopic, otologic, ophthalmic, dermatologic, and dental procedures, which do not expose internal organs or result in much edema formation. Losses may sometimes be estimated from suction and sponges, which must be weighed.

If the patient has an adequate oxygen-carrying capacity (Hct 25% or greater), loss of up to 10% to 15% of the estimated blood volume is tolerated if the volume of the estimated loss is replaced with 0.9% sodium chloride solution or 5% albumin at least milliliter for milliliter. With large estimated losses or low oxygen-carrying capacity (low Hct), replacement in the form of whole blood or packed RBCs reconstituted with 0.9% sodium chloride solution or 5% albumin must be given milliliter for milliliter. If excessive loss of protein-containing fluids occurs (ascites, peritonitis), a protein-containing solution such as 5% albumin or 25% albumin may be used. If blood is unavailable, rapid replacement may be achieved using a colloid (protein-containing) solution. Colloid solutions are particularly useful in neonates or patients with limited myocardial reserve since a smaller volume is needed to restore the circulating blood volume than if a crystalloid solution were used. Fresh frozen plasma, although of the appropriate composition for a replacement fluid for blood or protein-containing losses, incurs the risk of blood-borne infection (hepatitis, CMV, HIV) and should be used only to correct documented abnormalities of coagulation.

Peripheral perfusion, urinary output, vital signs, and other variables relating to volume status must be assessed continuously throughout the perioperative period to judge the adequacy of fluid administration. The need for more invasive monitoring of volume status may be indicated by the complexity of the surgery or the patient's health status.

For complex procedures with expected large third-space or blood loss, several secure IV routes will be needed to ensure that all fluids can be given as quickly as they are needed. Generally catheters in the upper extremities, neck, or right atrium perform best when large volumes must be given rapidly; in addition the central circulation is readily accessible for drug administration or central venous blood pressure monitoring.

Intraoperative blood glucose determinations tend to be higher than expected; possible explanations include stress-mediated release of glucocorticoids and catecholamines and low peripheral use of glucose as a result of decreased muscle activity and tone and interference with peripheral glucose uptake. Hypoglycemia is difficult to diagnose in the anesthetized patient because the usual signs and symptoms are absent. The developing brain is highly dependent on adequate glucose levels. For these reasons and in the absence of ongoing blood glucose monitoring, non-glucose–containing solutions are not given to infants less than 2 years of age or to those patients with nutritional deprivation or debilitating disease processes, particularly those involving the liver. Glucose is administered as 5% dextrose in water with 0.2%, 0.45%, or 0.9% sodium chloride solution or in a concentration sufficient to give 100 to 200 mg/kg/hr of glucose. Patients receiving TPN may have become accustomed to much higher glucose loads; discontinuing such solutions before surgery places the patients at risk for hypoglycemia. TPN must be continued at its usual rate, and other fluids for the placement of third-space or blood losses can be given through a second IV catheter. The most accurate way to follow glucose homeostasis throughout the perioperative period is with serial blood glucose or Chemstix determinations. Occasionally the blood glucose level exceeds the renal capacity for reabsorption, and osmotic diuresis occurs secondary to glucosuria. Decreasing the concentration or the administration rate of the glucose-containing solution will be necessary.

TERMINATING ANESTHESIA

At the termination of the procedure the patient should awaken without major changes in vital signs. During the patient's emergence from anesthesia, anesthetic agents are withdrawn, the effect of muscle relaxants reversed, and the endotracheal tube removed. If the patient's condition is unstable or potentially unstable or if he has had an extensive procedure, control of ventilation in the postoperative period may be desirable. In that instance neuromuscular blockade will not be reversed, and the patient will not be extubated. Critically ill patients may by-

pass the usual recovery process and may be taken directly to the PICU for stabilization and recovery, in which case monitoring of vital signs during the transport process is essential. Statistically, emergence is a high-risk period for patients with dysrhythmias, airway instability, hypotension, and hypertension, and monitoring for abnormalities of circulation and ventilation at this time is just as important as at the beginning of anesthetic induction.

MONITORING

Meticulous attention to detail and frequent assessment of vital signs will ensure a stable and reactive patient in the postoperative period. Anesthesia blunts all physiologic reflexes, including those concerned with maintenance of volume homeostasis and protection of the airway. Because of alteration of the patient's protective reflexes, the anesthesiologist must assume a protective function. Changes in the function of various organ systems must be recognized promptly and corrective action, if needed, instituted immediately. The more information available to the anesthesiologist, the more appropriate his corrective action can be. Critically ill patients, long procedures, invasive surgery, or surgery on essential systems such as the cardiorespiratory or central nervous systems mandate more extensive monitoring. All types of monitoring referred to in this text can be adapted successfully for intraoperative use; in many operating rooms the same systems are in use as in the PICU. The indications for invasive intraoperative monitoring are usually the same as for medical problems.

The basic intraoperative standards adapted by the ASA for all patients receiving general or major regional anesthetics are given on pp. 446-447. The most important technologic advance for intraoperative care has been the widespread introduction of oxygen saturation monitoring (see Chapter 122), or oximetry. Subtle changes in respiratory function are recognized early enough to prevent hypoxia from inadvertent esophageal intubation, circuit disconnection, or endotracheal tube occlusion. Oximetry has proved so effective that its use has been mandated by law in several states, and some malpratice carriers discount the cost of insurance in areas in which oximetry is in widespread use.

Other monitoring modes in frequent use in the operating room and their indications are listed in Table 59-7. Many of these monitoring capabilities are incorporated into computerized monitoring systems

Table 59-7 Frequently Used Intraoperative Monitoring Modes

Mode	Instrumentation	Invasive	Indication	Complication
CVP	Indwelling catheter	Yes	Unstable volume status	See Chapter 114
PAP, PWP	Indwelling catheter	Yes	Unstable volume status, cardiac dysfunction	See Chapter 116
LAP, RAP	Indwelling catheter	Yes	Cardiac dysfunction	See Chapter 116
Cardiac output	Indwelling catheter	Yes	Cardiac dysfunction	See Chapter 116
ICP	Indwelling catheter	Yes	Increased ICP	See Chapter 118
Urinary output	Indwelling catheter	Yes	Unstable volume status	Urethral stricture
Neuromuscular blockade	Nerve stimulator, externally applied leads	No	Need for continued paralysis	Painful if patient awake (see Chapter 130)
Processed EEG	Externally applied leads	No	Unstable CNS status	None
Somatosensory-evoked potential	Externally applied leads	No	Assessment of integrity of spinal pathways	None
Expired tidal volume, airway pressures	In-line sensors in ventilator circuits	No	Control of ventilation	Subject to mechanical disruption
End-tidal anesthetic gases	Expired gas analysis cannot be used effectively without endotracheal tube	No	Depth of anesthesia	Subject to individual variation and interpretation

that allow the setting of individual alarms for each patient; the systems store trended data for each variable monitored and display data in various formats. As the complexity of monitoring and anesthesia equipment increases, the anesthesiologist must be thoroughly familiar with his equipment and ensure its proper functioning before beginning a case. In the case of premature infants and neonates one must be certain that the equipment will function adequately for the size of the patient; often specialized equipment designed for use in nurseries is more appropriate for these patients. Finally, all this information must be recorded, along with anesthetic drugs and techniques used, to provide a permanent record of the intraoperative events.

MANAGEMENT OF SPECIFIC POSTOPERATIVE PROBLEMS
Airway Problems

Postintubation croup secondary to laryngeal or cricoid edema (see Chapter 36), upper airway obstruc-

tion from processes other than croup, and apnea secondary to oversedation or incomplete reversal of neuromuscular blockade constitute the most frequent airway problems that occur in the postoperative period. IV naloxone (Narcan) titrated in small incremental doses (0.002 to 0.004 mg/kg) is used to pharmacologically counteract the effects of narcotic anesthetics; a positive response includes increased respiratory rate and tidal volume and greater patient awareness. No pharmacologic reversal is available for nonnarcotic agents such as barbiturates, benzodiazepines, or phenothiozine; the sedative side effects resolve with time as the agent is metabolized. In general the younger the infant, the longer the elimination of sedative agents, and postoperative observation for respiratory obstruction and depression must be correspondingly lengthened. Inhalation anesthetic agents are stored in fatty tissue; however, an exposure of several hours must occur before such storage is a significant element in retarding arousal or prolonging sedation in the postoperative period. The anesthetic

ASA STANDARDS FOR BASIC INTRAOPERATIVE MONITORING
(Approved by House of Delegates on October 21, 1986)*

These standards apply to all anesthesia care, although in emergency circumstances appropriate life support measures take precedence. These standards may be exceeded at any time based on the judgment of the responsible anesthesiologist. They are intended to encourage high-quality patient care, but observing them cannot guarantee any specific patient outcome. They are subject to revision from time to time as warranted by the evolution of technology and practice. This set of standards addresses only the issue of basic intraoperative monitoring, which is one component of anesthesia care. In certain rare or unusual circumstances, (1) some of these methods of monitoring may be clinically impractical and (2) appropriate use of the described monitoring methods may fail to detect untoward clinical developments. Brief interruptions of continual† monitoring may be unavoidable. *Under extenuating circumstances, the responsible anesthesiologist may waive the requirements marked with a double dagger (‡); it is recommended that when this is done, it should be so stated (including the reason) in a note in the patient's medical record.* These standards are not intended for application to the care of the obstetric patient in labor or in the conduct of pain management.

Standard I   Qualified anesthesia personnel shall be present in the room throughout the conduct of general anesthesia, regional, and monitored anesthesia care.

OBJECTIVE   Because of the rapid changes in patient status during anesthesia, qualified anesthesia personnel shall be continuously present to monitor the patient and provide anesthesia care. In the event there is a direct known hazard (e.g., radiation) to the anesthesia personnel that might require intermittent remote observation of the patient, some provision for monitoring the patient must be made. In the event that an emergency situation requires the temporary absence of the person primarily responsible for the anesthetic, the best judgment of the anesthesiologist will be exercised in comparing the emergency with the anesthetized patient's condition and in the selection of the person left responsible for the anesthetic during the temporary absence.

Standard II   During use of all anesthetics, the patient's oxygenation, ventilation, circulation, and temperature shall be continually evaluated.

Oxygenation

OBJECTIVE   To ensure adequate oxygen concentration in the inspired gas and the blood during use of all anesthetics.

METHODS

1. Inspired gas: During every administration of general anesthetic using an anesthesia machine, the concentration of oxygen in the patient's breathing system shall be measured by an oxygen analyzer with a low oxygen concentration limit alarm in use.‡

2. Blood oxygenation: During use of all anesthetics, adequate illumination and exposure of the patient is necessary to assess color. Although this procedure and other qualitative clinical signs may be adequate, the use of quantitative methods such as pulse oximetry is encouraged.

---

*Modified from Anesthesia Patient Safety Foundation Newsletter 2:3, March 1987. Reprinted with permission from the American Society of Anesthesiologists, ASA, 515 Busse Highway, Park Ridge, Illinois 60068.
†*Continual* is defined as "repeated regularly and frequently in *steady* succession," whereas *continuous* means "prolonged without any interruption at any time."

Ventilation

Objective   To ensure adequate ventilation of the patient during use of all anesthetics.

Methods

1. Every patient receiving a general anesthetic shall have the adequacy of ventilation continually evaluated. Although the use of qualitative clinical signs such as chest excursion, observation of the reservoir breathing bag, and auscultation of breath sounds may be adequate, quantitative monitoring of the carbon dioxide content and/or volume of expired gas is encouraged.

2. When an endotracheal tube is inserted, its correct positioning in the trachea must be verified. Clinical assessment is essential, and end-tidal carbon dioxide analysis, in use from the time of endotracheal tube placement, is encouraged.

3. When ventilation is controlled by a mechanical ventilator, a device that is capable of detecting disconnection of components of the breathing system shall be in continuous use. The device must give an audible signal when its alarm threshold is exceeded.

4. During regional anesthesia and monitored anesthesia care, the adequacy of ventilation shall be evaluated at least by continual observation of qualitative clinical signs.

Circulation

Objective   To ensure the adequacy of the patient's circulatory function during use of all anesthetics.

Methods

1. Every patient receiving anesthesia shall have the ECG continuously displayed from the beginning of anesthesia until preparing to leave the anesthetizing location.‡

2. Every patient receiving an anesthetic shall have his arterial blood pressure and heart rate determined and evaluated at least every 5 minutes.

3. Every patient receiving a general anesthetic shall have, in addition to the above, his circulatory function continually evaluated through at least one of the following: palpation of a pulse, auscultation of heart sounds, monitoring of a tracing of intra-arterial pressure, ultrasound peripheral pulse monitoring, or pulse plethysmography or oximetry.

Body temperature

Objective   To aid in the maintenance of patient's appropriate body temperature during use of all anesthetics.

Methods   There shall be readily available a means to measure continuously the patient's temperature. When changes in body temperature are intended, anticipated, or suspected, the temperature shall be measured.

agent becomes available to the circulation for elimination as alveolar and blood levels decrease, and a concentration gradient is created favoring movement of the anesthetic agent from fatty tissue into the blood and then into the alveolar gas compartment for excretion. The patient may experience drowsiness for some hours postoperatively; hypoventilation can occur in this setting, particularly if narcotics are given for analgesia or if hypothermia causes decreased drug elimination. Respiratory insufficiency may occur in the heavily sedated patient for a number of reasons, including depressed central respiratory drive, upper airway muscle relaxation causing obstruction, or loss of protective airway reflexes with aspiration of secretions or stomach contents.

Premature infants less than 60 weeks after conceptual age often display apnea in the postoperative period, even when factors such as hypothermia, hypoxia, hypoglycemia, and electrolyte imbalances are eliminated. A predictable response of the immature CNS to sedation of any kind, including general anesthesia, may be a periodic respiratory pattern and apnea. This type of breathing pattern may be noted during induction and emergence from anesthesia, or it may not become manifest for some hours after the procedure. Patients less than 60 weeks after conceptual age, particularly those with history of significant apnea, those receiving theophylline or caffeine for treatment of apneic episodes, or those with abnormal sleep studies, cannot be treated as ambulatory patients. They must be monitored for apnea for at least 24 hours before discharge. Extubation may need to be delayed if any factors predisposing to prolonged neuromuscular blockade are present (Table 59-8).

Table 59-8   Factors Potentiating Neuromuscular Blockade

Condition	Mechanism of Action	Correction
Hypothermia	Delayed excretion	Withhold reversal agents until patient normothermic

Pharmacologic agents
  Aminoglycosides
  Propranolol
  Quinidine
  Procainamide
  Diphenylhydantoin
	Depolarization of neuromuscular membrane	Withhold drugs during surgery and in PARU if possible; some drugs may be reversed with calcium

Electrolyte imbalance
  Hypokalemia
  Hyperkalemia
  Hypocalcemia
  Hypermagnesemia
  Lithium treatment
  Hyponatremia
  Acidosis
	Changes in neuromuscular membrane potential	Correct imbalance

Abnormal neuromuscular membrane
  Myasthenia gravis
  Muscular dystrophy
  Lower motor neuron disease
	Interruption of depolarization-repolarization process	None

Prolonged administration of neuromuscular blocking drugs (chronic overdose)	Possible change in structure of membrane receptor sites	Monitor dose effect with nerve stimulator
Decreased levels of pseudocholinesterase	Decreased metabolism of succinylcholine	Provide ventilation until succinylcholine is metabolized

Reversal of Muscle Relaxants

Signs of inadequate reversal of neuromuscular block-ade include air hunger, poor air entry as determined by auscultation, floppy muscle tone, and uncoordi-nated semipurposeful movements; these signs are often mistaken for patient uncooperativeness rather than hypoxia. The work of breathing cannot be ac-complished because of weak and partially paralyzed muscles. A specific evaluation of muscle strength in older children will reveal an inability to lift the head off the bed or grasp a hand for more than 10 seconds and inability to generate a crying vital capactiy >15ml/kg or an inspiratory pressure > − 20 cm H_2O. Infants will be unable to lift hips and flex knees against gravity and will not exhibit abdominal muscle tone. Evaluation of blockade with a nerve stimulator will show decreased magnitude of a single twitch, with fading of that response after multiple stimuli. In response to a rapid rate of stimulation (tetanus) rapid decline of twitch magnitude is seen, followed by an increased magnitude of the twitch after tetanus (post-tetanic stimulation). These responses to applied stim-uli to a peripheral nerve are characteristic of a partial block that is caused by nondepolarizing muscle re-laxants.

Respiratory depression, regardless of the cause, must be treated immediately. Bag and mask ventila-tion with increased inspired oxygen must be begun; an unobstructed airway must be assured by use of proper head position and an oral or nasal airway. Reinsertion of the endotracheal tube and reinstitu-tion of mechanical ventilation may be necessary. After hypoxia and hypercarbia are controlled, the cause of respiratory depression may be investigated and treated.

Nondepolarizing neuromuscular blocking agents (*d*-tubocurarine, vecuronium, pancuronium, atracu-rium) act by occupying acetylcholine receptor sites on the neuromuscular membrane. The relaxant mol-ecule prevents neurotransmitter release, thereby preventing neurotransmitter-mediated membrane depolarization, which must occur to initiate the con-traction process; as long as sufficient relaxant mol-ecules are available to occupy membrane receptor sites, the action of acetylcholine and ultimately con-tractions are inhibited. The interaction at the receptor is competitive, however, and the presence of excess acetylcholine molecules will displace the relaxant and cause reinitiation of membrane depolarization.

Anticholinesterases are agents that prevent the en-zymatic clearance of acetylcholine molecules, thus creating an excess of neurotransmitter. When anti-cholinesterases are administered, excess acetylcho-line displaces relaxant molecules from neuromus-cular membrane receptor sites and allows restora-tion of muscle contractile function. The bond between the relaxant and the receptor is initially quite strong, and administration of anticholinester-ases will not disrupt it for a variable period after the relaxant is given; thereafter pharmacologic reversal of the effects of neuromuscular blockade can be at-tempted.

After displacement from their site of action by acetylcholine, muscle relaxant molecules must be physically changed by metabolic processes before they are rendered pharmacologically inactive and are excreted. Paralysis can recur if relaxant molecules gain access to unoccupied neuromuscular mem-brane receptors. Factors that predispose to inade-quate reversal of neuromuscular blockade include excess availability of relaxant (overdose); primary muscle disease such as myasthenia gravis, which may cause loss of receptor sensitivity to acetylcholine (end-organ dysfunction); or presence of a depolar-izing block secondary to succinylcholine. Excess drug may be present because of medication dose error, inability to break down the relaxant molecule (e.g., with renal or hepatic dysfunction or hypothermia), or large stores of protein-bound agent that have not been metabolized. Renal failure may increase serum proteins, which bind relaxant molecules and thus prevent breakdown and/or excretion. Factors that fa-vor recurarization after the initial block has been reversed, potentiate the action of relaxants, and lead to unintentional overdose are listed in Table 59-8.

Inadequate reversal of neuromuscular blockade results in inadequate ventilation, which should be treated as described previously. Reintubation and use of controlled ventilation are often needed until the partial paralysis characterized by incomplete reversal of neuromuscular blockade resolves. A second dose of anticholinesterases may be given under the fol-lowing conditions: (1) block is related to use of a nondepolarizing, not a depolarizing, muscle relaxant; (2) conditions known to potentiate neuromuscular blockade have been sought and treated if present; and (3) 20 minutes or more have passed since the initial attempt at reversal. Narcotic agents must be withheld until full muscle strength is established; depression of respiratory drive will compound the hypercarbia and hypoxia already present.

Anticholinesterases cause muscarinic side effects, including bradycardia, bronchorrhea, and excessive salivation; to prevent these effects anticholinergics are generally given at the same time. The usual reversal agents are pyridostigmine, 0.14 mg/kg, or neostigmine, 0.04 to 0.07 mg/kg, accompanied by glycopyrrolate, 0.005 to 0.006 mg/kg, or atropine, 0.01 mg/kg by IV push. If adequate reversal does not occur, support of the airway and ventilation must continue until full return of muscle strength is documented. At this point arterial blood gas and pH values should be within normal limits while the patient is breathing spontaneously, and safe extubation and withdrawal of ventilatory support can be accomplished (see also Chapter 12).

Hypotension

Hypovolemia is the usual cause of declining blood pressure in the postoperative period; vasodilation, usually drug induced, may cause a relative hypovolemia, whereas loss of circulating blood volume causes an absolute hypovolemia. This last situation can be caused by inadequate replacement of fluids intraoperatively and postoperatively or by acute hemorrhage. Restoration of volume must occur immediately, through rapid administration of Ringer's lactate, 0.9% sodium chloride, or 5% albumin solutions at 10 to 20 ml/kg while the cause of the hypovolemia is investigated. Hemorrhage may be secondary to inadequate surgical hemostasis or less commonly to a coagulopathy, particularly if the patient has received anticoagulants or massive transfusion therapy intraoperatively. Vasodilation may result from transfusion reaction, sepsis, or residual autonomic blockade accompanying epidural or spinal anesthesia or may be secondary to the action of drugs such as chlorpromazine, alcohol, narcotics, droperidol, and barbiturates. Patients with suspected hypovolemia should receive a decreased dose of drugs known to cause vasodilation, and these drugs should be administered in an incremental fashion to minimize changes in blood pressure. The blood pressure of all patients with hypovolemia must be frequently assessed; monitoring of other variables of volume status (perfusion, CVP, urinary output, state of consciousness) may be instituted to assure patient stability until the problem is corrected.

Hypothermia

The incidence of hypothermia is higher when the child is exposed to a cold environment, which may be common in the operating room with its usual ambient temperatures of 18° to 21° C. The reasons for low body temperature include prolonged exposure and decreased ability to conserve and generate heat (see Chapter 21), which may be compounded by use of anesthetics that promote vasodilation. Hypothermia is associated with increased caloric and oxygen consumption, particularly when shivering is present. All patients are subject to diminished rate of metabolic reactions, particularly hepatic degradative functions, which cause prolonged recovery from general anesthesia and longer drug serum half-life (particularly narcotics and muscle relaxants). Neonates are at high risk for development of hypoglycemia, apnea, and disturbances in peripheral perfusion.

Core temperature should be measured on every patient at the time of admission to the PARU and at regular intervals until temperature stability is assured. Abnormally low temperatures must be treated promptly with external warming procedures (warm blankets, radiant heaters, increased ambient temperature). In addition, fluids, particularly blood products, may be warmed. Until core temperature is >36° C, the patient must receive warmed, humidified oxygen at whatever inspired oxygen concentration is needed to keep an adequate saturation as measured by oximetry. Severely affected patients may need arterial blood gas alterations to assure adequate oxygenation since peripheral vasoconstriction may negate use of an oximeter and make estimation of extremity perfusion and color difficult. Glucose values must be determined in all neonates and low values treated promptly. The high incidence of respiratory instability coupled with an increased work of breathing and decreased levels of consciousness and movement usually make removal of the endotracheal tube and ventilatory support unwise. Respiratory support often must be increased in the patient who becomes hypothermic in the PARU.

Emesis

Emesis is a multifactorial problem that commonly occurs in the postanesthetic period. Causes may include (1) use of drugs known to stimulate vomiting centrally (narcotics, inhalational agents), (2) development of ileus after GI surgery, (3) surgical procedures that directly stimulate the semicircular canals (ophthalmologic, otologic), (4) retained blood in the stomach after oral procedures such as tonsillectomy or palatoplasty, (5) history of motion sickness or eustachian tube obstruction, or (6) swallowed air or other causes of gastric distention.

Treatment also takes multiple forms. Emptying the patient's stomach before emergence from anesthesia may be helpful in relieving distention and removing blood and secretions. In the immediate postanesthetic period vomiting can be a source of aspiration because protective airway reflexes may not be intact. When emesis occurs, the patient should be placed in the head down, lateral position so vomitus will be returned to the mouth and can be quickly removed by suctioning the mouth and posterior pharynx. Fluid losses secondary to persistent emesis should be replaced with appropriate IV fluids. Antiemetics such as droperidol, promethazine, metoclopramide, or chlorpromazine may be given through IV, oral, or rectal routes during either the intraoperative or postoperative periods to control emesis. It may be necessary to withhold oral fluids from ambulatory patients until nausea and emesis have subsided; this process may necessitate a longer period of PARU observation or admission overnight.

Pain

Although the anesthetic relieves pain and eliminates the attendant physiologic problems of hypertension, tachycardia, and agitation, pain may recur and become intense in the PARU as the primary anesthetic agents wear off. Patients who have received nerve blocks intraoperatively, particularly at the termination of the procedure, may need short-term control of pain until the block is well established. Emergence delirium will be decreased by reduction of pain, and nausea and vomiting may be diminished. Splinting may lead to decreased tidal breathing and ineffective coughing.

Pain should be assessed in the PARU setting to ensure that it is not greater than is expected (i.e., is not indicative of some related problem such as pneumothorax, muscular compartment compression, bladder distention, perforation of a viscus) and then treated promptly. Pain assessment may be difficult since self-reporting is not reliable until after 6 years of age. Before then behavior observation must be used and may be difficult to quantitate; physiologic variables such as tachycardia, hypertension, agitation, increased neuromuscular activity, and crying must be evaluated as possible indicators of pain. Several scoring systems have been developed to assist in quantitating such observations.

Besides the use of appropriate agents to relieve pain, treatment must be directed toward allaying the anxiety that surrounds the postoperative period, which may contribute to the behavioral response to pain events. This goal is best accomplished by explaining to the patient where he is and what has happened, by instituting measures designed to comfort a distraught child (cuddling, swaddling, giving clear liquids or pacifier, rocking), by providing distractions in the form of familiar toys, music boxes, or games, and by allowing early and frequent parental visitation. Anxiety and agitation that persist must be evaluated separately to rule out hypoxia, inadequate perfusion (decreased cardiac output), metabolic disturbances such as hypoglycemia or hypothermia, and drug effect.

The most commonly used agents for pain relief are narcotics, particularly short-acting ones for ambulatory patients; the most appropriate route is intravenous because most patients will already have IV catheters and IM injections may increase the patient's anxiety. If oral fluid can be tolerated, acetaminophen alone or combined with codeine may be used for moderate pain; if the patient is on an NPO regimen, rectal acetaminophen may be given. Routine PARU monitoring must be frequent and thorough enough to assess drug side effects (such as respiratory depression or changes in circulation) adequately after administration of patient pain relievers.

ADDITIONAL READING

Abramowitz MD, Oh, TH, Epstein BS, et al. The antiemetic effect of droperidol following strabismus surgery in children. Anesthesiology 59:579-583, 1983.

Barash PG, Ganz S, Katz JD, et al. Ventricular function in children during anesthesia: An echocardiographic evaluation. Anesthesiology 49:79-85, 1978.

Brandom BW, Rudd GD, Cook DR. Clinical pharmacology of atracurium in pediatric patients. Anesth Analg 63:309-312, 1984.

Brandom BW, Brandom RB, Cook DR. Uptake and distribution of halothane in infants: In vitro measurements and computer simulations. Anesth Analg 62:404-410, 1983.

Collins C, Koren G, Crian T, et al. Fentanyl pharmacokinetics and hemodynamic effects in preterm infants during ligation of patient ductus arteriosus. Anesth Analg 64:1078-1080, 1985.

• Cook DR, Marcy JH. Neonatal anesthesia. Pasadena: Appleton Davies, 1988.

Cook DR, Fischer CB. Neuromuscular blocking effects of succinylcholine in infants and children. Anesthesiology 42: 662-665, 1975.

• Eckenhoff JE. Some anatomic considerations of the infant larynx influencing endotracheal anesthesia. Anesthesiology 12:401-410, 1951.

Fisher DM. Pharmacodynamics of vecuronium in infants and children. Clin Pharmacol Ther 37:402-406, 1985.

Fisher DM, Cronelly R, Sharma M, et al. Clinical pharmacology of edrophonium in infants and children. Anesthesiology 61:428-433, 1984.

Friesen RH, Lichtor JL. Cardiovascular depression during halothane anesthesia in infants: A study of three induction techniques. Anesth Analg 61:42-45, 1982.

Friesen RH, Lichtor JL. Cardiovascular effects of inhalation induction with isoflurane in infants. Anesth Analg 62:411-414, 1982.

• Furman EB, Roman DG, Lemmer LAS, et al. Specific therapy in water, electrolyte and blood-volume replacement during pediatric surgery. Anesthesiology 42:187-203, 1975.

Goudsouzian NG. Maturation of neuromuscular transmission in the infant. Br J Anaesth 52:205-213, 1980.

Goudsouzian NG, Liu LMP, Savarses JJ. Metocurine in infants and children: Neuromuscular and clinical effects. Anesthesiology 49:266-269, 1978.

Goudsouzian NG, Ryan JE, Savarese JJ. Neuromuscular effects of pancuronium in infants and children. Anesthesiology 41:95-98, 1974.

Goudsouzian NG, Martyn J, Liu LMP, et al. Safety and efficacy of vecuronium in adolescents and children. Anesth Analg 62:1083-1087, 1983.

Goudsouzian NG, Dorion JV, Savarses JJ, et al. Re-evaluation of dosage and duration of action of *d*-tubocurarine in the pediatric age group. Anesthesiology 43:416-424, 1975.

Hickey PR, Hansen DD, Wessel D. Responses to high dose fentanyl in infants: Pulmonary and systemic hemodynamics. Anesthesiology 61:A445, 1986.

Hickey PR, Hansen DD, Cromolini GM. Pulmonary and systemic responses to ketamine with normal and elevated pulmonary vascular resistance. Anesthesiology 62:284-293, 1985.

Hickey PR, Hansen DD, Strafford M, et al. Pulmonary and systemic effects of nitrous oxide in infants with normal and increased pulmonary vascular resistance. Anesthesiology 65:374-378, 1986.

Ledez KM, Lerman J. The minimum alveolar concentration (MAC) of isoflorane in preterm neonates. Anesthesiology 67:301-207, 1987.

Lerman J, Robinson S, Willis MM, et al. Anesthetic requirements for halothane in young children 0-1 month and 1-6 months of age. Anesthesiology 59:421-424, 1983.

Liu LMP, Cote CJ, Gousouzian NG, et al. Life-threatening apnea in infants recovering from anesthesia. Anesthesiology 59:506-510, 1983.

Nicodemus HF, Nassiri-Rahimi C, Bachman L, et al. Median effective doses (ED50) of halothane in adults and children. Anesthesiology 31:344-348, 1969.

Pullertis JP, Burrows FA, Ray WL. Arterial desaturation in healthy children during transfer to the recovery room. Can J Anaesth 34:470-473, 1987.

• Ryan JF, Cote GI, Todres ID, et al, eds. A Practice of Anesthesia for Infants and Children. New York: Grune & Stratton, 1986.

• Salem MR, Wong AY, Collins V J. The pediatric patient with a full stomach. Anesthesiology 39:435-440, 1973.

Salem, MR, Bennett EJ, Schweiss JF, et al. Cardiac arrest related to anesthesia: Contributing factors in infants and children. JAMA 233:238-246, 1975.

• Stehling LC, Zauder HL, eds. Anesthetic Implication of Congenital Anomalies in Children. New York: Appleton-Century-Crofts, 1980.

Steward DJ. A simplified scoring system for the postoperative recovery room. Can Anaesth Soc J 22:11-115, 1975.

Steward DJ, Creighton RE. The uptake and excretion of nitrous oxide in the newborn. Can Anaesth Soc J 25:215-217, 1978.

Zaster M, Deshpand JK. Management of pediatric pain with opioid analgesics. J Pediatr 113:421-429, 1988.

60 Malignant Hyperthermia

Mary F. Harris

BACKGROUND AND PHYSIOLOGY

Malignant hyperthermia (MH), a frequently fatal condition, is a runaway hypermetabolic condition that can be triggered dramatically by certain agents given to induce and maintain general anesthesia.

Trigger agents

Succinylcholine
Halothane
Enflurane
Isoflurane
Methoxyflurane
Trichloroethylene
Chloroform
Diethyl ether
Ethylene
Cyclopropane
Halogenated x-ray contrast media (e.g., iodopyracet)
Amide local anesthetics (especially large doses with epinephrine)

Aggravating agents

Sympathomimetics
Parasympatholytics
Cardiac glycosides
Calcium
Potassium
MAO inhibitors

In 1960 the genetic nature of uncontrolled perianesthetic fever occurring in an Australian family was reported. The term "malignant hyperthermia" was coined in a review of a 1966 Canadian symposium devoted to this abnormal reaction to anesthetic agents. The estimated incidence varies from 1:15,000 pediatric patients to 1:150,000 adult patients. The apparent higher incidence in children may reflect the common use of mask induction with halothane, often followed by IM or IV succinylcholine to facilitate endotracheal intubation. IV inductions are preferred in adults.

During the early 1970s two laboratory developments enhanced our knowledge of the etiology, pathology, and diagnosis of MH. First, porcine stress syndrome was accepted as an animal model. This condition is widespread, especially in certain laboratory pig strains, and can be induced by high ambient temperature, emotional upset, overexertion, or anesthetic triggering agents. Second, the caffeine contracture test became and has remained the standard method of diagnosing MH. Unfortunately this test must be performed on fresh muscle still capable of contracting in response to electrical stimulation. The sample must weigh at least 2 g and is usually taken from the patient's vastus lateralis muscle. In MH-susceptible muscle a smaller dose of caffeine will induce baseline contractures than in normal muscle. Halothane will decrease the contracture dose of caffeine in MH-susceptible muscle and in severely affected muscle can cause contracture even in the absence of caffeine. This test is also used to identify pigs susceptible to porcine stress syndrome. Efforts are being made to improve the uniformity of this test worldwide and to find a less invasive, more easily performed test. The latest and most promising is a ionized calcium blood lymphocyte test, which reveals higher levels of ionized calcium in lymphocytes of susceptible pigs and people.

When MH was first recognized and studied, its mortality rate was >85%, but through use of the pig model, an effective therapeutic drug was found. IV dantrolene was introduced in 1979; since then, improvements in understanding, diagnosis, monitoring, and treatment have decreased the mortality rate for MH to <7%.

MH may represent the final outcome of a spectrum of biologic defects. Genetically, 50% of reported cases appear to be autosomal dominant; 20% have suggested recessive or multifactoral inheritance; another 20% have no detectable familial involvement;

453

and approximately 10% are too poorly documented to allow any conclusions. The clinical appearance also varies greatly. Myotonic or nonrigid forms, immediate or delayed onsets, variable cardiac involvements, and even variable temperature elevations are seen. MH does not occur with every anesthetic experience or only with anesthesia.

Malignant hyperthermic reactions are initiated by an elevation in myoplasmic calcium. This sudden and sustained elevation appears to be related to calcium-induced calcium release from the sarcoplasmic reticulum. Many causative defects have been proposed, including defects in (1) mitochondria, (2) sarcoplasmic reticulum, (3) excitation-contraction coupling, (4) calmodulin, (5) sarcolemma, and (6) adrenergic innervation of muscle.

Excessive myoplasmic calcium drives reactions within the cell. Calcium accelerates conversion of phosphorylase *b* to phosphorylase *a*, stimulating catabolism of glycogen to lactate, carbon dioxide, and heat. Phosphorylase *a* also drives electron transport in the mitochondria, increasing oxygen consumption. This process is accelerated even more when catecholamines activate phosphorylase kinase. Lactate is transported to the liver, where it is metabolized to carbon dioxide, water, and heat. Calcium combines with troponin to allow actinomyosin cross bridges to form. Myosin ATPase is also activated by calcium to generate ADP, phosphate, and heat. In healthy muscle formation of actinomyosin is reversed when myoplasmic calcium decreases. In the muscle of patients with MH there is no fall in myoplasmic calcium, and the process is sustained. Increased temperature eliminates the calcium requirements for myosin-actin interaction. ATP levels are depleted, and the process becomes irreversible.

Similar calcium-related biochemical defects may be present in cells or cell organelles other than muscle. These primary defects may account for some of the later signs of MH rather than being secondary effects of temperature elevation, electrolyte disturbances, acid-base imbalance, or hypoxia.

The diagnosis of MH can be made based on the following clinical signs.

Rising end-tidal carbon dioxide. The earliest metabolic change in a patient with MH is a marked increase in oxygen consumption and carbon dioxide production. End-tidal carbon dioxide will be elevated far above levels expected for the patient's tempera-

ture if ventilation is controlled. Tachypnea and hyperpnea will appear during spontaneous ventilation. Venous carbon dioxide tension will rise before arterial carbon dioxide tension because of respiratory compensation. Mixed venous oxygen saturation will fall before arterial oxygen tension decreases. As tissue demands exceed delivery, metabolic acidosis is added to the existing respiratory acidosis.

Tachycardia. Tachycardia is one of the earliest and most consistent signs of MH. Dysrhythmias, often ventricular extrasystoles progressing to ventricular tachycardia, are common. Tall, peaked T waves on the ECG may appear with hyperkalemia. A primary calcium-related defect of cardiac muscle, similar to that of skeletal muscle, is likely to play a role in early or refractory dysrhythmias. Cardiac impairment will progress to ultimate failure in later stages of MH.

Unstable systemic arterial blood pressure. Initially, as cardiac output increases to meet increased metabolic demands, systemic arterial blood pressure increases. An intense peripheral vasoconstriction may develop as the arteriovenous oxygen gradient widens. Hypotension appears with progressive cardiac impairment and dysrhythmias.

Mottled cyanosis. Profuse sweating and bright red flushing of the upper torso may be followed by mottled cyanosis as vasospasm intensifies despite good ventilation and arterial oxygenation.

Muscle rigidity. Rate of onset and degree of involvement of muscle rigidity vary markedly, depending on the severity of the disease, triggering and modifying anesthetic agents used, and presence of other muscle diseases or associated metabolic defects. The most fulminant onset occurs after administration of succinylcholine, especially if the patient was induced with halothane before use of this depolarizing muscle relaxant. Intense contractures can make intubation impossible and any type of ventilation difficult. The rigidity will not be relieved by administering more succinylcholine or any of the nondepolarizing muscle relaxants.

Occasionally only isolated masseter spasm develops after administration of succinylcholine. This spasm has been associated with a positive muscle contracture test rate of 50% in some centers and should be considered presumptive evidence of MH susceptibility. Other investigators have shown increased masseter tone is common in pediatric patients who have been given succinylcholine during use of halogenated agents. Isolated masseter spasm usually resolves in 20 minutes.

Elective surgery may be canceled and the patient observed for MH progression for 24 hours if muscle spasm occurs. If surgery must proceed, use of the anesthetic may continue with increased monitoring and withdrawal of all triggering agents. The end-tidal carbon dioxide and ECG must be monitored and the patient observed for other early warning signs. Muscle rigidity may develop insidiously, especially if a nondepolarizing muscle relaxant rather than a depolarizing muscle relaxant has been used during induction and maintenance of anesthesia. The level of intensity ultimately developed is unpredictable. In rare cases no rigidity is noted in patients. Release of myoglobin and potassium is more or less proportional to the severity of contracture. Soreness, swelling, and weakness persist after recovery.

Dark urine myoglobinuria. Myoglobin casts may obstruct urinary flow and must be differentiated from other causes of renal failure and anuria.

Body temperature elevation. Hyperthermia is a relatively late sign of MH metabolic abnormalities. Most of the excess heat production occurs in skeletal muscle and the liver. Temperature production parallels muscle contractures in a delayed manner. Once the core temperature begins to rise, it may do so rapidly (1° C every 5 minutes). If fever is not controlled, it can become an important contributor to permanent organ damage.

Coagulopathy. Excessive bruising or bleeding at sites of incisions or venipunctures may be noted. Thrombocytopenia and decreased coagulation factors suggest a consumptive process as the crisis develops.

Abnormal cerebral function. Stupor, coma, and convulsions are possible, and permanent neurologic impairment may develop. Cerebral edema may be caused by a defect of brain tissue or be secondary to high fever, hypoxia, and other biochemical derangements.

MONITORING AND LABORATORY TESTS

Monitoring must be started intraoperatively as soon as MH is suspected and continued until the crisis is resolved and circumstances make recrudescence unlikely. The patient must be monitored for at least 12 hours after receiving his last dantrolene dose. Sug-

---

MONITORING AND LABORATORY TESTS IN PATIENT WITH MH

Monitors	*Laboratory tests*
End-tidal carbon dioxide*	Serial arterial blood gases and pH; mixed venous blood gas and pH values may also be helpful in evaluating disease progression vs. compensation
Pulse oximeter*	
Direct systemic arterial blood pressure†	
ECG	
Urinary output (bladder catheter strongly recommended)	CPK
	Serum electrolytes (especially potassium)
Temperature—continuous core	Serum calcium
	Urinary myoglobin
CVP or PA catheter‡	PT, PTT, platelet count

*Transcutaneous oxygen and carbon dioxide measurements are less reliable because of intense cutaneous vasospasm and local metabolic derangements.
†Repeated systemic arterial blood pressures are not adequate measurements, and frequent blood samples are readily available.
‡Allows mixed venous sampling and improved assessment of fluid balance and cardiac status.

---

gested monitoring modalities and helpful laboratory tests are listed above.

TREATMENT

Stop anesthesia and surgery immediately. All known triggering agents must be discontinued. A ventilatory system free of contamination by halogenated hydrocarbons ("clean machine") should be substituted for the regular anesthetic machine. Elective surgery must be postponed or finished expeditiously. Emergency surgery may have to continue with use of a trigger-free technique and crisis treatment.

Hyperventilate the patient with 100% oxygen. Generous inspiratory flow rates (5 to 10 L/min) and two to three times the normal minute ventilation (even more as indicated by $Paco_2$) may be necessary. This is determined by blood gas values. Pulse oximetry and end-tidal carbon dioxide can provide constant trend monitors of ventilator adequacy.

Administer dantrolene sodium IV. Dantrolene should be given at a rate of 1 mg/kg/min with the patient monitored by ECG until $Petco_2$ declines, heart rate falls, muscle stiffness subsides, and temperature begins to fall. A dose of 2 to 3 mg/kg is usually enough. A maximum dose of 10 mg/kg of IV dantrolene may be given over a 15-minute period. Using 3 mg/kg will cause significant voluntary muscle weakness in healthy individuals. The IV loading dose must be repeated if the reaction recurs. Even in the absence of recurrence a maintenance infusion of 2 mg/kg every 4 hours can be given until all evidence of an active MH crisis is resolved. Because of its extreme insolubility, IV dantrolene is supplied in vials of 20 mg with 3 g of mannitol and sodium hydroxide to raise the pH to 9.5 when reconstituted with 60 ml of sterile water. Administration in a large-bore IV tube with D_5W solution is recommended since salts can increase precipitation. Because of the severe thrombophlebitis induced by this very alkaline, irritating solution, it should be replaced by oral dantrolene as soon as practical after the crisis. Oral dantrolene is approximately 70% absorbed, peaks in 4 hours, and has an elimination half-life of 8 hours. Its active metabolite, 5-OH dantrolene, has a half-life of 16 hours and may account for the prolonged subjective weakness reported by volunteers.

Dantrolene is a lipid-soluble hydantoin derivative that causes relaxation of skeletal muscle by inhibiting release of calcium from the sarcoplasmic reticulum. The mechanism of inhibition is unknown but apparently is postsynaptic, with depression of resting and twitch tensions without EMG changes. Dantrolene has a marked affinity for skeletal muscle and can cause profound weakness. Respiratory function is normally spared. However, in a patient already laboring from compromised respiratory reserves, any weakness in the accessory muscles of respiration might lead to respiratory failure requiring ventilatory assistance.

Dantrolene also interferes with calcium release in cardiac and smooth muscle but with less affinity than in skeletal muscle. Depression of contractility, automaticity, and conduction can occur in the myocardium. When dantrolene is combined with calcium channel blockers, greater than normal myocardial depression has occurred. Vascular smooth muscle tends to relax and is less responsive to norepinephrine. Genitourinary and GI effects seem minimal. Endocrine effects are poorly defined, but decreased insulin release is suggested. Minimal CNS effects have been reported despite a structural relationship to some anticonvulsants and anesthetics. Some depression of assorted liver oxidation reactions occur, plus long-term therapy has been associated with hepatic dysfunction.

Administer sodium bicarbonate. Two mEq/kg of sodium bicarbonate may be given by slow IV push, then administered as indicated by arterial blood gas and pH values. Increasing the serum pH drives potassium into cells and is highly effective in the temporary treatment of hyperkalemia. No more than 50% base deficit correction is warranted without reevaluation.

Actively cool the patient. Iced 0.9% sodium chloride solution, 10 ml/kg every 10 minutes for 1 hour if needed and tolerated, should be rapidly infused intravenously. Solutions containing calcium or potassium (e.g., lactated Ringer's solution) must not be used.

Available body cavities can be lavaged with iced 0.9% sodium chloride solution. Using the stomach via a nasogastric tube is particularly appropriate because it does not interfere with monitoring procedures. Also available are the bladder, rectum, and open surgical wounds.

Surface cooling with ice and a hypothermia blanket is effective in children, especially since their surface area to mass ratio is larger than that of adults. Extracorporeal circulation has been used to cool larger patients and unresponsive patients.

Maintain brisk urinary output. Use of a bladder catheter is mandatory for accuracy in monitoring urinary output. Urinary output >2 ml/kg/hr can help prevent myoglobin cast formation that can lead to obstructive renal failure. If urinary output is <1 ml/kg/hr and more than adequate IV fluids have been given (20 mg/kg/hr plus amount equal to the deficit, with good CVP and systemic arterial blood pressures), the patient may need furosemide, 1 mg/kg. Mannitol, 3 g, is added to every 20 mg vial of dantrolene, and the amount already given must be subtracted from any additional dose planned. Mannitol seems especially beneficial in treating muscle and cerebral edema. Doses of 0.25 to 0.5 g/kg are adequate.

Treat life-threatening dysrhythmias. Most dysrhythmias in patients with MH respond to treatment of acidosis and hyperkalemia. Procainamide, 1 mg/kg every 5 minutes up to 7 mg/kg given slowly to avoid systemic hypotension, may be necessary for short-term use. If hyperkalemia is not significantly improved with acidosis correction, 10 units of regular insulin in 10 ml of $D_{50}W$ solution may be infused intravenously as needed to help drive potassium into cells. Hypokalemia can result from overly vigorous treatment and resolution or worsening of the crisis. The severe, prolonged hypokalemia associated with unresolved crisis is difficult to correct.

Avoid sympathetic overstimulation. Sympathetic stimulation worsens and may even trigger MH crisis. Since catecholamines facilitate prejunctional acetylcholine release and increase cyclic AMP and calcium uptake and release from the sarcoplasmic agents, their use is not recommended during hyperthermic crisis. Phosphodiesterase inhibitors, which potentiate catecholamines, are also theoretically contraindicated.

Adrenergic blocking agents have had positive effects in the laboratory. However, they are not the best choice in a patient with a fluctuating systemic arterial blood pressure and cardiac function. Beta blockers combined with dantrolene can cause serious myocardial depression. A small dose of a short-acting beta blocker by IV infusion can be given to test for effect. Beta blockade without alpha blockade may cause an imbalance and not improve the chance for survival.

Digitalis raises the intracellular calcium level, and its use is best avoided. Calcium channel blocking drugs lack any therapeutic effect on patients with established MH syndrome. Verapamil enhances the myocardial depression caused by dantrolene. Very large doses of nifedipine have shown some efficacy in attenuating MH.

Local anesthetics may be used to decrease input from painful procedures. Amide local anesthetics have not triggered MH in swine even in toxic doses, and the clinical reports are not very straightforward.

Sedate with care. Narcotics will be needed before completing surgery after a crisis and to relieve any postoperative pain that might increase plasma catecholamine levels. Morphine can release histamine if given rapidly, and histamine can cause unwanted cardiovascular or respiratory problems. Meperidine is metabolized to normeperidine, which causes undesirable CNS stimulation. Fentanyl and its analogs can be given as loading doses and constant infusions to achieve constant blood levels without resulting in the stiff chest caused by large boluses. Ketamine has not been advocated because of increased catecholamine levels. However, it does not trigger MH in swine.

Barbiturates are often used as premedications and induction agents in MH-susceptible patients. Thio-

pental is thought to slow and attenuate the onset of crisis caused by halothane, but cardiovascular depression limits its usefulness. Chlorpromazine has been advocated to increase peripheral vasodilatation and decrease shivering. In addition it may have a depressant effect on phosphodiesterase activity and depress intracellular thermogenesis. Benzodiazepines are acceptable and effective.

Droperidol has been used without problems during anesthesia, especially as a low-dose antiemetic. However, the problem of neuroleptic malignant syndrome makes the use of butyrophenone, phenothiazine derivatives, tricyclics, monoamine oxidase inhibitors, and other antipsychotic drugs controversial. Neuroleptic malignant syndrome usually develops 24 to 72 hours after drug exposure. It is characterized by akinesis, muscle rigidity, hyperthermia, tachycardia, cyanosis, autonomic dysfunction, altered consciousness, diaphoresis, and increased levels of creatine kinase. It is thought to be caused by a central presynaptic defect involving dopamine-receptor blockade in the hypothalamus and basal ganglia. Amantadine and bromocriptine are dopamine antagonists that have been used successfully. Dantrolene, which blocks the calcium-induced muscle contractures peripherally, is effective in treating neuroleptic malignant syndrome. This is fortunate since the differential diagnosis would be difficult after a known MH crisis. Caffeine contracture tests show a variable relationship between MH and neuroleptic malignant syndrome. In one study five of seven survivors of the syndrome had positive contracture tests.

Observe CPK and serum calcium and potassium levels. These should be monitored until they are normal.

Observe the patient in a PICU setting after resolution of a crisis. Recrudescence of MH may occur, particularly in a patient who was difficult to treat. Transporting the patient stimulates recurrence with especially troublesome dysrhythmias, which will require immediate reinstitution of treatment, especially of dantrolene. An effective dose of IV dantrolene can be estimated from the dose required to reverse the crisis. This dose can be given every 8 to 12 hours prophylactically, especially if the patient is still experiencing stressful stimuli such as pain or infection. After an easily treated mild crisis one may elect to give no further dantrolene unless observation reveals recrudescence. Prophylactic oral dantrolene, 4 mg/kg/day for 1 to 2 days in divided doses every 6 to 8 hr in the form of 25 mg capsules, can be given in more difficult cases after crisis resolution with IV dantrolene. Continuous observation would be advisable for 12 to 24 hours after administration of the last dantrolene dose.

Counsel the family about further diagnostic workup. Until the diagnosis is confirmed by muscle biopsy with contracture testing, the patient and all his blood relatives should be treated as susceptible to MH, with strict avoidance of triggering agents and high levels of suspicion and monitoring so that dantrolene can be given as soon as indicated. Dantrolene can be given preoperatively in an attempt to prevent MH. Prophylactic preoperative dantrolene can cause weakness, dizziness, diplopia, dysarthria, nausea, abdominal pain, diarrhea, and elevated serum potassium levels. Oral dantrolene, 1 mg/kg every 6 hr for 24 to 48 hours, has been used for this purpose. Absorption can be unpredictable, especially if vomiting occurs. IV dantrolene, 2 to 3 mg/kg given 30 to 60 minutes before induction, is much more dependable but is damaging to veins. IV administration allows more intense monitoring and shorter duration of any unpleasant side effects. Opinions vary about the best plan for dantrolene administration, but watchful preparedness without prophylaxis is acceptable to many experts. When dantrolene is used in pregnant patients, the fetal/maternal ratio is approximately 1:2 and could contribute to infant hypotonicity.

NOTE: The family should be put in contact with the Malignant Hyperthermia Association of the United States (MHAUS), Box 3231, Daven, CT 06820. For further information about available treatment or patient referral call 1-203-655-3007. MHAUS also provides a hot line for questions about unresolving crisis and other emergency problems through Medic Alert Foundation International, 1-209-634-4917. Ask for INDEX ZERO, Malignant Hyperthermia Consult List.

ADDITIONAL READING

• Britt BA. Aetiology and pathophysiology of malignant hyperthermia. In Britt B, ed. Malignant Hyperthermia, United States and Canada. Boston: Kluwer Academic, 1987, pp 11-33.

• Britt BA. Dantrolene—an update. In Britt B, ed. Malignant Hyperthermia, United States and Canada. Boston: Kluwer Academic, 1987, pp 11-33.

Britt BA. Malignant Hyperthermia. Can Anaesth Soc J 32:666-677, 1985.

Caroff SM, Rosenberg H, Fletcher JE, Heiman-Patterson TD. Malignant hyperthermia susceptibility in necroleptic malignant syndrome. Anesthesiology 67:20-25, 1987.

Dershwitz M, Sréter F, Ryan JF. Ketamine does not trigger malignant hyperthermia in susceptible swine. Anesth Analg 69:501-503, 1989.

Flewellen EH. Malignant hyperthermia and associated conditions: Dilemma, controversy, unanswered questions. In IRAS Review Course Lectures. Cleveland: 1985, pp 76-83.

• Flewellen EH, Nelson TE, Jones WP, Areas JF, Wagner BA. Dantrolene dose response in awake man: Implications for management of malignant hyperthermia. Anesthesiology 59:275-280, 1983.

Gallant EM, Foldes FF, Rempel WE, Gronert GA. Verapamil is not a therapeutic adjunct to dantrolene in porcine malignant hyperthermia. Anesth Analg 64:601-606, 1985.

Glassenberg R, Cohen H. Intravenous dantrolene in a pregnant malignant hyperthermia susceptible patient. Anesthesiology 61:A404, 1984.

Harrison GG, Morrell DF. Response of MH swine to infusion of lignocaine and bupivicaine. Br J Anaesth 52:385-387, 1980.

Jones DE, Ryan JF. Treatment of acute hyperthermia crisis. In Britt B, ed. Malignant Hyperthermia, United States and Canada. Boston: Kluwer Academic, 1987, pp 393-405.

Karlow W. Inheritance of malignant hyperthermia—a review of published data. In Britt B, ed. Malignant Hyperthermia, United States and Canada. Boston: Kluwer Academic, 1987, pp 393-405.

Klip A, Ramal T, Walker D, Britt BA, Elliott ME. Selective increase in cytoplasmic calcium by anesthetic in lymphocytes from malignant hyperthermia-susceptible pigs. Anesth Analg 66:381-385, 1987.

Lynch C, Durbin CG, Fisher NA, Veselis RA, Althaus JS. Effects of dantrolene and verapamil on atrioventricular conduction and cardiovascular performance in dogs. Anesth Analg 65:252-258, 1986.

Nelson TE. Skeletal muscle sarcoplasmic reticulum in the malignant hyperthermia syndrome. In Britt B, ed. Malignant Hyperthermia, United States and Canada. Boston: Kluwer Academic, 1987, pp 43-75.

Steward DJ, O'Conner GAR. Malignant hyperthermia—the acute crisis. In Britt B, ed. Malignant Hyperthermia, United States and Canada. Boston: Kluwer Academic, 1987, pp 1-9.

VanDerSpek AFL, Fang WB, Ashton-Miller JA, Stohler CS, Carlson DS, Schork MA. Increased masticatory muscle stiffness during limb muscle flaccidity associated with succinylcholine administration. Anesthesiology 69:11-16, 1988.

Wingard DW, Bobko S. Failure of lidocaine to trigger porcine malignant hyperthermia. Anesth Analg 58:99-103, 1979.

61 Cardiothoracic Surgery: Perioperative Principles

Hisashi Nikaidoh · Steven R. Leonard · Michelle Morris-Copeland

BACKGROUND

The principal focus in caring for the patient undergoing cardiac or thoracic surgery must be the protection of cardiac and pulmonary function. Frequently the patient has multisystem involvement (e.g., renal, hepatic, hematologic, neurologic) in addition to cardiopulmonary dysfunction. Infections also have serious consequences in these patients.

Most important, these patients' hemodynamic, pulmonary, and metabolic functions must be monitored continuously and extensively. Direct physical examination is indispensable and must be performed only by the experienced critical care staff. Treatment consists of (1) recognition and correction of various preoperative dysfunctions, (2) intraoperative protection of all organs, and (3) postoperative support and management of the temporary dysfunction of vital systems. All these efforts should lead to successful cardiothoracic surgery.

PREOPERATIVE MANAGEMENT

Preoperative management begins with appropriate communication among the staff members involved in patient care, possibly including general pediatricians, specialized pediatricians such as cardiologists or pulmonologists, surgeons, anesthesiologists, intensivists, the nursing staff from various disciplines (admitting, operating room, intensive care), social workers, and hospital chaplains. Preoperative review conferences including these personnel provide an effective means of accomplishing this communication. The evaluation must include (1) routine physical examination, (2) laboratory tests, (3) a chest roentgenogram, and (4) pulmonary or cardiac evaluations (invasive and noninvasive).

Specific Problems

Nutritional problems. Nutritional condition is an important concern for all preoperative patients. If at all possible, establishing a positive preoperative nutritional balance is beneficial in a catabolic patient. This may necessitate supplementation with TPN or nasogastric tube feedings in certain patients. Building an adequate iron supply in the patient is also important for developing a higher level of hemoglobin preoperatively, thus possibly reducing the potential need for blood transfusion. In a patient with cyanotic heart disease a normal hemoglobin level may be inappropriately low, indicating the need for iron treatment before surgery.

Infections. Infections must be carefully sought and appropriately treated before surgical intervention. Viral upper respiratory infections can leave the respiratory epithelial lining abnormal for 2 to 3 weeks. Otitis media, pharyngitis, or urinary tract infection can be a source of bacteremia during the course of cardiac surgery in which the risk of endocarditis is not negligible. In some cases otitis media can be a recurrent problem that prevents appropriate timely surgical care. It can be managed by preparatory tympanostomy or with careful and limited use of suppressive antibiotic therapy. Superficial skin infections such as folliculitis (including acne), recent burns or wet eczematous lesions, infected lacerations, and wet diaper rashes are all potential hazards for inducing wound or deeper infections. Intraoral infections are often overlooked. Dental caries and associated gingivitis, usually seen in bottle-fed children, may cause bacteremia during intubation. Dental problems must be corrected before any elective cardiothoracic operation. If at all possible, it is wise to keep the infant or toddler out of day care centers, church nurseries, or crowded classrooms for approximately 2 weeks before the scheduled surgery to avoid exposure to various childhood infections.

Congestive heart failure. Congestive heart failure must be treated medically to obtain the best hemodynamic stability possible before surgery. This is ordinarily accomplished with digitalization and diuretic therapy. In a more acute and serious situation IV inotropic medications such as dopamine, dobutamine, isoproterenol, epinephrine, and amrinone may be used to improve cardiac function (see Chapter 11). Further relief may be obtained by using vasodilators, which decrease the cardiac work load by afterload reduction.

Hypoxemia. Hypoxemia is often a serious problem preoperatively, and administration of oxygen in a high concentration may be of benefit. Hypoxic patients are often tachypneic or dyspneic and consume additional oxygen during the increased respiratory effort, leading to further decompensation and metabolic acidosis. To decrease the work of breathing and oxygen consumption these patients can be pharmacologically paralyzed, intubated, and supported by mechanical ventilation. If the hypoxemia is primarily caused by the constriction of a patent ductus arteriosus in a newborn infant with cyanotic heart disease, dilation of the ductus with PGE_1 infusion must be attempted.

A severe hypoxic "spell" may occur in a patient with tetralogy of Fallot when the hyperdynamic constriction occurs in the outlet area of the right ventricle. In addition to conservative treatment with oxygen and sedation, administering propranolol will effectively reduce the infundibular spasm.

Aortic obstructions. Coarctation of the aorta or an interrupted aortic arch in a neonate may be treated temporarily by PGE_1 infusion, which reestablishes adequate blood flow to the lower part of the body by dilating the patent ductus arteriosus and nearby "ductal" tissue in the aorta. This preoperative treatment may be crucial in an infant with severe metabolic acidosis and congestive heart failure secondary to the aortic obstruction.

Metabolic abnormalities. Metabolic abnormalities may arise from various problems. Hypocalcemia is not unusual in small infants. The possibility of DiGeorge syndrome must be considered, especially in patients with aortic arch anomalies, tetralogy of Fallot, or pulmonary atresia. If DiGeorge syndrome is suspected, irradiated blood products must be used for blood replacement. The serum potassium level may be low in patients who are vigorously treated with diuretics. Metabolic acidosis must be corrected by infusion of sodium bicarbonate and by the improvement of other problems such as poor peripheral tissue perfusion and oxygenation. As previously mentioned in the discussion of hypoxemia, any acidotic patient should be treated with mechanical ventilation and muscle relaxants (paralysis) to reduce oxygen consumption from an inordinately high respiratory effort. Renal failure caused by decreased renal perfusion in patients with coarctation syndrome or critical aortic stenosis can be reversed temporarily by improving blood flow to the kidneys by dilating the patent ductus arteriosus with PGE_1 infusion. Serious hepatic failure has been seen in patients with low cardiac output associated with high central venous blood pressure such as occurs with coarctation syndrome. Normalization or improvement of the coagulation profile and platelet count with appropriate transfusion of blood products if possible is important in all patients.

Adjustment of Cardiac Medications

If the patient has been receiving digoxin and/or diuretics, these medications should be withheld starting the evening before surgery to avoid intraoperative or postoperative dysrhythmias and electrolyte imbalance. Short-acting antiarrhythmic medications should be continued until the time of surgery. If a patient is receiving propranolol for the prevention of hypercyanotic spells, the medication must be continued until the time of surgery to avoid critical hypoxemia before the initiation of cardiopulmonary bypass. Antiplatelet medications (e.g., aspirin), which are often given to patients with systemic-pulmonary artery shunts using graft material, should be discontinued 7 to 10 days before the scheduled date of surgery to prevent hemorrhagic complications.

Psychological and Emotional Preparation

The child must be prepared for surgery in a manner appropriate for his age and development. Older children (6 years of age and older) are allowed to tour the PICU if desired. Dolls are provided for surgical play. The family should meet with the surgeon and anesthesiologist preoperatively to discuss the planned operation, any anticipated or potential problems, and the expected outcome. Family members can be given a tour of the PICU and meet the child's admitting nurse whenever possible.

INTRAOPERATIVE MANAGEMENT
Monitoring and Laboratory Tests

Close and significantly invasive monitoring is needed in most of the cardiac surgical patients and some pulmonary surgical patients. The extent of monitoring must be tailored to the needs of the individual patient. However, the following guidelines are suggested. The minimal basic monitoring of all cardiac and thoracic surgical patients must include continuous observation by ECG, pulse oximetry, and in mechanically ventilated patients end-expiratory carbon dioxide monitoring. If the need for close systemic arterial blood pressure monitoring exists or frequent arterial blood gas and pH analysis is indicated, an arterial catheter must be placed. Left and/or right atrial monitoring catheters are indicated in any patient who may exhibit ventricular failure or atrioventricular valve dysfunction. In patients with preoperative pulmonary artery hypertension (systolic pulmonary/systemic blood pressure ratio greater than two thirds), use of a pulmonary artery monitoring catheter should be planned if at all possible. In some patients who may need close observation of cardiac output a thermal dilution cardiac output catheter can be inserted. See Table 61-1 for a summary of vascular monitoring guidelines. These invasive monitoring catheters can be placed with the cooperative effort of surgeons and anesthesiologists in the operating room only after the anesthesia is properly induced to reduce patient discomfort.

Monitoring of somatosensory-evoked potentials has been advocated in thoracic aortic surgery, es-

Table 61-1   Recommended Vascular Monitoring for Cardiothoracic Operations

Procedure	SAP	RAP/CVP	LAP	PAP	CO
Patent ductus arteriosus division	−	−	−	−	−
Coarctation repair	+	−	−	−	−
Pulmonary artery banding	+	±	−	−	−
Blalock-Hanlon atrial septostomy	+	±	−	−	−
Superior vena cava–right pulmonary artery (Glenn) shunt	+	+ (CVP)	−	−	−
Blalock-Taussig shunt	+	−	−	−	−
Central shunt	+	±	−	−	−
Division of vascular ring	+	−	−	−	−
Aortopulmonary window repair	+	+	±	+	±
Ventricular septal defect with pulmonary artery hypertension	+	+	+	+	+
Ventricular septal defect without pulmonary artery hypertension	+	+	−	−	−
Atrial septal defect secundum repair	+	+	−	−	−
Atrial septal defect primum repair	+	+	+	±	±
Complete atrioventricular septal defect repair	+	+	+	+	±
Truncus arteriosus repair	+	+	+	±	±
Norwood/Damus-Stansel procedure	+	+	−	−	−
Fontan procedure	+	+	+	−	−
Tetralogy of Fallot repair	+	+	+	±	±
Mustard/Senning procedure	+	+	+	−	−
Arterial switch operation	+	+	+	±	±
Aortic valvotomy/aortic valve replacement	+	+	±	−	−
Mitral valve repair/replacement	+	+	+	+	+
Total anomalous pulmonary venous return repair	+	+	+	+	±
Pulmonary valvotomy/right ventrical outflow tract repair	+	+	−	−	−
Supraaortic/subaortic stenosis repair	+	+	±	−	−

SAP = systemic artery blood pressure; RAP = right atrial blood pressure; CVP = central venous blood pressure; LAP = left atrial blood pressure; PAP = pulmonary artery blood pressure; CO = cardiac output.

pecially during coarctation repair in children beyond the neonatal stage.

Hemodynamics and Oxygenation
Closed heart operations

A midline incision (sternotomy) will usually cause the least hemodynamic disturbance since neither lung will be manipulated, compressed, or retracted during the procedure. However, the majority of closed heart operations are routinely performed through thoracotomy incisions because of the anatomic accessibility and future potential problems associated with a "re-do" midline sternotomy. Left posterolateral thoracotomy, usually through the fourth intercostal space, is used for patent ductus arteriosus division, coarctation repair, classic or modified Blalock-Taussig shunts, and division of the vascular ring. Left anterolateral thoracotomy is used for isolated pulmonary artery banding, and right anterolateral thoracotomy is used for a Blalock-Hanlon atrial septostomy and Glenn procedure (superior vena cava to right pulmonary artery anastomosis).

Retraction and compression of the exposed lung must be kept to a minimum, and injury to the various structures in the chest (vagus nerve, recurrent laryngeal nerve, phrenic nerve, major lymphatic ducts, esophagus, lung) must be avoided.

During the course of the operation various vascular structures must be either partially or totally occluded. The surgeon must minimize occlusion to maintain an acceptable circulatory state and oxygenation level. This requires careful planning and organization during the surgery. Temporary hypoxemia must be dealt with by delivering higher inspired concentrations of oxygen to the patient. A short episode of bradycardia during atrial manipulation in the Blalock-Hanlon procedure or Glenn procedure can be treated pharmacologically with atropine. Some temporary depression of cardiac function may need inotropic catecholamine infusion. Thoracic aortic occlusion must be kept to a minimum to avoid ischemic injury to the lower part of the body, especially the spinal cord. Total occlusion of the aortic arch can be tolerated as long as 20 minutes in the presence of normal systemic arterial blood pressure in a person without previously developed collateral vessels. Ischemic spinal cord injury is rare during coarctation repair in neonates but is a serious problem in older children, even if they have well-developed collateral vessels, if the aortic occlusion is prolonged.

Open heart operations

Stable hemodynamics must be maintained, and the myocardium should not be unduly overloaded during the course of open heart surgery. Cooperation among anesthesiologists, perfusionists, and surgeons is critical if this goal is to be achieved.

Cardiopulmonary bypass is not a physiologic system for perfusion and oxygenation. To reduce various injurious effects of cardiopulmonary bypass the following principles must be considered: (1) the circuit must contain a minimal amount of priming volume to avoid excessive hemodilution or need for transfusion; (2) the perfusion time must be short so that physiologic derangement will be minimal; and (3) unnecessary mechanical injury to the blood should be prevented, especially in complex cases that require longer perfusion time.

Myocardial protection can be provided by hypothermic cardioplegia induced by using cold hyperkalemic blood or crystalloid solutions injected into the aortic root when the aortic cross clamp is applied. Careful planning can minimize this critical period of myocardial ischemia. Low cardiac output syndrome in patients who have had anatomically appropriate repairs is often the result of inadequate myocardial protection.

Some surgical procedures are performed with the patient under hypothermic circulatory arrest. Absolute indications for the technique include (1) repair of total anomalous pulmonary venous return, (2) repair of an interrupted aortic arch with simultaneous closure of a ventricular septal defect, (3) Norwood procedure for hypoplastic left heart syndrome, and (4) difficulty in ordinary venous cannulation. Relative indications include (1) any small infant undergoing complex intracardiac repair (e.g., repair of complete atrioventricular septal defect, arterial switch operation for transposition of the great arteries, repair of truncus arteriosus), (2) expected massive hemorrhage from an ascending aortic aneurysm, and (3) division of a previous Potts' shunt. Hypothermic circulatory arrest is a distinct advantage to the surgeon in many technically difficult situations; however, it is no panacea and is not without complications if not used with care and for limited periods of time. The hypothermic state can be readily induced by cardiopulmonary bypass. The importance and value of surface-induced hypothermia may have been somewhat exaggerated in the past.

The postoperative consequences of prolonged

cardiopulmonary bypass are (1) decreased coagulation factors resulting from consumption and denaturation, (2) activation of the fibrinolytic system, (3) activation of the complement cascade, (4) consumption and deactivation of platelets, (5) pulmonary endothelial injury and increased capillary permeability, (6) generalized increase in vascular permeability secondary to toxic effect of bradykinin, and (7) damage to cellular components of blood, resulting in leukocytopenia and hemolysis. In contrast to the ordinary bubble oxygenators, the recently available hollow filter membrane oxygenators are less injurious to blood cellular components, including platelets. Major organ system injuries are usually induced by technical problems such as an inadequately low perfusion rate, air emboli, major breakdown of the cardiopulmonary bypass system, and inadequate anticoagulation (heparinization).

Discontinuation of cardiopulmonary bypass

At the completion of the intracardiac repair the patient is taken off cardiopulmonary bypass. In sequence (1) the body temperature is normalized; (2) the cardiovascular system is carefully de-aired, especially the left heart chambers and the pulmonary veins; (3) atrial and pulmonary arterial monitoring catheters are placed if their use is indicated; (4) an appropriate cardiac rhythm is restored either by medication or electrical pacing; (5) the ventilation is resumed; and (6) a gradual shift to partial bypass is accomplished by increasing the patient's own cardiac output. In general the transition from cardiopulmonary bypass to the patient's own intrinsic cardiac function is supported by appropriate oxygenation through ample pulmonary ventilation with high oxygen concentration, intravascular volume supplementation in small increments under careful atrial blood pressure monitoring, maintenance of appropriate acid-base balance, control of cardiac rhythm, and pharmacologic support of myocardial function if indicated. An early and aggressive pharmacologic manipulation within the first several minutes after discontinuing cardiopulmonary bypass can be detrimental to the myocardium, which is often in a precarious metabolic balance of supply and demand. Although IV use of calcium for the augmentation of cardiac action is commonly practiced, excessive calcium ions can cause serious myocardial injury in the unstable postischemic and postperfusion state.

In patients with preoperative pulmonary arterial hypertension, pulmonary vascular resistance can be the determinant of cardiac output. A maximum effort to reduce pulmonary vascular resistance includes hyperventilating the patient, providing a high alveolar oxygen concentration, and administering vasodilating agents (e.g., continuous infusions of nitroprusside or nitroglycerine or bolus injection of tolazoline if indicated). Vasoconstrictive catecholamines (e.g., epinephrine, dopamine) must be used judiciously, with attention given to their effects on pulmonary vascular resistance.

Ensuring hemostasis is most important since postoperative bleeding is the most common surgical complication in cardiac surgery. This must be accomplished both by surgical control of bleeding and by adequate supplementation of the coagulation system (e.g., platelets and/or fresh frozen plasma). If their use is indicated, appropriate temporary cardiac pacing leads are placed. Providing sequential atrioventricular pacing may be of importance in patients whose cardiac output may be marginal. Appropriate drainage tubes are inserted before closure of the chest. Before the transfer of the patient from the operating room, the nursing unit that will receive the patient must be advised about the patient's general and hemodynamic status and about details concerning his ongoing support (e.g., respirator settings, IV medications, cardiac pacing, monitoring, drainage systems).

Psychological and Emotional Support

Psychological support for the parents and other family members during the operation is a major concern, and frequent progress reports must be given to them by the operating room nurses. Other hospital personnel such as a social worker and/or hospital chaplain can also provide emotional support and can play a critically important role if any serious problem is encountered during the course of surgery. During these communications one must be absolutely honest, make clear statements, and show compassion for the anxious family members.

POSTOPERATIVE MANAGEMENT

The postoperative period for a cardiothoracic surgical patient requires meticulous attention to detail by personnel, and careful integration of information involving all the body systems is essential. The anatomy and physiology must be considered for the individual patient; a routine "cookbook" approach to patient care is inadequate. However, the following guidelines will help to provide uniform care.

Monitoring and Laboratory Tests

Continuous monitoring of the ECG, respiratory rate, heart rate, and systemic arterial blood pressure is mandatory. In most patients oxygen saturation will be continuously monitored by a pulse oximeter. In addition the catheters that have been placed in the operating room (CVP, Swan-Ganz, right and left atrial, pulmonary arterial) must be monitored. A Swan-Ganz catheter allows periodic measurement of cardiac output and calculation of the cardiac index as well as systemic and pulmonary vascular resistances. The patient's temperature must be recorded hourly. Accurate measurement of intake (IV and enteral) and output (urinary catheter, chest tubes, nasogastric tube) must be performed at least hourly. Blood samples must be checked often until the patient's condition is stable and acceptable values are obtained for arterial blood gas tensions and pH, hemoglobin and hematocrit, serum electrolytes (especially potassium and calcium), BUN, creatinine, glucose, and coagulation profile (PT, PTT, platelet count). Correction of metabolic or coagulation abnormalities must be done expeditiously to avoid serious complications.

A chest roentgenogram is taken immediately when the patient arrives in the PICU to confirm positions of the endotracheal tube, nasogastric tube, chest tubes, and intracardiac monitoring catheters. The chest roentgenogram is generally repeated daily or as indicated (for repositioning of the endotracheal tube or change in ventilatory or hemodynamic status). In addition pathologic conditions such as pneumothorax, pleural effusions, atelectasis, or lobar collapse must be ruled out or treated if diagnosed. The ECG is continuously monitored using a single lead. An ECG with multiple leads is indicated in case of dysrhythmia or suspected myocardial ischemia. Echocardiography is not routinely performed but may be helpful in the diagnosis of pericardial effusion, residual defects, intracardiac shunts, and valvar or ventricular dysfunction.

Fluids and Electrolytes

Patients who have had operations requiring cardiopulmonary bypass generally have a volume overload and need limited IV volume administration. Usually 5% dextrose in 0.2% NaCl is infused at one half the maintenance rate for the first 24 hours after surgery. In infants 10% (or sometimes 20%) dextrose solutions are used to prevent hypoglycemia. It is customary to add 20 to 40 mEq/L potassium chloride to the fluid when renal function is normal. Should increased volume be necessary to maintain adequate filling and perfusion pressures, colloid solution (5% albumin, fresh frozen plasma, whole blood, packed RBCs) is administered. After the first 24 hours fluid administration is increased toward the maintenance requirement, as indicated by hemodynamic stability. When the intravascular volume stabilizes, usually 24 to 48 hours postoperatively, IV diuretics (furosemide) are administered to reduce excess intravascular fluid. Patients who have undergone operations without cardiopulmonary bypass are given IV fluid at the maintenance rate, with boluses of colloid solution as needed for volume expansion.

The cavopulmonary connections (Glenn or Fontan procedure) will cause significant systemic venous hypertension, and patients who have had these procedures will need much higher fluid administration in the early postoperative period. Patients who have had systemic-pulmonary artery shunt procedures also need higher fluid volume infusion during the early postoperative period.

Serum electrolyte values (especially potassium and calcium) must be measured frequently after cardiac surgery and deficits replaced as indicated. Potassium and calcium infusions must be diluted in fluid and administered over several minutes to avoid sudden serum fluctuations that result in cardiac instability. In addition these electrolytes and vasoconstrictive inotropic agents must *not* be infused through peripheral venous sites because infiltration into subcutaneous tissue can cause significant morbidity. Infusion through central venous catheters prevents this problem.

Ventilatory Care

Most patients undergoing cardiothoracic surgery will remain intubated and will be mechanically ventilated. Frequent arterial blood gas and pH determinations are necessary to adjust the ventilator settings appropriately. Pressure or volume ventilators may be used; however, patients may suffer decreasing or changing pulmonary compliance when pulmonary or chest wall edema develops or when they have pulmonary artery hypertension, and these patients are best ventilated with volume ventilators. Ventilatory rate and/or tidal volumes are varied to produce arterial P_{CO_2} in the normal range and to maintain normal arterial pH. The F_{IO_2} is maintained at the lowest level that assures adequate arterial oxygen saturation. Ventilation with elevated Fio_2 should be avoided if possible because of the morbidity associated with oxygen toxicity. PEEP may be added to maximize oxygenation at the lowest possible Fio_2.

Manipulation of ventilation may be useful in managing some specific situations. Patients with excessive pulmonary blood flow (e.g., who have hypoplastic left heart syndrome, double-outlet right ventricle, unoperated truncus arteriosus, or aortopulmonary window) may benefit from efforts to increase pulmonary vascular resistance, thus decreasing pulmonary flow and increasing systemic flow. This is accomplished by avoiding hyperventilation (i.e., maintaining arterial Pco_2 at 40 to 45 mm Hg and arterial pH at 7.35 to 7.45) and using room air ventilation. Patients who are prone to postoperative pulmonary hypertension or vasospasm (e.g., who have ventricular septal defect, atrioventricular canal, repaired truncus arteriosus, or aortopulmonary window) will benefit from measures to decrease pulmonary vascular resistance, including hyperventilation (to maintain arterial Pco_2 at 25 to 30 mm Hg and arterial pH at 7.45 to 7.55) and the use of higher Fio_2 (0.40 to 0.50). The patients are usually given neuromuscular blocking agents to achieve muscle paralysis for the first 24 to 48 hours after surgery and are hyperventilated at an Fio_2 of 1.0 for at least 1 minute before and after suctioning of the endotracheal tube.

Some patients who have undergone palliative operations can be expected to retain right-to-left intracardiac shunts and remain cyanotic. For these patients arterial saturation of 80% or greater is acceptable.

The time and rate at which a child can be weaned from mechanical ventilation depends on many variables. Before extubation the patient's Fio_2 must be 0.40 or less, PEEP must be no greater than 2 to 4 cm H_2O, and the child must demonstrate adequate ventilation with minimal support (0 to 4 mechanical breaths per minute) by maintaining an acceptable pH and Pco_2. The patient's hemodynamic status must be stable with minimal support from vasoactive agents. After extubation supplemental humidified oxygen is usually administered via tent, hood, or face mask.

Pain Control and Comfort Measures

The child initially is given sedation and/or an analgesic as often as his condition permits. This is especially true of pharmacologically paralyzed patients. Morphine sulfate (0.1 mg/kg IV) is the preferred agent, but if this is not sufficient, diazepam (0.1 mg/kg IV) or chlorpromazine (0.2 mg/kg IV) may be added. As the child's condition improves, he will need less pain medication and can be weaned rapidly. Continuous IV administration of fentanyl (2 to 5 µg/kg/hr) is particularly useful in critically ill patients who may receive mechanical ventilation for more than 24 to 48 hours. This drug is especially effective in children likely to demonstrate pulmonary artery hypertension (e.g., after a Norwood procedure or repair of truncus arteriosus). These patients must be pharmacologically paralyzed because of potential chest wall rigidity caused by the fentanyl.

The child must be turned side to side to prevent skin breakdown. Since an unstable patient may not tolerate positional changes, he is placed on a foam egg-crate mattress and repositioned every 1 to 2 hours to the extent his condition allows. It may not be possible to do more than turn the patient's head side to side and tilt the body slightly. If the patient will be immobilized for more than a few days, a physical therapy program must be initiated.

Psychological and Emotional Support

The family members must be kept informed of the patient's postoperative progress. They must be notified immediately of any unexpected problems, complications, or significant changes in the child's condition in a straightforward and compassionate manner. As the patient improves, the family members need to be involved in his care as much as possible (e.g., feed or bathe the child, apply lotion to the skin, do range-of-motion exercises). Discharge may involve parent teaching about activities such as tube feedings, medication administration, chest physiotherapy, and cardiopulmonary resuscitation.

COMPLICATIONS
Postoperative Bleeding

Excessive bleeding is a risk in any patient who has undergone cardiopulmonary bypass. It is difficult to define "excessive," but certainly specific therapy or surgical exploration is warranted when chest tube output exceeds 3 to 5 ml/kg/hr for more than 3 to 4 hours. Significant accumulation of blood in the pericardial cavity may result in cardiac tamponade. If left untreated, bleeding may further compromise an unstable patient by reducing cardiac output.

Postoperative bleeding may be defined as "surgical" or "medical" (secondary to a coagulopathy). Surgical bleeding is a result of inadequate hemostasis at the time of closure. Virtually every possible site has been incriminated, but the most common ones are cardiac incisions, cannulation sites, sites of entry for intracardiac monitoring lines, periosteal vessels, pericardial edges, or dilated collateral vessels in severely cyanotic children. Patients who have had previous cardiac operations are particularly at risk for bleeding from lysed adhesions. Hemostasis may be adequate at the time of closure when the patient is anesthetized; however, as the patient awakens and begins to move or cough, bleeding may ensue. If bleeding persists despite correction of a coagulopathy, it must be assumed to be secondary to inadequate hemostasis, and urgent exploration is indicated.

Medical bleeding results from a coagulopathy. Cardiopulmonary bypass causes trauma to platelets and dilution of clotting factors, which may cause a coagulopathy. In addition reversal of heparinization may be incomplete or fibrinolysis may occur. Thus coagulation function must be assessed in every patient by determination of platelet counts, PT, PTT, and activated clotting time (ACT). If fibrinolysis is suspected, fibrin split products must be quantitated.

Therapy is directed at replenishing specific blood components. Thrombocytopenia (platelet count $<50,000/mm^3$) is treated by platelet infusion (1 to 2 units of platelets/10 kg body weight). Dilution of clotting factors (moderate to severe prolongation of both PT and PTT) is treated by administering fresh frozen plasma (10 to 20 ml/kg body weight), which must be done cautiously while right and left atrial pressures and systemic arterial blood pressure are monitored. If the filling pressures limit the amount of volume that can be infused, cryoprecipitate may be considered (1 to 2 units/10 kg body weight). Fibrinolysis (in a patient with normal PT and PTT but with the presence of fibrin split products and lysis of clot in a glass test tube) is treated with epsilon-aminocaproic acid (100 to 200 mg/kg initially, followed by 100 to 150 mg/kg every 2 hours while fibrinolysis persists). In any bleeding patient the chest tubes must be vigorously cleared of blood clots to maintain patency. Continuous administration of blood is necessary to prevent volume depletion and hypotension. One must always be certain adequate blood products are readily available in the blood bank. The use of fresh whole blood (<48 hours old) is most effective in reversing coagulopathy and maintaining adequate vascular volume. Blood products must be warmed during administration to prevent

hypothermia. Some blood products, especially platelets and fresh frozen plasma, can cause hypotension during administration (presumably from release of vasoactive substances and/or chelation of ionized calcium) and must be given slowly.

Cardiac Tamponade (see Chapter 40)

Accumulation of blood or fluid within the pericardial cavity can cause insufficient diastolic filling of the ventricles, resulting in low cardiac output. If the condition is not immediately treated, cardiac arrest and death may follow. Even though the pericardium may not have been completely closed and mediastinal tubes are in place, cardiac tamponade may still occur.

Cardiac tamponade may be difficult to diagnose since the findings may be subtle until cardiac output is severely depressed. It is also difficult at times to differentiate cardiac tamponade from hypovolemic shock or low cardiac output syndrome. The following indications are helpful but not necessarily diagnostic of cardiac tamponade: (1) excessive postoperative bleeding that stops suddenly, (2) signs of low cardiac output (hypotension, oliguria, poor peripheral perfusion), (3) equalization of filling pressures (right atrial, left atrial, pulmonary artery diastolic, and ventricular end-diastolic pressures), (4) enlarging cardiac silhouette on serial chest roentgenograms, and (5) distant or muffled heart sounds. Echocardiography may be helpful (see Chapter 119), but in an unstable patient time does not permit waiting for the results.

Treatment of cardiac tamponade involves drainage of the pericardium. When the patient's condition permits, this procedure is best done in the operating room. However, in a critical situation it may be necessary to perform the sternotomy in the intensive care unit. Sometimes all that is necessary is to open the lower portion of the wound and evacuate the blood with a sterile suction tip. The patient is then taken to the operating room for complete mediastinal exploration and control of hemorrhage. Pericardiocentesis is of no value in this situation.

Delayed cardiac tamponade can occur several days to weeks postoperatively as a result of accumulation of bloody or serous fluid within the pericardium. Its signs and symptoms may include weakness and fatigue, precordial pain or discomfort, dyspnea, edema, paradoxical pulse, oliguria, and enlarging cardiac silhouette on chest roentgenograms. Echocardiography is diagnostic. In older children and adults pericardiocentesis may be performed if the echocardiogram demonstrates a large anterior fluid collection within the pericardium (see Chapter 143). However, in infants and small children or in any patient in whom the fluid is located more posteriorly, pericardial drainage via a tube pericardiostomy is best done in the operating room.

Low Cardiac Output

Low cardiac output can result from dysrhythmias, decreased preload, increased afterload, or myocardial dysfunction. Indirect signs of low cardiac output include systemic hypotension, narrow pulse pressure, tachycardia, oliguria or anuria, poor peripheral perfusion (slow capillary refill, pale, cool extremities with weak pulses), and lethargy or stupor. Metabolic acidosis may occur. Direct measurement of cardiac output is possible using the thermal dilution technique. A cardiac index <2.0 L/min/m^2 is critically low and must be treated.

Management of low cardiac output first involves correction of contributing factors such as dysrhythmias, electrolyte disorders, acid-base disturbances, and hypothermia. Second, adequate preload must be provided. Preload is best determined by measurement of left atrial blood pressure and must be maintained at 10 to 15 mm Hg in most patients. Administration of crystalloid solution is only temporarily effective for volume expansion and is avoided in the early postoperative period. Packed RBCs or whole blood is used if the patient's hematocrit is low ($<35\%$ to 40%). If the hematocrit is adequate, intravascular volume may be expanded by infusing fresh frozen plasma (if clotting factors are needed) or 5% albumin.

Inotropic agents are used when preload is adequate but low cardiac output persists because of myocardial dysfunction. The most commonly used inotropic agents are dobutamine, dopamine, epinephrine, and isoproterenol (see Chapter 12). All have in common the capacity for increasing myocardial contractility (inotropism). Some also aid in reducing systemic and pulmonary vascular resistances (dobutamine, isoproterenol) and may thus increase cardiac output by altering afterload. Isoproterenol is a potent chronotropic agent and is particularly useful in treating patients with bradycardia or conduction delay. Dopamine has the advantage of improving renal blood flow in lower doses (3 to 6 μg/kg/min).

If low cardiac output persists despite optimal pre-

load and use of inotropic agents, afterload reduction with vasodilating agents can be initiated. Vasodilating agents must be added very carefully in a patient who may already be hypotensive because of a low cardiac output. Atrial pressures must be continuously monitored; rapid vasodilation may suddenly decrease preload, and the cardiac output may drop precipitously. It is often necessary to administer volume (whole blood, packed RBCs, plasma, albumin) as vasodilation occurs to maintain adequate preload.

Pulmonary Arterial Hypertension

Patients with high preoperative pulmonary vascular reactivity and/or resistance may have pulmonary hypertension or pulmonary vascular crises postoperatively. The only method for following pulmonary artery blood pressure is direct monitoring through either an indwelling catheter placed through the right ventricular outlet area into the pulmonary artery or a transvenous catheter such as a Swan-Ganz. With such monitoring it is possible to intervene when pulmonary artery blood pressure becomes dangerously elevated (usually greater than two thirds the systemic pressure). If this problem is not corrected, cardiac output may decrease precipitously and cause cardiac arrest.

The pulmonary vasculature is sensitive to hypoxia, hypercarbia, and acidosis. Patients who are at high risk are mechanically ventilated for the first 24 to 48 hours after surgery to maintain Pa$_{O_2}$ >100 mm Hg, Pa$_{CO_2}$ <40 mm Hg, and pH >7.40. This is usually best accomplished in a well-sedated and pharmacologically paralyzed patient. If this procedure is not effective, vasodilating agents such as nitroprusside (0.5 to 5.0 μg/kg/min), nitroglycerin (1.0 to 20.0 μg/kg/min), or chlorpromazine (0.1 to 0.2 mg/kg IV every 3 to 4 hours) should be administered. In the event of intense pulmonary arterial vasospasm, hyperventilation with 100% oxygen concentration (usually by hand ventilation) should be initiated. It may be necessary to administer tolazoline (1 mg/kg over several minutes) either intravenously or directly through the pulmonary arterial catheter to decrease pulmonary vascular resistance.

Weaning from mechanical ventilation must be carried out slowly in patients at risk for pulmonary arterial hypertension. Too rapid withdrawal of ventilatory support may precipitate pulmonary hypertension. The pulmonary artery blood pressure in these patients is usually highest on the first and second postoperative days. Pulmonary vasospasm may occur with suctioning or manipulation of the endotracheal tube. Such a crisis is best avoided by hyperventilating the patient with 100% oxygen concentration for 1 minute before and after the procedure.

Dysrhythmias

Dysrhythmias are not uncommon occurrences after cardiac surgery. Most are transient and may be surprisingly well tolerated by the patient. However, they may occasionally decrease cardiac output and cause significant morbidity or mortality. Most dysrhythmias occur as a result of metabolic disorders such as hypoxemia, metabolic acidosis, or electrolyte imbalances (especially potassium and calcium). Correction of these abnormalities is usually accompanied by the recurrence of normal cardiac rhythm. Ventricular (and occasionally atrial) pacing wires are placed at the time of surgery and can be used for treating any bradycardia that is compromising cardiac output. Sinus bradycardia or atrioventricular conduction delay can be treated by infusing isoproterenol at low doses (0.01 to 0.1 µg/kg/min).

Supraventricular tachycardias can adversely affect cardiac output by decreasing diastolic filling. If the tachycardia has a sinus node origin, precipitating causes such as pain, acidosis, hypovolemia, hypoxia, or tamponade must be ruled out. In addition high doses of inotropic agents can cause tachycardia. Atrial fibrillation or flutter can occur in any patient after cardiac surgery but is more likely after operations involving a great deal of atrial manipulation (e.g., Mustard, Senning, or Fontan procedure). If cardiac output is significantly depressed, DC countershock (1 watt-sec/kg) is indicated. In patients who are not severely compromised administration of digoxin may effectively lower heart rate and improve cardiac output. Verapamil should *not* be used to treat postoperative supraventricular tachycardia in children because of the risk of asystole.

Tachycardia originating in the atrioventricular node (so-called junctional ectopic tachycardia) is an ominous dysrhythmia that is accompanied by markedly decreased cardiac output, and it must be treated aggressively. The patient must be pharmacologically paralyzed and sedated, potassium and calcium levels must be kept in the high-normal range, and the body temperature must be cooled to approximately 36° C (as measured by esophageal or "core" temperature, not rectal temperature). In addition digoxin is ad-

ministered intravenously, and the use of inotropic agents is minimized or avoided if possible. Ventricular tachycardia is a very malignant dysrhythmia that almost always produces extremely low cardiac output. Treatment includes administration of IV lidocaine (1 mg/kg, followed by a continuous drip at 20 to 50 µg/kg/min) and DC countershock. Premature ventricular beats (more than five per minute, coupling, or multifocal) are also treated with lidocaine. Persistent ventricular irritability may require administration of procainamide.

Renal Failure

Acute renal failure (see Chapter 14) becomes manifest as oliguria or anuria, accompanied by rising BUN and creatinine levels. Renal failure is usually caused either by decreased renal perfusion (prerenal azotemia) or by damage to the nephrons (renal azotemia or acute tubular necrosis). Table 61-2 lists some guidelines that may assist in differentiating prerenal azotemia from acute tubular necrosis.

Prerenal azotemia is usually caused by decreased cardiac output and consequent low renal perfusion. Restoration of cardiac output through volume expansion and administration of inotropic and/or vasodilating agents will usually improve urinary output. If not, furosemide (1 to 3 mg/kg) may be given. If there is still no response, acute renal injury is confirmed, and measures must be taken to avoid fluid and metabolic imbalances. All potassium must be removed from IV fluids and fluid administration re-

---

Table 61-2   Differentiation of Renal Failure

	Prerenal Azotemia	Acute Tubular Necrosis
U/P creatinine ratio	>40	<10
U/P urea ratio	>20	<10
U/P osmolarity ratio	>1.1	<1.1
Urinary specific gravity	>1.015	<1.010
Fractional sodium excretion*	<1%	>2%
Urinary sodium concentration (mEq/1)	<10	>25

U/P = urine to plasma.

*Fractional sodium excretion =

$$\frac{U/P \text{ sodium concentration ratio}}{U/P \text{ creatinine concentration ratio}} \times 100$$

duced to 400 ml/m²/day (insensible water loss) without significant reduction in glucose intake. Serum electrolyte, BUN, and creatinine levels must be monitored closely. Hyperkalemia may develop rapidly with fatal consequences if not treated immediately. Once the serum potassium level exceeds 5.5 mEq/L, glucose (400 mg/kg IV bolus) and insulin (0.2 unit/kg IV bolus) should be given. Because this provides only temporary reduction of serum potassium, enemas with sodium ion-exchange resin (sodium polystyrene sulfonate [Kayexalate] 1 to 2 g/kg per rectum in 20% sorbitol every 4 to 6 hours) must be initiated. Inability to reverse hyperkalemia and/or severe volume overload may necessitate the use of peritoneal dialysis or hemodialysis. Fortunately most cases of postoperative renal failure are transient and resolve without the need for dialysis.

Wound Infection

Because of the length of most cardiac operations, multiple instrumentations, including intubations or catheter insertions, and the possible depression of host defense mechanisms, infection is a real threat to patients undergoing cardiac surgery. Strict adherence to sterile technique is the most important factor in preventing infection. In addition perioperative administration of IV antibiotics is used as a prophylactic measure. Since most postoperative infections are caused by gram-positive bacteria, the antibiotic chosen must be active against these organisms. We use a cephalosporin (cefuroxime or cefamandole). The first dose is given at the time of induction of anesthesia, and the antibiotic is continued until all intracardiac monitoring catheters are removed.

Despite these measures, wound infections occur in approximately 1% of patients. Infections may be superficial, involving only the soft tissue anterior to the sternum, or they may be deep, resulting in mediastinitis. Superficial wound infections usually respond to local care involving adequate drainage, debridement, and frequent dressing changes. Sternal instability in the presence of a wound infection usually represents involvement of the retrosternal space (mediastinitis). However, mediastinitis can exist without sternal instability and be difficult to diagnose. Noninvasive methods such as echocardiography or CT can be helpful in diagnosing this condition. Treat-

ment of mediastinitis, with or without sternal instability, requires surgical drainage and debridement. The wound can often be closed over catheters through which dilute (0.5%) povidone-iodine solution is used for irrigation. Extensive involvement of mediastinal tissues is best treated by debriding and packing open the wound, followed by delayed primary closure or healing by secondary intention.

Sternal dehiscence can occur *without* infection. It may manifest with instability of the sternal halves, serosanguineous drainage from the incision, or a visable or palpable defect. This complication requires prompt reclosure in the operating room.

Postpericardiotomy Syndrome

Some patients who have undergone cardiac surgery may develop a syndrome characterized by fever, pleural and pericardial effusions, pleuritic or precordial pain, and pleural or pericardial friction rubs. A pericardial effusion may enlarge enough to cause cardiac tamponade. The etiology of postpericardiotomy syndrome may be an autoimmune process with production of heart-reactive antibodies. It can occur after any operation in which the pericardial cavity has been entered. It usually occurs 1 to 3 weeks postoperatively but can occur as early as 48 to 72 hours after surgery or as long as a few months after surgery. The syndrome is usually self-limited, and significant relief may be provided by nonsteroidal anti-inflammatory drugs such as aspirin or indomethacin. If symptoms persist, a short course of steroids may be used, but steroid therapy should be avoided if possible. Large pleural or pericardial effusions may dictate needle aspiration or tube drainage.

ADDITIONAL READING

Hazinski MF. Cardiovascular disorders. In Hazinski MF, ed. Nursing Care of the Critically Ill Child. St Louis: CV Mosby, 1984, pp 63-252.

• Kirklin JW, Barratt-Boyes BG. Postoperative care. In Kirklin JW, Barratt-Boyes BG, eds. Cardiac Surgery. New York: John Wiley, 1986, pp 139-176.

• Sade RM, Cosgrove DM, Castaneda AR. Infant and Child Care in Heart Surgery. Chicago: Year Book, 1977.

Stark J. Postoperative care. In Stark J, de Leval M, eds. Surgery for Congenital Heart Defects. New York: Grune & Stratton, 1983, pp 135-163.

62 Neurosurgery

Kenneth Shapiro · Cole A. Giller

BACKGROUND AND PHYSIOLOGY

The perioperative care of the neurosurgical patient provides a special challenge to the clinician. Because the delicate tissues of the CNS are encased in an unyielding bony container, they are prone to both insidious and explosive changes that can lead to neurologic devastation. Furthermore, therapeutic maneuvers must be tailored to detect and prevent any potentially catastrophic effects on the CNS. For these reasons the proper care of these patients, which includes vigorous neurologic monitoring, is best accomplished in a PICU setting.

The nervous system is composed of soft tissues that have a high water content and subserve an intricate and fragile electrical function. The brain and spinal cord are protected by bony coverings that for the most part are unyielding to pressure. Therefore the nervous system is dependent not only on general physiologic variables such as systemic arterial blood pressure, electrolyte balance, and oxygen saturation, but also on mechanical forces such as ICP and local mass effect. For example, cerebral edema can lead to a rise in ICP, which can produce cerebral ischemia and infarction. The effect of any treatment modality on both the ordinary physiologic variables and on mechanical forces must be anticipated when planning therapy in the PICU.

MONITORING

Frequent and meticulous neurologic examinations remain the foundation of neurosurgical monitoring and can provide the only indication for admission to a PICU. Results of the examinations must be recorded as often as appropriate (usually hourly) and must include mental status, extraocular movements, pupillary equality and reactivity, and motor function (see Chapter 4). Other observations such as fontanelle tension and CSF leakage must be noted when applicable. Adequate analgesia can be achieved with

small doses of narcotics in the postoperative period, but oversedation, which might obscure changes in the neurologic status, should be avoided. At nursing shift changes it is helpful for the incoming and outgoing nurses to perform the neurologic examination together so that descriptive information is not lost or distorted.

TREATMENT
Patient Position

Elevating the head of the bed to 30 degrees promotes cerebral venous drainage and can, in itself, decrease ICP. For the same reason the head must be kept at midline and not flexed when intracranial hypertension is a concern in the pre- or postoperative period. The elevated position may prevent aspiration in the obtunded patient and may promote CSF drainage in a patient with hydrocephalus. Infants with hydrocephalus can be nursed at even greater angles on a foam wedge mattress supported by a Velcro harness arrangement.

To prevent pressure necrosis of the scalp, care must be taken to position small children and infants so that they do not lie on their wounds. Special attention is needed when a shunt device lies directly under the skin, particularly in the thin-skinned premature infant.

Children with spinal injuries may need specialized positioning to provide immobilization. Careful attention must be paid to pressure points and frequent turning to avoid decubitus ulceration. Patients with tears of the thoracolumbar dura must be nursed prone with the head of the bed down to minimize CSF leakage.

Hemodynamics and Volume

Under normal circumstances cerebral blood flow is autoregulated so that perfusion is maintained relatively constant under moderate systemic arterial hypotension or hypertension. This autoregulation can be impaired when the brain is injured or is harboring a mass. In such a patient cerebral perfusion pressure (CPP) may be directly related to systemic arterial blood pressure. Even transient hypotension may lead to ischemia, and moderate hypertension may promote bleeding into an operative site. Therefore meticulous attention to systemic arterial blood pressure control is important while treating the neurosurgical patient. Position changes must be monitored to prevent orthostatic hypotension. The postoperative patient must be given adequate analgesia and, if necessary, antihypertensive agents to ensure normotension. Patients with elevated ICP present special problems since an elevated systemic arterial blood pressure may be needed to maintain adequate cerebral perfusion but at the same time can cause intracranial hypertension. It is crucial to monitor CPP as the systemic arterial blood pressure is manipulated by directly monitoring ICP and calculating CPP ($CPP = MAP - ICP$).

In general a neurosurgical patient should be maintained euvolemic or slightly hypovolemic. Even when ICP control necessitates vigorous use of hyperosmotic agents such as mannitol, fluid losses can be routinely replaced with colloid solution to maintain euvolemia and perfusion without the addition of free water. When vasospasm occurs, volume expansion and, if necessary, induced hypertension are used, but this event is unusual in children.

Ventilation

Neurosurgical patients often need ventilatory assistance to support the airway in cases of severe obtundation or to provide hyperventilation to control ICP. Appropriate narcotic sedation allows patient comfort; prevents straining, which can lead to reflex tachycardia, and hypertension, which can elevate ICP; and usually does not interfere with the neurologic examination. Pulmonary compliance must be measured and tidal volumes adjusted to reduce high intrathoracic inspiratory pressures, which can impair cerebral venous return and, in turn, cause intracranial hypertension. Moderate levels of PEEP (5 to 10 cm H_2O) probably do not significantly affect ICP. For older children the intermittent mandatory ventilation (IMV) mode is used to minimize straining against the ventilator and to avoid the unwanted hyperventilation that frequently occurs in obtunded patients on controlled ventilation.

Hyperventilation is a mainstay of ICP control, and the desired P_{CO_2} is 25 to 30 mm Hg when intracranial hypertension is a concern. Occasionally even lower levels of P_{CO_2} are needed for adequate ICP control, and monitoring jugular blood gas levels to calculate arteriovenous differences can be helpful to avoid excessive hypocarbia. Intermittent vigorous hand ventilation with a breathing bag attached to an oxygen source may be necessary to reduce sharp peaks in ICP.

Weaning from ventilatory support can be prolonged in the unconscious patient. Use of the IMV mode with intermittent continuous positive airway pressure (CPAP) (5 cm H_2O for 15 minutes every 2 hours) may be helpful in prolonged weaning and allows careful attention to changes in mental status, tidal volumes, respiratory rate, and peak inspiratory pressures. Hyperventilation is best slowly decreased with an ICP monitor in place to avoid rebound ICP. The occasional neurosurgical patient will need a tracheostomy.

Intracranial Pressure

ICP is monitored in patients with a variety of neurosurgical conditions, including traumatic injuries, hydrocephalus, and encephalopathy, and during the postoperative period. Cerebral edema and hyperemia occur after head trauma, and an ICP monitor is frequently placed to guide therapy. Monitoring also forewarns of an increased mass effect and impending cerebral herniation in a patient with a tumor or hematoma. Posterior fossa masses can lead to obstructive hydrocephalus, and a ventriculostomy is often used to monitor ICP and provide CSF drainage. A ventriculostomy may also be placed after a craniotomy when postoperative cerebral edema or hydrocephalus is anticipated (see Chapters 7 and 118).

Electrolytes

Electrolytes must be closely monitored in the neurosurgical patient since fluid shifts occurring after trauma or operative procedures can lead to profound neurologic sequelae unless recognized and corrected. Diabetes insipidus and SIADH accompany many neurosurgical diseases and can occur de novo in the postoperative patient. Diabetes insipidus not uncommonly occurs intermittently and transiently in the postoperative period, and frequent checks of serum and urinary electrolytes and urinary specific gravity must be made to correct these fluctuations.

The patient with elevated ICP is best kept hypertonic and needs close electrolyte and osmolar monitoring during diuresis and fluid replacement. Infants with significant CSF drainage through a ventriculostomy or lumbar drain can become hyponatremic unless sodium lost in the CSF is replaced. Finally, the occurrence of hypernatremia with hypokalemia can indicate adrenal insufficiency, which can occur after prolonged courses of steroid administration.

Nutrition

Early nutritional supplements may be an important factor in recovery from any surgical procedure but especially after neurosurgery. Head trauma in particular produces exceedingly high metabolic demands. Enteral nutrition is desirable whenever possible, reserving parenteral nutrition for the patient with prolonged ileus or other GI disorder. If the patient is obtunded, feeding tubes can be placed in the duodenum to avoid aspiration. When nutritional components are selected, hyponatremia and even minor hypotonicity must be avoided for the patient with elevated ICP.

Hematologic Factors

Although significant intraoperative blood loss and fluid shifts during neurosurgical procedures can decrease the hematocrit level, blood flow through the microcirculation may be augmented by the resulting decrease in blood viscosity. Some studies suggest that the optimal adult hematocrit level, which balances oxygen-carrying capacity with viscosity, may be 30% to 33%. The optimal hematocrit level for perfusing the brains of infants and children is not known, but experience indicates that hematocrit levels of 10% to 15% below the normal range are tolerated.

Brain tissue contains large amounts of tissue thromboplastin, which can be released by extensive brain trauma and can produce disseminated intravascular coagulopathies (see Chapter 19). Low-grade coagulopathies are thus not uncommon after neurosurgical procedures. Careful monitoring and replacement of clotting factors must be done frequently, particularly if further operative procedures or placement of ICP monitors is planned. Because of the grave consequences of even small intracranial hemorrhages, clotting factors must be replaced for patients with even mildly prolonged coagulation times or for a platelet count of $<80,000/mm^3$.

Seizures

Seizures can occur before and after neurosurgical operations and may herald intracranial hemorrhage or a change of intracranial dynamics. Accordingly, the evaluation of new seizures in a neurosurgical patient must include a CT scan, especially when the postictal state clouds the neurologic examination. Status epilepticus is life threatening and must be aggressively and quickly controlled as described in Chapter 9, particularly since epileptiform activity with or without motor manifestations can increase the cerebral metabolic rate and elevate ICP. One pitfall in controlling seizure in the intubated patient is extreme hyperventilation; simply allowing the Pco_2 to rise 5 to 8 mm Hg may make difficult seizure control possible. Seizures are protean in presentation and must be suspected with any sudden change in mental status, including presumed herniation.

Antiepileptic agents are given routinely whenever the cerebral cortex is opened during a surgical procedure, the exceptions being routine ICP monitor or ventricular shunt placement.

Fever

Fever may indicate infection but also follows the introduction of blood and other irritants into the subarachnoid space. Temperature elevations commonly occur after neurosurgical procedures; these fevers are not treated with antibiotics unless there is a suspected or documented source of bacterial infection or a change in the CSF glucose and white blood cell count. Since fever produces cerebral vasodilation and elevated ICP and can cloud the neurologic examination, aggressive treatment with acetaminophen or cooling blankets is indicated.

Infection

Neurosurgical patients are subject to the same kinds of infection experienced by other critically ill patients. Meningitis is an added danger, and monitoring must include an examination and culture of CSF before antibiotics are started or changed. Lumbar puncture in the neurosurgical patient must be preceded by CT scanning to assess mass effect unless ICP monitors or fontanelle pressure convincingly indicates lack of cerebral shift. If mass effect is present, a ventricular tap may be indicated (see Chapter 118).

Neurosurgical infections are commonly caused by staphylococci, streptococci, or gram-negative organisms, and antibiotics must be chosen for broad-spectrum coverage and their ability to penetrate the blood-brain barrier.

Transportation

Transportation of neurosurgical patients in the PICU to and from other areas in the hospital (e.g., the CT suite) is common and potentially hazardous. Elective studies must be scheduled during daytime hours when nursing and support personnel are available. ECG and systemic arterial blood pressure monitoring are needed for most patients, and the respiratory therapist must be instructed and reminded to maintain hyperventilation if appropriate. Infants and small children often need active warming (especially while in cold CT machines), and all IV drips must be carefully watched. Although ICP monitors are routinely clamped during transport, the occasional patient may need intermittent CSF drainage during prolonged transit or procedures.

ADDITIONAL READING

Cooper KR, Boswell PA, Choi SC. Safe use of PEEP in patients with severe head injury. J Neurosurg 63:552-555, 1985.

Frankel LR. The evaluation, stabilization, and transport of the critically ill child. Int Anesthesiol Clin 25:77-103, 1987.

Gadisseix P, Ward JD, Young HF, et al. Nutrition and the neurosurgical patient. J Neurosurg 60:219-232, 1984.

Green BA, Marshall LF, Gallagher TJ. Intensive Care from Neurological Trauma and Disease. New York: Academic Press, 1982.

Kaufman HD, Hui KS, Mattson JC, et al. Clinicopathological correlations of disseminated intravascular coagulation in patients with head injury. Neurosurgery 15:34-42, 1984.

Kee DB, Wood JH. Rheology of the cerebral circulation. Neurosurgery 15:125-131, 1984.

Kvan DA, Loftus CM, Copeland B, et al. Seizures during the immediate postoperative period. Neurosurgery 12:14-17, 1983.

Landesman S, Rechtman D, Cooker P. Infectious complications of head injury. In Cooper PR. Head Injury, ed 2. Baltimore: Williams & Wilkins, 1987, pp 422-440.

Lederman RJ. Status epilepticus. Cleve Clin Q 51:261-266, 1984.

Levin AB. Intensive care. In Wilkins RH, Ringachary SS, eds. Neurosurgery. New York: McGraw-Hill, 1985.

Marsh ML, Marshall LF, Shapiro HM. Neurosurgical intensive care. Anesthesiology 47:149-163, 1977.

63 Major Craniofacial Surgery

Douglas P. Sinn · Maria Ortega · H. Steven Byrd ·
Frederick H. Sklar

BACKGROUND

In approximately 1:1000 births in the United States the infant has a variant of some facial, skeletal, or craniofacial deformity. If the more common deformities of cleft lip and cleft palate are included, the incidence is far greater.

In general cranial and facial deformities can be divided into three subgroups: (1) those involving the cranial skeleton only (coronal, sagittal, metopic, lambdoidal synostosis), (2) those involving the cranial and facial skeleton (Crouzon's, Apert's, and Pfeiffer's syndrome), and (3) those involving the facial skeleton only (Treacher Collins syndrome, hemifacial microsomia, cleft lip/cleft palate, Pierre Robin anomalad). In all of these deformities maldevelopment of the skeleton may directly and significantly affect the overlying soft tissue.

The surgical approach to these congenital deformities was radically changed by techniques introduced by Paul Tessier in France in 1967. From his imaginative intracranial and extracranial approaches, numerous advances have been made that facilitate the care of the majority of these children. The specific surgical techniques and approaches rather than the diagnosis determine most management considerations in the immediate postoperative period. Those approaches limited to an extracranial alteration of the facial skeleton necessitate emphasis on the management of fluid and electrolytes, blood volume, and the airway. Since bone graft or alloplast infections, although rare, may occur after the third or fourth postoperative day, evaluation of fever occurring at that time must take into consideration these possibilities. Intracranial procedures with manipulation and retraction of the brain necessitate careful monitoring of fluids and electrolytes, airway, blood volume, signs of increased ICP, and life-threatening CNS infection. Some procedures involve both an intra-cranial and extracranial approach and, in addition to the concerns indicated, introduce considerations related to ocular compression and potential CSF leaks from injury to the cribriform plate. The surgery may be limited to a sterile intracranial/extracranial approach or may extend into the nasal cavities and midfacial area, creating contamination of the wound with pathogens from the nasal and pharyngeal areas.

Timing of the surgical management of these patients has been advocated from the first few weeks after birth until well into the second decade. Many of these patients will need multiple, staged procedures involving movements of bone and soft tissue from both an intracranial and extracranial approach. On occasion posterior cranial access will be indicated, as will removal or addition of bone and soft tissue components necessary to correct the pathologic craniofacial skeleton.

SPECIFIC SURGICAL/ANESTHETIC CONSIDERATIONS
Oral and Maxillofacial Surgery

The diagnosis and management of skeletal facial, craniofacial, and dentofacial deformities should include input from each of the surgical specialists and the anesthesiologist. Decisions are based on the deformity, age, and general health of the patient, with associated cardiac, respiratory, and neurologic problems excluded or addressed in planning decisions.

Surgery of the upper and lower jaws necessitating maxillomandibular fixation (stabilization achieved by wiring the upper and lower teeth together) eliminates access to the oral cavity and airway, which can create multiple problems postoperatively in the PICU. With the advent of rigid internal fixation, the use of maxillomandibular fixation has been eliminated and some of the postoperative airway problems substantially reduced. Careful management of fluids, including free water restriction to decrease airway edema, slow, careful introduction of oral intake, and frequent suctioning, will allow these patients to tolerate the PICU phase with little difficulty.

Oral incisions generally are performed in the sulcus between the maxillary and mandibular alveolus and cheek. Postoperatively this means the patient must receive good oral hygiene, including oral rinses after oral intake and intermittently throughout the day in the early postoperative stages. A liquid diet is generally offered during the first 2 to 3 days, and the patient is then advanced to a soft diet when possible. Diet considerations in these instances are based on the fixation and stability of the facial skeleton.

Special dietary considerations for patients after surgical cleft lip/cleft palate correction with pharyngeal flaps include a diet of liquid consistency administered via a cup or a catheter-tip syringe. To avoid injury to the repair in patients with a cleft lip, suctioning must be done only if the airway is compromised. The common clear-liquid and full-liquid diets (e.g., Popsicles, hard ice cream, congealed Jell-O) must be avoided. Gavage feedings are contraindicated in patients with cleft palate if they can be avoided.

Plastic Surgery

The incisions involved in gaining access to the craniofacial skeleton are multiple and varied. The typical scalp incision is a coronal incision and passes behind the hairline from just in front of one ear to the opposite side. Through this incision the forehead and soft tissues of the face are reflected away from the cranial and facial skeleton, thereby allowing access for surgical osteotomies. When an extracranial approach through this incision is used, a strip of hair is shaved, leaving hair both in front of and behind the incision. Many surgeons favor completely shaving the head for combined extracranial and intracranial surgery.

Suction drains are almost always used to evacuate blood and serum from potential dead spaces in and around the osteotomies. These drains are typically removed within 48 hours unless ouput is excessive, and removal is almost always followed by an increase in periorbital edema, which is related to the gravitational effect on fluid and settling of residual blood and serum. It is not infrequent for the eyes to swell completely shut the day after drain removal. When a combined intracranial and extracranial procedure

such as in the correction of hypertelorism has been performed, the use of suction drains may be complicated by an air leak caused by sucking ambient air or nasal secretions through the nose and ethmoid sinus area into the cranial dead space. When this occurs, the drains must be disconnected from negative suction pressure and allowed to act as passive conduits. In this situation the surgeon must anticipate prolonged serous drainage from the nose after the drain is moved.

Fluid leaking from the nose after removal of the drain is frequently confused with CSF rhinorrhea and necessitates a careful evaluation. If the drainage is gravitational flow of blood and serum from the surgical site out of the ethmoid space through the nose, the morbidity and risk are minimal. If, however, the fluid is CSF leaking from an unrepaired dural tear or cribriform injury, the risk of meningitis is significant.

Periorbital incisions include incisions beneath the lower lid (subciliary), brow incisions, and inner canthal incisions. When these incisions are present, a greater risk of exposure keratitis can be anticipated, and the need for lubrication and protection of the eye is paramount. A temporary tarsorrhaphy stitch is sometimes placed. When permanent sutures are used in and around the eyelids, early removal on the third to fifth postoperative day is advised.

Nasal incisions are typically made inside the nose and have few management requirements. Postoperative bleeding from the nasal area can be treated initially with Afrin nasal spray and humidification. If attempts at vasoconstriction are not successful after one or two applications, consideration must be given to tamponade of the bleeding site.

Neurosurgery

Surgical procedures to correct the various cranial deformities caused by synostosis are numerous. They involve the occiput to correct the deformities of lambdoid synostosis and both the parietal and occipital areas with skull reshaping for sagittal synostosis. Metopic or coronal suture fusion involves reshaping the forehead and advancing the supraorbital rims to establish a more normal relationship between the brow and the eyes. Multiple suture synostosis or marked distortion of the cranial configuration may necessitate extensive reworking of the entire cranial vault.

Despite the often dramatic degree of cranial skeleton alteration, these surgeries usually do not involve significant manipulation of the brain. Accordingly, postoperative problems with cerebral edema, intracranial hypertension, bleeding, and other complications of major intracranial surgery are infrequent. Nonetheless, in addition to the airway problems already discussed, the most common postoperative problems in patients undergoing craniofacial surgery are neurosurgical in nature.

Before the patient's eyes swell shut, an initial evaluation of vision, pupillary response, and extraocular movements must be performed. Injury to the optic nerve and orbital contents is an unusual operative complication, but it can occur. Direct injury of the optic nerve is a rare complication of hypertelorism surgery and is presumably related to stretching, kinking, or bony compression of the nerve in the orbit or optic canal. Early recognition of complications can lead to surgical reexploration in the hope of restoring vision. Postoperative strabismus, although also uncommon, occurs on occasion.

CSF rhinorrhea may occur in craniofacial patients in whom the anterior fossa dura has been dissected away from the cranial base. In the PICU the first task is to attempt to clarify whether or not the leaking fluid is CSF or innocent epidural serous drainage; both may be glucose positive. CSF is more waterlike, and drainage volumes usually will be significant. Alternatively, serous drainage tends to be a self-limited process. CSF rhinorrhea is treated initially by positioning the patient upright, using gravity to reduce the fluid pressure promoting the leak. Persistent leak will necessitate placement of a lumbar subarachnoid catheter to drain CSF. Overdrainage of CSF can result in symptomatic intracranial hypotension, as evidenced by systemic arterial blood pressure and/or pulse changes, headache, and perhaps alteration in the level of consciousness. When hypotension occurs, the use of intermittent drainage may be necessary. Usually these nonoperative measures will suffice to stop the rhinorrhea. Infrequently reoperation to repair and reinforce the dural defect will be necessary.

Postoperative fever is common in the craniofacial patient, although persistent fever will indicate the need to search for an infectious origin. Perioperative prophylactic antibiotics are used routinely for cranial procedures that do involve concurrent nasal or oral exposure at the University of Texas Southwestern Medical Center. In these latter cases the patients are maintained on antibiotics for 5 days.

There may be a significant oozing from the dura and bone in the early postoperative period that, in the infant undergoing craniofacial surgery, may necessitate transfusion replacement therapy. For this reason frequent measurements of hematocrit and hemoglobin values and subgaleal wound drainage are needed during the first 24 hours after surgery. Assessment of adequate vascular volume (heart rate, systemic arterial blood pressure, peripheral perfusion, urinary output) must be done frequently.

Finally, the patient undergoing craniofacial surgery may experience problems related to fluid and electrolyte balance, postoperative seizures, intracranial hypertension, and brain edema. These problems are discussed in detail in Chapters 7 and 62.

Anesthesia

Although anesthetic techniques used for these patients do not differ significantly from those for other children, the potential for large blood loss and prolonged surgical time necessitate special preparation. Major craniofacial reconstruction can take 3 to 10 hours and longer. Hypotensive anesthesia with induced low systemic arterial blood pressure can be advantageous from the standpoint of both decreased blood loss and specific control of the vascular components of the craniofacial skeleton. Our choice is to use hypotensive anesthesia when possible.

PREOPERATIVE MANAGEMENT

In addition to the deformity itself, preoperative considerations in these patients include an assessment of the cardiopulmonary, neurologic, endocrine, and renal systems as well as the airway.

Airway. A significant percentage of children undergoing craniofacial surgery will have airway problems. The physical examination must focus on the upper airway to obtain airway control and intubation. Assessment must include the following:

Facial asymmetry
Micrognathia
Range of motion of jaw and neck
Tongue anatomy, including glossoptosis, hypoplasia, bifid tongue
Dental integrity
Cleft palate and its repair (pharyngeal flap)
Position of larynx and trachea
Nasal patency

Any pertinent airway history, especially evidence of airway obstruction, must be obtained during the interview. The following list includes important historical points in airway assessment:

Mouth breathing

Snoring

Sleep apnea

Feeding difficulties (e.g., problems swallowing, choking)

Poor sucking and gag reflexes

Recurrent upper airway infections, including croup, chronic nasal discharge, otitis media

Tonsillar/adenoidal hypertrophy

Previous anesthetic history (e.g., difficult intubation, emergency tracheostomy)

Cardiopulmonary assessment. Certain craniofacial syndromes are known to be associated with congenital heart disease (e.g., Apert's, Carpenter's, Goldenhar's, Down, Treacher Collins syndromes). In addition chronic upper airway obstruction may result in pulmonary arterial hypertension and cor pulmonale. At best the cardiac lesion may be hemodynamically insignificant and necessitate only antibiotic prophylaxis for subacute bacterial endocarditis. At worst the condition may have such profound physiologic effects as to determine the entire anesthetic management, including induction, choice of technique, monitoring, and ventilation. The cardiopulmonary status may also preclude the use of adjuvant techniques such as controlled systemic arterial hypotension and osmotic diuresis. The cardiac lesion may be so severe that the child has an unacceptable anesthetic risk for a complex and lengthy procedure and the operation must be scaled down to only that intervention necessary to relieve airway obstruction or intracranial hypertension.

Neurologic assessment. Although single-suture synostoses are not invariably associated with intracranial hypertension, the presence of multiple-suture synostoses should alert the physician to the possibility of increased ICP. The management of all these children is designed on the assumption that they have or are at risk for increased ICP.

Preexisting neurologic deficits are documented preoperatively, and special note is made of neurologic problems of airway control and protection. This becomes most important in the postoperative period when the child is at risk for airway obstruction, apnea, and aspiration. Children with a history of seizures are maintained on their routine anticonvulsant regimen, assuming the seizures are controlled. If the seizures are not well controlled, blood levels of the anticonvulsants are obtained and the levels increased before surgery.

Renal assessment. If the systemic arterial blood pressure and serum creatinine level are normal, renal function is considered adequate. Renal function must be adequate to permit the intraoperative use of controlled hypotension. Certain syndromes and conditions, including Chotzen's syndrome, orofacial-digital syndrome, and neurofibromatosis associated with renal artery stenosis and pheochromocytoma, are seen in conjunction with renal anomalies and impaired renal function.

Endocrine assessment. Hypopituitarism is not infrequently encountered. The patient must be euthyroid at the time of surgery, and adrenal steroids sufficient to meet stress needs are administered perioperatively (see below). Adrenal suppression also may be assumed to be present if the patient has been on exogenous steroids for more than 2 weeks within the preceding year. When in doubt, steroids must be administered.

Laboratory Tests and Radiologic Evaluation

In an otherwise healthy child the preliminary laboratory workup and radiologic evaluation need not be extensive. Often the only laboratory tests ordered are a CBC and type and crossmatch. In the event the child has associated medical problems or intraoperative problems are anticipated, other preoperative evaluations may be indicated, including the following.

Complete blood count. Except for the infant in the "physiologic trough" (6 to 12 weeks), a healthy child should have a minimum hemoglobin level of 10 g/dl. A craniofacial procedure is a major surgical undertaking, and the potential for severely stressing the cardiopulmonary and neurologic systems exists; thus the availability of adequate oxygen-carrying capacity is essential. Although a child with chronic anemia may readily tolerate his lowered hemoglobin level when not stressed, he may not readily tolerate the stresses imposed by surgery and anesthesia.

The possibility of unsuspected hemoglobinopathies, chronic occult losses, or chronic renal disease must be considered and adequately investigated. If time permits, iron is added to the diet, and the child is reevaluated in 1 to 2 months. If the anemia will not respond to iron therapy or time is short, the child is given a transfusion of 10 ml packed RBCs/kg body weight at least 12 hours before surgery, and it may need to be repeated to achieve a hemoglobin value of 10 g/dl. The remainder of the blood unit is then used intraoperatively.

White blood count. Any evidence of current infection must be thoroughly evaluated. Viral upper respiratory infections are relative contraindications to surgery. A mild upper respiratory infection can become a major problem intraoperatively and postoperatively because of the following factors:

Airway irritability, including laryngospasm in the already difficult airway

Bronchospasm

Increased secretions, mucous plugs, atelectasis

Difficulty with ventilation and oxygenation

Increased brain volume because of inability to control Pco_2 and because of increased peak inspiratory pressure needed for ventilation

Increased surgical bleeding because of increased intrathoracic pressures needed for ventilation

Postoperative croup

Increased risk of postoperative pneumonia, atelectasis, and respiratory insufficiency

Need for postoperative intubation and mechanical ventilation

Postoperative fever, which necessitates complete laboratory and radiologic evaluation

A low WBC (e.g., in a patient with a recent viral infection) may be present occasionally. An absolute neutrophil count of $500/mm^3$ or greater is a prerequisite for surgery.

Platelets. The platelet count may be elevated to $>500,000/mm^3$ in patients with conditions other than myeloproliferative disorders. Chronic anemias such as iron deficiency anemia and hemolytic anemias and acute-phase reactions associated with either acute infection or chronic inflammatory states may have associated thrombocytosis. Counts $<100,000/mm^3$ must also be investigated preoperatively. A platelet count $>100,000/mm^3$ is necessary for surgical hemostasis during performance of an extensive procedure. The platelet count must be obtained again before initiating an extensive workup since the presence of a small clot in the specimen or a technical problem with the slide preparation may result in a grossly inaccurate count.

PT/PTT. Major blood loss can be anticipated because of the extensive surgical dissection over a long period in areas where bleeding may be difficult to control. Although the presence of hemophilia is rare and is usually well known to the family, undiagnosed von Willebrand's disease has been diagnosed in preoperative evaluations.

Electrolytes. Electrolyte determinations are not done unless there is some indication there may be an abnormality (e.g., with digoxin and diuretic therapy, feeding difficulties, vomiting, SIADH, adrenal steroid replacement therapy).

Creatinine. If a controlled systemic arterial hypotension technique is planned, a baseline serum creatinine determination is requested. Renal anomalies and renal dysfunction may be associated with certain craniofacial syndromes.

Urinalysis. Urinalysis is routinely done for all patients for whom surgery is planned.

Chest roentgenogram. A preoperative chest roentgenogram is not routinely ordered. However, there often is so much upper airway noise from the distorted anatomy that chest auscultation is difficult. A chest roentgenogram must be obtained in any child with a history of chronic pulmonary disease, recurrent pulmonary infection, or chronic upper airway obstruction (cor pulmonale).

ECG. This test is usually requested in conjunction with a pediatric cardiology evaluation.

Type and crossmatch. Packed RBCs are prepared since they will be needed in the majority of patients.

Bacterial cultures. Any purulent discharge from the nose, eyes, throat, or sputum is cultured preoperatively. If onset of the discharge is recent, cancellation of surgery must be considered. If the discharge is chronic and the surgeon does not consider the condition a contraindication to surgery, topical or systemic antibiotics should be started preoperatively to treat the most likely organisms (see below).

Informed Consent

The preoperative visit represents a time for the exchange of information between the child, parents, and physicians. The child gives information about himself through the physical examination; his parents provide information by giving the child's medical and surgical history, and the physicians explain the preoperative preparation, intraoperative anesthetic management, and expected postoperative course.

Contrary to the fear of some that this information will promote anxiety in the child and the parents, usually the reverse is true. Information presented in a calm, unhurried, and compassionate manner reassures the parents and affords them the opportunity to become informed participants in their child's care.

INTRAOPERATIVE MANAGEMENT
Induction

Venous access is secured with the child awake. Once access is obtained, the choice of induction technique is determined by the needs of the patient, including control of the airway, anticipated difficulty of intubation, and complicating medical conditions. A functioning IV line is essential when an inhalation induction is planned because of a difficult airway.

When no significant problems with airway control and intubation are anticipated and no other contraindications exist, thiopental (4 to 5 mg/kg), vecuronium (0.2 mg/kg), and fentanyl (2 μg/kg) are used for induction. This technique is rapid and well tolerated and allows immediate control of the airway, hyperventilation, and ICP.

Anesthetic Maintenance Technique

Any number of anesthetic agents and drug combinations are acceptable choices as long as the following requirements are met: (1) cardiovascular stability, (2) compatibility with the use of epinephrine, (3) control of ICP with preservation of adequate cerebral perfusion, and (4) rapid emergence. The combination of isoflurane, vecuronium, and fentanyl almost invariably is well tolerated and meets all the requirements for an anesthetic technique.

Fluid Management and Blood Replacement

Maintenance and deficit fluids are initially given as lactated Ringer's solution. Changes to 0.9% sodium chloride or 0.45% sodium chloride solutions are made if so indicated by electrolyte determinations. Hourly maintenance (and deficit) fluids are calculated for body-weight increments using the following regimen:

1. 4 ml/kg/hr for the first 0 to 10 kg
2. 2 ml/kg/hr for the next 10 to 20 kg
3. 1 ml/kg/hr for weight >20 kg

Example: 38 kg child

$$4 \text{ ml/kg/hr} \times 10 \text{ kg} = 40 \text{ ml/hr}$$
$$2 \text{ ml/kg/hr} \times 10 \text{ kg} = 20 \text{ ml/hr}$$
$$1 \text{ ml/kg/hr} \times 18 \text{ kg} = 18 \text{ ml/hr}$$

Hourly maintenance for 38 kg = 78 ml/hr

Fluid deficit is replaced over the first 2 to 3 hours and more rapidly if the child is clinically hypovolemic. However, since this calculation of fluid deficit represents fluid not given rather than fluid lost (except for urinary output and insensible losses), this volume need not be completely replaced. If clinical assessment shows the child is well hydrated and urinary output is adequate (1 to 2 ml/kg), completely correcting the deficit is not necessary.

CSF loss is not replaced since this loss is usually minimal and CSF itself is not acutely replaced but rather produced continuously at approximately 0.3 ml/kg/hr. CSF replacement does become necessary postoperatively if there are continued losses from a CSF leak or spinal or ventriculostomy drainage. It is then replaced "milliliter for milliliter" with 0.9% sodium chloride solution over 8 hours for losses incurred over the previous 8-hour period.

Crystalloid solutions are used to replace modest blood losses (<5% estimated blood volume). Larger losses are replaced one for one with a colloid-containing solution (5% albumin in normal saline or lactated Ringer's solution) until transfusion becomes necessary. The decision to start replacement with blood is influenced by many factors, including the preoperative hemoglobin level, anticipated losses, the preexisting medical illness, and intraoperative clinical status. Blood units are split into approximately 100 ml packets so that only that blood needed intraoperatively is warmed and used. Those packets not used are available for postoperative replacement, thus minimizing the number of units (donors) to which the child is exposed. Significant postoperative blood loss may occur, and further transfusion is often needed.

Glucose is administered as a separate constant infusion at 100 mg/kg/hr in the infant under 6 months of age and 50 mg/kg/hr or less in the older child. Because of decreased metabolic demands, decreased glycogen production, use of steroids, and the stress response to surgery, hyperglycemia with fluid shifts and glycosuria may develop if glucose administration is not regulated and glucose levels not monitored.

Controlled Hypotension

Because craniofacial surgery can incur large blood loss, a hypotensive technique is often of advantage since it (1) reduces the patient's need for blood and blood products, (2) facilitates the surgery, and (3) reduces the operative times. Isoflurane and labetalol have become the preferred agents for inducing hypotensive anesthesia. Labetalol is a selective, competitive α_1-adrenergic blocking agent and a nonselective, noncompetitive β-adrenergic blocking agent. The ratio of α to β blockade is approximately 1:7 for IV administration. Elimination half-life is 5½ hours after IV administration and is not altered by hepatic or renal dysfunction. It is metabolized by glucuronide conjugation and can cause orthostatic hypotension as most α-blockers do. A loading dose of 0.25 mg/kg IV of labetalol is given over a 5-minute period. The onset of action is rapid (5 to 10 minutes) but not precipitous. If after 10 minutes the degree of hypotension is judged inadequate, an additional dose is administered. Once an adequate degree of hypotension is achieved, the drug may be administered as intermittent boluses or as a continuous infusion.

Diuretics

Although the need for brain relaxation is not as great as in a neurosurgical procedure, some degree of brain relaxation is necessary during craniofacial surgery. A tense brain interferes wtih the intracranial approach used with these procedures, and excessive pressure on the brain tissue from retractors is a risk. A tight dura is more likely to be torn than one not under tension. Intracranial hypertension is more than an inconvenience to the surgeon—it is a threat to the patient and must be controlled.

Diuresis is achieved with the use of furosemide, 0.25 to 0.5 mg/kg, followed 15 minutes later by mannitol, 0.5 to 1.0 g/kg. A reduction in ICP will occur within 10 to 15 minutes, but obvious bulk shrinkage does not become optimal for 45 minutes. The agents are administered 45 minutes before the skull flap is turned and the dura exposed.

Antibiotics

Prophylactic antibiotic therapy is begun at the time of surgery and is continued for 48 hours into the postoperative period. Antibiotics are continued postoperatively because a number of factors contribute to decreased host resistance: (1) a poor host, including marginal nutritional status and associated medical illness, (2) a catabolic state postoperatively, and (3) immunosuppression caused by the use of steroids and anesthesia.

The choice of drug is determined by the surgical site to provide adequate coverage against the most likely contaminating organisms (Table 63-1). A bolus antibiotic is given at the time of closure to promote a high antibiotic level in any resulting hematoma.

Steroids

Methylprednisolone sodium succinate, 2 mg/kg IV, is administered every 4 hours intraoperatively and continued postoperatively for 48 hours. When IV steroids are discontinued, a single dose of methylprednisolone acetate, 1 mg/kg IM, is administered. Methylprednisolone stabilizes cell membranes, which results in decreased postoperative swelling at the surgical site. This will have a number of advantages in the postoperative period, including aesthetic considerations, improved patient comfort, decreased

Table 63-1   Perioperative Antibiotics Used in Patients Undergoing Craniofacial Surgery*

Antibiotic	Dosage
Intraoral	
Aqueous penicillin G	50,000 U/kg IV q 4 hr intraoperatively
	25,000 U/kg IV q 4 hr postoperatively
Intranasal (includes ear and sinuses)	
Cefuroxime	50 mg/kg IV q 6 hr intraoperatively
	25 mg/kg IV q 6 hr postoperatively
Skin	
Methicillin or	50 mg/kg IV q 6 hr intraoperatively
	25 mg/kg IV q 6 hr postoperatively
Cefazolin	25 mg/kg IV q 6 hr intraoperatively
	25 mg/kg IV q 8 hr postoperatively
Intradural	
Methicillin or cefuroxime plus gentamicin	2 mg/kg IV q 8 hr intraoperatively and postoperatively

*Variable resistance patterns in an institution will necessitate individualization of these recommendations.

tension on suture lines, and decreased incidence of airway obstruction.

POSTOPERATIVE MANAGEMENT

Extubation and pulmonary care. Most patients are extubated in the operating room at the end of the surgical procedure since the vast majority of cases proceed uneventfully and the patient is judged able to maintain and protect his own airway. Each case is judged inidividually, and the decision to extubate is made after the patient emerges from anesthesia. The decision to keep the patient intubated, however, may be made at any point during the procedure for the following conditions:

Very difficult intubation (increased likelihood of trauma to the airway)

Prior airway compromise not corrected as part of the procedure

Cardiovascular instability

Problems with oxygenation and ventilation

Intracranial hypertension

Massive blood loss and massive transfusion do not influence the decision to extubate as long as the patient is hemodynamically stable and normothermic and has neither a metabolic acidosis nor alkalosis at the end of the procedure.

Humidified supplemental oxygen is continued for 12 to 24 hours postoperatively. Frequent, gentle chest percussion therapy may be indicated to help mobilize secretions and prevent (treat) atelectasis. Incentive spirometry is ordered if the patient is old enough to cooperate. Postoperative mechanical ventilation may be necessary for airway management or control of ICP.

Bleeding. Blood loss will continue into the postoperative period, and frequent hemoglobin/hematocrit determinations are obtained for 24 hours postoperatively. Clinically significant losses are replaced with packed RBCs, with the aim to achieve euvolemia and adequate oxygen-carrying capacity (Hb ≥ 10 g/dl).

Intracranial hypertension. Intracranial hypertension, although uncommon is managed as follows:

Fluid restriction to 70% of maintenance dose

Diuretics

Mannitol, 0.5 mg/kg q 2-4 hr IV

Furosemide, 0.5-1 mg/kg q 4-6 hr IV

Steroids: dexamethasone, 1 mg/kg/24 hr IV

Ventriculostomy: used both for monitoring of ICP and for venting of CSF (CSF losses may become significant, and CSF is replaced milliliter for milliliter with 0.9 sodium chloride solution over 8 hours for losses incurred over the previous 8-hour period)

Mechanical ventilation (for hyperventilation, see Chapter 7)

Thirty-degree head-up position to maintain cerebral profusion pressure by keeping mean arterial pressure within adequate range; avoidance of noxious stimuli (e.g., suctioning), which may cause changes in ICP

SIADH. SIADH, a frequent occurrence in the postoperative period (especially after combined intracranial/extracranial procedures involving retraction of the frontal lobes), can be managed with (1) fluid restriction, including insensible losses (300 ml/m^2/24 hr) plus urinary output over the previous hour, and (2) small doses of furosemide (0.1 mg/kg q 6 to 8 hr IV) if hyponatremia is pronounced or diuresis is otherwise indicated (see also Chapter 57).

ADDITIONAL READING

Artru A, Wright K, Colley P, et al. Cerebral effects of hypocapnia plus nitroglycerin-induced hypotension in dogs. J Neurosurg 64:924-931, 1986.

Bedford R, Colley P. Intracranial tumors: Supratentorial and intratentorial. Clinical case studies in neuroanesthesia and neurosurgery. New York: Grune & Stratton, 1986, pp 135-179.

Bourke D, Smith T. Estimating allowable hemodilution. Anesthesiology 4:609-612, 1975.

Buckland RW, Manners JM. Venous air embolism during neurosurgery. Anesthesiology 31:633-643, 1976.

• Diaz JH, Lockhart CH. Hypotensive anesthesia for craniectomy in infancy. Br J Anaesth 51:233-235, 1979.

Edwards H, King T. Cardiac tamponade from central venous catheter. Arch Surg 117:965-967, 1982.

Miller R. Complications of massive blood transfusions. Anesthesiology 39:82-91, 1973.

• Munro I. Orbito-cranio-facial surgery: The team approach. Plast Reconstr Surg 55:170-176, 1975.

Rogers M, Nugent S, Traystman R, et al. Control of cerebral circulation in the neonate and infant. Crit Care Med 8:570-574, 1980.

64 Organ Transplantation: Liver

Elizabeth A. Wanek · Walter S. Andrews

BACKGROUND

The first liver transplantation was performed in the United States in 1963. With immunosuppression therapy limited to prednisone, azathioprine, and later antilymphocyte globulin, however, the 1-year survival rate was only 30%. With the introduction of the lymphokine-inhibitor cyclosporine A (CyA) in 1980, the 1-year survival rate has increased dramatically to 70% to 80%, allowing liver transplantation to become a therapeutic alternative for children with irreversible liver failure.

A National Institute of Health Consensus Development Conference on Liver Transplantation (1983) established guidelines regarding indications for transplantation and the timing of surgery. The diseases considered amenable to transplantation included extrahepatic biliary atresia, chronic active hepatitis, primary biliary cirrhosis, inborn errors of metabolism, hepatic vein thrombosis, sclerosing cholangitis, primary hepatic malignancy confined to the liver but not amenable to resection, and alcohol-related liver cirrhosis. Surgery should be considered when death is imminent, when irreversible damage to the CNS is inevitable, or when the quality of life has deteriorated to unacceptable levels.

In children the primary indication for liver transplantation is biliary atresia. Other indications, in decreasing order of frequency, are inborn errors of metabolism (Wilson's disease, α_1-antitrypsin deficiency, tyrosinemia, glycogen storage disease, familial hypercholesterolemia), familial cholestasis, acute hepatic failure, congenital hepatic fibrosis, neonatal hepatitis, secondary biliary cirrhosis, sclerosing cholangitis, Budd-Chiari syndrome, idiopathic purpura, primary biliary cirrhosis, primary liver tumors, toxic hepatitis, and trauma.

A child is considered for transplantation when there is evidence of deterioration of metabolic function (increasing PT or PTT or decreasing serum albumin level), uncontrollable ascites with or without recurrent pleural effusions, recurrent and persistent biliary sepsis, variceal hemorrhage, encephalopathy, or uncontrollable pruritus. A multivariate analysis of these risk factors has shown that children with cholesterol levels <100 mg/dl, a bilirubin level >6 mg/dl, or a PT >20 seconds are at risk of imminent death from liver failure and must be considered as high-priority candidates. Patients who have become social invalids because of incapacitating pruritus or uncorrectable metabolic bone disease must also be considered high-priority candidates. Patients are excluded from transplantation if they have anatomic abnormalities (thrombosis of the portal vein or lack of a superior mesenteric vein–splenic vein confluence), metastatic tumor from or to the liver, advanced nonhepatic disease (severe cardiac or pulmonary disease), an underlying disease uncorrectable by transplantation, or any active infection. The presence of stage IV hepatic coma is a relative contraindication to liver transplantation.

THE PROCEDURE

Three phases are involved in transplantation: (1) organ retrieval and recipient preparation, (2) the anhepatic phase, and (3) revascularization of the donor liver.

A surgical team removes the donor liver in a 2- to 4-hour operation during which the hepatic arterial and venous anatomy is carefully defined. Organ preservation is accomplished by using a 4° C solution that is flushed into the liver through the hepatic artery and portal vein. The organ is then stored on ice while the recipient operation is in progress.

The initial phase of the recipient operation is the preparation of the recipient's liver for removal. This can take 2 to 5 hours, depending on the number of

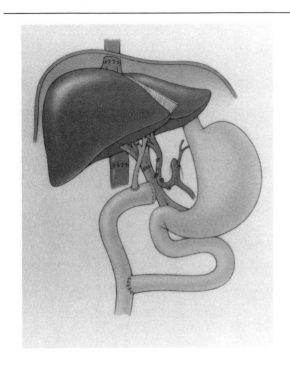

Fig. 64-1 Vascular reconstruction for liver transplant: suprahepatic CAVA, infrahepatic caval, portal vein, and hepatic artery.

previous operations and the density of the adhesions. Next is the anhepatic phase in which the diseased liver is removed and the donor liver is connected by the sequential anastomosis of the suprahepatic vena cava, the infrahepatic vena cava, the portal vein, and finally the hepatic artery (Fig. 64-1). During the anhepatic phase the patient's glucose and electrolytes, clotting factors, blood gases, pH, and Hct are serially monitored. Blood and clotting factors are administered as necessary, and any metabolic abnormalities are corrected. The cold ischemic time (time out of the donor) for the liver is generally limited to 24 hours. The anhepatic phase includes 1½ to 2 hours for the completion of the vessel anastomoses.

The final phase is the revascularization of the graft and the biliary reconstruction. The biliary anastomosis is accomplished with a Roux-en-Y choledochojejunostomy (duct to small bowel) in those patients whose original bile duct is not usable or via a choledochocholedochostomy (duct to duct) in older patients whose own bile duct is large enough to be used (Fig. 64-2). T tubes are used as external drains in the duct-duct groups, and internal stents (feeding tubes) are used in the Roux-en-Y group. Both of these stents are radiopaque and can be seen in the right upper quadrant on a plain abdominal film.

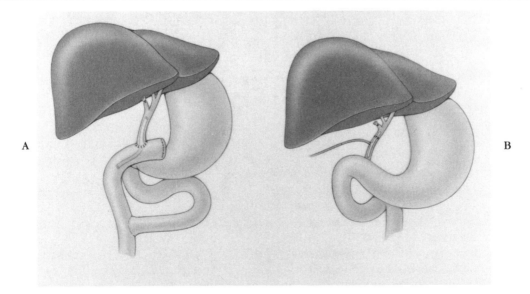

Fig. 64-2 **A,** Biliary reconstruction with a Roux-en-Y choledochojejunostomy using an internal stent. **B,** End-to-end choledochocholedochostomy with T-tube stenting biliary anastomosis.

LABORATORY TESTS

Postoperatively the patient is taken to the PICU, and the following laboratory values are obtained every 6 hours: Hb, Hct, glucose, electrolytes, ionized calcium, phosphorus, PT, and PTT. Liver function tests (ALT, AST, GGT, bilirubin) are performed daily or more often if there is a question of a severe harvest injury or technical difficulty with the graft. CyA is given every 8 hours and trough whole blood CyA levels are drawn 1 hour before the morning dose and assayed daily using high-pressure liquid chromatography (HPLC). Initially the CyA levels are kept at 250 to 350 ng/ml.

IMMUNOSUPPRESSION

The immunosuppressive armamentarium of the liver transplant surgeon consists of four types of drugs: steroids, CyA, azathioprine, and antilymphocyte agents.

Prednisone and CyA are the modern cornerstones of immunosuppressive therapy. Steroids (1 g of methylprednisolone) are given intraoperatively after revascularization of the graft. All patients are then placed on a steroid recycle regimen based on their weight. Patients <40 kg receive methylprednisolone, 25 mg intravenously, every 6 hours for four doses, which is then tapered by 20 mg/day to prednisone, 20 mg/day. Patients >40 kg are given methylprednisolone, 50 mg IV every 6 hours for four doses, which is then tapered by 40 mg/day to prednisone, 20 mg/day. The prednisone is tapered to 0.2 mg/kg/day according to the child's clinical status.

CyA (2 mg/kg) is begun intravenously in the operating room and continued postoperatively at 6 mg/kg/day in three divided doses. Azathioprine (1 mg/kg/day) is added orally on the fifth postoperative day and is increased to 2 mg/kg/day, providing the WBC count does not fall below 4000 cells/mm³. Minnesota antilymphocyte globulin (MALG) and OKT3 monoclonal antibody (Orthoclone OKT3) are used for treating steroid-resistant rejection episodes. These agents are directed against the cells that cause rejection—MALG against thymocytes and OKT3 against T cells with the T_3 marker.

The major complications of immunosuppression include an increased susceptibility to bacterial, fungal, and viral infections; possible mild growth retardation; and possible drug reactions to MALG and OKT3 if they are used.

DETECTION AND MANAGEMENT OF SPECIFIC POSTOPERATIVE PROBLEMS

Routine postoperative monitoring includes hourly recordings of CVP, systemic arterial blood pressure via an arterial catheter, Dynamap blood pressure, heart rate, respiratory rate, urinary output, and abdominal drain output. Abdominal girth and weights must be recorded twice a day.

Neurologic Function
Monitoring

The postoperative neurologic status must be monitored every 2 hours using a routine neurologic examination that includes an assessment of sensory and motor function.

Management

The best evidence of good graft function is a progressive improvement in neurologic status, culminating in the child's being awake and alert within 48 hours after transplantation. Persistent neurologic depression can be related to several problems: (1) persistent muscle blockade, (2) persistent effect of narcotic analgesics and/or other sedatives, (3) impaired hepatic function, (4) a structural CNS lesion, or (5) metabolic abnormalities.

A persistent effect of muscle relaxants postoperatively is not unusual because of decreased metabolism by the new liver. Additional muscle blockade is not routinely used unless it is needed to ensure adequate ventilation. All patients must be monitored with a nerve stimulator for twitch response to document the return of normal muscle function. If continued paralysis is necessary, additional muscle relaxants must be given when movement returns (bolus method) or must be regulated to one or two twitches (continuous infusion method) (see Chapter 130). Regardless of the technique used, paralytic agents must be withheld once a day to assess the patient's neurologic status.

Sedation and pain relief are needed after transplantation. Children, as they awaken from anesthesia, often become extremely restless and agitated, increasing the risks of inadvertent line loss or premature extubation. We advocate the use of narcotic agents (meperidine, 1 mg/kg IV q 6 hr) for pain relief and diphenhydramine (1 mg/kg IV q 4 to 6 hr) or midazolam (0.1 mg/kg IV q 4 to 6 hr) for agitation. Frequent use of narcotic agents in children with imperfect hepatic function will lead to a depressed neurologic status. If this occurs, the narcotic agents can be reversed with naloxone (0.1 mg/kg IV).

Impaired hepatic function can cause persistent coma. If impaired hepatic function is considered as a cause, other signs of graft dysfunction should be present, including elevated PT (>18 seconds), elevated fasting arterial blood ammonia, or elevated total bilirubin values. If the coma is secondary to hepatic dysfunction, the child will need a new organ emergently. Additional experimental and as yet unsubstantiated supportive measures while awaiting a new organ would include plasmapheresis (see Chapter 142) and charcoal hemoperfusion (see Chapter 147).

Structural reasons for persistent coma must always be excluded if no other obvious causes of coma are apparent. Intracranial hemorrhage or infarctions can occur (albeit rarely) during the operative procedure. The neurologic examination may suggest a localized lesion, which can be confirmed with a CT scan. Management is specific to the identified lesion. A patient who is in stage IV hepatic coma at the time of transplant is at increased risk for increased cerebral edema during the operation. This edema can cause herniation during or shortly after completion of the operation. Unfortunately this is a lethal condition.

Metabolic causes of coma in the immediate postoperative period include hypoglycemia and electrolyte imbalance (hyponatremia). Management would be directed toward each problem.

Seizures

Approximately 20% of children undergoing liver transplantation will experience a grand mal seizure. These seizures are most commonly associated with an elevated CyA level (>600 ng/ml HPLC). Seizures, however, can also be caused by metabolic derangements, most of which are poorly defined.

Monitoring. Patients must have their CyA level, along with serum electrolyte, glucose, calcium, phosphorus, and magnesium levels, measured at the time of the seizure.

Management. The initial seizure activity must be controlled in the usual fashion (see Chapter 9). Maintenance therapy includes oral phenobarbital (5 mg/kg/day), with dosage adjustments according to the serum phenobarbital level. Phenobarbital is chosen for its ease of administration and good absorption in children. Phenobarbital and phenytoin, however, decrease serum CyA levels by stimulating the cytochrome P-450 system in the liver. The CyA level, therefore, must be closely monitored and its dose increased to compensate for increased metabolism. All other metabolic abnormalities detected must also be corrected (e.g., hypoglycemia, hyponatremia, hypophosphatemia).

All patients who have had a seizure need a neurologic consultation and a CT scan and/or MRI of the head. Patients must be maintained on phenobarbital therapy for a minimum of 2 weeks. If repeat CT or MRI scanning at this time continues to show structural defects, anticonvulsant therapy must be continued. If, however, any previously noted defects have resolved, the phenobarbital can be discontinued. We have seen recurrent seizures in those patients with persistent structural lesions who have been removed from anticonvulsive therapy.

Respiratory Function
Monitoring

An end-tidal carbon dioxide or transcutaneous carbon dioxide monitor can be used for monitoring in conjunction with a pulse oximeter and arterial blood gas and pH determinations. A pitfall in monitoring these patients is that a discrepancy can exist between the oxygen saturation measured by pulse oximeter and the oxygen saturation directly measured from the blood gas sample. The oxygen saturation measured peripherally is always higher (10% to 40%) than the saturation measured directly from the blood gas sample. The exact cause of this discrepancy is under investigation; however, it is not related to the patient's perfusion status or serum bilirubin level.

Management

Routine management is directed toward extubating the patient as soon as possible. Several factors may preclude extubation, especially a depressed respiratory drive, which can occur because of excessive sedation, impaired hepatic recovery, persistent paralysis, or a persistently elevated P_{CO_2}.

Children needing more than one blood volume transfusion using acid citrate dextrose blood products have an elevated serum citrate level. As the liver begins to function, the citrate is converted into bicarbonate, thereby elevating serum bicarbonate levels. As the patient becomes alkalotic, a compensatory respiratory acidosis develops, resulting in decreased respiratory drive and increased Pco_2, which delays extubation.

Respiratory complications

Pulmonary edema. Pulmonary edema in the immediate postoperative period is most always secondary to fluid overload and is usually accompanied by decreased urinary output and weight gain. Initial corrective steps include the administration of diuretics (furosemide, 2 mg/kg IV) and fluid restriction.

A pulmonary edema pattern that occurs after the initial extubation is a more complex problem. The necessity for reintubation in this situation is assessed using standard respiratory criteria. Fluid overload is considered if the patient has decreased urinary output with an associated weight gain and peripheral edema. Acute management consists of using diuretics and fluid restriction as described previously, but other causes must be investigated.

Pulmonary edema can occur as the result of depressed myocardial function from myocardial ischemia. The onset of this myocardial dysfunction can be from 5 days to 2 weeks after transplantation and initially is seen as the sudden onset of pulmonary edema. It can be associated with ventricular ectopy, an injury pattern visible on ECG, and/or depressed myocardial contractility apparent on an echocardiogram. The pathogenesis apparently is a type of Prinzmetal ischemia. In a few cases the ECG and echocardiographic abnormalities are improved by using IV nitroglycerin. Pathologic studies of patients who died with this problem have shown no evidence of coronary artery disease.

A roentgenographic "pulmonary edema" can be seen with adult respiratory distress syndrome caused by systemic sepsis or a primary pulmonary infection (see Chapter 35). An aggressive search must be instituted for a systemic infection using serial blood cultures, urine cultures, a careful physical examination (fever, localized abdominal tenderness), and radiographic studies (ultrasound, CT, MRI). If these studies are not productive, a primary pulmonary infection must be considered.

Opportunistic infections (CMV, *Pneumocystis carinii,* fungal pneumonitis) are the most common sources of primary pulmonary disease in immunosuppressed patients; however, the more routine bacterial infections must not be overlooked. Initially a sputum sample, free of mouth flora, must be obtained using either an endotracheal tube, transtracheal as-

piration, or bronchoscopy. If a Gram stain of the specimen shows no bacteria and the fluorescent antibody staining for *Legionella* is negative, an open lung biopsy must be performed for diagnosis. Treatment for some opportunistic infections includes IV trimethoprim/sulfamethoxazole at 20 mg/kg/day, divided q 6 hr, for *Pneumocystis;* IV erythromycin at 20 mg/kg/day, divided q 6 hr, for *Legionella;* the appropriate antifungal agent for fungal infections; and ganciclovir at 10 mg/kg/day IV, divided q 12 hr, for CMV pneumonitis.

Acute pulmonary edema is also associated with severe hepatic failure. This problem is unremitting and responds only to retransplantation. In this situation retransplantation must not be withheld because of pulmonary disease unless the patient cannot be mechanically ventilated adequately.

Pleural effusion. It is not uncommon to see a right-sided pleural effusion in association with volume overload and/or significant ascites. This effusion represents a transudation of fluid from the abdomen into the right side of the chest through the denuded diaphragmatic surface. Diuretics usually can decrease the ascites and reduce the pleural effusion. If they are not effective or if the pleural effusion causes respiratory embarrassment, a percutaneous pigtail catheter can be inserted into the chest using the Seldinger technique. Using chest tubes in liver transplant patients can be complicated by severe bleeding. It is easy to lacerate one of the chest wall collateral veins that are present because of the patient's liver disease. If a vein is injured, blood will track along the chest tube and spill into the chest. Chest tube placement, if needed, must be done under direct vision with electrocautery.

Atelectasis. All liver transplant patients need vigorous chest physiotherapy. If atelectasis occurs that does not respond to chest physiotherapy and/or increased ventilation, a bronchoscope must be used on the child both for diagnostic and therapeutic reasons. Flexible bronchoscopy can be used in a child whose endotracheal tube will allow the passage of the scope. If the patient is already extubated, we recommend rigid bronchoscopy with aggressive suctioning, lavage, and insufflation.

Cardiovascular Function
Monitoring

Cardiovascular status is monitored using a CVP catheter, a systemic arterial catheter, Dynamap systemic arterial blood pressures, and an ECG.

Management

The most common cardiovascular problem after liver transplantation is systemic hypertension, which can begin immediately when the patient arrives in the PICU. The most common cause of hypertension in a patient who is emerging from anesthesia is pain; however, if analgesics do not resolve the problem, volume overload is considered. Supportive evidence includes decreased urinary output (<1 ml/kg/hr), increased CVP (>12 to 15 mm Hg), or edema (periorbital or pedal). IV furosemide (2 mg/kg) can be given when volume overload is detected. If the patient appears pain free or if diuretic management does not lower the systemic arterial blood pressure, IV hydralazine (0.2 to 0.5 mg/kg) can be given as a single IV bolus. If it is not effective or if the child needs hydralazine dosing (more frequent than every 4 hours), IV nitroprusside (1 μg/kg/min) must be started and the dose adjusted to keep the systemic arterial blood pressure normal. The patient must be weaned from nitroprusside as rapidly as possible to avoid toxicity. Nitroglycerin is also an effective agent, but it requires both a larger dilution volume and higher doses to achieve the same results as nitroprusside.

Hepatic Function

Laboratory tests

Pertinent laboratory studies include liver function tests (bilirubin, AST, ALT, GGT, PT, PTT) and determination of the CyA level.

Monitoring

Evaluation of abdominal girth, measurement of drain outputs, and a description of the liver size and character must be noted at every shift.

Management

The best indicator of improving hepatic function is the resolution of coma, which should occur in the first 24 to 36 hours after transplantation. During this time the liver is manufacturing clotting factors, as evidenced by the PT and PTT returning to normal. Immediately postoperatively, fresh frozen plasma is given as replacement for abdominal drain output on a milliliter-for-milliliter basis. It supplies clotting factors and albumin during the time when the graft is not producing these proteins. When the clotting studies return to normal, administration of fresh frozen plasma is stopped. IV vitamin K (0.2 mg/kg/day) is also given to supply substrate for the new clotting factors.

The initial set of liver function tests (bilirubin, AST, ALT, GGT) reflects harvest and implantation injury. Unfortunately the degree of enzyme elevation does not correlate with subsequent hepatic function except that the higher the elevations, the greater will be the risk for an unrecoverable hepatic injury (primary nonfunction). The serum bilirubin level should start to decline by day 3 to 5 after transplantation. When a large amount of blood is needed during the transplant (more than three blood volumes), it is not unusual to see an initial decrease in the total bilirubin level (washout), only to see it rebound the next day; however, this is not an indicator of poor hepatic function.

Postoperative bleeding

Immediate postoperative bleeding can occur if there is a leak from a suture line, most commonly at the suprahepatic or infrahepatic vena caval anastomosis. This possibility must be considered when a rapidly falling Hct level is coupled with an increasing output of blood from the drain. A check of the abdominal drain Hct level will give a rapid indication of rate of bleeding (i.e., the closer the Hct level is to the arterial Hct level, the more rapid the bleeding). Often this bleeding can be controlled nonoperatively through the replacement of blood, fresh frozen plasma, and platelets. If bleeding persists for more than 6 hours and/or the patient becomes hemodynamically unstable, reoperation is necessary.

Ascites

Ascites is a common problem after transplantation. The degree of postoperative ascites accumulation can be related to the degree of ascites the child had before transplantation; children with ascites before transplantation tend to have ascites after transplantation. Initially ascites formation is related to the disruption of the perihepatic lymphatics during the hepatectomy; therefore the degree of initial ascites accumulation is directly related to the patient's volume status. Diuretics may be helpful in the first 24 hours, but complete resolution of the ascites is uncommon. Aggressive diuretic management to eliminate the ascites must not be attempted in the early posttransplant period because the child will become intravascularly depleted before the ascites resolves. Albumin is not indicated in the first 24 to 36 hours because it will also leak into the ascites fluid. Aggressive management of the initial ascites must be undertaken only if there is respiratory embarrassment; otherwise careful fluid managment and/or fluid restriction is the best therapy.

Rejection

Rejection is rare in the first days after transplantation because the child is on high-dose CyA and steroid immunosuppression therapy. Rejection is the diagnosis when there is a sudden increase in the total bilirubin, AST, ALT, or GGT level and is often accompanied by systemic signs such as fever and malaise. Liver biopsy provides confirmatory evidence by showing a mixed cellular infiltrate that is centered in the portal areas. Treatment of rejection is accomplished by either an increase in the baseline steroid dose or the use of an antithymocyte globulin or OKT3.

Vascular thrombosis

An orthotopic liver transplant requires four vascular anastomoses: suprahepatic vena cava, infrahepatic vena cava, portal vein, and hepatic artery.

Vascular thrombosis of the suprahepatic or infrahepatic vena cava is rare. A patient with suprahepatic vena caval thrombosis has hepatic enlargement, rapidly increasing ascites, and liver function derangements. A patient with infrahepatic vena caval thrombosis has edema of the lower extremities and potential renal vein thrombosis if clot extension occurs.

Portal vein thrombosis also occurs rarely and has two different presentations, depending on when the thrombosis occurs. Thrombosis occurring in the first 1 to 2 weeks after transplant will result in acute hepatic necrosis and graft loss. In contrast portal vein thrombosis that occurs months after transplantation is initially seen as the return of portal hypertension (esophageal variceal bleeding).

Diagnosis of a vena caval or portal vein thrombosis is confirmed with ultrasonography coupled with Doppler imaging. The portal vein and vena cava are readily seen with ultrasound, and the absence of Doppler flow in the portal vein or retrohepatic vena cava provides conclusive evidence of a thrombosis.

Patients with vena caval thrombosis are at risk for developing pulmonary emboli and must receive anticoagulants, provided there are no mitigating factors. If anticoagulation is too risky or if a pulmonary embolus appears imminent, a direct operative approach can be considered. The only therapy for acute portal vein thrombosis is emergency transplantation. Delayed portal vein thrombosis that presents as portal hypertension without hepatic failure can be ade-

quately treated with endoscopic sclerotherapy and/ or a distal splenorenal shunt.

Hepatic artery thrombosis is a troublesome and often devastating complication after orthotopic liver transplantation. The hepatic artery supplies blood to both the major and minor hepatic ductal systems. When hepatic artery thrombosis occurs, the ductal system undergoes necrosis, resulting in any of the following: (1) common bile duct necrosis with intra-abdominal biliary leakage; (2) single or multiple infected bilomas with minimal damage to the ductal system; (3) necrosis of the intrahepatic biliary system with large bilomas associated with extensive damage to the biliary system; or (4) acute or subacute hepatic necrosis with marked derangement in liver function and multiple intrahepatic abscesses.

No definite pattern of signs or symptoms is diagnostic of hepatic artery thrombosis. The most suggestive presentation is a spiking fever curve, usually occurring approximately 14 days after the transplant, and positive blood cultures for enteric organisms. Alterations in liver function tests can, but do not always occur.

The presence of intrahepatic air on an abdominal plain film is highly suggestive of hepatic artery thrombosis. The absence of a Doppler hepatic artery pulse during ultrasonography of the liver is also highly suggestive and should lead to arteriography, which confirms thrombosis of the donor hepatic artery.

Management. Once hepatic artery thrombosis is diagnosed, the patient's management depends on the reaction of the liver to the loss of arterial flow. If the patient does not develop intrahepatic air and/or acute or subacute hepatic necrosis, conservative management can be attempted. It includes (1) supplemental oxygen to keep the patient's oxygen saturation at 100% to maximize portal venous Po_2; (2) IV antibiotic therapy, including coverage for gram-negative bacteria, anaerobes, and enterococci; and (3) serial ultrasound examinations and/or CT scans to diagnose intrahepatic abscesses or bilomas. These children can have persistent fevers and positive blood cultures despite adequate antibiotic therapy if infected bilomas occur. Once a biloma is detected by ultrasonography or CT scan and is adequately drained (we advocate percutaneous drainage), the patient's temperature will rapidly fall. Once adequate drainage is achieved, long-term drainage of the biloma becomes an important issue. (Further information is included in the article by Rollins et al. cited at the end of this chapter). If the child has acute or subacute hepatic necrosis or suffers irreparable biliary damage, retransplantation will be necessary.

Renal Function

Venoveno bypass, which decompresses the mesenteric venous system and inferior vena cava, is not used in most centers for children <40 kg. Therefore the suprarenal vena cava is occluded 1½ to 2 hours during the implantation of the new liver, causing a transient decrease in urinary output. Mannitol is given before restoration of hepatic blood flow in an attempt to increase urinary output and decrease any renal injury that results from cross clamping.

Laboratory tests

BUN and creatinine levels are the primary laboratory tests obtained. A 4-hour creatinine clearance test is helpful if a more detailed analysis is desired.

Monitoring

Urinary output is measured hourly using an indwelling bladder catheter connected to a urometer. The urine is checked for specific gravity every 6 hours by using a dipstick. CVP is monitored for central filling pressures.

Management

Urinary output commonly decreases in the first 24 to 48 hours after transplantation. This decrease is usually a multifactorial problem and can be related to (1) the presence of renal disease before transplantation; (2) the use of nephrotoxic antibiotics before and/or after transplantation; (3) vena caval occlusion during graft implantation; (4) intraoperative insults such as hypotension; and/or (5) CyA given either intraoperatively or postoperatively.

The initial management of oliguria is an assessment of the child's intravascular volume status. The CVP must be maintained at 8 to 10 mm Hg using fresh frozen plasma or 5% albumin. If adequate intravascular volume does not result in diuresis, a single dose of furosemide (2 mg/kg IV) can be administered. If this fails to establish diuresis, further attempts at volume loading in the presence of a normal CVP or administration of higher doses of furosemide will not be effective. At this point a renal failure protocol must be instituted, replacing insensible losses and urinary output on a milliliter-for-milliliter basis.

Usually CyA-induced renal dysfunction will im-prove within 48 hours after transplantation. However, if the patient has sustained a severe renal insult and the urinary output has not improved after 48 hours, the patient will need additional support. We advocate the use of continuous arteriovenous hemofiltration with predilution (see Chapter 148), which allows excellent control of the patient's volume status and electrolyte and BUN values with minimal cardiovascular effects. Our preferred site of cannula placement in small children is the femoral artery and femoral vein on opposite sides. In larger children we place a shunt (Scribner) in the foot. Hemodialysis is rarely needed and should be reserved for those circumstances in which the patient needs long-term renal support.

Hemoglobinuria

Hemoglobinuria is the presence of hemoglobin in the urine without the presence of RBCs. The most common cause of hemoglobinuria is a transplant performed in the presence of a minor ABO incompatibility (placement of an O liver into either an A or B recipient). The mechanism is a minor graft-vs.-host reaction in which passenger lymphocytes from the donor (carried in the liver) begin to make anti-A or anti-B antibodies. These antibodies subsequently attack the recipients RBCs, causing hemolysis.

Laboratory tests. Characteristically the hemolysis occurs 7 to 14 days after transplantation, and it must be considered a possibility when there are a sudden increase in the total bilirubin level with minimal parenchymal enzyme changes, a sudden drop in the Hct and Hb levels, an elevated reticulocyte count, and hemoglobinuria and an ultrasound shows no biliary tract obstruction. Serial Hb and Hct determinations, total, direct, and indirect bilirubin levels, reticulocyte count, urinalysis, and the appropriate anti-A or anti-B titers are useful in establishing the diagnosis. The serum haptoglobin level is not helpful since it is a hepatic-manufactured protein and its level depends on hepatic function.

Management. The hemolysis can be stopped rapidly by transfusing the patient with type O blood. Serial reticulocyte counts are a sensitive indicator of ongoing hemolysis and must be obtained every 12 hours. As long as hemolysis is present, the patient should receive type O blood. The hemolysis is self-limited, usually lasting 2 to 4 weeks. A major pitfall is to confuse this clinical picture with that of rejection or biliary tract obstruction, thereby initiating inappropriate therapy.

Nutritional Status

Laboratory tests needed for determining the patient's nutritional status include total protein, albumin, prealbumin, cholesterol, triglyceride, retinal binding protein, and transferrin levels.

Monitoring

Monitoring includes careful caloric measurements and, when feasible, metabolic cart monitoring.

Management

By the time patients need liver transplantation they are protein/calorie malnourished. Therefore nutritional supplementation must be stated as soon as possible after transplantation (i.e., as soon as the patient is hemodynamically stable). IV hyperalimentation is often begun in the PICU, and the child is later switched to enteral tube feedings if his oral caloric intake is not adequate. In almost all patients we aim for a calorie intake of 100 kcal/kg/day (see Chapters 149 and 150).

Several problems can occur early after transplantation that make alimentation difficult. Glucose intolerance can occur in the first 5 to 6 days secondary to the high-dose steroids that are given for immunosuppression and is manifested as glycosuria and hyperglycemia. If it seriously impairs nutritional repletion, IV insulin can be started with an initial carbohydrate/insulin ratio of 10:1. As the steroid dose is reduced, glucose tolerance will increase, thereby decreasing the need for insulin. Serum glucose must be carefully monitored using Dextrostix/Chemstrips every 6 hours while an insulin drip is used.

Liver transplant patients also have elevated serum triglyceride levels. Before IV lipids are begun, the serum triglyceride level must be checked; IV lipids are not started until the triglycerides fall below 200 mg/dl.

Fluid and Electrolyte Balance

Laboratory tests

Serum electrolytes, calcium (total and ionized), phosphorus, magnesium, and osmolality must be checked every 6 hours.

Monitoring

Monitoring includes CVP, urinary output, urinary specific gravity, abdominal girth, systemic arterial blood pressure, and body weight.

Management

Postoperative fluid management is a dynamic problem requiring careful monitoring and frequent adjustment. Fluid in the immediate postoperative period is given at 80% of maintenance. The patient also receives milliliter-for-milliliter replacement of abdominal drain outputs with fresh frozen plasma, which compensates for the intra-abdominal third-space losses that occur as a result of intraoperative lymphatic disruption. Fluid management must be adjusted every 6 hours so that the CVP is maintained at 8 to 10 mm Hg, the urinary output at 1 to 2 ml/kg/hr, the systemic arterial blood pressure at normal for age, and the ascites at a minimum.

Unfortunately the above-mentioned factors are not mutually exclusive. To maintain an adequate CVP and urinary output, increased fluid administration may be needed, which can result in increased ascites accumulation and increased systemic arterial blood pressure. Alternatively, isolated postoperative hypertension is usually related to volume overload, and a reduction in the amount of fluid administered may be necessary despite a normal CVP. If the urinary output remains low despite a fluid challenge or apparent euvolemia and the patient is unresponsive to diuretics, a renal-failure regimen will be necessary.

Electrolytes

Sodium management. Hyponatremia usually is related to excessive free-water administration and is a common problem after liver transplantation. Ascites results in decreased intravascular volume, resulting in increased salt and water reabsorption. Hyponatremia is treated optimally with fluid and sodium restriction, which will result in both an increase in serum sodium level and a decrease in ascites. For a more rapid correction of the serum sodium level, furosemide, with or without an infusion of 25% albumin, can be used to increase free-water loss with a milliliter-for-milliliter urinary output replacement with 0.9% sodium chloride solution.

Hyponatremia also can result from excessive diuretic usage, especially of metolazone (Zaroxolyn). Ceasing administration of this diuretic will rapidly increase the patient's serum sodium level.

Hypocalcemia. Hypocalcemia is also a common finding after liver transplantation and is determined by monitoring the ionized serum calcium level every 6 hours. When poor hepatic function exists, calcium chloride must be used for repletion (10 mg/kg/dose) since calcium gluconate must be metabolized by the liver before the calcium is available. If hepatic function is improving, IV calcium gluconate can be safely used (100 mg/kg/dose). Repeated doses are often necessary, and calcium infusions must be given *only* through a central venous catheter. Calcium extravasation from a peripheral vein can lead to calcification in the subcutaneous tissue with overlying skin necrosis and ulcer formation.

Hypokalemia. Hypokalemia is common and is usually related to the aggressive diuresis required to maintain urinary output, to achieve ascites control, or to maintain the patient at a stable weight. It is readily treated with an IV infusion of potassium chloride over 1 hour (0.2 to 0.3 mEq/kg). Concentrated potassium infusions cause intense thrombophlebitis and must be administered only through a central venous catheter.

Acid-base management

Metabolic alkalosis. Any patient receiving more than one blood volume of banked blood receives a large citrate load. As the new liver begins to function, the citrate is converted to bicarbonate, resulting in an increased serum bicarbonate level, which can reach as high as 40 mEq/L. The child attempts to compensate for the metabolic alkalosis by hypoventilation, causing a respiratory acidosis, often to such a degree that it prohibits weaning from the ventilator.

The metabolic alkalosis is self-limited, lasting approximately 24 to 36 hours before the bicarbonate level returns to normal. These patients do not need acid infusions unless the metabolic alkalosis is so severe that it cannot be compensated for by respiratory acidosis.

Metabolic acidosis. Metabolic acidosis in the immediate postoperative period is usually due to renal or hepatic failure. Metabolic acidosis associated with renal failure can be controlled with continuous arteriovenous hemofiltration and predilution with added bicarbonate. We also have controlled the acidosis of hepatic failure in a similar fashion with high-dose predilutional bicarbonate and continuous hemofiltration. Acidosis coupled with evidence of a nonfunctioning graft indicates that the graft has been irreversibly damaged, and immediate retransplantation is the only hope for patient survival.

Hyperkalemia. Hyperkalemia is associated with a decreased urinary output and renal impairment. Hyperkalemia can be treated with sodium polystyrene enemas (1 g/kg) in a 70% sorbitol solution administered through a catheter placed in the rectum. All potassium-containing solutions must be immediately stopped. If these measures are not successful, the use of continuous hemofiltration will be necessary. Sudden hyperkalemia in the presence of a failing graft is an ominous sign because hepatocellular necrosis and cell death cause intracellular potassium release and unremitting, untreatable hyperkalemia.

Acute, life-threatening hyperkalemia can be treated with a calcium chloride (10 mg/kg) infusion or a glucose and insulin infusion (1 unit of insulin per 4 g glucose). These methods are only useful in controlling the acute hyperkalemia; chronic control requires administration of sodium polystyrene or dialysis (see Chapter 14).

Metabolic abnormalities. Hypophosphatemia is a common occurrence after liver transplantation. Its cause is multifactorial and is related to poor vitamin D absorption, high parathormone levels (favors phosphate excretion), increased renal phosphate excretion (high-dose steriod administration), increased phosphate uptake by the new liver, and decreased total body phosphate stores secondary to malnutrition.

Hypophosphatemia leads to depletion of intracellular ATP and tissue hypoxia secondary to decreased erythrocyte levels of 2,3-DPG. These metabolic disturbances are clinically manifested as paresthesia or weakness, which may progress to ataxia; seizures; coma; decreased myocardial contractility, which may progress to congestive cardiomyopathy; hemolysis; diminished platelet aggregation; decreased affinity of hemoglobin for oxygen, resulting in tissue hypoxia; and poor neutrophil chemotaxis and phagocytosis.

Acute correction of hypophosphatemia is accomplished through IV administration of 0.3 to 0.6 mmol/kg sodium phosphate over 6 hours, depending on the severity of the hypophosphatemia (potassium phosphate can be used if the serum potassium is low), with monitoring of the serum phosphate level. Once the serum phosphate level reaches 3.0 to 3.5 mg/kg, oral supplementation may be used if the patient is able to tolerate enteral medication. Oral phosphate is given as capsules. Each capsule must be diluted in 75 ml of water or juice, and a portion, depending on the phosphate level and the child's weight, is given to the child. Serial phosphate measurements (at least q 12 hr) are necessary to adjust the oral dose appropriately. Calcium supplementation may also be needed during phosphate repletion to avoid hypocalcemic tetany. Hyperkalemia and hyponatremia are associated with phosphate repletion; therefore serum electrolytes must be carefully monitored during phosphate therapy.

ADDITIONAL READING

Esquivel CO, Iwatsuki, S, Gordon RD, et al. Indication for pediatric liver transplantation. J Pediatr 111:1039-1045, 1987.

• Malatack JJ, Schaid DJ, Urbach AH, et al. Choosing a pediatric recipient for orthotopic liver transplantation. J Pediatr 111:479-489, 1987.

McHugh MJ. Intensive care aspects of organ transplantation in children. Pediatr Clin North Am 34:187-201, 1987.

National Institutes of Health Consensus Development Conference statement: Liver transplantation—June 20-23, 1983. Hepatology 4:107S-110S, 1984.

Rollins N, Andrews W, Currarino G, et al. Nonsurgical management of infected bile lakes following pediatric liver transplantation. Radiology 166:169-171, 1988.

Staff JS. Phosphate homeostasis and hypophosphatemia. Am J Med 72:489-495, 1982.

• Winter PM, Kang YG, eds. Hepatic Transplantation: Anesthetic and Perioperative Management. New York: Praeger, 1986.

65 Nursing Aspects of Liver Transplantation

Elizabeth Brunetti-Fyock · Susan A. Gray

BACKGROUND

As discussed in the previous chapter, pediatric liver transplantation has become a therapeutic modality for children suffering from terminal liver disease. Immediate posttransplant PICU nursing care is similar to the care of any child following a major abdominal operation. Caring for these children, however, can be quite exciting and also quite challenging should complications arise. This chapter focuses on the nursing implications involved in caring for a child after liver transplantation.

PHYSIOLOGY AND MONITORING

Refer to Chapter 4 for routine PICU monitoring protocols.

Neurologic Status

Preoperatively the child's neurologic status may vary from awake and alert to stage 1 to stage 4 hepatic coma, depending on the severity of the child's liver disease. Thus postoperatively it is important to monitor the child's neurologic status. For the most accurate assessment the child is allowed to recover from anesthesia as soon as possible. Most children begin spontaneous respiration and movement 4 to 6 hours after the transplant. The responsiveness of the child is a good gauge as to whether or not the new liver is beginning to function well.

When the child is admitted to the PICU, the nurse must check his pupils and note movements as he begins to awaken. Using restraints is a must for these children to prevent their pulling out catheters or removing their endotracheal tube before the appropriate time. Medication for pain and/or sedation is administered as needed (usually meperidine, 1 mg/ kg IV q 6 hr, or diphenhydramine, 1 mg/kg IV q 4 to 6 hr, for agitation).

If a child needs to continue receiving neuromuscular relaxants during the initial postoperative period, the nurse must continue to observe his pupillary responses; these agents are withheld once a day in order to assess neurologic status.

Respiratory Function

In most instances the patient will be orally intubated when admitted to the PICU and will be placed on a volume-controlled ventilator. The nurse must observe the patient's chest for equal lung expansion and must auscultate breath sounds bilaterally, making note of any wheezing, rales, rhonchi, or inequality of air movement. Also, the child's nail beds must be observed for signs of decreased oxygenation.

The use of aggressive chest physiotherapy with vibration and tracheal suctioning is important during the initial postoperative period to correct atelectasis and plugging that occurs as a result of the long anesthetic and surgical procedure. The oral tracheal tube needs suctioning every 1 to 2 hours or as needed; the nasopharynx must be suctioned gently as needed.

Because of the increased risk of infection the child is weaned from the ventilator as soon as he is fully awake and able to maintain adequate ventilation on his own. Oxygenation is assessed with the use of a pulse oximeter and an end-tidal carbon dioxide monitor, and this information is correlated with arterial blood gas values. Arterial blood gas and pH values are determined every 6 hours and/or with ventilator changes or changes in the patient's clinical status. Once the child is extubated, he will receive oxygen by face mask for 12 to 24 hours to maintain a 95% to 100% oxygen saturation, which is of the utmost importance to the newly transplanted organ.

While the patient is in the PICU, daily chest roentgenograms must be obtained to monitor for signs of early complications such as atelectasis, pulmonary edema, or pleural effusions. Nursing management of these complications include the following: for atelectasis, changing a patient's position at least every 2 hours, suctioning the endotracheal tube every 1 to 2 hours and as needed, carefully noting the color and the amount of secretions, and making certain aggressive chest physiotherapy is performed at least every 4 hours; for pulmonary edema, which is usually secondary to volume overload, administering diuretics properly and maintaining the child's fluid restriction as ordered; for pleural effusions, administering diuretics and assisting the physician in placement of a chest tube if needed.

With careful monitoring the nurse will be alert to sudden changes in the patient's respiratory status and can notify the physician so that proper treatment measures may be instituted.

Cardiac Function

The cardiovascular system of the child who has received a liver transplant is monitored with the use of an indwelling arterial catheter, a CVP catheter, a noninvasive blood pressure device, and a routine cardiorespiratory monitor.

The child's vital signs must be monitored every hour, including the apical pulse, systemic arterial blood pressure, and CVP readings. Accurate measurement of the child's intake and output is also necessary. Another method for assessing cardiac function is to check capillary refill and to check for coolness of the extremities.

The most common cardiovascular problem after the transplant is systemic arterial hypertension. Some theories about its cause include fluid overload secondary to the use of large volumes of intraoperative fluids, decreased urinary output secondary to the introduction of cyclosporine A, and/or the use of a combination of high doses of cyclosporine A and steroids during the initial postoperative period. Once the nurse notes hypertension in the child, he or she must contact the physician so that appropriate medications may be ordered; these medications are discussed in the previous chapter.

Another potential problem affecting the cardio-vascular system after liver transplantation is bleeding. The newly transplanted liver has four vascular anastomoses: the suprahepatic vena cava, the infrahepatic vena cava, the portal vein, and the hepatic artery. Until the newly transplanted liver is functioning normally, the action of the child's clotting factors may be prolonged, and oozing may occur from any of the above-mentioned anastomoses or any of the insertion sites of invasive catheters. For this reason no heparin is used in any of the catheters, including the arterial catheter.

Three abdominal drains, generally J-vac drains, are inserted at the end of the surgical procedure. These drains are placed in the right subphrenic space, the right subhepatic space, and the left subphrenic space. When the patient is admitted to the PICU, the nurse must label these drains either 1,2,3 or A,B,C and must observe and record the amount of drainage every 4 hours from each drain and be alert for signs of bleeding. The amount of J-vac drainage will vary from patient to patient and may vary from serosanguineous to a straw color. If bright red blood appears in the J-vac drain, the nurse must aspirate a small amount of the fluid and spin it to determine the Hct level.

Bleeding from the J-vac drain may indicate a leak from one of the vascular anastomosis sites. If necessary the child can receive a transfusion of packed red cells. The amount of J-vac drain output is routinely replaced milliliter for milliliter with fresh frozen plasma over 4 hours during the first 24 to 48 hours after the transplant.

In addition to monitoring vital signs the nurse must be alert for signs and symptoms of bleeding and shock, must monitor the child's CBC and PT/PTT results every 6 hours, and must maintain accurate J-vac drainage output records.

Hepatic Function

The transplanted liver invariably undergoes some damage during the process of being removed from the donor and implanted into the recipient. As discussed earlier, the best indicator of good graft function is improvement of the child's neurologic status. In addition, the child's liver function, including bilirubin, AST, ALT, alkaline phosphatase, GGT, and PT/PTT, must be monitored daily. In some children a T tube is inserted when a duct-to-duct anastomosis of the bile duct is possible, and monitoring the amount of the bile drainage from the T tube is also a good indication of liver function. The tube must be taped securely, and an occlusive dressing needs to be present at the insertion site. If liver function decreases, it is not unusual for the bile drainage to decrease and for its color to become light. The nurse must be certain blood for the liver function tests is drawn in the morning so that the results will be ready that same day. These and other daily laboratory results are normally recorded on a large chart kept at the patient's bedside.

Renal Function

When the child reaches the PICU, a bladder catheter with gravity drainage will be in place. Maintaining accurate records of intake and output and daily weights is of utmost importance in the assessment of the child's renal function, and urinary output is recorded on an hourly basis. The physician must be notified if the urinary output falls below 2 ml/kg/hr. A decrease in urinary output is not uncommon in the first 2 days after the transplant. Diuretics must be administered as ordered and the patient's response recorded. If the patient has a large amount of ascites, albumin infusions followed by IV furosemide (1 to 2 mg/kg) may be instituted in an attempt to establish diuresis.

The child's BUN and creatinine levels are monitored every 6 hours. If fluid management and diuretic therapy do not result in an adequate urinary output and the BUN and creatinine levels continue to rise, further measures to support the patient must be instituted. Low-dose dopamine (5 to 8 μg/kg/hr) infusion may be used to increase renal blood flow. Renal dysfunction may persist, however, especially if the child had the hepatorenal syndrome before the transplant. If so, continuous arteriovenous hemofiltration can be instituted (see Chapter 148). Meticulous care of the catheters inserted for hemofiltration is necessary to prevent infection, and they must be cared for in the same manner as the central catheters.

Nursing management of renal function includes weighing the patient every day, recording urinary output every hour, administering fluids and medications as ordered, and monitoring the BUN and creatinine levels every 6 hours.

GI/Nutritional Status

Children who undergo liver transplantation have various degrees of malnutrition secondary to end-stage liver disease. Aggressive nutritional support, there-fore, must be instituted as soon as possible after the liver transplant.

On arrival at the PICU the child will have a NG tube placed on low intermittent suction. The quantity, color, and consistency of gastric secretions must be monitored every 4 to 8 hours. IV fluid will be ordered to replace the volume of drainage. Because of the stress of illness, surgery, and high-dose steroids, the patient is at risk for developing stress ulcers. Any bleeding through the NG tube must be reported immediately. Gastric pH must be checked and recorded every 4 hours. An antacid is administered via the NG tube every 4 hours and the tube clamped for 30 minutes after each dose.

The nurse must auscultate the child's bowel sounds when he arrives in the PICU and then every shift. Bowel sounds usually return within 12 to 36 hours postoperatively. Once the child has a bowel movement, the NG tube is placed to gravity drainage, and if no nausea or vomiting occurs within 8 hours, the NG tube will be removed. The nurse must record stool output, describing the color and consistency of the stool. It is not uncommon for the first few stools to contain some old blood or to be diarrheal in nature. If GI function returns while the child is in the PICU, enteral feedings will be started. Clear fluids will be given first, and if they are tolerated, the diet will be advanced to a no-added-salt diet. The salt intake is limited while the child is on high-dose steroids to help prevent fluid retention and systemic arterial hypertension. Initially many children do not have much appetite, and tube feedings with an isotonic formula and a low content of medium-chain triglycerides will be needed to ensure adequate protein/calorie intake. If tube feedings are instituted, a soft Silastic tube is inserted and secured with transparent dressing material such as OpSite or Tegaderm. The insertion guidewire must be saved in case the tube is pulled out and must be reinserted. Calorie counts are instituted and the feedings decreased as the child's oral intake improves. Some children do not tolerate enteral feedings; therefore IV hyperalimentation must be started in these patients and continued until feedings are tolerated.

Immune System

Although the transplant patient is receiving immunosuppressive medications, isolation of the child is not necessary. Good handwashing, however, is vital. Common immunosuppressants will be discussed.

MEDICATIONS
Steroids

During surgery the child receives a bolus of IV methylprednisolone sodium succinate, 500 to 1000 mg, depending on body weight. On arrival in the PICU he is placed on IV steroids in sequentially decreasing doses. Methylprednisolone will be ordered as follows:

Patient weight <40 kg

25 mg IV q 6 hr × 4 doses, then
20 mg IV q 6 hr × 4 doses, then
15 mg IV q 6 hr × 4 doses, then
10 mg IV q 6 hr × 4 doses, then
 5 mg IV q 6 hr × 4 doses

Patient weight >40 kg

50 mg IV q 6 hr × 4 doses, then
40 mg IV q 6 hr × 4 doses, then
30 mg IV q 6 hr × 4 doses, then
20 mg IV q 6 hr × 4 doses, then
10 mg IV q 6 hr × 4 doses

After the last IV dose of steroids, the child will be started on methylprednisolone, 20 mg PO once a day. If the child experiences rejection at a later date, this IV steroid dosage schedule may be repeated.

Cyclosporine A

IV cyclosporine A administration is begun during surgery and is continued postoperatively. The usual dosage is 2 mg/kg IV every 8 hours. The IV dose will be decreased as oral cyclosporine A is introduced and absorbed adequately. Oral cyclosporine A is usually begun at 20 mg/kg/day and is given every 12 hours. The IV dose is changed to every 12 hours at corresponding times. Important aspects of cyclosporine A administration are indicated below.

IV cyclosporine A

250 mg ampules (50 mg/ml)
Minimum dilution of 2.5 mg/ml
Infused over a minimum of 2 hr
No filter on line

Oral cyclosporine A

50 ml bottle (100 mg/ml) comes with own measuring burette.
It must be diluted at least 10:1 in milk, chocolate milk, or juice (if dose must be taken in clear liquid, root beer is acceptable).

It should be mixed in glass container.
Mixture will clump and become unpalatable if not taken immediately after mixing.
Bottle's contents expire 2 mo after opening.
Extra fluid (e.g., milk) should be used to "rinse" residual from container and taken immediately after dose.

Cyclosporine trough levels are drawn each day so that the child's dosage can be adjusted appropriately. The nurse must be certain the blood is drawn before the morning IV and oral doses are administered. A level as measured by the whole blood high-performance liquid chromatography (HPLC) method is usually maintained at 250 to 350 μg/L. Lower levels may put the child at risk for rejection. Levels >350 μg/L are considered toxic and can cause an elevation in the child's liver enzymes, BUN, and creatinine levels and, in some cases, seizures.

Minnesota Antilymphocyte Globulin

Minnesota antilymphocyte globulin (MALG) is sometimes used for maintenance immunosuppression, especially if the child has compromised renal function and cannot tolerate the nephrotoxic effects of cyclosporine A. In most instances, however, it is used for the treatment of rejection. The antilymphocyte globulin is made from either horse or goat serum; because an anaphylactic reaction to the animal antigens can occur, the child must be monitored in the PICU when receiving the first dose.

A skin test is performed subcutaneously with equine MALG before administration of the first dose. If a reaction occurs, the goat serum preparation may be used instead of the equine. A negative reaction, however, does not guarantee the child will not have an anaphylactic reaction. The child may experience fever and malaise during the course of therapy.

The following information pertains to the administration of MALG:

1. It must be administered via a central venous catheter.
2. The dose is diluted 10 mg/ml in 0.9% sodium chloride solution (dosage range, 5 to 15 mg/kg/dose/day).
3. Once diluted the dose must sit for 2 hours before administration.
4. The child must be premedicated with acetaminophen (1 mg/year of age) PO or rectally and diphenhydramine (1 mg/kg) IV or PO.

5. The dose is infused over 6 hours (given as one dose per day).
6. Vital signs must be monitored every 15 minutes × 4, every 30 minutes × 4, and every hour × 4.

The child is usually treated with a 10- to 14-day course of MALG. Only the first dose must be given in the PICU. To help prevent herpes and possibly Epstein-Barr virus, the child must be given IV acyclovir (5 mg/kg/dose) every 8 hours during the course of treatment. In addition IV immune globulin (IgG) is administered to help prevent cytomegalovirus infection.

OKT3 Monoclonal Antibody

OKT3 is a monoclonal antibody that is used to treat steroid-resistant rejection. It is currently approved for for treating rejection in renal transplant patients and should soon be approved for use in liver and heart transplant recipients. Until approval, however, a consent form must be signed before starting therapy. Also, the doses must be administered by a physician until approval is granted by the Food and Drug Administration.

Unlike MALG, OKT3 may be given via a peripheral IV line. The dose is 2.5 mg/dose for children <30 kg and 5 mg/dose for children >30 kg. One dose is given per day for 10 to 14 days. The first dose is preceded by the administration of IV steroids (see below).

OKT3 is a mouse antibody and occurrence of an anaphylactic reaction is possible. Therefore the child must receive the first two doses in the PICU. The child must remain in the PICU for 2 hours after each of the doses; he may then return to the general ward if other PICU care is not needed.

IV acyclovir and IV IgG are administered during the course of treatment as described for MALG. Other information regarding OKT3 follows:

1. Draw up with filter supplied with ampule.
2. Administer 1 mg/ml (supplied in 5 mg ampules).
3. Give by slow IV push (over 5 minutes).
4. Premedicate patient before each dose with acetaminophen (1 mg/yr) PO or rectally and diphenhydramine (1 mg/kg) PO or IV.
5. Give IV steroids before first dose. Administer methylprednisolone (250 mg if patient's weight is <30 kg, 500 mg if weight is >30 kg) 6 to 12 hours before administration of OKT3; or administer hydrocortisone (500 to 1000 mg if weight is <30 kg, 1 g if weight is >30 kg) 1 hour before administration of OKT3.

Vital signs must be monitored every 15 minutes × 4, then every 30 minutes × 2, and then every hour × 2. If the first two doses are administered without incident, the remaining doses may be given on the general ward.

ADDITIONAL READING

Traiger GL, Bohachick P. Liver transplantation care of the patient in the acute postoperative period. Crit Care Nurse 3:96-103, 1983.

Williams L, Rzucidlo SE. Care of the pediatric liver transplant patient in the ICU. Crit Care Q 8:13-23, 1985.

66 Renal Transplantation

Steven R. Alexander

BACKGROUND

Renal transplantation has become widely accepted as the treatment of choice for children with irreversible renal failure. Recent advances in chronic dialysis techniques have proved particularly beneficial to pediatric end-stage renal disease (ESRD) patients, almost all of whom can now be safely maintained on dialysis until conditions for renal transplantation in the individual child are as favorable as possible. In the comprehensive management of children with ESRD dialysis serves as a bridge that carries children to (and between) renal transplantation. Thus, to be most effective in children, dialysis and transplantation should be designed as complementary elements in a life-long treatment plan.

More than twice as many children in Europe and North America currently receive renal allografts each year than was the case only a decade ago. It is unlikely that this doubling of the annual pediatric renal transplantation rate correlates with an increased incidence of ESRD among children, although this possibility has not been studied systematically. A more plausible explanation for rising pediatric renal transplantation rates is the increasing number of children with ESRD who have *access* to renal transplantation. During the past 10 years advances in dialysis have allowed more (primarily younger) children to be accepted for ESRD treatment. In addition the practice of "preemptive" transplantation (i.e., transplantation without prior dialysis) has gained in popularity, and it has been shown that children who have previously rejected one or more renal allografts can be successfully retransplanted.

Despite steadily increasing annual pediatric renal transplantation *rates,* the actual number of renal transplants performed in children each year is still relatively small, constituting <10% of the total renal transplants performed yearly in Europe and North America. For example, of the 8331 renal transplants reported to the United States Renal Data System (USRDS) in 1987, only 679 recipients were less than 19 years of age at the time of transplantation. Pediatric transplantation in North America is also widely and somewhat unevenly distributed among many centers. According to data collected by the North American Pediatric Renal Transplant Cooperative Study (NAPRTCS) from 71 participating pediatric centers during the period January 1, 1987, to February 16, 1989, each of the five most active pediatric renal transplant centers in North America performed 15 to 25 transplants per year in recipients less than 18 years of age. The average for the 30 busiest participating NAPRTCS centers was approximately 10 renal transplants per year (range 5 to 25/yr). In our own center (Children's Medical Center of Dallas) 35 children less than 18 years of age received renal transplants from January 1, 1987, to December 31, 1988. During this same 2-year period the most active adult renal transplant program in Dallas performed more than 200 renal transplants in patients over 18 years of age.

Thus renal transplants are relatively infrequent events in even the most active pediatric centers. In addition most children require only a brief period of PICU care after renal transplantation. Typically, a child spends only the initial 24 to 72 postoperative hours in the PICU. Perhaps it is this brief and relatively infrequent exposure to pediatric renal transplant patients that leads many PICU physicians to consider the management of renal transplant recipients the exclusive province of the transplant nephrology and surgery team. The PICU nursing care of even the most "routine" pediatric renal transplant recipient is complex and demanding (see Chapter 67), but all too often busy PICU house staff and attending physicians develop a hands-off attitude toward renal transplant patients, an attitude that is likely to be encouraged (covertly or overtly) by the transplant team. This is unfortunate. When the child with a renal transplant develops life-threatening complications, the role of the pediatric critical care specialist becomes increasingly important, and the PICU physician who has become familiar with the renal transplant patient through routine involvement in his care will have more to offer this child in a crisis.

Specific treatment recommendations in this chapter are examples of the way selected problems were approached in our center in 1989.

Historical Context

A complete history of renal transplantation in children has not been compiled and is beyond the scope of this chapter. A few vignettes from the rich history of renal transplantation are presented to illustrate the role played by pediatric patients in the early development of this therapy, and the turbulent state of current clinical practice that has resulted from recent developments is briefly described.

The first experiments in organ transplantation were performed in animals at the beginning of the twentieth century when pioneering surgeons developed the necessary vascular suturing techniques. The kidney, with its simple vascular arrangement, was an obvious subject for these early experiments. A Viennese surgeon, Emerich Ulmann, is credited with performing the first successful organ transplant. In 1902 Professor Ulmann auto-transplanted the kidney of a dog to the vessels in the animal's neck, briefly obtaining some urinary output. Also during 1902 Alexis Carrel described the technique for suturing one blood vessel to another, a technique that is used almost unchanged today. In 1902 Carrel's vascular anastomosis method requires careful dissection, control of bleeding from both vessels, precise identification of the various layers of the vessels to be connected, and sewing the vessels together with fine needles and thread in a manner that everts the intima. Carrel left France for America; during the next 10 years he perfected the vascular anastomosis technique by performing many dog-to-dog and cat-to-cat renal allografts, work for which he received a Nobel prize in 1912.

These early animal experiments stimulated interest in renal transplantation as a treatment for renal failure in humans. The first kidney transplants in humans were xenografts (i.e., transplants between different species) performed in Lyon, France, by Jaboulay. In 1902 Jaboulay reported the transplantation of kidneys from pigs and goats to the arm or thigh of human patients suffering from chronic renal failure. None of the xenografts functioned for more than 1 hour. A few years later a Berlin surgeon, Ernst Unger, attempted to transplant a kidney from a stillborn infant into a baboon. The baboon died, but the vascular anastomosis was patent at the time of death. Bolstered by this relative surgical "success" and stimulated by the new information that monkeys and man were serologically similar, Unger next attempted to save the life of a young girl dying of renal failure by transplanting the kidney of a small ape to the vessels of the child's thigh. No urine was produced despite a successful vascular anastomosis. Similar repeated failures eventually led Unger, Jaboulay, Carrel, and their contemporaries to conclude that although renal transplantation was technically possible, there was a "biologic barrier" to successful transplantation that could not be surmounted.

By the end of World War I little interest remained in clinical kidney transplantation. Of the many gifted investigators frustrated by consistent graft failures, only Carrel had glimpsed the solution to the biologic barrier that prevented successful organ transplantation. In an astounding paper read before the International Surgical Association in 1914, Carrel called attention to recent work by Murphy, who had found that radiation treatment could increase the success of tumor grafts in rats. Based on Murphy's findings, Carrel postulated that the " . . . power of the organism to eliminate foreign tissue was due to organs such as the spleen or bone marrow, and that when the actions of these organs (is) less active a foreign tissue can develop rapidly after it has been grafted. . . . The surgical side of the transplantation of organs is now completed. . . . All our efforts must now be directed toward the biological methods which will prevent the reaction of the organism against foreign tissue and allow the adapting of homoplastic grafts to their hosts. . . ."

Although a few unsuccessful human kidney allografts were performed in the Union of Soviet Socialist Republics in the 1930s and 1940s and a transiently successful cadaveric renal allograft was placed in the antecubital fossa of a patient with acute renal failure in Boston in 1946, little real progress was made until the early 1950s when the immunologic mechanisms responsible for the destruction of allografts began to be understood. Improvements in the surgical technique were also made during this period when it became clear that the pelvic placement of the graft was superior to a superficial site. Much of the success of these early efforts came from centers in Paris and Boston, where hemodialysis was first used in the 1950s to prepare and sustain patients before transplantation.

The first living-related kidney transplant (thus probably the first pediatric renal allograft) was reported by Michon and associates in 1953. The donor was the mother of a boy whose solitary kidney had been crushed in a motor vehicle accident. The allograft functioned well for 22 days, at which point it abruptly failed, and the boy died soon thereafter. In 1954 the first renal transplant between identical twins was performed in Boston. The tenth such twin-to-twin renal transplant was performed at the University of Oregon Medical School in Portland in 1955 between 13-year-old identical twin sisters. Both sisters are alive and well today, making this the longest known surviving pediatric renal allograft.

Extending transplantation beyond genetically identical individuals required the development of potent inhibitors of the immune response. Total body irradiation was attempted in the late 1950s with limited success in non-twin sibling allografts. The introduction of 6-mercaptopurine (6-MP) and later azathioprine (Imuran), a less toxic derivative of 6-MP, by Calne in 1960 to 1962 heralded the modern era of immunosuppression. Earlier clinical experiments using ACTH and other corticosteroid derivatives had been inconclusive, if not outright failures; but when azathioprine was routinely combined with prednisone by Starzl in Denver and Hume in Richmond and live, related donors (LRDs) were used, long-term renal allograft survival became a reality.

Improvements in tissue typing and pretransplant screening (crossmatching) of potential recipients for antibodies against donor tissue, coupled with improvements in cadaver kidney harvesting and preservation techniques, led to increased emphasis on cadaver donors during the 1970s. Unfortunately the long-term results of cadaveric renal transplantation using prednisone and azathioprine immunosuppression did not live up to expectations. The rejection of more than two thirds of all cadaveric allografts in <5 years led to reluctance on the part of many internist-nephrologists to subject their stable adult dialysis patients to the rigors and risks of renal transplantation for what were perceived as, at best, only short-term

benefits. In contrast, pediatric nephrologists recognized that the quality of life experienced by children receiving chronic hemodialysis was generally poor and inferior to the life provided by a successful renal transplant; thus pediatric dialysis patients were still considered candidates for transplantation even when a family donor was not available. However, children less than 1 to 5 years of age (depending on the individual program) were generally excluded from ESRD treatment when a family donor was not available because of severe technical difficulties associated with attempts to maintain small children on chronic hemodialysis and the abysmal results of cadaveric renal transplantation when performed in very young children.

During the 1980s two dramatic advances have taken place in the care of children with ESRD: continuous peritoneal dialysis (see Chapter 145) and cyclosporine. The introduction of continuous peritoneal dialysis (CPD) to pediatrics in 1979 made it possible to offer chronic renal replacement therapy to children of all ages and sizes (including newborn infants) who could be supported with CPD until they reached a size at which renal transplantation could be comfortably accomplished. Since its introduction in the late 1970s (widespread use in the United States began in 1984), cyclosporine has substantially improved renal allograft survival rates, at least in the short term. Even more important has been the effect cyclosporine has had on the pace of developments in transplantation immunobiology. The advent of cyclosporine seemed to rescue renal transplantation from the scientific doldrums of the 1970s, perhaps because with cyclosporine it became possible to transplant other solid organs. Worldwide interest in research on transplantation biology is currently at an all-time high and is continuing to grow, fueled by clinical accomplishments in solid organ transplantation that were inconceivable before the introduction of cyclosporine. Much current research has focused on understanding the phenomenon of allograft rejection, Carrel's biologic barrier to transplantation, and from this research have come additional potent antirejection agents such as the monoclonal antibodies (e.g., OKT3) directed against specific populations of cells (e.g., T cells [thymic-derived lymphocytes] bearing the CD-3 surface antigen), which are intimately involved in the destruction of the allograft by the new host.

As is true for most periods of rapid medical advances, the field of pediatric renal transplantation is currently rife with controversies. Many widely held tenets of clinical practice are being questioned and have become the subjects of much intense debate and some research. Unfortunately the current emphasis is more on debate than research, but this may be changing as the importance of obtaining better information on which to base pediatric transplant patient decisions becomes more widely appreciated. It can be said that no prior notion about clinical pediatric renal transplantation should be considered sacred. For example, there is vigorous disagreement about such basic clinical issues as the relative advantages of LRD vs. cadaveric transplantation, the optimal timing of transplantation in young children, and the most effective and safest immunosuppressive regimen for children of different ages. Consensus no longer exists on the use of pediatric cadaveric donors in pediatric recipients; the approach to the child with a dysfunctional lower urinary tract; the role of human leukocyte antigen (HLA) histocompatibility matching in short- and long-term graft survival; the use of living *non*related donors; the potential impact on allograft survival of recurrence of the primary renal disease in the allograft; the relative risks of life-threatening infections and malignancies that may accompany the use of more potent antirejection agents; the importance of pretransplant blood transfusions; and which, if any, pediatric patients should *not* be considered candidates for transplantation (e.g., severely brain-damaged neonates). These and other important issues must be addressed scientifically during the coming years if renal transplantation is to become an effective and reliable *long-term* treatment for children with irreversible renal failure.

Incidence of ESRD

A precise determination of the incidence of ESRD in pediatric patients is difficult to obtain from published information, partly because of inconsistencies in both the upper and lower age limits used in reports from various regional pediatric ESRD referral centers and groups of such centers. Moreover, the incidence of ESRD in children based on surveys of ESRD treatment centers depends on decisions made by primary physicians to refer children for ESRD treatment. Early surveys clearly underestimated the incidence of ESRD among infants and young children, for whom dialysis and transplantation were widely considered futile and inappropriate therapies. A more accurate

estimate of ESRD incidence among pediatric patients may now be possible in those areas of the world (e.g., Canada, United States, Western Europe) in which treatment is generally sought for almost all children with irreversible renal failure, regardless of age. Prematurely born infants with ESRD may constitute the remaining exceptions to this practice.

Based on the best currently available information, the incidence of ESRD among children less than 18 years of age is estimated at three to five children per 1 million total population per year. The regional and national differences in reported pediatric ESRD incidence that still exist reflect either the persistence of variable criteria for referral for treatment or actual differences in population characteristics and/or prevalence of specific disorders that cause ESRD in children. The fact that variable access to ESRD treatment still exists in many parts of the world is suggested by the annual reports of the European Dialysis and Transplant Association (EDTA), in which the overall acceptance rate for new pediatric ESRD patients is consistently at least 20 times greater in countries with the highest acceptance rates compared to those with the lowest.

Access to Renal Transplantation

Most pediatric patients begin chronic renal replacement therapy (RRT) with either hemo- or peritoneal dialysis. For more than 20% of U.S. children with ESRD the first chronic RRT is a renal transplant, an approach that differs markedly from many other countries. For example, a renal transplant is the first chronic RRT for <1% of children receiving ESRD treatment in the 22 member countries of the EDTA. This difference is in part due to the fact that nearly half of the pediatric renal transplants performed in the United States (e.g., 46% in 1987) are from living donors. Only 17% of the 1151 pediatric transplants performed in the period 1984 to 1986 in the member countries of the EDTA were from living donors. The willingness to use family members as donors for children in the United States and the relative reluctance to do so in most of the rest of the world have not been explained. The use of a living donor allows scheduling of the transplant before the need for dialysis in some children who have slowly progressive chronic renal insufficiency. The same approach to preemptive transplantation may be taken with some children who do not have a living donor, although the timing is obviously more difficult since the period spent by the child on the cadaver-recipient waiting list is unpredictable.

Time spent on the cadaver-recipient waiting list varies widely. Data from the EDTA show a mean waiting time of more than 2 years, but there are large differences among member countries. Waiting times have generally been much shorter for North American children, although this favorable condition may currently be changing as donor organs become scarcer and total waiting lists (adult plus pediatric) grow longer in most centers. Many different factors influence the length of time that any individual child will remain on the waiting list, the most important of which is the overall availability of donor organs. Recipient blood type (type A is statistically favored over type O; type B is most difficult to find) and the degree of presensitization to human tissue antigens are also important determinants of waiting time. The relative strictness of criteria used by different centers to assess acceptability of donated organs can influence waiting time. Some centers will not accept kidneys from infants or young children; others require that donor and recipient share a minimum number of HLA antigens. What is known about the relative importance of these and other factors that might influence the outcome of pediatric renal transplantation is briefly presented later in this chapter.

Etiology of ESRD in Children

Several large surveys have shown that approximately half of the children needing treatment for ESRD have a congenital or hereditary renal disorder and half an acquired renal lesion. The large number of children who have congenital/hereditary renal disorders is in striking contrast to the adult ESRD patient population, in which more than 80% of patients have acquired renal diseases.

The etiology of renal failure is important information to most pediatric ESRD patients for several reasons. The proper identification of a hereditary renal disease has obvious implications for other family members who may themselves have occult disease and/or may wish to be considered as kidney donors. Certain renal diseases tend to recur in the allograft; information on recurrence risk can be important in the choice of a LRD vs. a cadaveric donor and can influence the timing of transplantation. Finally, knowledge about the primary renal disease can be helpful in pre- and posttransplant patient care. For example, children whose primary renal disorder was

congenital renal dysplasia or obstructive uropathy often remain polyuric despite very low glomerular filtration rates. In these patients polyuria persists after the transplant, even when the allograft itself is not functioning well due to acute tubular necrosis or acute rejection. Thus the value of urinary output as an indicator of allograft function is lost. These children may also continue to waste large amounts of sodium chloride in their urine. The stringent dietary salt restriction routinely imposed on children after

Table 66-1 Primary Renal Diagnoses in Pediatric Renal Transplant Recipients Enrolled in the NAPRTCS, January 1, 1987, to February 16, 1989*

Diagnosis	N	%
Aplastic/hypoplastic/dysplastic kidneys	131	18.1
Obstructive uropathy	116	16.0
Focal segmental glomerulosclerosis	87	12.0
Systemic immunologic disease	34	4.7
Reflux nephropathy	30	4.1
Hemolytic-uremic syndrome	28	3.9
Congenital nephrotic syndrome	28	3.9
Chronic glomerulonephritis	27	3.7
Syndrome of agenesis of abdominal musculature	26	3.6
Familial nephritis	22	3.0
Pyelonephritis/interstitial nephritis	21	2.9
Medullary cystic disease/juvenile nephronophthisis	21	2.9
Cystinosis	19	2.6
Renal infarct	16	2.2
Idiopathic crescentic glomerulonephritis	14	1.9
Membranoproliferative glomerulonephritis type I	14	1.9
Polycystic kidney disease	13	1.8
Membranoproliferative glomerulonephritis type II	10	1.4
Oxalosis	7	1.0
Wilms' tumor	5	0.7
Drash syndrome	4	0.6
Membranous nephropathy	3	0.4
Diabetic glomerulonephritis	0	0
Sickle cell nephropathy	0	0
Other	25	3.5
Unknown	24	3.3

*From the Second Annual Report, North American Pediatric Renal Transplant Cooperative Study, May 1989.

the transplant to reduce the incidence and severity of hypertension may lead to serious electrolyte and volume depletion in children with persistent sodium chloride wasting due to their primary disease.

The primary renal disease diagnoses for 701 patients enrolled in the NAPRTCS from January 1, 1987, to February 16, 1989, for whom a diagnosis was reported are listed in Table 66-1 in order of the frequency of reported diagnoses. This table reflects a larger proportion of congenital/hereditary disorders (61%) than acquired renal diseases (39%). It represents a large sample of the North American children who received a renal transplant during the study period, whereas previously reported surveys of pediatric primary renal disease diagnoses (in which patients were more evenly divided between congenital/hereditary disorders and acquired renal diseases) were based on children who received either dialysis or transplantation.

THE TRANSPLANT
Factors Influencing Pediatric Renal Transplantation
Recipient age

The optimal form of therapy for the *infant* with ESRD is highly controversial. Advocates of early renal transplantation (i.e., before 1 to 2 years of age) point to the permanently debilitating effects of the uremic state on the growth and neurologic development of many infants treated with either conservative management alone or in combination with dialysis. The results of chronic hemodialysis in this age group are uniformly abysmal, but treatment with continuous ambulatory peritoneal dialysis (CAPD) or continuous cycling peritoneal dialysis (CCPD) has been more successful, especially when dialysis is instituted early and is combined with controlled enteral nutrition (i.e., tube feeding). However, even the most aggressive use of CAPD or CCPD and tube feeding has not eliminated the problems of growth failure and delayed development seen in some infants with ESRD. Mortality rates are more than three times greater among infants treated with CAPD or CCPD compared to older children receiving the same treatment, and infants who begin dialysis before 3 months of age fall an average of 1 SD further below the mean for length during the first year of treatment. Some of these infants also demonstrate poor growth in head circumference, reflecting subnormal brain growth and predicting adverse neurologic consequences. A

successful renal transplant can prevent further harmful effects of uremia on the young infant and to some extent reverse those already present. It is not surprising that the restoration of near-normal renal function after successful transplantation results in a better outcome than is possible with CAPD or CCPD; even the most effective dialytic therapy currently available can only maintain the infant in a condition of chronic renal insufficiency, still exposed to the effects of the uremic state during this critical period of growth and development. Renal transplantation would seem the obvious treatment of choice for the infant with ESRD.

Unfortunately early experience with renal transplantation in young infants was dismal. Of the first 13 infants who were reported to have received renal allografts during the first year of life, only one survived for more than 12 months. Generally poor (but less uniformly fatal) outcomes were also reported in several series published before 1984 for children who received transplants before the age of 5 years.

However, there is a clear difference in outcome, depending on donor source. When LRDs are used in children less than 5 years of age, short-term outcome is dramatically superior compared to the use of cadaveric donors in this age group. Excellent patient and graft survival results have also been reported from a few centers when infants less than 1 year of age have received a kidney from a LRD (usually a parent). Technical problems inherent in the transplantation of the adult kidney into an infant can be overcome in most experienced pediatric transplant centers when the infant recipient weighs at least 8 kg. A few centers have reported successful transplantation of adult LRD kidneys into infants weighing as little as 5 kg.

It appears that recipient age is a more important consideration when only cadaveric transplantation is possible; most centers now prefer to maintain infants who require renal replacement therapy during the first year of life on continuous peritoneal dialysis (CAPD or CCPD) for 1 or 2 years before seeking a cadaver transplant. If a family member is available as a donor, the timing of LRD transplantation is highly variable from center to center, with most centers waiting until the infant weighs at least 8 kg before proceeding with transplantation. These practices may change dramatically as more information becomes available on all aspects of the management of the infant with ESRD, a patient group about which little information existed before the present decade.

Donor age

To be considered as a living kidney donor an individual must be at least 18 years of age. The exception to this general practice occurs when an identical twin sibling is medically suitable as a donor. Outcome in such twin-to-twin transplants is uniformly so successful that siblings as young as 9 years of age have been allowed to serve as donors.

Potential living donors must be highly motivated. For parent-to-child transplants, which constitute the majority of pediatric LRD grafts, motivation is rarely questioned. When sibling donors are being considered, however, it is important to evaluate the level of motivation of the potential donor carefully. Family pressure to donate can be intense, leaving the sibling little perceived choice to refuse. The medical team must first provide a setting in which potential donors (siblings or parents) can make informed decisions that reflect an honest self-appraisal of their motives and that are in their own best interests. The medical team must also provide full support to the individual who decides not to be a donor and must be prepared to assist the family's efforts to come to terms with that decision.

The influence of the age of the donor on the outcome of *cadaveric* renal transplantation in children is currently a subject of growing controversy. Until very recently the general practice throughout the world has been to transplant pediatric patients with kidneys from pediatric cadaver donors whenever possible, primarily reflecting technical concerns. That this practice is still widespread is apparent from the 1989 annual report of the NAPRTCS.* Of the 441 cadaver transplants performed in pediatric recipients at participating North American centers from January 1, 1987, to February 16, 1989, 41% were from donors less than 11 years of age. Infant donors (less than 24 months of age) accounted for 5.1% (22/441) of these cadaveric transplants. Donor age significantly influenced 1-year graft survival in these children, with donors 0 to 5 years, 6 to 10 years, and more than 10 years of age associated with 1-year probabilities of graft survival of 55% ± 0.06 (SE), 67% ± 0.07, and 79% ± 0.03, respectively. Similar results have recently been reported from a large European multicenter study.

*Available from Clinical Coordinating Center, SUNY Health Science Center at Brooklyn, Box 49, 450 Clarkson Ave., Brooklyn, NY 11203 (Atn: Dr. Amir Tejani, Director).

The combination of very young cadaver donors and young recipients appears to have particularly adverse effects on outcome. Arbus and associates at The Hospital for Sick Children in Toronto were the first to document this association. In their patients the use of a cadaver kidney from a donor less than 4 years of age in a recipient less than 3 years of age was associated with a 1-year graft survival rate of only 33%; the 1-year graft survival rate was 74% when donors were more than 9 years of age and recipients more than 3 years of age.

Why kidneys from young cadaver donors do not fare as well in pediatric recipients as kidneys from older donors is not understood. Technical problems resulting from the anastomoses of small blood vessels are unlikely to be the most important determinants of poor outcome since these anastomoses are routinely performed using portions of the walls of the donor aorta and vena cava (Carrel patch), thereby avoiding the need for microvascular surgery.

Anencephalic donors

More than 30 cases of pediatric patients receiving one or both kidneys from anencephalic donors have been reported. In 50% of these cases the grafts never functioned due to vascular thrombosis. A slightly higher incidence of renal and urogenital malformations has been reported in anencephalic infants (11.5% vs. 8.4%). Ethical and legal issues have also made the use of the anencephalic infant as an organ donor less attractive. Many anencephalic infants do not meet the usual criteria for brain death until their cardiopulmonary condition has deteriorated to such a degree that suitability as an organ donor becomes questionable. Efforts to alter brain-death criteria to allow earlier organ harvest from anencephalic infants have been met with general disfavor. These concerns, combined with the high rate of primary nonfunction of the renal allograft, have dissuaded most pediatric centers from using kidneys from anencephalic donors.

Malignancy

The renal malignancy most often associated with ESRD in children is Wilms' tumor, which is bilateral in >80% of such cases. Transplantation within 1 year of diagnosis has been associated with development of recurrent or metastatic disease in nearly 50% of reported cases. However, when transplantation is delayed for at least one recurrence- and metastasis-free year, outcome has been uniformly good, with no additional malignant disease yet reported in these children.

Inadequate information is available on the outcome of renal transplantation in children with preexisting nonrenal malignancies. At least three children with nonrenal malignancies have been successfully transplanted without recurrence of the primary malignancy.

Potential for recurrence of primary renal disease in the allograft

The recurrence of the primary renal disease in the allograft is a disheartening phenomenon that may be of particular importance to pediatric recipients of renal transplants. Before the introduction of cyclosporine, it was generally observed that histologic recurrence of primary disease only rarely resulted in graft loss. Rejection, either acute or chronic, almost always destroyed the graft before damage attributable to recurrent primary disease could do so. Recent improvements in antirejection therapy have stimulated renewed concern for the potential impact of recurrent disease on graft survival.

Focal segmental glomerulosclerosis. Focal glomerulosclerosis (FGS) is the most common glomerular disease causing ESRD in children (Table 66-1). Recurrence of FGS in the allograft has been reported in 5% to 50% of cases. Graft loss due to recurrence of FGS may be as high as 50% in patients who suffer recurrent disease. The reason(s) for the wide disparity in recurrence rates among reported series is unknown. Factors that may be predictive of a high likelihood of recurrence of FGS include onset of the original disease during the first 3 years of life, progression to ESRD within less than 3 years after onset of FGS, and appearance of mesangial proliferation in the native kidney biopsy. The histocompatibility between donor and recipient may also be important. Several series have reported a high incidence of recurrence when LRD kidneys were used. However, these same series reported recurrence in subsequent cadaver retransplants, suggesting that these patients would have experienced recurrence of FGS regardless of donor source.

Graft loss due to recurrence of FGS frequently occurs when the patient develops massive proteinuria and resulting nephrotic syndrome within the first 2 weeks after transplant. Successful treatment of this "malignant" form of recurrent FGS using very high-dose cyclosporine and/or plasmapheresis has recently been described. Additional experience is needed before this approach can be generally recommended.

The variability in recurrence rates and the inability to predict the clinical importance of recurrent FGS to graft survival in the individual patient make denial of renal transplantation to children whose primary renal disease is FGS untenable at this time.

Hemolytic-uremic syndrome. Hemolytic-uremic syndrome (HUS) has been reported to recur in up to 50% of children after renal transplantation. HUS has also been seen de novo in association with high-dose cyclosporine (CyA) therapy and in some patients receiving polyclonal antilymphocyte globulin (ALG). Some authorities suggest avoidance of CyA and ALG in patients whose primary renal disease was HUS. In contrast, others have reported a much lower incidence of recurrent HUS and have also noted successful use of both ALG and CyA in this setting. The only area of general agreement appears to be the timing of transplantation, which should be delayed until all manifestations of the original disease have been absent for 6 to 12 months.

Membranoproliferative glomerulonephritis types I and II. Membranoproliferative glomerulonephritis types I and II both recur in renal allografts, with type II appearing in 100% of allograft biopsies and type I in 50% to 70% of biopsies. However, the histologic recurrence of membranoproliferative glomerulonephritis is not associated with graft loss in the majority of patients. Similar conclusions can be drawn for systemic lupus erythematosus (SLE) and IgA or Henoch-Schönlein purpura (HSP) nephropathy. Recurrence of SLE nephritis has been reported in adults but not in pediatric allograft recipients. Both IgA and HSP nephropathy have been found in allograft biopsies in children, but clinically important allograft dysfunction resulting from recurrence of these primary nephropathies has not been described.

Cystinosis. Cystinosis is an inherited metabolic disorder that frequently results in ESRD. Despite the histologic appearance of cystine crystals in renal allograft biopsies of children with cystinosis, graft dysfunction due to cystinosis does not occur. In fact, cystinosis has been associated with an improved outcome in cadaver transplantation in some series, an observation attributed to the reduced immunocompetence of cystinotic lymphocytes. The successful treatment of ESRD in children with cystinosis has allowed these children to survive for extended periods. Unfortunately the extrarenal manifestations of cystinosis persist after successful transplantation and are allowed to reach levels of severity previously unseen when most of these children died early from renal failure. A recent survey documented the long-term extrarenal consequences of cystinosis in 80 children who had received a successful renal transplant. Hypothyroidism (75%), photophobia (82%), hepatomegaly (43%), splenomegaly (27%), decreased visual acuity (32%), corneal ulcerations (15%), insulin-dependent diabetes mellitus (2.5%), and various neurologic abnormalities (7.5%) characterized this group. All were moderately to severely growth retarded. This study has led to a clinical trial of cystine-depleting agents in transplant recipients.

Oxalosis. Oxalosis is another inherited metabolic disorder that has a much different outcome after transplantation. Recurrence of oxalosis in the allograft was so frequently associated with allograft destruction that, until recently, children with oxalosis were excluded from renal transplant programs. An aggressive approach to pre- and posttransplant management of hyperoxaluria has yielded encouraging results in a few centers, although the majority of children with this disease still lose their grafts to recurrence. Combined liver and kidney transplantation may offer the best hope for these children in the future.

Abnormalities of the lower urinary tract

The frequency with which children (usually boys) reach ESRD with dysfunctional lower urinary tracts has prompted the development of innovative approaches to urologic surgical management that has yielded excellent results. The presence of abnormalities of the lower urinary tract is not a contraindication to transplantation. Reconstruction of a previously diverted urinary tract before transplantation is recommended by most authorities. Various techniques to enhance function of the bladder in such cases can be tried, including surgical augmentation at the time of reconstruction. Every effort is made to use the bladder, even if to do so requires intermittent clean catheterization after transplantation, as in the case of a neurogenic bladder. When the bladder cannot be used, several diversionary options remain, including various ileal and colonic conduits. Although an increased incidence of urinary tract infec-

tions after transplantation has been reported in these patients, overall graft survival rates have been no different from those seen in children with normal lower urinary tracts.

Pretransplant Dialysis

Children treated with peritoneal dialysis (PD) before transplantation have comparable graft survival rates to children treated with hemodialysis. When children maintained on PD receive a renal transplant, the peritoneal catheter is usually left in place for variable periods until good graft function has been demonstrated. For most centers this period lasts 2 to 6 weeks. Placement of the allograft in an extraperitoneal location allows use of the peritoneal cavity for dialysis during periods of early graft dysfunction or severe episodes of rejection. The catheter may also be used to drain posttransplant ascites, an uncommon complication of transplantation in patients receiving PD.

Several large series of pediatric patients report that the presence of the peritoneal catheter and the use of PD after transplantation have not adversely affected outcome. The incidence of posttransplant infectious complications related to PD (e.g., peritonitis, exit site/tunnel infections) has been low, and response to appropriate antibiotic therapy for peritonitis and antibiotic therapy plus catheter removal for exit site/tunnel infections has been reliable.

The approach to the child on PD varies widely among pediatric ESRD centers. The following, largely arbitrary guidelines are currently in use in my center:

1. A recent episode of peritonitis does not disqualify a child for transplantation as long as (a) the peritoneal fluid has been documented to be sterile by culture obtained while he was receiving intraperitoneal antibiotics (peritoneal fluid cultures must be incubated for at least 5 days) and (b) peritoneal fluid cell count and differential count obtained at the time of final crossmatch (i.e., about 4 hours before transplant) do not suggest the continued presence of peritonitis.

2. The presence of a typical mild exit site/tunnel infection does not disqualify a child for transplantation. The catheter is removed at the time of transplantation, and appropriate antibiotics are continued for a minimum of 10 additional posttransplant days. More severe tunnel infec-

tions such as those caused by *Pseudomonas* and other gram-negative organisms usually require prompt removal of the catheter and constitute a contraindication to transplantation.

3. The PD catheter is usually removed at the time of LRD transplantation to save the child a second operation. The catheter is left in place for 2 to 6 weeks following cadaveric transplantation, depending on graft function.

4. PD is performed when needed after transplantation, often using reduced exchange volumes to avoid abdominal discomfort and minimize tension on abdominal wounds. Intraperitoneal placement of the allograft is generally considered a contraindication to posttransplant PD. However, such situations must be individualized.

5. Routine flushing of the dormant PD catheter is avoided after transplantation. Samples of peritoneal fluid are obtained for culture via the PD catheter when evaluating a child with fever.

Preemptive Transplantation

Transplantation without prior dialysis has been termed preemptive transplantation by Kahan and others. The increasing popularity of this approach is indicated by the fact that of the 761 transplants reported by the NAPRTCS, 21% were preemptive. Whether or not a child had received dialysis before transplantation did not influence 1-year graft survival probabilities in these children. However, these are only short-term results. There is growing evidence that noncompliance with immunosuppressive medication regimens is a factor in graft loss in a large number of pediatric patients. This problem is thought to be more widespread among adolescents. Although there are currently no data about children to support insistence on a pretransplant period of "punitive" dialysis as a means of increasing compliance, the potential relationship between preemptive transplantation and an increased incidence of noncompliance must be kept in mind. Additional counseling and more careful follow-up may be warranted in such patients, especially adolescents.

ABO Blood Group Compatibility

ABO-incompatible transplants were originally performed by mistake, and almost all resulted in hyperacute or acute vascular rejection. These observations led to the general rule that renal transplantation should be performed only between an ABO-compatible donor and recipient (the presence or absence of the Rh antigen was observed to be unimportant).

Recent efforts to transplant "across the ABO barrier" have had limited success, usually with plasmapheresis to reduce ABO isoagglutinin titers in the recipient. Splenectomy has also been used to increase graft survival. These measures carry substantial risks and can only rarely be justified in individual cases.

HLA Matching

The genes coding for the expression of the HLA antigens are located on the short arm of chromosome number 6. Six loci have been identified: HLA-A, HLA-B, HLA-C, HLA-DP, HLA-DQ, and HLA-DR, each containing multiple alleles. The large number of alleles make the HLA system the most polymorphic genetic system found in man. HLA-A, HLA-B, and HLA-C are known as class I antigens, and they are distributed ubiquitously, occurring on the surface of cells of all transplantable organs such as kidney, heart, liver, and pancreas. Class I antigens are found on the endothelium of all blood vessels within the kidney, as well as on tubular and mesangial cells. B and T lymphocytes also express class I antigens. Class II antigens (HLA-DR, HLA-DP, HLA-DQ) are confined mainly to endothelium and dendritic cells in most nonlymphoid tissues. They also occur on B and activated T lymphocytes. Widespread expression of class II antigens on many kidney cells can be induced after transplantation and may correlate with rejection.

HLA genes are usually inherited en bloc from each parent. The HLA antigens coded for by the genes of one chromosome are known collectively as a haplotype, and each individual inherits one haplotype from each parent. Thus parent-to-child transplants are one haplotype matches, and sibling transplants can range from HLA-identical matches (i.e., two haplotype matches) to total HLA mismatches.

The role of HLA matching in LRD transplantation was previously well defined: HLA-identical transplants enjoyed 1-year graft survival rates of 90% to 95%, with haploidentical grafts at 70% to 80% and completely mismatched grafts at 60% to 70%. The introduction of donor-specific blood transfusions and the use of CyA have each individually resulted in marked improvement in graft survival in haplo-identical and completely mismatched LRD transplants. A small effect of HLA matching on outcome in LRD transplantation can still be detected by large multicenter studies, but in general the use of donor-specific blood transfusions or CyA will minimize this effect in the individual patient.

The role of HLA matching in cadaveric transplantation is highly controversial. It is believed that only HLA-A, HLA-B, and HLA-DR are important, but there is little information available on this subject in pediatric patients. Large multicenter studies involving thousands of patients (of whom <5% are children) continue to show an effect of HLA matching on cadaveric transplant outcome, with 0- and 1-antigen mismatched grafts faring better than 5- and 6-antigen mismatched grafts. There is some evidence to support the notion that matching for the HLA-DRs is most important in pediatric cadaver transplantation. However, this evidence is presently inconclusive and at times conflicting. The logic inherent in obtaining the best possible HLA matching when kidneys are transplanted in children is compelling, but at the present time the magnitude of the HLA matching effect on outcome is yet to be clearly demonstrated.

Immunosuppression

Conventional immunosuppression (i.e., prednisone, azathioprine). Before the introduction of Cya pediatric patients were treated with various maintenance immunosuppression regimens using prednisone and azathioprine. Results varied from center to center, but overall outcome appeared to be no worse among pediatric recipients compared to adults when "conventional" immunosuppression was used. Unfortunately, for cadaver grafts, results were relatively discouraging for all groups, with 2-year allograft survival rates rarely exceeding 50% using prednisone and azathioprine. In addition the side effects of prolonged corticosteroid use in high doses were particularly harmful to children who continued to suffer poor growth and sexual maturation despite the presence of a functioning transplant. Steroid side effects could be reduced by conversion to alternate-day prednisone therapy once graft function had been stable for approximately 1 year, but in the experience of some centers this maneuver was too often followed by rejection episodes. Only well-matched LRD grafts (haploidentical or at least one haplotype match) resulted in acceptable long-term (i.e., >3

years) graft survival rates using standard immunosuppression in pediatric recipients, and only in HLA-identical grafts were 3-year survival rates reliably >75%.

Deliberate blood transfusions. Anemia is a consistent feature of ESRD in patients of all ages. During the 1960s potential renal transplant patients were freely given blood transfusions when needed to treat clinically significant anemia. It became apparent that frequent transfusions promoted the development of circulating antibodies directed against human tissue antigens (now termed preformed or panel-reactive antibodies and expressed as %PRA). The %PRA is determined by testing the potential recipient's serum for circulating antibodies against lymphocytes obtained from a panel of blood donors representing a wide variety of HLA tissue types. When the %PRA was high, as was often the case in frequently transfused patients, it was proportionally more difficult to find a donor whose kidney would not be destroyed by humoral (hyperacute) rejection caused by the presence in the recipient of circulating antibodies formed as a result of sensitization by blood transfusion. These observations led to the adoption in the early 1970s of an almost universal policy of withholding blood transfusions from dialysis patients. This policy added greatly to the morbidity associated with chronic hemodialysis for children, who often were forced to tolerate hematocrit levels of 14% to 15% for protracted periods.

The startling observations by Opelz and Teresaki that graft survival was substantially better in patients who had received prior blood transfusions compared to nontransfused patients swung the transfusion pendulum back in favor of not only the free use of blood products for clinically significant anemia, but the deliberate exposure of potential transplant recipients to a minimum number of random blood transfusions as part of the overall immunosuppression strategy. The beneficial effect of blood transfusions is clearly seen in virtually every large series of cadaver graft recipients treated with conventional immunosuppression. The mechanism by which this effect is achieved is unknown.

Salvatierra and Potter and their associates in San Francisco discovered that the outcome in LRD transplantation could also be improved when blood from a potential living donor was deliberately transfused into the recipient. These investigators originally proposed donor-specific transfusions for donor-recipient pairs whose mixed lymphocyte culture results predicted a poor outcome despite the absence of preformed antibodies. (The mixed lymphocyte culture is a more precise method of in vitro testing of recipient and donor histocompatibility than the standard crossmatch, which looks only for circulating antibodies against donor lymphocytes.) Various donor-specific transfusion protocols were developed that were associated with improved LRD graft survival rates, approaching those seen in HLA-identical transplants.

Unfortunately the use of donor-specific transfusions resulted in sensitization of the recipient to the potential donor in more than 20% of cases, thereby rendering transplantation from that donor impossible. Various modifications to the donor-specific transfusion protocol, including the use of azathioprine during donor-specific transfusion exposure, has reduced the sensitization rate to approximately 10% in most series.

The introduction of CyA has provided an alternative to deliberate donor-specific transfusion and random donor blood transfusions. Although blood transfusions probably still have a beneficial effect on outcome in CyA-treated patients, the incremental gain is small at best, and for most centers the risks of sensitization (by donor-specific transfusion) or transmission of viral diseases (HIV; non-A, non-B hepatitis) from random donor transfusions outweigh their potential benefits when CyA is used. Thus the pendulum has again swung away from the use of deliberate transfusions as immunosuppressive therapy. The introduction of recombinant human erythropoietin will likely soon eliminate the need for blood transfusions altogether for most ESRD patients, and as more and more of these never-transfused patients receive transplants, the beneficial immunosuppressive effects of blood transfusions on graft survival may become easier to define in their absence.

Cyclosporine. CyA was discovered in 1972 by chemists at Sandoz, Ltd., in Switzerland who were actually looking for new antimicrobial agents. CyA is a metabolite of the fungal species *Tolypocladium inflatum,* which is dissolved in olive oil for oral use. The resulting concoction has the taste one might expect from a rotting fungus mixed in olive oil, a problem of no small consequence when attempting to treat children twice daily with the drug.

A review of the vast literature on the use of this powerful immunosuppressive agent is beyond the

scope of this chapter. The beneficial effects on short-term renal allograft survival, both LRD and cadaveric, have been so well demonstrated that controversies currently are focused not on whether to use CyA, but when and how to use it and how best to minimize its nephrotoxic and other side effects, which are considerable. One of the unique features of CyA among the immunosuppressive agents commonly used in renal transplantation is the ability to monitor therapy by measuring blood levels of the drug. Unfortunately the pharmacokinetics of CyA in children are highly variable and rarely remain the same in the same child. Thus frequent CyA blood levels are needed to adjust therapy, especially during the initial posttransplant period. Even with frequent blood levels the use of CyA in children can be extremely difficult. This is largely due to our poor understanding of the pharmacodynamics of this agent in the individual child. The CyA blood levels below which therapeutic effect becomes inadequate and above which nephrotoxicity develops can only be roughly predicted at the present time. Although there is no doubt that several thousand children have been the direct beneficiaries of the discovery of CyA, there are times when the complexities, controversies, apparent contraindications, and outright confusion that accompany the use of CyA in children make the task much more demanding than it was in the days of conventional immunosuppression.

Antilymphocyte antibodies. There are two main types of antilymphocyte antibody preparations in widespread use today: polyclonal antibodies (e.g., Minnesota ALG, Atgam) and monoclonal antibodies (e.g., OKT3). These agents are most often used to treat acute rejection episodes. Concerns about the exposure of the new allograft to the nephrotoxic effects of CyA during the period of marginal allograft function that often follows engraftment have prompted development of sequential induction immunosuppression strategies that replace CyA with an antilymphocyte preparation (e.g., ALG, OKT3) for the first few days after transplantation until the allograft is functioning well. An example of such an induction protocol currently in use in this center for cadaver graft recipients is given in Table 66-2.

Combination immunosuppression strategies. Excellent results can be obtained with the use of CyA alone or in combination with either corticosteroids (e.g., prednisone [pred]) or azathioprine (AZA). Toxicity due to these potent agents is a common prob-

Table 66-2 Cadaver Donor Renal Transplant: Immunosuppression Schedule for Children *With* Statural Growth Potential

Name _____   Transplant Date _____   *Schedule 2*

Time After Treatment	Date	Weight	ALG	Prednisone	Azathioprine	Cyclosporine (CyA)
On Call to OR				Prednisone 2.5 mg/kg IV = ___ mg	2.5 mg/kg/day IV = ___ mg	
Day 0			*15 mg/kg =	Methylprednisolone 1 mg/kg at 7 hr postop = ___ mg/dose	Wt >25 kg = 25 mg/day* Wt ≤25 kg = 12.5 mg/day	
1, 2			15 mg/kg =	2 mg/kg ÷ bid = ___ mg =		
3, 4			15 mg/kg =	1.75 mg/kg = ___ mg ÷ bid = /↓		
5, 6			†15 mg/kg =	1.6 mg/kg = ___ mg ÷ bid = /↓		Begin on day 5† at 15 mg/
7-9				1.5 mg/kg = ___ mg ÷ bid = /↓	2.5 mg/kg/day (max dose	kg ÷ bid = ___ mg/kg
10-12				1.25 mg/kg = ___ mg ÷ bid = /↓	150 mg/day)	Adjust dose to give a whole
13-15				1.0 mg/kg/day = ___ mg		blood trough HPLC
16-18				0.75 mg/kg/day = ___ mg		level of 100 to 200 ng/ml
19-29				0.6 mg/kg/day = ___ mg		(sustain these levels
30-89				0.5 mg/kg/day = ___ mg		until 12 mo)
90-96				0.7 mg/kg alt 0.4 = ___ mg/ ___ mg		
97-103				0.7 mg/kg alt 0.3 = ___ mg/ ___ mg		
104-110				0.7 mg/kg alt 0.2 = ___ mg/ ___ mg		
111-4 mo				0.7 mg/kg alt 0.1 = ___ mg/ ___ mg		
4-5 mo				0.7 mg/kg every other day = ___ mg		
5-6 mo				0.6 mg/kg every other day = ___ mg		
6-10 mo				0.5 mg/kg every other day = ___ mg		
10-12 mo				0.4 mg/kg every other day = ___ mg		At 12 mo, reduce CyA
12 mo...				0.3 mg/kg every other day = ___ mg		dosage to give trough
						level of 50 to 100 ng/ml

↓ = Decrease P.M. dose *only*.

*Give day 0 ALG and azathioprine on evening of transplant day.

†If poor graft function due to acute tubular necrosis persists at day 5, delay CyA and continue ALG until days 10 and 12, respectively, or until creatinine is ≤2.0 mg/dl, whichever comes first. Always continue ALG for 2 days after starting CyA. Do not delay CyA beyond day 10 regardless of graft function.

Revised 3/11/88

lem, however. By combining three agents (CyA + AZA + Pred) lower doses of each individual drug can theoretically be used, thereby reducing the risks of individual drug toxicity. These goals have been generally met in adult renal transplantation in which relatively low doses of prednisone and CyA are rapidly achieved after transplantation. Fig. 66-1 depicts the combinations of immunosuppressive agents used in the patients enrolled in the NAPRTCS. Note that "triple therapy" (CyA + Pred + AZA) is clearly the most popular regimen currently in use in North American pediatric renal transplant centers. Average doses used in these children were relatively greater on a weight basis than typical triple-therapy regimens used in adults. The need for more immunosuppressive medication may be a reflection of the increased immunocompetence of young children with ESRD, as demonstrated by in vitro studies of immunologic cell functions performed by Ettenger and associates. Higher doses on a weight basis also reflect the in-

creased metabolic rates of children compared to adults. The fact remains, however, that the use of combination strategies have not had the same dose-lowering effect in children as in adults, and immunosuppressive drug toxicity remains a major concern in pediatric renal transplant recipients.

Practical Considerations in the Perioperative Period

General considerations

The overriding management goal for children with irreversible renal insufficiency is to initiate RRT (dialysis or transplantation) *before* the child experiences any serious consequences of the uremic state. Earlier and more aggressive use of dialysis and transplantation is believed to be of particular importance to children for whom the deleterious effects of chronic uremia on growth and development are often permanent.

One additional benefit of this aggressive approach to RRT can be a generally improved physical condition at the time of renal transplantation. Unlike children with end-stage hepatic or cardiac disease who often come to transplantation seriously, if not critically ill, the child with ESRD should be in stable condition at the time of the transplant. Gone are the days of the emergency renal transplant performed on a child who was, in effect, rapidly dying on dialysis. More than 98% of transplanted children survive beyond 3 months after transplantation, and death in the immediate postoperative period is rare. The generally improved clinical condition of pediatric renal transplant recipients at the time of surgery may be an important contributor to such excellent survival statistics.

Obviously the posttransplant management of the dialysis-dependent child differs substantially from that of the child receiving preemptive transplantation. All hinges on early allograft function. When the allograft functions well from the time of reanastomosis, as is the case with almost all LRD transplants, postoperative management is obviously much easier. Early graft nonfunction results in the need for dialysis not only in dialysis-dependent patients, but in many patients receiving preemptive transplantation whose native kidney function is marginal and often inadequate to sustain the child through the hypercatabolic postoperative period. Thus contingency plans for dialysis are made for all patients before transplantation should early graft function prove inadequate.

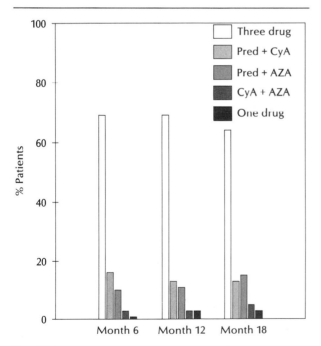

Fig. 66-1 Maintenance immunosuppression therapy patterns in pediatric renal transplant recipients at 6, 12, and 18 months after transplant. (From the Second Annual Report, North American Pediatric Renal Transplant Cooperative Study, May 1989.)

Preoperative dialysis

Children must be adequately dialyzed before undergoing renal transplantation. For the child receiving chronic hemodialysis this often means that a 3- to 4-hour hemodialysis treatment is needed before surgery. CPD patients rarely need additional dialysis before surgery. An attempt should be made to avoid overly aggressive fluid removal in all pediatric patients during pretransplant dialysis. Similarly, the polyuric child cannot be put on an NPO regimen unless adequate IV fluids are provided to maintain a well-hydrated state.

Intraoperative fluid management

Maintenance of an adequate vascular volume throughout the operative procedure is essential to successful renal transplantation in children. When an adult kidney is placed in a small child, intraoperative fluid management is especially critical. Continuous monitoring of the CVP and systemic arterial pressure are essential guides to fluid therapy in the operating room. Most pediatric centers require a CVP >10 cm H_2O and a systolic BP >110 mm Hg before the vascular clamps are removed to allow perfusion of the transplanted kidney. Even then, the anesthesiologist must be prepared to rapidly infuse another 250 to 300 ml of isotonic fluid (preferably 5% albumin solution or blood) as soon as the vascular clamps are removed. The additional volume is needed to prevent an acute hypotensive episode that can rapidly develop when the vascular capacity of the adult renal allograft is added to the circulatory capacity of the child.

Such aggressive fluid therapy can obviously be harmful, especially in children whose myocardial function has been adversely affected by chronic hypertension. These children often need an intraoperative dopamine infusion (at 5 μg/kg/min) as a precautionary measure before signs of congestive heart failure actually develop. Some centers advocate the *routine* intraoperative use of dopamine infusions in all pediatric allograft recipients to help maintain an adequate systemic arterial blood pressure, improve cardiac output, and increase perfusion of the allograft.

Postoperative fluid management

Management of fluid replacement therapy in the first 24 to 48 hours after transplantation is frequently a challenging clinical problem. When the allograft functions well, a brisk diuresis usually ensues, which is driven by the osmotic effects of the patient's total body urea load (which can now be excreted by the allograft) and by the new kidney's attempt to excrete the volume load received by the patient during surgery. During this initial period the allograft is exquisitely sensitive to even brief episodes of hypoperfusion. Renal vascular hemodynamic autoregulatory mechanisms may be unstable and unreliable. For pediatric patients who have received an adult kidney, it is particularly important to maintain a generous intravascular volume and an adequate blood pressure.

Close monitoring of CVP and aggressive milliliter-for-milliliter replacement of urinary output is usually needed for at least the initial 24 hours after transplantation. Total urinary replacement may not be sufficient to maintain the CVP in the target range (e.g., 8 to 12 cm H_2O) because of third-space fluid losses into the operative site and/or development of occult postdialysis ascites in patients previously maintained on peritoneal dialysis. Supplemental fluid therapy (usually 5% albumin solution infusions in 5 to 10 ml/kg doses) are often needed during this period to maintain the desired CVP and to support BP. A systolic BP of at least 110 mm Hg is mandatory.

At the same time the cardiopulmonary status of the patient must be carefully monitored. Some children will be intolerant of such aggressive fluid loading, and dopamine or dobutamine will be needed to sustain cardiac output and avoid congestive heart failure. Fortunately cardiac decompensation is an uncommon event, although the risk is present in all of these children. Occasionally a child will return from the operating room with an obvious fluid overload. If the allograft is functioning, it is a simple matter to replace only a portion of the brisk urinary output for a few hours until signs of congestive heart failure have resolved and intravascular volume status has become more nearly normal, after which milliliter-for-milliliter urinary replacement can be resumed. It may be necessary to keep these symptomatically fluid-overloaded children intubated for several additional hours in the PICU while fluid overload is resolving. Early institution of dialysis is recommended for oliguric children with symptomatic posttransplant fluid overload, but fluid removal by dialysis must be done with great care. Hypotension during dialysis as a result of too aggressive ultrafiltration can result in thrombosis of the allograft.

Urinary output can reach staggering hourly volumes during the immediate posttransplant period. Replacement fluid should be 0.45% saline solution *without dextrose* to avoid development of hyperglycemia. A second IV line containing dextrose is conveniently run at a rate calculated to replace insensible water losses (see Chapter 15).

At some point during the second postoperative day it is appropriate to begin replacing only a portion of the urinary output to avoid driving a diuresis indefinitely. Most patients with good allograft function will be manageable on routine maintenance fluid volumes by the third postoperative day.

Problems during initial 24 to 48 hours after transplantation

Oliguria. A brisk urinary output is the hallmark of good graft function (except in patients whose primary renal disorder is characterized by polyuria). When urinary output falls below 1 to 2 ml/kg/hr, the most likely cause is a decreased intravascular volume. After irrigating the urinary catheter to be sure that drainage is not impeded by clots, the CVP should be measured and a fluid bolus given (5 to 10 ml/kg of 5% albumin solution is preferred in this center) if the CVP is <10 cm H_2O. Persistent oliguria despite adequate systemic arterial blood pressure and CVP may herald a more ominous problem. Delayed onset of acute tubular necrosis (ATN) can occur at any time during the initial 24 posttransplant hours. Obstruction of the transplant ureter can occur early, and development of a urinary leak can also occur, although this is more typically a late complication resulting from ischemia and necrosis of the transplanted ureter. Early acute allograft rejection is also a possibility, and acute CyA nephrotoxicity may mimic ATN, especially when the drug is given intravenously. The onset of oliguria resistant to volume and pressors in an allograft that previously had good urinary output is an urgent situation necessitating prompt evaluation by ultrasound and radionucleotide scan. Fluid management must be adjusted to replace only measured losses plus insensible water losses. If ATN is suspected, one to three doses of furosemide (see Chapter 14) may be tried but should not be continued if response is poor since furosemide can be a potent nephrotoxin in this situation. Dialysis may be needed if fluid loading in an effort to stimulate diuresis has been too aggressive. Early allograft biopsy is often helpful when the clinical picture is not clear.

Hypotension. The maintenance of systolic BP >110 mm Hg is essential to early management of the adult kidney placed in a small child. Volume is given until the CVP is at least 10 cm H_2O, after which dopamine at 5 to 10 μg/kg/min should be used.

Hypertension. Mild degrees of hypertension (i.e., within 10% to 15% of the 95th percentile for age and sex) are frequently tolerated during the immediate posttransplant period. Higher BPs are often due to pain and can be successfully controlled by more aggressive use of analgesics. The choice of an analgesic must be made with the level of allograft function in mind. Potent metabolites of morphine sulfate have been shown to accumulate in the circulation of patients with decreased renal function and can potentially cause respiratory depression. Levorphanol tartrate (Levo-Dromoran) may be a better choice for patients whose allografts are not functioning well. When hypertension is due to causes such as high-dose steroids or preexisting hypertensive renal disease, the blood pressure can rapidly reach dangerous levels. Nifedipine (0.15 to 0.3 mg/kg per dose) given sublingually has been an effective agent in this setting (see Chapter 53). Nifedipine also has theoretically beneficial effects on blood flow within the allograft.

Fever. Early fever is most often a consequence of the use of an antilymphocyte immunosuppressive agent such as ALG. Postoperative atelectasis is another frequent cause. A patient with acute rejection may also present with fever. Thorough evaluation with appropriate cultures of blood, urine, and peritoneal fluid must be obtained and a diligent search made for a focus of infection. Broad-spectrum antibiotics are routinely given for at least 72 hours after transplantation and may be continued for longer periods when the child is febrile for unknown reasons.

Acidosis. A moderate metabolic acidosis frequently occurs in the first few hours after transplantation, especially in small children. This is due at least in part to the dilutional effects of large volumes of crystalloid solutions given perioperatively but may be enhanced by poor graft function. If the graft is functioning well, the acidosis usually resolves in a few hours without specific therapy.

Hypophosphatemia. Phosphate wasting by the renal allograft can rapidly result in phosphate depletion with serum phosphate levels <2.0 mg/dl. Frequent monitoring is needed (see below). Phosphate supplementation (usually as IV potassium or sodium phosphate) should be instituted when serum phosphate levels fall to <4.0 mg/dl.

Hemorrhage. Bleeding from the vascular anastamosis is a very rare complication, but when present, hypotension and a rapidly declining hematocrit level are the cardinal signs. Sonography will be useful in some cases, but most transplant surgeons who suspect postoperative hemorrhage return the patient to the operating room for another look without delay. Failure to respond aggressively in this situation dooms the graft and places the child in some danger.

Monitoring during initial 24 to 48 hours after transplantation

The following laboratory tests must be performed immediately when the patient is admitted to the PICU: (1) CBC with differential and platelet count; (2) serum sodium, potassium, chloride, carbon dioxide, BUN, creatinine, calcium, and phosphorus; and (3) urine for sodium and potassium. Tests 1 and 2 should be repeated q 8 hr times 3, then q 12 hr.

An immediate portable chest roentgenogram (to confirm CVP placement) and a KUB must be performed on admission of the patient to the PICU. Additional studies performed daily include the following values: magnesium, alkaline phosphatase, ALT, and AST.

The physician must be notified if any of the following occur:

Urinary output <50% of previous hour's output
Urinary output <____ ml (1 to 2 ml/kg during previous hour)
CVP <____ (8 to 10 cm H₂O) or >____ (12 to 14 cm H₂O)
Systolic BP <110 mm Hg or >____ (130 to 140 mm Hg)
Axillary temperature >38° C
Heart rate >____ (110 to 140 bpm, depending on age)

A renal transplant sonogram and radionuclide scan must be obtained within 12 to 24 hours of admission to serve as a baseline for future comparison.

COMPLICATIONS OF TRANSPLANTATION
Rejection

There are at least three main clinical rejection syndromes: hyperacute, acute, and chronic rejection.

Hyperacute rejection is mediated by preformed cytotoxic antibodies against donor tissue antigens. The process begins as soon as the graft is revascu-

larized; the kidney literally turns black before the surgeon's eyes. There is no treatment. Fortunately improved histocompatibility laboratory methods have all but eliminated hyperacute rejection.

The immunobiology of *acute (cellular) rejection* is complex and incompletely understood. Acute rejection can occur at any time after transplantation but rarely begins before the third or fourth posttransplant day. Before the introduction of CyA, acute rejection was typically characterized by fever, graft pain and tenderness, reduced urinary output, weight gain, hypertension, increasing BUN and creatinine levels, and occasionally hematuria and proteinuria. CyA-treated patients often demonstrate only an increase in serum creatinine level. This can be extremely subtle when an adult kidney has been placed in a small child; for this patient a rise in serum creatinine from 0.3 to 0.4 mg/dl accompanied by a low-grade fever is acute rejection until proved otherwise.

Diagnosis of acute rejection can be difficult. The differential diagnosis includes acute urinary obstruction, CyA nephrotoxicity, urinary extravasation, and persistent ATN. A sonogram will rule out obstruction, and a radionuclide scan will demonstrate extravasation. If both of these studies are unrevealing, a biopsy of the transplant is often needed to differentiate acute rejection from CyA nephrotoxicity and ATN.

Treatment of acute rejection is routinely begun with large daily or alternate-day doses of IV methylprednisolone (10 to 30 mg/kg per dose) for three to five doses. More than 60% of acute rejection episodes are completely reversed by IV methylprednisolone. For those rejection episodes resistant to IV methylprednisolone, an antilymphocyte preparation such as OKT3 or ALG may be used.

Chronic rejection is an inexorable process of graft destruction that is poorly understood. Renal function slowly deteriorates over time despite apparently adequate maintenance immunosuppression. Allograft biopsies show arteriolar and interstitial fibrosis. There is no effective treatment.

Opportunistic Infection

The most common cause of death in pediatric renal transplant recipients is infection. The immunocompromised transplant recipient is at risk for a wide variety of infections, as is shown in Fig. 66-2, which also gives a representative time of onset (after the transplant) of the more common infections. As immunosuppressive regimens become more potent in an effort to suppress or reverse rejection, the risk of opportunistic infection obviously increases. The ability to determine for each child the fine line between adequate immunosuppression to prevent rejection and excessive immunosuppression leading to potentially life-threatening opportunistic infection is one of the major challenges of clinical transplantation.

Hypertension

Hypertension occurs in more than 70% of children who have received a renal transplant. The etiology of hypertension is often difficult to determine in the individual patient, perhaps because multiple causative factors may be involved. The following potential etiologic factors should be considered:

1. Side effect of CyA
2. Acute and/or chronic rejection
3. Transplant artery stenosis
4. Recurrence of primary renal disease
5. Ischemia/fibrosis of native kidneys
6. Side effect of prednisone
7. Excessive sodium chloride and fluid retention
8. Side effect of antihistamines and other nonprescription medications

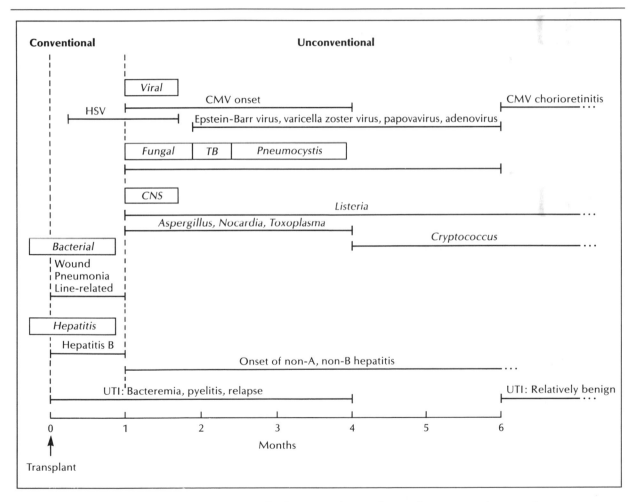

Fig. 66-2 Timetable for occurrence of infection in the renal transplant patient. (From Rubin RH, Wolfson JS, Losini AS, Tolkoff-Rubin NE. Infection in the renal transplant recipient. Am J Med 70:405, 1981.)

Effective treatment for posttransplant hypertension is essential (see Chapter 53) since poor control of hypertension can cause accelerated deterioration of graft function.

Other Complications

The following complications are listed to call attention to the wide array of problems that can be encountered by children after renal transplantation.

CyA side effects

Hypertrichosis
Tremor
Gingival hypertrophy
Hypertension
Nephrotoxicity
Interaction with other drugs

Corticosteroid side effects

Cataracts
Aseptic necrosis at hips and knees
Retardation of growth and sexual maturation
GI bleeding (gastritis, peptic ulcer)
Pancreatitis
Hyperlipidemia
Hyperphagia/obesity
Hypertension
Diabetes mellitus
Cushingoid facies
Acne
Emotional lability

Malignancy (de novo)

Psychosocial maladjustment and noncompliance

RESULTS OF RENAL TRANSPLANTATION IN PEDIATRIC PATIENTS

Short-term results in the 754 children who received 761 renal transplants from January 1, 1987, to February 16, 1989, at the 71 participating centers in the NAPRTCS are summarized as follows:

1. Survival probabilities for LRD and cadaver grafts are plotted in Fig. 66-3. One-year graft survival was 88% for LRD and 71% for cadaver grafts.
2. Causes of graft failure are listed in Table 66-3. Note the large number of grafts lost to vascular thrombosis, a problem encountered much less often in adult transplantation.
3. Thirty-five of 754 children in the NAPRTCS study died after receiving a renal transplant. One-year patient survival probabilities for LRD and cadaver transplant recipients were 96% and 92%, respectively. The main cause of death was infection (16/35). Five children died from hemorrhages and four from malignancy that either was unrecognized before transplantation or developed after transplantation. Eight deaths occurred during the first 30 days after transplantation, with two of them in the first postoperative week.

These results represent pooled data from multiple centers. Much higher graft and patient survival rates have been reported by individual pediatric centers. One-year cadaveric graft survival rates of >90% have recently been reported from large pediatric transplant centers in Southern California and West Germany. However, the explanation for such spectacular

Table 66-3   Causes of Graft Failure*

Cause	Index Graft Failures (n = 139)	Second Failures (n = 13)	Total (N = 152)(%)
Primary nonfunction	6	0	6 (4)
Vascular thromboses	21	4	25 (16)
Other technical problems	5	0	5 (3)
Hyperacute rejection, <24 hr	3	0	3 (2)
Accelerated acute rejection, 2-7 days	15	1	16 (11)
Acute rejection	38	5	43 (28)
Chronic rejection	19	0	19 (13)
Recurrence of original disease	6	1	7 (5)
Death	12	1	13 (9)
Other	14	1	15 (10)

*From the Second Annual Report, North American Pediatric Renal Transplant Cooperative Study, May 1989.

results remains unclear, even to those who practice in these centers. Similar beneficial "center effects" have been noted in a small number of adult transplant centers, but the source of the improved outcomes reported by these adult centers is also obscure. It is encouraging that such excellent results are clearly attainable in pediatric renal transplantation, but widespread achievement of these optimum outcomes will not be possible without a better understanding of the many complex factors involved in the treatment of these children.

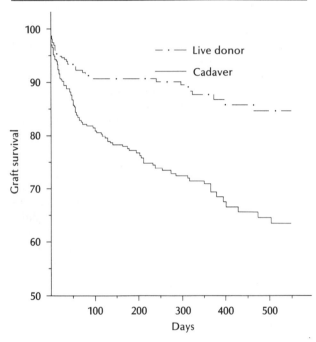

Fig. 66-3   Probability of renal allograft survival in pediatric recipients of cadaver and LRD transplants. NOTE: Graft-survival range plotted from 50% to 100%. (From the Second Annual Report, North American Pediatric Renal Transplant Cooperative Study, May 1989.)

ADDITIONAL READING

Ehrich JHH, Rizzoni G, Broyer M, et al. Combined report on regular dialysis and transplantation of children in Europe, 1987. Berlin: Springer-Verlag, 1988, pp 33-41.

Fine RN. Renal transplantation of the infant and young child and the use of pediatric cadaver kidneys for transplantation in pediatric and adult recipients. Am J Kidney Dis 12:1-10, 1988.

• Fine RN, Ettenger RB. Renal transplantation in children. In Morris PJ, ed. Kidney Transplantation, 3rd ed. Philadelphia: WB Saunders, 1988, pp 635-691.

Leone MR, Alexander SR, Barry JM, et al. OKT3 monoclonal antibody in pediatric kidney transplant recipients with recurrent and resistant allograft rejection. J Pediatr 111:45-50, 1987.

Offner G, Hayer PF, Brodehl J, et al. Cyclosporin A in pediatric kidney transplantation. Pediatr Nephrol 1:125-130, 1987.

Potter D, Garavoy M, Hopper S, et al. Effect of donor-specific transfusions on renal transplantation in children. Pediatrics 76:402-405, 1985.

• Second Annual Report, North American Pediatric Renal Transplant Cooperative Study, May 1989. Pediatr Nephrol (in press).

Sheldon C, Najarian J, Mauer S. Pediatric renal transplantation. Surg Clin North Am 65:1589-1621, 1985.

Simmons RL, Najarian JS, Finch ME. Kidney transplantation in infants and small children. In Simmons RL, Finch ME, Ascher NL, et al, eds. Manual of Vascular Access, Organ Donation and Transplantation. New York: Springer-Verlag, 1984, pp 324-328.

67 Nursing Care of the Renal Transplant Patient

Debbie L. LeVasseur

BACKGROUND

Pediatric transplant nursing is a specialized and challenging profession that encompasses all aspects of medical care, including pediatrics, surgery, medicine, psychology, patient education, and social work. In the PICU objectivity and astute observation skills are necessary as is compassion for a family whose lives have been in turmoil.

The family of a child with end-stage renal disease (ESRD) is faced with complex decisions. The treatment options include chronic hemodialysis, chronic peritoneal dialysis, transplantation, or death without treatment or transplantation. In most cases the family that chooses a transplant for the child has already experienced one of the available chronic treatment modalities. If ESRD has been gradually approaching, a "primary" transplant may be possible, in which case the transplant would take place before any dialysis has been initiated. When the family chooses transplantation, there are two potential donor sources— a live, related donor (LRD) or a cadaver.

PREPARATION FOR TRANSPLANTATION

In preparation for transplantation the patient and all potential ABO-compatible donors in the immediate family are tissue typed to identify their histocompatibility antigens (HLAs). Tissue typing enables close matching of the donor's antigens with those of the recipient. Each person inherits four HLAs (a haplotype) from each parent; therefore each parent is always at least one haplotype, or half identical, to his child. A haplotype is considered a very good match for transplantation. Siblings may inherit the same or different haplotypes and thus be either a very good match or a complete mismatch with each other. LRD transplantation offers the highest expectation for a successful outcome statistically. Since it is an elective scheduled surgical procedure, renal transplantation with an LRD organ permits optimal preparation for the recipient and donor. However, for many potential recipients an LRD transplant is not available, and they must rely on the use and availability of a cadaveric kidney.

When cadaveric transplantation is the option chosen, the patient is placed on a list with other ESRD patients awaiting transplantation. When a kidney becomes available, it is tissue typed and matched against ABO-compatible patients on the list. Once a recipient is selected, he is brought into the hospital for further testing. In addition a final "crossmatch" is performed immediately before surgery by incubating the recipient's serum with lymphocytes from the donor. If the donor lymphocytes are killed by the recipient's serum, the crossmatch is positive, indicating that the recipient has preformed antibodies against that donor's cells and a transplant with that kidney must not be done because of the risk of hyperacute rejection. A positive crossmatch may occur from the presence of preformed cytotoxic antibodies. Cytotoxic antibodies may be produced any time a potential recipient is exposed to antigens other than his own (e.g., blood transfusions, pregnancy, previous transplants). Frequent serum samples are obtained from potential transplant recipients and kept frozen for crossmatching against available cadaveric donor lymphocytes. The greater the number of circulating cytotoxic antibodies, the higher is the risk of a positive final crossmatch and therefore cancellation of the transplant. If the crossmatch is negative and the patient is medically stable, the transplant may proceed.

PRETRANSPLANT EVALUATIONS

All recipients

Day 1

Skin tests placed (mumps, tuberculin, *Candida*)
Chest roentgenogram
ECG
Bone age evaluation
Stool guaiac test × 2
Dental evaluation
Ophthalmologic evaluation
Laboratory tests
    Tissue typing
    Urinalysis
    Urine culture
    Blood work
        ABO group and Rh
        BUN, creatinine
        Na, K, Cl, CO_2, Ca, P
        Alkaline phosphatase, AST/ALT, bilirubin (total and direct)
        Albumin, total protein, cholesterol, fasting blood glucose, amylase, Mg
        CBC—differential, platelet count, PT, PTT
        Serial WBCs until WBC >6000 mm^3 or three have been done
        Parathormone—N-terminal
        CMV titer, herpes titer, EBV titer, varicella titer
        Hepatitis B surface antigen, antibody and CORE antibody, hepatitis A Ab, HIV-ab, VDRL

Day 2

24-hr urine for volume, protein, and creatinine
Voiding cystourethrogram
Urology evaluation
Obtain immunization and communicable disease records
Read and record skin test results

Live, related donor

Tissue typing has already been performed.

Day 1

History and physical examination
ECG
Chest roentgenogram

Laboratory tests
    Glofil clearance test
    Urinalysis
    Urine culture
    24-hr urine for volume, protein, and creatinine
    CBC
    SMA-12
    Renal panel
    Lipid panel
    Liver panel
    VDRL
    Amylasc
    Lipase
    CMV titer
    HIV antibody
    ABO group and Rh
    Hepatitis B surface antigen

Day 2

Psychiatric evaluation
Renal CT scan

Day 3

Renal arteriogram

Final pretransplant testing for all recipients
(immediately before transplantation)

Final crossmatch of donor with recipient is performed (if positive, transplant is canceled).
Chest roentgenogram
ECG
Urinalysis
Urine culture
Blood culture
Stool culture
Nasopharyngeal culture
Peritoneal dialysis fluid culture (if PD catheter is in place)
BUN, creatinine, Na, K, Cl, CO_2, Ca, P, CBC with differential, PT/PTT, AST/ALT, alkaline phosphatase, amylase, bilirubin, Mg, LDH
CMV titer, EBV titer
HBsAb, HB CORE Ab, HBsAg
HIV-ab

TRANSPLANT PROCEDURE

All renal transplants are performed with the patient under general anesthesia and usually take 3 to 4 hours. The kidney is stored in a sterile iced electrolyte slush solution during transport. Still cold, the kidney is placed in the extraperitoneal space in the right or left iliac fossa. The donor's renal artery usually is anastomosed to the recipient's hypogastric or iliac artery and the donor's renal vein to the recipient's iliac vein (Fig. 67-1). The donor's ureter is tunneled below the mucosa of the recipient's bladder and is implanted into the posterior bladder wall. Occasionally, if the donor's ureter is short, it may be attached to the patient's ureteral stump if nephrectomies of the patient's own kidneys have previously been performed.

The recipient's own kidneys are not removed at the time of transplantation. Preferably, the patient's kidneys remain in place unless there has been recurrent or chronic infections, hydronephrosis, or vesicoureteral reflux or there is uncontrollable hypertension. If the patient's kidneys are removed, dialysis

---

INDWELLING BLADDER CATHETER CARE

I. *Purpose*

   A. To prevent complications of infection associated with an indwelling bladder catheter.

   B. To evaluate and cleanse site of insertion and adjacent catheter exterior.

II. *Policy*

   A. Bladder catheter care is given every shift and after fecal incontinence.

III. *Equipment*

   A. Soap, water, washcloth

   B. Gloves

IV. *Essential steps*

   A. Prepare patient and family by explaining the process and purpose.

   B. Prepare equipment.

   C. Use the following method:

     1. Wash hands and don gloves.

     2. Clearly visualize site of catheter insertion and surrounding skin area to be cleansed.

     3. Clean area with soap and water.

       Girls: Separate labia minora and gently cleanse from above meatus downward toward rectum.

       Boys: Gently retract foreskin and cleanse glans and penis using circular motion.

     4. Cleanse exterior of catheter from point of insertion outward approximately 2-4 inches.

     5. Keep level of drainage bag lower than patient's bladder to prevent retrograde flow toward bladder. Teach parents and other caregivers correct positioning of tubing and drainage bag.

     6. Place excessive tubing on bed to prevent a U-loop and to facilitate gravitational drainage. U-loops allow stasis of urine.

     7. Support drainage tube to prevent pull on catheter. Bag should always remain lower than child's bladder.

     8. Consult with physician about changing catheter after 7 days. Consider changing catheters if catheter concretions are felt or if urine contains visible precipitates. Silastic catheters may remain in place for prolonged periods of time.

     9. An obstructed catheter may be irrigated or removed only by physician order. (Contact transplant surgeon before performing any irrigation.)

    10. Change drainage system and bag if/when changing catheter.

    11. Empty bag following the directions for each type of bag. It is important to empty the bag using aseptic technique; avoid touching drain to cup.

V. *Charting*

   Record on Nurse's Progress Record:

   1. Time of catheter care

   2. Secretions: color, consistency, amount

   3. Skin condition

   4. Appearance of urine: color, consistency, odor, amount

Table 67-1   Postoperative Care of the Renal Transplant Patient

Nursing Diagnosis	Goal/Objective Criteria	Nursing Interventions
Potential for infection related to: Renal failure Immunosuppression Malnutrition Break in skin integrity	The patient will remain free of infection as evidenced by: Lack of fever Incisions free of erythema, tenderness, and/or drainage Clear breath sounds Sputum clear and odorless Clear urine, free of bacteria	Perform thorough handwashing between patient contacts to prevent cross contamination. Monitor and record temperature q 2 hr for 24 hr, then every 4 hr. Use sterile technique with all dressing changes (wound, puncture sites, catheters). When changing incision dressing, assess and report signs of infection (erythema, drainage, tenderness, swelling). Maintain pulmonary hygiene: (a) turn, cough, and deep breathe; (b) encourage use of incentive spirometer; (c) encourage early ambulation. Maintain a closed urinary drainage system. (If system must be opened, use strict sterile technique.) Observe for signs and symptoms of urinary tract infection. Perform perineal/bladder catheter care q 8 hr. If peritoneal dialysis catheter is in place, assess for development of peritonitis, exit site/tunnel infection, or ascites. Restrict visitation; infected visitors, patients, and personnel are restricted. Keep patient in private room. Encourage adequate nutritional intake to promote healing of wounds and incisions.
Fluid volume excess related to renal failure and/or intraoperative fluid administration Fluid volume deficit related to dialysis and serum electrolyte imbalance	The patient will remain in proper fluid and electrolyte balance as evidenced by: Weight maintained ± _____ kg (age dependent) Minimal peripheral edema Urinary output >1 ml/kg/hr Blood pressure within normal limits for age Moist mucous membranes, good skin turgor, and no weight loss Electrolytes, calcium, and phosphorus within normal limits	Record daily weights. Monitor and record intake and output (I&O). Record I&O from surgery and q 1 hr thereafter. Notify physician if urinary output <50% of previous hour's output. Notify physician if urinary output <1 ml/kg/hr. Maintain indwelling catheter patency (with drainage collection system below the level of the bladder). Replace previous hour's urinary output over the following hour (per physician's orders). Assess skin turgor and mucous membranes for hydration. Assess for periorbital or dependent edema and weight gain. Draw laboratory work on patient's arrival to PICU and q 8 hr × 2, q 12 hr × 2, then every morning. Review and record. Administer phosphorus binders or supplements as needed.

Continued.

Table 67-1   Postoperative Care of the Renal Transplant Patient—cont'd

Nursing Diagnosis	Goal/Objective Criteria	Nursing Interventions
Fluid volume deficit related to dialysis and serum electrolyte imbalance—cont'd		Monitor the patient's vital signs closely. The newly transplanted kidney must be well perfused. Notify physician if: Temperature >38.3° C Pulse > _____ or < _____ bpm (age dependent) BP > _____ or < _____ mm Hg (age dependent) CVP >8 or <10 mm Hg If hemodialysis access (AV fistula or graft) is present, assess bruit and thrill with each set of vital signs. Notify physician if bruit or thrill is absent or diminished.
Potential for impaired kidney function related to ATN, obstruction, and/or rejection	The patient will maintain adequate/optimal kidney function as evidenced by: Urinary output ≥1 ml/kg/hr Negative urinary protein Declining creatinine and BUN levels Systolic BP <_____ mm Hg (age dependent) Diastolic BP <_____ mm Hg (age dependent) Weight gain <_____ kg/day (age dependent) Minimal peripheral edema	Obtain baseline renal scan/Doppler sonogram 12-24 hr after transplantation. Monitor temperature, pulse, BP, and CVP closely; report any sudden changes immediately. Monitor urinary output hourly; assess volume and color. Urine is usually bloody because of surgical procedure but should be clear within 24-48 hr. Notify physician of volume <1 ml/kg/hr or <50% of previous hour's output or if urine suddenly becomes bloody. See p. 528 for causes of oliguria/anuria. If bladder catheter obstruction is suspected, notify renal transplant resident. Monitor daily creatinine and urine protein values. Creatinine level should steadily decline after transplantation and should be almost normal by fourth postoperative day if there is no ATN, rejection, or obstruction. Urine protein value should be negative by fourth postoperative day. Differentiate between incisional pain and tenderness over upper pole of kidney, which may indicate rejection. Administer daily immunosuppressive medication as ordered. Assess patient for edema and/or weight gain. If rejection occurs: Administer anti-rejection drugs as ordered. Observe for side effects of antirejection therapy (Table 67-2). If hemodialysis is necessary, "hold" antihypertensive medications before hemodialysis treatments.

Table 67-1   Postoperative Care of the Renal Transplant Patient—cont'd

Nursing Diagnosis	Goal/Objective Criteria	Nursing Interventions
Ineffective breathing pattern related to anesthesia and pain	Patient will have adequate ventilation and oxygenation as evidenced by: Respiratory rate within normal limits Clear breath sounds Pink mucous membranes O_2 saturations >90%	Maintain adequate airway; if patient is intubated, keep airway free of secretions. Assess respiratory status hourly (skin color, respiratory rate, breath sounds, capillary refill). Provide oxygenated mist after extubation. Encourage incentive spirometry q 2 hr. Encourage turning, coughing, and deep breathing q 2 hr. Medicate for pain prn before respiratory treatments. Encourage early ambulation.
Anxiety related to unknown outcome and fear of rejection and/or return to dialysis	Patient and family will experience minimal anxiety and be emotionally prepared for all procedures and outcomes as evidenced by: Verbalization by family and patient Constructive participation within plan of care and use of specialized auxillary personnel	Explain the PICU visitation hours and policy. Assess the patient's and family's knowledge. Discuss and reinforce any physician's explanations. Explain all procedures before they are performed. Involve patient and/or family in daily care and decision making if possible. Encourage patient and family to verbalize feelings and fears and provide emotional support. Answer questions honestly (contact transplant coordinator for assistance; these are chronic patients and presence of a familiar person can be comforting, especially at difficult times). Involve social work, child life, and pastoral care personnel.

treatments are more difficult, bone disease is more severe, and the patient needs more frequent blood transfusions. If nephrectomies are necessary, they are performed as an elective procedure before transplantation.

After transplantation a bladder catheter is kept in place for several days to facilitate urinary drainage and to keep the bladder decompressed, reducing leaks at the ureteral anastomosis.

The patient goes from the operating room directly to the PICU or intermediate PICU where he is weighed and monitoring begins (Table 67-1). The early success of the transplant may depend on the PICU nurse's rapid and appropriate response to early signs of complications.

POSTOPERATIVE COMPLICATIONS
Immunosuppression/Infection

In an immune response the body can recognize a foreign substance and produce antibodies to fight it. Immunosuppressive therapy in renal transplantation involves administering medications (e.g., azathioprine, prednisone, cyclosporine, ALG, OKT3) (Table 67-2) that block or decrease the intensity of the body's immune response to the transplanted organ.

After transplantation the recipient is given large doses of immunosuppressant drugs that will be tapered slowly over the next several months to smaller daily maintenance doses. If an acute rejection occurs, additional immunosuppression (bolus steroids, ALG, OKT3) is used to destroy the T cells that are attacking

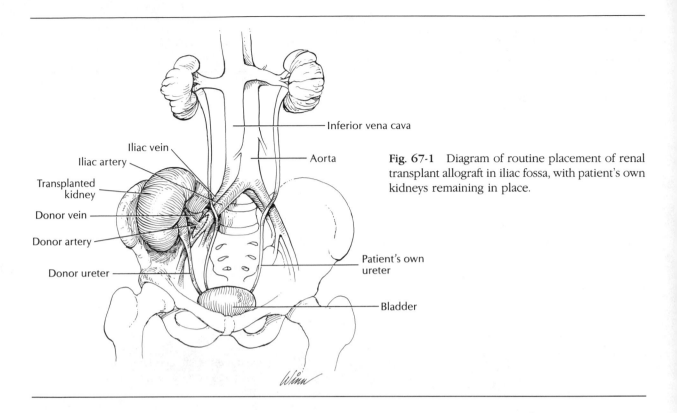

Iliac vein
Iliac artery
Transplanted kidney
Donor vein
Donor artery
Donor ureter

Inferior vena cava
Aorta
Patient's own ureter
Bladder

Fig. 67-1   Diagram of routine placement of renal transplant allograft in iliac fossa, with patient's own kidneys remaining in place.

Table 67-2   Commonly Used Immunosuppressive Agents

Agent	Action	Dose	Side Effects	Comments
Prednisone Prednisolone Methylprednisolone	Anti-inflammatory; reduces number of circulating T lymphocytes	Initial dose: 0.5 to 2 mg/kg/day IV, tapered slowly to maintenance dose of 0.15 mg/kg/day or 0.3 mg/kg PO every other day at 12 months Rejection dose: 10 to 30 mg/kg/day on days 1, 2, 4, and 6 or 1, 2, 3, 5, 7 of rejection episode to maximal dose of 1 g/day	Increased sodium absorption Increased appetite Hypertension Impaired wound healing Predisposition to infection Steroid-induced diabetes Cushingoid effects Gastric ulcers Acne Softening and destruction of weight-bearing joints	Many side effects decrease with tapering dose

Table 67-2   Commonly Used Immunosuppressive Agents—cont'd

Agent	Action	Dose	Side Effects	Comments
Azathioprine (Imuran)	Cytotoxic to cells that initiate immune response (interferes with proliferation of leukocytes and synthesis of nucleic acid)	2.5 mg/kg IV/PO	Bone marrow suppression Leukopenia; increased liver enzymes Hair loss	Adjust dose according to WBC count and weight; maintain WBC >4000/mm^3
Antilymphoblast globulin (ALG) from horse, goat, and/or rabbit antibodies	Inhibits and destroys circulating human lymphocytes (T and B cells); antibodies in ALG bind with lymphocytes, which are then phagocytized and eliminated	15 mg/kg/day IV through a central line *only* (give over 4-6 hr); observe platelet count and lymphocyte count daily; adjust dose accordingly Acute rejection dose: dose varies among centers (given mg/kg of body weight for 10-21 days)	Local reactions: pain, swelling, erythema Systemic reactions: fever, dyspnea, chills, arthralgias, hypotension, dizziness, anaphylaxis, thrombocytopenia, serum sickness	Skin test *must* be done before administration of first dose. Pretreat each dose with diphenhydramine and acetaminophen. (ALG is made by injecting human lymphocytes into horses, goats, rabbits; the animals make antibodies to human lymphocytes, and globulin fraction of serum is extracted to produce ALG)
Cyclosporine A (Sandimmune)	Fungal metabolite with selective action against T-cell lymphocyte production	Dose is blood-level dependent; initial dose: 5 to 15 mg/kg/day divided into BID dose (PO); follow with levels to maintain trough level at 100-200 ng/ml HPLC; after 12 mo maintain trough level at 50-100 ng/ml	Hypertension Nephrotoxity Hirsutism Tremors/seizures Hepatoxicity GI ulcers Lymphomas	Must mix in glass; adheres to plastic
OKT3 monoclonal antibody	Blocks generation and function of cytotoxic T cells (lymphocytes)	Patients <30 kg, 2.5 mg/day; >30 kg, 5 mg/day, IV push for 10- to 14-day course (may double dose if necessary)	Fever, chills Dyspnea Pulmonary edema Chest pain Wheezing Nausea, vomiting Diarrhea Headache Tremor	Pretreat first two doses with diphenhydramine and acetaminophen 3% weight gain in last 7 days contraindicates use of OKT3 Cyclosporine is discontinued until day 8 of OKT3 administration

the allograft. At times of peak immunosuppression the patient is at greatest risk for infection, which is by far the most common extrarenal complication of renal transplantation. Although all surgical patients are at risk for nosocomial infections postoperatively, additional risk for transplant patients lies in the severity and potential outcome of these infections. The transplant recipient may undergo a more serious, prolonged, or even lethal infection because of his altered immune response. The organisms involved are not only the typical bacterial agents found in hospitals (e.g., *Staphylococcus, Pseudomonas*), but also viral agents (e.g., CMV) as well as fungal *(Candida)* and opportunistic agents (e.g., *Pneumocystis carinii*).

Very often pediatric patients have not previously had CMV infections and therefore lack the antibody to CMV. If these patients receive a kidney from a donor who is positive for the CMV antibody, they are at high risk for developing a CMV infection. To reduce their risk for developing severe CMV infections, this high-risk group of patients may be treated with prophylactic IV-CMV immune globulin. Licensure of IV-CMV has been in process at the FDA since 1986. Programs in which this drug has not been approved for use are using commercial forms of IV immune globulin (e.g., Sandoglobulin, Gammagard). The patient receives the first dose within 72 hours of transplant (in LRD transplants it is often given the day before transplant), then 2, 4, 6, 8, 12, and 16 weeks after the transplant.

The dose of IV-CMV Ig will vary during the total treatment period from 150 to 50 mg/kg and is administered per protocol.

Preoperatively or within 72 hr post-operatively	150 mg/kg IV
Second, fourth, sixth, and eighth wk	100 mg/kg IV
Twelfth and sixteenth wk	50 mg/kg IV

Assessment of the transplant patient for infection must be systematic, ongoing, and well documented. Subtle changes must be detected since steroids often mask typical signs and symptoms of infection. Aseptic technique, thorough handwashing both before and between patient contacts, and meticulous wound and catheter care are imperative. Because urinary tract infections are the most common bacterial infections in renal transplant recipients, prevention must be a major focus of nursing care and includes keeping urinary drainage bags below bladder level at all times; not disconnecting the system except when absolutely necessary; and using aseptic technique to prevent contamination. Bladder catheter and perineal care must be performed every shift.

Postoperative atelectasis and pneumonia must be prevented by diligent monitoring and vigorous pulmonary toilet starting as soon as the patient awakens. Early ambulation helps prevent pneumonia as well as pulmonary emboli and thrombophlebitis.

Fluid Management

Accurate recording of fluids and fluid balance is essential since the hourly urinary volume and the electrolyte content determine the type and volume of fluid replacement necessary. IV fluids must be adjusted hourly according to the patient's urinary output and state of hydration. Routine postoperative management includes using two IV lines, one of which must be a central catheter. One IV line contains D_5W solution for replacing insensible losses.

Insensible water loss (IWL) is the evaporative loss from the skin and lungs that cannot be directly measured (does not include sweating).

Skin losses	30 ml/kcal/day
Pulmonary losses	15 ml/kcal day
	45 ml/kcal day*

The other IV line contains 0.45% sodium chloride solution to replace the previous hour's urinary output milliliter for milliliter. Replacement volume may vary, depending on the patient's volume status.

Other guidelines for fluid management depend on the assessment of vital signs. Monitoring of systemic arterial blood pressure, central venous blood pressure, and pulse rate is important since these patients can be extremely sensitive to volume changes. If there is some renal tubular dysfunction from ischemia, a large osmotic diuresis may occur and may be misinterpreted as good renal function. Polyuria may also cause bladder spasms since often the bladder has not been distended for a long time (i.e., months).

Hypovolemia resulting in hypotension must be prevented to maintain adequate systemic arterial blood pressure, especially to perfuse the new allo-

---

*In actual practice, the IWL of hospitalized children varies from 35-45 ml/kcal/day.

graft. The allograft has been cold and ischemic for many hours and has areas of poor perfusion, which are more susceptible to injury from decreased blood flow than normal organs.

Reestablishing renal function and the subsequent polyuria often results in lowering BUN and serum creatinine levels to nearly normal by the third or fourth postoperative day. Proteinuria is often present immediately postoperatively because of hematuria and/or ischemic changes in the renal tubules and should diminish or disappear within a few days. Its reappearance signifies that a different process is occurring (e.g., rejection, renal vein thrombosis, recurrent disease).

Both calcium and phosphorus homeostasis is regulated by the parathyroid gland. Normally an increase or decrease in serum calcium is associated with the opposite change in serum phosphorus. Excess calcium is largely eliminated in the feces, whereas phosphorus is mostly excreted in the urine. As the kidney function increases after transplantation, the excretion of phosphorus in the urine increases, thereby helping to normalize the serum calcium and phosphorus levels. If hyperparathyroidism preexists, as often is the case, hypophosphatemia and hypercalcemia may occur postoperatively. Oral phosphate supplements such as Neutra-Phos can be given until this problem is corrected.

Acute Tubular Necrosis

Diminished or absent urinary output after transplantation may occur as a result of prolonged graft ischemia during the organ retrieval and preservation process, resulting in ATN. This is much more common with a cadaveric than an LRD transplant. The cold ischemic time in a LRD transplant kidney is generally 1½ to 2 hours since the donor and recipient are in adjoining operating rooms and there is no delay in implanting the organ. Cadaveric transplants may have an ischemic time of 24 hours or more from the time of harvest to the time of implantation. Also, the cadaveric donor may have been hypotensive before the nephrectomy, resulting in hypoperfusion of the kidney. Dialysis may be necessary for days or weeks postoperatively until ATN has resolved.

Oliguria or anuria must not be dismissed as ATN because they can be caused by many different factors, each of which must be investigated systematically (Table 67-3).

Obstruction to Urinary Flow

The bladder catheter must be checked for patency since a simple kink can obstruct urinary flow. If the urine is bloody, the catheter may be obstructed by a clot. Gentle irrigation may be needed; if so, sterile technique must be used. To avoid damage to any suture line, check with the surgeon before performing any irrigation.

Hypovolemia

Hypovolemia may be due to blood loss during surgery or postoperatively, and an abdominal roentgenogram or sonogram can help exclude a hematoma. Alternatively, in the absence of bleeding the patient may need more crystalloid fluids. Measurement of CVP and systemic arterial blood pressure can help determine if the patient is hypovolemic. A challenge with a bolus of IV fluids may increase urinary output if the patient is hypovolemic.

Renal Artery Stenosis

Although complete obstruction is rare in children, partial obstruction can occur from kinking or torsion of the vessels. Clinically, renal artery stenosis may present as unexplained systemic hypertension with decreased renal function. A renal scan and arteriogram confirm the diagnosis. If stricture or occlusion is present, the patient is returned to the operating room for reexploration, resection, and anastomosis of the vessels.

Renal Vein Thrombosis

Persistence of gross hematuria and enlargement of the graft, along with gradually diminishing renal function, are clinical signs of renal vein thrombosis. Occasionally kinking of the iliac-renal vein anastomosis or a clot within the iliac vein itself will impair iliac vein drainage and lead to engorgement or edema of the lower extremity on that side. An arteriogram may be suggestive, but venography is diagnostic of the condition. Generally renal vein thrombosis results in loss of the graft and is treated by transplant nephrectomy.

Ureteral Leaks

Although the ureteral implant site is checked for leaks at the time of surgery, occasionally the distal ureter becomes necrotic from ischemia. Extravasation becomes evident after the urethral catheter is removed.

Table 67-3 Posttransplant Oliguria/Anuria

Causes	Observations/Interventions
Prerenal	
Hypovolemia	Assess volume status by monitoring pulse rate, systemic arterial BP, CVP, and skin turgor. Institute volume expansion if necessary; obtain abdominal roentgenogram or sonogram if hematoma or bleeding is suspected.
Congestive heart failure	Monitor breath sounds, heart sounds, CVP, systemic arterial BP, and pulse rate; obtain chest roentgenogram. Treat with diuretics and/or ultrafiltration as necessary.
Renal artery lesion	Monitor systemic arterial BP and urinary output (an unexplained increase in BP and decrease in urinary output may occur). Observe for sudden abdominal pain. Obtain renal scan and/or arteriogram for diagnosis.
Renal	
Rejection	Watch for decreased volume of urine with low sodium concentration, proteinuria, increased systemic arterial BP, pain, firmness, tenderness over graft site, rising BUN/creatinine levels, and edema/weight gain. Obtain renal sonogram/scan.
ATN	Watch for small quantities of urine with high sodium content; note long ischemic time of donor kidney. Obtain renal sonogram/scan. Dialysis and fluid restriction may be necessary until resolved.
Postrenal	
Bladder catheter obstruction	Check bladder catheter for patency, kinking, and clots. Call transplant surgeon to irrigate bladder if necessary.
Ureter obstruction	Rarely occurs; if urinary output is minimal, is extremely bloody, and contains clots, ureter may be obstructed; ultrasonography may show hydronephrosis. Call transplant surgeon.
Ureteral leak	Watch for feeling of fullness or pain in lower abdomen, urgency, and sudden decrease in urinary output from bladder catheter. If drain is present and an increase in drainage is seen, obtain sonogram and scan.
Renal vein thrombosis	Allograft becomes larger; persistent hematuria, massive proteinuria, and diminished urinary output are present (engorgement or edema of leg on same side as transplant may be present). Obtain sonogram and arteriogram/venogram for diagnosis.

Decreased urinary output, pain in the lower abdomen, and urgency are common. The leak can be readily seen on an intravenous pyelogram or renal scan. A urinary leak can lead to infection and death and must be treated promptly. Placement of a ureteral stent or a nephrostomy tube or reimplantation of the ureter may be necessary. If the ureteral leak is very small, a bladder catheter can provide adequate drainage until the site has healed; otherwise surgical repair is needed.

Rejection

In all transplant patients except identical twins the patient's immune response is aimed at rejecting the newly transplanted organ. Rejection is classified into different categories based on its clinical manifestations.

Hyperacute rejection. Hyperacute rejection occurs at the time blood flow to the kidney is established or up to several hours after surgery. The fulminant event destroys the kidney with diffuse thrombosis, and the kidney must be removed immediately. Hyperacute rejection is thought to be caused by preformed circulating antibodies to antigens in the donor kidney.

Delayed hyperacute rejection. Delayed hyperacute rejection is similar to hyperacute rejection, but it can occur 2 to 10 days after the transplant. Urinary volume declines suddenly, and the patient develops fever and experiences pain at the site of the new kidney. Vascular occlusion must be ruled out. Diagnosis must be made promptly because if the kidney is left in place, severe leukopenia and thrombocytopenia develop and could result in death.

Acute rejection. This is the most common type of rejection, and most transplant patients will undergo at least one episode. Although it can occur at any time after transplantation, acute rejection most commonly occurs during the first few weeks; it is usually reversible if identified and treated early. The signs and symptoms of acute rejection are as follows:

1. Fever
2. Increased creatinine and BUN levels
3. Decreased urinary output
4. Tenderness or swelling over graft site
5. Increased systemic arterial blood pressure
6. Rapid weight gain
7. Peripheral edema
8. General malaise
9. Proteinuria

Renal ultrasonography and renal scans are useful in the diagnostic process if baseline studies were performed before the rejection episode. Treatment of acute rejection must be started promptly after diagnosis and consists first of administering high-dose IV bolus steroids on days 1, 2, 4, and 6 (or days 1, 2, 3, 5, and 7) of the rejection episode. Some centers give boluses for 3 to 5 consecutive days. OKT3 and ALG are also used to treat acute rejection episodes, most commonly episodes that are resistant to steroids (Table 67-2).

Chronic rejection. Chronic rejection is an insidious process characterized by a gradual rise in the serum creatinine level, decreasing creatinine clearance, hypertension, and proteinuria. However, the patient may feel fine. Chronic rejection is a constant immunologic conflict between the transplanted kidney and its new environment. The graft gradually loses glomerular function as fibrosis and scar tissue develop, and the patient eventually returns to ESRD and dialysis.

Emotional support of the patient and the family is essential. During the early postoperative period both the patient and the family are anxious about the level of kidney function. They are concerned about immediate rejection as well as the longevity of the kidney function. The PICU staff must be particularly aware of these concerns to have effective interactions with the patient and family.

DISCHARGE TEACHING

The goal of postoperative teaching is to ensure that by the time of discharge the patient and the family are familiar with the administration of all of their medications, indications, and side effects. The necessity and importance of taking the immunosuppressive drugs and the signs and symptoms of rejection as well as urinary tract infection must be stressed. If they understand that frequent laboratory tests are necessary to evaluate renal function and the effectiveness of immunosuppressive therapy, compliance with the regimented follow-up schedule will be improved. The patient and family are given dietary instruction and information about the patient's resumption of normal activities and schooling. Special precautions are given about immunizations and vaccinations since no live viruses may be given to these immunosuppressed children. On discharge they are given a schedule of the required routine laboratory tests and follow-up visits to the transplant clinic. If age permits, the child is encouraged to be an active participant in all of his care.

ADDITIONAL READING

Bass M. Common complications of immunosuppression in the renal transplant patient. ANNA J 13:196-200, 1986.

Harwood CH, et al. Cyclosporine in transplantation. Heart Lung 14:529-540, 1985.

Hollander LA. Renal transplantation in school-age children: Beyond physiologic care. ANNA J 12:252-254, 264, 1985.

Kegg DL. My kidney transplant—a preoperative teaching tool. J Nephrol Nurs 2:268-270, 1985.

Leatherwood J, et al. Tools for educating transcultural patients. ANNA J 13:26-28, 1986.

Lee D. General aspects for consideration in renal transplant patients. Nephrol Nurs 5:15-16, 1983.

• Moir E. Nursing care of patients receiving orthoclone OKT3. ANNA J 16:327, 328, 366, 1989.

Oyler-Mooney J, et al. Care of the renal transplant patient receiving cyclosporine. J Nephrol Nurs 2:274-276, 1985.

• Prewitt D. Post-operative [sic] complications—an overview. Nephrol Nurs 5:27, 30-32, 1983.

Rawbaks I. Posttransplant hypertension. J Nephrol Nurs 2:115-118, 1985.

Remai JM. Cyclosporine for organ transplantation. Matern Child Nurs J 10:237, 1985.

• Richard AB, et al. Renal transplantation. Nursing management of the recipient. AORN J 41:1022-1036, 1985.

• Richard C. Comprehensive Nephrology Nursing. Boston: Little, Brown, 1986.

Schoenberg L, et al. Using cyclosporine in renal transplantation. ANNA J 11:9-12, 1984.

68 Heart and Heart-Lung Transplantation

W. Steves Ring · Lynn Mahony

BACKGROUND

The first heterotopic heart and heart-lung transplants were performed in dogs in 1905. However, it was more than 50 years before the first successful orthotopic heart transplant was reported in 1960, with dogs surviving for up to 21 days without immunosuppression. In 1964 the first xenograft was attempted in a human when the heart of a chimpanzee was transplanted into a patient in cardiogenic shock. However, the small size of the donor heart and probable hyperacute rejection prevented weaning the patient from cardiopulmonary bypass.

The first "successful" orthotopic heart transplant in man was performed at the University of Capetown, South Africa, on December 3, 1967. The patient survived for 18 days before succumbing to infection, but this transplant clearly indicated the feasibility of orthotopic heart transplantation in man. Several days later the first pediatric heart transplant was attempted in New York. Using deep hypothermia and total circulatory arrest the heart from an anencephalic donor was placed into an 18-day-old infant with severe heart failure caused by Ebstein's anomaly.

Over the next year more than 100 heart transplants were performed worldwide with a <10% survival rate. This poor initial experience prompted most programs to discontinue heart transplantation. In the United States only Stanford University and the Medical College of Virginia continued to perform transplants during the early 1970s, at a rate of fewer than 25 transplants per year. By 1978 the Stanford group reported a 1-year survival rate of 66% prompting several other centers to resume their heart transplant programs.

The introduction of cyclosporine-based immunosuppression in 1982 has resulted in a significantly improved survival rate and an exponential growth of heart transplantation in the 1980s (Fig. 68-1). Pediatric heart transplantation has seen a similar exponential rise over the past decade, with more than 100 transplants performed in children less than 18 years of age in 1988. In the 5-year period from 1984 through 1988 more than 60 heart transplants were performed in infants less than 1 year old, and more than 200 were performed in children less than 10 years of age (Fig. 68-2).

Heart-lung transplantation can also trace its roots back to the early work at the University of Chicago in 1905 and in Russia in the 1940s using heterotopic dog allograft models. The first human heart-lung transplant was performed in 1968 in a 2-year-old girl with an atrioventricular canal defect and pulmonary vascular disease. However, the patient died several hours after surgery from severe pulmonary insufficiency. In 1980 the first long-term successful orthotopic heart-lung transplant using a primate model was reported in animals. This research led to the first successful heart-lung transplant on March 9, 1981, in a 45-year-old woman with primary pulmonary hypertension. From 1981 through 1988 more than 500 heart-lung transplants have been performed worldwide, with more than 200 performed in 1988. However, fewer than 20 have been performed in children less than 10 years old.

HEART TRANSPLANTATION
Recipient Selection

Selection of potential heart transplant recipients necessitates a careful pretransplant evaluation to achieve optimal long-term results. The goals of the pretransplant evaluation are to (1) determine the need for transplantation, (2) determine the feasibility

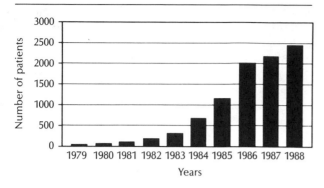

Fig. 68-1 Number of heart transplantations performed per year. (From Heck CF, Shumway SJ, Kaye MP. The Registry of the International Society for Heart Transplantation: Sixth official report—1989. J Heart Transplant 8:271-276, 1989.)

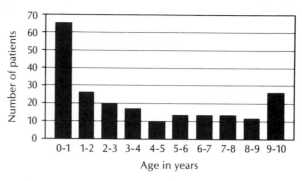

Fig. 68-2 Age distribution of pediatric heart transplant recipients, 1984-1988. (From Heck CF, Shumway SJ, Kaye MP. The Registry of the International Society for Heart Transplantation: Sixth official report—1989. J Heart Transplant 8:271-276, 1989.)

of transplant, (3) minimize perioperative and postoperative management problems, and (4) establish a baseline database for long-term follow-up.

Indications and medical necessity

Heart transplantation may be considered for any patient whose functional capacity or expected long-term survival is severely limited by end-stage heart disease and for whom no satisfactory medical or surgical alternative therapy is available.

The selection criteria for heart transplantation in children are as follows:

Primary heart disease
   End-stage cardiomyopathy
   End-stage ischemic heart disease
   End-stage congenital heart disease
   Intractable life-threatening dysrhythmias
   Primary cardiac tumor
   Allograft rejection
Severe limitation of function and/or expected survival
No adequate medical or surgical alternative therapy
No contraindication to heart transplant

As in adults, primary cardiomyopathy is the major indication for heart transplantation in children. During evaluation treatable causes of cardiomyopathy and congestive heart failure such as incessant tachycardia, myocarditis, carnitine deficiency, endocrine

cardiomyopathy, coronary anomalies, constrictive pericarditis, and high cardiac output states must be excluded. Natural history studies of medically treated primary cardiomyopathy have demonstrated a poor prognosis, with only 50% of the patients surviving for 1 year from the time of diagnosis, although children less than 2 years of age have a somewhat better prognosis. An aggressive attempt at medical therapy with inotropic agents, diuretics, and afterload reduction is necessary in all patients. Transplantation should be considered only if there are signs of progressive clinical deterioration in the presence of optimal medical therapy.

Cardiac transplantation may also be considered for selected children with congenital heart disease, including patients who have severe ventricular dysfunction and congestive heart failure following multiple palliative procedures and those for whom further surgical intervention would carry a prohibitive operative risk or be unlikely to result in clinical improvement. Recently heart transplantation has been advocated for neonates with hypoplastic left heart syndrome because of the historically poor results with efforts to palliate this condition. However, the improved results reported by Norwood have resulted in controversy about the best way to manage this difficult group of patients. Patients with other congenital heart defects such as Ebstein's anomaly with pulmonary atresia, in which the palliative or corrective surgery is associated with an unacceptable mortality rate, may also be considered for transplant.

Relative contraindications

Since more potential heart transplant recipients die on the waiting list for a transplant than after a transplant, donor availability is the major limiting factor. Therefore it is ethically necessary to ensure optimal use is made of every donor heart. This implies that recipients must be selected to maximize the likelihood of long-term survival. Therefore any factor that would significantly impair long-term survival or functional status after transplantation is considered a relative contraindication. These factors include (1) ABO incompatibility or preformed lymphocytotoxic antibodies, which could result in hyperacute rejection; (2) elevated pulmonary vascular resistance (>6 to 8 Wood units or >480 to 640 dsc^{-5}), which could cause acute right heart failure in the deconditioned donor heart; (3) noncardiac factors that could limit survival or rehabilitation potential (e.g., neurologic dysfunction, malignancy, major systemic illness, active infection, severe nutritional deficiency); (4) irreversible major organ dysfunction (CNS, renal, hepatic, pulmonary) that could deteriorate with immunosuppressive therapy; (5) psychosocial factors that would lead to medical noncompliance with a rigid follow-up protocol (e.g., recreational drug or alcohol abuse, history of medical noncompliance, lack of adequate social support structure, psychopathic or sociopathic behavior); and (6) financial factors that would impair the ability to maintain rigid medication and follow-up protocols. It must be emphasized that each case must be evaluated carefully and independently by all members of the transplant team before a decision is made about suitability for heart transplantation.

Pretransplantation evaluation

To facilitate determination of the indications and contraindications and to provide a baseline database for long-term follow-up, exhaustive cardiac, major organ, immunologic, psychosocial, and financial evaluations are performed before final patient selection for transplantation.

After a detailed history and a thorough physical examination an extensive cardiac evaluation is performed to determine if a heart transplant is needed and whether alternative medical or surgical therapies exist. This evaluation usually includes cardiac cath-eterization for angiographic and hemodynamic assessment, including determination of pulmonary vascular resistance. If pulmonary vascular resistance is elevated (>4 Wood units or >320 dsc^{-5}), pharmacologic intervention with inotropes (dobutamine, amrinone) and vasodilators (nitroprusside, nitroglycerin) should be attempted to determine reversibility of the elevated pulmonary vascular resistance. A functional assessment of the myocardium may be obtained using metabolic stress testing, rest and exercise MUGA scan, or possibly a thallium stress examination.

Routine pretransplant evaluation of major organ function includes (1) renal tests (BUN, creatinine, creatinine clearance), (2) pulmonary tests (chest roentgenogram, pulmonary function tests, pulmonary consultation), (3) hepatic tests (liver function tests, hepatitis screen, coagulation profile), (4) neurologic tests (head CT or MRI, EEG, neurologic consultation), (5) musculoskeletal tests (bone age, densitometry, skeletal survey), (6) endocrine/metabolic tests (serum glucose, calcium, and magnesium levels, thyroid function tests), (7) dental tests (examination, roentgenograms), and any other tests indicated by history or examination.

Immunologic evaluation includes (1) ABO blood typing, (2) a transfusion and pregnancy history, (3) antileukocyte antibody screen (panel-reactive antibodies [PRA]), (4) HLA typing, and (5) serologic testing for viral (HIV, CMV, Epstein-Barr virus, herpes simplex virus, varicella zoster virus), fungal (toxoplasmosis), and mycobacterial (tuberculin skin test) exposures.

A careful psychosocial evaluation of the patient, parents, and family is made by each member of the transplant team and includes a careful assessment of (1) availability and adequacy of family and parental support, (2) intelligence and comprehension, (3) psychiatric history, (4) history of medical noncompliance, and (5) history of substance abuse (tobacco, alcohol, drugs). This assessment is of particular importance in older children and teenagers who tend to have a high incidence of late medical noncompliance, which results in late rejection and death.

The financial evaluation is important to ensure the patient's ability to adhere to the extensive and unfortunately costly medication and follow-up protocol. Experience has shown that survival is impaired because of noncompliance when adequate financial support is not available for follow-up.

Donor Selection
Donor suitability

The criteria most frequently used to determine suitability for organ donation are listed below:

> Brain death certification
> Age less than 50 years
> ABO compatible/identical
> Size match
> Crossmatch negative for PRA (>5%)
> Normal heart function
> HIV and HBsAg negative

Under the Uniform Anatomical Gift Act, which has been adopted in all 50 states, the legal criteria for brain death must be satisfied before organ donation can occur. However, the legal criteria for brain death may vary since not all states have adopted the guidelines outlined in the Uniform Determination of Death Act, which defines death as (1) the irreversible cessation of circulatory and respiratory function or (2) the irreversible cessation of all brain function, including brain stem activity. Therefore, under current legal constraints, anencephalic infants with persistence of brain stem function must be considered unsuitable for organ donation. This issue remains a controversial topic with strong ethical and emotional arguments on each side. Legislative and judicial clarification is needed before most anencephalic infants may be used as organ donors.

After obtaining information about the donor's age, sex, race, height, weight, and ABO blood type, a careful history is probably the most important tool in screening for suitable donors. Emphasis must be placed on (1) the mechanism of brain death (trauma, intracranial hemorrhage, anoxia, primary CNS tumor); (2) past medical history (heart disease, hypertension, diabetes, other cardiac risk factors, malignancy, hepatitis, infection); (3) family history (coronary disease); (4) social history (alcohol, tobacco, drug abuse), (5) medications (inotropes, pressor agents, antibiotics), and (6) clinical course since admission (hemodynamic instability, cardiopulmonary resuscitation, cardiac arrest, diabetes insipidus, dysrhythmias, transfusions, infection, clinical sepsis).

Laboratory evaluation includes (1) serology (HIV, HBsAg, CMV, VDRL), (2) immunology (ABO blood typing, HLA tissue typing), (3) hematology (CBC, PT, PTT), (4) biochemistry (serum electrolytes, glucose, BUN, creatinine, liver function tests, arterial blood gases, pH), and (5) microbiology (blood, sputum, urine cultures; sputum Gram stain).

Evaluation of the heart and cardiovascular system includes (1) analysis of cardiac history and risk factors, (2) assessment of hemodynamic instability and need for pressor support, (3) ECG, (4) echocardiogram, (5) cardiology consultation, and, most important, (6) direct inspection of the heart by the procurement team. A thermodilution pulmonary artery pressure catheter is not routinely needed but may be quite helpful in both the evaluation and long-distance management of the hemodynamically unstable donor.

The only absolute exclusionary criteria for organ donation are clinical sepsis, active tuberculosis, non-CNS malignancy, IV drug abuse within the past year, hepatitis, active viral infection, and positive HBsAg or HIV serology. However, the decision regarding suitability for organ donation in brain-dead patients should always be deferred to the local organ procurement agency and should not be made by the referring hospital or physician.

Donor allocation

After matching for ABO blood type and size range, donor hearts are distributed according to guidelines approved by the United Network for Organ Sharing. In general donor hearts are allocated to recipients within the local region first on the basis of clinical status and second on the basis of time on the waiting list. ABO-identical matches take precedence over ABO-compatible matches to prevent shortchanging the blood group O recipient pool. Recipients with elevated PRA (preformed cytotoxic antibodies) should also have preference over low PRA recipients. However, regional allocation policies may vary.

Surgical Technique

Orthotopic heart transplantation in most centers is performed using minor modifications of the technique first described by Lower and Shumway. The recipient is placed on cardiopulmonary bypass through a median sternotomy, taking care to place the arterial cannula high on the aorta and the selective vena caval cannulas posteriorly and remote from the atrioventricular groove. Deep hypothermia and total circulatory arrest using a single right atrial cannula is used for infants. The aorta is cross-clamped, and the heart is removed by incising the atria just above the atrioventricular valves and the great vessels just above the semilunar valves. The ventricles, all four valves, and the atrial appendages are thus excised, leaving most of the right and left atria joined at the atrial septum. The donor heart is implanted by first anastomosing the donor left atrium to the recipient left atrial cuff. This is followed by anastomosing the pulmonary artery and aorta. After extensive de-airing maneuvers, the aortic cross-clamp is removed and the right atrial anastomosis completed. Temporary atrial and ventricular pacing wires are left in all patients to facilitate postoperative management.

Bailey's technique is used in neonates with the hypoplastic left heart syndrome. The descending aorta is cannulated through the pulmonary artery and ductus arteriosus to initiate cardiopulmonary bypass for hypothermic total circulatory arrest. After excision of the donor heart as described previously, the underside of the aortic arch is incised, and all ductal tissue is removed. The donor aortic arch is first anastomosed to the recipient aortic arch, extending beyond the ductus to correct any coarctation, which occurs in up to 85% of neonates with the hypoplastic left heart syndrome. Following arch reconstruction the left atrial, right atrial, and pulmonary arterial anastomoses are completed. The right atrial cannula is placed into the donor right atrial appendage, and the aortic cannula is inserted into the new aorta for resuming cardiopulmonary bypass. Again, careful de-airing of the heart is essential to prevent neurologic complication and right heart dysfunction.

Heterotopic heart transplantation has been used in some centers for isolated right or left heart assist and for selected patients with elevated pulmonary vascular resistance or an inadequately sized donor heart. The technique of heterotopic heart transplant most commonly performed for biventricular assist was described by the Cape Town group. The donor heart is positioned in the right chest with direct anastomosis of the two left atria, followed by the right atrial anastomosis, direct end-to-side aortic anastomosis, and end-to-side pulmonary artery anastomosis using a prosthetic conduit. This procedure is more frequently associated with technical anastomotic complications, pulmonary problems, and thromboemboli from the poorly contractile recipient left ventricle than orthotopic heart transplantation.

Immunosuppression

The number of different immunosuppressive protocols is as varied as the number of transplant centers,
with each center having its own peculiar "recipe." However, most protocols are based on cyclosporine in combination with steroids and/or azathioprine, with or without induction antibody therapy.

Cyclosporine

Cyclosporine is a small lipophilic cyclic polypeptide derived from a fungal extract that was noted to have unique immunosuppressive properties. The principal immunologic effect of the drug is to block the production of interleukin-2 (IL-2) by helper (CD-4) T cells, thus inhibiting the proliferation of cytotoxic (CD-8) T lymphocytes. Cyclosporine may be administered orally or as a continuous IV infusion. Careful monitoring of blood levels is essential to ensure adequate immunosuppression and to minimize toxicity. Cyclosporine has many potential side effects, hypertension and nephrotoxicity being the most common serious ones. Hypertension occurs in more than 90% of adult heart transplant recipients, and multiple drugs are usually needed to control blood pressure. However, hypertension is less common in pediatric patients. Acute nephrotoxicity seems to be caused by renal arteriolar constriction and can usually be reversed by reducing the cyclosporine blood levels and by using calcium antagonists. Prolonged usage causes interstitial fibrosis and impaired glomerulotubular function, but the mechanism of this chronic nephrotoxicity remains unclear. Symptoms of neurotoxicity include seizures, tremors, paresthesias, cerebellar syndromes, and mental status changes. Cyclosporine can produce hypomagnesemia, which can potentiate the neurotoxic side effects. Hirsutism is an annoying side effect of the drug, particularly among girls and teenagers.

Prednisone

Corticosteroids have a wide variety of effects on different cell populations, resulting from their ability to alter the availability or function of cellular receptors as well as to influence the synthesis and release of mediators such as hormones, peptides, vasoactive substances, eicosanoids, and lymphokines. The immunosuppressive effects of corticosteroids result primarily from the blockage of interleukin-1 (IL-1) production by macrophages. IL-1 is needed in the presence of a stimulating antigen for the activation of T-helper (CD-4) lymphocytes, a key initial step in cellular rejection.

When used, steroids are usually administered on

a rapidly tapering dosage schedule during the first month, followed by a slow tapering over the first year and then a very low (<0.15 mg/kg/day) maintenance dose. Chronic steroid administration is associated with many potentially serious side effects. Growth retardation is seen in prepubertal patients, but these effects can be minimized with rapid tapering to very low levels or by using an alternative-day dosage schedule after the first year. Some centers advocate not using routine steroids unless the recipient experiences multiple rejection episodes, whereas others have found that half the patients can be weaned totally from steroids within the first 4 to 6 months after transplantation.

Azathioprine

Azathioprine is a purine analog that interferes with DNA synthesis and cell proliferation. This results in a very generalized nonspecific effect on any replicating cell line. Leukopenia, hepatic dysfunction, and

susceptibility to viral infections are the major side effects and are usually dose related. Other antimetabolites such as cyclophosphamide and vincristine have been used, but experience with these agents is limited.

Antibody therapy

Polyclonal antibody induction therapy with antilymphocyte globulin (ALG) or antithymocyte globulin (ATG) has been used for nearly 20 years by the Stanford group as a routine part of their conventional immunosuppressive protocols. Since these agents are produced in animals, they are foreign proteins, and their administration in humans may be associated with serum sickness or even anaphylaxis. These antibodies are used for the first 5 to 14 days after surgery, either in addition to cyclosporine for greater immunosuppression or temporarily in place of cyclosporine to prevent perioperative nephrotoxicity.

The recent introduction of monoclonal antibodies

IMMUNOSUPPRESSIVE DRUG SIDE EFFECTS

Cyclosporine
Hypertension
Nephrotoxicity
Seizures
Tremors, paresthesias
Hepatotoxicity
Hirsutism
Gingival hyperplasia
Lymphoproliferative disorders

Prednisone
Infection
Delayed wound healing
Cushingoid features, acne
Obesity
Diabetes, hyperlipidemia
Hypertension, hyperkalemia
Pancreatitis
Acute psychosis
Proximal muscle weakness
Osteoporosis, avascular necrosis
Growth retardation
Cataracts

Azathioprine
Leukopenia
Thrombocytopenia
GI distress
Infection
Hepatotoxicity
Alopecia
Stomatitis

OKT3
Fever, chills
Headache
Nausea, vomiting
Diarrhea, abdominal pain
Hypotension
Dyspnea, chest pain
Pulmonary edema
Aseptic meningitis
Anaphylaxis
Infection

ALG and ATG
Fever, chills
Serum sickness
Anaphylaxis
Thrombocytopenia
Phlebitis
Infection

directed against specific antigenic markers on lymphocytes represents the most important advancement in immunosuppression since the discovery of cyclosporine. OKT3 is a murine monoclonal antibody directed against the CD-3 antigen marker present on all T lymphocytes and is the first monoclonal antibody approved for clinical use. OKT3 binds to the CD-3 antigen, which is part of the T-cell receptor present on all T lymphocytes, activating the T cell but blocking the major antigen recognition site. Lymphokines and vasoactive substances are transiently released from T lymphocytes, producing a systemic flulike syndrome characterized by fever, chills, malaise, arthralgias, diarrhea, nausea, vomiting, and headache. Hypotension and acute pulmonary edema have also have been reported, prompting most centers to withhold therapy for 24 to 48 hours after transplantation until cardiovascular stability is achieved. Antibodies against these murine proteins can develop in 10% to 15% of patients and render the proteins ineffective for later rejection therapy. T cells must be monitored during administration of OKT3 to determine efficacy of treatment.

Perioperative Management and Complications

In general the postoperative management of heart transplant recipients is similar to that for most other open-heart procedures. However, some early complications more commonly occur in heart transplant recipients.

Cardiovascular complications

Cardiovascular problems are common, and most patients are given several days of inotropic support. Vasodilating inotropes such as dobutamine, isoproterenol, and amrinone are frequently used, more for their effects on the pulmonary circulation and support of the right ventricle than for support of the systemic circulation. Right ventricular dysfunction is much more commonly observed because of elevated pulmonary vascular resistance, problems with preservation of the right heart, and the predilection for any intracardiac air to embolize preferentially to the right coronary artery. Sinus node dysfunction can occur due to denervation, trauma to the sinus node or nodal artery, and problems with preservation. Since the cardiac output in transplant recipients is highly rate-dependent, prolonged atrial pacing may be needed. The sinus node usually recovers spontaneously, although to do so may take several weeks.

COMPLICATIONS OF HEART TRANSPLANTATION

Early complications

Cardiac dysfunction
    Right ventricle more than left ventricle dysfunction
    Dysrhythmias
    Sinus node dysfunction
    Pericardial effusion
Reversible renal insufficiency
Hepatic dysfunction
Neurologic dysfunction
    Seizure
    Stroke
Infection
    Bacterial
    Fungal
    Viral
Side effects of immunosuppressive drug

Late complications

Infection
Rejection
    Acute rejection
    Chronic vascular rejection
Side effects of immunosuppressive drug
Malignancy
Psychiatric complications
Medical noncompliance

Permanent pacemaker insertion is usually not needed. Frequently, two P waves are seen on the ECG, one from the donor atrium and one from the remaining recipient atrium. Other dysrhythmias occur approximately as frequently as they do after conventional open-heart surgery. Pericardial effusions can occur more commonly because of the redundant pericardium, with dilated lymphatics and elevated right heart filling pressures.

Renal complications

Renal dysfunction is commonly seen in the early postoperative period in patients receiving cyclosporine, particularly in those with significant prerenal insufficiency before the transplant. This is due to renal arteriolar constriction caused by cyclosporine and can usually be minimized by the addition of calcium antagonists such as nifedipine or diltiazem. However, most patients are discharged with better renal function than they had before the transplant.

Neurologic complications

Neurologic complications have been reported in up to 15% of patients after heart transplantation. In addition to the rare (<1%) ischemic complications that occur after conventional open-heart surgery, an increased incidence of seizures, tremors, and psychiatric abnormalities have been reported. Cyclosporine, steroids, and hypomagnesemia have been implicated in the pathogenesis of posttransplant seizures. However, the seizures apparently are not a dose-related phenomenon and are usually self-limited. Magnesium replacement or anticonvulsant therapy may be indicated, but the interactions of anticonvulsants with cyclosporine must be considered.

Infectious complications

Infection is the major cause of mortality after heart transplantation, accounting for 38% of all deaths. The risk of infection increases significantly with antirejection therapy. Therefore most infections occur during the first 3 months after transplantation when immunosuppressive and antirejection drug doses are greatest. In a recent review of patients treated with cyclosporine the most common bacterial infections were from gram-negative enteric organisms, *Legionella, Nocardia,* and *Staphylococcus. Candida* and *Aspergillus* account for most fungal infections, whereas *Pneumocystis carinii* and *Toxoplasma gondii* account for most protozoal infections. The most common viral agents include CMV, herpes simplex, varicella zoster, and hepatitis B. HIV seroconversion after heart transplantation has also been reported from the Pittsburgh group.

The introduction of cyclosporine has permitted the reduction of steroid dosage and has reduced the risk of bacterial and fungal infections. Although the overall incidence of infection has been reduced only slightly, the risk of serious infection has been significantly decreased. Antimicrobial prophylaxis with trimethoprim and sulfamethoxazole (Bactrim), acyclovir, nystatin, and perioperative systemic antibiotics has been recommended by several centers for use in these immunocompromised patients. Routine surveillance cultures for bacterial, fungal, and viral cultures can be obtained to facilitate early diagnosis and treatment of infection. CMV and fungal infections are particularly lethal, and treatment necessitates the use of toxic drugs such as amphotericin and ganciclovir.

Rejection
Hyperacute rejection

Hyperacute rejection usually occurs within the first few minutes to hours after heart or heart-lung transplantation. It is humorally mediated because of the presence of preformed cytotoxic antibodies to ABO, HLA, or tissue-specific antigens such as vascular endothelial cell (VEC) antigens. Screening for PRA or performing a lymphocyte crossmatch before the transplant can minimize the risk. However, logistical considerations prevent a prospective lymphocyte crossmatch in most cases. Patients who have received prior transfusion or have been pregnant are at higher risk for developing preformed antibodies.

Clinically, hyperacute rejection is characterized by early or immediate graft failure caused by IgG-complement–mediated vascular endothelial cell damage, resulting in microvascular fibrin-platelet thrombi, infarction, and necrosis. Although plasmapheresis has been used to remove antibodies, it is usually too late, and the only effective treatment is insertion of a mechanical support device followed by retransplantation.

Acute rejection

Acute rejection usually occurs from 1 week to 6 months after the transplant. However, it may occur even later after events such as altered immunosuppression or nonspecific stimulation of the immune system caused by infection or surgery. Acute allograft rejection is a complex and incompletely understood process that involves both cellular and humoral immune responses. Rejection is initiated by the recognition of foreign histocompatibility antigens. Although numerous minor antigens may play a lesser role, ABO blood type antigens and HLAs are the major antigenic stimuli leading to transplant rejection. HLAs are coded within the genes of the major histocompatibility complex on chromosome 6 and can be identified serologically. Class I (HLA-A, HLA-B, and HLA-C) antigens are expressed to varying degrees on most tissue parenchymal cells, B and T lymphocytes, and platelets. Class II (HLA-DR, HLA-DQ, HLA-DP) antigens are normally expressed only on B lymphocytes, dendritic cells (monocytes), and some endothelial cells. Normal cardiac myocytes usually do not express either class I or II antigens, and their expression during rejection remains controversial. Macrophages and helper T cells interact with antigen-presenting cells within the graft, causing release of IL-1 from the macrophages. This activates helper T cells, stimulating them to release a variety of lymphokines, chemoattractants, and stimulating factors that result in the recruitment and proliferation of antibody-producing B cells, cytotoxic and helper T cells, other cytocidal macrophages, and natural killer cells. One of these factors, IL-2, causes the proliferation of both helper T cells, which respond primarily to class II antigens, and antigen-specific cytotoxic T cells, which respond predominantly to class I antigens.

Clinical symptoms of acute cardiac rejection are nonspecific, characterized by fatigue, malaise, dyspnea, irritability, poor feeding, and dizziness. Physical signs of rejection are predominantly those of right heart failure and diastolic dysfunction (e.g., weight gain, peripheral edema, hepatomegaly, S_3 gallop, jugular venous distention). Dysrhythmias or signs of systolic dysfunction (e.g., hypotension, low output) occur late and carry an ominous prognosis.

A variety of laboratory tests have been used for the noninvasive diagnosis of cardiac rejection. A chest roentgenogram may show evidence for cardiac enlargement, pulmonary vascular congestion, or increasing pleural effusions. The ECG may demonstrate new dysrhythmias, conduction abnormalities, and reduced QRS voltage. However, these ECG changes have become less reliable during the cyclosporine era. Recent reports of using heart rate power spectral analysis and frequency analysis for diagnosing rejection have been encouraging but unconfirmed. Alterations in echocardiographic indices of left ventricular mass and diastolic function correlate reasonably well with histologic evidence for rejection. The isovolemic relaxation time, mitral pressure half time, and early peak mitral flow velocity seem to be the most sensitive indices. MRI and indium-111–labeled antimyosin imaging have been used. Cytoimmunologic monitoring has also been attempted. This technique involves the morphologic detection of activated lymphocytes in peripheral blood and the determination of lymphocyte subsets using serologic typing. A wide variety of substances (e.g., neopterin, prolactin, β_2-microglobulin, IL-2 receptor, polyamines) found in peripheral blood and urine have also been examined and reported to correlate with rejection. Unfortunately no single noninvasive parameter of rejection is sufficiently sensitive or specific that it can replace endomyocardial biopsy for the diagnosis of acute rejection.

Endomyocardial biopsy remains the standard for diagnosis of acute cardiac rejection. Routine biopsies are usually obtained on a protocol basis during the first year following transplant, although some centers forego biopsy in small children and infants because of the increased risk. Acute rejection of the heart is generally characterized by the presence of perivascular and interstitial mononuclear cell infiltrates, with or without myocyte necrosis. However, the interpretation of biopsy specimens varies widely, with no universally accepted criteria for acute rejection.

Treatment for moderately severe acute rejection usually consists of an initial trial of pulsed steroids (methylprednisolone), which is effective in approximately 80% of cases. If this fails to control or reverse the rejection, if the rejection is severe, or if there is hemodynamic compromise, antibody therapy with ALG, ATG, or OKT3 should be promptly instituted. OKT3 has been shown to be effective in controlling approximately 90% of refractory rejection episodes. For mild-to-moderate rejection, high-dose oral cyclosporine has also been effective in some patients. Experience has shown that most rejection episodes can be easily reversed with early diagnosis and initiation of appropriate therapy.

Chronic vascular rejection

Since the earliest days of heart transplantation, accelerated coronary artery disease has been recognized as a major impediment to long-term survival. Histologically, graft atherosclerosis is characterized by mild mononuclear cell infiltrates, lipid deposition, and myointimal hyperplasia resulting in luminal narrowing. This prompted the recommendation that all patients have routine coronary angiography after a heart transplant. Angiography usually demonstrates a mixture of the more proximal lesions of typical atherosclerosis along with the more diffuse concentric narrowing and pruning of distal vessels, with a lack of collaterals found in graft atherosclerosis. Angiographic abnormalities are observed in approximately 10% of transplant recipients at 1 year, increasing to approximately 40% by 5 years. They remain the major late cause of death following heart transplantation.

Clinically, graft atherosclerosis may present as a silent myocardial infarction, progressive congestive heart failure resulting from repeated microinfarcts, or sudden death presumably due to dysrhythmias. Early clinical signs of ischemia are absent since angina does not occur in the denervated heart. Although antiplatelet agents have been helpful in preventing the lesions, once they have developed conventional forms of therapy such as angioplasty and revascularization are generally ineffective. Retransplantation remains the only effective means of treatment.

The etiology of accelerated graft atherosclerosis is unknown, although an immunologic mechanism is favored by most. Factors that have been implicated in the development or progression of accelerated coronary artery disease include elevated cholesterol or triglycerides, multiple rejection episodes, the development of circulating B-cell or anti-HLA cytotoxic antibodies, and CMV infection. The immunosuppressive protocol does not appear to significantly alter the incidence of graft atherosclerosis.

Results

As recently as 1983 an editorial suggested that heart transplantation was not suitable for children less than 15 years of age. In 1984 there were only nine published cases of successful heart transplantation in children, the youngest 10 years old. By 1985 review of the data obtained from a questionnaire and from the Heart Transplant Registry indicated 95 pediatric patients from 15 centers. The 3-month survival rate for all patients was 62% and was not significantly affected by age, but only 14 patients were less than 10 years of age. The survival rate beyond 3 months for pediatric heart transplants performed in 1984 was 84%, not significantly different from the data for adults during the same time period. The major causes of death were infection and rejection, similar to the experience in adults.

Heart transplantation for congenital heart disease has a significantly decreased survival rate as compared to transplantation for other forms of end-stage heart disease. This probably reflects the risks associated with pulmonary vascular disease, multiple prior surgeries, and technical problems such as pulmonary artery abnormalities or anomalous venous return to the heart. Data from the Registry of the International Society for Heart Transplantation reveal

a perioperative (30-day) mortality rate of 25% in children less than 10 years of age, which is significantly higher than the 10% perioperative mortality for all older age groups.

Individual centers have recently begun reporting their experiences with small series of children and infants. The preliminary observations have been encouraging, with excellent survival and rehabilitation. The Stanford group has reported actuarial survival rates of 75% at 4 years, comparable with their experience in adults (Fig. 68-3). The risk of rejection has also been similar in adults and children (Fig. 68-4). The personal experience of this author (Ring) in 16 pediatric patients at the University of Minnesota and at the University of Texas Southwestern Medical Center, compared with 120 adults, has been similar (Fig. 68-5). The recent experience of Bailey in neonates with hypoplastic left heart syndrome has been very encouraging, with 40 out of 45 recipients surviving, the longest over 4 years. When transplanted as neonates, these infants appear to develop some degree of immune tolerance, requiring minimal immunosuppression with only low-dose cyclosporine beyond the first year. However, the long-term outlook for heart transplantation in children must be viewed with caution because of the progressive risk of graft atherosclerosis.

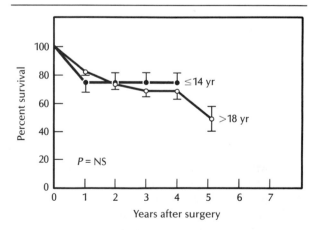

Fig 68-3 Actuarial survival after pediatric vs. adult heart transplantation. (From Starnes VA, Bernstein D, Dyer PE, et al. Heart transplantation in children. J Heart Transplant 8:20-26, 1989.)

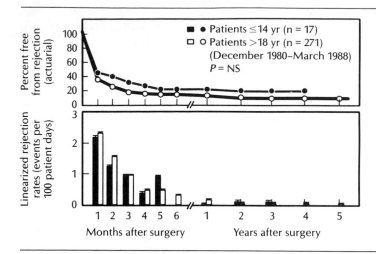

Fig. 68-4 Actuarial incidence of acute rejection and linearized rejection rate after pediatric vs. adult heart transplantation. (From Starnes VA, Bernstein D, Dyer PE, et al. Heart transplantation in children. J Heart Transplant 8:20-26, 1989.)

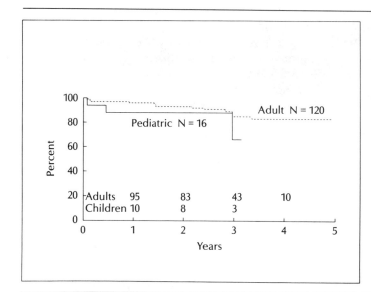

Fig. 68-5 Actuarial survival after pediatric vs. adult heart transplantation. Experience of author (Ring) at University of Minnesota and University of Texas Southwestern Medical Centers.

Growth of the graft, anastomoses, and linear bone growth have been major concerns for infants and young children following transplant. Preliminary experimental and clinical results suggest normal growth of the graft without stenosis of the anastomoses. However, recurrent coarctation can develop in children with a hypoplastic left heart if the arch reconstruction is not carried well beyond the area of coarctation. Preliminary observations in prepubertal children receiving steroids for immunosuppression

or rejection therapy suggest that growth retardation will be a problem in pediatric heart transplantation, even with relatively low-dose steroid administration.

In summary, the early results of heart transplantation in children have been quite encouraging, with excellent short-term results in terms of survival and quality of life. However, significant progress needs to be made in several areas. First, newer immunosuppressive agents with fewer side effects must be developed. Second, more sensitive and specific noninvasive techniques for diagnosing rejection must be found. Third, the mechanism of chronic vascular rejection must be elucidated and a means for its prevention developed. Finally, the problems of donor availability must be overcome, both by enhanced organ donation and by continued research into the use of xenografts.

HEART-LUNG TRANSPLANTATION
Recipient Selection

The indications for heart-lung transplantation are evolving, particularly with the development of isolated lung and double-lung transplantation. Based on data from the Registry of the International Society for Heart Transplantation, the most common indications are primary pulmonary hypertension and Eisenmenger's syndrome (Table 68-1). The selection criteria for a heart-lung transplant are listed below.

> End-stage pulmonary vascular or parenchymal lung disease
> Severe limitation of function and predicted survival
> Criteria as a suitable heart recipient satisfied
> Relative contraindications
> > More than 50 years of age
> > Prior major thoracotomy
> > Tracheostomy
> > Malnutrition
> > Ventilator dependence
> > Steroid dependence

Heart-lung transplant candidates should be less than 50 years of age and must satisfy the usual criteria for heart transplant recipients except for low pulmonary vascular resistance.

Although the experience with heart-lung transplantation in children is limited, the most likely indications would be for uncorrectable congenital heart disease, cystic fibrosis, and hereditary pulmonary disorders. Unfortunately uncorrectable congenital heart disease is usually cyanotic and is frequently complicated by multiple prior surgical procedures, with the development of adhesions and numerous collateral vessels. This significantly increases the risk of bleeding complications and mortality, making prior surgery a relative contraindication for heart-lung transplantation. The indications for heart-lung and double-lung transplantation in patients with cystic fibrosis include stable (nonventilator-dependent) respiratory failure with a $Pao_2 < 55$ torr on room air, severe obstructive lung disease ($FEV_1 < 30\%$ to 40%

Table 68-1   Indications for Heart-Lung Transplantation

Condition	%
Primary pulmonary hypertension	39
Eisenmenger's syndrome	24
Congenital heart disease	13
Pulmonary parenchymal disease	13
Cystic fibrosis	8
Cardiomyopathy	3

predicted), requirement for continuous or intermittent oxygen therapy, and a predicted survival of 12 to 18 months. Relative contraindications include severe malnutrition, prior chemical or surgical pleurodesis, tracheostomy, ventilator dependence, and steroid dependence.

Donor Selection

The selection criteria for heart-lung donors are quite stringent.

> Acceptable heart donor
> Age less than 45 years
> No chest trauma
> No pulmonary disease (e.g., asthma, heavy smoking)
> No pulmonary infection
> No prolonged mechanical ventilation
> Normal chest roentgenogram
> Normal lung function
> > Peak airway pressure <25 mm Hg for tidal volume of 15 ml/kg
> > $Pao_2 > 100$ torr on Fio_2 of 0.40

Less than 10% of acceptable heart donors are suitable for heart-lung donation. In addition to satisfying the usual criteria for heart donation, heart-lung donors must have normal lung function, no history of lung disease, a minimal smoking history, no thoracic trauma, a limited period of ventilatory support, and no evidence of infection. The evaluation of normal lung function requires a normal chest roentgenogram, a $Pao_2 > 100$ torr on 0.40 oxygen, and normal lung compliance, with a peak airway pressure <25 mm Hg on a tidal volume of 15 ml/kg. Size match is more critical than for heart transplantation since a donor lung that is too large can lead to atelectasis and infection and one that is too small can result in pleural fluid collection necessitating prolonged chest tube drainage. To prevent serious CMV infection, CMV seronegative recipients should probably receive organs and blood transfusions only from seronegative donors.

In contrast to heart donors, excessive volume resuscitation must be avoided in heart-lung donors. The FiO_2 must be kept <0.40 and the donor maintained on 3 to 5 cm H_2O PEEP, with periodic sighing to prevent atelectasis. Frequent samples of tracheal aspirates for Gram staining are obtained to detect pathogenic bacteria, fungi, and white blood cells. The final decision about heart-lung donor suitability is not made until the procurement team arrives at the donor hospital. With the possibility of the donor's heart-lung being turned down at the last minute, a heart recipient must be made ready as a backup to the heart-lung recipient candidate.

Surgical Technique
Donor operation
Donor procurement is begun through a sternotomy incision with removal of the thymus and pericardium, including phrenic nerves to the level of the hilum. Care is taken to avoid manipulation or damage to the lungs. Preservation of the heart-lung block is accomplished using either autoperfusion, pulmonary artery flush plus aortic root cardioplegia, or core cooling with cardiopulmonary bypass. With autoperfusion the lung remains ventilated, whereas with the static flush or core-cooling techniques the lungs are left moderately inflated with the trachea stapled. The trachea is divided above the staple line, and the heart-lung block is excised by dividing the mediastinal attachments to the esophagus. The heart-lung block is transported in a container that holds cold physiologic crystalloid solution.

Recipient operation
The technique of heart-lung transplantation begins with excision of the recipient heart as for a conventional heart transplant. The left atrium is then transected at the atrial septum. The pericardium is incised posterior to the phrenic nerves from the diaphragm to the top of the pulmonary artery bilaterally, taking care to avoid injury to either the phrenic or recurrent laryngeal nerve. After the branch pulmonary arteries are divided, the right and left mainstem bronchi are stapled and divided. Each lung is then removed separately with its pulmonary veins and a cuff of the left

atrium. Meticulous hemostasis of the posterior mediastinum and chest cavities is essential. The heart-lung block is carefully positioned in the thorax by passing each lung posterior to the phrenic nerve pedicle. The recipient's tracheal bifurcation is resected and anastomosed directly to the donor trachea above the carina. The aortic anastomosis is then completed, followed by the right atrial anastomosis as in a heart transplant.

Immunosuppression
In general the immunosuppressive protocols for heart-lung transplantation are similar to those for a heart transplant. However, steroids are usually avoided during the first 2 weeks after the transplant to allow for adequate healing of the tracheal anastomosis. To avoid rejection during this early period, azathioprine and cyclosporine are administered. The cyclosporine dosage is often increased more rapidly and to higher levels than with a heart transplant. Antibody therapy with ATG, ALG, or OKT3 is also commonly used until low-dose steroids can be started.

Pulmonary Rejection
Acute pulmonary rejection
Acute pulmonary rejection occurs after a heart-lung transplant but often takes place in the absence of simultaneous endomyocardial biopsy evidence of acute cardiac rejection. Acute rejection usually occurs 7 to 21 days after transplantation. Clinically, it is characterized by low-grade fever, leukocytosis, cough, dyspnea, and hypoxemia. Careful monitoring of pulmonary function often reveals a decline in FEV_1 or FVC as a sign of rejection. Although the development of a new infiltrate on chest roentgenogram suggests rejection, this is a rather nonspecific finding and may represent either the implantation response, infection, or rejection. Bronchoalveolar lavage has been useful for the identification of opportunistic infections but has not been specific enough for the diagnosis of rejection. Transbronchial biopsy has been helpful in distinguishing rejection from infection.

Chronic pulmonary rejection
Progressive airflow obstruction commonly occurs late following heart-lung transplantation and is associated with histologic evidence for bronchiolitis obliterans. This is the major cause of late death following heart-lung transplant, accounting for approximately 50% of all deaths beyond 4 months. The cause

of obliterative bronchiolitis is unknown. Both infection and rejection have been implicated. The common association of bronchiolitis obliterans, pulmonary arteriosclerosis, and accelerated graft atherosclerosis suggests a possible common mechanism. Although isolated cases have been reported that respond to increased immunosuppression, clinical improvement is usually transient, and the disease tends to be progressive. A recent report suggests that the development of donor-specific alloreactivity correlates with the development of obliterative bronchiolitis.

Results

More than 500 heart-lung transplants have been performed worldwide since 1981 with more than 200 performed in 1988. The 1-year actuarial survival rate is approximately 60%, with infection accounting for approximately half the deaths. The largest experience from a single institution has a 62% 2-year survival rate in 157 patients. Stanford University has reported a 65% 1-year survival rate, but the long-term survival rate continues to decline to approximately 25% at 5 years, with most late deaths caused by obliterative bronchiolitis. No data are available for the results in children because of very small numbers.

A total of 50 heart-lung transplants have been performed in the United States and the United Kingdom for cystic fibrosis with 35 survivors. The longest survivor is 3 years past transplantation, but approximately 25% of the late survivors have developed evidence of obliterative bronchiolitis.

In summary, the long-term results of heart-lung transplantation are somewhat discouraging when compared to those for heart transplantation. Although it is likely that the 30-day mortality rate, currently approximately 20%, can be reduced, the problem of obliterative bronchiolitis must be solved before significant improvement in the long-term results can be expected.

ADDITIONAL READING

ACS/NIH Organ Transplant Registry. First Scientific Report. JAMA 217:1520, 1971.

Ahmed-Ansari A, Tadros TS, Knopf WD, et al. Major histocompatibility complex class I and class II expression by myocytes in cardiac biopsies post transplantation. Transplantation 45:972-978, 1988.

Andreone PA, Olivari MT, Elick B, et al. Reduction of infectious complications following heart transplantation with triple-drug immunotherapy. J Heart Transplant 5:13-19, 1986.

Arras JD, Shinnar S. Anencephalic newborns as organ donors: A critique. JAMA 259:2284-2285, 1988.

Bailey LL, Wood M, Razzouk A, et al. The Loma Linda University Heart Transplant Group. Heart transplantation during the first 12 years of life. Arch Surg 124:1221-1226, 1989.

Bailey LL, Assaad AN, Trimm RF, et al. Orthotopic transplantation during early infancy as therapy for incurable congenital heart disease. Ann Surg 3:279-286, 1988.

Bailey LL, Concepcion W, Shattuck H, et al. Method of heart transplantation for treatment of hypoplastic left heart syndrome. J Thorac Cardiovasc Surg 92:1-5, 1986.

Bailey LL, Nehlsen-Cannarella SL, Doroshow RW, et al. Cardiac allotransplantation in newborns as therapy for hypoplastic left heart syndrome. N Engl J Med 315:949-951, 1986.

Bailey LL, Roost H, Li ZJ, et al. Host maturation after orthotopic cardiac transplantation during neonatal life. J Heart Transplant 3:265-267, 1984.

Baldwin JC, Frist WH, Starkey TD, et al. Distant graft procurement for combined heart and lung transplantation using pulmonary artery flush and simple topical hypothermia for graft preservation. Ann Thorac Surg 43:670-673, 1987.

Barnard CN. A human cardiac transplant: An interim report of a successful operation performed at Groote Schuur Hospital, Cape Town. S Afr Med J 41:1271-1274, 1967.

Barnard CN, Losman JG. Left ventricular bypass. S Afr Med J 49:303-312, 1975.

Baum D, Stinson EB, Shumway NE. The place for heart transplantation in children. Pediatr Cardiol 4:741-747, 1981.

Baumgartner WA, Reitz BA, Bieber CP, et al. Current expectations in cardiac transplantation. J Thorac Cardiovasc Surg 75:525-530, 1978.

Baumgartner WA, Williams GM, Fraser CD, et al. Cardiopulmonary bypass with profound hypothermia. Transplantation 47:123-127, 1989.

Bieber CP, Hunt SA, Schwinn DA, et al. Complications in long-term survivors of cardiac transplantation. Transplant Proc 13:207-211, 1981.

Bieber CP, Stinson EB, Shumway NE, et al. Cardiac transplantation in man. VII. Cardiac allograft pathology. Circulation 41:753-771, 1970.

Billingham ME. Diagnosis of cardiac rejection by endomyocardial biopsy. J Heart Transplant 1:25-30, 1982.

Bonser RS, Fragomeni LS, Kriett JM, et al. Technique of clinical double-lung transplantation. J Heart Transplant 7:298-303, 1988.

Borel JF, Feurer C, Gubler HU, et al. Biological effects of cyclosporin A: A new antilymphocytic agent. Agents Actions 6:468-475, 1976.

Bricker JT, Frazier OH. Preoperative evaluation of the pediatric heart transplant candidate. Clin Transplant 1:164-168, 1987.

Bristow MR, Gilbert EM, Renlund DG, et al. Use of OKT3 monoclonal antibody in heart transplantation: Review of the initial experience. J Heart Transplant 7:1-11, 1988.

Burke CM, Morris AJR, Dawkins DK, et al. Late airflow obstruction in heart-lung transplantation recipients. J Heart Transplant 4:437-440, 1985.

Burke CM, Theodore J, Dawkins DK, et al. Post-transplant obliterative bronchiolitis and other late lung sequelae in human heart-lung transplantation. Chest 86:824-829, 1984.

Carrel A, Gutherie CC. The transplantation of veins and organs. Am Med 10:1101, 1905.

Chartrand C, Dumont L, Stanley P. Pediatric cardiac transplantation. Transplant Proc 21:3349-3350, 1989.

Cooley DA, Bloodwell RD, Hallman GL, et al. Organ transplantation for advanced cardiopulmonary disease. Ann Thorac Surg 8:30-42, 1969.

Cooper JD, Pearson FG, Patterson GA, et al. Technique of successful lung transplantation in humans. J Thorac Cardiovasc Surg 93:173-181, 1987.

Dal Col RH, Rabinowich H, Herlan DB, et al. Donor-specific cytotoxicity testing: An advance in detecting pulmonary allograft rejection. Ann Thorac Surg (in press).

Dawkins KD, Oldershaw PJ, Billingham ME, et al. Changes in diastolic function as a noninvasive marker of cardiac allograft rejection. J Heart Transplant 3:286-294, 1984.

Demikhov VP. Experimental Transplantation of Vital Organs. Moscow: Medgiz State Press for Medical Literature in Moscow, 1960. Translated by Haigh B, Consultants' Bureau, New York, 1962.

Desruennes M, Corcos T, Cabrol A, et al. Echocardiography for the diagnosis of acute cardiac allograft rejection. J Am Coll Cardiol 12:63-70, 1988.

Dresdale AR, Drusin RE, Lamb J, et al. Reduced infection in cardiac transplant recipients. Circulation 72:II237-II240, 1985.

Drummer JS, Erb S, Breinig MK, et al. Infection with human immunodeficiency virus in the Pittsburgh transplant population. Transplantation 47:134-139, 1989.

Dunn JM, Cavarocchi NC, Balsara RK, et al. Pediatric heart transplantation at St. Christopher's Hospital for Children. J Heart Transplant 6:334-342, 1987.

English TAH. Is cardiac transplantation suitable for children? Pediatr Cardiol 4:57-58, 1983.

Fieguth HG, Haverich A, Schafers HJ, et al. Cytoimmunologic monitoring in early and late acute cardiac rejection. J Heart Transplant 7:95-101, 1988.

Fiel S, Baldwin J, Rosenstein BJ, et al. Heart-Lung transplantation in cystic fibrosis—overview. Clin Transplant 3:162-163, 1989.

Fragomeni LS, Kaye MP. The registry of the international society for heart transplantation: Fifth official report—1988. J Heart Transplant 7:249-253, 1988.

Fricker FJ, Griffith BP, Hardesty RL, et al. Experience with heart transplantation in children. Pediatrics 72:138-146, 1987.

Frist W, Yasuda T, Segall G, et al. Noninvasive detection of human cardiac transplant rejection with indium-111 antimyosin (Fab) imaging. Circulation 76(Suppl 5):81-85, 1987.

Gao SZ, Alderman EL, Schroeder JS, et al. Accelerated coronary vascular disease in the heart transplant patient: Coronary arteriographic findings. J Am Coll Cardiol 12:334-340, 1988.

Gao SZ, Schroeder JS, Hunt S, et al. Retransplantation for severe accelerated coronary artery disease in heart transplant recipients. Am J Cardiol 62:876-881, 1988.

Gao SZ, Schroeder JS, Alderman EL, et al. Clinical and laboratory correlates of accelerated coronary artery disease in the cardiac transplant patient. Circulation 76(Suppl 5):56-61, 1987.

Grattan MT, Moreno-Cabral CE, Starnes VA, et al. Cytomegalovirus infection is associated with cardiac allograft rejection and atherosclerosis. JAMA 261:3561-3566, 1989.

Griepp RB, Stinson EB, Bieber CP, et al. Control of graft arteriosclerosis in human heart transplant recipients. Surgery 81:262-269, 1987.

Griepp RB, Wexler L, Stinson EB, et al. Coronary arteriography following cardiac transplantation. JAMA 221:147-150, 1972.

Griffin ML, Hernandez A, Martin TC, et al. Dilated cardiomyopathy in infants and children. J Am Coll Cardiol 11:139-144, 1988.

Griffith BP. Heart-lung transplantation. Tex Heart Inst J 14:364-368, 1987.

Griffith BP, Hardesty RL, Trento A, et al. Heart-lung transplantation: Lessons learned and future hopes. Ann Thorac Surg 43:6-16, 1987.

Griffith BP, Hardesty RL, Trento A, et al. Asynchronous rejection of heart and lungs following cardiopulmonary transplantation. Ann Thorac Surg 40:488-493, 1985.

Grigg MM, Costanzo-Nordin MR, Celesia GG, et al. The etiology of seizures after cardiac transplantation. Transplant Proc 20:937-944, 1988.

Haberl R, Weber M, Reichenspurner H, et al. Frequency analysis of surface electrocardiogram for recognition of acute rejection after orthotopic cardiac transplantation in man. Circulation 76:101-108, 1987.

Hakim M, Higenbottam T, Bethune D, et al. Selection and procurement of combined heart and lung grafts for transplantation. J Thorac Cardiovasc Surg 95:474-479, 1988.

Hardesty RL, Griffith BP. Autoperfusion of the heart and lungs for preservation during distant procurement. J Thorac Cardiovasc Surg 93:11-18, 1987.

Hardesty RL, Griffith BP. Procurement for combined heart-lung transplantation. J Thorac Cardiovasc Surg 89:795, 1985.

Hastillo A, Thompson JA, Lower RR, et al. Cyclosporine-induced pericardial effusion after cardiac transplantation. Am J Cardiol 59:1220-1222, 1987.

Haverich A, Scott WC, Jamieson SW. Twenty years of lung preservation—a review. J Heart Transplant 4:234-240, 1986.

Haverich A, Kemnitz J, Fieguth HG, et al. Non-invasive parameters for detection of cardiac allograft rejection. Clin Transplant 1:151-158, 1987.

Heck CF, Shumway SJ, Kaye MP. The Registry of the International Society for Heart Transplantation: Sixth official report—1989. J Heart Transplant 8:271-276, 1989.

Hess ML, Hastillo A, Mohanakumar T, et al. Accelerated cytotoxic B-cell antibodies and hyperlipidemia. Circulation 68(Suppl 2):94-101, 1983.

Hess ML, Hastillo A, Wolfgang TC, et al. The noninvasive diagnosis of acute and chronic cardiac allograft rejection. J Heart Transplant 1:31-38, 1981.

Higenbottam T, Stewart S, Wallwork J. Transbronchial lung biopsy to diagnose lung rejection and infection of heart-lung transplants. Transplant Proc 20:767-769, 1988.

Higenbottam T, Hutter JA, Stewart S, et al. Transbronchial biopsy has eliminated the need for endomyocardial biopsy in heart-lung recipients. Transplantation 7:435-439, 1988.

Higenbottam T, Stewart S, Penketh A, et al. Transbronchial lung biopsy for the diagnosis of rejection in heart-lung transplant patients. Transplantation 46:532-539, 1988.

Hutter JA, Stewart S, Higenbottam T, et al. Histologic changes in heart-lung transplant recipients during rejection episodes and at routine biopsy. J Heart Transplant 7:440-444, 1988.

Jamieson SW, Stinson EB, Oyer PE, et al. Operative technique for heart-lung transplantation. J Thorac Cardiovasc Surg 87:930-935, 1984.

Jamieson SW, Stinson EB, Oyer PE, et al. Heart-lung transplantation for irreversible pulmonary hypertension. Ann Thorac Surg 38:554-562, 1984.

Joss DV, Barrett AJ, Kendra JR. Hypertension and convulsions in children receiving cyclosporine A. Lancet 1:906, 1982.

Kahan BD. Pharmacokinetics and pharmacodynamics of cyclosporine. Transplant Proc 21:9-15, 1989.

Kanakriyeh MS, Mullins CE, Parisi F, et al. Late hemodynamic results after orthotopic heart transplantation in early infancy. Circulation 78(Suppl 2):294, 1988.

Kantrowitz A, Haller JD, Joos H, et al. Transplantation of the heart in an infant and an adult. Am Coll Cardiol 22:782-790, 1968.

Kaye MP. The Registry of the International Society for Heart Transplantation: Fourth official report—1987. J Heart Transplant 6:63-67, 1987.

Kemnitz J, Choritz H, Cohnert TR, et al. Predictive implications of bioptic diagnosis in cardiac allografts. J Heart Transplant 8:315-329, 1989.

Keren A, Gillis AM, Freedman RA, et al. Heart transplant rejection monitored by signal-averaged electrocardiography in patients receiving cyclosporine. Circulation 70(Suppl 1):124, 1984.

Kobashigawa J, Stevenson LW, Moriguchi J, et al. Randomized study of high dose oral cyclosporine therapy for mild acute cardiac rejection. J Heart Transplant 8:53-58, 1989.

Kosek JC, Bieber C, Lower RR. Heart graft arteriosclerosis. Transplant Proc 3:512-514, 1971.

Landwirth J. Should anencephalic infants be used as organ donors? Pediatrics 82:257-259, 1988.

Lawrence KS, Fricker FJ. Pediatric heart transplantation: Quality of life. J Heart Transplant 6:329-333, 1987.

Linder J. Infection as a complication of heart transplantation. J Heart Transplant 7:390-394, 1988.

Lower RR, Shumway N. Studies on orthotopic homotransplantation of the canine heart. Surg Forum 11:18-19, 1960.

Lund G, Morin RL, Olivari MT, et al. Serial myocardial T2 relaxation time measurements in normal subjects and heart transplant recipients. J Heart Transplant 7:274-279, 1988.

McAllister HA, Schnee MJM, Radovancevic B, et al. A system for grading cardiac allograft rejection. Tex Heart Inst J 13:1-3, 1986.

McDonald K, Rector TS, Braunlin E, et al. Association of coronary artery disease in cardiac transplant recipients with cytomegalovirus infection. Am J Cardiol 64:359-362, 1989.

McGregor CGA, Baldwin JC, Jamieson SW, et al. Isolated pulmonary rejection after combined heart and lung transplantation. J Thorac Cardiovasc Surg 90:623-626, 1985.

McGregor CGA, Jamieson SW, Baldwin JC, et al. Heart-lung transplantation for end-stage Eisenmenger's syndrome. J Thorac Cardiovasc Surg 91:443-450, 1986.

Mason JW, Stinson EB, Hunt SA, et al. Infections after cardiac transplantation: Relation to rejection therapy. Ann Intern Med 85:69-72, 1976.

Mavroudis C, Harrison H, Klein JB, et al. Infant orthotopic cardiac transplantation. J Thorac Cardiovasc Surg 96:912-924, 1988.

Migliori RJ, Simmons RL. Infection prophylaxis after organ transplantation. Transplant Proc 3:395-399, 1988.

Novitzky D, Cooper DKC, Barnard CN. The surgical technique of heterotopic heart transplantation. Ann Thorac Surg 36:476-482, 1983.

Olivari MT, Antolick A, Ring WS. Arterial hypertension in heart transplant recipients treated with triple-drug immunosuppressive therapy. J Heart Transplant 8:34-39, 1989.

Olivari MT, Homans DC, Wilson RF, et al. Coronary artery disease in cardiac transplant patients receiving triple-drug immunosuppressive therapy. Circulation 80(Suppl III):III-111–III-115, 1989.

Otulana BA, Higenbottam TW, Scott JP, et al. Pulmonary function monitoring allows diagnosis of rejection in heart-lung transplant recipients. Transplant Proc 21:2583-2584, 1989.

Oyer PE, Stinson EB, Bieber CP. Diagnosis and treatment of acute cardiac allograft rejection. Transplant Proc 11:296-303, 1979.

Oyer PE, Stinson EB, Jamieson SW, et al. Cyclosporine-A in cardiac allografting: A preliminary experience. Transplant Proc 1:1247-1252, 1983.

Oyer PE, Stinson EB, Jamieson SW, et al. One year experience with cyclosporine A in clinical heart transplantation. J Heart Transplant 1:285-290, 1978.

Pahl E, Fricker FJ, Trento A, et al. Late follow-up of children after heart transplantation. Transplant Proc 20(Suppl 1):743-746, 1988.

Patterson GA, Cooper JD, Dark JH, et al. Experimental and clinical double lung transplantation. J Thorac Cardiovasc Surg 95:70-74, 1988.

Penkoske PA, Freedom RM, Rowe RD, et al. The future of heart and heart-lung transplantation in children. J Heart Transplant 3:233-236, 1984.

Pennington DG, Codd JE, Merjavy JP. The expanded use of ventricular bypass systems for severe cardiac failure and as a bridge to cardiac transplantation. J Heart Transplant 4:441-445, 1985.

Pigott JD, Murphy JD, Barber G, et al. Palliative reconstructive surgery for aortic atresia. Ann Thorac Surg 45:122-128, 1988.

Radovancevic B, Frazier OH. Treatment of moderate heart allograft rejection with cyclosporine. J Heart Transplant 5:307-311, 1986.

Reitz BA, Burton NA, Jamieson SW, et al. Heart and lung transplantation, autotransplantation in primates with extended survival. J Thorac Cardiovasc Surg 80:360-371, 1980.

Reitz BA, Wallwork JL, Hunt SA, et al. Heart-lung transplantation, successful therapy for patients with pulmonary vascular disease. N Engl J Med 306:557-564, 1982.

Renlund DG, O'Connell JB, Gilbert EM, et al. Feasibility of discontinuation of corticosteroid maintenance therapy in heart transplantation. J Heart Transplant 6:71-78, 1987.

Revel D, Chapelon C, Mathieu D, et al. Magnetic resonance imaging of human orthotopic heart transplantation: Correlation with endomyocardial biopsy. J Heart Transplant 8:139-146, 1989.

Rose EA, Addonizio LJ, Smith CR. Optimal timing of pediatric heart transplantation. Circulation 78(Suppl 2):278, 1988.

Rose EA, Smith CR, Petrossian GA, et al. Humoral immune responses after cardiac transplantation: Correlation with fatal rejection and graft atherosclerosis. Surgery 106:203-208, 1989.

Rose ML, Coles MI, Griffin RJ, et al. Expression of class I and class II major histocompatibility antigens in normal and transplanted human heart. Transplantation 41:776, 1986.

Sands KEF, Appel ML, Lilly LS, et al. Power spectrum analysis of heart rate variability in human cardiac transplant recipients. Circulation 79:76-82, 1989.

Scott JP, Higenbottam TW, Clelland C, et al. Natural history of obliterative bronchiolitis and occlusive vascular disease of patients following heart-lung transplantation. Transplant Proc 21:2592-2593, 1989.

Sell KW, Tadros T, Wang YC, et al. Studies of major histocompatibility complex class I/II expression on sequential human heart biopsy specimens after transplantation. J Heart Transplant 7:407-418, 1988.

Sibley RK, Olivari MT, Ring WS, et al. Endomyocardial biopsy in the cardiac allograft recipient. Ann Surg 203:177-187, 1986.

Simmons RL, Migliori RJ. Infection prophylaxis after successful organ transplantation. Transplant Proc 6:7-11, 1988.

Solis E, Kaye MP. The Registry of the International Society for Heart Transplantation: Third official report—June 1986. J Heart Transplant 5:2-5, 1986.

Starnes VA, Bernstein D, Oyer PE, et al. Heart transplantation in children. J Heart Transplant 8:20-26, 1989.

Starnes VA, Stinson EB, Oyer PE, et al. Cardiac transplantation in children and adolescents. Circulation 76(Suppl 5):43-47, 1987.

Stinson EB, Dong E, Bieber CP. Cardiac transplantation in man. II. Immunosuppressive therapy. J Thorac Cardiovasc Surg 58:326-337, 1969.

Suitters A, Rose ML, Higgins A, et al. MHC antigen expression in sequential biopsies from cardiac transplant patients: Correlation with rejection. Clin Exp Immunol 69:575, 1987.

Taliercio Cp, Seward JB, Driscoll DJ, et al. Dilated cardiomyopathy in the young: Clinical profile and natural history. Am J Cardiol 6:1125-1131, 1985.

Thomson JG. Production of severe atheroma in a transplanted human heart. Lancet 1:1088-1092, 1978.

Toronto Lung Transplant Group. Unilateral lung transplantation for pulmonary fibrosis. N Engl J Med 18:1140-1145, 1986.

Uniform Anatomical Gift Act. 8a Uniform Law Annot 270(Suppl), 1985.

Uniform Determination of Death Act. 12 Uniform Law Annot 270(Suppl), 1985.

Uretsky BF, Murali S, Reddy PS, et al. Development of coronary artery disease in cardiac transplant patients receiving immunosuppressive therapy with cyclosporine and prednisone. Circulation 76:827-834, 1987.

Uzark K, Crowley D, Callow L, et al. Linear growth after pediatric heart transplantation. Circulation 78(Suppl 2):492, 1988.

Valentine HA, Fowler MB, Hunt SA, et al. Changes in Doppler echocardiographic indices of left ventricular function as potential markers of acute cardiac rejection. Circulation 76(Suppl 5):86-92, 1987.

Valentine HA, Hunt SA, Gibbons R, et al. Increasing pericardial effusion in cardiac transplant recipients. Circulation 79:603-609, 1989.

Vandenberg BF, Mohanty PK, Craddock KJ, et al. Clinical significance of pericardial effusion after heart transplantation. Transplantation 7:123-134, 1988.

Wisenberg G, Pflugfelder PW, Kostuk WJ, et al. Diagnostic applicability of magnetic resonance imaging in assessing human cardiac allograft rejection. Am J Cardiol 60:130-136, 1987.

Yacoub M. Cardiac transplantation with cyclosporine and azathioprine double drug therapy. Transplant Immunol 3:2-6, 1986.

Yousem DA, Conor BM, Billingham ME. Pathologic pulmonary alterations in long-term human heart-lung transplantation. Hum Pathol 16:911-923, 1985.

Yousem SA, Paradis IL, Dauber JH, et al. Late airflow obstruction in heart-lung transplantation recipients. Transplantation 47:564-569, 1989.

Zeluff B, Gentry L. Management of infection in the post-cardiac transplant patient. Tex Heart Inst J 14:247-251, 1987.

Zerbe TR, Arena V. Diagnostic reliability of endomyocardial biopsy for assessment of cardiac allograft rejection. Hum Pathol 19:1307-1314, 1988.

Zerbe TR, White L, Zeevi A, et al. Tissue expression of major histocompatibility complex (HLA) antigens in cardiac allograft recipients. Transplant Proc 20(Suppl 1):72-73, 1988.

Zusman DR, Stinson EB, Oyer PE, et al. Determinants of accelerated graft atherosclerosis (AGAS) in conventional and cyclosporine treated heart transplant recipients. Heart Transplant 4:587, 1985.

69 Congenital and Neonatal Bowel Disorders

Theodore P. Votteler · William Dammert

Esophageal Atresia

Theodore P. Votteler

BACKGROUND AND PHYSIOLOGY

In esophageal atresia there is an abnormal separation of the esophagus from the trachea some time after the twenty-fourth day of gestation. There are four anatomic configurations (Fig. 69-1); the most common form (87%) is proximal esophageal atresia, with a fistula between the distal esophageal segment and the trachea just superior to the carina.

During fetal life the normal mechanism for swallowing amniotic fluid may be disrupted, and approximately 35% of these infants have a maternal history of polyhydramnios. Shortly after birth they develop respiratory difficulties from an inability to swallow oral secretions, inhalation of these secretions into the lungs, and regurgitation of stomach contents through the distal fistula into the trachea. Infants may also have respiratory distress caused by associated cardiac (25%) and pulmonary anomalies or prematurity and hyaline membrane disease. Attempts to feed these infants produce dysphagia, aspiration of the feeding, and exacerbation of the respiratory distress. It may be difficult to provide adequate alveolar ventilation in patients with decreased lung compliance since the gas can flow more easily through the fistula into the more compliant stomach rather than the lung.

Esophageal atresia occurs in approximately 1 out of 3000 live births and is frequently associated with cardiac defects (25%), imperforate anus (12%), agenesis or hypoplasia of the lung (4%), and GI anomalies (4%). In addition patients with identifiable chromosomal abnormalities such as a trisomies 13, 18, and 21; polysplenia syndrome; and VATER syndrome (vertebral anomalies, anal atresia, tracheoesophageal fistula, radial dysplasia, renal dysplasia) have a high incidence of esophageal atresia. These associated anomalies may need evaluation before definitive surgery for the esophageal atresia. Patients who have cyanotic congenital heart disease, especially those who have lesions that may need immediate attention such as D-transposition of the great vessels (balloon atrial septostomy) or pulmonary atresia (PGE_1 infusion followed by systemic-pulmonary shunt), and patients in whom a lesion potentially incompatible with survival such as aortic atresia is suspected must be evaluated before correction of the esophageal atresia.

In addition to the clinical signs the diagnosis is established by the inability to pass an NG tube and by roentgenographic identification of the blind esophageal pouch. Although the use of a radiopaque NG tube and air contrast may be adequate in establishing the diagnosis roentgenographically, it is important to identify an upper pouch fistula if one is present. An experienced radiologist can carefully install 1 ml of contrast material (thin barium) into the proximal pouch using fluoroscopic control with the patient in the lateral position. The contrast material must be aspirated from the pouch after adequate roentgenograms are obtained to minimize the chance of accidental introduction of barium into the lungs. Air in the stomach and intestine revealed by a roentgenogram indicates the presence of a tracheoesophageal fistula in addition to esophageal atresia.

Occasionally a tracheoesophageal fistula may be present without esophageal atresia (H-type fistula). These patients have cough or apnea when given liquid feedings, abdominal distention with crying, and/ or unexpected pneumonia. Since the presence of

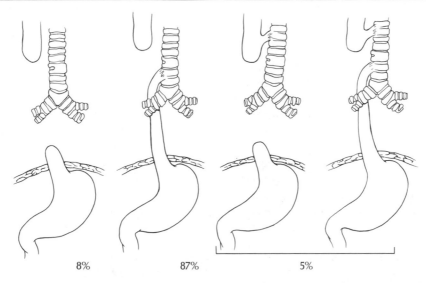

8%   87%   5%

Fig. 69-1 The usual anatomic configurations of esophageal atresia and tracheoesophageal fistula in infant with necrotizing enterocolitis.

multiple H-type fistulas is a possibility, the diagnosis is best established through an esophagram with cinefluoroscopy. If the esophagrams do not establish the diagnosis, endoscopy with bronchoscopy and esophagoscopy may be necessary. In some cases the findings of an increased gastric oxygen concentration may be helpful. A posterior laryngeal cleft may be characterized by similar clinical signs.

MONITORING AND LABORATORY TESTS

See Chapter 4. Special attention must also be given to signs of respiratory distress and signs of cardiac abnormalities.

TREATMENT
Gastrointestinal System
Preoperative management

The patient is placed in the head-up position to minimize aspiration of gastric contents through the tracheoesophageal fistula into the lungs, and a double-lumen tube with multiple vents at the tip (Replogle tube) is inserted into the esophagus to suction and empty the blind upper pouch. The tube is set on low continuous suction to minimize aspiration of oral secretions, and the patient cannot be fed. Instead, maintenance fluids, minerals, and glucose are given

through an IV catheter. Both the quality and quantity of his oral secretions must be noted.

Preliminary gastrostomy

In patients with severe respiratory distress that does not improve with initial management by suctioning, tracheal intubation, and mechanical ventilation, a gastrostomy and fistula ligation may be done as initial steps to avoid worsening pulmonary status with aspiration of stomach contents and to provide better alveolar ventilation by not allowing gas to go to the highly compliant stomach instead of the low-compliance lungs.

Patients with multiple severe congenital anomalies may need gastrostomy only for feeding purposes, and patients with associated distal GI obstruction may need gastrostomy for decompression.

Postoperative management

The quality and character of oral secretions must be noted. The NG tube or gastrostomy tube is aspirated for gastric residuals every 4 hours, but the NG tube must not be removed if it is being used for feedings because passing it over the anastomotic site may disrupt the suture line. The patient must be carefully observed for signs of breakdown of the esophageal anastomosis, including mediastinitis (temperature instability, elevated WBC count, abnormal chest roentgenogram with pneumothorax and/or pneumomediastinum).

The pharynx is suctioned with a catheter marked in such a manner that if it is inserted orally, the tip will not be introduced into the esophagus and disrupt or stress the suture line. The anastomosis between the upper and the lower esophagus is often taut and can be easily disrupted.

On the fifth to seventh postoperative day a hypaque esophagram is performed to establish the integrity of the esophageal anastomosis. Minimal esophageal leaks may be present, but if there is a retropleural loculation, they do not need treatment other than delayed feedings. Alternatively, large esophageal leaks of air, if they are intrapleural, need reoperation or drainage.

Feedings are begun 2 to 3 days after surgery by slow continuous infusion into an NG tube placed at the time of surgery. The tube position must be checked roentgenographically before feedings are started. If the tip is not in the stomach, the tube cannot be manipulated across the esophageal suture line except by the responsible surgeon. If the esophagram is normal, oral (nipple) feedings may begin on the fifth or sixth day.

Cardiorespiratory System
Preoperative management

Severe respiratory distress may necessitate tracheal intubation, suctioning, and mechanical ventilation. A chest roentgenogram must always be obtained and examined for signs of atelectasis, pneumonia, and associated cardiac or pulmonary anomalies. Arterial blood gas tensions and pH must be measured to assess the degree of respiratory dysfunction.

Postoperative management

A nasotracheal tube may remain in place for one night after surgery to provide an adequate means of suctioning. The use of high CPAP must be avoided unless specifically indicated by the patient's severe respiratory distress. Should the endotracheal tube become dislodged, a careful assessment must be done to determine if it absolutely must be replaced. If replacement is necessary, reintubation must be performed by skilled personnel to avoid undue stretch on the esophagus or esophageal intubation and rupture of the suture line.

Alternatively, patients with pulmonary parenchymal disease may need prolonged ventilatory support (see Chapters 30 and 128). Vigorous suctioning, chest physiotherapy, and, when feasible, placing the patient in a lateral-prone position to prevent atelectasis may be needed for 2 to 3 days after surgery. If chylothorax occurs, continued drainage of the chest through a thoracostomy tube is needed. Small holes in the thoracic duct may seal spontaneously if flow through the defect is decreased by use of either an enteral diet free of fat or total parenteral nutrition. If this treatment is unsuccessful, surgical closure may be attempted.

Surgical or medical management of congenital cardiac anomalies may be necessary.

Other Systems
Preoperative management

Serum creatinine and BUN values must be measured and indicated imaging studies obtained if a renal anomaly is suspected. The use of chromosome analysis may be considered if indicated by physical examination.

Intestinal Atresia and Imperforate Anus
Theodore P. Votteler

BACKGROUND AND PHYSIOLOGY

Intestinal atresia is a lack of patency of a segment of bowel, single or multiple, of varying length. The atretic segment usually occurs as the result of insufficient vascular supply. Duodenal (1:3500), jejunal (1:5000), and ileal atresias (1:4000) are not rare, but colonic atresia (1:20,000) is exceptional. A high atresia must be suspected in infants with lack of progression of air to the rectum as shown by appropriate roentgenograms and repeated bile-stained vomiting. These infants may pass small volumes of meconium. The more distal the obstruction is, the more distention and delay in vomiting. Abdominal supine and erect roentgenograms show an obstructed pattern with dilated loops of bowel and air-fluid levels. Special positional views of the abdomen with air or radiopaque material in the colon may be needed to define the exact point of atresia. These views must be obtained only after consultation with a pediatric radiologist and pediatric surgeon.

Imperforate anus includes a spectrum of findings from a single membrane covering the anal orifice to rectal atresia. The bowel terminates at a level either proximal or distal to the puborectalis muscle sling of the levator musculature. The diagnosis is established by careful inspection of the perineum during the initial newborn examination. Approximately 70% of affected males will have a fistulous connection to the urethra, and 90% of the females have a fistula to the perineum or the vagina. Roentgenographic studies establish the level of the atresia, the presence and location of a fistula, and associated anomalies such as renal, vertebral, or esophageal defects.

MONITORING AND LABORATORY TESTS

See also Chapter 4.

GI System
Preoperative management

The color and quantity of the vomitus must be noted in addition to the presence of meconium on the perineum or in the urine.

Postoperative management

The color and quantity of NG aspirate and specifically the presence of stools must be noted. It is helpful to measure the abdominal girth every 8 hours and auscultate for bowel sounds at the same time. If stools are loose or excessive, TesTape may be used to determine excess glucose loss.

Renal-Metabolic System
Preoperative management

Serum sodium, potassium, chlorine, calcium, and glucose levels must be noted. Infants, especially those with repeated vomiting, may become dehydrated, electrolyte depleted, and alkalotic. If they have not been given an IV glucose solution, they will almost certainly be hypoglycemic. Arterial or venous blood gas tensions and pH must be measured to document acid-base status. Vomiting may result in metabolic alkalosis and dehydration, and underperfusion can result in metabolic acidosis. An IV pyelogram and a cystogram are performed in patients with an imperforate anus.

Postoperative management

Sodium, potassium, and chlorine concentrations in gastric secretions must be measured if electrolyte imbalance occurs or output is excessive.

TREATMENT
GI System
Preoperative management

An NG tube must be placed for gastric decompression (a double-lumen tube of adequate size). The tube is attached to continuous or intermittent low-pressure suction. The tube must be irrigated every 2 hours with 2 to 3 ml of 0.9% sodium chloride solution to remove plugs. The infant cannot be fed, but venous access is provided for appropriate fluid replacement, including glucose.

Postoperative management

The double-lumen NG tube must be left in place and irrigated as described previously. The position of the tip of the tube is checked roentgenographically. If the patient vomits or becomes distended, the patency of the tube and the adequacy of suction is checked first. The NG drainage must be measured and the amount recorded every 4 hours. The presence of green (biliverdin) gastric secretions is due to stasis and is a contraindication to removal of the NG tube. Patients with duodenal atresia with an incompetent pylorus postoperatively are exceptions to this rule. When the patient passes stool or air (per rectum or ostomy sites), the NG tube may be removed. Gastric residuals of up to 6 ml every 4 hours are acceptable after the NG tube has been removed. Feedings are begun after the patency and function of the GI tract have been established as indicated previously, using dilute electrolyte solutions with glucose.

Renal-Metabolic System

Maintenance fluids, minerals, and glucose are administered as indicated in Chapter 15. Additional fluids and minerals must be given to correct deficits, to account for postoperative losses, and to replace NG drainage. Excessive loss of protein or blood is not usually a problem with these patients.

Necrotizing Enterocolitis
William Dammert

BACKGROUND AND PHYSIOLOGY

The term "necrotizing enterocolitis" (NEC) was first coined in 1953. Since then this disease has reached epidemic proportions; it is now one of the most frequent GI diseases seen in newborn ICUs and is a common surgical emergency.

The pathogenesis is unclear, although the integrity of the intestinal mucosa plays a pivotal role. The intestinal mucosa's protection can be breached either directly through local mucosal cell injury (e.g., bacteria, hypertonic oral solutions) or indirectly by mucosal cell hypoxia. The latter can occur during generalized hypoxia as encountered in patients with severe respiratory or cardiac problems, low cardiac output states, vascular obstruction, and hyperviscosity. After loss of the mucosal cell barrier, intramural invasion with bacteria will cause further tissue injury. Certain bacterial elements seem to predominate: clostridia sp, *Pseudomonas* sp, *Escherichia coli, Bacteroides* sp, and some viral elements, especially rotavirus.

The degree of GI tract maturation is a risk factor since the mean gestational age of patients developing NEC is 31 weeks. Eighty percent of cases are encountered in premature infants <2500 g and 50% in infants <1500 g. Oral feedings apparently increase the risk in these infants.

MONITORING AND LABORATORY TESTS

A triad of abdominal distention, rectal bleeding, and bilious vomiting (or increasing volumes of gastric residuals) in a lethargic and unstable neonate, with typical radiologic findings of pneumatosis intestinalis (Fig. 69-2), provides the diagnosis. A useful clinical staging system has been developed.

NEC STAGING SYSTEM BASED ON HISTORICAL, CLINICAL, AND RADIOGRAPHIC DATA*

Stage I (suspect)

a. Any one or more historical factors producing perinatal stress
b. Systemic manifestations include temperature instability, lethargy, apnea, bradycardia
c. GI manifestations include poor feeding, increasing pregavage residuals, emesis (may be bilious or test positive for occult blood), mild abdominal distention; occult blood may be present in stool (no fissure)
d. Abdominal radiographs show distention with mild ileus

Stage II (definite)

a. Any one or more historical factors
b. Above signs and symptoms plus persistent occult or gross GI bleeding; marked abdominal distention
c. Abdominal radiographs show significant intestinal distention with ileus; small bowel separation (edema in bowel wall or peritoneal fluid), unchanging or persistent "rigid" bowel loops, pneumatosis intestinalis, portal vein gas

Stage III (advanced)

a. Any one or more historical factors
b. Above signs and symptoms plus deterioration of vital signs, evidence of septic shock, or marked GI hemorrhage
c. Abdominal radiographs may show pneumoperitoneum in addition to others listed in IIc

---

*From Bell MJ, Ternberg JL, Feigin RD, et al. Neonatal necrotizing enterocolitis: Therapeutic decisions based upon clinical staging. Ann Surg 187:1, 1978.

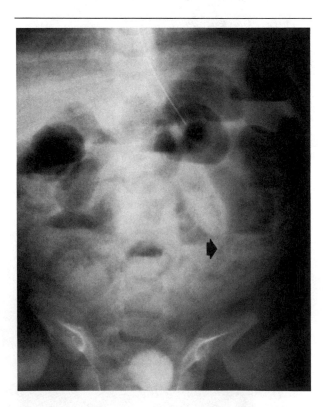

Fig. 69-2 Abdominal roentgenogram demonstrating pneumatosis intestinalis (arrow).

Laboratory abnormalities include decreased platelet count, increased or decreased WBC, increasing metabolic acidosis, hyponatremia, and stool positive for reducing substances and blood.

Radiologic abnormalities include air-fluid levels, persistent dilated bowel loops, portal vein gas (Fig. 69-3), free peritoneal fluid, and pneumoperitoneum.

TREATMENT

The initial nonoperative therapy includes parenteral nutrition, NG suction, and broad-spectrum antibiotics for 10 to 14 days (see Chapters 42 and 45).

Surgical intervention is indicated if pneumoperitoneum is present. Sound surgical judgment based on clinical, laboratory, and radiologic findings is necessary to determine which child would benefit from surgery. The object of surgery is to remove necrotic bowel and create stomas at the viable ends. Stomal closure is done electively 6 to 12 weeks later. The survival rate approaches 60% to 70%, but the long-term morbidity is high and includes short-bowel syndrome, fat malabsorption, vitamin B_{12} deficiency, and, in approximately 10% of patients, intestinal strictures,

of which 75% are colonic. This last complication occurs even in patients treated medically; therefore a barium enema is recommended 4 to 6 weeks after recovery in all patients.

Omphalocele

William Dammert

BACKGROUND AND PHYSIOLOGY

Omphalocele is a congenital herniation of intra-abdominal organs into the usually intact umbilical cord (Fig. 69-4). The size of the defect varies widely from small to giant, in which most of the abdominal organs can be herniated. Significant associated anomalies are present in a large percentage of patients, including cardiac anomalies (tetralogy of Fallot [most frequent], atrial septal defect), trisomies D, E, and 21, diaphragmatic hernias, bladder extrophy, and spina bifida. A diligent search for these anomalies is necessary since the prognosis will be greatly influenced by their presence as well as by the size of the defect.

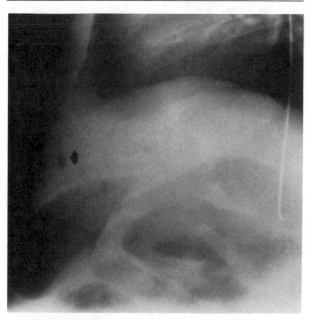

Fig. 69-3 Lateral abdominal roentgenogram in infant with NEC demonstrating portal vein gas (arrow).

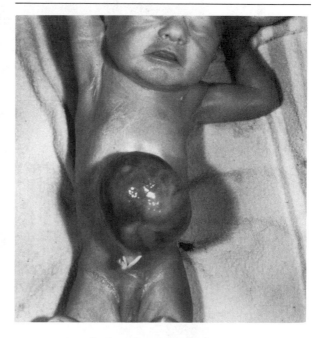

Fig. 69-4 Infant with omphalocele.

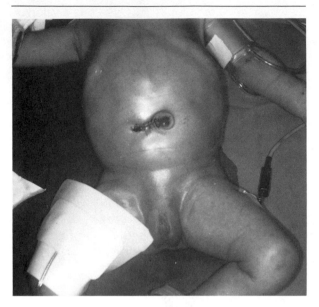

Fig. 69-5 Infant with omphalocele after primary closure. Note suture line to right of patient's umbilical cord stump.

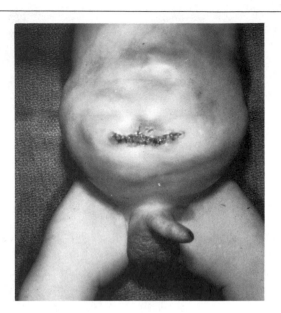

Fig. 69-6 Infant with omphalocele after skin closure only.

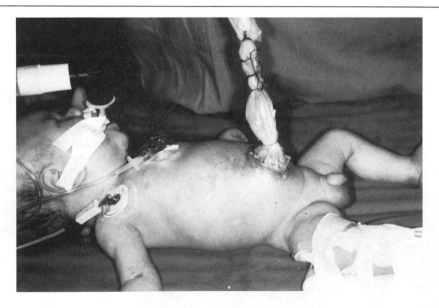

Fig. 69-7 Infant with omphalocele after Silon pouch placement. The individual silk knot lines represent progressive, sequential days of squeezing the abdominal contents back into the abdominal cavity.

MONITORING AND LABORATORY TESTS

See Chapter 4. Particular attention must be paid to the infant's temperature and fluid status since heat and water can be lost in large quantities and rapidly through the omphalocele covering.

TREATMENT

Preoperative management

An NG suction tube must be placed to prevent further abdominal distention. IV fluids with dextrose must be administered to prevent hypoglycemia (see Chapter 15), and the omphalocele must be covered with warm moist 0.9% sodium chloride solution dressings enclosed in an intestinal bag to prevent both thermal loss and contamination.

Operative management

Ideally, primary closure of both fascia and skin can be accomplished, although in patients with large omphaloceles this may compromise the abdominal contents as well as respiratory function (Fig. 69-5). In these instances mechanical ventilation and expansion of the circulating blood volume may be necessary until cardiorespiratory homeostasis is restored, generally on the second to third postoperative day. If primary closure is not feasible, skin coverage alone is attempted, which can provide a skin barrier for fluid homeostasis and infection control, and the re-

sulting ventral hernia can be closed at a later date (Fig. 69-6). If closure with the patient's natural tissues is impossible, a Silon pouch is sutured circumferentially to the fascia with the herniated abdominal contents contained within the pouch; and the pouch is squeezed down daily until fascia and skin closure becomes feasible (Fig. 69-7). This delayed closure process is usually accomplished in <10 days because of gradual expansion of the abdominal cavity and a decrease in edema in the herniated tissues.

Postoperative management

An NG suction tube is used until bowel function returns, as evidenced by passage of meconium and stools and a decrease in NG drainage. Broad-spectrum antibiotics are administered for 5 days postoperatively (see Chapters 42 and 45).

Gastroschisis

William Dammert

BACKGROUND AND PHYSIOLOGY

Gastroschisis is a congenital defect of the anterior abdominal wall, approximately 4 to 5 cm in diameter, most frequently occurring to the right of the intact umbilical cord (Fig. 69-8). A nonrotated intestine her-

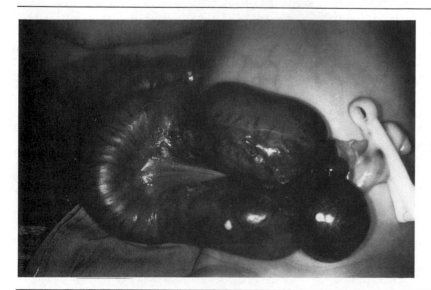

Fig. 69-8 Infant with gastroschisis.

niates through this defect and has no covering, rendering it susceptible to chemical damage by the acidic amniotic fluid while in utero. At the time of birth it is leathery, thick, and edematous and has temporarily lost its peristaltic action. The abdominal cavity fails to grow and at birth is small. Associated anomalies are rare, with the exception of intestinal atresias (or stenosis) caused by mechanical vascular compromise of the bowel segment.

MONITORING AND LABORATORY TESTS

See Chapter 4. Special attention must be paid to the infant's temperature and fluid status. In addition the herniated abdominal contents must be frequently observed for signs of ischemia since the vascular supply to them may become compromised and may lead to infarction.

TREATMENT

The same principles that apply to patients with omphalocele should be followed, with additional emphasis on the following aspects.

Preoperative management

There is even greater potential for thermal and fluid loss and bacterial contamination because of the absence of a hernia sack.

Operative management

The use of warm 0.9% sodium chloride solution enemas and retrograde decompression of intestinal gas and fluids into the NG tube can decrease the volume of the herniated bowel and therefore facilitate closure.

Postoperative management

There is almost always a need for total parenteral nutrition since return of peristalsis is usually delayed for several weeks in these patients (see Chapter 149). A central venous catheter is usually placed 2 to 3 days after the original surgery.

ADDITIONAL READING
Esophageal Atresia

Abe K, Shimada Y, Takezawa J, et al. Long-term administration of prostaglandin E₁: Report of two cases with tetralogy of Fallot and esophageal atresia. Crit Care Med 10:155-158, 1982.

Barry JE, Auldist AW. The VATER association. Am J Dis Child 128:769-771, 1974.

Bedard P, Trivan DP, Shanding B. Congenital H-type tracheoesophageal fistula. J Pediatr Surg 9:663-668, 1974.

• Blair GK, Filler RM, Theodorescu D. Neonatal pharyngoesophageal perforation mimicking esophageal atresia: Clues to diagnosis. J Pediatr Surg 22:77-774, 1987.

Cumming WA. Esophageal atresia and tracheoesophageal fistula. Radiol Clin North Am 13:277-295, 1975.

David TJ, O'Callaghan SE. Cardiovascular malformations and oesophageal atresia. Br Heart J 36:559-565, 1974.

• Day DL. Aortic arch in neonates with esophageal atresia: Preoperative assessment using CT. Radiology 155:99-100, 1985.

German JC, Mahour GH, Woolley MM. Esophageal atresia and associated anomalies. J Pediatr Surg 11:299-306, 1976.

Greenwood RD, Rosenthal A. The cardiovascular malformations associated with tracheoesophageal fistula and esophageal atresia. Pediatrics 57:87-90, 1976.

• Holder TM, Ashcraft KW, Sharp RJ, et al. Care of infants with esophageal atresia, tracheoesophageal fistula, and associated anomalies. J Thorac Cardiovasc Surg 94:828-835, 1987.

Kimura K. Nishijima E, Tsugawa C, et al. A new approach for the salvage of unsuccessful esophageal atresia repair: A spiral myotomy and delayed definitive operation. J Pediatr Surg 22:981-983, 1987.

• Kluth D. Atlas of esophageal atresia. J Pediatr Surg 11:901-919, 1976.

Koop CE, Schnaufer L, Broennle AM. Esophageal atresia and tracheoesophageal fistula: Supportive measures that affect survival. Pediatrics 54:558-564, 1974.

Korones SD, Evans LG. Measurement of intragastric oxygen concentration for the diagnosis of H-type tracheoesophageal fistual. Pediatrics 60:450-452, 1977.

• Meyers NA. Oesophageal atresia: The epitome of modern surgery. Ann R Coll Surg Engl 54:277-287, 1974.

Schneeberger AL, Scott RB, Rubin SZ, et al. Esophageal function following Livaditis repair of long gap eosphageal atresia. J Pediatr Surg 22:779-783, 1987.

Intestinal and Imperforate Anus

Adkins JD, Kieswetter WB. Imperforate anus. Surg Clin North Am 56:379-394, 1976.

• deVries P, Pena A. Posterior sagittal anorectoplasty. J Pediatr Surg 17:638-643, 1982.

Santulli TV, Kieswetter WB, Bill AH. Anorectal anomalies: A suggested international classification. J Pediatr Surg 5:281-287, 1970.

Santulli TV, Schullinger JN, Kieswetter WB, et al. Imperforate anus: A survey from the members of the surgical section of the American Academy of Pediatrics. J Pediatr Surg 6:484-487, 1971.

• Stephens FD, Smith ED. Classification, identification, and assessment of surgical treatment of anorectal anomalies. Pediatr Surg Int 1:200-205, 1986.

Stephens DG Smith ED. Anorectoal Malformations in Children. Chicago: Year Book, 1971.

Wangensteen DG, Rice CO. Imperforate anus: A method of determining the surgical approach. Ann Surg 92:77-81, 1930.

Necrotizing Enterocolitis

Bell MT, Fernberg JL, Askin FB, et al. Intestinal stricture in necrotizing enterocolitis. J Pediatr Surg 11:319, 1976.

Bell MT, Kosloske AM, Benton C, et al. Neonatal enterocolitis: Prevention of perforation. J Pediatr Surg 8:601, 1973.

Book LS, Herbst JJ, Jung Al. Carbohydrate malabsorption in necrotizing enterocolitis. Pediatrics 57:201, 1976.

Kirks DR, O'Byrne SA. The value of the lateral abdominal roentgenogram in the diagnosis of neonatal hepatic portal venous gas. Am J Roentgenol Radium Ther Nucl Med 122:153, 1974.

• Musemeche CA, Kosloske AM, Ricketts RR. Enterostomy in necrotizing enterocolitis: An analysis of techniques and timing of closure. J Pediatr Surg 22:479, 1987.

Oldham KT, Coran AG, Drongowski RA, et al. The development of necrotizing enterocolitis following repair of gastroschisis: A surprisingly high incidence. J Pediatr Surg 23:945, 1988.

• O'Neill JA, Jr. Neonatal necrotizing enterocolitis. Surg Clin North Am 61:1031, 1981.

Rotbart HA, Levin MJ, Yolken RH, et al. An outbreak of rotavirus associated neonatal enterocolitis. J Pediatr 103:454, 1983.

• Ryder RW, Shelton JD, Guinan ME. Necrotizing enterocolitis: A prospective multicenter investigation. Am J Epidemiol 112:113, 1980.

Schmid O, Quaiser K. Ueber eine besondere schwere verlaufende Form von Enteritis bein Saugling. Oesterr Z Kinderh 8:114, 1953.

Omphalocele

• Girvan DP, Webster DM, Shandling B. The treatment of omphaloceles and gastroschisis. Surg Gynecol Obstet 139:222, 1974.

• Shuster SR. A new method for the staged repair of large omphaloceles. Surg Gynecol Obstet 125:837, 1967.

Gastroschisis

• Di Lorenzo M, Yazbeck S, Ducharme JC. Gastroschisis: A 15-year experience. J Pediatr Surg 22:71, 1987.

Wesson DE, Baesl TJ. Repair of gastroschisis with preservation of the umbilicus. J Pediatr Surg 21:764, 1986.

70   Congenital Diaphragmatic Hernia

Daniel L. Levin

BACKGROUND AND PHYSIOLOGY

In a patient with a congenital diaphragmatic hernia abdominal contents are displaced through the diaphragmatic defect into the thoracic cavity. There are five types of congenital diaphragmatic hernia (Fig. 70-1).

Bochdalek's Hernia

A Bochdalek hernia is a posterolateral defect. It is the most common diaphragmatic defect and is on the left side in 85% to 90% of patients. A sac covers the abdominal contents in only 10% to 15% of patients. The defect probably results from a failure of the triangular pleuroperitoneal canal to close. However, it has been suggested that the primary embryologic defect is not a failure of closure of the diaphragm but a defect in the embryonic lung bud; in this proposed scheme the diaphragmatic defect is secondary. Much evidence, however, in experimental animals based on measurement of both lung volume and weight indicates pulmonary hypoplasia can be caused by creating a surgical defect in the fetal diaphragm. The histologic appearance of the ipsilateral lung in these animals is immature also in both the parenchymal architecture and pulmonary vessel development and is consistent with the gestational age of the animal at the time of the surgery.

If the diaphragmatic defect is a primary one and if abdominal organs migrate into the thoracic cavity early in gestation, the left lung can fail to develop and can be extremely hypoplastic. The heart is pushed to the right, and the right lung is smaller than normal. Clinically these patients are in respiratory distress from birth, have dextroposition of the heart, and have a scaphoid abdomen. If a roentgenogram is obtained early in the course, the left hemithorax is opaque; but as the patient swallows air, bowel loops may be seen in the chest (Fig. 70-2). Patients with hypoplastic lungs have small pulmonary vascular beds, a decreased number of pulmonary resistance vessels per unit of lung tissue, increased pulmonary vascular smooth muscle, peripheral extension of muscle in normally muscularized arteries, and muscularization of arteries not normally muscularized. The excess of muscle in the already small pulmonary vascular bed is more than enough to cause a physiologically significant decrease in the cross-sectional area of the vascular bed and therefore a physiologically significant increase in pulmonary vascular resistance. In addition to the anatomic abnormalities,

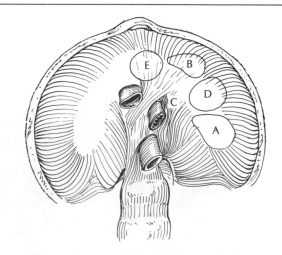

Fig. 70-1   Five types of congenital diaphragmatic hernia: *A,* Bochdalek; *B,* Morgagni; *C,* esophageal hiatus; *D,* congenital absence of one diaphragm; *E,* central tendon defect.

hypoxemia, hypercarbia, and acidosis further increase pulmonary vascular resistance, all leading to a significant right-to-left shunt through the patent ductus arteriosus (PDA) and the patent foramen ovale even after the diaphragmatic defect is repaired. In many cases infants with severe pulmonary hypoplasia who are operated on in the first few hours of life, either with or without a postoperative "honeymoon period" of increased PaO_2 values, have an extremely poor prognosis.

If the abdominal organs do not migrate upward through the diaphragmatic defect until later in gestation, lung development may proceed relatively normally. Although the defect can be large, these infants tend to have less distress than do those with hypoplastic lungs, present slightly later (many hours to days of life), and do better postoperatively.

Between these two extremes, some infants with moderate-to-severe hypoplasia and prolonged post-

operative courses can survive. They exhibit some increase in lung volume with age but may still have diminished pulmonary vascular supply to the affected lung.

In 10% to 15% of patients with Bochdalek's hernia the defect is on the right. In most of these patients the liver fills the defect and roentgenographically appears as a mass in the right lower lobe (Fig. 70-3). These patients usually have mild respiratory distress

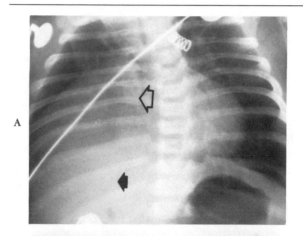

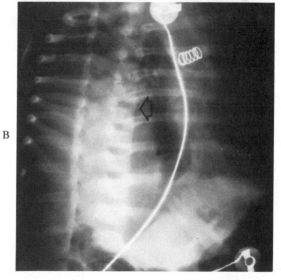

Fig. 70-3 Anterior (**A**) and oblique (**B**) chest roentgenograms of infant with right-sided diaphragmatic hernia. Open arrow indicates what was interpreted as "infiltrate" of pneumonia. Closed arrow shows abnormally cephalad abdominal gas pattern.

Fig. 70-2 Roentgenogram of infant with left-sided congenital diaphragmatic hernia with air-filled loops of bowel in the left hemithorax.

and develop symptoms at several days or weeks of life or even later. Some patients with right-sided diaphragmatic hernia have large defects with bowel loops in the chest, have pulmonary hypoplasia and experience the same problems as patients with left-sided defects, and show signs of respiratory distress at birth. Rarely the defects are bilateral, and these infants are moribund at the time of delivery.

Malrotation of the gut commonly occurs in association with diaphragmatic hernia. The differential diagnosis of congenital diaphragmatic hernia includes eventration of the diaphragm and adenomatoid cystic lung malformation.

Morgagni's Hernia

A Morgagni hernia is a parasternal defect. Although there is a higher incidence of this lesion in patients with Down syndrome, this is a rare lesion (2% of all hernias). The defect is usually on the right, and a sac usually covers the abdominal organs. The lesion results from a failure of complete muscularization of the diaphragm. Signs of distress are usually mild or absent.

Esophageal Hiatus Hernia

Esophageal hiatus hernia is a common lesion in which the stomach can migrate upward through the esophageal opening of the diaphragm. Eighty percent of them are sliding lesions, and thus the stomach may be partially in the mediastinum or may return completely to the normal position; the other 20% are paraesophageal because the short esophagus pulls the stomach up into the mediastinum. Signs include vomiting and a parasternal mass seen on a chest roentgenogram. Silent aspiration of gastric contents may occur when severe gastroesophageal reflux is present. Accompanying esophagitis may cause substernal pain and/or irritability in young infants.

Congenital Absence of the Diaphragm

Congenital absence of the diaphragm is usually unilateral and is most commonly located on the left. It is a rare lesion and is clinically similar to Bochdalek's hernia.

Central Tendon Defect

Central tendon defect occurs in the tendinous (nonmuscular) portion of the diaphragm. It is a rare lesion.

Acquired Diaphragmatic Hernia

Acquired diaphragmatic hernias may be caused by trauma (see Chapter 89) or pulmonary infection. The latter occurs in infants who are born with a normal diaphragm and lungs but have a neonatal group B β-streptococcal infection, particularly in the lower lobe of the lung. It apparently causes a secondary diaphragmatic defect and subsequent herniation of abdominal viscera through the defect into the thorax.

MONITORING AND LABORATORY TESTS

See also Chapter 4. Arterial blood gas tensions and pH must be measured every 1 to 2 hours via an intraarterial catheter. Continuous pulse oximetry and transcutaneous carbon dioxide monitoring are particularly helpful in treating these sensitive and unstable patients. Since there may be a large right-to-left shunt through a PDA, simultaneous arterial blood samples must be obtained from both pre- and postductus arteriosus sites (see Chapter 39). A ($P[A-a]O_2$) >500 mm Hg has been correlated significantly with a poor prognosis, although these studies were done by obtaining blood samples from a postductus arteriosus (lower body) site.

Considerable interest exists in defining predictive criteria for survivors vs. nonsurvivors. The interest has been heightened by the availability of extracorporeal membrane oxygenation (ECMO) for these patients (see Chapter 137). Since ECMO is an invasive, hazardous, and potentially harmful procedure, it would be ideal if accurate predictive criteria could limit its use to patients with the worse prognosis. One such predictor is the ventilatory index (VI) (VI equals mean airway pressure [MAP] times respiratory rate [RR]). Since VI multiplies MAP by RR, it takes both the degree of difficulty in oxygenation (MAP) and the degree of difficulty in carbon dioxide elimination (RR) into account. In one study of congenital diaphragmatic hernia all nonsurvivors had persistent hypoxemia and hypercarbia despite a high VI with a MAP ≥20 cm H_2O and a RR of ≥60/min (VI ≥1200).

If a congenital diaphragmatic hernia is suspected, the diagnosis can be made even prenatally through contrast fetography or sonography. A postoperative abdominal roentgenogram is taken to look for signs of bowel obstruction.

Since DIC is commonly associated with shock and respiratory failure (see Chapter 19), a platelet count, PT, and PTT must be obtained before or soon after the patient goes to the operating room. A type and crossmatch must be done before the operation.

TREATMENT

Although some authors suggest waiting to perform surgery until the infant's condition is stable, this remains a controversial approach. The suggestion is based on the finding that those patients with large defects who do poorly after surgery actually have a decrease in total pulmonary compliance postoperatively caused by surgical tethering of the chest to the diaphragm. In addition the same workers believe that although the primary reason for infants not surviving this lesion is pulmonary hypoplasia, not pulmonary arterial hypertension, much of the instability both pre- and postoperatively is due to increased pulmonary vascular resistance that is potentially reversible with good medical and ventilatory management. Therefore, they argue, surgery can be delayed until maximum medical management of pulmonary hypertension is achieved. Delaying surgery may, however, be dangerous. For example, in infants in whom the diagnosis is missed and thus surgery is delayed, the intrathoracic bowel can strangulate and become infarcted.

Since the safety and efficacy of delayed surgery are not (at the time of this writing) firmly established, surgical correction of the lesion is still of immediate importance.

With Bochdalek's hernias the patients are usually in respiratory distress, and surgery usually must be performed as an emergency procedure. If signs of malrotation exist, surgical correction of the bowel will be necessary before feeding is attempted.

If the patient is in respiratory distress, he must be intubated, and an NG tube must be inserted to prevent accumulation of air in the bowel, which would further impair pulmonary function. The use of bag and mask ventilation, which further distends the bowel entrapped in the chest, must be avoided as much as possible, especially in infants who will be transported by air to a referral center because the volume of gas in the intrathoracic bowel will expand at high altitudes, causing a worsening of the infant's condition.

Metabolic acidosis (pH <7.10 to 7.20) must be corrected by administering sodium bicarbonate, by giving one half the calculated deficit ($\frac{1}{2}$ deficit = 0.3 × body weight in kg × base deficit) at a rate of 1 mEq/kg/min, and by providing oxygenation, ventilation, and volume. Respiratory acidosis ($Paco_2$ >45 mm Hg) must be corrected with mechanical ventilation. The lungs are hypoplastic, and the risk of pneumothorax is great, especially on the side of the more compliant lung. To decrease the risk of pneumothorax (1) paralyze the patient with vecuronium, 0.1 mg/kg, or pancuronium (Pavulon), 0.1 mg/kg; (2) use low peak inspiratory and low end-expiratory pressures (e.g., 20/2 cm H_2O); and (3) use fast respiratory rates, as high as 100 breaths/min, to provide adequate alveolar ventilation.

If right-to-left shunting via a PDA is documented by simultaneous preductus and postductus arteriosus arterial blood oxygen samples (see Chapter 39), several regimens have been suggested and have had variable success. In most patients the success of treatment is determined by the size of the pulmonary vascular bed, more so than by reversal of the pulmonary hypertension with vasodilators, and just about every one imaginable has been tried. The old standard is the alpha blocker tolazoline at 1 to 2 mg/kg/hr by continuous IV infusion. Recently a lower dose has been recommended. Use of vasoactive agents that increase pulmonary vascular resistance must be avoided (see Chapter 12).

Many people currently accept the concept of using heavy sedation for these patients as routine management. The rationale is as follows: although hypoxia and hypocarbia are potent stimulators of pulmonary vasoconstriction, the endogenous release of catecholamines in response to noxious stimuli (e.g., pain, instrumentation, particularly suctioning, mechanical ventilation) can also cause increases in pulmonary arterial pressure and pulmonary vascular resistance, which may not be compensated by the accompanying potential increase in cardiac output. Elimination of the infant's ability to respond to such stimuli may make the overall management easier by eliminating some of the wide swings in pulmonary arterial blood pressure. The most efficacious ways to do this are to (1) decrease noxious stimuli as much as possible (e.g., draw all blood from an indwelling arterial catheter and eliminate as many venipunctures and heelsticks as possible, provide a quiet environment, minimize suctioning and passage of NG tubes) and (2) provide heavy continuous sedation via a fentanyl infusion. Fentanyl will not adversely alter hemodynamic stability, but if high doses (>5 μg/kg/hr) are needed, neuromuscular blocking agents must be used to prevent chest wall rigidity. Infusions are usually started with a loading dose of 2 to 3 μg/kg IV bolus, followed by 3 to 30 μg/kg/hr. To blunt all responses to noxious stimuli high doses may be necessary; the infusion must be titrated to the patient's response to suctioning or other known painful events (see Chapter 129).

As indicated previously, there is a great deal of interest in using unconventional means of management in the high-risk, high-mortality groups of infants with congenital diaphragmatic hernia. These unconventional therapies include high-frequency ventilation (HFV) and ECMO. HFV has not shown much promise in improving outcome, but ECMO apparently has. Clinicians are currently awaiting publication of results from the clinical ECMO trials.

Although ligation of the PDA with infusion of vasodilators into the pulmonary artery has been suggested in the past, this regimen has no place in the management of these patients.

Patients are frequently hypotensive secondary to hypovolemia and hypoproteinemia. Postoperative fluid management may necessitate providing 1½ to 2 times maintenance rates to maintain urinary output at a minimum of 1 ml/kg/hr. Protein given in the form of 5% albumin, 10 ml/kg over 1 hour, to maintain adequate preload is used unless clotting factors are needed, in which case fresh frozen plasma, 10 ml/kg over 1 to 2 hours, is used. When the patient starts to recover and mobilize fluid sequestered in tissues, furosemide, 1 mg/kg IV, may be necessary to increase urinary output and reduce edema. Shock and hypoxia may have resulted in acute tubular damage and may complicate the fluid management (see Chapter 14). Patients are frequently hypocalcemic and may need large doses (200 to 400 mg/kg/24 hr) of IV calcium gluconate to maintain total serum calcium levels >8.0 mg/dl or ionized calcium levels >4.5 mg/dl.

Patients in cardiorespiratory distress need to be provided with an optimal oxygen-carrying capacity (HC plus ≥45%). DIC must be diagnosed promptly and managed vigorously (see Chapter 19).

Nutritional support in the form of total parenteral fluids (administered via centrally placed catheter) can be considered for those infants with bowel defects.

ADDITIONAL READING

Akierman AR, Mayock DE. Group B streptococcal septicemia and delayed-onset congenital right-sided diaphragmatic hernia. Can Med Assoc J 129:1289-1290, 1983.

Bell MJ, Ternberg JL. Antenatal diagnosis of diaphragmatic hernia. Pediatrics 60:738-740, 1977.

Bloss RS, Turmen T, Beardmore HE, Arand JV. Tolazoline therapy for persistent pulmonary hypertension after congenital diaphragmatic hernia repair. J Pediatr 97:984-988, 1980.

• Bohn D, Tamura M, Perrin D, Barker G, Rabinovitch M. Ventilatory predictors of pulmonary hypoplasia in congenital diaphragmatic hernia, confirmed by morphologic assessment. J Pediatr 111:423-431, 1987.

Cartlidge PHT, Mann NP, Kapila L. Preoperative stabilization in congenital diaphragmatic hernia. Arch Dis Child 61:1226-1228, 1986.

Chinn DH, Filly RA, Callen PW, Nakayama DK, Harrison MR. Congenital diaphragmatic hernia diagnosed prenatally by ultrasound. Radiology 148:119-123, 1983.

• Geggel RL, Murphy JD, Langleben D, Crone RK, Vancanti JP, Reid LM. Congenital diaphragmatic hernia: Arterial structural changes and persistent pulmonary hypertension after surgical repair. J Pediatr 107:457-464, 1985.

Hickey PR, Hansen DD, Wessel P. Responses to high dose fentanyl in infants: The blunting of stress responses in the pulmonary circulation. Anesthesiology 61:A446, 1984.

Hickey PR, Hansen DD, Wessel P. Responses to high dose fentanyl in infant with pulmonary and systemic hemodynamics. Anesthesiology 61:A445, 1984.

Langham MR, Krummel TM, Greenfield LJ, Drucker DEM, Tracy TF, Mueller DG, Napolitans A, Kirkpatrick BV. Extracorporeal membrane oxygenation following repair of congenital diaphragmatic hernias. Ann Thorac Surg 44:247-252, 1987.

Levin DL. Congenital diaphragmatic hernia: A persistent problem. J Pediatr 111:390-392, 1987.

• Levin DL. Morphologic analysis of the pulmonary vascular bed in diaphragmatic hernia. J Pediatr 92:805-809, 1978.

Levy RJ, Rosenthal A, Freed MD, Smith CD, Eraklis A, Nadas AS. Persistent pulmonary hypertension in the newborn with congenital diaphragmatic hernia: Successful treatment with tolazoline. Pediatrics 60:740-752, 1977.

Naeye RL, Shochat SJ, Whitman V, Maisels MJ. Unsuspected pulmonary vascular abnormalities associated wth diaphragmatic hernia. Pediatrics 58:902-906, 1976.

Ohi R, Susuki H, Kato T, Kasai M. Development of the lung in fetal rabbits with experimental diaphragmatic hernia. J Pediatr Surg 11:955-959, 1976.

Raphaely RC, Downes JJ. Congenital diaphragmatic hernia: Prediction of survival. J Pediatr Surg 8:815-823, 1973.

Sakai H, Masanori T, Hoskawa Y, Bryan AC, Barker GA. Effect of surgical repair on respiratory mechanics in congenital diaphragmatic hernia. J Pediatr 111:432-438, 1987.

Stolar CJH, Dillon PW, Stalcup SA. Extracorporeal membrane oxygenation and congenital diaphragmatic hernia: Modification of the pulmonary vasoactive profile. J Pediatr Surg 20:681-683, 1985.

Tholkes DR. Air transport of the neonate with a congenital diaphragmatic hernia. Aviat Space Environ Med 57:183-185, 1986.

Trento A, Griffith BP, Hardesty RL. Extracorporeal membrane oxygenation experience at the University of Pittsburgh. Ann Thorac Surg 42:56-59, 1986.

Ward RM, Daniel CH, Kendig JW, Wood MA. Oliguria and tolazoline pharmacokinetics in the newborn. Pediatrics 77:307-315, 1986.

Weber TR, Connors RH, Pennington G, Westfall S, Keenan W, Kotagal S, Lewis JE. Neonatal diaphragmatic hernia. Arch Surg 122:615-618, 1987.

Wohl MEB, Griscom NT, Strieder DJ, Schuster SR, Treves S, Zwerdling RG. The lung following repair of congenital diaphragmatic hernia. J Pediatr 90:405-414, 1977.

71 Gastrointestinal Bleeding

Judy B. Splawski

BACKGROUND AND PHYSIOLOGY
General Approach

In the pediatric patient suspected of having GI bleeding one first must confirm that the patient actually is bleeding. Red material in vomitus or stools may be due to ingestion of food coloring, beets, or tomatoes and black stools to ingestion of bismuth, charcoal, licorice, or iron. False positive Hemoccult tests on stool are seen after the ingestion of red fruits and meat.

If it appears likely that actual blood loss has occurred, an estimate of the amount must be made. The history is often unreliable since GI bleeding is frightening and exaggeration is common. In addition, if blood loss is rapid, it may be difficult to quantify. The informant must be asked to estimate the amount lost in terms of concrete measures such as a cup or a tablespoon. The character of the bleeding may be helpful in assessing the amount of blood lost. Lower GI bleeding is usually not as voluminous as upper GI bleeding; however, large amounts of bright red blood per rectum may suggest massive upper intestinal bleeding. It is easy to underestimate blood loss in children based on their physical examination because of their amazing ability to compensate by vasoconstriction. Pallor, tachycardia, poor capillary filling, and decreased urinary output may be better indicators than systemic arterial blood pressure. A drop in the systemic arterial blood pressure indicates a loss of more than 20% of the blood volume. The hematocrit value is misleading acutely because both plasma and red blood cells are lost, resulting in proportionately low red blood cell count and low plasma volume and therefore a normal hematocrit value until the plasma volume has reequilibrated. Calculation of the blood volume based on the body weight in kilograms is helpful in determining the significance of the blood loss. (Blood volume in ml = 80 ml × body weight in kg [85 ml/kg in infants and neonates].) The volume of blood lost need not be large in a small child to be significant.

Signs of an acute condition of the abdomen requiring surgery such as a mass, guarding, rebound tenderness, abdominal distention, or fluid will change the approach to the patient. A history of abdominal trauma would suggest a duodenal hematoma or hematobilia. An abdominal roentgenogram must be obtained to determine if free air, intraluminal air, or a pattern of bowel obstruction is present.

Evidence of a systemic disease, such as Henoch-Schönlein purpura, hemolytic-uremic syndrome, or liver disease will have major implications for the diagnostic workup and treatment. Petechiae, bruises, or bleeding from multiple sites suggests a hemato-

---

GENERAL APPROACH TO GI BLEEDING

1. Document blood loss.
2. Quantitate the amount of blood lost.
3. Rule out an acute condition of the abdomen requiring surgery.
4. Evaluate for possible trauma.
5. Examine for signs of systemic disease.
6. Question the family about a history of coagulopathy.
7. Rule out ingestion of a drug, toxin, or foreign body.
8. Determine the site of blood loss (extragastrointestinal vs. upper, lower, or middle GI bleed).

logic problem. A family history of a bleeding disorder must be sought. Jaundice, hepatosplenomegaly, spider angiomas, prominent abdominal veins, clubbing, and ascites are clues to liver disease. These patients have multiple etiologies of GI bleeding, including deficient clotting factors, decreased platelets, esophageal or gastric varices, and hemorrhoids.

Knowledge that the patient ingested a drug or toxin known to be associated with bleeding such as aspirin, corrosives, iron, nonsteroidal anti-inflammatory medications, boric acid, or heavy metals will alter how aggressively other causes are sought.

It is important to determine the site of bleeding since different diagnostic and therapeutic techniques are needed. Extragastrointestinal sources of bleeding such as swallowed blood from a nasal or pharyngeal lesion or hemoptysis must be considered. Hematemesis, a positive gastric aspirate, or melena usually indicates an upper GI hemorrhage. Bright red or maroon-colored blood per rectum usually indicates lower intestinal bleeding.

Diagnosis

The age of the patient is an important diagnositic clue in determining the etiology of GI bleeding in childhood (Table 71-1). Causes of upper GI bleeding in the neonate include swallowed maternal blood, hemorrhagic disease from vitamin K deficiency, maternal ingestion of aspirin or anticoagulants, hemorrhagic gastritis, or stress ulcer. Spontaneous perforation of the esophagus or stomach may also occur in newborns, in which case surgery is urgently needed. Swallowed maternal blood can be differentiated from fetal blood by the Kleinhauer Betke or Apt tests, which are accurate only on grossly bloody stool or gastric aspirate in the first 24 hours of life. Tarry stools test falsely for adult hemoglobin.

Important causes of lower intestinal bleeding in the newborn that necessitate surgical intervention include necrotizing enterocolitis and Hirschsprung's disease with colitis and malrotation with midgut volvulus. These diagnoses must be considered in any sick neonate with vomiting and abdominal distention. Bleeding from colitis is suggested by small, frequent loose stools with blood mixed in the stool. Inflammatory cells are generally found on the stool smear. The most frequent causes are infectious or protein intolerance. Infectious causes of colitis include *Escherichia coli, Salmonella, Campylobacter, Shigella,* and *Yersinia*. Pseudomembranous colitis caused by

Clostridium difficile can occur in the newborn period. Colitis due to protein intolerance usually occurs at the end of the first month of life and responds to withdrawal of the offending protein.

Two important causes of rectal bleeding in toddlers are Meckel's diverticulum and intussusception. Meckel's diverticulum is a remnant of the omphalomesenteric duct, which occurs approximately 2 feet from the ileocecal valve. In lesions that bleed the presence of ectopic gastric mucosa that secretes acid results in an ulcer in the adjacent small intestine. The bleeding can manifest as hematochezia that is bright red to maroon in color or as a frankly melenotic stool. The diagnosis can be made promptly with a Meckel scan. Intussusception presents with abrupt onset of abdominal pain, an abdominal mass in the right lower quandrant, and bloody "currant jelly"–colored stool. If intussusception is suspected, an abdominal radiograph should be obtained immediately, followed by a barium enema that is both diagnostic and potentially therapeutic. The presence of gross blood in the stools and fever in this situation may indicate necrotic bowel, which decreases the opportunity for nonsurgical reduction of the intussusception.

In preschool-age children polyps, vasculitis, esophageal varices, and foreign bodies must be considered as causes of GI bleeding. Juvenile polyps result in painless rectal bleeding associated with the passage of stool; 20% to 30% of these lesions can be palpated on rectal examination. Proctoscopy may be sufficient for diagnosis and removal of distal sigmoidal polyps; otherwise an air-contrast barium enema, followed by polypectomy during colonoscopy, will be necessary. Juvenile polyposis coli, in which the colon is studded with juvenile polyps, is associated with severe bleeding and hypoalbuminemia despite the benign histologic character of the polyps. Melanotic spots on the buccal mucosa suggest that bleeding is from the small intestinal hamartomatous polyps of underlying Peutz-Jeghers syndrome. Efforts to obtain a family history of colonic polyposis are indicated because adenomatous polyps are present in several familial syndromes; since these lesions are associated with an increased incidence of colonic cancer, colectomy is ultimately needed. Henoch-Schönlein purpura is a systemic vasculitis characterized by abdominal pain, purpuric rash on the lower extremities, arthritis, and nephritis. Hemolytic-uremic syndrome, also a systemic vasculitis, is

Table 71-1   Diagnosis of GI Bleeding by Age

Causes	Signs and Symptoms	Tests
Neonate (upper GI)		
Swallowed maternal blood	First 24 hr	Kleinhauer Betke and Apt tests
Hemorrhagic disease of the newborn	Oozing from multiple foci	PT/PTT, platelet count
Gastritis, stress ulcer	Difficult delivery, CNS injury, sepsis	Chest x-ray, KUB, upper endoscopy
Esophagitis	Irritability, respiratory distress, poor feeding, end of first month of life	Upper GI, pH probe, upper endoscopy
Neonate (lower GI)		
Anal fissure	Bright red blood on outside of stool	Inspection, anoscopy
Colitis	Small frequent stools with blood mixed in stool	Stool smear for polymorphonuclear leukocytes, proctoscopy
Infectious	Associated with fever, vomiting	Culture, *Clostridium difficile* toxin, Rotazyme, ova and parasites
Milk/soy protein intolerance	Occurs at 1 month of age	Withdrawal of protein
Hirschsprung's disease	Failure to pass meconium, abdominal distention, sepsis	KUB, barium enema, rectal biopsy
Necrotizing enterocolitis	History of compromised infant, first week of life, vomiting, abdominal distention	Serial KUBs for free air, air in bowel wall or biliary tree
Malrotation with volvulus	Bile-stained vomitus, shock	KUB, upper GI
Toddler		
Meckel's diverticulum	Painless passage of maroon to melanotic stools	Meckel scan
Duplications	Mass, crampy abdominal pain	Meckel scan, barium studies
Intussusception	Acute onset of abdominal pain, right lower quadrant mass; currant jelly stools	KUB, barium enema

associated with a preceding episode of diarrhea or upper respiratory infection. Patients present with pallor, edema, hemolytic anemia, thrombocytopenia, and seizures. Ischemia of the colon may occur, resulting in lower intestinal bleeding in patients with this disease.

In the school-age child peptic ulcer disease and inflammatory bowel disease begin to appear. Peptic ulcers predominate in boys, and duodenal ulcers predominate over gastric ulcers. The symptoms include pain, vomiting, anemia, and occult blood loss. There is usually a strong family history of ulcer disease. A third of the patients present with a complication such as a massive hemorrhage or perforation necessitating

surgery. Although these lesions are generally responsive to medical care, vagotomy, pyloroplasty, and, if necessary, oversewing the ulcer are the surgical procedures of choice in patients in whom bleeding cannot be medically controlled. Multiple large ulcers should suggest Zollinger-Ellison syndrome, and fasting serum gastrin levels must be obtained.

Bleeding from Mallory-Weiss esophageal mucosal tears, stress ulceration, acute gastritis, and vascular malformations can occur at any age. Mallory-Weiss lesions are characterized by a history of nonbloody emesis followed by hematemesis. Stress ulcers occur in neonates and burn patients, after major head trauma or surgery, in association with high-dose cor-

Table 71-1   Diagnosis of GI Bleeding by Age—cont'd

Causes	Signs and Symptoms	Tests
Preschool-age child		
Juvenile polyps	Painless rectal bleeding after bowel movement	Proctoscopy, air-contrast barium enema, colonoscopy
Henoch-Schönlein purpura	Purpuric rash on lower extremities and buttocks, abdominal pain, vomiting, hematuria, hypertension	Physical examination, barium studies
Hemolytic-uremic syndrome	Antecedent diarrhea, pallor, petechia, oliguria	CBC and differential, BUN
Esophageal varices	Massive hematemesis, associated ascites, splenomegaly, chronic liver disease	Endoscopy
School-age child		
Peptic ulcer disease	Abdominal pain and vomiting, occult blood to melanotic stools	Hb, Hct, reticulocyte, upper endoscopy
Inflammatory bowel disease	Crampy abdominal pain, weight loss, poor growth, occult to moderate blood	Fecal leukocytes, CBC and differential, sedimentary rate, barium studies, endoscopy with biopsy
Any age child		
Swallowed blood	Oral, pharyngeal, or pulmonary lesion, usually bright red	ENT examination, chest x-ray
Mallory-Weiss tear	Nonbloody emesis, followed by bloody emesis	History, upper endoscopy
Stress ulcers	Sick patient, burn, head injury, sepsis, steroids	Upper endoscopy
Gastritis, esophagitis	Chest and/or abdominal pain, vomiting	Upper endoscopy
Vascular malformations	Associated cutaneous lesions, Turner's syndrome, hemihypertrophy	CBC and differential, barium studies, endoscopy, angiography
Trauma, ingestion, foreign body	History	Chest x-ray, KUB, upper endoscopy, proctoscopy

ticosteroid therapy, and in patients with acute respiratory or renal failure. In short, they should be considered in any patient in the intensive care setting who has a bloody gastric aspirate or hematemesis. Stress ulceration may occur anywhere in the gastric mucosa but most commonly occurs in the proximal stomach. The ulcerations range in severity from superficial erosions to deep ulcerations that can erode into a major blood vessel. Several good studies suggest that stress ulcers can be prevented by maintaining a gastric pH of 4.0 or greater in patients at risk. The cause of stress ulcers is suggested to be a combination of decreased cytoprotection and increased gastric acidity.

MONITORING AND LABORATORY TESTS
Laboratory Evaluation

Laboratory evaluation of patients with GI bleeding need not be extensive but should include a complete blood and differential count to provide a baseline hematocrit value and to check the platelet count, white blood cell count, and red blood cell morphology. PT and PTT are necessary to evaluate clotting function. If DIC is suspected, serum fibrinogen and fibrin split products must be evaluated. The patient can be screened for liver disease by obtaining serum transaminases (AST, ALT). Renal function can be assessed by serum creatinine and BUN tests. An elevated BUN value with a normal creatinine level

---

**LABORATORY EVALUATION OF PATIENT
WITH GI BLEEDING**

Blood studies

Complete blood count and differential, reticulocyte
   count
Prothrombin time (PT) and partial thromboplastin
   time (PTT)
Type and crossmatch

Miscellaneous studies

Alanine transaminase (ALT)
Aspartate transaminase (AST)
Ammonia
Creatinine
Blood urea nitrogen (BUN)
KUB roentgenogram
Chest roentgenogram

---

indicates absorption of blood proteins from the GI tract. A type and crossmatch must be obtained and blood products made available. An abdominal roentgenogram must be obtained to rule out obstruction, an inflammatory mass, or bowel perforation.

Diagnostic Workup by Location of Bleeding

Hematemesis or a grossly bloody nasogastric aspirate suggests bleeding proximal to the ligament of Treitz. An upper endoscopic examination is most valuable in determining the cause of upper GI bleeding. Since the equipment is portable, the examination can be performed in the PICU. The esophagus, stomach, and upper duodenum can be examined without interfering with later studies. The patient must be fully volume resuscitated before the procedure and before the use of sedation or anesthesia can be considered; adequate red blood cell volume for oxygen-carrying capacity is essential. For optimal examination the bleeding should be stopped and the stomach lavaged until clear. Upper endoscopy cannot be considered therapeutic except for sclerosing esophageal varices. However, it is often helpful to know the site of bleeding to anticipate the patient's needs better or to determine whether surgical intervention will be necessary.

If lower intestinal bleeding is suspected, proctoscopy must be done. It may demonstrate colitis, a polyp, telangiectasia, hemorrhoids, or a more proximal lesion. Colonoscopy is rarely helpful on an emergency basis because it requires a stable patient and a prepared colon. This modality is most useful for diagnosis of chronic bleeding or for performing polypectomy.

If a midintestinal hemorrhage is suspected and the patient is believed to be bleeding briskly, a bleeding scan must be considered. These studies can indicate an active bleeding site if the rate of blood loss is >0.5 ml/min. Two scans are available: technetium-labeled sulfur colloid and labeled red blood cells. The sulfur-colloid scan is more sensitive; however, since the sulfur-colloid complex is picked up by the reticulo-endothelial system in the liver and spleen, large portions of the GI tract are obscured. Also, the circulating half-life is 30 to 60 minutes, and the bleeding source must be identified within that time period. The red blood cell scan is slightly less sensitive because of higher background activity; the images, however, can be obtained over a 24-hour period. This scan will interfere with a Meckel scan for approximately 1 week. Therefore a Meckel scan must be done first unless the patient is bleeding briskly. If a site is demonstrated by the red cell scan, it may indicate a general anatomic area for use of a selective arteriogram, which can be therapeutic as well as diagnostic.

If the patient's bleeding has stopped and a midintestinal site is suspected, a Meckel scan should be done first. The radioisotope used is cleared rapidly so it does not interfere with the other radionucleotide studies. Barium interferes with this scan by sequestering the technetium pertechnetate; therefore barium contrast studies must be performed after this scan. The technetium pertechnetate is picked up by mucus-secreting gastric cells; therefore duplications with gastric mucosa will show up as well. Pentagastrin administration increases the uptake of the pertechnetate; glucagon and cimetidine decrease secretion and thus also enhance the examination. Aluminum-containing antacids interfere with the examination for several days. False negative tests are obtained when there is no gastric mucosa, when there is decreased blood flow to the lesion from bowel torsion or intussusception, or when brisk bleeding rapidly washes away the pertechnetate. False positive results occur with inflammation, vesicular ureteral reflux, and hemangiomas.

INVESTIGATION FOR SUSPECTED CAUSE OF BLEEDING

Upper GI bleeding (hematemesis, bloody gastric aspirate, melena): Esophagogastroduodenoscopy

Lower GI bleeding (red blood in or on stool): Proctoscopy

Midintestinal bleeding (actively bleeding): Technetium-labeled red cell scan; arteriogram

Midintestinal bleeding (not actively bleeding): Meckel scan; barium enema; upper GI examination with small bowel follow-through; upper endoscopy; colonoscopy; arteriogram

Intussusception: Barium enema

Malrotation with midgut volvulus: Water-soluble contrast study

---

VOLUME RESUSCITATION

Establish and maintain a circulating blood volume.
Provide supplemental oxygen.
Protect the airway.
Correct clotting deficiencies.
Monitor adequacy of replacement therapy.
    Central venous catheter
    Bladder catheter
Monitor for ongoing blood loss or rebleeding.
Evaluate for sepsis.
Monitor the neurologic status.
Notify the surgical service.

The use of barium studies is of questionable value in patients with acute GI bleeds unless intussusception or midgut volvulus is suspected; in such cases they must be done promptly. Intussusception can be reduced and surgery avoided by a barium enema. Rapid diagnosis of volvulus, followed by surgical correction, is essential to reduce intestinal loss from ischemia.

In cases of chronic GI bleeding that have eluded diagnosis by other modalities, an arteriogram must be done to rule out arteriovenous malformations or telangiectasia.

TREATMENT
Volume Resuscitation

To establish and maintain a circulating blood volume the patient must have a large-bore venous catheter in place. Either a 0.9% sodium chloride solution or lactated Ringer's solution is readily available and should be the first fluid given. If the patient continues to bleed, whole blood replacement is necessary. If the bleeding has stopped, packed red blood cells are preferred. Fresh frozen plasma and platelets must be considered after transfusion of more than 50% to 100% of the blood volume acutely.

Hemorrhage results in an acute loss of oxygen-carrying capacity; therefore supplemental oxygen must be given. Tracheal aspiration of gastric contents can lead to morbidity and mortality; thus the use of endotracheal intubation must be considered to protect the airway in patients with massive upper bleeding and in patients with an altered mental status. A central venous catheter may be necessary to monitor replacement in patients with other complicating factors such as liver disease or renal impairment. If bleeding esophageal varices are considered likely, a hematocrit value of no more than 30% is the goal since vigorous expansion of the intravascular compartment may result in continued bleeding or increase the risk of rebleeding. To assess the adequacy of blood volume replacement the patient's urinary output must be carefully monitored; to do so, use of an indwelling urinary catheter may be necessary. Rebleeding may occur in as many as 50% of patients with a major upper GI bleed; therefore these patients must be monitored until it is reasonably certain that they will not rebleed. Sepsis is a common complicating factor and appropriate cultures must be taken, although antibiotics are not routinely administered. In patients with liver disease GI bleeding may precipitate hepatic encephalopathy. Neurologic status and ammonia levels must be monitored and therapy in the form of lactulose enemas or neomycin instituted when necessary (see Chapter 16). Specific clotting deficiencies associated with liver failure must be corrected with platelets or fresh frozen plasma. Since many of these patients may need surgery acutely, it is prudent to notify the surgical service to achieve cooperative management.

Decreasing Bleeding

Management of upper GI bleeding includes the following: using saline solution lavage, decreasing acidity, increasing cytoprotection, and providing vasoconstriction.

After perforation and intestinal obstruction have been ruled out, gastric lavage through a NG tube is used in patients with GI bleeding. Although the therapeutic efficacy of this procedure has not been established, it does clear the stomach of blood so further diagnostic studies can be performed and allows quantitation of ongoing bleeding. In children a 0.9% sodium chloride solution must be used to avoid electrolyte abnormalities; the amount of saline solution lavaged varies from 20 to 50 ml per pass, depending on the size of the child, and its use continues till the return is clear. Iced saline solution must be used with caution because it can induce hypothermia in small children.

Reduction in gastric acidity is the cornerstone of therapy for acute upper GI bleeding (Table 71-2). Administration of antacids titrated every hour to maintain a gastric pH >4 is used to prevent rebleeding and should be started after gastric lavage. If the patient is to undergo endoscopy, the administration of antacids is delayed because they interfere with the examination. The use of aluminum- and magnesium-containing antacids can lead to toxicity in patients with renal failure. The diarrhea induced by magnesium can be avoided by alternating magnesium- and aluminum-containing antacids. Aspiration of antacids must be avoided. For chronic suppression of gastric acidity, histamine H_2-receptor antagonists generate better compliance. Side effects of H_2 blockers include diarrhea, dizziness, confusion, gynecomastia, leukopenia, increased transaminase values, and decreased clearance of phenytoin, diazepam, and theophylline. Ranitidine has fewer side effects and a longer half-life than cimetidine. Unfortunately there is less experience with this drug in children.

Recent attention has focused on increasing gastric cytoprotection. The one drug available at present is sulcralfate (Table 71-2). Some evidence suggests that it may be beneficial in the prevention of stress ulcers by acting locally to form a protective barrier. It also increases cytoprotection by stimulating prostaglandins and inactivating pepsin. There is no systemic absorption, and complications are limited to constipation. It can be dissolved in water for administration to children and for administration by NG tube.

Infusion of vasopressin or somatostatin has been recommended to control persistent GI bleeding (Table 71-2). Vasopressin is a potent vasoconstrictor that decreases splanchnic blood flow and thereby decreases portal hypertension. However, its effects are not limited to the splanchnic circulation, and there is a high incidence of systemic hemodynamic effects, including an increase in systemic arterial and venous blood pressure, a decrease in cardiac output, and peripheral ischemia. Simultaneous administration of nitroglycerin has been proposed to decrease the myocardial ischemia and systemic side effects of this drug, but therapeutic trials are limited. Somatostatin appears to be more selective for the splanchnic circulation, resulting in decreased portal hypertension with minimal side effects. Preliminary results in adults are encouraging; however, these drugs have not been studied in children. In children who do not stop bleeding with conservative treatment vasopressin or somatostatin may decrease GI bleeding so that more definitive measures such as sclerosis of varices, arteriography, or surgery can be undertaken. These drugs should not be used for more than 24 hours.

Variceal bleeding should be suspected in patients with upper GI bleeding and chronic liver disease. However, in as many as one third of adult patients with liver disease and upper GI bleeding, a lesion other than varices is identified; therefore the presence of bleeding varices must be documented. Therapy for variceal bleeding includes the following:

Acute	Vasopressin/somatostatin
	Balloon tamponade/sclerosis
	Surgery
Chronic	Sclerotherapy
	Propranolol/somatostatin
	Shunt
	Liver transplant

Vasopressin or somatostatin may be tried acutely as above. Although balloon tamponade is effective, it is associated with major complications, including perforation or erosion of the esophagus and stomach. In addition pulmonary aspiration is a major problem with this form of therapy, and deflation of the balloon is frequently associated with rebleeding. The balloons are not intended for use beyond 24 hours. Endoscopic variceal sclerosis is effective but is also associated with complications, including esophageal ulceration with rebleeding, perforation, and future stricture formation. An anaphylactic response to the sclerosant is also possible. Once started, sclerotherapy is continued until all of the varices are obliterated, and even though multiple endoscopies are necessary, it is probably the treatment of choice. Emergency shunt surgery or surgery to devascularize the distal esophagus is associated with a mortality rate in excess of 30%. Percutaneous transhepatic, transumbilical, or transjugular variceal obliteration is

Table 71-2 Pharmacologic Management of Acute Upper GI Bleeding

Drug	Dosage	Warning	Indications
Antacids			
Aluminum hydroxide Magnesium hydroxide Calcium carbonate	0.5 ml/kg/dose PO q 2 hr Maximal single dose, 30 ml	Aluminum and magnesium toxicity in patients with renal impairment Monitor sodium content	Prevention of stress ulcers, gastritis, esophagitis
H_2-receptor antagonists			
Cimetidine	30-40 mg/kg/day PO or IV divided q 6 hr Maximal dose, 2400 mg/day	Altered mental status Decreased clearance of phenytoin, diazepam, and theophylline	Therapy for stress ulcers, gastritis, esophagitis, peptic ulcers
Ranitidine	2 mg/kg/dose IV or PO q 8 hr Adults: 150 mg PO bid		Same as above
Cytoprotective agents			
Sulcralfate	Adults: 1 g PO or NG qid	Constipation	Prevention of stress ulcers, gastritis, esophagitis, peptic ulcers
Vasoconstrictors			
Vasopressin	Bolus: 0.3 U/kg (maximal dose, 20 U) in 2 ml/kg of 5% dextrose IV over 10-20 min; infusion rate 0.2 to 0.4 U/1.73 m²/min for 12-24 hr; taper	Hypotension, myocardial ischemia, dysrhythmia, decreased cardiac output, increased BP, peripheral ischemia, hyponatremia	Uncontrolled GI bleeding, esophageal or gastric variceal bleeding
Somatostatin	0.5 to 1.0 µg/kg IV bolus; infusion rate 7.5 µg/min	Fewer systemic side effects than vasopressin	Same as above
Vasodilator			
Nitroglycerin	0.2 µg/kg/min IV	Few theurapeutic trials—none in children	Systemic side effects of vasopressin
Beta-adrenergic blocker			
Propranolol	0.5-1.0/kg/day PO divided q 6 hr Maximal daily dose, 60 mg	Asthma, bronchospasm, heart block, sinus bradycardia, metabolic acidosis, hypoglycemia; not studied in children	To prevent rebleeding from varices

associated with multiple complications, is technically difficult, and probably should not be considered as a first choice or emergency procedure.

Chronic treatment with propranolol to decrease portal blood flow may be helpful in preventing bleeding from esophageal varices and may be a useful adjunct to sclerotherapy (Table 71-2). It cannot be administered until the bleeding is stopped and the systemic arterial blood pressure is restored to normal. It is contraindicated in the presence of circulatory failure, heart block, sinus bradycardia, or bronchospasm.

Surgical shunts are most appropriate when there is preservation of the hepatic parenchyma and portal hepatopedal blood flow is demonstrated. Shunts decrease the possibility of rebleeding but increase hepatic encephalopathy. Patients need to have generous vessels to maintain patency; thus they generally must be >6 years of age to receive a shunt.

If cirrhosis is present, liver transplantation should be considered (see Chapter 64).

ADDITIONAL READING

Bosch J. Effect of pharmacological agents on portal hypertension: A haemodynamic appraisal. Clin Gastroenterol 14:169-184, 1985.

• Hyams JS, Leichtner AM, Schwartz AN. Recent advances in diagnosis and treatment of gastrointestinal hemorrhage in infants and children. J Pediatr 106:1-9, 1985.

Lacroix J, Infante-Rivard C, Gauthier M, et al. Upper gastrointestinal tract bleeding acquired in a pediatric intensive care unit: Prophylaxis trial with cimetidine. J Pediatr 108:1015-1018, 1986.

• Oldham KT, Lobe TE. Gastrointestinal hemorrhage in children. Pediatr Clin North Am 32:1247-1263, 1985.

Priebe HJ, Skillman JJ, Bushnell LS, et al. Antacid versus cimetidine in preventing acute gastrointestinal bleeding. N Engl J Med 302:426-430, 1980.

Steer MJ, Silen W. Diagnostic procedures in gastrointestinal hemorrhage. N Engl J Med 309:646-649, 1983.

Winzel GC, Forelich Jw, McKusick KA, et al. Scintigraphic detection of gastrointestinal bleeding: A review of current methods. Am J Gastroenterol 78:324-347, 1983.

72 Gastroesophageal Reflux

Robert H. Squires, Jr. · *William M. Belknap*

BACKGROUND AND PHYSIOLOGY

Gastroesophageal reflux (GER) is the movement of gastric contents from the stomach into the esophagus. Reflux is usually brief, asymptomatic, and self-limited; it commonly occurs in healthy infants, children, and adults. In contrast to adults, however, infants may have greater frequency and duration of reflux episodes during both the sleeping and awake conditions. The basis for these episodes is physiologic, since the mechanisms for normal motility and gastroesophageal sphincter control appear to be immature in early infancy. Moreover, although reflux in infancy is generally benign, complications may occur and cause significant morbidity. These patients may, therefore, initally be seen in the PICU in such a morbid state.

The mechanism for GER is a transient or fixed incoordination of esophago-gastro-duodenal motility. GER, therefore, is a general term for a condition in which one of the three following mechanisms may be dominant: distal esophageal dysmotility, altered gastroesophageal sphincter function, or delayed gastric emptying. The control and function of this complex motor function requires the integration of neural pathways and sequential muscle contraction; hormonal modulation probably also occurs. Normal swallowing initiates this process; this coordinated motor process is necessary for safe passage of a solid or liquid bolus from the mouth through the pharynx and cricopharyngeus muscle into the proximal esophagus. Swallowing dysfunction manifested as nasopharyngeal reflux, hypopharyngeal incoordination, or cricopharyngeal malfunction can result in a food bolus lingering in the pharynx over the airway. Coughing, choking, and aspiration, which are symptoms often attributed to GER, often result.

The bolus is then propelled smoothly from the proximal one third of the esophagus to the distal esophagus and quickly into the stomach through a relaxed lower esophageal sphincter (LES). Esophageal motor dysfunction can occur and disturb this orderly process. This abnormality can be seen in patients with Down syndrome, collagen vascular disease, esophagitis, achalasia, and severe neurologic impairment. Once the bolus passes into the stomach, the LES becomes hypertonic before returning to its baseline pressure; thus the sphincter acts as a functional barrier to the backflow of gastric contents. The stomach stores the bolus until it eventually passes into the duodenum through the pylorus, aided by propulsive waves through the gastric antrum. An incompetent LES is often thought to be the "cause" of GER; LES pressure, however, is usually normal in patients with significant GER. The combination of transient LES relaxations and delay in gastric emptying, which occurs in many patients, suggests a more

---

DOCUMENTED COMPLICATIONS OF GASTROESOPHAGEAL REFLUX IN INFANTS

Failure to thrive
Esophagitis
   Blood loss
   Protein loss
Esophageal stricture
Aspiration pneumonia
Apnea
   Obstructive
   Central
Bradycardia
Barrett's esophagus (mucosal metaplasia)

global dysfunction in motility as the primary cause of GER.

Clinically, GER most commonly occurs in infants as passive regurgitation ("spitting") and is generally harmless. In contrast, vomiting in an infant usually signals a problem and must never be presumed to be GER. Vomiting is a common presenting sign in infants for a number of potentially serious conditions. All of these entities must be considered in the infant or young child presenting to the intensive care setting with new-onset or unexplained vomiting.

Pathologic GER occurs when the frequency or duration of reflux episodes results in a defined complication. It has been suggested that premature in-

---

CAUSES OF VOMITING IN INFANTS

Diseases of the CNS

Increased intracranial pressure
Infections (meningitis, encephalitis)
Intracranial mass
Hemorrhage (subdural hematoma)
Head trauma

Metabolic diseases

Acidosis
Hyperammonemia

Drug toxicity

Salicylism
Others

GI/hepatic diseases

Gastroenteritis
Obstruction (pyloric stenosis, malrotation)
Appendicitis
Gastroesophageal reflux
Hepatitis
Hepatic failure
Pancreatitis
Intussusception

Infections

Otitis media
Pneumonia
Urinary tract infection

---

fants, particularly those with bronchopulmonary dysplasia, have a greater propensity for complicated reflux. Patients with congenital heart disease and congestive heart failure may also be troubled by concomitant reflux. Since the energy needs for such patients are high, they cannot tolerate any compromise in the ability to sustain enteral intake.

Recently the cause of a number of cardiorespiratory conditions in pediatric patients, including obstructive and centrally mediated apnea, bradycardia, sudden infant death syndrome, and bronchospasm has been attributed to GER. It appears likely that frequent or long-duration reflux can result in obstructive apnea. The evidence for mechanisms of reflux mediating the other clinical events cited here is less well defined. Nevertheless, the use of sleep studies or a pneumocardiogram has been added to the diagnostic armamentarium for evaluating the patient with complicated reflux in an effort to demonstrate a cause-and-effect relationship between reflux and its reported cardiorespiratory sequelae.

GER is particularly severe in the patient with a repaired tracheoesophageal fistula. Emptying of the distal esophagus is virtually nonexistent in these patients; as a result, esophagitis and stricture formation may ensue. Furthermore, formation of a new fistula because of reflux and improper healing of the esophageal anastomosis may occur. Thus patients presenting after the repair of a tracheoesophageal fistula with pulmonary signs and symptoms must be carefully evaluated for these complications.

The older child with severe asthma may have reflux resulting from the effects of bronchodilator therapy on LES function or secondary to frequent coughing. Although it has been suggested that reflux may precipitate episodes of bronchospasm in asthmatic children, confirmatory data are lacking.

Reflux is documented by a compatible history of regurgitation or by distal esophageal pH monitoring. The infant who regurgitates and who also has hematemesis, poor weight gain, unexplained bronchospasm, apnea, or documented aspiration pneumonia needs further investigation (see below). Swallowing dysfunction must also be considered, particularly in the infant or child with static encephalopathy or other major neurologic disease. The other diseases cited previously should be thoroughly investigated. Empiric treatment for presumed reflux in such settings is never warranted.

MONITORING AND LABORATORY TESTS

GER generally is easy to define clinically, but its nearly universal occurrence in infants makes it difficult to define a cause-and-effect relationship between reflux and the child's other symptoms. Although rigorous care must be taken not to assume that reflux is the sole cause of conditions such as failure to thrive, severe asthma, or recurrent pneumonia, extensive investigation must be curtailed in a growing and otherwise healthy infant with GER.

A number of investigative tools are available to assess patients suspected of having significant gastroesophageal reflux. A thorough history is indispensable in gaining insight into parental concerns and perceptions. An upper GI series with barium swallow is useful to ensure normal anatomy. A detailed videotaped recording of the swallowing of barium, the cine-esophagram, will define the completeness and efficiency of the patient's swallowing function. However, the upper GI series is not reliable in defining the occurrence of GER and its frequency, duration, and relationship to meals and sleep.

The most sensitive test for documenting these variables is the 24-hour esophageal pH study. It can determine if the precise type and time of symptoms that occur during the 12- to 24-hour study are associated with episodes of reflux. Esophageal motility studies, performed with a soft, water-perfused triple-lumen catheter, are useful in characterizing the function of the LES and for proper pH probe placement. Abnormal distal esophageal motility can be defined in patients with esophagitis. Gastroesophageal scintiscanning using a ^{99m}Tc–sulfur colloid–labeled meal has aided in defining the rate of gastric emptying in the reflux patient. Moreover, this study may demonstrate the occurrence of pulmonary aspiration of the radiolabeled gastric contents. Upper endoscopy or blind-suction biopsy is used to assess esophageal mucosal integrity; inflammation may be evident either grossly or histologically on biopsy of areas above the LES and always indicates significant reflux. Rarely, in patients with chronic pneumonia of unknown cause it may be necessary to perform bronchoscopy to rule out a small H-type tracheoesophageal fistula or to obtain bronchial washings to stain for lipid-laden macrophages often seen in patients with chronic aspiration. Specific investigations aimed at quantifying reflux or defining one of its complications include those listed in the accompanying box.

MONITORING AND LABORATORY EVALUATION

Complete history and physical examination

Laboratory studies

Complete blood count
Serum electrolytes
Serum glucose
BUN, creatinine
Urinalysis
Liver function
Total serum protein and albumin

Radiographs

Chest
    Acute or chronic infiltrate in dependent lobes
    Recurrent pneumonia in multiple sites
Barium esophagram and upper GI series
    Rule out swallowing dysfunction
    Achalasia
    Gastric antral web
    Pyloric stenosis
    Intestinal malrotation

Esophageal pH probe study

Continuous (24 hr) pH monitoring
Document frequency, duration of reflux
Define relationship to cardiorespiratory events

Esophageal manometry

Lower esophageal sphincter position
Esophageal propulsive waves (motility)

Endoscopy, esophageal biopsy

Confirm absence of anomalies
Document esophagitis

To rule out aspiration secondary to reflux

^{99m}Tc-sulfur colloid scintiscanning
    Rapidity of gastric emptying
    Visualize aspiration event(s)
Bronchoscopy
    Bronchial washings
    Rule out tracheoesophageal fistula (H-type)

TREATMENT

Therapy for GER is multitiered. The simplest, but most time-consuming therapy is to provide reassurance to the family of the uncomplicated patient. In the vast majority of cases symptoms resolve by 12 to 18 months of age without specific therapy. The next therapy includes providing thickened feedings and elevating the head of the bed. Thickened feedings are not "heavier" and thus more likely to remain in the stomach; rather, it is more likely that the increased caloric density of the formula allows the infant to consume less formula and thus tend not to be overfed. The ideal position for the infant with GER after feeding and during sleep is prone with the head elevated approximately 30 degrees; ensuring this position safely can be a challenge.

Antacids, bethanechol, and metoclopromide are the only medications that are currently available to treat reflux. Neutralizing gastric acid helps in reducing esophagitis, thus improving distal esophageal mo-

tility and LES pressure. Bethanechol, an anticholinergic, improves esophageal clearing and increases LES pressure. Possible side effects include fatigue, blurred vision, lower abdominal cramps, and irritability. Metoclopromide is a dopamine antagonist that improves gastroduodenal motility and gastric emptying and has a minor effect on increasing LES pressure. Its side effects can be quite disturbing and include oculogyric crisis, tremor, agitation, extreme irritability, and intestinal cramping; infants are particularly prone to these side effects.

Surgery should be reserved for those patients who are suspected of having a significant sequela from their reflux such as recurrent pneumonia or esophageal stricture and who have not responded adequately to intense medical therapy of at least 6 to 8 weeks' duration. A Nissen fundoplication is the surgical procedure of choice. However, even under optimal conditions, the complication rate with surgical fundoplication is 10% to 20%, and freedom from

---

THERAPY FOR GASTROESOPHAGEAL REFLUX

Provide reassurance (uncomplicated patients)

Minimize reflux episodes

Position infant
  Prone
  Head of bed up 30 degrees
Thickened feedings (15 ml rice cereal per ounce formula)

Treat esophagitis

Antacids
  0.5 ml/kg/dose
  Four doses per day, 1 hour after feedings
  Avoid inducing diarrhea
  Monitor serum magnesium (small infants)
H_2-receptor blocker (cimetidine)
  5-10 mg/kg/dose
  Four doses per day
  Monitor CBC, CNS, liver and renal functions

Enhance gastroduodenal motility

Bethanechol
  0.1-0.15 mg/kg/dose
  Four doses per day, 30-60 minutes before feeding
  Side effect: colic
Metoclopramide
  0.1 mg/kg/dose
  Four doses per day, 30-60 minutes before feeding
  Side effects: restlessness, oculogyric crisis

Perform anti-reflux surgery

Generally not advocated
Decision made on individual basis
  Neurologic devastation
  Recurrent aspiration pneumonia
  Esophageal stricture
Procedure: Nissen fundoplication, often accompanied
  by pyloroplasty
Postoperative complications
  Intestinal obstruction (9%)
  Gas-bloat syndrome
  Dumping syndrome

reflux cannot be guaranteed. Surgical intervention, therefore, is rarely indicated in the patient who is not neurologically devastated.

Most patients with GER improve by 6 months of age, and 90% have resolution of their symptoms by 18 months of age. Those patients with an underlying neurologic disorder are more likely to have continued symptoms. Therapy must be individualized based on the severity of the child's symptoms and the age of the patient and includes those modalities listed on p. 576.

ADDITIONAL READING

• Dedinsky GK, Vane DW, Black T, et al. Complications and reoperation after Nissen fundoplication in childhood. Am J Surg 153: 177-183, 1987.

Jolley SG, Johnson DG, Roberts CC, et al. Patterns of gastroesophageal reflux in children following repair of esophageal atresia and distal tracheoesophageal fistula. J Pediatr Surg 15:857-862, 1980.

• Orenstein SR, Orenstein DM. Gastroesophageal reflux and respiratory disease in children. J Pediatr 112:847-858, 1988.

Richter JE, Castell DO. Gastroesophageal reflux. Pathogenesis, diagnosis, and therapy. Ann Intern Med 97:93-103, 1982.

Weihrauch TR. Gastroesophageal reflux—pathogenesis and clinical implications. Eur J Pediatr 144:215-218, 1985.

Wilkinson JD, Dudgeon DL, Sondheimer JM. A comparison of medical and surgical treatment of gastroesophageal reflux in severely retarded children. J Pediatr 99:202-205, 1981.

73 Hyperbilirubinemia

William M. Belknap

BACKGROUND AND PHYSIOLOGY

Bilirubin is the normal metabolic breakdown product of the heme moiety of hemoglobin and is generated during the destruction of senescent RBCs. The multistep metabolic pathway for the conversion of heme to bilirubin is located in the reticuloendothelial system of the spleen and bone marrow. Once formed, bilirubin enters the plasma, is bound to albumin, and is transported to the liver. Since bilirubin is quite lipophilic and incapable of renal clearance, it is taken up by the liver for biotransformation to a mono- or diglucuronide conjugate. In this water-soluble form conjugated bilirubin is rapidly transported into its ultimate excretory pathway, the bile.

Bilirubin accumulation, or hyperbilirubinemia, occurs in the body only during specific abnormal circumstances: (1) increased production, (2) reduced uptake from blood by the liver, (3) reduced conjugation in the liver, and (4) reduced excretion of conjugated bilirubin from liver to bile. These conditions become clinically apparent as jaundice, the yellow staining of skin and organs, which becomes manifest when the total serum bilirubin exceeds 3 mg/dl. In the PICU hyperbilirubinemia is not an infrequent occurrence as either overt jaundice or an unexpected laboratory finding. Hyperbilirubinemia falls into two general categories, unconjugated and conjugated. In the discussion that follows the conditions causing these two entities are defined.

Increased bilirubin production is principally caused by the premature intravascular or extravascular destruction of RBCs by a congenital or acquired hemolytic disease. These disorders exhibit an age-related preponderance; isoimmunization disorders such as ABO incompatibility and Rh disease are present at birth. Certain other familial disorders such as hemoglobinopathies, structural defects, or metabolic diseases such as glucose-6-phosphate dehydrogenase (G6PD) deficiency may be seen in infancy or later.

Acquired disease may manifest as hemolysis alone or as a complicating feature of an infectious disease or a multisystem collagen vascular disease.

Unconjugated hyperbilirubinemia may occur on a physiologic basis in infancy (Table 73-1). In this instance bilirubin production is high, whereas its conjugation and excretion are functionally deficient. This phenomenon is of short duration and only occurs in a discrete period during the first week of life. Persistence of unconjugated hyperbilirubinemia beyond this specific period (days 2 to 5 of life) always must be evaluated since a serious underlying disease such as congenital hypothyroidism or hemolytic disease may be present. In the breast-fed infant remarkable jaundice may occur and persist; although commonly raising alarm, it has no deleterious effect. An occasional infant may initially be seen with unconjugated hyperbilirubinemia as the major manifestation of an underlying urinary tract infection. Inborn errors of the enzyme responsible for bilirubin conjugation, glucuronyl transferase (Crigler-Najjar syndrome; Table 73-1), exist in two forms. Serum unconjugated bilirubin has a major toxic effect on the CNS when it exceeds a given range (usually 20 to 25 mg/dl) in the term infant. In those instances the unbound lipid-soluble pigment moves from the blood into the basal ganglia of the brain and causes an irreversible toxicity, resulting in devastating motor and intellectual deficits. This permanent CNS toxicity from marked elevation in serum unconjugated bilirubin is known as kernicterus.

Conjugated hyperbilirubinemia results from impaired hepatic excretory function. Intra- or extrahepatic diseases of several types result in either interruption of normal cellular bile formation or obstruction of biliary flow from the liver. This phenomenon, known as cholestasis, is generally only one facet of more generalized liver cell dysfunction; primary obstruction of small or large ducts is less common.

Cholestasis is particularly common in neonates. The most common cause is neonatal hepatitis, a stereotypic form of hepatic disease peculiar to infants that is usually idiopathic in origin but may be caused by any one of several insults such as congenital infections, metabolic disease, or drug or nutrient toxicity. Metabolic diseases or sepsis may also occur during infancy as cholestasis alone in the absence of more generalized liver dysfunction. Since many of these conditions are treatable, their rapid identification is necessary to treat and reverse hepatic injury or prevent further toxicity (Table 73-2).

Once the intrahepatic and treatable causes of neonatal cholestasis are ruled out, careful investigation for the presence of extrahepatic obstruction must be undertaken. Biliary atresia, a focal or diffuse inflam-

---

UNCONJUGATED HYPERBILIRUBINEMIA CAUSED BY HEMOLYTIC DISEASES

Familial

Hemoglobinopathies
   Sickle cell anemia (hemoglobin SS and SC diseases)
   Hemoglobin C disease
   Homozygous β-thalassemia
   Heterozygous β-thalassemia
   Hemoglobin S-β-thalassemia
Defects of red blood cell structure
   Hereditary spherocytosis
   Hereditary elliptocytosis
   Acanthocytosis (abetalipoproteinemia)
Enzyme defects in red blood cells
   Glucose-6-phosphate dehydrogenase (G6PD) deficiency
   Pyruvate kinase deficiency
   Others

Acquired

Newborn
Rh isoimmunization (only Rh)
Autoimmune hemolytic anemia
Acanthocytosis (secondary to liver disease)
Vitamin E deficiency
Infections
   Haemophilus influenzae
   Streptococcus pneumoniae
   Staphylococcus aureus
   Escherichia coli
   Clostridium welchii
   Malaria
Blood transfusion reaction
Collagen-vascular diseases
Snake and spider venoms
Hemolytic-uremic syndrome

NEONATAL CHOLESTASIS

Extrahepatic ("surgical jaundice")

Biliary atresia
Biliary hypoplasia
Spontaneous perforation of the common bile duct
Choledochal cyst
Bile duct stenosis
Bile plug
Choledochal-pancreatic ductal junction obstruction

Intrahepatic (NOTE: Largest group is idiopathic, neonatal "hepatitis")

Infections
   Viral hepatitis (hepatitis B, non-A, non-B)
   Systemic viral infection (CMV, rubella, herpes, *Enterovirus,* varicella)
   Bacterial (syphilis, listeriosis, tuberculosis)
   Parasitic (toxoplasmosis)
Toxic
   Drug related
   Endotoxemia
   Total parenteral nutrition
Metabolic
   Galactosemia
   Hereditary fructose intolerance
   Tyrosinosis
   α_1-Antitrypsin deficiency
   Glycogen storage disease, type IV
   Cystic fibrosis
   Lipidoses (Niemann-Pick disease, Gaucher's disease)
   Zellweger syndrome
   Others*
Idiopathic familial
   Arteriohepatic dysplasia
   Biliary hypoplasia
   Others*

---

*See references listed in Additional Reading for further information.

matory-fibrotic obliteration of the biliary tree, is the diagnosis that causes overwhelming concern. Biliary atresia is a progressive disease; unless identified and treated before the infant is 8 to 12 weeks old, it will inexorably lead to biliary cirrhosis, end-stage liver disease, and death. The evaluation for biliary atresia is focused first on documenting obstruction (e.g., acholic stools) and later on demonstrating a compatible liver biopsy. Diagnosis is confirmed by operative cholangiography and complete dissection of the biliary tree; surgical palliative repair is undertaken during the same procedure through construction of a Roux-en-Y portoenterostomy (Fig. 73-1).

Cholestasis in the older infant and child has a different differential diagnosis. Although acute viral hepatitis is most commonly not associated with jaundice in pediatric patients, it should be considered first, not only because of its endemic nature and the necessity for the prophylactic administration of gamma globulin to family members and contacts to prevent further cases, but also because patients with icteric hepatitis occasionally develop acute hepatic

Table 73-1 Unconjugated Hyperbilirubinemia Secondary to Hepatic Physiologic Immaturity or Metabolic Defects

Unconjugated	Serum Bilirubin (mg/dl)
Neonatal physiologic jaundice (days 2-6)	6-12
Breast milk jaundice (days 10-90)	10-20
Upper GI obstruction (days 3-14)	5-10
Congenital hypothyroidism (days 6-42)*	6-20
Familial syndromes (glucuronyl transferase)	
Crigler-Najjar, type I (severe)	13-50
Crigler-Najjar, type II (moderate)	8-22
Gilbert's disease	1.5-3.0
Urinary tract infection	
Conjugated (familial only)	
Dubin-Johnson syndrome	Normal to 19 (60% is conjugated)
Rotor's syndrome	Normal to 9

*If untreated, irreversible brain damage after day 21 of life.

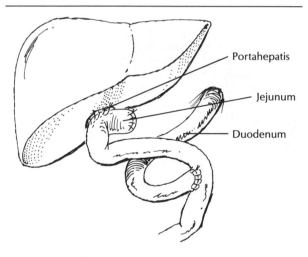

Fig. 73-1   Portoenterostomy.

Table 73-2   Treatable Causes of Neonatal Cholestasis

Condition	Diagnosis	Treatment
Sepsis	Clinical suspicion, cultures	Antibiotics
Galactosemia	(+) Reducing substance in urine	Elimination of lactose from diet
Panhypopituitarism	Hypoglycemia, low cortisol level	Hormone replacement
Congenital infection	Syphilis, toxoplasmosis, herpes	Antimicrobial therapy

failure (see Chapter 16). A history of blood or blood product transfusion or intravenous drug abuse must be sought to implicate non-A, non-B or type B hepatitis. Liver injury from drugs or toxins may cause generalized cellular injury or, as with phenothiazines or estrogen, cholestasis exclusively. Patients with chronic liver disease usually have a history of compatible symptoms or physical findings such as firm or nodular hepatomegaly or splenomegaly. Conjugated hyperbilirubinemia may also occur after liver injury from shock or ischemia.

The disorders causing extrahepatic biliary obstruction in the older infant or child are also listed below. Once intrahepatic causes have been considered and excluded, biliary obstruction must be ruled out. If abdominal pain accompanies jaundice, obstruction must be carefully sought; the additional presence of fever adds further urgency to this evaluation since suppurative, ascending cholangitis may be present. Finally, the postoperative patient may acutely develop hyperbilirubinemia that is either conjugated or unconjugated.

The primary diseases causing hyperbilirubinemia are frequently encountered in the intensive care setting. Furthermore, the degree of jaundice is enhanced by the presence of associated factors such as anemia, fever, sepsis, hypoxemia, and vascular collapse. It is essential, therefore, that a focused evalu-

---

CONJUGATED HYPERBILIRUBINEMIA IN OLDER INFANTS AND CHILDREN

Intrahepatic

Infections
  Viral hepatitis
  Fungal hepatitis
  Mycobacteria
  Rickettsia
Toxic
  Endotoxemia
  Pneumonia *(S. pneumoniae)*
  Cholestatic drugs (phenothiazines, estrogens)
  Total parenteral nutrition
  Hepatotoxic drugs (INH, acetaminophen, aspirin, others)
Chronic liver disease
  Chronic hepatitis (viral)
  Chronic hepatitis (autoimmune)
  α_1-Antitrypsin deficiency
  Wilson's disease
Collagen-vascular disease
  Sarcoidosis
  Juvenile rheumatoid arthritis (with aspirin or gold therapy)
  Systemic lupus erythematosus (with aspirin therapy)
Shock, hypoxemia
Anatomic
  Caroli's disease
Metastatic disease

Extrahepatic (biliary)

Congenital anomalies: choledochal cyst
Hydrops of the gallbladder: *Str. pyogenes, S. aureus,* leptospirosis, Kawasaki disease
Gallstones: total parenteral nutrition and furosemide use, hemolytic disease, cystic fibrosis
Cholecystitis
Pancreatitis (secondary to common bile duct swelling)
Suppurative ascending cholangitis (also intrahepatic)
Tumor: rhabdomyosarcoma, lymphoma
Sclerosing cholangitis

Postoperative jaundice

Unconjugated hyperbilirubinemia from large bilirubin load (physiologic overload)
  Hemolysis
  Transfusion of stored blood
  Hematoma (resorption)
  Blood absorbed from pleural and peritoneal cavities
Conjugated hyperbilirubinemia from intrahepatic insults
  Liver cell injury: hypotension, hypoxia, shock, halothane, other drugs, viral hepatitis
  Cholestasis: sepsis, drugs
Conjugated hyperbilirubinemia from extrahepatic injury related to specific surgery performed in right upper quadrant

ation of the patient based on age, history, physical findings, and the type of hyperbilirubinemia be made.

MONITORING AND LABORATORY TESTS

As implied in the previous discussion, a carefully directed evaluation based on age, symptoms, and signs is indicated in cases of hyperbilirubinemia. The majority of patients are asymptomatic; those infants and children with signs and laboratory evidence of liver disease must be monitored for progression (rapid rise in bilirubin or coagulopathy) and the onset of encephalopathy (see Chapter 16). In cases of unconjugated hyperbilirubinemia during the first 2

weeks of age, the patients must be carefully monitored for the rate of rise and peak in the serum bilirubin level (Table 73-3). All infants with unconjugated hyperbilirubinemia must be examined for clinical neurologic signs of kernicterus. Within a given range of serum bilirubin (Fig. 73-2), a theoretically toxic threshold may be crossed that creates a risk for permanent brain injury from kernicterus. The fundamental aspect in the laboratory evaluation of the jaundiced infant or child is first to fractionate the serum bilirubin to differentiate unconjugated from conjugated hyperbilirubinemia or to document the presence of bilirubin in the urine in the patient with conjugated hyperbilirubinemia.

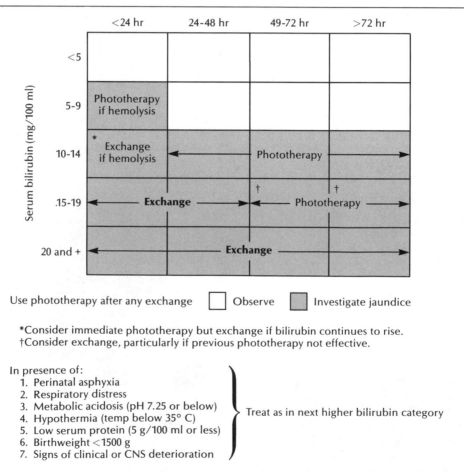

Fig. 73-2   General guidelines for the management of unconjugated hyperbilirubinemia. (Modification reproduced by permission from Brown AK. Jaundice. In Berman RE, ed. Neonatology: Diseases of the Fetus and Infant. St. Louis: CV Mosby, 1973.)

LABORATORY EVALUATION OF HYPERBILIRUBINEMIA

Unconjugated hyperbilirubinemia
Infants (general guide)

a. Hematologic
   Complete blood counts
   Blood smear (spherocytes, others)
   Reticulocyte count
   Blood type, Rh, Coombs' test
   Sickle test*
   Osmotic fragility*
   Hemoglobin electrophoresis*
   G6PD screen*
b. Infectious disease
   Urinalysis, urine culture
   Blood culture
c. Hepatic
   Daily or twice daily bilirubin level
   Total, conjugated, unconjugated
d. Metabolic, endocrine
   Urine for reducing substances
   Thyroid studies: T_3, T_4, TSH
   Maternal drug screen

Children

Follow *a, c* above

Conjugated hyperbilirubinemia
Infants (identify treatable disorders)

a. Rule out sepsis
   Complete blood counts
   White cell differential
   Blood culture
   Urine culture
b. Rule out metabolic causes
   Urine-reducing substances
   Erythrocyte galactose-1-uridylyltransferase
   Quantitative amino acids (urine, serum)
   Blood glucose
   T_3, T_4, TSH
   Sweat chloride
   Cortisol
   α_1-Antitrypsin level

c. Check for congenital infection
   VDRL (blood, CSF)
   Urine for cytomegalovirus
   Rubella titer†
   Toxoplasmosis titer†
   Viral cultures
d. Identify biliary atresia
   Stool bilirubin (i.e., negative or acholic)
   Urinary bilirubin (positive)
   Ultrasound (fasted, gallbladder present?)
   Duodenal aspiration for bile
   Biliary scintigraphy
   Liver biopsy (obstruction vs. hepatitis)
   Operative cholangiography
e. Evaluate hepatic function in all patients
   Coagulation profile
   AST, ALT
   Alkaline phosphatase
   γ-Glutamyl transpeptidase
   Bilirubin
   Total protein, albumin
Evaluate nutritional status
   Serum calcium, phosphorus
   Serum vitamins A, E, D

Children

a. Follow *a* (if febrile, *e, f,*) above.
b. Screen for hepatitis (see Chap. 16).
c. Consider chronic liver disease.
d. Check for toxins
   Drug screen (serum, urine)
   Acetaminophen level (serum)
e. Check for obstruction
   Ultrasound (mass, dilated ducts)
   CT scan
   MRI
f. Perform liver biopsy

*As needed or indicated.
†Titers of all infants must be paired with maternal titers.

Table 73-3   Monitoring of Patients With Hyperbilirubinemia (see also Chapter 4)

Unconjugated	Conjugated
Infants; observe for the following:	Infants
Rise in bilirubin	Lethargy
Lethargy	Hypotonia
Hypotonia	Fever
Fever	Ascites
Input, output	Hemorrhage
Children	Children (see Chap. 16)
No specific monitoring	Fever
	Encephalopathy

The onset of conjugated hyperbilirubinemia in the second to fourth week of life may be more indicative of vertical infections such as congenital varicella, herpes simplex, *Enterovirus,* or Ebstein-Barr virus (see Chapter 16).

TREATMENT

The principles of therapy are matched to age, diagnosis, and type of hyperbilirubinemia. Treatable causes, especially congenital hypothyroidism or sepsis, need a high index of suspicion for both early diagnosis and prompt initiation of specific therapy. For all causes of unconjugated hyperbilirubinemia in infancy the level of serum bilirubin on a particular

---

TREATMENT OF HYPERBILIRUBINEMIA

Unconjugated hyperbilirubinemia
Infants

a. Hydration
b. Enhancement of bile flow
   Encourage feeding
c. Transfusion for anemia
d. Phototherapy (see Fig. 73-2)
   Observe specific indications
   Provide hydration (100-150 ml/kg/day)
   Monitor serum albumin
   Shield eyes
   Monitor temperature
   Repeat serum bilirubin test 4 hr later
e. Exchange transfusion
   Determine blood volume
   Provide fresh whole blood
   Provide packed RBCs, reconstituted fresh frozen plasma
   Maintain normal serum albumin
   See Chapter 141

Children

a. General supportive care
b. Treatment of primary illness

Conjugated hyperbilirubinemia

Infants (NOTE: *e* and *f* apply to patients with chronic cholestasis)

a. Infectious disease
   Ampicillin (50-100 mg/kg/day)
   Aminoglycoside

b. Congenital infection
   Syphilis: penicillin
   Herpes: acyclovir
c. Metabolic, endocrine disorders
   Hypothyroidism: thyroxine
   Panhypopituitarism: hydrocortisone
   Galactosemia: removal of dietary lactose
d. Biliary atresia (Fig. 73-1)
   Portoenterostomy
   Nutritional care
   Prophylactic antibiotic for cholangitis
e. Nutrition (monitor vitamin levels)
   Formula containing medium-chain triglyceride (100-130 kcal/kg/day)
   Vitamin K (2.5 mg/day)
   Vitamin A (5000-25,000 units/day)
   Vitamin D (3500 units/day)
   Vitamin E—*d*-α-tocopherol (50-200 IU/kg/day)
   Calcium, phosphate supplements as needed
f. Enhancement of bile flow
   Phenobarbital (5 mg/kg/day)
   Cholestyramine (8 g [two packets] per day)

Children

a. See above and Chapter 16
b. Provide nutritional support (individualize to patient needs)
c. Treat primary illness
d. Reserve use of phenobarbital, cholestyramine for chronic cholestasis
e. Monitor serum levels of fat-soluble vitamins carefully

day of life will indicate the need for intervention and whether such therapy must be in the form of phototherapy or exchange transfusion. Treatment of the symptomatic infant with unconjugated hyperbilirubinemia is mandatory, regardless of the level of the serum bilirubin. The use of phenobarbital for the general therapy of hyperbilirubinemia is not advised.

In a patient with conjugated hyperbilirubinemia or cholestasis, nutritional support for all conditions is essential. Fat malabsorption from reduced bile flow is universal; fat-soluble vitamin as well as dietary long-chain triglyceride malabsorption occurs. Therapy for specific metabolic diseases is outlined in the references cited at the end of this section.

ADDITIONAL READING

Balistreri WF. Liver and biliary system. In Behrman RE, Vaughn VC, eds. Nelson Textbook of Pediatrics. Philadelphia: WB Saunders, 1987, pp 821-850.

Gartner LM, Morecki R, Lee R, Lee KS. Jaundice and liver disease. In Fanaroff AA, Martin RJ, eds. Neonatal-Perinatal Medicine. Disease of the Fetus and Infant. St. Louis: CV Mosby, 1987, pp 946-980.

74 Starvation in the PICU

Ricardo Uauy · Charles E. Mize

BACKGROUND AND PHYSIOLOGY

Intensive care may preclude normal modes of feeding or nutritional support, despite the recognition that increased metabolic demands are usually present. Endogenous body stores may be utilized effectively for a period of days without overt body wasting in patients who were previously well nourished and not chronically ill. Preexisting undernutrition from any cause shortens this period of endogenous supply, however, and the risk of significant body mass wasting, even during initial PICU management, is increased. Anthropometric and biochemical parameters that help define in-hospital undernutrition indicate that nutritional depletion in the PICU may affect up to 50% of the hospitalized population. Repetitive stress periods necessitating prolonged PICU hospitalization without adequate substrate support can clearly contribute to this occurrence. The low birthweight infant and the malnourished infant possess diminished reserves to handle acute substrate demands and may exhaust those reserves rapidly. Consequently, the risk of an evolving substrate deficit or unnoticed relative starvation based on protein-energy malnutrition may be high even during acute PICU management.

Factors Contributing to Malnutrition in the PICU

Specific conditions that contribute to the potential for malnutrition in the PICU include host, environmental, and dietary factors.

Host	Physiologic (age, activity, growth) and pathologic (infections, trauma, stress, surgery, GI disease, depleted nutrient reserves, genetic and metabolic disease, anorexia, neoplasia, burn, drug-nutrient interaction)
Environment	Thermal, psychological (stress), microbiologic, iatrogenic semistarvation
Agent—diet	Chemical composition, bioavailability and utilization of nutrient, metabolic and GI tolerance, balanced supply of essential nutrients

Host factors include both physiologic and pathologic conditions that modify nutrient requirements, including increased basic nutritional needs secondary to increased metabolic requirements of severe illness (e.g., respiratory insufficiency with increased work of breathing, fever, infection, trauma, surgery); protracted nutrient losses (e.g., short-bowel syndromes, chronic diarrhea, Fanconi's syndrome); significant preexisting low body weight or recent weight loss of 10% or more (e.g., small-for-gestational-age infant, tumor, cachexia); and intake of drugs with catabolic or nutrient-antagonist properties (e.g., tetracyclines, antimetabolite agents). All of these conditions increase nutrient requirements in the PICU patient.

Environmental factors include the thermal environment (of special relevance for the newborn, malnourished infants, and burn patients); stress, including pain (affecting nutrient utilization through increased catecholamine and corticosteroid secretion); and microbiologic conditions that increase nutrient needs. Iatrogenic semistarvation is all too traditional a practice in the PICU setting when there are prolonged periods of zero enteral intake while a patient is receiving extremely low-substrate-density IV solutions (e.g., only 5% glucose-electrolyte solutions).

Finally, dietary-related factors are important and include both the quality and quantity of the nutrient supply. Note that it is the careful balance of all essential nutrients that determines nutrient utilization.

Table 74-1   Estimating Protein-Energy Requirements in Disease Conditions

Category	Clinical Status	Percent of Resting Metabolic Energy	Percent of Protein RDA
Well child	Normal population	100	100
Low stress	Anemia, fever, mild infection, elective minor surgery	100-120	150-180
Medium stress	Skeletal trauma, debilitating chronic disease	120-140	200-250
High stress	Sepsis, severe musculoskeletal trauma, major surgery	140-170	250-300
Severe stress	Burns, rapid recovery from malnutrition	170-200	300-400

For example, if a protein lacks one essential amino acid, the utilization of nitrogen will be limited by the deficient amino acid. Furthermore, the relative excess of the remaining amino acids will be catabolized to urea. Hence not only will protein synthesis be impaired, but a greater metabolic load will be imposed on kidney and liver. In early infancy the chemical nature of the nutrient supply is critical for GI tolerance (enteral osmolar load); for renal handling of catabolic products (renal osmolar load); and for adequate bone mineralization (calcium and phosphorous product balance). The balance in the supply of all essential nutrients is critical for optimal utilization; for example, if zinc is deficient, protein utilization and growth will be restricted.

Estimation of Nutritional Needs in Disease States

The first approximation of nutritional need is based on standard recommendations, which must be adjusted for degree of depletion, increased losses, and decreased utilization in the individual patient. Under optimal conditions the individual needs of the patient can be established by calorimetry, nitrogen balance, and substrate fluxes using stable isotope tracers. These approaches serve as an initial assessment of nutritional needs. The next step is to monitor the patient's nutritional state and reserves and modify nutrient supply accordingly.

The quantitative needs for nitrogen, energy (calorie and protein requirements), and cofactors may be unexpectedly high during physiologic response to stress and disease. Increased resting energy expenditures may double, ranging from 20% to 100% above basal level, in almost all PICU patients as a consequence of hypermetabolic states associated with surgery and severe medical illness (Table 74-1).

Catabolism of body tissue can provide substrates to support this exaggerated metabolic response, which may in turn support initial tissue repair, wound healing, and key protein synthesis. This occurs because the turnover of body protein proceeds whether the patient is malnourished or not. In a patient with severe childhood protein-energy malnutrition the rates of total body protein synthesis and degradation approximate 4 to 6 g/kg/day; they rise to 9 to 10 g/kg/day in a rapid rebuilding state and stabilize at 6 to 7 g/kg/day in a postrecovery state. An important feature of protein dynamics, nonetheless, is that as exogenous protein input declines, the rate of body protein catabolism appears to increase, with an unchanged protein synthesis rate. Relative immobilization can induce net nitrogen loss. Thus the body protein pool and the closely correlated muscle mass can be significantly depleted when inadequate precursors for new protein are provided. Moreover, in patients in relatively acute hypermetabolic states, protein turnover is increased, even though there are generally increased protein synthetic demands of stress, and flux leading to potential nitrogen depletion can thus be accelerated.

Other body constituents that are essential for tissue synthesis and breakdown (e.g., minerals) may reflect similar turnover kinetics. Vitamins and essential cofactors in this metabolic flux cannot be synthesized, and although prior storage of some of them is possible, relative starvation for these nutrients will rapidly deplete the stores. Clinical vitamin and mineral deficiencies subsequently develop. The water-soluble vitamins (niacin, thiamin, riboflavin, pyridoxine, folate, cyanocobalamin, and ascorbic acid) are easily depleted, and the minerals calcium, phosphorous, sodium, potassium, chloride, and zinc are frequently affected.

The energy base for these reactions, ATP production, comes from the oxidation of glucose and fatty acid. Endogenous fatty acid derives indirectly from a quantitatively variable adipose triglyceride store, providing free fatty acids as a major transported fuel for peripheral tissue oxidation. This lipid oxidation, associated with elevated blood catecholamines and cortisol, appears to continue even when glucose is available in critically ill patients. Endogenous glucose derives directly from a minimal glycogen store and indirectly via gluconeogenesis from gluconeogenic amino acid primarily derived from skeletal muscle. The latter source, when used for glucose production, can effectively remove gluconeogenic amino acids from the amino acid pool used for protein synthesis. This loss results in a progressive quantitative loss of muscle protein. If insufficient glucose is provided to maintain glucose requirements during relative starvation periods, this loss of nitrogen can account for continuing body-protein depletion and ultimately for declining rates of endogenous protein synthesis. Lipid does not serve as a source of net carbohydrate production. Unless adequate nutritional intervention ultimately provides these several resources exogenously, the rates of other metabolic functions in the cell economy are altered, a net body mass depletion commences, and a variety of organ system deficits attendant to starvation or selective undernutrition develops. The general clinical consequences of the metabolic changes that evolve in association with suboptimal nutritional input may modify resistance to infection, specific protein synthesis, oxygen delivery to tissues, and individual organ functioning capacity.

Functional significance of starvation

Altered host defense mechanisms
Nutrition-infection interactions
Muscle wasting and decreased ventilatory function
Delayed repair process and recovery
Altered neurotransmitter formation
Decreased hepatic drug metabolism
Cardiac dysfunction
Intestinal malabsorption

Functional Significance of Starvation in the PICU

Changes that occur in general organ function during mild-to-moderate undernutrition can reflect significant and occasionally major dysfunction, depending on the severity and selectivity of the nutritional deficit. Marasmus and kwashiorkor as pure clinical syndromes are rare, but a marginal protein-energy deficit, with or without selective nutrient, mineral, or cofactor deficits, may account for a variety of suboptimal organ system dysfunctions.

Intestinal dysfunction and/or deficient intestinal surface area, either of which may be a primary cause of inability to absorb sufficient substrates enterally, may become more severe as a consequence of ongoing malnutrition that diminishes intestinal muscle mass and microvillus protein synthesis. Villus transport may be seriously diminished. Cellular immunity specifically, but also secretory and humoral immunity, may be depressed or aberrantly expressed; for example, antibody response to new antigens can be impaired. Bacterial or fungal overgrowth within the intestine may emerge, and the risk for sepsis, specific localized infections, and delayed healing of local infections and wounds increases with even relative starvation.

Respiratory capacity diminishes, with diminished and weakened respiratory accessory and intercostal muscle mass; diminished gas flow rates and lessened ability to mobilize lung secretions may contribute to a heightened risk for pneumonitis. In addition impaired muscle work performance, lower functional residual capacity, and altered response to carbon dioxide result in the hypoventilation typical of malnourished patients. It is commonly observed that unless the patient is anabolic, he will fail to wean effectively from the ventilator. Hematopoietic stem cell maturation is retarded, anemia and diminished oxygen-carrying capacity occur, and diverse hematologic aberrations can appear (e.g., altered erythrocyte membrane transport, increased susceptibility to DIC associated with enhanced antithrombin activity).

Peripheral nerve conduction may be slowed, and over even relatively short periods, head growth may be retarded. Brain neurotransmitters are affected by lack of amino acid precursors. Tryptophan is necessary for serotonin production and phenylalanine or tyrosine for production of catecholamines. In addition glutamine and glycine play roles in nervous conduction.

Hepatic albumin synthesis ultimately can be reduced, resulting in hypoalbuminemia and clinical edema. Functional hepatic metabolic adaptations such as hepatic drug handling may be significantly

Table 74-2   Basic Calorimetric and Energy Data: Infants (calories per gram)

	Gross Energy*	Digested Energy†	Metabolizable Energy (oral)‡	Metabolizable Energy (IV)
Glucose	3.74	3.7	3.7	3.4
Starch	4.18	4.1	4.1	—
Long-chain triglyceride (average)	9.45	8.0	8.0	9.4
Medium-chain triglyceride	8.75	7.5	7.5	8.0
Protein (average)	5.65	5.1	4.0	4.4
Glycine	3.12	3.0	2.1	2.2

*Bomb calorimetry.
†Digested energy equals gross energy minus fecal energy loss.
‡Metabolizable energy equals digested energy minus urinary energy loss.

altered when selective hepatic drug-metabolizing enzyme systems manifest reduced activity, yielding longer biologic drug half-lives or altered pharmacokinetic clearances for diverse drugs ranging from cefoxitin and chloramphenicol to phenobarbital and thiopental.

Blood volume increase occurring with severe protein deprivation will enhance the risk for heart failure. Cardiac hemodynamics may be further affected as myocardial mass is depleted with significant protein starvation. Pancreatic exocrine dysfunction, selective endocrine changes (e.g., increased thyroxine-binding globulin), renal dysfunction with increased risk for bacteriuria, aberrant body temperature control, and psychomotor changes have all been variously reported in long-term nonselective pediatric undernutrition. In some instances these effects may only reflect different aspects of disordered separate nutritional factors, but in other instances severely suboptimal nutrition may allow many of them to be evident sequentially and/or concomitantly. Superimposed on these symptom complexes specific vitamin and/or mineral deficiency syndromes may be seen.

Special Situations

The low birthweight infant presents special nutritional problems, since the infant has not accrued the full complement of body minerals and stores of the full-term infant, and depletion of these body reserves occurs relatively rapidly compared to full-term infants and older infants and children. The maturing organ systems of low birthweight infants may metabolize minerals and substrates at varying rates, and absorption of nutrient materials is generally less efficient than in more mature infants and children. Recognition of these differences in net metabolizable energy from respective energy resources will help define nutrition restitution needs more accurately (Table 74-2).

The caloric equivalent of weight gain in the normal low birthweight infant has been estimated at approximately 4.5 to 5.5 kcal/g weight gain. Adult estimates average 3 to 4 kcal/g during early weight loss, and 6 to 8 kcal/g during progressive weight loss. The energy cost of depositing adipose tissue is estimated at 7 to 8 kcal/g. When patients are severely ill and manifest a hypermetabolic state, additional input of energy and nutrients must be supplied. Even without evident initial undernutrition, large numbers of calories are needed to provide the energy for the hypermetabolism engendered by the illness. Direct measurements in severely ill pediatric patients are not generally available, but extrapolation from adult data yields estimates that can be applied to the PICU population. The caloric needs appear to vary, depending on the particular pathophysiolgic state (Table 74-1).

The energy needs have been reasonably well established clinically for recovery from classic childhood marasmus (150 or more kcal/kg/day). Increased oxygen consumption and increased metabolic flux or turnover of body components have furnished estimates of the energy needs during severe illness (Table 74-1). The addition of appropriately balanced exogenous amino acid mixtures to resupply the pool for new synthesis and to reduce the net conversion of amino acids to catabolic end products will most efficiently bring about protein sparing and positive nitrogen balance. The need for additional levels of some trace minerals has been established (zinc, 200 μg/kg/day; copper, 80 μg/kg/day enterally), but the specific metal-substrate interactions or competitions that affect gut absorption of these minerals have not been fully defined. The importance of these trace minerals is illustrated by the role that one such mineral, zinc, plays in cellular immunity. Enzymic cofactor and structural roles exist for other trace minerals, and kinetic fluxes dictate the need for nutritional repletion and maintenance, although at requirement levels that are poorly defined at present. Essential fatty acid needs are similarly recognized for precursor and possibly structural membrane roles; the recommended daily requirement is 2% to 4% of the net daily enteral caloric intake (for normal metabolic processes) and is based on normal intestinal absorption; more may be necessary during nutritional restitution.

MONITORING AND LABORATORY TESTS

Optimally, assessment of nutritional status is initiated when the patient is first seen. This assessment must be repeated at regular intervals at least every 3 to 4 days during a protracted hospitalization and should include the following steps.

1. Clinical history, with an estimate of the duration of stress and nutritional deprivation and an estimate of actual nutrient intake over a defined period (monthly or more frequently) (Special arrangements with the dietary department may be necessary to achieve accurate recording of caloric intake.)
2. Physical clues to nutritional integrity (continuous observation)
   a. Energy and/or protein: Estimate of adipose mass and muscle mass (separately) by clinical examination and by objective anthropometric measures.
   b. Cofactors (vitamins, minerals, essential fatty acids): Hair character, mucous membrane and skin changes, nail bed and ear cartilage changes.
3. Objective anthropometric measurements (weekly)
   a. Simple grid-charted percentiles for height, weight, head circumference, and length (and the age at which the measurement coincides with the 50th percentile).
   b. Percentage of expected weight adjusted for length and/or age. An estimate of expected weight (kg) for length (when length is 50 to 95 cm) may be derived as follows:

   $$\text{Male weight} = (0.24 \times \text{Length}) - 8.28$$
   $$\text{Female weight} = (0.24 \times \text{Length}) - 8.13$$

   For example, a boy 81.9 cm long would be expected to have a weight of 11.4 kg (50th percentile).
   c. Standard deviation (Z scores) units away from mean expected for age: observed value minus expected value/standard deviation (SD) for given age and gender. If values of weight for length are lower than minus 1 SD, consider as evidence for acute depletion of a moderate degree; if values are minus 2, consider possibility of severe depletion. Weight for age is a sensitive indicator of nutritional status in infants but not for children more than 2 years old. Length for age and weight for age may be compromsied by early malnutrition; stunting may be partially responsive to administration of aggressive nutritional support. Linear growth is usually not responsive to good nutrition if stunting occurred in the first 2 years of life. The minimal goal for nutritional therapy in the PICU setting is normalizing weight for length or preventing drops beyond minus 0.5 SD away from mean.
   d. Midarm circumference/head circumference ratio (each measured in centimeters). The norm from infancy to age 4 years is 0.33 or greater.
   e. Triceps skinfold thickness. Compare with graphs of norm for age.
   f. Consider, if available, tomography and total body potassium, water, or electrical conductivity measurements to estimate more accurately lean body mass.
4. Laboratory indices
   a. General: Hb, serum albumin, glucose, potassium, and phosphorus values must be assessed frequently (at least weekly).
   b. Specific: Measure serum proteins with shorter half-lives than albumin to assess more rapid

changes in hepatic protein synthesis (e.g., prealbumin, retinol-binding protein), and measure blood levels of trace minerals (e.g., zinc, copper, manganese, selenium, iodine, chromium) to assess unexpectedly large losses or unusual requirements.

c. Timed urine collections (continuing at least 24 hours) for urinary urea nitrogen value to estimate gross nitrogen balance, urinary creatinine excretion to estimate sequential muscle mass restitution, and urinary methylhistidine excretion (on exactly known intake) to estimate gross muscle catabolism.

d. Blood drug levels to estimate biologic serum decay or half-life (e.g., blood levels two or more times after the drug injection to calculate logarithmic blood concentrations as a function of time).

e. Periodic long-bone roentgenograms and alkaline phosphatase levels to assess the occurrence of osteopenia or rickets.

f. Antigen skin tests of cellular immunity (when prior antigen exposure can be expected to have sensitized the patient adequately) to assess immune competence.

5. Continuing estimates of metabolic energy requirements (daily)

a. Percentage increments for degree of expected hypermetabolic status if present (Table 74-1).

b. Amounts attributed to presence of fever (12% increase in energy needs per degree Centigrade), muscular activity, and respiratory (muscle) efforts.

c. Ongoing normal growth and development of organ systems (4 to 5 kcal/g weight gain).

TREATMENT

The clinical goals of nutritional intervention therapy include wound healing, nonfluid weight gain associated with positive nitrogen balance and protein accretion, brain growth, and normal mental and motor development. The management decisions to achieve these ends must be based on a plan that progresses through the following steps on a regular and recurring basis:

1. Nutritional evaluation (assessment of status)
2. Diagnosis of qualitative and quantitative nutritional deficits (energy, protein, minerals, vitamins)
3. Detailed determination (qualitative and quantitative) of substrate needs
4. Nutritional therapy implementation by the enteral and/or parenteral route (see Chapters 149 and 150)

Complications of Nutritional Support

Complications and risks for morbidity and mortality are associated primarily with parenteral nutrition, but some risks such as aspiration of formula or gastric contents occur with enteral hyperalimentation. The complications may be categorized in three groups:

1. Infection, which is primarily associated with parenteral catheter
2. Metabolic alterations such as vitamin or mineral imbalances, hypophosphatemia, hypercalciuria, osteopenia, metabolic bone disease, lactic acidosis (with increased glucose load), cardiac overload/failure, cholestasis, nitrogen imbalance, hyper- or hypoglycemia
3. Technical difficulties, which are primarily mechanical problems with catheter such as breakage, blockage, perforation, or tissue migration.

Infectious complications can occur with total parenteral nutrition (TPN), and minimizing the risk of infection and sepsis should be the first priority for TPN programs.

Metabolic risks of nutritional restitution often result from a need for a different balance of nutrients during repletion than during normal nutrition. This need is either not perceived or not easily achieved. For example, during active anabolism, the requirement for macrominerals (e.g., potassium, phosphorus) may significantly increase. If exogenous supplies are not increased, plasma levels of these minerals may fall to low levels. A requirement for administration of extra tocopherol if unsaturated essential fatty acids (EFA) (ratio of tocopherol/EFA >0.5) are given has long been recognized. Insufficient provision of either may be associated with the development of mild-to-severe essential fatty acid deficiency or with hemolysis. Occasional patients receiving a high glucose input develop lactic acidosis. Patients with severe pulmonary function abnormalities may be particularly sensitive to high glucose input either enterally or parenterally and have increased risk for hypercarbia because of the oxidation of glucose to carbon dioxide. Critically ill patients may have glucose intolerance as a result of an apparent insulin resistance, with hyperinsulinemia and elevated catecholamine and/or cortisol blood levels; exogenously provided insulin may help overcome this resistance (see Chapter 150).

Moreover, when it may not be possible to initiate nutritional support with high-caloric enteral or parenteral solutions, too great an input of nutrient solutions or formula (of low-caloric density) given in a legitimate attempt to provide sufficient net nutrients may increase the risk for fluid overload. Such risk is enhanced by increased intravascular volume, which develops in patients with severe protein malnutrition. Cardiac muscle wasting, which can develop during malnutrition, may also predispose the patient to heart failure if too rapid refeeding is instituted.

Osteopenia, which may be evident in low birthweight infants, may evolve into overt rickets in the absence of sufficient mineral deposition as growth occurs. Cholestasis can develop in the course of TPN but rarely occurs with total enteral nutrition support (see Chapter 149). Finally, technical problems of nutrient supply occasionally contribute to morbidity associated with nutritional support but can generally be anticipated or readily recognized for corrective intervention (see Chapters 149 and 150).

ADDITIONAL READING

Beisel WR. Nutrition and infection. In Linder MC, ed. Nutritional Biochemistry and Metabolism. New York: Elsevier, 1985, pp 369-394.

Castillo-Duran C, Fisberg M, Valenzuela A, Egana JI, Uauy R. Controlled trial of copper supplementation during the recovery from marasmus. Am J Clin Nutr 37:898-903, 1983.

Castillo-Duran C, Heresi G, Fisberg M, Uauy R. Controlled trial of zinc supplementation during recovery from malnutrition: Effects on growth and immune function. Am J Clin Nutr 45:602-608, 1987.

Dhopeshwarkar GA. Effects of malnutrition on brain development. In Dhopeshwarkar GA. Nutrition and Brain Development. New York: Plenum, 1983, pp 49-83.

• Merritt RT, Suskind RM. Nutritional survey of hospitalized patients. Am J Clin Nutr 32:1320-1326, 1979.

• Mize CE, Cunningham C, Teitell BC, Strickland AD, Dickey E, McCarty C, Parker T. Undernutrition of pediatric inpatients: Repeated nutrition status evaluation. Nutr Support Serv 4:27-39, 1984.

Parsons HG, Francoeur TE, Howland P. The nutritional status of hospitalized children. Am J Clin Nutr 33:1140-1146, 1980.

Pollac M, Wiley J, Kanter R, Holbrook R. Malnutrition in critically ill infants and children. JPEN 6:26-24, 1982.

• Stewart S, Uauy R, Kennard B, Waller DA, Andrews W. Mental and motor development correlates in patients with end-stage biliary atresia awaiting liver transplantation. Pediatrics 79:882-888, 1987.

Vesell ES. Effect of dietary factors on drug disposition in normal human subjects. In Finley TW, Schwass DE, eds. Xenobiotic Metabolism—Nutritional Effects. Washington, D.C.: American Chemical Society, 1985, pp 61-75.

75 Poisoning: General Considerations

Frances C. Morriss

BACKGROUND

Although accidental ingestion of nonnutritional substances is common among children, most of these incidences are not serious enough to warrant a visit to an emergency department. The most recent statistics available from the National Clearing House of Poison Control Centers indicate that approximately 130,000 pediatric ingestions occur each year; 86,500 occur in children less than 5 years of age. The peak age for ingestion is 2 years. The most common agents are easily found in the home and include medications, particularly benzodiazepines, antidepressants, salicylates, theophylline, and antihistamines, cleaning agents, cosmetics, plants, ethanol, insecticides, and petroleum products. Almost all are ingested orally.

Management by telephone is sufficient for 85% of these ingestions. Standard protocols developed by poison control centers can determine the potential severity of the ingestant, whether or not hospitalization is indicated, and what type of therapy to institute at home. In addition to a child who has ingested a potentially lethal amount of an agent, any child less than 6 months of age, any child known to have been the victim of a previous ingestion, or any child for whom the reliability of the history seems in question should be evaluated in an emergency department. For children treated at home an essential part of the management must be follow-up at regular intervals during the first 24 hours after the initial call to determine the ongoing status of the patient and the effects of therapy. Acute intoxication or substance abuse withdrawal must be suspected in any patient presenting in the emergency department with unusual symptoms or multiple system involvement.

Recently poisonings severe enough to necessitate a PICU admission have been examined. Over a 3-year period the 105 patients admitted for acute ingestions represented 3.1% of the total PICU admissions; 42% of these children were less than 3 years of age, and 33% were more than 12 years of age. These admissions represented 0.4% of annual ingestions evaluated by a poison control center serving a population of 2 million persons and 15% of patients requiring hospitalization because of the ingestion. No child died of an ingestion despite the severity of symptoms necessitating admission (Table 75-1). In general treatment was supportive, nonspecific, and interventionist, and discharge occurred within 48 hours of admission. Children older than 12 years were more likely to have attempted suicide than to have suffered an accidental ingestion.

Table 75-1 Indications for PICU Admission for 105 Cases of Poisoning*

Indication	Cases
Coma	55
Respiratory insufficiency	13
Ingestion of a potential lethal dose	13
Cardiac monitoring for asymptomatic tricyclic antidepressant overdose	12
Arrhythmias	6
Convulsions	3
Shock	1
Hepatic failure	1
Extreme agitation	1

*From LaCroix J, Gaudveault P, Gauthier M. Admission to a pediatric intensive care unit for poisoning: A review of 105 cases. Crit Care Med 17:749, 1989. Copyright by Williams & Wilkins.

MONITORING AND LABORATORY TESTS

Multisystem involvement is common in severe intoxications, and multiple organ failure may occur (see Chapter 22). Symptoms referable to specific organs should be monitored as they occur, with particular attention paid to cardiorespiratory and renal function. A scoring system such as the Glasgow Coma Scale can be extremely helpful in assessing CNS function over time. Monitoring and observation should be continuous initially and then decrease as the stability of various organ systems is known.

Assessment of the respiratory system should include a chest roentgenogram to assess for possible aspiration, particularly if the patient has a history of emesis, choking, cyanosis, or apnea, and an arterial blood gas and pH determination. Until adequacy of ventilation is known, continuous oxygen saturation monitoring and/or transcutaneous oxygen and carbon dioxide monitoring will be helpful. Close observation for increased work of breathing (grunting, use of accessory muscles of respiration, tachypnea) and for changes in respiratory rhythm and auscultation for abnormal breath sounds, rales, or wheezing must also be done.

Cardiovascular function should be assessed in the usual ways (see Chapters 11 and 12); if hypovolemia exists, placement of central venous, intra-arterial, and bladder catheters will allow more precise monitoring, particularly in situations in which there is little or no response to volume resuscitation.

Frequent neurologic examinations are mandatory; findings must be recorded so that subtle changes in consciousness and activity can be followed by multiple observers. EEG and ICP monitoring, cranial CT scan or MRI, and CSF analysis may be indicated.

If symptoms persist, GI function must be assessed through frequent abdominal examinations, including girth measurements, the output of the nasogastric tube, serial abdominal roentgenograms, and analysis of gastric contents for pH, blood, electrolyte content, and toxins. Hepatic and pancreatic function may need to be evaluated as well. Gastroscopy and esophagoscopy may be needed for evaluation of GI mucosal damage.

Urinary output must be measured hourly until adequacy of renal function is established or if forced diuresis is used as a therapeutic mode. Routine urinalysis must be done.

Skin and mucous membranes must be inspected closely for burns, bruises, puncture wounds, bites,

Table 75-2 Additional Laboratory Tests

Suspected Toxin or Specific Problem	Laboratory Determination
Hepatotoxin	Hepatic enzymes (ALT, AST, GGT, alkaline phosphatase)
	Albumin
	Ammonia
	Bilirubin
	Serum drug half-lives
	Lactate, pyruvate
	Glucose
	PT, PTT
	Amylase
Nephrotoxin	BUN, creatinine
	Serum electrolytes (Na, K, Cl, Mg, Cu, PO_4)
	Serum and urinary osmolality
Myocardial injury	Serial ECG
	Echocardiogram
	Serial cardiac enzymes
Rhabdomyolysis	Serum and urinary myoglobin
	CPK
Carbon monoxide	CO, oxygen saturation
	P_{50}
Hemolysis	Serial hematocrit
	Coombs' test
	Type and crossmatch
Persistent acidosis	Serial venous or arterial blood gas and pH determination
	Serum and urinary organic acids
	Glucose, amylase
	Urinary pH
	Serum and urinary osmolality
Uncontrolled bleeding/anticoagulant	PT, PTT
	Platelets
	Bleeding time
	Fibrinogen
	Fibrin split products
	Type and crossmatch
Coma	Toxicology screen for narcotics, sedatives
	Serum electrolytes
	Ammonia
	Glucose
	Serum ethanol
	CT scan
	CSF analysis
	Heavy metal screening

Table 75-3   Frequently Found Drugs (1982) Listed in Order of Decreasing Frequency*

| Police Laboratory | Coroner's Laboratory | | Reference Laboratory |
	All Cases	Poisonings	
Cannabis	Ethanol	Benzodiazepines	Benzodiazepines
Tripelennamine	Benzodiazepines	Carbon monoxide	Ethanol
Pentazocine (Talwin)	Lidocaine	Ethanol	Barbiturates
Cocaine	Acetaminophen	Tricyclic antidepressants	Acetaminophen
Benzodiazepines	Salicylate	Opiates	Salicylate
Phencyclidine (PCP)	Tricyclic antidepressants	Barbiturates	Sympathomimetic
	Barbiturates	Acetaminophen	amines
	Opiates		Phenothiazines
	Carbon monoxide		Tricyclic antidepressants
			Opiates

*From Sunshine I. Analytic toxicology. In Klassen CD, Amdur MO, Doull J, eds. Casarett's and Doull's Toxicology. The Basic Science of Poisons, 3rd ed. New York. Macmillan, 1986, p 859.

and other signs of trauma. Fluorescent ophthalmic examination can diagnose a corneal abrasion or laceration or other injury. Musculoskeletal examination for possible limb trauma must be done; appropriate skeletal films must be obtained as indicated.

Hypothermia and hyperthermia must be followed closely, and continuous temperature monitoring may be needed.

Table 75-2 lists other screening tests that may be useful for specific conditions.

POISON IDENTIFICATION

Every effort should be made to identify the ingestant. The family or caretaker must be questioned closely to determine if the suspected agent is known. The types of medications available in the home and their whereabouts must be determined. Any substance found near the patient should be brought in for identification. Other helpful information includes estimated time of the ingestion, probable amount taken if it can be estimated, time of last meal, type of therapy already tried and results of such therapy, and ongoing changes in the child's status from the time of the first symptom. Features that affect absorption of an orally ingested substance include presence of food in the stomach (impedes absorption), pH of agent ingested (acids more rapidly absorbed than bases), and form of the agent (liquids absorbed more rapidly). The agent's container can provide information since the Federal Hazardous Substance Act of 1960 requires

that labels for dangerous household chemicals list ingredients. Information on labels about possible antidotes and treatment regimens may be misleading, and a more definitive source such as a poison control center must be consulted for treatment.

Urinary, blood, and gastric content samples must be sent for toxicology screening as well as any agent, if unknown, brought in with the victim. The more accurate the information that accompanies any of these samples about the suspected nature of the ingestion, the more likely the toxicology screening will be able to provide useful information. Qualitative information is more helpful in planning initial therapy than quantitative levels of drug; however, quantitative information may be more useful in predicting outcome, particularly if lethal levels of the drug are documented. The clinician must be aware of what drugs the toxicologic screening actually examines; a negative screening result does not necessarily indicate the absence of all toxic agents. Several studies, including one from the National Institutes of Health, have shown that 80% to 90% of all acute poisonings involve approximately 20 substances (Table 75-3); analysis for these agents should be available from the toxicology laboratory. Furthermore, comprehensive analysis is likely to be time consuming and nonproductive unless very specific information is being sought. Often a reliable reference laboratory may be used for more exotic analyses.

Even if only one agent is suspected in an acute

intoxication, screening for multiple agents should be done since studies have shown that as many as 25% of victims may have ingested more than a single agent.

TREATMENT

Treatment must be dual, but the first step must be to assure patient stability. Supportive therapy for life- or limb-threatening conditions in the form of ventilation, volume resuscitation, treatment of dysrhythmias or seizures, and care of wounds or other trauma must be instituted immediately (see Chapters 8-10, 14, 16, and 23). The second step, when the patient's vital functions are stabilized, should include measures to decrease toxin absorption, increase toxin elimination, and administer any known specific antidotes that are indicated. Nonspecific antidotes in particular and medullary stimulants such as caffeine, picrotoxin, doxapram, and nikethamide are not recommended to reverse CNS depression. Doses necessary to achieve respiratory stimulation approach toxic drug levels associated with seizure activity. Severe side effects such as hypertension, bradycardia, hyperthermia, psychosis, and emesis are common. In most cases the stimulating effect is short lived, and multiple doses would be needed to sustain any positive effect. Support of the airway and mechanical ventilation are safer forms of treatment.

Decreasing Absorption of Toxin

Emptying the stomach is the traditional method of limiting absorption of a toxic ingestant; however, some controversy exists as to whether this is more efficacious than using an agent to bind the ingested toxin. Much of the evidence is anecdotal or based on adult or animal experimentation and may not be relevant to clinical pediatric problems. The most commonly used emetic produces a mean recovery of approximately 30% of stomach contents. The amount of ingested material recovered is usually <50% and is highly variable. Therefore reliance on induced emesis to limit absorption of a toxin is often not justified, and other measures must be used in addition to emptying the stomach.

Activated charcoal

Use of activated charcoal as a binder of toxin reduces absorption of remaining stomach contents by a greater amount than all other methods; it is unclear whether a combination of methods is superior to use of activated charcoal alone. Gastric lavage after administration of activated charcoal may be better than either procedure by itself. One of the side effects of induced emesis may be persistent vomiting, which might interfere with subsequent retention of charcoal. In favor of induced emesis is the fact that ipecac can be obtained inexpensively without a prescription and can be given at home, thus decreasing the period of time from ingestion to the initiation of therapy designed to reduce absorption.

Emesis

Gastric emptying is accomplished by either induction of emesis or by gastric lavage. Many products ingested by children are nontoxic and require no treatment or removal from the stomach. Solid objects (unless accompanied by symptoms suggestive of gastric perforation or obstruction), petroleum distillates, and acidic or alkaline corrosives should not be removed from the stomach. Endoscopy may be needed, however, to assess the integrity of esophageal or gastric mucosa (see Chapter 84) or to remove a foreign body. Induction of emesis is also contraindicated if the patient is less than 6 months of age or if the patient is obtunded, comatose, convulsing, or likely to become so within 30 to 60 minutes. In all these instances there is a risk of aspiration of stomach contents secondary to decreased ability to protect the airway (i.e., weak or absent protective airway reflexes). Emesis can be induced with an ipecac preparation or apomorphine (Table 75-4), both of which stimulate vomiting by a CNS mechanism. Some concern exists about the toxicity of ipecac, which contains emetine, an alkaloid that in large doses can cause cardiac dysrhythmias. Abuse of ipecac by anorectic or bulimic patients has caused severe myocardial toxicity. Used as directed (small doses, not repetitively) ipecac is safe; the American Academy of Pediatrics recommends ipecac as one of five home measures for anticipatory poison prevention and treatment in small children. As stated previously, one obvious advantage of ipecac is that it can be given at home. It has proved to be a very safe drug in this setting; emesis is induced on an average within 20 to 30 minutes in 96% of patients.

Apomorphine, a derivative of morphine, is as effective as ipecac in producing emesis (98% of patients), usually within 5 minutes of administration. There can be significant respiratory depression with therapeutic doses, especially in children, and a nar-

Table 75-4   Use of Emetics

Emetic	Dose	Side Effects	Comments
Ipecac preparation	<6 mo: do not use 6-12 mo: 5-10 ml PO with 2-4 oz fluid 1-12 yr: 15 ml PO with 4-8 oz fluid >12 yr: 30 ml PO with 8-16 oz fluid	Protracted emesis (5%) Diarrhea (16% to 20%) Drowsiness (20%) Diaphoresis Fever Irritability	Nonprescription drug; may be given at home Bound by charcoal May repeat dose if no emesis in 30 min Milk and food delay onset of emesis Large volumes or cold fluids promote gastric emptying
Apomorphine	0.07 mg/kg SC	Respiratory depression CNS depression	Cannot be given at home Antidote: naloxone, 0.2 mg/kg IV or IM Do not use if ingestant is CNS depressant No oral preparation

cotic antagonist should be given after emesis occurs. Other disadvantages of apomorphine include the absence of an oral preparation; therefore the patient must be brought to an emergency department to receive the drug parenterally. Since the antiemetic effect depends on dopaminergic pathways, it may be ineffective with ingestion of phenothiazines or other dopamine blockers.

The efficacy of other emetics such as mechanical stimulation of the posterior pharynx and ingestion of diluted dishwashing detergent solutions remains unclear.

Gastric lavage

Gastric lavage is indicated if induction of emesis fails, the patient cannot protect his airway (comatose or convulsing), and removal of stomach contents is deemed necessary because of ingestion of a highly toxic substance such as camphor or strychnine or a very large amount of toxin. The yield will be affected by the physical form of the ingested toxin (solid, liquid), how rapidly it is absorbed from the stomach, whether gastric emptying is inhibited by the ingestant, and the time since the ingestion. To minimize the chances of aspiration the patient must be placed in the left lateral position with the head down. If there is an absent gag reflex, the patient must be intubated, preferably with a cuffed endotracheal tube, before lavage. Studies have shown that the most effective emptying occurs with use of large volumes of lavage fluid and the largest tube that can be passed into the stomach. Since nasogastric tubes are limited

in size by the size of the nares, a large oral single-lumen tube (32 to 40 F) is preferred. After the tube is inserted, gastric contents should be aspirated and the first sample saved for toxicologic laboratory analysis. Lavage fluid should be warm 0.9% sodium chloride solution to prevent loss of electrolytes and body heat. Lavage is performed with aliquots of 15 ml/kg until the return fluid is clear or until 5 to 10 L have been used. Larger aliquots may encourage gastric emptying. Care must be taken to retrieve all fluid instilled into the stomach to prevent distention. The most common complication of lavage is aspiration pneumonitis; esophageal trauma and laryngospasm with desaturation have also been reported. If appropriate, a specific antidote or activated charcoal and a cathartic may be instilled at the completion of the procedure and the lavage tube removed.

Antidotes

Antidotes change the nature of a poison by rendering it less toxic or by preventing its absorption. Activated charcoal is the most commonly used nonspecific antidote. Several specific antidotes are as follows*:

1. Ammonia (5 ml in 100 ml of water) reacts with formaldehyde to form a nontoxic product, hexamethylenetetramine. Ammonia solution must be instilled first, followed by lavage as described previously.

*Modified by permission from Levin DL, Morriss FC, Moore G. A Practical Guide to Pediatric Intensive Care, 2nd ed. St. Louis: CV Mosby, 1984, p 393.

2. Sodium bicarbonate 5% solution can be used to combine with ferrous sulfate to form an insoluble salt, ferrous carbonate, which must be mechanically removed by lavage. Otherwise bicarbonate is *not* recommended for neutralizing acid products; the production of carbon dioxide may cause gastric distention, and the production of heat may damage an already irritated mucosa.

3. Starch solution, 80 g in 1 L of water, neutralizes iodine; lavage should be performed until there is loss of blue color in the return fluid.

4. Dairy or evaporated milk may be used as a demulcent to coat the gastric mucosa and decrease irritation; however, the presence of such a material may hinder endoscopic evaluation if it is needed. General lavage is not indicated for ingestion of corrosives (see Chapter 84).

5. The universal antidote (a mixture of charcoal [burned toast], tannic acid [tea], and magnesium oxide [Milk of Magnesia]) is ineffective, may be harmful, and must not be used.

6. Baking soda, lemon juice, and vinegar should never be given in an effort to neutralize an ingested acid or alkali. The ensuing exothermic reaction can cause further mucosal damage and promote emesis with reexposure of the esophageal mucosa to caustic agents.

The most commonly used and readily available antidote is activated charcoal, prepared by pyrolysis of organic material and activation with an oxidizing gas flow at a high temperature to produce a fine network of pores. It is an inert, nontoxic, and nonabsorbable material of vast surface area that absorbs a wide variety of organic substances. Agents not well absorbed include mineral acids, strong bases, boric acid, cyanide, ferrous sulfate, lithium, and other ionized small molecules. If the ingestion does not fall into one of the above categories, it is safe to assume that activated charcoal will be effective. Toxin absorption depends on the ratio of activated charcoal to toxin (10:1) on a weight basis. The amount of ingested toxin is often unknown; therefore a large dose of charcoal is recommended. In vivo observations document the efficacy of a relative charcoal excess as opposed to a calculated dose, possibly because food, digestive fluids, and other by-products may compete with the toxin for binding sites on charcoal. Absorbed material is retained tenaciously until the charcoal is eliminated from the GI tract. The rec-

ommended dose is 25 to 30 g for a child less than 12 years of age and 50 to 180 g for older children and adults. Charcoal is available as a powder (1 tablespoon equals 3 to 6 g), a premixed aqueous solution, or a suspension in 10% sorbitol. Charcoal capsules and tablets, which may not contain the activated form, are not recommended. Charcoal is usually administered as a slurry; poor palatability may be a problem, although in one study 86% of children presenting with an ingestion drank all of it. In general flavorings or food added to charcoal to make it more acceptable have decreased its absorbency. Acceptance may be increased by placing the slurry in an opaque container or a bottle with an enlarged nipple opening. If charcoal is not taken within a reasonable time, it should be given via a nasogastric or orogastric tube. A recently introduced superactivated charcoal (Superchar), which has a surface area and absorptive capacity three times that of the usual preparation, can be given in a smaller dose and volume with equal results. Adverse effects are minimal; rapid administration may cause gagging and emesis. Repeated doses may cause constipation.

In recent years multiple-dose charcoal therapy (GI dialysis) has been demonstrated as more effective than a single dose for a number of drugs, including theophylline, phenobarbital, digoxin, aspirin, and tricyclic antidepressants. Significantly shorter half-lives for drugs are seen with this method. Increased drug excretion may occur by any of the following mechanisms: interruption of the enterohepatic drug cir-

---

**GUIDELINES FOR
MULTIPLE-DOSE CHARCOAL***

Administer routine initial charcoal/cathartic dose at presentation.
Administer one half of the above dose (without cathartic) every 4 hr.
Cathartic may be administered every 12 hr if patient has not had a stool.
Endpoint: nontoxic blood levels or lack of symptoms or signs of clinical toxicity after 12-24 hr.

---

*From Tenenbien M. Pediatric toxicology—current controversies and recent advances. Curr Probl Pediatr 16:214, 1986.

culation (drug reentry into GI tract via biliary excretion), interruption of the enterogastric drug circulation (drug reentry into GI tract from blood perfusing intestinal organs, often aided by acidic gastric pH), and diffusion of drug back into the bowel lumen because the continued presence of charcoal produces a low ultraluminal concentration gradient. This third mechanism is probably the most significant one. Serum drug levels of ingestants have been shown to increase when multiple-dose charcoal therapy is stopped. Since this type of intervention can be started easily and quickly, it should be used even if a more invasive procedure such as dialysis or hemoperfusion is indicated.

Cathartics

If the activated charcoal was not mixed with sorbitol, saline cathartics are usually administered to prevent constipation and increase elimination of the charcoal-toxin complex. The mechanism of action of the saline cathartics depends on the poor absorbability of certain salts. When these salts are introduced into the GI tract, increased intraluminal osmolality causes retention of water and indirectly stimulates peristalsis and defecation. Used alone cathartics do not consistently decrease drug absorption. Cathartics are contraindicated following ingestion of caustic agents, following bowel surgery, or in the presence of ileus. Sodium-containing agents must be avoided in patients with hypertension and congestive heart failure; magnesium-containing cathartics are contraindicated in patients with renal insufficiency, ingestion of a nephrotoxic agent, or presence of myoglobinuria. Increased GI fluid and electrolyte losses may occur, and close monitoring of the patient's volume status is necessary. Serial electrolyte monitoring must include calcium, phosphate, and magnesium determinations. Magnesium sulfate (250 mg/kg PO), sodium sulfate (250 mg/kg PO), and magnesium citrate (4 ml/kg PO) as single or multiple doses are commonly used. Osmotic catharsis will be induced when sorbitol is the emulsicant for activated charcoal, and in this case a saline cathartic is unnecessary. Enemas do not enhance removal of orally ingested agents since absorption occurring in the small bowel is not affected.

Endoscopy has been used to remove agents, primarily gastric concretions, bezoars, and foreign bodies, from the GI tract. Whole-bowel irrigation, developed as a preparation for colonoscopy, has been used as a method of bowel decontamination, and anecdotal reports suggest it is efficacious. The procedure involves the administration of large amounts of a special electrolyte solution (GoLYTELY) orally. Fluid and electrolyte imbalances have been reported, and the usefulness of this method is yet to be determined.

Increasing Toxin Elimination
Urinary excretion

Increased urinary output or a change in urinary pH may be used to increase elimination of certain toxic ingestants. For drugs that are excreted in proportion to urinary output (alcohols, barbiturates, salicylates, amphetamines, bromides), increasing urinary output from 3 to 6 ml/kg/hr is helpful. Decreased distal tubular reabsorption occurs because exposure of the toxin to the absorptive sites is shortened and because in the presence of high urinary flow the blood-urine osmotic gradient diminishes. Parenteral administration of fluids at volumes sufficient to provide one and one half times the maintenance rate will produce a copious dilute urine. Care must be taken to monitor serum electrolyte, osmolality, and glucose values closely (every 4 to 6 hours) to detect and treat any abnormalities; CVP monitoring may be helpful, and a bladder catheter must be used. The patient should not have any underlying cardiac, pulmonary, or renal disease that would make the development of congestive heart failure secondary to fluid overload or pulmonary or cerebral edema more likely. Osmotic diuretics such as mannitol (0.5 to 1 g/kg IV) may be useful in treating pending water intoxication; otherwise diuretics are not recommended unless some other aspect of the patient's condition indicates their use.

Changing the pH of the urine causes drugs with an appropriate pK_a to ionize after being filtered by the glomerulus. Since only nonionized drugs can be reabsorbed in the distal tubule, manipulation of pH can trap drugs in urine when reabsorption is prevented. Classic examples of increased elimination by pH alteration are barbiturates and salicylates, which are ionized in an alkaline medium, and amphetamines, phenothiazines, and phencyclidine, which are ionized in an acid medium. Even though an agent may have a favorable pK_a (acids, 3.0 to 7.5; bases, 7.5 to 10.5), increased elimination may be prevented by the degree of protein binding, lipid solubility, or volume of distribution of the toxin.

Alkalinization of the urine occurs with administration of a base such as sodium bicarbonate, tromethamine (Tham) buffer, or sodium lactate. Sodium bicarbonate (2 mEq/kg IV as a bolus followed by a constant IV infusion of 2 mEq/kg over 6 hours) can be used. Urinary pH should be >7.0. Before alkalinization is attempted, serum electrolyte, ionized calcium, blood pH, and osmolality values must be known and any abnormalities corrected. Alkalinization will be unsuccessful if either hypokalemia or systemic alkalosis is present. The dangers of this type of therapy include hypernatremia, hyperosmolality, and systemic alkalosis, which may precipitate symptomatic hypocalcemia. It is not appropriate for patients with impaired cardiac or renal function or any patient with impaired CNS autoregulation. Serum electrolyte, pH, osmolality, and urinary electrolyte values must be monitored frequently. If a brisk diuresis is present, acetazolamide (5 mg/kg IV) may be used; carbonic anhydrase inhibitors act by blocking the renal absorption of sodium bicarbonate and retention of hydrogen ion. Existing metabolic acidosis that may occur with salicylate ingestion can be exacerbated, and increased excretion of sodium, potassium, and water can occur. Systemic acidosis is a contraindication to the use of acetazolamide.

Acidification of urine to promote base elimination occurs with use of ascorbic acid and ammonium chloride, although there has been some question about the efficacy of using ascorbic acid and urinary pH must be checked periodically during its use. Ascorbic acid is sometimes given concomitantly with deferoxamine to increase ion excretion. Doses range from 50 to 200 mg/kg daily in four divided oral doses. Should the oral route be contraindicated, it may be given parenterally; the intramuscular route is preferred because utilization of the drug is best via this route. Ammonium chloride is a more potent urine acidifier, but it will exacerbate systemic acidosis. Contraindications to its use include hepatic dysfunction, metabolic or respiratory acidosis, renal dysfunction, and cardiac impairment. The drug must be administered slowly enough to allow hepatic metabolism of the ammonium ion and to prevent development of ammonia toxicity. Signs of this toxicity include diaphoresis, respiratory irregularity, emesis, dysrhythmias (particularly bradycardia), seizures, and coma. Ammonium chloride may be given orally or by slow IV administration (rate not to exceed 0.007 ml/kg/min of a dilute solution). The oral dose is 75 mg/kg/day in four divided doses. For IV administration 100 to 200 mEq of ammonium chloride should be diluted in 500 to 1000 ml of 0.9% sodium chloride solution and given in the same dose; the total dose must not exceed 4 to 6 g. Monitoring should include serum electrolyte and pH, serum ammonia, and urinary pH determinations at regular intervals.

The time to discontinue therapy for forced diuresis or pH manipulation is when the levels of the drug decrease in either the urine or serum as determined by the toxicology laboratory.

Dialysis

For more severe intoxicants with which fatal outcome or major organ damage seem likely or conservative management is unsuccessful as evidenced by clinical deterioration of the patient, more invasive types of drug elimination are available. They include peritoneal dialysis, hemodialysis, hemoperfusion, lipid dialysis, and exchange transfusion (see Chapters 141 and 145-147); continuous arteriovenous hemoperfusion is usually not helpful because only agents of small molecular weight can be removed.

The most appropriate methods of elimination for a number of commonly ingested agents are listed on p. 601. Of these techniques peritoneal dialysis requires the least expertise for use, and it can be instituted earlier than the other methods. It is not quite as efficient as hemodialysis. Contraindications to peritoneal dialysis include peritoneal infection, recent abdominal surgery, or bleeding diathesis. Hemodialysis, although requiring more expertise and equipment, is a more efficient way of removing many toxins. Updated recommendations about dialysis for intoxications can be obtained from the Proceedings of the American Society for Artificial Internal Organs (ASAIO). Lipid dialysis is a technique developed to remove lipid-soluble drugs that will not concentrate in aqueous medium, and it uses an oil instead of a water-based dialysate. It has not proved as efficacious as hoped because lipophilic drugs have a large volume of distribution and even prolonged dialysis may not accomplish much removal of the drug.

Charcoal hemoperfusion uses a column of charcoal or absorbent resin to remove toxic agents from extracorporeally circulated blood. This technique requires placement of arterial and venous catheters for circulation of blood; it may be limited by the absorptive capacity of the column, the volume of distribution of the agent, and the degree of protein or tissue binding of the drug. As with all techniques requiring anticoagulation, thrombocytopenia, bleeding, and hypotension may be a problem.

Techniques for displacement of toxins from tissue- or protein-binding sites are poor, and patients who have ingested agents bound to these sites may require long periods of supportive care before the intoxicant is eliminated.

Exchange transfusion

An exchange transfusion may be used to assist with the elimination of toxins bound to RBCs (carbon monoxide) or that produce methemoglobinemia (aniline dyes, nitrates, nitrites, chlorates, nitrobenzine). It will also restore normal oxygen-carrying capacity. Availability of large volumes of blood, size of

the child, and adequate IV access are limiting factors (see Chapter 141).

• • •

Toxins may also be absorbed from body surfaces such as skin or pulmonary membrane.

Inhaled toxins

Inhaled toxins may be absorbed directly by diffusion and can elicit several pulmonary responses, depending on the nature of the inhalant (particulate vs. vapor), site of deposition (proximal vs. distal airway), degree of clearance from the lung, type of exposure (acute vs. recurrent), and chemical form of the toxin. Responses can include irritation of the tracheobronchial tree with development of bronchospasm,

---

DRUG TOXIN REMOVAL BY DIALYSIS, INTENSIVE SUPPORTIVE CARE, AND USE OF ACTIVATED CHARCOAL*

Dialysis indicated on basis of condition of patient

Amphetamines	Calcium	Meprobamate	Potassium
Anilines	Chloral hydrate	(Equanil; Miltown)	Quinidine
Antibiotics	Fluorides	Paraldehyde	Salicylates
Boric acid	Iodides	Phencyclidine	Strychnine
Bromide	Isoniazid	Phenobarbital	Thiocyanates

Dialysis not indicated except for support in the following poisons: therapy is intensive supportive care

Antidepressants (tricyclic and MAO inhibitors also)	Ethchlorvynol (Placidyl)	Nodular (Methyprylon)
Antihistamines	Glutethimide (Doriden)	Oxazepam (Serax)
Chlordiazepoxide (Librium)	Hallucinogens	Phenothiazines
Digitalis and related agents	Heroin and other opiates	Synthetic anticholinergics and belladonna compounds
Diphenoxylate (Lomotil)	Methaqualone (Quaalude)	

Well absorbed by activated charcoal

Amphetamines	Digitalis	Nicotine	Potassium permanganate
Antimony	Glutethimide	Opium	
Antipyrine	Iodine	Oxalates	Quinine
Atropine	Ipecac	Parathion	Salicylates
Arsenic	Malathion	Penicillin	Selenium
Barbiturates	Mercuric chloride	Phenol	Silver
Camphor	Methylene blue	Phenolphthalein	Stramonium
Cantharides	Morphine	Phenothiazine	Strychnine
Cocaine	Muscarine	Phosphorus	Sulfonamides

*From Rumack BH, Lovejoy FH. Clinical toxicology. In Klassen CD, Amdur MO, Doull J, eds. Casarett's and Doull's Toxicology: The Basic Science of Poisons, 3rd ed. New York: Macmillan, 1986, p 882.

edema, and secondary infection, cellular damage, and necrosis to tissues lining the airway, resulting in intraluminal edema and production of fibrosis and evoking allergic mechanisms and oncogenesis. Asphyxiation with hypoxia occurs when 20% to 30% of the inhaled gas is replaced by toxic fumes; at an inspired oxygen concentration of <10%, the inhalation may be fatal. Commonly inhaled toxins include smoke, steam, dust, carbon monoxide, ammonia, volatile petroleum distillates, and hydrogen sulfide.

Treatment consists of removing the patient to an environment free of the inhaled gas and administering 100% oxygen to dilute toxic gas in the lung. Since gases can be absorbed from alveolar air spaces into the blood, dilution of the offending gas in the alveolus will create a concentration gradient favoring movement into the alveolus. Oxygen must be administered until the patient is asymptomatic and all toxin is likely to be eliminated. Ventilatory support may be necessary if pulmonary edema, chemical pneumonitis, or other pulmonary damage has occurred. Bronchoscopy may be needed for removal of particulate matter from the airway.

Contact toxins

Toxins coming in contact with the skin or mucous membranes must be removed mechanically. After all contaminated clothing has been removed, copious amounts of water must be applied to exposed skin surfaces and any needed therapy for burns or dermatitis instituted. Transcutaneous absorption sufficient to cause systemic toxicity can occur with chlorinated and inorganic phosphate insecticides, halogenated hydrocarbons, caustics, and corrosives. Chemical antidotes must not be applied to the skin; heat released by the chemical interaction, particularly between acids and bases, may initiate further skin damage.

Ophthalmic toxins

Toxins introduced via the eyes must be lavaged from them with large volumes of water. If the patient is at home, tap water is suitable; in the emergency department flushing may be done with 0.9% sodium chloride solution for 1 to 2 minutes. Application of a local anesthetic drop may facilitate this process and allow more detailed ophthalmologic examination. Prolonged flushing of an eye irritant is indicated only for a chemically active agent or one that has a lipid or viscous base. If a caustic has entered the eye, flushing must be continued until the pH is 8.0 to 8.5 (normal pH of tears is 7.0). Corneal erosion, scarring, and opacity can occur from introduction of alkaline (pH 11.0 to 12.0) substances such as phosphate-free detergents, lye, or hair neutralizer. Fluorescein examination with ultraviolet light will reveal any epithelial damage. Solid particles can be removed by continuous irrigation or with a cotton-tipped applicator moistened with antibiotic ointment. An ophthalmologist should be consulted for further care and treatment of affected eyes.

Toxins and Specific Antidotes

Specific antidotes are not numerous and can be identified by a poison control center. Even though an antidote is available, supportive therapy remains the most important form of therapy, and treatment of life-threatening organ failure should never be deferred. Table 75-5 lists toxins that have specific antidotes.

Opiates

Opiates are administered for pain relief, for antitussive effect, and to slow GI motility in addition to having an illicit use. Overdose of opiates can cause life-threatening respiratory depression and coma. The antidote of choice is naloxone (Narcan), which competes with the opiate molecule for binding at all receptor sites without having any agonist activity at that receptor site. After parenteral administration effects are seen immediately; the plasma half-life is 1 hour and duration of action 1 to 4 hours. Depending on the degree of excess opiate available to bind opiate receptors, naloxone administration may result in no response or an initial response followed by recurrence of symptoms. In overdose situations the "correct" naloxone dose may be variable and is that which is required to reverse symptoms.

As an antidote naloxone may be used in several ways. First, it may be used empirically to determine if coma and respiratory depression are opiate related. In this case a parenteral dose of 0.05 mg/kg should be given, followed by 0.1 mg/kg in 5 minutes if there is no response and then by 0.2 mg/kg for continued lack of expected response. If the third dose fails to reverse or alter symptoms, an alternative diagnosis for coma must be considered.

For reversal of known opiate overdose, the same

Table 75-5   Antidotes

Toxin	Antidote	Mechanism of Action
Opiates	Naloxone	Competitive antagonism at μ, δ, κ, and σ receptors
Organophosphate insecticides	Atropine	Pharmacologic antagonist of acetylcholine
	Pralidoxime	Reactivation of cholinesterase
Heavy metals	Dimercaprol, calcium disodium edetate, deferoxamine	Chelation of metal ion
Carbon monoxide	100% oxygen	Displacement of carbon monoxide from hemoglobin
Warfarin (Coumadin)	Vitamin K (phytonadione)	Restoration of activity of vitamin K–dependent clotting factors
Cyanide	Sodium nitrite, amyl nitrite	Production of methemoglobin
	Sodium thiosulfate	Provision of substrate for hepatic enzyme rhodanese
	Available from Eli Lilly as Cyanide Poisoning Kit (Stock No. M76)	
Belladonna alkaloids	Physostigmine	Prevention of breakdown of acetylcholine by inhibition of cholinesterase
Nitrites	1% methylene blue solution	Promotion of reduction of methemoglobin to hemoglobin
Nitrates		

See accompanying text and Chapters 85 and 86.

empiric regimen may be used to establish a reasonable dose. The American Academy of Pediatrics' recommendation for naloxone as an emergency drug is as follows:

> Dose: (Intoxication with opiates) IV, intratracheal— 0.1 mg/kg from birth including premature infants until age 5 years or 20 kg of weight at which time a minimum 2 mg dose should be used. These doses may be repeated as needed to maintain opiate reversal.
>
> The use of neonatal naloxone (Narcan 0.02 mg/kg) is no longer recommended because unacceptable fluid volume administration will result especially to small neonates. Preparations containing 0.4 mg/ml or 1 mg/ml are available and can be accurately dosed with appropriate sized syringes (1 ml).*

Recurrence of symptoms, particularly respiratory depression and apnea, after the initial naloxone dose has been metabolized may place the patient at risk for continued hypoxia. A more reasonable use of naloxone may be a constant infusion. This form of

*American Academy of Pediatrics. Emergency drug doses for infants and children and naloxone use in neonates: Clarification. Pediatrics 83:803, 1989.

dosing should be considered under the following circumstances: the need for repeat boluses of naloxone to relieve symptoms, ingestion of a long-acting opiate, ingestion of a large dose of opiate, and decreased ability to metabolize opiates (hepatic dysfunction). The dose for an infusion is empiric and is based on the initial naloxone dose required to reverse opiate toxicity. Tenenbien gives the following guidelines for a continuous infusion:

> Administer as a loading dose the previously successful bolus dose.
> Administer as an hourly infusion dose the above loading dose.
> Be prepared to increase the infusion dose if the patient's condition warrants it.
> Attempt to discontinue infusion every 12 hours.

Patients requiring this type of therapy must be closely monitored for respiratory function in an area in which airway stabilization and mechanical ventilation are immediately available.

Although naloxone has no agonist properties with respect to opiate receptors, intense pressor responses secondary to endogenous catecholamine release have been reported after its use. This is particularly evident if the patient has restoration of pain appreciation. Of particular concern is the occurrence of hypertension, increased myocardial oxygen consumption, and dysrhythmias; fulminant pulmonary edema has also been identified after naloxone administration.

Alcohols

Alcohols and their derivatives are metabolized by the hepatic enzyme alcohol dehydrogenase, and the preferred substrate even in the presence of other alcohols is ethanol. Very small amounts of methanol or ethylene glycol, whether introduced through the GI tract, the lungs, or the skin, can be fatal since the by-products of their metabolism include formaldehyde, formic acid, glyoxylic acid, and other organic acids. Patients present with either inebriation unassociated with characteristic ethanol breath odor or coma accompanied by a profound metabolic acidosis and a large anion gap. Complaints of visual disturbances accompanied by optic disc hyperemia, pericapillary edema, and decreased pupillary responsiveness suggest methanol intoxication. Supportive therapy, especially correction of the severe acidosis, must begin immediately.

Since alcohol dehydrogenase has an affinity for ethanol 100 times greater than that for other alcohols, saturation of the enzyme with ethanol will inhibit metabolism of methanol and ethylene glycol to their more toxic metabolities. Ethanol may be given orally or intravenously to maintain a blood ethanol level of 100 mg/dl, a level at which the enzyme is fully inhibited. A loading dose of 7 to 10 ml/kg IV of 10% ethanol in D_5W, followed by a continuous infusion of 1.4 ml/kg of the same solution, should be administered. Alternatively, 0.8 to 1 ml/kg of 95% ethanol diluted in a palatable liquid may be administered orally, followed by 0.15 ml/kg/hr. Blood concentrations must be monitored and the infusion or oral dose adjusted to maintain a stable blood ethanol level. This regimen will increase the half-life of methanol from 8 to 35 hours and of ethylene glycol to 17 hours. For ingestions characterized by severe persistent acidosis, blindness, methanol or ethylene glycol serum levels >50 mg/dl, and/or prolonged coma, concomitant hemodialysis to remove the intact alcohols is recommended. This combined therapy decreases methanol half-life to 2 to 3 hours and significantly decreases the time patients require intensive support and monitoring. Peritoneal dialysis is inef-

fective. Folate supplementation may decrease the accumulation of formate, thus decreasing the severity of the metabolic acidosis. The recommended dose is 1 mg/kg IV (maximum single dose, 50 mg). Every 4 hours for a total of six doses thiamine and pyridoxine may be given empirically to help decrease oxalate production and thus avoid the renal toxicity seen with ethylene glycol intoxication.

Cyanide

Free cyanide groups (CN^-) from ingested plant products (cherry, apricot, peach pits), pesticides, or pharmacologic sources (laetrile, sodium nitroprusside) have an affinity for the iron moiety of the cellular respiratory enzyme cytochrome oxidase equal to that of oxygen for the enzyme. Binding of excess cyanide results in anaerobic metabolism with lactic acid production by interference with oxidative phosphorylation and ATP production. The signs of toxicity include development of metabolic acidosis, increased mixed venous oxygen content in the absence of increased cardiac output, hypotension, seizures, and eventually cardiac arrest unresponsive to CPR. The patient may report dizziness, dyspnea, palpitations, and headache. Free cyanide ions are bound preferentially by methemoglobin, forming cyanmethemoglobin; the cyanide ion, although bound, must still be metabolized and excreted to avoid toxicity. Cyanide ions are metabolized by the hepatic enzyme rhodanese, a sulfydryl transferase, which adds a sulfur ion to cyanide to form thiocyanate, a less toxic, renally excreted compound with a half-life of 12 to 23 days. The limiting factor in the conversion of cyanide to thiocyanate is the availability of a suitable sulfur donor (usually sodium thiosulfate [$NaSSO_4$]), although cysteine can act as a donor. Rhodanese is an abundant enzyme, and hepatic disease does not affect the ability to metabolize cyanide, although it may affect levels of suitable sulfur donors.

Therapy for cyanide toxicity is twofold: (1) increasing immediate binding sites for free cyanide ions by promoting the formation of methemoglobin and (2) providing a sulfur donor to drive the reaction to metabolize cyanide to thiocyanate. If successful, these two measures cause cyanide ions to be driven off cytochrome oxidase and bring about restoration of cellular respiratory processes. Chemical reactions that bind cyanide ions are shown on p. 605

Administration of sodium nitrite (5 mg/kg by slow IV bolus) promotes conversion of hemoglobin to

REACTIONS TO BIND CYANIDE IONS

Conversion of hemoglobin to methemoglobin

$$HbFe^{2+} + NaN_2O_2 \rightleftharpoons HbFe^{3+} + Na$$

Binding of cyanide by methemoglobin

$$CN^- + HbFe^{3+} \rightleftharpoons HbFeCN$$

Metabolism of bound cyanide

$$HbFeCN^- + NaSSO_4 \underset{}{\overset{rhodanese}{\rightleftharpoons}}$$
$$NaSCN + SO_4^{2-} + HbFe^{3+}$$

Binding of cyanide by cytochrome oxidase

$$CN^- + Cytochrome\ oxidase \rightleftharpoons$$
$$CN\ cytochrome\ oxidase$$

NaN_2O_2 = sodium nitrite; CN^- = cyanide ion; $NaSSO_4$ = sodium thiosulfate; $NaSCN$ = sodium thiocyanate; $HbFe^{2+}$ = oxyhemoglobin; $HbFe^{3+}$ = methemoglobin; $HbFeCN$ = cyanomethemoglobin.

methemoglobin. Nitrites are systemic vasodilators, and careful monitoring of systemic arterial blood pressure and peripheral perfusion must be done. Methemoglobin will also be produced by amyl nitrite; an ampule of it can be broken into an anesthesia breathing bag or mask and the patient ventilated until an IV can be started. Next a sulfur donor must be provided; sodium thiosulfate (150 mg/kg IV) must be given rapidly and repeated every 10 minutes for three or four doses. Both agents should be given during CPR, and administration should not await confirmation of toxicity with elevated cyanide levels (>3 to 5 µg/ml; lethal at 6 to 8 µg/dl). Cyanide and thiocyanate levels as well as arterial pH determination and mixed venous oxygen content may be monitored during the course of therapy. Thiocyanate levels are not predictive for the degree of cyanide toxicity but reflect only the adequacy of sulfur donors. Thiocyanate levels may be increased if a source of cyanide is ingested chronically or if therapy continues over a long time period. Increased levels are associated with toxic psychosis.

Anticholinergics

Physostigmine, an anticholinesterase, is a tertiary amine capable of crossing the blood-brain barrier and entering the CNS. It inhibits the enzymatic hy-drolysis of the neurotransmittor acetylcholine in the synaptic cleft at the neuromuscular junction and at all cholinergic nerve synapses. The central effect is one of continuous cholinergic stimulation.

Toxic doses of belladonna alkaloids (scopolamine, hyoscine, atropine) result in both central and peripheral anticholinergic signs and symptoms, including dysarthria, disorientation, delirium, hallucinations, somnolence, convulsions, and coma centrally, as well as dilated pupils, tachycardia, inhibition of sweating, flushing, and atonic bowel peripherally. The central and peripheral symptoms can be reversed only with physostigmine, 0.02 mg/kg IV at a rate of 0.01 mg/kg/min every 5 minutes until the desired response is observed or until a maximum dose of 0.2 mg is given. The half-life is short, and a second dose or a continuous infusion at 1 to 10 µg/kg/min may be necessary if symptoms recur within 30 to 60 minutes. Side effects may include bradycardia, mydriasis, urinary retention, hypotension, and dysrhythmias; physostigmine should be withheld from patients with severe asthma, urinary obstruction, poor myocardial function, and signs of cholinergic toxicity.

Because of its central cholinergic stimulation, some authors recommend the use of physostigmine for the treatment of overdose secondary to sedatives and CNS depressants whose actions may include central acute cholinergic activity. It has been used in the treatment of phenothiazine and tricyclic antidepressant toxicity (see Chapter 78) for unresponsive or life-threatening symptomatology. Use of physostigmine as a diagnostic aid is not recommended since CNS arousal or stimulation is a nonspecific action of the drug. Reversal of respiratory depression and cardiac dysrhythmias or return of obtunded reflexes may not necessarily occur, and all usual supportive measures must be used.

Nitrates and nitrites

Compounds containing nitrates and nitrites (adulterated food and water, aniline dyes, silver nitrate, nitroglycerin) cause the production of methemoglobin by oxidation of ferrous ion to ferric ion. Methemoglobinemia can impair molecular oxygen transport in blood and distort the oxygen dissociation curve with resulting tissue hypoxia. Symptomatic patients present with cyanosis unresponsive to oxygen administration. The major system responsible for metabolism of methemoglobin in erythrocytes is methemoglobin reductase, a cytochrome B5 enzyme. This reaction requires NADH as a cofactor. Treatment of acute symptomatic methemoglobinemia (levels >30% to 40% methemoglobin blood concentration; lethal at 70%) in intact erythrocytes (i.e., hemolysis has not accompanied development of methemoglobinemia) is reduction of the concentration of the abnormal pigment. A 1% methylene blue solution (1 to 2 mg/kg IV) should be given over 5 minutes. This dose may be repeated in 1 hour if no response occurs; the total dose should not exceed 7 mg/kg, or new production of methemoglobin will occur. Methylene blue enhances the production of NADP and conversion of methemoglobin to hemoglobin by methemoglobin reductase through the stimulation of the monophosphate shunt and methylene blue reductase (see Chapter 49).

ADDITIONAL READING

Berg MJ, Berlinger WG, Goldbery MJ, et al. Acceleration of the body clearance of phenobarbital by oral activated charcoal. N Engl J Med 307:642-643, 1982.

Fozen LE, Lovejoy FH, Crane RK. Acute poisoning in a children's hospital: A 2 year experience. Pediatrics 77:144-148, 1986.

• Goldfrank L, Brismitz E. Toxic inhalants. Hosp Physician 15:54-60, 1979.

• Handbook of Common Poisonings in Children. FDA-76-7004. Rockville, Md.: U.S. Department of Health Education and Welfare, 1976.

Klassen CD, Amdur MO, Doull J, eds. Casarett's and Doull's Toxicology: The Basic Science of Poisons, 3rd ed. New York: Macmillan, 1986.

Lacroix J, Gaudreault P, Gauthier M. Admission to a pediatric intensive care unit for poisoning: A review of 105 cases. Crit Care Med 17:748-750, 1989.

Mafenson HC, Greenshaw J. Physostigmine as an antidote: Use with caution. J Pediatr 87:1010-1011, 1975.

Moore RA, Rumack BH, Connu CS, et al. Naloxone: Underdosage after narcotic poisoning. Am J Dis Child 134:156-158, 1980.

Post KM, Jaeger RW, deCastro FJ. Eye contamination: A poison center protocol for management. Clin Toxicol 14:295-300, 1979.

• Rogers GC, Matyunas NJ. Gastrointestinal decontamination for acute poisoning. Pediatr Clin North Am 33:261-285, 1986.

Rumack BH. Poisondex. Denver, Colo.: Nicromedix, 1986.

Rumack BH, Temple AR, eds. Management of the Poisoned Patient. Princeton, N.J.: Science Press, 1977.

• Tenenbein M. Pediatric toxicology: Current controversies and recent advances. Curr Probl Pediatr 26:187-233, 1986.

Thompson DF, Trammel HL, Robertson NJ, et al. Evaluation of regional and non-regional poison centers. N Engl J Med 308:191-192, 1983.

76 Aspirin Ingestion and Toxicity

Frances C. Morriss

BACKGROUND AND PHYSIOLOGY

The incidence of salicylate poisoning in children has been decreasing since 1965 for a number of reasons, including voluntary limitation by manufacturers of the number of tablets in bottles containing children's aspirin, widespread use of childproof packaging for both pediatric and adult preparations, more accurate labeling of proprietary combination products containing aspirin, and widespread publicity concerning the relationship between aspirin intake and Reye's syndrome. Even so, the majority of cases still occur in children. In 1978 ingestions numbered 3575 as compared to 16,887 in 1967; deaths in children under 5 years of age had decreased 70%, from 46 in 1972 to 12 in 1978. The epidemiology of these deaths (most of which occurred at home in infants less than 12 months of age) suggests dosing errors rather than accidental ingestions. In 1986 ingestions in children under 5 years of age numbered 5883 and in children 5 to 17 years 3523, for a total of 9406. There were no deaths in children under 5 years; six deaths in older children were all listed as intentional suicide. There has also been a shift, particularly in older children and adults, toward greater morbidity from chronic salicylate exposure. The zero-order kinetics characteristic of salicylates favors disproportionately large increases in serum and tissue levels after small dose changes in patients on daily therapy.

Salicylates are rapidly absorbed from the stomach because the low gastric pH causes weak acids such as aspirin to remain in the nonionized form that crosses cell membranes by passive diffusion along a concentration gradient. Ionized salicylate is biologically inactive. Topically applied salicylates (salicylic acid, methylsalicylate, oil of wintergreen) are well absorbed from intact skin and mucous membranes. All salicylates are biotransformed to salicylic acid in the liver; distribution to various tissues then becomes a pH-dependent process. At a normal serum pH (7.4) most salicylate is ionized; a fall in pH to 7.2 will double the number of nonionized molecules available to cross cell membranes. Acidemia promotes intracellular salicylate deposition; alkalemia causes retention of salicylate in extracellular fluids. The other factor that alters body distribution of salicylate is protein binding of the drug since only unbound molecules are capable of diffusing into cells regardless of the state of ionization. With large doses of salicylate the available binding sites become occupied and more unbound drug is available. This saturation phenomenon accounts in part for the higher than expected tissue levels of salicylate seen with ingestion of large amounts of drug.

Salicylate is metabolized to salicylic acid, gentistic acid, and salicylic or phenolic or acyl glucuronides, which are rapidly excreted by the kidney. At high plasma levels of salicylate the appropriate hepatic enzymes function at capacity, and plasma half-life may become prolonged from an expected 3 to 6 hours to as long as 15 to 30 hours. At this point the majority of salicylate is excreted unchanged in the urine. Excretion of unmetabolized salicylate will be influenced by the same pH considerations as plasma salicylate; that is, more salicylate will be excreted if the urine is alkalotic and the salicylate remains in an ionized inactive state. Saturation of the two major hepatic metabolic pathways can occur in patients receiving therapeutic doses of the drug chronically. If this occurs, small changes in the usual aspirin dose may result in large changes in plasma salicylate concentration, resulting in intoxication. One can see that ingestion of large doses of aspirin will cause higher than expected drug levels because of the development of a characteristic metabolic acidosis (favoring tissue deposition rather than excretion), saturation of hepatic enzymes needed to biotransform salicylate, and saturation of available binding sites on plasma protein.

Toxicity from salicylates, defined as a serum level >30 mg/dl, particularly from a single large dose, can be predicted from a nomogram (Fig. 76-1) if the time since the ingestion and the plasma salicylate level are known. Lethal overdoses result in brain death when a critical cerebral tissue level is reached; this can occur with serum concentrations from 45 to 195 mg/dl. Essential to successful treatment is prevention of equilibration between plasma (extracellular) salicylate and cerebral tissue (intracellular) salicylate concentrations.

Salicylate functions intracellularly as an enzyme inhibitor. (1) Uncoupling of oxidative phosphoryla-

tion, (2) inhibition of Krebs cycle enzymes, and (3) inhibition of amino acid metabolism by interference with aminotransferases occur. These inhibitions result in decreased adenosine triphosphate (ATP) production and increased anaerobic glycolysis in an attempt to increase ATP levels. Excess energy released from these processes produces heat as oxygen consumption and carbon dioxide production increase. Tissue glycolysis results in increased gluconeogenesis and an elevation of serum glucose; intracellular glucose depletion occurs despite normal or elevated serum glucose. A metabolic acidosis characterized by a large anion gap results from increased ketone production associated with interference in Krebs cycle enzyme function, from increased production associated with pyruvate acid and lactate (anaerobic glycolysis), and from increased levels of serum amino acids. In 78% of ingestions metabolic acidosis will be exhibited sometime during the course regardless of age. The most common presentation, however, is respiratory alkalosis, a conse-

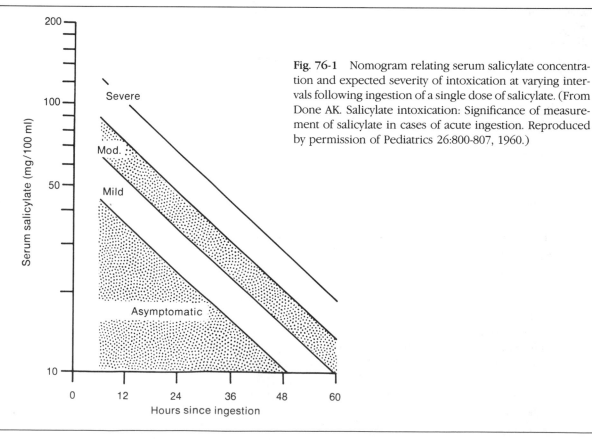

Fig. 76-1 Nomogram relating serum salicylate concentration and expected severity of intoxication at varying intervals following ingestion of a single dose of salicylate. (From Done AK. Salicylate intoxication: Significance of measurement of salicylate in cases of acute ingestion. Reproduced by permission of Pediatrics 26:800-807, 1960.)

quence of direct central stimulation of the respiratory center. Glycolysis stimulates lipid metabolism and ketone production. Even though intracellular glucose depletion is common, hyperglycemia is documented more often than hypoglycemia.

The clinical correlates of these metabolic derangements are multiple, as summarized in Table 76-1. Patients often experience profound disturbances of fluid and electrolyte homeostasis, resulting in dehydration, hypovolemia, hypotension, and loss of sodium and potassium. Associated with hyperpnea and a greater than normal minute ventilation is increased insensible water loss from the respiratory tract. Increased heat production and fever cause increased skin and sweat losses of water and electrolytes. Nausea and vomiting are common with serum salicylate in excess of 50 mg/dl. Renal wasting of bicarbonate and potassium accompanies the initial respiratory alkalosis and continues as buffers are required to excrete increased amounts of organic acids (pyruvate, lactate, amino acids, ketones, salicylate).

The ability to compensate for metabolic acidemia becomes severely compromised. There may also be bleeding abnormalities because salicylate inhibits platelet aggregation, causes local irritation to the gastric mucosa, and produces hypoprothrombinemia as a result of decreased factor VII synthesis. DIC is seen rarely.

Profound CNS disturbances can develop and include lethargy, confusion, coma, and death. Seizures occur as a preterminal event and are a poor prognostic sign. Although the CNS manifestations can be exacerbated by fever, dehydration, bleeding, and electrolyte abnormalities, their cause is intracellular metabolic dysfunction resulting in glucose depletion.

Occasionally salicylate ingestion may be complicated by pulmonary edema, ARDS bronchospasm, renal failure, inappropriate ADH secretion, and hemolysis. Tables 76-2 and 76-3 correlate the ingested dose with observed levels of clinical toxicity and correspond well to the nomogram (Fig. 76-1) relating toxicity and serum salicylate level. (Remember the

Table 76-1   Clinical and Metabolic Derangements Characteristic of Salicylate Toxicity

Biochemical Abnormality	Clinical Correlate	Laboratory Correlate
Direct stimulation of respiratory center	Hyperpnea Dehydration	Respiratory alkalosis ($\uparrow$ pH, $\downarrow$ Paco$_2$), $\uparrow$ minute ventilation Alkalotic urine pH
Uncoupling of oxidative phosphorylation	Hyperthermia Dehydration Hypovolemia Oliguria Hypotension	Metabolic acidosis ($\downarrow$ pH, $\uparrow$ anion gap) $\uparrow$ CO$_2$ production $\uparrow$ O$_2$ consumption
Inhibition of Krebs cycle enzymes		Metabolic acidosis Lactic and pyruvic acidemia Ketosis $\uparrow$ Urine sodium and potassium
Inhibition of amino acid metabolism		Metabolic acidosis $\uparrow$ Serum amino acids Aminoaciduria $\uparrow$ Urine bicarbonate

Abnormal glucose homeostasis
  Stimulation of gluconeogenesis
  Increased anaerobic tissue glycolysis
  Increased lipid metabolism
	CNS disturbances (depletion of intracellular glucose)	Hypo/hyperglycemia
		$\downarrow$ CSF glucose
		Abnormal EEG
		Ketosis

Interference with hemostatic mechanisms	Bleeding Gastritis	Hypoprothrombinemia $\uparrow$ Bleeding time $\uparrow$ PT

Table 76-2   Usual Clinical Manifestations With Various Levels of Severity of Salicylate Intoxication*

Symptom Category	Types of Symptoms Expected
Asymptomatic	None
Mild	Mild to moderate hyperpnea, sometimes with lethargy
Moderate	Severe hyperpnea, prominent neurologic disturbances (marked lethargy and/or excitability), but not coma or convulsions
Severe	Severe hyperpnea, coma, or semicoma, sometimes with convulsions

*From Temple AR. Acute and chronic effects of aspirin toxicity and their treatment. Arch Intern Med 141:364-369, 1981. Copyright 1981, American Medical Association.

Table 76-3   Assessment of Severity of Salicylate Intoxication Based on the Estimated Dose Ingested*

Ingested Dose (mg/kg†)	Estimated Severity
<150	No toxic reaction expected
150-300	Mild to moderate toxic reaction
300-500	Serious toxic reaction
>500	Potentially lethal toxic reaction

*From Temple AR. Acute and chronic effects of aspirin toxicity and their treatment. Arch Intern Med 141:364-369, 1981. Copyright 1981, American Medical Association.
†Number of tablets ingested times the milligrams of aspirin per tablet divided by patient weight in kilograms equals the acute ingested dose. If a patient has been receiving aspirin therapeutically during the previous 24 hours, the potential toxicity of the acutely ingested dose will be increased.

nomogram is useful only for ingestions of a single dose where the approximate time of ingestion is known and not for chronic salicylism). Discordance between the expected severity of symptoms, salicylate levels, and the amount thought to have been ingested should alert the caregiver to the possibility of other diagnoses such as chronic salicylism rather than an acute ingestion, Reye's syndrome, malignant hyperpyrexia, toxic hepatitis of other etiologies, or ingestion of other agents in addition to aspirin. In 1986 ingestions of aspirin as a single agent in patients 17 years or less totaled 9406; aspirin in combination with narcotics or other analgesics accounted for an additional 2391 incidents in the same age group.

MONITORING AND LABORATORY TESTS

To document the peak and fall of the salicylate level a toxicology screen needs to be done in addition to measuring serum salicylate. Arterial blood gas tensions and especially pH are important to document and follow if abnormal. Obtain a Hct, PT, PTT, bleeding time, and platelet count if bleeding is present or surgery must be performed. Check for gastric bleeding and stool guaiac. Measure serum Na, K, Cl, and HCO_3 initially and if alkaline therapy is instituted.

Strict monitoring of intake and output is essential for instituting forced diuresis and bicarbonate therapy; a bladder catheter may be needed. Invasive monitoring of systemic arterial blood pressure and central venous blood pressure will be necessary for severe ingestions.

TREATMENT

Treatment of salicylism should include efforts to diminish drug absorption, particularly if a large single dose has been ingested, to increase drug elimination, and to minimize tissue accumulation. Induced emesis and/or gastric lavage to empty the stomach followed by oral activated charcoal to bind salicylate in the GI tract is indicated to decrease absorption. Efforts to enhance drug elimination should include measures to alkalinize the urine while increasing urine output. Raising urine pH to 8.0 will trap salicylate in the ionized state in the urine and result in a four-fold increase in salicylate elimination for each 1 unit rise in urine pH. Alkalinization is accomplished by administering an IV sodium bicarbonate infusion and increasing IV fluids to a greater than maintenance rate. Severe potassium depletion must be corrected before bicarbonate will be effective. Alkalinization is contraindicated if systemic alkalosis, renal failure, or pulmonary edema is present (see Chapters 10, 14, and 15 for details). Acetazolamide is contraindicated since it may contribute to high brain salicylate levels. Of the two measures, alkalinization of the urine is more effective than forced diuresis. Repeated oral doses of activated charcoal (GI dialysis; see Chapter 75) have been shown to enhance salicylate clearance;

apparent salicylate half-life values have decreased from 15 to 8 hours. Experience with this technique is limited but promising. In the event of severe intoxication unresponsive to conventional therapy (deteriorating clinical state, serum salicylate >100 mg/dl, failure to alkalinize the urine with bicarbonate, or presence of conditions that preclude bicarbonate therapy), alternate methods for elimination must be considered. These include peritoneal dialysis, hemodialysis, and charcoal or resin hemoperfusion.

Minimizing intracellular drug accumulation depends on manipulation of the serum pH with IV sodium bicarbonate therapy to trap salicylate in the serum and in the extracellular fluid spaces so it can be excreted via the kidneys. The success of this therapy depends on maintaining extracellular fluid pH greater than intracellular pH; a serum pH of 7.50 to 7.55 is usually adequate. Tromethamine (THAM) is less useful than sodium bicarbonate since it raises intracellular and extracellular pH, thus creating less of a gradient between the two. Sodium bicarbonate increases extracellular fluid pH more than intracellular pH because it remains confined to the extracellular space.

Supportive measures include aggressive rehydration and correction of electrolyte abnormalities, particularly hypokalemia. Fluid deficits can be large (as much as 4 to 6 L/m^2 of body surface). Despite documentation of normal serum glucose, glucose-containing solutions need to be given and the amount of glucose in the infusion adjusted to maintain normoglycemia. Hyperthermia needs to be treated by external cooling measures outlined in Chapter 21. If needed, stabilize the patient's airway, particularly if seizures unresponsive to anticonvulsant therapy occur. Hemorrhagic problems are treated as they occur; hypoprothrombinemia will be corrected by parenteral administration of vitamin K. Successful recovery will depend on ongoing assessment of the patient's volume status, frequent determination of serum electrolytes, glucose osmolality and pH, urine pH, and salicylate levels. With complicating pulmonary, renal, and cerebral problems, invasive monitoring (CVP, arterial and pulmonary blood arterial pressure) will be needed to guide fluid administration, particularly if forced diuresis is employed in addition to alkalinization of serum and urine.

The prognosis is excellent, especially in patients who have ingested a single dose of salicylate.

All intracellular abnormalities are reversible unless severe CNS disturbances are present or the course is complicated by major organ failure. Chronic salicylism carries a worse prognosis because of unexpectedly high serum salicylate levels and because the diagnosis is often delayed. Sequelae of salicylate intoxication include CNS deficits. Intoxication complicated by seizures, particularly if volume, temperature, glucose, and electrolyte abnormalities have been corrected, indicate the possibility of lethal ingestion; the most aggressive measures should be undertaken for treatment.

ADDITIONAL READING

Done AK. Salicylate intoxication: Significance of measurement of salicylate in cases of acute ingestion. Pediatrics 26:800-807, 1960.

Gaudreault P, Temple AR, Lovejoy FH. The relative severity of symptoms of acute versus chronic salicylate poisoning in children: A clinical comparison. Pediatrics 70:566-569, 1982.

• Hell JB. Salicylate intoxication. N Engl J Med 288:1110-1113, 1973.

• Levy G. Clinical pharmacokinetics of aspirin. Pediatrics 62(Suppl):867-872, 1978.

Litovitz TL, Martin TG, Schmitz B. 1986 annual report of the American Association of Poison Control Centers National Data Collection System. Am J Emerg Med 5:405-445, 1987.

• Snodgrass WR. Salicylate toxicity. Pediat Clin North Am 33:381-391, 1986.

Snodgrass WR, Rumack BH, Peterson RY, et al. Salicylate toxicity following therapeutic doses in young children. Clin Toxicol 18:247-259, 1981.

• Temple AR. Pathophysiology of aspirin overdose toxicity with implications for management. Pediatrics 62:843-876, 1978.

Vertus JE, McWilliams BC, Kelly HW. Repeated oral administration of activated charcoal for treating aspirin overdose in young children. Pediatrics 85:594-598, 1990.

Winters RW, White JS, Hughes MC, et al. Disturbance of acid-base equilibrium in salicylate intoxication. Pediatrics 23:260-285, 1965.

77 Acetaminophen Poisoning

Robert H. Squires, Jr.

BACKGROUND AND PHYSIOLOGY

Acetaminophen (Anacin, Tylenol, Tempra) is a non-prescription analgesic/antipyretic that can be found in more than 200 medications. When administered in recommended doses (15 mg/kg/dose q 4 hr), acetaminophen is safe; however, if taken in excessive amounts, this agent has the potential to produce fatal hepatic, renal, and rarely myocardial necrosis.

After ingestion acetaminophen is rapidly absorbed into the systemic circulation; peak plasma concentrations occur in 30 to 60 minutes. The major pathway of detoxification of acetaminophen is in the hepatocyte, in which the drug is conjugated with either glucuronide or sulfate and is then excreted in the urine. A fraction of the acetaminophen is also eliminated through the cytochrome P-450 mixed-oxygenase system, resulting in the creation of reactive metabolites, which are initially conjugated with glutathione and then converted to cysteine and mercapturic acid. Depletion of glutathione allows the reactive metabolite to combine covalently with essential hepatic proteins and enzymes, resulting in cell death and necrosis.

The toxicity of acetaminophen depends upon the balance between the formation of the reactive metabolite and the availability of glutathione. It is uncommon to see significant hepatic injury with acute ingestions <125 mg/kg; most patients show signs of toxicity when 250 mg/kg is ingested, and virtually all patients are affected by a dose >350 mg/kg. Toxicity can be potentiated by drugs such as phenobarbital, which stimulate the microsomal enzyme system, and by disease states such as malnutrition, chronic liver disease, and alcohol abuse, which decrease the amount of available glutathione.

The clinical course of acetaminophen toxicity de-velops over 3 to 7 days. Initial symptoms of nausea, vomiting, and anorexia are nonspecific and resolve within 12 to 24 hours. In untreated patients biochemical evidence of hepatic injury occurs within 48 to 72 hours and is manifested by high transaminase levels, modest hyperbilirubinemia, and coagulopathy. If the cause of hepatic injury is in question, the differential diagnosis must include the following: Reye's syndrome, acute viral hepatitis, an acute manifestation of a chronic liver disease (Wilson's disease, chronic active hepatitis, α_1-antitrypsin deficiency), or other drugs (valproic acid, isoniazid, halothane, toxic mushrooms). Death occurs in 1% to 2% of patients within 4 to 18 days.

Histologically, there is centrilobular necrosis without steatosis. In patients who survive the liver is histologically normal after 3 to 4 months, and there are no reports of long-term sequelae.

MONITORING AND LABORATORY TESTS

Determining the exact time of the acetaminophen ingestion is important and must be documented carefully. It is also important to determine other medications that could have been taken. The nomogram frequently used to assess the potential of acetaminophen hepatotoxicity is based on serum levels obtained in adult patients who took a single large dose of acetaminophen (Fig. 77-1). Patients with liver disease or malnutrition may experience liver injury at lower serum levels. The nomogram is not useful in patients who have taken excessive amounts of acetaminophen over a period of days.

The plasma acetaminophen level must be determined 4 hours after ingestion or within 18 hours of ingestion baseline. Liver function tests, PT/PTT, CBC, BUN and glucose values, urinalysis, gastric aspirate

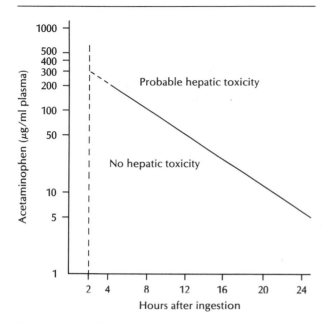

Fig. 77-1 Semilogarithmic plot of plasma acetaminophen levels vs. time. (From Rumack BH. Acetaminophen poisoning and toxicity. Reproduced by permission of Pediatrics 55:871-876, 1975.)

and urine for toxicology screen, and serum electrolyte and ammonia values must be obtained and repeated at least daily if hepatic injury from acetaminophen ingestion is feared.

TREATMENT

Treatment is directed toward reducing the toxic effects of acetaminophen by neutralizing the active metabolite either by providing glutathione precursors (cysteine or methionine) or by providing other sulfhydryl compounds (*N*-acetylcysteine). IV cysteamine, intramuscular dimercaprol, and oral methionine have been used for this purpose, but the large incidence of adverse side effects and limited protection from toxicity have made their use unattractive. *N*-Acetylcysteine is the treatment of choice for acute acetaminophen overdose. This agent is most effective when it is administered within the first 18 hours after the toxic ingestion has occurred. The therapeutic window that exists after the acute ingestion is likely related to the rate of glutathione depletion. For reasons that are not clear, children seem less prone to

severe hepatic injury than adults. In addition there is experimental evidence that cimetidine can reduce acetaminophen toxicity by inhibiting cytochrome P-450–mediated drug metabolism.

Treatment is based on early recognition, administration of *N*-acetylcysteine within 18 hours of ingestion, and supportive care for hepatic insufficiency or failure. Careful attention to fluids must be given since patients may develop renal tubular injury.

For appropriate general and supportive care see Chapters 4 and 75. Gastric aspiration and lavage should be performed if they have not already been done. Activated charcoal must not be administered if *N*-acetylcysteine is to be given enterally since the charcoal will interfere with its absorption. Ideally, *N*-acetylcysteine therapy is initiated within 10 to 18 hours of ingestion. *N*-Acetylcysteine could be given up to 24 hours after acetaminophen ingestion, but there is no specific therapy for patients initially seen more than 24 hours after ingestion or for patients who have ingested a high dose on a chronic basis. Therapy is initiated after blood for determining the drug level is obtained from patients who have ingested >125 mg/kg (do not await the test result). A decision to continue therapy may be made after the level is known.

If the plasma acetaminophen level is >200 μg/ml at 4 hours or >50 μg/L at 12 hours after ingestion or if the plasma $t_{1/2}$ is >4 hours or if >125 mg/kg of acetaminophen was ingested, the patient is at risk for developing hepatotoxicity. *N*-Acetylcysteine is formulated in the following manner: *N*-acetylcysteine 20% is diluted to a 5% solution with water or with 0.9% sodium chloride solution if given through a nasogastric tube. It is mixed with soda or juice if given by mouth. A loading dose of 140 mg/kg of *N*-acetylcysteine is given initially, followed by a maintenance dose of 70 mg/kg every 4 hours for an additional 17 doses. If vomiting occurs within 1 hour after administration of a dose, the dose must be repeated. If protracted vomiting precludes enteral administration of *N*-acetylcysteine, recommendations for altering the standard protocol and centers approved for IV use of *N*-acetylcysteine are available through the Rocky Mountain Poison Center in Denver, Colorado (1-800-525-6115).

Liver transplantation can be considered if the patient has a fulminant course and was initially seen >24 hours after acetaminophen ingestion.

ADDITIONAL READING

Agran PF, Zenk KE, Romansky SG. Acute liver failure and encephalopathy in a 15-month-old infant. Am J Dis Child 137:1107-1114, 1983.

• Black M. Acetaminophen hepatotoxicity. Gastroenterology 78:382-392, 1980.

Black M, Cornell JF, Rabin L, Schacter N. Late presentation of acetaminophen hepatotoxicity. Dig Dis Sci 27:370-374, 1972.

Currey RW Jr, Robinson JD, Sughrue MJ. Acute renal failure after acetaminophen ingestion. JAMA 247:1012-1014, 1982.

Greene JW, Craft L, Ghishan F. Acetaminophen poisoning in infancy. Am J Dis Child 137:386-387, 1973.

Mitchell AA, Lovejoy FH, Slone D, Shapiro S. Acetaminophen and aspirin. Am J Dis Child 136:976-979, 1982.

Mitchell MC, Schenker S, Avant GR, Speeg KV Jr. Cimetidine protects against acetaminophen hepatotoxicity in rats. Gastroenterology 81:1052-1060, 1981.

• Prescott LF, Critchley JAJH. The treatment of acetaminophen poisoning. Annu Rev Pharmacol Toxicol 23:87-101, 1983.

Rumack BH. Acetaminophen overdose in young children. Am J Dis Child 138:428-433, 1984.

Rumack BH, Matthew H. Acetaminophen poisoning and toxicity. Pediatrics 55:871-876, 1975.

Rumack BH, Peterson RC, Koch GG, Amara IA. Acetaminophen overdose. Arch Intern Med 141:380-385, 1981.

Smith DW, Isakson G, Frankel LR, Kerner JA Jr. Hepatic failure following ingestion of multiple doses of acetaminophen in a young child. J Pediatr Gastroenterol Nutr 5:822-825, 1986.

78 Tricyclic Antidepressant Overdose

W. Gary Reed · Ron J. Anderson

Tricyclic antidepressants (amitriptyline, imipramine, desipramine, nortriptyline) are drugs commonly encountered in accidental as well as intentional overdose situations because the drugs are commonly prescribed for many conditions. This section reviews the presentation and treatment of overdoses of these drugs.

BACKGROUND AND PHYSIOLOGY

As a class, tricyclic antidepressants are lipophilic drugs that are quickly absorbed from the GI system and have a large volume of distribution. When toxic doses (usually >20 mg/kg) are ingested, symptoms generally appear within 1 to 4 hours. Some patients, however, absorb the drug very rapidly and exhibit severe symptoms of toxicity within 30 minutes of ingestion.

Tricyclics block uptake of norepinephrine and/or serotonin or dopamine in presynaptic nerve endings, causing an increase in central and peripheral adrenergic tone. There are also moderate central and peripheral anticholinergic effects. Tricyclics may also cause induction of adrenergic-receptor hyperactivity.

All tricyclics increase (2 to 10 times) the pressor response to injected direct-acting sympathetic agonists, including norepinephrine, epinephrine, and phenylephrine, which can lead to hyperthermia, tachycardia, severe hypertension, and death. This interaction may extend to other drugs with less well-known sympathetic actions such as ketamine and pancuronium.

Concomitant use of other drugs such as atropine with anticholinergic properties may cause additive side effects, particularly of the central side effects, and may precipitate central anticholinergic syndrome (confusion and delerium). It may be necessary to decrease the doses of narcotics and barbiturates since tricyclics are known to potentiate the side effects, including respiratory depression, of these agents.

Symptoms of mild toxicity are due primarily to the anticholinergic properties of the drugs and include sinus tachycardia, flushing, dry skin, agitation, adynamic ileus, and urinary retention.

Serious toxicity of tricyclic antidepressants involves primarily the cardiac and neurologic systems. Because the drugs are distributed unevenly between the plasma and different tissues, serum levels are difficult to interpret.

Major cardiac toxicity is due to a quinidine-like effect that results in a slowing of intracardiac conduction and myocardial depression, causing prolongation of the PR and QRS intervals, dysrhythmias, and hypotension. Prolongation of the QRS interval signifies a severe overdose, but its prognostic significance is not clear since this interval may vary significantly over short periods of time, especially with changes in acid-base status. Serious toxicity may occur in patients with a normal QRS duration. Prolongation of the QT interval may occur with therapeutic levels and consequently is not a reliable predictor of toxicity. Death in cases of serious overdose is usually due to cardiac toxicity, with ventricular dysrhythmias, bradycardias, or idioventricular rhythms as terminal events.

Delayed cardiac toxicity occurs rarely and unpredictably in the form of sudden cardiac death in patients 2 to 5 days after ingestion when serum levels of the drug have returned to nontoxic levels. The etiology of this syndrome is unknown but may be related to the accumulation of toxic metabolites of the parent drug, and many times this syndrome occurs in patients receiving other cardiotoxic drugs such as phenothiazines.

Neurologic complications in patients also complicate serious overdoses of tricyclic antidepressants. Early symptoms include agitation, delirium, and hallucinations. With severe toxicity, coma, myoclonus, and seizures dominate the neurologic picture. Seizures frequently are associated with a poor prognosis because the accompanying metabolic acidosis makes the amount of drug ingested more cardiotoxic. The level of consciousness of the patient is a good indicator of outcome.

MONITORING AND LABORATORY TESTS

Serum levels of the ingested drug and metabolites of the drug must be monitored serially if possible. Arterial pH must be measured if significant acidosis is suspected. Neurologic status must be monitored carefully, with special attention to myoclonus, the level of consciousness, the degree of respiratory depression, and seizures. All patients with seizures or significant depression of mental status must be admitted to the hospital.

Cardiac status can be monitored with frequent measurements of systemic arterial blood pressure and heart rate. A 12-lead ECG must be obtained on admission. Continuous ECG monitoring is mandatory to detect tachycardia, ventricular dysrhythmias, and conduction delays, including QRS prolongation. Any significant abnormality in rate, rhythm, or conduction is an indication for admission to the hospital.

Patients with trivial overdoses and no evidence of significant cardiac or neurologic toxicity can be monitored for at least 6 hours for the development of toxicity; if none is observed, the patient can be discharged. Patients with significant overdoses must have their ECG and neurologic status monitored for at least 24 hours after toxic manifestations have disappeared.

TREATMENT

Good supportive care is the mainstay of treatment, with special attendance to cardiac status, the airway, and ventilation. All patients with depressed ventilation or gag reflex and patients who are seizing must have their airway protected by tracheal intubation. Further support in the form of assisted ventilation may be required. Hypotension can be treated with fluids and Trendelenburg positioning if possible. Unabsorbed drug in the stomach must be removed. The use of ipecac in these patients is controversial since the mental status of the patient can deteriorate rapidly before vomiting is produced. Consequently, many authorities recommend gastric lavage in all patients, with or without endotracheal intubation. After the stomach is cleared, activated charcoal (1 g/kg) can be given with a cathartic such as sorbitol (1 to 1.5 g/kg as a 35% solution, with a maximum dose of 50 g) if bowel sounds are present. The initial dose of charcoal can be repeated at 2- to 6-hour intervals.

Seizures can be treated with diazepam (0.25 mg/kg IV, with a maximum dose of 5 mg if the patient is <5 years of age or 10 mg if patient is >5 years of age). If refractory seizures develop, phenytoin (15 mg/kg, maximum infusion rate of 0.5 mg/kg min, with a maximum dose of 1000 mg) and/or phenobarbital (10 to 15 mg/kg infused at 25 to 50 mg/min) can be used.

Conduction defects (QRS duration >0.12 msec or AV conduction abnormalities) should be treated with alkalinization of the blood to an arterial pH of approximately 7.5 by controlled hyperventilation if the patient is intubated or by the administration of sodium bicarbonate (1 to 2 mEq/kg). Alkalinization apparently decreases the toxicity of tricyclic antidepressants by increasing protein binding and thereby decreasing the amount of free drug available to cause toxicity. Phenytoin (12 to 15 mg/kg, maximum infusion rate of 0.5 mg/kg/min, with a maximum dose of 1000 mg) may counteract the cardiac effects of tricyclics. Ventricular dysrhythmias should be treated by alkalinization of the blood to a pH of approximately 7.5 with hyperventilation and sodium bicarbonate (dose as above). Refractory dysrhythmias can be treated with phenytoin (same dose as above) or lidocaine (1 mg/kg/bolus, with continuous rate of 3 μg/kg/min). Quinidine and procainamide should not be used since they potentiate the cardiac toxicity of the tricyclic antidepressants.

Physostigmine can reverse many of the neurologic manifestations of tricyclic overdose, but its use is not recommended because of its propensity to cause seizures. It does not reverse the cardiac effects of the tricyclic antidepressants.

ADDITIONAL READING

• Boehnert MT, Lovejoy FH. Value of the QRS duration versus the serum drug level in predicting seizures and ventricular arrhythmias after an acute overdose of tricyclic antidepressants. N Engl J Med 313:474-479, 1985.

• Brown TCK. Sodium bicarbonate treatment for tricyclic antidepressant arrhythmias in children. Med J Aust 2:380-382, 1976.

Emerman CL, Conners AF Jr, Burma GM. Level of consciousness as a predictor of complications following tricyclic overdose. Ann Emerg Med 16:326-330, 1987.

Foulke GE, Albertson TE. QRS interval in tricyclic antidepressant overdosage: Inaccuracy as a toxicity indicator in emergency settings. Ann Emerg Med 16:160-163, 1987.

Litovitz TL, Troutman WG. Amoxapine overdose. JAMA 250:1069-1701, 1983.

Mayron R, Ruiz E. Phenytoin: Does it reverse tricyclic antidepressant-induced cardiac conduction abnormalities? Ann Emerg Med 15:876-880, 1986.

• Nattel S, Keable H, Sasyniuk BI. Experimental amitriptyline intoxication: Electrophysiologic manifestations and management. J Cardiovasc Pharmacol 6:83-89, 1984.

79 Methylxanthine Toxicity

Frances C. Morriss

BACKGROUND AND PHYSIOLOGY

The methylxanthines comprise a group of closely related alkaloids occurring naturally in plants with worldwide geographic distribution, namely, *Thea sinensis,* the source of tea; *Theobroma cacao,* the source of chocolate; *Cola acuminate,* the source of cola; and *Coffea arabica,* the source of coffee. The popularity of these products derives from the belief that they are potent stimulants with the ability to elevate mood, decrease fatigue, and increase work capacity.

Pharmacologically significant methylxanthines for the pediatric age group are caffeine, used in the treatment of neonatal apnea and readily available in many common beverages (coffee, tea, cola drinks), and theophylline (or aminophylline), used as a bronchodilator in patients with reactive airways disease. They share a number of physiologic actions, which are summarized in Table 79-1. The cellular mechanisms of action of methylxanthines include translocation of intracellular calcium, increased levels of cyclic nucleotides, particularly 3′,5′-cyclic adenosine monophosphate (cyclic AMP), and blockade of adenosine receptors. In addition they may potentiate inhibitors of prostaglandin synthesis and reduce uptake of catecholamines.

Methylxanthines are well absorbed from the oral, parenteral, and rectal routes and are widely distributed to all body compartments. They are protein bound, theophylline more than caffeine. A number of conditions affect the half-life and elimination of theophylline, as outlined in Table 79-2.

Pharmacokinetic studies in children and neonates have revealed significant age-related differences in the handling of methylxanthines, particularly caffeine. Protein binding of theophylline is 25% to 36% in neonates as compared to 70% in children and adults, thus making the volume of distribution larger in neonates. These compounds are metabolized by the hepatic mixed-function mono-oxidase system; different forms of cytochrome P-450 (i.e., different pathways) are involved with the metabolism of theophylline and caffeine. Caffeine is excreted largely unchanged in the urine of neonates up to 3 to 4 months of age, as opposed to adults in whom 98% of caffeine is handled by demethylation to other metabolites. Theophylline is oxidized and demethylated to caffeine by a unique pathway in the neonates; this reaction does not occur in infants older than 16 months or in children, in whom theophylline metabolism is controlled by a separate portion of the P-450 mono-oxygenase system. In addition theophylline metabolism varies widely from patient to patient and from time to time in the same patient. The only accurate way to determine dose requirements is by obtaining serial serum levels.

Toxicity from methylxanthines can occur in several ways, namely, ingestion or accidental administration of a single large dose; accumulation of the drug after multiple doses, particularly with repetitive use of the rectal route of administration; interaction with other drugs; and too rapid administration of a single dose. Because of the large number of events that can affect theophylline levels, a wide variety of drug levels can exist in the same patient on a stable dose regimen. Sudden death secondary to dysrhythmias has been reported with too rapid IV administration. Signs of acute toxicity associated with levels >25 to 40 µg/ml include emesis, restlessness progressing to delirium, dysrhythmias, hyperreflexia, and convulsions. Patients with seizures secondary to theophylline toxicity have a poor prognosis; 50% may experience permanent neurologic sequelae. These seizures may be refractory to the usual anticonvulsants (phenytoin, barbiturate, benzodiazepines). Signs of chronic toxicity in neonates may be subtle, may occur in the therapeutic range, and may manifest as failure to gain weight, restlessness, irritability, diuresis, hyperglycemia, and tachycardia. At serum the-

ophylline levels >20 μg/ml neonates as well as older children have gastroesophageal reflux. Caffeine levels >40 to 50 μg/ml are associated with jitteriness in neonates and levels >100 μg/ml with glycosuria and tachycardia. The toxic range for caffeine in neonates has not been as well established as the toxic level for theophylline; tachypnea, hyperglycemia, ketonuria, and diuresis to the point of dehydration have all been reported at serum levels <40 μg/ml in in-

Table 79-1 Physiologic Effects of Methylxanthines

System	Physiologic Effects	Toxic Effects*
Central nervous system	Stimulation manifested as follows: Increased capacity for intellectual effort Nervousness, restlessness Tremors Increased sensitivity of all respiratory centers Increased cerebrovascular resistance, decreased cerebral blood flow Alteration of sleep state (increased REM sleep)	Insomnia Delirium (caffeine >15-30 μg/ml) Seizures (theophylline >25-40 μg/ml) Opisthotonus (caffeine >40 μg/ml)
Cardiovascular	Increased heart rate Decreased peripheral vascular resistance Increased myocardial contractility	Tachycardia (theophylline >10-20 μg/ml) Dysrhythmias (theophylline >40 μg/ml; caffeine >100 μg/ml) Death (theophylline >40 μg/ml; caffeine >80-100 μg/ml)
Respiratory	Bronchial smooth muscle relaxation Increased vital capacity Inhibition of mast cell secretion	
Skeletal muscle	Increased work capacity Augmented contractility, especially of diaphragm	
Renal	Diuresis (inhibition of solute reabsorption in proximal tubules and collecting ducts)	Dehydration
Gastrointestinal	Increased secretion of gastric acid (maximal response at caffeine level of 20 μg/ml)	Emesis (theophylline >20 μg/ml) Hematemesis of gastroesophageal reflux ? Necrotizing enterocolitis
Endocrine	Increased levels of circulating catecholamines Increased basal metabolic rate Increased levels of gastrin Hyperglycemia Decreased levels of thyroid-stimulating hormone and growth hormone (animal models)	Failure to gain weight Osmotic diuresis

*For most effects, the therapeutic index is larger for caffeine than theophylline.

fants receiving multiple dose therapy. An association between methylxanthine therapy for apnea and development of necrotizing enterocolitis may exist.

MONITORING

For asymptomatic patients receiving constant infusions of the drug or on a stable dosing schedule, only careful monitoring of cardiovascular variables, in-

Table 79-2   Conditions and Drugs that Affect Theophylline Clearance*

	Decreased Clearance	Increased Clearance
Age	Prematurity Neonates Aging	1-16 yr
Diet	High carbohydrate, low protein Caffeine Theobromine	Low carbohydrate, high protein Charcoal cooking
Smoking		Cigarettes Marijuana
Diseases	Hepatic diseases Congestive heart failure (moderate to severe) Acute pulmonary edema Severe airflow obstruction Pneumonia Acute viral illness	
Drugs	Oral contraceptives (smokers only) Cimetidine Macrolide antibiotics Erythromycin Lincomycin Troleandomycin (TAO) Thiabendazole ? Long-term theophylline therapy	Phenobarbital Benzodiazepines Alcohol

*From Plummer AL. Bronchodilator drugs in the cardiac patient. In Kaplan J, ed. Cardiovascular Anesthesia, vol 2, Cardiovascular Pharmacology. New York: Grune & Stratton, 1983, p 491.

cluding urinary output and urinary glucose concentrations in younger patients, and dose reduction may be all that is necessary. Monitoring during the use of multiple-dose charcoal therapy must include frequent evaluation of theophylline levels and of fluid and electrolyte status since excess losses can occur from both the GI tract and secondary to drug-induced or glucose-induced diuresis. Continuous ECG monitoring is needed for detection of dysrhythmias until the theophylline level is in a therapeutic range (<20 $\mu g/ml$). Procedures such as hemodialysis and charcoal perfusion must be performed in a PICU where close monitoring of CVP, systemic arterial blood pressure, urinary output, and other cardiovascular variables can be done.

TREATMENT

Treatment for methylxanthine overdose particularly depends on the circumstances and whether the patient is symptomatic. Asymptomatic patients need no specific therapy. In the event of an acute ingestion the usual measures of emptying the stomach and clearing the drug from the GI tract should be followed (see Chapter 75). Repeated doses of charcoal (GI dialysis) have been shown to be a very effective way to remove theophylline from the system. Serial serum levels demonstrate consistent lowering of theophylline, even in cases in which the overdose occurred from an IV route. Serial levels must be monitored after charcoal administration is stopped since a rebound phenomenon can occur.

For life-threatening intoxications both hemodialysis and charcoal hemoperfusion can be used effectively. Hemoperfusion, if available, is a somewhat simpler procedure. If possible these techniques must be instituted before the onset of dysrhythmias and seizures and must be based on the amount ingested and/or highly toxic serum levels (theophylline, >40 $\mu g/ml$, or caffeine, >80 to 100 $\mu g/ml$). Either technique necessitates adequate intra-arterial and IV access. While the appropriate catheters are placed and equipment readied, GI dialysis with multiple doses of charcoal can be started since this method will begin to bring down theophylline levels immediately and will supplement the more definitive therapy. Supportive therapy must include IV hydration and treatment of dysrhythmias and convulsions, although a specific recommendation for an anticonvulsant is difficult because of the refractory nature of seizures.

ADDITIONAL READING

Abramowicz M, ed. Hemoperfusion for removal of toxins. Med Lett 28:80, 1986.

Ginoza GW, Strauss AA, Lskra MK, et al. Potential treatment of theophylline toxicity by high surface area activated charcoal. J Pediatr 111:140-142, 1987.

Grosfield JL, Dalsing MC, Hull M, et al. Neonatal apnea, xanthines and necrotizing enterocolitis. J Pediatr Surg 18:80-82, 1983.

• Howell J, Clozel M, Aranda JV. Adverse effects of caffeine and theophylline in newborn infants. Semin Perinatol 5:359-382, 1981.

Kerbo M, Odajima Y, Ishizake T, et al. Intraindividual changes in theophylline clearance during constant aminophylline infusions in children with acute asthma. J Pediatr 108:1011-1018, 1986.

Park GD, Spector R, Roberts RJ, et al. Use of hemoperfusion for treatment of theophylline intoxication. Am J Med 74:961-966, 1983.

Shannon M, Amitar Y, Lovejoy FH. Multiple dose activated charcoal for theophylline poisoning in young infants. Pediatrics 80:368-370, 1987.

• Sullivan JL. Caffeine poisoning in an infant. J Pediatr 90:1022-1023, 1977.

Walther FJ, Sims ME, Siassi B, et al. Cardiac output changes secondary to theophylline therapy in preterm infants. J Pediatr 109:874-876, 1986.

80 Acute Digoxin Poisoning

David E. Fixler

BACKGROUND

Acute digoxin poisoning in childhood may have potentially lethal complications. Although elevated digoxin levels are most commonly the result of therapeutic overdosing, acute poisonings are usually the result of accidental ingestion. Mild cases of intoxication may cause GI complaints such as nausea and vomiting, mild conduction disturbances, and neurologic symptoms that dictate general supportive care and close monitoring. Severe overdoses can lead to life-threatening cardiac dysrhythmias such as ventricular tachycardia, ventricular fibrillation, high-grade atrioventricular (AV) block with marked bradycardia and CNS complications ranging from lethargy to coma, and generalized seizures.

Historical information is of the utmost importance since it may determine the type of therapy needed. The time of the ingestion must be determined and the amount ingested estimated.

MONITORING AND LABORATORY TESTS

A 12-lead ECG and rhythm strip must be obtained, and the patient must be continuously observed with ECG monitoring in the PICU until the serum digoxin levels have fallen within the normal range and/or no abnormal rhythm has been observed for at least 12 hours.

TREATMENT

If on admission the patient shows no evidence of lethargy or CNS complications, ipecac should be administered to facilitate gastric emptying. Following emesis a nasogastric tube of the largest possible caliber must be placed for gastric lavage to remove any remaining tablet particles.

Dysrhythmias usually occur within 1 to 2 hours after ingestion. Rhythm disturbances that compromise cardiac output must be treated promptly. Sec-

Table 80-1 Dosage of Digoxin Immune Fab Based on Estimated Ingestion

No. of 0.25 mg Digoxin Tablets Ingested	Digoxin Immune Fab Dose	
	mg	No. of Vials
5	70	1.7
10	140	3.4
15	200	5.0
20	275	7.0
25	340	8.5

ond-degree AV block and ventricular tachycardia may respond to IV phenytoin (15 mg/kg) given over a 60-minute period. Because IV phenytoin precipitates if diluted, the undiluted solution must be injected, giving one twelfth of the total dose every 5 minutes, followed by an IV flush of 0.9% sodium chloride solution to ensure the tube is cleared of drug. Phenytoin cannot be given as a continuous IV infusion. If ventricular tachycardia persists, lidocaine (1 mg/kg) should be infused as an IV bolus, which may be repeated. With ventricular fibrillation administration of IV lidocaine should be followed by DC defibrillation. Severe bradycardia secondary to sinus bradycardia should be treated with atropine (0.01 to 0.02 mg/kg, with a minimum dose of 0.1 mg). With second- and third-degree AV block, pacing must be initiated transcutaneously or transvenously.

A potassium chloride infusion need not be started unless significant hypokalemia is documented. Lethal hyperkalemia is most frequently associated with digoxin intoxication because of inactivation of sodium-potassium adenosine triphosphate. Therefore admin-

Table 80-2   Dosage of Digoxin Immune Fab Based on Serum Digoxin Level

Child's Weight (kg)	Serum Digoxin Level					
	2 ng/ml	4 ng/ml	8 ng/ml	12 ng/ml	16 ng/ml	20 ng/ml
3	2 mg	5 mg	9 mg	13 mg	18 mg	22 mg
5	4 mg	8 mg	15 mg	22 mg	30 mg	40 mg
10	8 mg	15 mg	30 mg	40 mg	60 mg	80 mg
20	15 mg	30 mg	60 mg	80 mg	120 mg	160 mg

istration of potassium supplements may be hazardous in these patients. After treatment with digoxin-specific antibody fragments (see below), potassium shifts back inside the cell, resulting in a fall in the serum potassium concentration. Therefore serum potassium must be measured repeatedly during the first few hours of treatment.

A preparation of digoxin-specific antibody fragments obtained from immunized sheep, digoxin immune Fab (Digibind), is now commercially available for treatment of life-threatening digoxin poisoning. Digoxin immune Fab binds molecules of digoxin, making them unavailable at their sites of action and resulting in a shift of the equilibrium away from the digoxin receptors, thereby reversing its effect. The serum digoxin concentration abruptly rises after administration of digoxin immune Fab because its bound fragments remain in the blood until excretion by the kidney. Therefore, after infusion of digoxin immune Fab, serum digoxin levels may be misleading until the elimination of the Fab digoxin fragments, which may occur over several days. As mentioned previously, serum potassium concentrations must be followed closely since, with the reversal of the effect of digoxin by the Fab fragments, potassium shifts back into the cell and serum potassium levels fall.

Indications for using digoxin immune Fab include the occurrence of life-threatening dysrhythmias, the ingestion of 4 mg or more of digoxin by a child, or serum digoxin levels associated with a high risk of developing life-threatening dysrhythmias. Digoxin immune Fab is administered IV over a 30-minute period. If cardiac arrest is eminent, it can be given as a bolus injection. The amount given depends on the estimated amount of digoxin ingested and the resulting serum digoxin concentration. When the serum digoxin level is not available, digoxin immune Fab can be administered on the basis of the estimated amount ingested (Table 80-1). The total body load of digoxin in milligrams will be approximately equal to 80% of the dose ingested in milligrams (allowing for incomplete absorption of tablets). The dosage of digoxin immune Fab may also be based on serum digoxin levels (Table 80-2). It is best to calculate the dosage based on both the amount ingested and on the serum concentration and to administer an amount based on the higher calculation.

Following infusion of the digoxin-specific antibodies, changes in cardiac dysrhythmias should occur within 15 to 30 minutes. If no clinical effect is obtained, administration of a second infusion must be considered.

ADDITIONAL READING

Murphy DJ, Bremner WF, Haber E, et al. Massive digoxin poisoning treated with Fab fragments of digoxin-specific antibodies. Pediatrics 70:472-473, 1982.

Smith TW, Butler VP, Haber E, et al. Treatment of life-threatening digitalis intoxication with digoxin-specific Fab antibody fragments. N Engl J Med 307:1357-1362, 1982.

Zucker AR, Lacina SJ, DasGupta DS, et al. Fab fragments of digoxin-specific antibodies used to reverse ventricular fibrillation induced by digoxin ingestion in a child. Pediatrics 70:468-471, 1982.

81 Antihypertensive Agent Ingestions

Frances C. Morriss

BACKGROUND AND PHYSIOLOGY

Because of the prevalence of chronic hypertension, antihypertensive medication is commonly available in many households. Antihypertensive drugs may be categorized by their mechanism of action; common types include diuretics, direct-acting vasodilators, calcium channel blocking agents, drugs that interfere with or modify adrenergic neuronal transmission, β-adrenergic antagonists, and angiotensin-converting enzyme inhibitors (Table 81-1). Diuretics are not discussed in this chapter, nor are agents such as nitroprusside and diazoxide that are used parenterally. Patients with chronic hypertension often receive more than a single type of antihypertensive medication, and ingestion of more than one type of drug may produce symptoms that appear to be atypical.

Specific Agents and Treatment
Direct Vasodilators

Direct-acting vasodilators such as hydralazine (Apresoline) and minoxidil (Loniten) inhibit vascular smooth muscle by direct action on the cell; the mechanism of action involves inactivation of guanylate cyclase, with accumulation of guanosine 3′,5′-cyclic monophosphate. Diastolic blood pressure is decreased more than systolic blood pressure; compensatory increases in heart rate, stroke volume, and cardiac output occur. Peripheral vasodilation is widespread, with increased splanchnic, coronary, cerebral, and renal blood flow. Compensatory mechanisms responding to the lowered blood pressure may also include increases in plasma renin activity, which can cause fluid retention. The more potent agent, minoxidil, triggers the release of systemic catecholamines as well. Overdoses of these agents are usually well tolerated; exaggerated hypotension is most likely to occur in conjunction with ingestion of another agent that blocks sympathetic nervous system input and inhibits the usual compensatory mechanisms that maintain systemic arterial blood pressure in the normal range.

Calcium channel blocking agents

Calcium channel blocking agents such as nifedipine, (Procardia), diltiazem (Cardizem), and verapamil (Isoptin) antagonize the movement of extracellular calcium across cellular membranes. In smooth muscle cells the flow of calcium ions from the sarcoplasmic reticulum to the cytoplasm is inhibited; consequently, activation of tropomyosin and the interaction between actin and myosin do not occur. Smooth muscle contraction is inhibited. Vasodilation occurs in the coronary and peripheral vascular systems, producing afterload reduction. Significant reduction in pulmonary vascular resistance without decreases in oxygenation has been noted.

The potential toxicity of these drugs as acute overdoses in children is not well documented. In general calcium channel blockers are well tolerated, and the most common side effects are headaches, dizziness, flushing, GI distress, and hypotension. As with other antihypertensives, exaggerated hypotension may occur with concomitant ingestion of other antihypertensives. Life-threatening bradycardia and asystole have been reported in young infants receiving IV verapamil; complete heart block and asystole have been reported in patients who have received β-blocking agents and verapamil.

Intravenous calcium chloride in doses of 10 to 20 mg/kg given over 30 minutes along with volume ex-

Table 81-1 Classes of Antihypertensives

Class of Drug	Example	Mechanism of Action
Diuretics	Chlorothiazide Furosemide	Prevention of sodium and water reabsorption
Direct vasodilators	Hydralazine Minoxidil	Smooth muscle relaxation
Calcium channel blockers	Verapamil	Inhibition of calcium movement from sarcoplasmic reticulum to cytoplasm
Peripheral adrenergic sympatholytics	Guanethidine Prazosin Reserpine	Inhibition of neurotransmitter reuptake α-Adrenergic blockade Depletion of catecholamines and 5-hydroxytryptamine
Central sympatholytics (adrenergic agonist)	Methyldopa Clonidine	Inhibition of central efferents at α-receptors
β-Adrenergic blockade	Propranolol	Competitive inhibition of β-agonist at receptor sites
Angiotensin-converting enzyme inhibitor	Captopril	Inhibition of conversion of angiotensin I to angiotensin II

pansion has been used to treat the toxic effects of verapamil. If no response occurs, atropine, 0.01 mg to 0.02 mg/kg IV, and an isoproterenol infusion, 0.05 to 0.1 μg/kg/min, can be tried. In the event of continued bradycardia pacemaker therapy may be considered.

Peripheral and central sympatholytics

The sympatholytic agents interfere with adrenergic transmission by several mechanisms, including (1) inhibition of neuronal reuptake of norepinephrine, an adrenergic neurotransmitter, (2) central adrenergic antagonism, (3) peripheral adrenergic blockade, and (4) β-adrenergic receptor antagonism.

Inhibition of reuptake of neurotransmitter is the mechanism of action of guanethidine (Ismelin) and probably of guanadrel (Hylorel). The agent itself is taken up and stored in the intraneuronal presynaptic storage granule and subsequently released. Although the agent acts as a false transmitter, the major effect derives from absence of norepinephrine. Responses to direct stimulation of adrenergic nerves and indirect stimulation from circulating catecholamines are diminished or inhibited. The initial action of the drug is release of norepinephrine from storage granules,

producing a transient increase in systemic arterial blood pressure and heart rate. Release of the agent from storage granules occurs slowly over several days once it is discontinued. The presence of guanethidine can cause an acute increase in tissue sensitivity to catecholamines, probably secondary to competition for an amine transport mechanism in the nerve membrane.

Acute overdoses with guanethidine have been associated with postural and exertional hypotension, syncope, shock, bradycardia, and diarrhea secondary to GI hypermotility. These symptoms will be aggravated by any condition such as fever or alcohol ingestion that promotes vasodilation. Treatment is directed toward restoring an adequate circulating blood volume, assuring a supine position to prevent orthostatic symptoms, and restoring heart rate through the administration of atropine. GI motility problems may also respond to atropine given in usual doses. Hypertension secondary to the initial release of norepinephrine either does not occur or is transient. Because of the slow release of stored guanethidine, observation and monitoring of cardiovascular variables must continue for several days after ingestion. If the use of pressor agents is necessary, direct-acting vasoconstrictors such as phenylephrine and methoxamine will be more efficacious than those agents that depend on release of neurotransmitter.

Reserpine (Serpasil) acts by depleting catecholamine and 5-hydroxytryptamine in many organs, including the central nervous system and the adrenal medulla, and by antagonizing reuptake. Norepinephrine synthesis is decreased because of the blockage of dopamine uptake into storage granules. Depletion is complete within 24 hours of administration, and restoration of tissue catecholamine occurs slowly. A transient sympathomimetic effect can occur initially, followed by a fall in blood pressure, sometimes accompanied by bradycardia. Decreased peripheral resistance is most marked in the skin. Cardiac output is reduced and accounts for the major reduction in blood presssure; normal pressor responses may be inhibited. Central effects include sedation and indifference to external stimuli, often accompanied by psychic phenomenon (nightmares, severe depression). GI tone increases, and cramping with diarrhea is common. Massive overdoses have been reported in children, although there have been no known fatalities. Signs and symptoms of overdose include reflex parasympathomimetic effects such as impairment of consciousness (including coma), flushing, pupillary constriction, hypotension, hypothermia, bradycardia, central respiratory depression, increased salivary and gastric secretions, and diarrhea. Treatment is supportive. Observation for at least 72 hours is recommended because of the long-acting nature of reserpine.

Central adrenergic neuronal antagonism can occur either through inhibition of a norepinephrine-mediated facilitatory pathway (β-receptors) or through stimulation of a lower brain stem regulatory system that inhibits sympathetic output. This second system is activated by lower brain stem α-adrenoreceptors, methyldopa (Aldomet) and clonidine (Catapres), both of which are potent central α-adrenergic agonists. In the synthesis of norepinephrine the enzyme dopa decarboxylase catalyzes the conversion of dopa to dopamine. Methyldopa competes with dopa for the enzyme site and inhibits the action of dopa decarboxylase so that α-methylnorepinephrine is produced instead of norepinephrine. It acts as an α-adrenoreceptor agonist, inhibiting central sympathetic output. Total peripheral resistance and systemic blood pressure decreases, whereas cardiac out-

put remains unchanged. Most side effects occur with chronic use; acute intoxication is well tolerated and requires only symptomatic treatment.

Clonidine, a powerful α₂-adrenoreceptor agonist, causes decreased release of norepinephrine from peripheral adrenergic nerves. In addition it has a central presynaptic effect in the brain stem where inhibition of efferent central impulses occurs, and stimulation of the baroreflexes from enhanced vagal excitation leads to slowing of the heart rate. An increase in blood pressure is sometimes noted after therapy is begun and is thought to be mediated by direct peripheral α-adrenergic stimulation. Circulating plasma renin secretion is inhibited centrally, and renal blood flow remains unchanged despite a lowered blood pressure.

Clonidine ingestions in children have been reported; symptoms include drowsiness, coma, contracted pupils, hypotension, bradycardia, hypothermia, and respiratory depression leading to apnea. Rhythm disturbances primarily related to enhanced vagal (parasympathetic) activity may include exaggerated sinus dysrhythmia, sinus bradycardia with premature atrial contractions, and atrioventricular (AV) conduction block. The amount ingested does not correlate well with the severity of symptoms, and all children ingesting clonidine must be observed using appropriate cardiovascular monitoring until stable. Treatment of ingestions is supportive; fluids are administered to maintain an adequate circulating volume and to support cardiac output. Ventilation is instituted as needed. IV atropine, 0.01 to 0.02 mg/kg, may be used for treating isolated bradycardia. Severe hypotension may necessitate the use of a vasopressor; good support of the cardiovascular system has been achieved with dopamine infusions at doses of 2 to 10 μg/kg/min. The role of tolazoline in treating clonidine ingestions remains unclear, and it should not be considered a specific antidote.

Peripheral α-adrenergic blockade can be produced by prazosin (Minipres), an α₁-adrenergic blocker. Prazosin, a quinazoline derivative, produces vascular smooth muscle relaxation by competitive inhibition of peripheral postsynaptic α₁-receptors. Since there are both α₁- and α₂-postsynaptic vascular receptors, the efficacy of this agent depends on the ratio of one subtype of receptor to the other subtype. The affinity of the drug for the α₁-receptor is high, and interference with neurotransmitter action on the

α_2-receptor is low. Peripheral resistance and mean arterial blood pressure are reduced, with no reflexively mediated increase in heart rate. Exercise and exposure to cold and other conditions associated with reflex vasodilation do not cause further hypotension. The first dose of the drug can cause profound changes in blood pressure; dizziness and syncope are not uncommon. Subsequent doses are not accompanied by similar symptoms. Since the drug requires hepatic glucuronidation for excretion, lower and less frequent doses must be used in neonates or patients with impaired hepatic function. Overdoses in children have been associated with prolonged drowsiness, diminished consciousness, hypotension, and diminished reflexes. Apnea has not been seen. Treatment is symptomatic and supportive; since the drug is highly protein bound, it cannot be removed by dialysis.

β-Adrenergic Blockade

β-Adrenergic antagonists compete with neurotransmitter at β-adrenergic receptors for occupation of the cellular membrane site. The competition is based on a structural affinity between the antagonist and isoproterenol. Changes in the structure of the antagonist molecule have allowed further selection for β_1-receptors (responsible for cardiac stimulation and lipolysis) and not β_2-receptors (responsible for bronchodilation, glucose mobilization, and catecholamine-induced insulin release), which propranolol (Inderal), the prototype β-blocking agent, does not have.

In the treatment of hypertension β-blocking agents act by reducing cardiac output (inhibition of central β-adrenergic stimulation and of peripheral cardiac receptors to reduce heart rate) and plasma renin activity that is adrenergically mediated. Renin secretion mediated by sodium imbalance or changes in renal perfusion or posture is unaffected. The most likely site of action for these changes is the peripheral β-receptor. Inhibition of centrally generated β-adrenergic impulses is not essential to the hypotensive action of the drug group; atenolol and practolol, which do not cross the blood-brain barrier, lower blood pressure adequately. It is unknown whether the central action is necessary for long-term maintenance of blood pressure control.

Predictable side effects of β-blockade include bradycardia, decreased cardiac output, bronchocon-

striction, impaired recovery from hypoglycemia, and vasoconstriction. Adverse reactions usually constitute more pronounced side effects such as bronchospasm in susceptible patients, congestive heart failure, symptomatic bradycardia or intensification of AV block, and augmentation of the action of insulin or hypoglycemia, particularly in infants. Propranolol is metabolized by the liver; it is not removed by dialysis.

Treatment is supportive and symptomatic. Atropine should be used to treat symptomatic bradycardia; if the patient has persistent slowing of the heart beat, use of an isoproterenol infusion or pacemaker therapy should be considered. β-Blockade is competitive, and a larger amount of isoproterenol may be needed to achieve a desired response (i.e., to counteract the structurally similar molecule occupying receptor sites). Aerosolized β-agonists and IV aminophylline, which has a mechanism of action on airway membrane receptors separate from β-agonists, should be used to treat symptomatic bronchoconstriction. Hypotension unresponsive to cautious fluid expansion should be treated with an epinephrine infusion of 0.05 to 0.1 μg/kg/min.

The following β-agonist–drug interactions should be kept in mind: rate of absorption decreases with ethanol ingestion and the presence of aluminum hydroxide gel; lidocaine and aminophylline clearances are reduced in the presence of propranolol; cimetidine decreases hepatic degradation, leading to an increase in plasma levels of propranolol; concomitant chlorpromazine administration causes increased plasma levels of both drugs; and phenytoin, barbiturates, and rifampin cause increased clearance and low serum levels.

Angiotensin-Converting Enzyme Inhibition

Renin is a proteolytic enzyme secreted by the renal juxtaglomerular apparatus in response to changes in renal perfusion. It acts on hepatically produced angiotensin substrate to produce angiotensin I. Angiotensin-converting enzyme located in pulmonary epithelial cells catalyzes formation of angiotensin II, which stimulates contraction of vascular smooth muscle, promotes aldosterone production with retention of sodium and water, and acts directly on renal tubules to cause sodium and water retention. Captopril (Capoten) and enalapril (Vasotec) are specific competitive inhibitors of angiotensin-converting enzyme. In addition conversion of bradykinin to an inactive metabolite is inhibited, and increased levels of bradykinin may contribute to the acute hypotensive effect through release of prostaglandins. Peripheral vascular resistance is lowered, with little effect on cardiac output or heart rate; in patients with congestive heart failure increased cardiac output and decreased left ventricular end-diastolic pressure may occur. Aldosterone production may be decreased, resulting in mild hyperkalemia. Cough is a very common side effect. Severe neutropenia, agranulocytosis, proteinuria, and azotemia are the most serious side effects seen in children. Overdoses are usually well tolerated; the primary treatment is supportive with maintenance of an adequate blood volume. Dialysis can be used for removal of the drug if necessary.

MONITORING

Even though the antihypertensive medications are drugs that have diverse mechanisms of action, the end result is a reduction in systemic arterial blood pressure. Monitoring begins with blood pressure determinations. Care must be taken that an appropriate-sized cuff is selected so that falsely high or low pressures do not confuse caretakers. An appropriate cuff has a bladder that encompasses three fourths of the circumference of the arm and a length that is approximately two thirds to three fourths of the distance from the elbow to the shoulder. Noninvasive blood pressure determinations through an automatic device equipped to cycle at specific intervals and equipped with alarms will ensure frequent and consistent monitoring.

Because many of the agents described previously cause relative hypovolemia, usually through alteration of peripheral resistance, repetitive evaluation of volume status by physical examination is necessary. This includes assessment of capillary refill, presence and character of pulses, warmth of extremities, and level of consciousness. In addition urinary output must be monitored if possible through use of a bladder catheter. If severe hypotension is present or anticipated, beat-to-beat intra-arterial pressure monitoring is needed (see Chapters 108 and 115). Vigorous fluid therapy to reestablish an effective blood volume must be guided by central venous blood pressure monitoring (see Chapter 114), particularly if the initial response to fluids is poor. Most of these patients are not dehydrated or having excessive fluid losses, but the normal blood volume is inadequate for the expanded vascular space and fixed peripheral resistance.

Patients who have ingested agents that act on the central or peripheral nervous system may have impaired vascular responses to lowered blood pressure, stress, cold, other medications, and diuresis. The usual reflex responses to lowered arterial blood pressure include (1) baroreceptor stimulation to increase heart rate and promote vasoconstriction; (2) carotid and aortic chemoreceptor reflexes that excite the vasomotor center to elevate pressure when arterial flow decreases, arterial oxygen decreases, or hydrogen ion or carbon dioxide levels increase; (3) atrial and pulmonary arterial stretch receptor (low-pressure receptors) response that increases pressure via the vasomotor center and via secretion of antidiuretic hormone (promotion of water and sodium retention); and (4) CNS ischemic response that occurs when cerebral perfusion pressure drops, promoting intense systemic vasoconstriction. All mechanisms for autoregulation of blood flow in various vascular beds may be impaired. In addition, in the patient with an unresponsive peripheral vasculature, heat loss will be accentuated, and frequent temperature determinations are necessary to follow existing or anticipated hypothermia. Centrally acting agents also possess the potential for a wide range of neurologic manifestations such as drowsiness, coma, tremors, delirium, hallucinations, agitation, impaired or altered reflexes, and impaired neuromuscular function. Maintenance of central cardiac and respiratory drive may be affected; therefore frequent neurologic examinations must be done and cardiorespiratory monitoring for dysrhythmias and apnea instituted.

SUPPORTIVE THERAPY

Supportive therapy must initially be directed toward treatment of orthostatic symptoms, which predictably occur with many of these drugs. An initial maneuver of placing the patient in the Trendelenburg position may restore blood pressure and cerebral blood flow sufficiently for the patient to regain consciousness and to allow IV access to be secured. Even though his initial blood pressure determinations are normal, the patient should probably be confined to a supine position during the initial observation period. Many of the agents in question cause an initial release of neurotransmitter that will support blood pressure for a short period of time (i.e., a biphasic blood pressure response can occur). Although the patient has a normal blood volume, a relative hypovolemia may exist. Cautious volume expansion with 0.9% sodium chloride solution, lactated Ringer's solution, or a 5% albumin solution, 10 to 20 ml/kg, should be started; failure of the blood pressure to respond indicates a need for central venous blood pressure monitoring to guide further fluid therapy. Unremitting hypotension may also result from depressed cardiac output (e.g., negative inotropy that occurs with β-blockade) or severe rhythm disturbances (e.g., bradycardia, AV dissociation that occurs with use of clonidine). Vasopressor or antidysrhythmic therapy may be needed to restore adequate cardiac output; direct measurement of cardiac output and changes after institution of therapy can be done with either a pulmonary artery catheter containing a thermistor or through a dye-dilution technique using arterial and central venous catheters.

The patient must be provided an environment that promotes heat retention; the use of warming devices such as fluid warmers, overhead radiant heaters, and heating blankets may be needed to ensure normal body temperature, particularly if the patient must be exposed for catheter placement or cardiopulmonary resuscitation. Use of drugs known to cause vasodilation (sedatives, narcotics, tranquilizers, antihistamines, some antibiotics, neuromuscular blocking agents that release histamine) should be avoided. Ventilatory support must be provided as needed for treating respiratory depression and loss of protective airway reflexes. In small infants glycogen depletion may occur, and serial glucose determinations may be needed to guide glucose administration.

All the usual measures directed toward removal of the ingested agent, prevention of absorption, and increase in clearance should be instituted (see Chapter 75). More invasive measures to further eliminate the drug (forced diuresis, dialysis, exchange transfusion) are rarely necessary. Many of these agents have a prolonged duration of action, particularly in peripheral and central nervous system sites, and the period of patient observation must be long enough to assure continued hemodynamic stability despite apparent lack of symptoms.

ADDITIONAL READING

Abramowicz M, ed. Drugs for hypertension. Med Lett 29:1-6, 1987.

Cardiovascular drugs. In Roberts RJ. Drug Therapy in Infants: Pharmacologic Principles and Clinical Experience. Philadelphia: WB Saunders, 1984, pp 173-205.

• Cho C, Pruitt SW. Therapeutic uses of calcium channel-blocking drugs in the young. Am J Dis Child 10:360-365, 1986.

• Conner CS, Watanabe AS. Clonidine overdose: A review. Am J Hosp Pharm 36:906, 1979.

Lloyd TR, Mahony LT, Koedel D, et al. Orally administered enalopril for infants with congestive heart failure: A dose-finding study. J Pediatr 114:650-654, 1989.

Llisson JM, Pruett SW. Management of clonidine ingestion in children. J Pediatr 103:646-650, 1983.

Passal DB, Crispin FH. Verapamil poisoning in an infant. Pediatrics 73:543-545, 1984.

Perlman JM, Volpe JJ. Neurologic complications of captopril treatment of neonatal hypertension. Pediatrics 83:47-52, 1989.

Rao PS, Andaya WG. Chronic afterload reduction in infants and children with primary myocardial disease. J Pediatr 108:530-534, 1986.

• Rudd P, Bloschke TT. Antihypertensive agents and the drug therapy of hypertension. In Gillman AG, Goodman LS, Rall TW, eds. Goodman and Gillman's the Pharmacologic Basis of Therapeutics, 7th ed. New York: Macmillan, 1985, pp 784-805.

Sinaiko AR, Mirkin BC, Hendrick DA, et al. Antihypertensive effect and elimination. Kinetics of captopril in hypertensive children with renal disease. J Pediatr 103:799-805, 1983.

• Williams GH. Converting-enzyme inhibitors in the treatment of hypertension. N Engl J Med 319:1517-1525, 1988.

82 Plant Poisoning

Frances C. Morriss

BACKGROUND

Accidental ingestions of plants or plant material remain the most common ingestion seen in children less than age 3 years. Of all inquiries to poison control centers, 5% to 10% involve plants. Most of these questions can be handled through phone instructions and reassurance; mortality is low, hospitalization infrequent, and side effects minimal.

However, some plant toxins can produce severe symptoms and death; to predict the likelihood and severity of symptoms and the need for other than supportive management, the plant must be identified, which is difficult for the following reasons: the treating physician is probably not versed in toxonomic plant identification, incomplete specimens may be presented (i.e., seed, flower, leaf instead of whole plant), and often only a vague description or a common name is given.

In addition to providing referral to the local poison control center it may be necessary to locate a trained toxonomic botanist to identify the plant. The local college department of biology, agriculture, or botany and staff members of arboretums or botanical gardens may act as consultants. The following is a poison control center that specializes in plant toxicology:

Texas State Poison Center
University of Texas Medical Branch
Galveston, TX
(409)765-1420

PLANT IDENTIFICATION

Standard references that may be useful in identifying plants are as follows:

Common Poisonous and Injurious Plants. HHS Pub #(FDA) 81-7006. Washington, D.C.: U.S. Government Printing Office, 1981. *(This is a color illustrated bulletin written for lay readers.)*

Ellis MD. Dangerous Plants, Snakes, Arthropods and Marine Life. Toxicity and Treatment. Hamilton, N.Y.: Drug Intelligence Publications, 1978.

Hardin JW, Arena JM. Human Poisonings from Native and Cultivated Plants, 2nd ed. Durham, N.C.: Duke University Press, 1974. *(This is intended for camp, school, and scout groups.)*

Lampe KF, McCann MA. AMA Handbook of Poisonous and Injurious Plants. Chicago: Chicago Review Press, 1985. *(Excellent photographs make this useful as a field guide.)*

Mitchell J, Rook A. Botanical Dermatology, Plants and Plant Products Injurious to the Skin. Vancouver: Grunglass, 1979.

In addition to identification of the plant the following information may be vital to predicting whether a severe reaction may occur: What part of the plant was ingested? In what quantity? By what route (oral, rectal, through the skin)? In what form was the plant (dried, ripe or unripe, whole, chewed, raw or cooked)? Was anything else consumed at the same time? Where was the plant located (in house, garden, woods, health food store)? Knowing the age of the patient is important as well; plants that may cause few symptoms in adults or teenagers may be fatal for the very young child. Toxicity may differ for the same plant, depending on factors such as the time of year, the part of the country, and the type of growing conditions in effect during any particular year. In addition plant material from widespread areas, including areas outside the United States, are now available through health food stores; these products are often not properly labeled and may contain mixtures from several sources. If the symptom complex does not seem to fit a known ingestion and the plant was consumed as food, the possibility of other contaminants such as pesticides, insecticides, or bacterial toxins must be considered.

PLANT TOXIN SYMPTOMATOLOGY

The common types of plant toxins that induce symptoms are listed in Table 82-1; many plants may contain more than one type of toxin, and several symptom groups may be encountered.

GI irritation is the most common symptom after plant ingestion and ranges from local mucous membrane irritation to severe enteritis with emesis, diarrhea, mucosal sloughing, severe bleeding, and volume depletion (Table 82-2). Plants such as rhubarb that contain calcium oxalate crystals cause burning, edema, and pain when the sharp crystals are driven into mucous membranes, but only local treatment is

necessary. For most ingestions symptomatic therapy is all that is required. Fatalities are usually secondary to fluid depletion, cardiovascular collapse, or secondary renal failure. Patients ingesting plants causing release of hydrocyanic acid must be treated for cyanide poisoning (see Chapter 75).

SPECIFIC PLANT TOXINS
Glycosides

Table 82-3 lists plants containing glycosides, the primary action of which is directed toward cardiac smooth muscle. Intoxication resembles digitalis overdose (see Chapter 80), with the most common dysrhythmias being bradycardia and atrial conduction defects. Only symptomatic dysrhythmias must be treated (see Chapter 23); atropine and phenytoin may be particularly useful in treating dysrhythmias and block; demulcents are helpful in treating GI symptoms from saponins, and CNS disturbances must be managed supportively.

Table 82-1   Common Plant Toxins

Class of Toxins	Characteristics	Examples
Alkaloids	Crystalline organic compounds having an alkaline pH; usually pharmacologically active; belladonna alkaloids are associated with anticholinergic effects; others have both central and peripheral acetylcholine receptor agonist-antagonist effects	Atropine Cholchicine Nicotine Solanine Gelsemine
Glycoside	A plant product that, through hydrolytic cleavage, releases a sugar and an aglycon (nonsugar component); usually toxic	
Irritant glycosides	Glycosides that act as vesicants	Daphnin Protoanemonin
Cardiac	Primary effect on cardiac smooth muscle; pacemaker fibers are markedly affected	Digoxin Digitoxin
Cyanogenic	On hydrolysis yields hydrocyanic acid	Sambinigen Amygdalin
Hematologic	Affects the coagulation system	Coumarin
Saponins	Steroidal glycosides hydrolyzed to active tripertene compounds, often severe GI irritants; form a durable foam in agitated water solutions	Diosmine Phytolaccatoxin
Phylotoxin	A plant exotoxin; large protein molecule related to bacterial toxins and snake venom; highly toxic, resistant to proteolytic digestion; some are capable of inhibition of ribosomal protein synthesis; includes toxalbumins	Ricin Robin Abrin
Oxalates	Insoluble calcium oxalate crystals that are not absorbed and cause mechanical irritation	
Resinoids	Semisolid plant products associated with CNS effects	Podophyllin

Table 82-2   Plants Causing Gastrointestinal Symptoms

Plants	Toxic Part	Toxin	Fatal	Comments
Amery uidaceae sp (narcissus, jonquil, amaryllus)	Bulb	Lycorine (alkaloid)	No	—
Abrus sp (rosary bean)	Seed	Abrin (phytotoxin)	Yes	Seed must be chewed to release toxin; seeds used to make jewelry in tropics
Aesculus sp (horse chestnut)	Seed	Saponins	No	—
Arnica sp	Flowers, roots	Unknown	No	House plants
Arum sp (calla lily, caladium, Diffenbachia philodendron)	All parts	Oxylate crystals, proteolytic enzymes, toxic resinoids	No	Common house plants
Barosma betulina	Leaves	Diosmin (saponin), volatile oils	No	Herbal use as diuretic
Blighia sapida (akee)	Fruit capsule	Hypoglycin A and B	Yes (within 24 hr)	Unripe fruit is cause of "Jamaican vomiting sickness"; depletion of liver glycogen with hypoglycemia
Buxus sempervirins (box)	Leaves	Daphnin (irritant glycoside)	Yes	—
Caltha palustris (cowslip)	Leaves, stems	Protoanemonin (irritant glycoside)	No	Vesicants blister mucous membranes
Clematis sp	Bulb	Protoanemonin (vesicant glycoside)	No	—
Daphne sp (spurge laurel)	All parts, especially berries	Daphnin (glycoside), phorbol	Yes	—
Euphorbia marginata	All parts	Diterpenes (saponin)	No	Sap is skin irritant as well
Hedera helix (English ivy)	All parts	Hederin (saponin)	No	—
Ilex sp (holly)	Berries	Ilicin (alkaloid)	Yes (20-30 berries in a child)	—
Iris sp (iris)	Bulb	Iridin	No	—
Lathyrus odorathus (sweet pea)	All parts	Toxic amines	Yes	—
Ligustrum sp (privet)	Berries	Grayanotoxin	No	—
Mentha pulegium (pennyroyal)	Leaves	Pulegone (volatile oil)	No	Used as abortifacient
Parathenocissus quinquefolia (American ivy)	Leaves, berries	Oxalic acid	No	Systemic oxalic poisoning
Phytolacca sp (pokeweed)	Berries, roots, leaves	Phytolaccatoxin	Yes	—
Podophyllum peltatum (may apple)	Leaves, roots, unripe fruit	Podophylloresin	No	Ripe fruit edible; peripheral neuropathy

Table 82-2 Plants Causing Gastrointestinal Symptoms—cont'd

Plants	Toxic Part	Toxin	Fatal	Comments
Prunus sp (cherries, apricots, plums, peaches)	Leaves, bark, stems, seed pits	Amygdalin (cyanogenic alkaloid), prunasin	Yes	Fruit edible
Ranunculus sp (buttercup)	All parts	Protoanemonin (vesicant glycoside)	No	—
Rheum rhaponticum (rhubarb)	Leaves	Oxalates	No	Cooked stems edible
Ricinus communis (castor bean)	Seeds	Ricin (phytotoxin)	Yes (one seed)	Seed must be chewed to release toxin; symptoms may be delayed
Robinia sp (black locust)	Bark, seeds, foliage	Robin (phytotoxin)	No	—
Sambucus sp (elderberry)	Leaves, shoots, bark	Sambinigen (cyanogenetic glycoside)	Yes	—
Senecio sp (ragwort)	All parts	Senecionine (pyrrolizidine)	Yes	Toxin metabolized to carcinogenic pyrroles; causes hepatic veno-occlusive disease
Solanum sp (woody nightshade, Jerusalem cherry, European bittersweet, horse nettle)	Leaves, fruit	Solanine (alkaloid)	Yes	—
Symplocarpus foetidus (swamp cabbage)	All parts	—	No	—
Veratrum sp (false hellebore, bear grass)	Leaves, roots	Veratrum (alkaloid)	No	Hypertension and tachycardia occur with large ingestion
Wisteria sinensis (wisteria)	Seeds, pods	Wistarine resinoids	No	—

Table 82-3 Plants Containing Cardiac Glycosides

Plants	Toxic Part	Toxin	Fatal	Comments
Convallaria (lily of the valley)	All parts	Convallarin	Yes	—
Digitalis purpurea (foxglove)	All parts	Digoxin,* digitoxin, saponins	Yes	Hemodialysis ineffective
Nerium oleander (oleander)	All parts	Oleandrin, nerioside	Yes	Ingestion of water from vases holding flowers can be fatal
Thevetia peruwiania (yellow oleander)	All parts	Cardiac glycoside	Yes	—

*Digoxin and digitoxin antibodies in RIA assays cross-react with other cardioactive glycosides to produce a positive response.

Belladonna Alkaloids

Anticholinergic symptoms suggestive of atropine overdose typify ingestion of plants containing belladonna alkaloids (Table 82-4). Signs of parasympathetic antagonism include mydriasis, loss of accommodation, dryness of mouth, dysphagia, flushed dry skin, and tachycardia. Ingestions of large amounts of these alkaloids can produce central anticholinergic effects such as hyperpyrexia, delerium, hallucinations, convulsions, and coma. Fatalities, although reported, are uncommon. Physostigmine, a tertiary amine capable of crossing the blood-brain barrier and an anticholinesterase inhibiting the breakdown of acetylcholine, the parasympathetic receptor agonist, may be used to antagonize atropine-like effects in severe cases.

Alkaloids With Autonomic Ganglion-Stimulating Properties

A second group of alkaloids whose symptoms may superficially resemble those caused by the parasympathetic antagonists cause stimulation of autonomic ganglia, which can produce emesis (central), salivation, diaphoresis, headache, confusion, incoordination, muscle weakness, hyperpyrexia, tachycardia, mydriasis, and occasionally convulsions or various combinations of these symptom complexes. Fatalities occur secondary to respiratory failure either from paralysis of respiratory muscles or secondary to hypoxia and prolonged seizures. Cardiac conduction defects may also occur. The most common alkaloids include nicotine, veratridine, anabasine, conium, jessamine, and aconitine; plants causing this group of problems are listed in Table 82-5. Treatment is supportive, with conservative management as symptoms occur. Patients suspected of ingesting this group of alkaloids must be carefully watched for respiratory failure; onset of muscle paralysis is often delayed and may be difficult to recognize initially.

Convulsants, Anticoagulants, and Hallucinogens

Table 82-6 lists miscellaneous plants associated with other toxic properties. These plants contain naturally occurring convulsants, anticoagulants, and hallucinogens.

Mushrooms

Mushrooms are the plants that "traditionally" cause fatalities, and their identification may be very difficult. If identification is in doubt, ingestion of wild mushrooms must be treated as serious until a nontoxic nature is established. The patient's stomach must be emptied and activated charcoal given, even if it is some hours past ingestion, to prevent enterohepatic reuptake of potential toxins. Intoxications have been

Table 82-4   Plants Containing Belladonna Alkaloids

Plants	Toxic Part	Toxin	Fatal	Comments
Atropa belladonna (deadly nightshade)	All parts; highest in roots	Hyoscyamine, solanine	Yes in children	—
Colchicum autumnale (autumn crocus)	Bulb	Cholchicine (mitotic poison)	No	Delayed onset of symptoms
Datura stramonium (jimson weed, thorn apple)	Seeds, flowers, roots	Hyoscyamine, scopolamine	No	—
Hyoscyamus niger (henbane)	All parts	Hyoscyamine	No	—
Lantana camara (wild sage)	Unripe berries	Lantanine	Yes	Delayed onset of symptoms; photosensitization of skin
Myristica fragrens (nutmeg)	Seeds	Myristicin, elemicin	No	—

divided into two subgroups based on the appearance of symptoms in relation to the time of ingestion and on the type of clinical presentation. Symptoms (usually suggestive of gastroenteritis) that appear within 6 hours of ingestion or within several hours of ingesting alcohol are rarely serious. The shorter the interval between ingestion and onset of symptoms, the less toxic the mushroom is likely to be. Coprine, a disulfiram-like toxin that blocks acetaldehyde de-hydrogenase and that remains active for up to 3 days after intake, causes symptoms occurring after alcohol has been ingested. An initial presentation of CNS disturbances or peripheral or central symptoms related to acetylcholine receptors (agonist or antagonist actions), never associated with fatal cyclopeptide or gyromitrin toxins, also indicates a probably favorable outcome.

Many mushrooms contain muscarine, the effects

Table 82-5　Plants Containing Alkaloids With Autonomic Ganglia-Stimulating Properties

Plants	Toxic Part	Toxin	Fatal	Comments
Aconitum (monkshood)	Leaves, seeds, roots	Aconitine	Yes	Dysrhythmias usual cause of death; toxin inhibits repolarization of membranes
Conium maculatum (poison hemlock)	Leaves, seeds	Coniine	Yes	Alkaloids resemble nicotine; death from respiratory muscle paralysis
Delphinium sp (larkspur)	Leaves, seeds, roots	Diterpenoids	Yes	Respiratory paralysis
Dicentra sp (bleeding heart)	All parts	Apomorphine, isoquinoline	No	Convulsant
Gelsemium sempervirens (jessamine)	All parts, nectar	Gelsemine	No	Most children poisoned by sucking nectar from flower; symptoms secondary to antagonism of central and peripheral acetylcholine receptors (muscarinic, nicotinic)
Laburnum anagyroides (golden chain tree)	Seeds	Nicotine	Yes	—
Lobelia sp (cardinal flower)	All parts	Lobeline	Yes	Death secondary to respiratory muscle paralysis
Nicotiana sp (weed tobacco)	All parts, concentrated in leaves	Nicotine, anabasine	Yes	Death secondary to respiratory failure
Rhododendron sp (rhododendron, azalea, laurels)	All parts	Grayanotoxins	Yes	Actions of toxin similar to aconitine; honey made from nectar is poisonous
Taxus sp (yew)	All parts, concentrated in seeds, bark	Taxine	Yes	Death secondary to respiratory failure
Veratrum sp (green hellebores)	Leaves, roots	Veratridine	Yes	Actions similar to aconitine
Zigadenus sp (deathcamus)	Bulb	Grayanotoxins	Yes	Action similar to *Aconitum;* hypotension

of which (profuse sweating, salivation, colic, rales) can be treated with atropine to provide comfort. Other mushrooms, notably *Amanita muscaria,* contain muscimol, a γ-aminobutyric acid (GABA), that causes drowsiness and sleep, followed by elation, tremors, illusions, and manic excitement. No therapy is needed; atropine is contraindicated. Psilocybin, a nonlethal hallucinogen of short duration, is derived from mushrooms. Adults need no treatment after its ingestion, but children may show persistent neurologic disturbances, including seizures, for up to 12 hours. Table 82-7 lists characteristics of mushroom intoxications.

Fatal poisonings occur with ingestion of *A. phalloides* species and *Gyromitra species.* With ingestion of both species the onset of symptoms is delayed, and no neurologic derangements are seen. *A. phalloides* contains two classes of thermostable cyclic octapeptides known as amatoxins. They bind and inhibit RNA polymerase II, preventing elongation of messenger RNA and resulting in a block of intracellular protein synthesis and subsequent necrosis. This is a dose-dependent process. Clinically, GI disturbances occur after a 12-hour latent period and subside, to be followed in 3 to 5 days by an intoxication resembling acute fulminant hepatitis or acute renal tubular

Table 82-6   Miscellaneous Toxic Plants

Plants	Toxic Part	Toxin	Fatal	Comments
Catharanthus roseus (periwinkle)	Dried whole plant	Indole and dihydroindole alkaloids, including vincristine	No	GI symptoms and seizures; long-term effects unknown
Cicuta maculata (water hemlock)	All parts, concentrated in roots	Cicutoxin (an unsaturated higher alcohol)	Yes	Plant is commonly mistaken for a wild parsnip; onset of convulsions with rapid death secondary to respiratory arrest; rhabdomyolysis also occurs
Corynanthe yohimbe	Leaves, roots, bark	Yohimbine (alkaloid)	Yes	Toxin is adrenergic-receptor antagonist, causing hallucinations, hypertension, paralysis
Coumarouna odorata (tonka bean)	Seeds	Coumarin	No	Seeds contain 1%-3% coumarin; anticoagulant
Oenananthe crocata (water dropwort)	Root	Resembles cicutoxin	Yes	Convulsant
Ipomoea purpurea (morning glory)	Seeds	Lysergic acid isoergine	No	Related to LSD; hallucinogenic
Karwinskia humboldtiana (coyotillo)	Fruit	Anthracenones	Yes	Paralysis after 4-5 wk secondary to demyelination
Melilotus officinalis (clover)	Flowers	Bishydroxycoumarin	No	Anticoagulant
Nepeta cataria (catnip)	Leaves	Acetic, butyric, valeric acids	No	Hallucinogenic
Panax quenquefolius (ginseng)	Roots	Panax acid, panaquilin, saponin	No	Insomnia, hypertension
Phoradendron flavescens (mistletoe)	Berries, stems, leaves	Phoratoxins, viscotoxins	Yes	Hallucinogenic, hypertension, bradycardia
Rauwolfia serpentina	All parts	Yohimbine	Yes	See above

necrosis. The toxin has a high affinity for hepatic cells, and increased enterohepatic uptake of excreted toxin occurs. Toxin is also filtered at the glomerulus and is reabsorbed by the tubules to produce necrosis. The fatality rate is 50% to 90%; the toxin can be removed through hemoperfusion (see Chapter 147). After the onset of symptoms, particularly hepatic, transplantation may be the only form of treatment.

The *Gyromitra* species contain gyromitrin, a toxin metabolized to a monomethalhydrazine, which inhibits pyridoxal phosphate–dependent enzymes. The patient's previous exposure to gyromitrins may induce the necessary hepatic enzymes needed to transform the toxin to its toxic metabolite. The water-soluble toxin may be attenuated by drying the mushroom before ingestion or by boiling it and dis-

Table 82-7   Mushroom Toxicity*

Genus	Toxin	Onset of Action Postingestion	Site of Toxicity	Symptoms	Mortality	In Addition to Standard and Supportive Therapy
Amanita sp, *Galerina* sp	Cyclopeptide, camatoxin	10-20 hr	Hepatic and renal cytotoxicity	Phase 3: hematuria, proteinuria, gastroenteritis, jaundice; increased AST, increased ALT, mixed muscarinic and atropinic effects	50%-90% (toxic at 0.1 mg/kg)	Thioctic acid† (alpha-lipoic acid), 50-150 mg q 6 hr IV
Gyromitra (*Helvella*)	Monomethylhydrazine (gyromitrin)	6-10 hr	Hepatic and renal cytotoxicity	Hemolysis, abdominal pain, hepatorenal failure, weakness	15%-40%	Pyridoxine, 25 mg/kg IV
Coprinus	Coprine	20 min to 2 hr	Autonomic nervous system	Antabuse-like effect	Rare	Avoid alcohol
Clitocybe, Inocybe sp	Muscarine	20 min to 2 hr	Autonomic nervous system	Muscarinic effects— SLUD (salivation, lacrimation, urination, and defecation)	5%-10%	Atropine, 2 mg IV as indicated
Amanita muscaris	Ibotenic acid, muscimol	20 min to 2 hr	CNS	Anticholinergic effects, rare delirium, dizziness, ataxia	Rare	Physostigmine salicylate, 2 mg IV as indicated
Psilocybe, Panaeolus	Psilocybin, psilocin (indoles)	15-30 min	CNS	Ataxia, hyperkinetic state, hallucination, atropine-like effects	Rare	—
Diverse	Multiple irritants	30 min to 3 hr	GI	Gastroenteritis	Rare	—

*Modified from Lincoff G, Mitchel DH. Toxic and Hallucinogenic Mushroom Poisoning: A Handbook for Physicians and Mushroom Hunters. New York: Van Nostrand Reinhold, 1977, pp 246-247.
†Available from Bartter FC, ACOS for Research, Audie Murphy Memorial VA Hospital, 7400 Merton Minton Blvd, San Antonio, TX 78284. (512)696-9660.

carding the broth. Symptoms of toxicity include GI complaints (nausea, emesis, diarrhea) and headache with dizziness 6 to 8 hours after ingestion, with recovery in 2 to 6 days. However, acute hepatitis with fatal hepatic failure may develop; rarely, hemolysis with secondary renal failure occurs. The fatality rate is 2% to 6%; treatment is supportive.

TREATMENT

Treatment, which in general can be accomplished at home, should be aimed at decreasing absorption by emptying the stomach and increasing elimination by using activated charcoal and a cathartic (see Chapter 75 for general guidelines of care of ingestion). Since the primary symptom complex usually involves GI symptoms, providing adequate intake to replace extra volume losses from diarrhea and emesis and to ensure urinary output is crucial.

ADDITIONAL READING

Mofenson HC, Cataccio TR. Poisonous plants. Pediatr Therap Toxicol 2 (Suppl): S9-S12, 1988.

Rumack BH, Salzman E, eds. Mushroom Poisoning Diagnosis and Treatment. New York: Van Nostrand Reinhold, 1977.

83 Hydrocarbon Ingestions

Kathy Amoroso · Charles M. Ginsburg

BACKGROUND AND PHYSIOLOGY

Hydrocarbons, by-products of the fractional distillation and catalytic "cracking" of crude petroleum and oil shale, account for 3% to 5% of all accidental poisonings in children who are less than 5 years old. Petroleum-based products such as gasoline, kerosene, furniture polish, and paint thinner are ubiquitous in homes and, as such, are potential hazards to children. The primary target organ for the toxic effects of these agents is the respiratory system. Additionally, some petroleum-based products contain heavy metals or organophosphates that also are potentially toxic to other organ systems.

Respiratory System

The major route for toxicity of hydrocarbons is pulmonary aspiration rather than GI absorption. Studies in experimental animals have demonstrated that instillation of hydrocarbons into the stomach after esophageal ligation is not associated with pneumonitis; only small amounts of these agents are absorbed into the systemic circulation from the gastric and intestinal mucosa. The risk for pulmonary damage correlates directly with the volatility, viscosity, and surface tension of the product. Agents with low viscosity and low surface tension spread rapidly over surfaces and quickly penetrate distal airways. Petroleum distillates may chemically irritate the bronchi, resulting in bronchospasm. In the alveoli these agents interact with surfactant, diminishing its effectiveness and resulting in alveolar instability, atelectasis, and ultimately ventilation-perfusion mismatch.

Pneumonitis occurs in 12% to 40% of patients and is the most common cause of morbidity and mortality. After ingestion of a petroleum distillate, the child experiences a burning sensation in the mouth and then gags, chokes, and coughs. Because of the noxious taste of most petroleum-based products the volume ingested is generally small, and spontaneous vomiting occurs in 20% to 50% of patients. Respiratory symptoms generally appear within 30 to 60 minutes after ingestion but may be delayed for up to 6 to 12 hours. A nonproductive cough, tachypnea, and tachycardia are the earliest signs of pulmonary involvement. Fever is present within hours after ingestion in up to two thirds of patients with pulmonary involvement and is indicative of chemical irritation rather than infection. In one study 64% of patients with hydrocarbon pneumonia had temperatures >38° C at the time of medical evaluation. Respiratory symptoms generally worsen during the first 24 hours, reach a plateau, and then gradually subside over 2 to 5 days. Children who have had hydrocarbon pneumonitis may have long-term sequelae and continue to have abnormal pulmonary function tests for years after ingestion.

The effect of hydrocarbons on the immune system is poorly understood. Studies performed in laboratory animals indicate that hydrocarbon pneumonitis may predispose them to bacterial infection as a result of impaired clearance of microorganisms from the tracheobronchial tree. This effect is greatest 24 to 36 hours after exposure and persists for up to 5 days.

The initial radiographic findings after hydrocarbon ingestion are variable but most often consist of fine, punctate densities in the perihilum, which gradually evolve into areas of patchy infiltrate and finally large areas of consolidation. The densities are usually bilateral, involving multiple lobes. Pulmonary effusions, pneumatoceles, pneumothorax, pneumomediastinum, and subcutaneous emphysema have been reported in patients with hydrocarbon pneumonitis (Fig. 83-1). Resolution of abnormal chest roentgenograms often lags behind clinical improvement, and the roentgenogram may remain abnormal for weeks to months after the result.

639

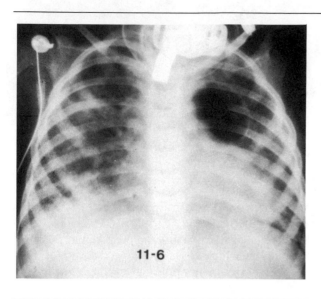

Fig. 83-1   Chest roentgenogram reveals patchy, diffuse infiltrates seen in patients after hydrocarbon ingestion. Pneumatocele, seen in left upper lobe, may also occur.

Prosection of lung tissue in patients who have succumbed to hydrocarbon aspiration correlates with the aforementioned mechanisms. Hyaline-like membranes similar to those found in infants with respiratory distress syndrome, constricted bronchioles, and atelectasis are present. It is not known whether the inflammation, vascular thrombosis, hemorrhage, and necrosis of lung tissue that are frequently observed are the result of the direct toxic effect of the hydrocarbon or a secondary effect of hypoxia.

Central Nervous System

CNS toxicity is the second major effect of hydrocarbon ingestion. Symptoms include lethargy and irritability, or less frequently, seizure and coma. Although animal studies using labeled hydrocarbons demonstrate only minimal GI absorption of these substances after ingestion, some patients manifest transient neurologic signs and symptoms within minutes after ingestion. In these cases neurologic effects are ascribed to direct CNS toxicity of the hydrocarbon and are related to the small concentrations of the substances that are absorbed into the systemic circulation. Subsequent neurologic signs and symptoms later in the course are much more common and result from hypoxia and acidosis.

Cardiac System

Although tachycardia is a common early finding, it is generally transient; persistent tachycardia is usually related to respiratory compromise. Myocardial irritability, manifested by an increased sensitivity to epinephrine and other catecholamines, has been reported, but the incidence of this finding is not known.

MONITORING AND LABORATORY TESTS

See also Chapters 4 and 75. The signs and symptoms and the subsequent course in children who ingest hydrocarbons vary widely. Because many children are asymptomatic after the ingestion, some authorities have recommended evaluation and management by telephone for children who initially appear well and whose caretakers are especially observant and reliable. We and others advocate careful physical examination and chest roentgenogram for each patient.

Patients who are asymptomatic at the time of initial evaluation do not need immediate hospitalization but must be monitored for the onset of pulmonary involvement for at least 6 and, preferably, 8 hours. A paradigm for evaluating the necessity for hospitalization is presented in Fig. 83-2.

Monitoring of these patients must be focused on the respiratory system and CNS.

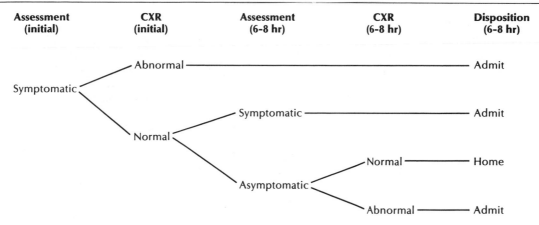

Fig. 83-2   A paradigm, which may be used to determine the necessity of hospitalizing a patient after hydrocarbon ingestion.

TREATMENT
Specific Measures

Inducing emesis is generally contraindicated in patients who have ingested hydrocarbons because it increases the risk for aspiration and pneumonitis. Hydrocarbons may contain insecticides, heavy metals, or other harmful substances that may be absorbed and cause systemic toxicity. In these instances the risk of inducing emesis and potentiating aspiration must be weighed against the toxicity of the contaminating substance. If removal of the ingested substance is deemed necessary and the patient is alert, the use of syrup of ipecac is preferred to gastric lavage. It must be administered under carefully monitored conditions in a hospital setting. If the patient is not alert but the ingested substance must be removed, we recommend gastric lavage using large volumes of 0.9% sodium chloride solution. The patient's trachea must first be intubated to minimize the risk of aspiration.

Despite their widespread use, corticosteroids have never been shown to be efficacious for the treatment of hydrocarbon aspiration. Further, studies performed in animals demonstrate that corticosteroids increase the incidence of positive lung cultures and may therefore increase the risk of secondary bacterial infection.

Prophylactic antibiotics have not been shown to be efficacious in treating hydrocarbon pneumonitis. Patients typically develop fever within hours of ingestion secondary to chemical irritation; in this case the use of antibiotics is not indicated. In addition use of prophylactic antibiotics has never been shown to prevent secondary bacterial infection in patients with hydrocarbon pneumonitis. Patients who develop fever several days into their course may be superinfected with a variety of organisms, including *Haemophilus influenzae, Staphylococcus aureus, Streptococcus pneumoniae,* or group A streptococcus, and antibiotic treatment must be undertaken after blood and sputum cultures are obtained.

Supportive Measures

Providing supportive care with particular attention to the respiratory system is critical (see Chapter 10). The use of positive end-expiratory pressure (PEEP) helps stabilize airways, recruit areas of atelectasis, and redistribute lung fluid from the alveoli to peribronchial areas, thus reducing intrapulmonary shunting. PEEP cannot be withdrawn until 48 to 72 hours into the course of treatment when the lungs begin to heal. Although bronchodilators have been shown to be efficacious in studies performed in animals, these agents have not been rigorously evaluated in children with hydrocarbon pneumonitis. Clinical experience, however, has indicated that they may be beneficial for the treatment of bronchospasm, particularly during the first few hours after onset of pulmonary symptoms (see Chapter 133).

ADDITIONAL READING

• Anas N, Namasonthi V, Ginsburg C. Criteria for hospitalizing children who have ingested products containing hydrocarbons. JAMA 246:840-843, 1981.

Brown J, Burke B, Dajani AS. Experimental kerosene pneumonia: Evaluation of some therapeutic regimens. J Pediatr 84:396-401, 1974.

Eade NR, Taussig LM, Marks MI. Hydrocarbon pneumonitis. Pediatrics 54:351-357, 1974.

Giammona ST. Effects of furniture polish on pulmonary surfactant. Am J Dis Child 113:658-663, 1967.

• Klein BL, Simon JE. Hydrocarbon poisonings. Pediatr Clin North Am 33:411-419, 1986.

Marks MI, Chicoine L, Kegere G, Hillman E. Adrenocorticosteroid treatment of hydrocarbon pneumonia in children—a cooperative study. J Pediatr 81:366-369, 1972.

Ng RC, Darwish H, Stewart DA. Emergency treatment of petroleum distillate and turpentine ingestion. Can Med Assoc 11:537-538, 1974.

Press E. Cooperative kerosene poisoning study. Evaluation of gastric lavage and other factors in the treatment of accidental ingestion of petroleum distillate products. Pediatrics 29:648-674, 1962.

Steele RW, Conklin RH, Mark HM. Corticosteroids and antibiotics for the treatment of fulminant hydrocarbon aspiration. JAMA 219:1434-1437, 1982.

Wolfsdorf J. Kerosene intoxication: An experimental approach to the etiology of the CNS manifestations in primates. J Pediatr 88:1037-1040, 1976.

Zucker AR, Berger S, Wood LDH. Management of kerosene-induced pulmonary injury. Crit Care Med 14:303-304, 1986.

84 Injuries From Corrosive Agents

Edward J. Lose · Charles M. Ginsburg

BACKGROUND AND PHYSIOLOGY

Corrosive injuries cause substantial immediate and long-term morbidity in the pediatric population. Common household items such as cleaning agents, drain cleaners, and disk batteries are potential hazards for the inquisitive child. Although the majority of caustic ingestions occur in children who are less than 5 years of age, the morbidity associated with corrosive ingestions is greater in older children since they generally ingest larger amounts of the corrosive agents.

Corrosive Ingestions

Acids (Table 84-1)

Acids that are readily available to the consumer and are therefore available in households include hydrochloric acid, sulfuric acid, chloroacetic acid, formic acid, oxalic acid, and salicylic acid. The severity of acid-induced injury is related to the concentration of the agent ingested, duration of contact, and the availability of a buffer. Acids tend to have a lower viscosity and specific gravity than alkalis, and as a result they have a propensity to produce skip injuries of the upper GI tract. On contact with tissue acids produce coagulation necrosis; therefore acid penetration is generally reduced by the coagulum. Burns of the oropharynx and esophagus occur with acid ingestions; however, the gastric antrum is usually the most severely affected. Stomach and proximal intestine injuries range from mucosal edema to perforation.

Pain, vomiting, and oropharyngeal lesions may be absent in children who have ingested acid-containing products. Thus fiberoptic endoscopy should be performed as soon as possible to assess the degree of involvement in any child who has ingested substantial quantities of an acid product. The usual appearance of an acid-induced injury comprises erythema, edema, and streaks of necrosis along the greater curvature and antrum of the stomach; the lesser curvature is generally not involved.

Oxalic acid, in addition to causing local contact injury, may produce signs of hypocalcemia because of its ability to chelate calcium ions. Systemic manifestations of salicylate toxicity are discussed in Chapter 76.

Alkalis

Alkalis are responsible for the majority of corrosive ingestions in children that result in significant morbidity. Sodium hydroxide, potassium hydroxide, and ammonium hydroxide are the most frequent alkalis involved in corrosive injuries to children. Because alkaline agents produce liquefactive necrosis with denaturation of proteins and saponification of fats, a large potential for perforation of the injured tissue exists. As with other corrosives, the extent of injury is related to the agent involved, the concentration of the agent, and the contact time.

The acute phase of an alkaline injury (first 24 to 48 hours) is characterized by marked edema of the mucosa and an extensive inflammatory response. If the burn is sufficiently deep, the inflammation may penetrate the muscularis layer of the esophagus, causing perforation. The subacute phase occurs after several days and lasts up to the second week. During this period the edema resolves, and necrotic tissue is sloughed. The last phase of injury is the cicatrization phase, which generally begins in the third week after injury. This phase is characterized by fibroblast replacement of the submucosa and the muscularis mucosa; adhesions and stricture formation may occur during this period. The overlying epithelium is regenerated within 6 weeks and consists of squamous epithelium.

Liquid forms of alkalis usually produce pain on mucosal contact, generally limiting the amount of toxic substance ingested. By contrast, crystalline preparations must dissolve on the mucosal surface before there is a sensation of pain. Because crystals tend to stick to the mucosal surface, they are often spit out before the individual swallows them. Although oropharyngeal lesions may not be present after ingestion of a concentrated alkali, a substantial number (up to 20% in some series) of patients have an esophageal injury.

The findings at the time of initial physical examination generally correlate with the duration of time that has lapsed since the injury. Early after the ingestion there may be a paucity of abnormal findings. Drooling generally antedates the appearance of edema, erythema, and white plaques or ulcers on the mucous membranes. Later a brownish discoloration of the mucous membrane lesions may occur, and ulcers are present. Drooling or the inability to clear secretions is often a sign of posterior pharyngeal or upper esophageal injury. Upper airway involvement produces respiratory distress. Vocal cord involvement must be suspected if there is dysphonia.

Ingestion of disk batteries poses a related problem. Gastric secretions may corrode the battery's seal, precipitating production of an electric current. Hydroxides and mercury salts, internal contents of the battery, are released and may produce local and systemic symptoms. If sufficient quantities of mercury have been released into the circulation, chelation therapy must be instituted.

The role of steroids and prophylactic antibiotics in the treatment of patients with corrosive injuries is controversial. Studies performed in experimental animals indicate that early administration of steroids reduces the incidence of stricture formation; however, the data from these studies indicate that corticosteroid-treated animals were at greater risk for secondary infection than were untreated controls. No information is available from randomized controlled trials in humans to ascertain the efficacy, the dosage, or the duration of corticosteroid therapy. The use of lathyrogens, agents that inhibit cross-linking of col-

Table 84-1   Common Household Corrosives*

Type	Brand Name	Corrosive Chemical
Acids	Mister Plumer (K-Lan Co.) (liquid)	Concentrated sulfuric acid
	Quaker House steam iron cleaner	Hydrochloric acid
	Sno Bol liquid toilet bowl cleaner	Hydrochloric acid, 15%
	Lysol liquid toilet bowl cleaner	Hydrochloric acid, 8.5%
		Ammonium chloride, 1%
	ZUD rust and stain remover (granular)	Oxalic acid
	Sani-Flush toilet bowl cleaner (granular)	Sodium bisulfate, 75%
	Vanish toilet bowl cleaner (granular)	Sodium acid sulfate, 62%
	Rooto	Sulfuric acid
Alkalis	Liquid Drano	Sodium hydroxide
		Ammonium hydroxide
	Drano (granular)	Sodium hydroxide
	Easy-Off liquid oven cleaner (liquid)	Sodium hydroxide
	Mr. Muscle overnight oven cleaner (liquid)	Sodium hydroxide
	Liquid Plumr	Sodium hypochlorite, potassium hydroxide, and sodium hydroxide
	Minute mildew remover	Calcium hypochlorite, 48%
	Comet liquid disinfectant bathroom cleaner	Tripotassium phosphate, 1.8%
		Sodium hypochlorite, 0.5%
	Westley Bleche-White whitewall cleaner	Sodium metasilicate

*From Graham DY. Corrosive injury to the stomach: The natural history and role of fiberoptic endoscopy. Am J Surg 137:803-806, 1979.

lagen fibers, has been studied in animals; however, their toxicity to humans has limited their study, and they should not be administered to humans.

Clinical experience indicates that the incidence of secondary infection in patients with corrosive injuries of the esophagus decreases with the use of antimicrobials. However, this has not been studied in a prospective manner. Gram-positive cocci and, rarely, anaerobic organisms are the usual infecting agents; therefore antimicrobial therapy should be directed against these organisms as well as against anaerobic flora. Brain abscesses caused by unusual organisms

have been reported after dilation procedures; however, no data are available to justify the administration of prophylactic antimicrobials before the procedure.

Nonionic Detergents (Table 84-2)

Ingestion of compounds containing nonionic detergents represents the majority of ingestions that occur in homes. Alcohols, monostearates, polyether sulfates, and sulfonates are the major active ingredients in laundry products and toilet soaps. These chemicals generally have low toxic potential because no reactive ions or pH changes are produced when they are

Table 84-2 Soaps, Detergents, Cleaners, and Bleaches*

Toxicity	Product	Toxic Ingredient or Effect	Treatment†
High	Electric dishwasher granules‡	Caustic (may be severe)	Treat as caustic burn‡
	Ammonia‡	Caustic; coma and convulsions	As caustic‡; supportive
	Bleach, commercial	Boric acid or oxalate poisoning	Milk; calcium; supportive
	Bleach, oxygen	Boric acid poisoning	Supportive
Medium	Bleach, chlorine	GI irritation, some causticity	Demulcents ± treat as caustic burn
	Borax	Boric acid poisoning	Supportive
	Water softeners‡ (soluble)	Some caustic; hypocalcemia and acidosis possible	Milk; as for caustic‡; supportive
	Liquid general cleaners:		
	Kerosene	Pneumonia, systemic toxicity	As for petroleum distillates§
	Pine oil	GI and genitourinary irritation; depression and weakness	Supportive; demulcents
	Detergent granules‡ for laundry, dishes, and general use	GI irritation to causticity (some frankly caustic and have higher toxicity)	Demulcents; treat as caustic burn‡
Low	Detergent powders‡	GI irritation (causticity possible, but unlikely)	Demulcents ± treat as caustic burn‡
	Liquid detergents	GI irritation	Demulcents
	Toilet soap	GI irritation	Demulcents
	Fabric softeners	None	None
	Window cleaners (liquid)	Alcohol	Demulcents
Inhalation hazard	Chlorine bleach mixed with:		
	Strong acid (bowl cleaner)	Chlorine gas (intense respiratory irritation)	Oxygen
	Ammonia	Chloramine fumes (respiratory irritation, nausea)	Terminate exposure; supportive

*From Done AK. Poisoning from household products. Pediatr Clin North Am 17:577, 1970.
†In addition to evacuation of stomach (except with caustic burn) or removal from skin when indicated.
‡Products threatening caustic effects will be identified with a *caution* label. Details of treatment can be found elsewhere.
§Details of treatment can be found elsewhere.

dissolved. Ingestion of a large volume of a nonionic detergent may produce gastric irritation that can be relieved with use of a demulcent such as milk or olive oil. Transient diarrhea is a common problem in patients who have ingested soaps and detergents.

Anionic Detergents

Anionic detergents are common constituents of "low-sudsing" laundry soaps and other biodegradable soaps. These agents contain ammonium, potassium, or sodium salts of fatty acids and phosphorylated or sulfurated hydrocarbons. Bleach is occasionally added but is generally of insufficient concentration to cause tissue damage. Coloring agents, perfumes, or surface-active agents, other common additives to detergents and soaps, are generally nontoxic; however, agents containing petroleum distillates such as pine oil place the child at potential risk for pneumonitis (see Chapter 83).

Ingestion of detergents containing ammonia can result in mucous membrane irritation without burns. Treatment consists of administering water to dilute the detergent, followed by administration of a demulcent such as milk.

Electric dishwasher granules and tripolyphosphate soaps are capable of causing esophageal injury because of their high pH. Ingestion of these substances must be treated as an alkaline ingestion.

Cationic Detergents

Cationic detergents are commonly included in antiseptics, bactericides, disinfectants, and deodorizers. Quaternary ammonium cations (i.e., benzalkonium chloride) and bromide, iodide, chloride, and nitrate anions are the major toxic components in these substances. Toxicity is produced by the cation's ability to inhibit cellular metabolism. Additional toxicity occurs with the addition of ingredients such as acids, hydrocarbons, and phenols.

Symptoms of cationic substance ingestion include vomiting and/or epigastric pain. Seizures, coma, cardiovascular compromise, and hepatic or renal failure may occur in patients who have ingested large quantities of these substances. Prompt treatment is indicated for patients who have ingested moderate quantities of concentrated products; fatalities have been reported after ingestion of only 20 to 30 ml of these substances. Gastric emptying may be attempted if no corrosive agent is involved, and further treatment is directed toward multisystem support. Water or de-

mulcents may be given, but weak alkali and soap administration is no longer recommended.

Bleach

Sodium or potassium hypochlorite–containing products are ubiquitous in households. Data from studies performed in animals indicate that household bleaches are capable of mucosal irritation, but large concentrations and prolonged contact time are required before injury occurs. Some of the newer bleaches may be fortified with more concentrated alkalis; thus the manufacturer must be consulted if the contents and the concentration of the product are not identified on the label.

Most children are asymptomatic after ingestion of a household bleach. Some children experience mild pain as a result of mucosal irritation, but these symptoms are generally relieved by dilution with water or a demulcent. Significant injury rarely occurs after bleach ingestion; however, if the bleach has been mixed with another cleaner, chlorine gas, which has the potential to cause respiratory tract inflammation, may be liberated. Treatment is supportive.

MONITORING AND LABORATORY TESTS

See also Chapters 4 and 75. In a patient with esophageal perforation or pneumonitis, a chest roentgenogram must be obtained. Arterial blood gas tensions and pH must be measured every 4 to 6 hours, or noninvasive $tcCO_2$ and O_2 saturation monitors must be used. Surgical consultation is mandatory if perforation is suspected.

TREATMENT

See also Chapter 75. The ingested agent must be identified and the amount ingested estimated. If no esophageal or gastric injury is present, oral administration of a demulcent or water is the only treatment necessary. If toxic additives are present, specific therapy is directed by the additive, and hospitalization may be necessary. Administration of neutralizing agents is no longer recommended.

Absorption of the agent must be reduced. Emesis induction and lavage are contraindicated since they may reintroduce corrosives into the esophagus and protective airway reflexes may be absent. Perforation may result from attempts to pass a nasogastric tube. Water may be given to alert patients to dilute remaining corrosives in the oropharynx, esophagus, or stomach. All the patient's clothing must be removed and areas with evidence of contact bathed with copious amounts of water. The eyes must be thoroughly irrigated until the pH is near neutral, and an ophthalmologist must be consulted if an eye injury has occurred.

Further treatment includes examination of the esophagus in most patients with corrosive ingestions. Esophagoscopy must be performed as soon as the patient is stable. The esophagus must be examined to the level of the first burn. Advancing the endoscope beyond the first burn may cause perforation. If no esophageal or gastric injury is noted, the patient may be discharged when oral intake is satisfactory; a barium esophagram must be obtained in 1 to 2 months to detect strictures.

Documented esophageal injury is an indication for steroid therapy. Prednisone, 2 mg/kg/day, or its equivalent must be given for 3 weeks, depending on the extent of injury. The use of prophylactic antibiotics is controversial. Clindamycin phosphate, 20 to 40/mg/kg/day IM or IV in three or five divided doses, provides adequate coverage for the most common organisms. Placement of a Silastic stent during the initial esophagoscopy is also controversial. If placed, the stent must remain in place for 3 weeks.

Esophagoscopy and cinefluoroscopy must be done 3 weeks after injury. The presence of a stricture without a lumen may be an indication for performing colonic interposition or gastrostomy with feeding tube placement. Esophageal dilation can be performed when strictures are evident. Bougienage is a relatively safe procedure; however, perforation is an immediate complication of the procedure. Brain abscesses have occurred in some patients after dilation procedures; therefore the cause of fever associated with CNS signs must be investigated thoroughly.

Treatment of gastric injuries includes withholding oral fluids and giving IV hydration. The role of steroids and antibiotics is unknown, and their use cannot be recommended at this time. Performing follow-up endoscopy and radiographic examinations is necessary to assess antrum and pyloric function.

ADDITIONAL READING

Arena JM. Treatment of caustic alkali poisoning. Mod Treatment 8:613-618, 1971.

Crain EF, Gershel JC, Mezey AP. Caustic ingestions: Symptoms as predictors of esophageal injury. Am J Dis Child 138:863-865, 1984.

• Done AK. Poisoning from household products. Pediatr Clin North Am 17:569-581, 1970.

• Gaudreault P, Parent M, McGuigan MA, Chicoine L, Lovejoy FH. Predictability of esophageal injury from signs and symptoms: A study of caustic ingestion in 378 children. Pediatrics 71:767-770, 1983.

National Clearinghouse Poison Control Centers Bull 23:1-2, 1979.

Rothstein FC. Caustic injuries to the esophagus in children. Pediatr Clin North Am 33:665-674, 1986.

• Wasserman RL, Ginsburg CM. Caustic substance injuries. J Pediatr 107:169-174, 1985.

85 Organophosphate and Carbamate Poisoning

Robert Jeffrey Zwiener · Charles M. Ginsburg

BACKGROUND AND PHYSIOLOGY

Organophosphates and carbamates are powerful inhibitors of carboxylic ester hydrolases, including the enzyme acetylcholinesterase. Acetylcholinesterase (true cholinesterase), an enzyme present in nervous tissue, skeletal muscle, and erythrocytes, hydrolyzes the neurotransmitter acetylcholine to acetic acid and choline. Intoxication with organophosphates or carbamates inhibits the conversion of acetylcholine to its by-products, resulting in the accumulation of the neurotransmitter at synapses throughout the central and peripheral nervous systems. As a result, initially there is excitation and then depression of neurotransmission at the synapses.

The most common route of exposure to organophosphates and carbamates in children is ingestion; however, intoxication may also occur as a result of inhalation or transcutaneous absorption. The onset of signs and symptoms of organophosphate and carbamate toxicity depends on the dose, route of exposure, inherent potency, and solubility characteristics of the offending agent. In general signs and symptoms occur within minutes to hours after exposure; however, in instances in which exposure to

---

AVAILABLE ORGANOPHOSPHATE AND CARBAMATE INSECTICIDES*

Organophosphate insecticides

Abate, azinphos-methyl (Guthion), carbophenothion (Trithion), chlorithion, ciodrin, coumaphos, DEF, demeton (Systox), diazinon (Basudin), dicapthon (Di-Captan), dichlorvos (DDVP), dicrotophos (Bidrin), dimethoate (Cygon), dioxathion (Delnav), disulfoton (Disyston), Dursban, echothiophate (Phospholine), EPN, ethion (Nialate), fenthion (Baytex), malathion (Malathon, Cythion), menazon, merphos, methyl demeton (Meta-Systox), methyl-parathion, methyltrithion, mevinphos (Phosdrin), monocrotophos (Azodrin), mipafox, naled (Dibrom), paraoxon (Mintacol), parathion, phosphamidon (Dimecron), phorate (Thimet), Phostex, ronnel (Korlan), Ruelene, schradan (Sytam, Pestox), TEPP (Bladan, Tetron), trichlorfon (Dipterex, Tugon)

Carbamate insecticides

Aldicarb (Temik), aminocarb (Matacil), bendiocarb (Ficam), aprocarb (Baygon), Bux, carbaryl (Sevin), carbofuran (Furaxdan), dimetan, dimetilan, dioxacarb, fenethcarb, formetanate, landrin, meobal, methomyl (Lannate, Nudrin), mexacarbate (Zectran), propoxur (Unden), tirpate, tsumacide

---

*From Goldfrank LR, Bresnitz EA, Kirstein RH, et al. Organophosphates. In Goldfrank LR, Flomenbaum NE, Lewin NA, et al, eds. Goldfrank's Toxicologic Emergencies, 3rd ed. Norwalk, Conn.: Appleton-Century-Crofts, 1986, pp 686-696.

one of the new lipophilic agents has occurred, the onset of signs and symptoms may be delayed 24 to 48 hours, and toxic symptoms may persist for 5 to 48 days because of the slow release of the agent from lipid reservoirs.

The signs and symptoms of 37 children (median age 22 months) with organophosphate or carbamate poisoning are summarized in Table 85-1. The diverse location and function of cholinergic receptors explains the complex response to intoxication with these agents. Cholinergic synaptic transmission is compromised in the CNS, somatic nerves, autonomic ganglia, parasympathetic nerve endings, and some sympathetic nerve endings (sweat glands). Muscarinic signs (postganglionic parasympathetic synapses to effector organs and postganglionic sympathetic synapses to sweat glands) include miosis, increased production of secretions, bronchoconstriction, and bradycardia. Nicotinic manifestations (motor nerve synapses to striated muscle and the synapses of autonomic ganglia) include muscle weakness, paralysis, tachycardia, hyperglycemia, pallor, and hypertension. Lethargy, ataxia, depressed mental status, and coma are the most common CNS manifestations (poorly defined receptors, both nicotinic and muscarinic, are present). Seizures occur in 5% to 22% of patients and are most likely secondary to the combined effects of hypoxia and the toxin. In patients with severe poisoning death occurs from respiratory arrest secondary to the combination of bronchoconstriction, bronchorrhea, weakness or paralysis of respiratory muscles, depressed mental status, and poor respiratory effort.

The diagnosis of organophosphate or carbamate poisoning is frequently delayed, particularly when severe respiratory distress or altered mental status dominates the clinical situation. This diagnosis must be suspected in all children with acute onset of symptoms and respiratory and CNS signs (coma), even if there is no history of exposure to one of these agents. The smell of insecticide on the child may be the first clue.

The diagnosis of organophosphate and carbamate toxicity is confirmed by assays for serum and/or erythrocyte cholinesterase activity and by toxicologic assays of blood, urine, and gastric contents. Although the laboratory assay for erythrocyte cholinesterase activity is technically more difficult to perform than the serum assay, its use is preferable

Table 85-1 Signs and Symptoms in 37 Children With Organophosphate or Carbamate Toxicity*

Affected Organ or System	Signs and Symptoms	No. (%) of Patients
Muscarinic		
Pupils	Miosis (can be unequal)	27 (73)
Salivary glands	Excessive salivation	26 (70)
Gastrointestinal	Nausea/vomiting	12 (32)
	Diarrhea/defecation	10 (27)
Cardiovascular	Bradycardia	7 (19)
Pulmonary	Wheezing, increased secretions	7 (19)
	Respiratory distress†	22 (59)
	Respiratory insufficiency‡	14 (38)
Sweat glands	Diaphoresis	5 (13)
Lacrimal glands	Excessive lacrimation	4 (11)
Bladder	Urinary incontinence	4 (11)
Ciliary body	Blurred vision	1 (3)
Nicotinic		
Striated muscle	Muscle weakness	25 (68)
	Hyporeflexia	15 (41)
	Hypotonia	13 (35)
	Fasciculations	8 (22)
Autonomic ganglia	Tachycardia	18 (49)
	Hyperglycemia	9 (22)
	Pallor	4 (11)
	Hypertension	3 (8)
Central nervous system	Lethargy	20 (54)
	Ataxia	9 (24)
	Seizures§	8 (22)
	Coma	8 (22)
	Depressed mental status	7 (19)
	Emotional lability	1 (3)
	Slurred speech	—
	Headache	—

*Modified from Zwiener RJ, Ginsburg CM. Organophosphate and carbamate poisoning in infants and children. Reproduced by permission of Pediatrics 81:121-126, 1988; and Namba T, Nolte CT, Jackrel J, et al. Am J Med 50:475-492, 1971.

†A consequence of bronchoconstriction, bronchorrhea, weak muscles of respiration, depressed central nervous system, and diminished respiratory effort.

‡Necessitating ventilatory support.

§A result of hypoxia and direct toxic effect.

to the latter because it measures "true" cholinesterase activity, which better reflects the concentration of acetylcholinesterase present at the synapse. The serum assay measures the concentrations of "pseudocholinesterase," an enzyme that may be decreased in patients with a number of acquired medical disorders or because of a congenital enzyme deficiency. The serum assay is therefore less specific and may be misleading.

In patients with severe organophosphate poisoning cholinesterase activity is usually less than 50% of the lower limits of normal. In patients with moderate toxicity the activity is 50% to 75%. On rare occasions the cholinesterase activity may be normal if the patient is examined shortly after exposure. Obtaining serial (once or twice a day) determinations of cholinesterase activity is not useful. After organophosphate (not carbamate) poisoning the enzymes and measurable activity may be depressed for 2 to 6 weeks (longer for lipophilic products like fenthion). By contrast, after carbamate toxicity acetylcholinesterase is rapidly and spontaneously reactivated as the poison is cleared. Cholinesterase activities therefore may be normal if determined several hours after the patient's exposure. In unusual cases it is wise to document the normalization of enzyme activity 2 to 3 months after the poisoning to rule out ongoing exposure or congenital enzyme deficiency.

MONITORING AND LABORATORY TESTS

Because of the frequency of respiratory failure all children with organophosphate or carbamate poisoning must be admitted to the PICU.

Respiratory System

The respiratory rate must be monitored continuously with an audible electronic apnea alarm. The respiratory status must be reassessed continually for signs of respiratory insufficiency, including cyanosis, retractions, wheezing, decreased respiratory effort, and increased secretions. Continual transcutaneous monitoring of carbon dioxide concentrations and pulse oximetry for oxygen saturation are indicated for any patient with respiratory symptoms. Arterial blood gases and pH should be measured as indicated. Measurements of vital capacity or forced inspiratory pressure may be helpful if progression of symptoms is slow, but they are of limited value in the very young, uncooperative, or comatose patient. A chest roentgenogram must be obtained. Many insecticides are petroleum distillate based, and hydrocarbon pneumonitis may occur concomitantly.

Cardiovascular System

The heart rate must be monitored continuously with an electronic monitor, and systemic arterial blood pressure must be measured hourly until stable. The patient must be reassessed frequently by skin appearance and capillary refill for adequate peripheral pulses and peripheral perfusion.

Renal-Metabolic System

The patient's body temperature must be measured hourly until it is stable and at least every 4 hours thereafter.

Central and Autonomic Nervous Systems

The patient must be monitored for the following signs and symptoms and the observations recorded hourly (these findings may indicate that current therapy is becoming inadequate and that further intervention is needed): worsening level of consciousness, seizures, miosis, increasing secretions (i.e., salivation, sweating), and persistent bradycardia or tachycardia.

Neuromuscular System

The patient must be observed for fasciculations and checked for muscle weakness with the following tests: hand grip, head control, ability to hold head off bed, general tone, and reflexes. A peripheral nerve stimulator can be used to monitor return of striated muscle function in the uncooperative young patient.

TREATMENT

Rapid implementation of therapy for organophosphate and carbamate poisoning is essential to avoid unnecessary morbidity and mortality. The three fundamentals of therapy are supportive care, removal of the intoxicant, and the administration of antidotes.

Supportive Care

Respiratory insufficiency is a frequent complication of anticholinesterase poisoning. Thus care must be provided in an area (PICU) capable of responding immediately to airway management emergencies and of providing assisted ventilation (see Chapters 127 and 128). General supportive therapy may also be needed to manage coma and seizures. Dysrhythmias, especially profound bradycardia, affecting cardiac output and systemic arterial blood pressure may also occur.

Removal of Intoxicant

An extensive effort must be made to avoid ongoing exposure to the poison. All clothing must be removed and discarded. The patient must be bathed and his eyes lavaged liberally. The usual methods of emptying the stomach can be employed with caution. Vomiting must not be induced in patients with depressed mental status or respiratory compromise or in those who have ingested an insecticide with a petroleum distillate base. Gastric lavage can be instituted only after the airway is protected; lavage is effective only if instituted soon after a liquid ingestion. In contrast, solid pellets or granules can be retained in the stomach for hours, and lavage must be done in these instances. Catharsis with magnesium citrate and activated charcoal must be provided.

Antidotes

Pharmacologic management of intoxication with anticholinesterase agents involves the administration of two complimentary drugs, atropine sulfate and pralidoxime chloride.

Atropine sulfate

Atropine sulfate, a muscarinic cholinergic-blocking agent, is the mainstay of therapy. It is a competitive antagonist of acetylcholine and in therapeutic doses ameliorates the effects of excess acetylcholine at parasympathetic neuroeffector junctions (muscarinic effects). The CNS effects of anticholinesterase poisoning are, however, only partially alleviated, reflecting the relative impermeability of the blood-brain barrier to the drug. Atropine has no effect on nicotinic cholinergic receptors, including those of the neuromuscular junction. Therefore, despite the use of atropine, patients may progress to respiratory arrest because of progressive paralysis of the muscles of respiration.

There is a tendency to undertreat patients with atropine because of the large doses that are sometimes needed. The goal is to administer atropine often enough in large enough doses to maintain signs of "atropinization" (dilated pupils, diminished secretions, decreased bowel sounds, improved breath sounds, cutaneous flushing). Tachycardia may be present as a sign of autonomic stimulation (a direct effect of the toxin); therefore atropine must not be withheld or administered in subtherapeutic doses

because of tachycardia in an otherwise symptomatic child. The following regimen for the administration of atropine is recommended.

1. The initial dose is 0.02 mg/kg. A dose up to 0.05 mg/kg (maximum dose, 2 to 4 mg) may be needed to produce atropinization and may be repeated as often as every 10 minutes until the desired effect is attained. Atropine may be given SC, IM, or IV.

2. The atropine effect may last 1½ to 4 hours. Full atropinization is continued for 24 to 48 hours or until signs and symptoms no longer recur.

3. Alternatively, continuous infusions of atropine may offer the advantages of a constant level of drug and efficient dosage adjustment. After a loading dose the initial infusion is administered at 0.02 to 0.05 mg/kg/hr (depending on previous bolus requirements) and adjusted as needed. This approach is particularly useful for treatment of severe toxicity and after poisoning with a lipophilic organophosphate (fenthion) when prolonged therapy is anticipated.

Pralidoxime chloride

Pralidoxime chloride (Protopam) is a cholinesterase reactivator. This agent greatly accelerates the hydrolytic reactivation of acetylcholinesterase that has been phosphorylated by an organophosphate. It competes with acetylcholinesterase for the phosphorus group on organophosphates, thus liberating active enzyme and detoxifying remaining poison. Because phosphorylated acetylcholinesterase undergoes a conversion to an irreversible bond with time, it is most effective as an antidote if administered within the first 24 to 48 hours after the patient's exposure. For the same reason pralidoxime has limited, if any, efficacy when administered after chronic exposure. The exception is intoxication that results from the lipophilic organophosphates (fenthion), which are distributed in adipose tissue and are gradually released into the circulation over many days. In these cases pralidoxime administration may be needed for up to 3 weeks.

The nicotinic receptors are most affected by reactivation of acetylcholinesterase by pralidoxime. Restoration of skeletal muscle strength (particularly respiratory muscles) often occurs within minutes after the administration of this agent. The effects of pralidoxime are less noticeable at autonomic effector sites and within the CNS.

The toxicity of pralidoxime is minimal at recommended doses. Overdoses can, however, produce neuromuscular blockade. If this drug is infused too rapidly, headache, nausea, vomiting, blurred vision, diplopia, dizziness, tachycardia, and hyperventilation may occur.

The following are recommendations for the administration of pralidoxime for organophosphate poisoning in children.

1. The initial dose is 25 to 50 mg/kg IV (maximum dose, 1 to 2 g) as a 5% solution given over no less than 5 minutes. This dose can be repeated in 1 hour if there is no improvement in muscle weakness or if fasciculations are noted. This dose is then repeated every 8 to 12 hours as needed for relief of nicotinic signs and symptoms.
2. Oral administration of repeat doses of pralidoxime is acceptable if toxicity is mild and if GI symptoms are absent.
3. Pralidoxime must be administered until symtoms no longer occur.
4. The dosage of pralidoxime must be decreased for the patient with renal insufficiency.
5. Pralidoxime enhances the response to atropine, often necessitating a decrease in the dosage of atropine.
6. Pralidoxime may be effective as an antidote even if administered at a time remote from the exposure and should, therefore, be given at least as a trial to all patients with organophosphate poisoning.
7. The use of pralidoxime in patients with carbamate poisoning is unnecessary because the carbamate-acetylcholinesterase bond is unstable and rapid spontaneous reactivation of acetylcholinesterase occurs. Furthermore, there are animal data that report increased mortality in carbaryl-poisoned laboratory animals (no data for humans) after administration of a pralidoxime-like agent. In situations in which the specific type of insecticide is unknown, pralidoxime should be administered if signs of cholinergic excess are progressive despite the use of atropine.
8. Alternatively, pralidoxime can be administered as a continuous infusion. After atropine, a loading dose of pralidoxime is given, followed by a pralidoxime continuous infusion, with close monitoring of plasma levels. An initial IV bolus dose of 10 to 15 mg/kg, followed by a continuous infusion of pralidoxime for 36 to 48 hours at 10 to 20 mg/kg/hr to maintain plasma pralidoxime levels of 20 to 40 mg/L, is recommended.

Other drugs

Diazepam is the drug of choice for treating seizures. The effects of phenobarbital are potentiated by anticholinesterases, and it must be used cautiously. Morphine, theophylline-like compounds, succinylcholine, reserpine, and phenothiazine-type tranquilizers must be avoided in these patients.

ADDITIONAL READING
• Goldfrank LR, Bresnitz EA, Kirstein RH, et al. Organophosphates. In Goldfrank LR, Flomenbaum NE, Lewin NA, et al, eds. Goldfrank's Toxicologic Emergencies, 3rd ed. Norwalk, Conn.: Appleton-Century-Crofts, 1986, pp 686-696.
McNabb SD, Kearns GL, Fiser DH. Continuous infusion pralidoxime (CIP) for treatment of organophosphate poisoning. Clin Res 36:56A, 1988.
Mortensen ML. Management of childhood poisoning caused by selected insecticides and herbicides. Pediatr Clin North Am 33:421-445, 1986.
Taylor P. Anticholinesterase agents. In Gilman AG, Goodman LS, Rall TW, et al, eds. The Pharmacologic Basis of Therapeutics, 7th ed. New York: Macmillan, 1985, pp 110-129.
Zwiener RJ, Ginsburg CM. Organophosphate and carbamate poisoning in infants and children. Pediatrics 81:121-126, 1988.

86 Heavy Metal Intoxication

Frances C. Morriss

BACKGROUND

Intoxications related to heavy metals involve multiple organ systems because metals bind to tissue ligands to form soluble, dissociable complexes. Ligands are molecules capable of functioning as a donor partner in one or more bonds. The most common preferential binding sites are those containing oxygen, nitrogen, sulfur, and phosphates (i.e., $OH-$, $COO-$, PO_4H_2-, SH, NH_2); the most stable complexes are formed with sulfur and hydrogen. Many of the toxic effects of heavy metal–ligand complexes derive from inactivation of the sulfhydryl groups essential to activity of many enzymes.

At the cellular level toxicity is related to availability, so the chemical form of the metal and the degree of binding are important. Liquid-soluble alkyl compounds (organic metal complexes) pass across biologic membranes and are slowly dealkylated or metabolized to inorganic salts, which can bind intracellular ligands. This prolongs excretion as compared to inorganic metal salts and may change the pattern of toxicity. Different metals may have different tissue affinity or different body distributions (e.g., gold accumulates in bone, cadmium in renal tissue, alkyl compounds of lead and mercury in CNS tissue).

In general inorganic salts are more toxic than organic compounds on a milligram/kilogram basis. Other factors influencing toxicity include age, diet, concurrent exposure to other metals, route of introduction of metal, and length of exposure. In addition many metals can provoke immune reactions, tumor formation, or teratogenic changes. Table 86-1 lists heavy metals and information about their toxicity.

DIAGNOSIS

Because of multiple-system effects, especially from chronic and usually industrial exposures, which can mimic many disease processes, diagnosis of metal intoxications can be difficult. Blood, urine, and hair are the most accessible tissues in which to measure metal levels. Blood and urine usually reflect recent exposure; hair is more useful for the assessment of long-term exposure. In some instances other tissues may show indirect evidence such as intracellular inclusion bodies, lead lines on roentgenograms, typical skin lesions, or pulmonary deposits.

TREATMENT

In addition to the usual symptomatic support, management may involve use of chelating agents that bind relatively tightly to the metal and prevent or reverse binding to tissue ligands. A chelate is a complex formed between the metal and a compound that contains two or more preferential binding sites that have a stronger affinity for the metal than the tissue-binding sites. The end product, usually a stable heterocyclic ring, can be excreted unchanged in the urine. Chelating agents are generally nonspecific in their affinity for metals and can enhance mobilization and excretion of a wide variety of metals, including essential ones such as zinc and calcium. Both free and soft tissue metal can be removed. These agents are most effective for treating acute intoxications; irreversible damage to enzyme systems can occur with prolonged exposure as well as storage of metal in tissues (e.g., hair, bone) that are inaccessible to chelation agents. Inadequate doses of chelators can cause redistribution of the metal and may increase some manifestations of toxicity. Chelation is less likely to be successful in cases of massive exposure because it becomes impossible to chelate excess metal. For these reasons therapy must be aimed at providing an excess of chelation agents so that all the heavy metal can be bound and excreted. Patients who are known to have ingested large doses or highly toxic sub-

Text continued on p. 661.

Table 86-1　Heavy Metals Toxicity

Metal	Source	Indicator of Toxicity	Target (acute)	Organs (chronic)	Mechanism of Action	Therapy (first agent listed is agent of choice)
Aluminum (Al)	Oral antacids Chronic hemodialysis	Brain tissue, 4-8 µg/g	GI tract: constipation	CNS: dementia, seizures, myoclonus Pulmonary: fibrosis (inhaled Al fumes)	Ingested Al inhibits fluoride, decreases Ca and Fe absorption Binds intraluminal phosphates Inhibits acetylcholine-induced contractions Competes with silicic acid for reactive sites in oxidative phosphorylation pathway	Deferoxamine
Antimony (Sb)	Manufacture of metal alloys, pigment, ceramics	—	GI tract: emesis	Respiratory: rhinitis, tracheobronchitis	—	Dimercaprol DMPS
Arsenic (As)	Manufacture of pesticides, herbicides Paint Trivalent compounds most toxic	Blood, >50 µg/L Urine, >100 µg/L (best indicator of acute exposure) Hair, 1 µg/kg	Systemic: fever, anorexia Cardiovascular: dysrhythmia CNS: coma, seizures Hematopoietic: anemia, granulocytopenia GI: bloody diarrhea, stomatitis Renal: hematuria, anuria	Skin and hair: melanosis, verrucosis, hyperkeratosis, alopecia Cardiovascular: endarteritis Hepatic: cirrhosis, angiosarcoma Pulmonary: (?) carcinogenesis Skin: carcinoma CNS: peripheral neuropathy, encephalopathy	Alters sulfhydral-containing proteins Inhibits mitochondrial enzymes concerned with NAD-linked substrates	Dimercaprol DMPS

Metal	Source/Use	Diagnostic level	Acute toxicity	Chronic toxicity	Mechanism	Treatment
Barium (Ba)	Insecticide	—	GI tract: gastroenteritis Cardiovascular: dysrhythmia Musculoskeletal: paralysis Other: potassium deficiency	—	—	IV potassium
Beryllium (Be)	Coal combustion Alloy manufacture Ore extraction	—	Pulmonary: fulminating pneumonitis from fume inhalation	Pulmonary: chronic granulomatous disease (berylliosis)	Induces cell-mediated hypersensitivity after combination with skin	—
Bismuth (Bi)	Antacids Cosmetics Antidiarrheals	Blood, >10 µg/dl	Renal: acute failure	Systemic: anorexia Musculoskeletal: arthritis, weakness Renal: nephropathy Skin and mucous membranes: gingivitis, dermatitis CNS: encephalopathy	Concentrated in kidneys and liver	Dimercaprol
Cadmium (Cd)	Electroplating Pigments Zinc and lead mining Soil and water	Renal tissue, >200 µg/g Ingestion of 200-300 µg/dl Urine, >2 µg/dl	GI tract: nausea, emesis, diarrhea Pulmonary: chemical pneumonitis	Pulmonary: obstructive pulmonary disease Renal: proximal tubular dysfunction (proteinuria, aminoaciduria, glycosuria) Musculoskeletal: osteoporosis Cardiovascular: hypertension Genital: Leydig cell tumors	Decreases α_1-antitrypsin activity Development of circulating antiglomerular basement membrane antibodies Interferes with Ca metabolism	Exposure to small doses of metal, particularly dietary Zn, Co, or Se, induces production of metallothionein, which binds Cd Chelation therapy of questionable use except for ingestion DMPS and calcium disodium edetate Dimercaprol contraindicated

Continued.

Table 86-1   Heavy Metals Toxicity—cont'd

Metal	Source	Indicator of Toxicity	Target (acute)	Organs (chronic)	Mechanism of Action	Therapy (first agent listed is agent of choice)
Chromium (Cr)	Ore smelting Pigment production Manufacture of stainless steel Chrome plating Hexavalent form most toxic	Blood, 20-30 μg/L Urine, >10 μg/dl	Renal: acute tubular necrosis	Respiratory: carcinoma Skin: chronic ulceration	Produces cellular hypersensitivity	Dimercaprol
Cobalt (Co)*	By-product of copper smelting	—	GI tract: nausea, emesis	Hematopoietic: polycythemia Cardiovascular: cardiomyopathy Endocrine: goiter	Toxicity may be increased with chronic alcohol ingestion	Penicillamine
Copper (Cu)	Fungicides Paints	Ingestion of 200 mg/kg	Systemic: ingestion of copper salts GI tract: hematemesis CNS: coma Cardiovascular: hypotension	Hematopoietic: hemolytic anemia Hepatic: failure	Centrilobular hepatic necrosis	Penicillamine DMPS Dimercaprol
Gold (Au)	Medicinal	Accumulation of gold in amorphous phagolysosomes and mitochondria		Renal: nephrotic syndrome Skin: dermatitis Hematopoietic: thrombocytopenia	Acts as hapten to generate production of antibodies Direct toxicity to mitochondria	Dimercaprol
Iron (Fe)*	Medicinal (ferrous sulfate) Multiple transfusions Mining and processing of iron ore	Ingestion of >2.5 g ferrous sulfate	GI tract: emesis, hemorrhagic gastroenteritis, duodenal stenosis Cardiovascular: collapse and shock Hematopoietic: coagulation defects Hepatic: necrosis	Pulmonary: interstitial fibrosis Hepatic: cirrhosis Endocrine: diabetes mellitus	Acute mucosal cell damage, capillary endothelial cell damage Hemosiderin deposition chronically in liver, pancreas, endocrine organs, heart	Deferoxamine Ascorbic acid increases Fe excretion

Metal	Source	Diagnosis		Clinical manifestations	Mechanism	Treatment
Lead (Pb)	Paint Industrial and car emissions Food	Blood, >10 μg/dl (subacute); >80 μg/dl (overt clinical symptoms) Nuclear inclusion bodies Lead lines in epiphyseal margins of long bones by roentgenogram	Renal: reversible tubular dysfunction	Renal: nephropathy CNS: peripheral neuropathy, encephalopathy, increased ICP Hematopoietic: anemia	Lipid peroxidation with membrane damage to intracellular organelles Impairment of heme synthesis; inhibition of RBC ATPase Inhibition of cholinergic function and dopamine uptake (γ-aminobutyric) function Schwann cell degeneration leading to demyelination Enhanced toxicity with dietary deficiencies of Fe, Ca, Zn	With CNS toxicity: dimercaprol and calcium disodium edetate Without CNS toxicity, calcium disodium edetate, followed by penicillamine Remove environmental source DMPS
Lithium (Li)	Medicinal Manufacture of ceramics, lubricants, alloys	Serum, >1.5 mEq/L	Skin: burns (lithium hydride) CNS: coma, seizures Cardiovascular: dysrhythmias Renal: tubular dysfunction GI tract: nausea, emesis	Renal: interstitial nephritis, diabetes insipidus CNS: tremor, ataxia, seizures, psychosomatic retardation Cardiovascular: dysrhythmias	Competition with potassium	Diuretics
Magnesium (Mg)*	Alloy manufacture Antacids CNS depressants	—	CNS: depression, muscle paralysis Cardiovascular: hypotension	Mucous membranes: conjunctivitis, rhinitis	Toxicity enhanced in renal failure Absorption inhibited by excess GI Ca	—

*Denotes essential metal.

Continued.

Table 86-1 Heavy Metals Toxicity—cont'd

Metal	Source	Indicator of Toxicity	Target (acute)	Organs (chronic)	Mechanism of Action	Therapy (first agent listed is agent of choice)
Manganese (Mn)*	Manufacture of alloys, dry cell batteries, dyes, ceramics, matches Fertilizers	—	Pulmonary: pneumonitis	CNS: psychiatric disorders, Parkinson-like syndrome Hepatic: cirrhosis	Decreases in CNS dopamine and serotonin levels; degeneration of basal ganglia	L-Dopa Chelating agents (calcium disodium edetate) unsuccessful
Mercury (Hg)	Inorganic Mining, smelting Manufacture of paper pulp, felt Combustion fossil fuels	Inorganic Air, 0.05 mg/m³ Blood, 3.5 µg/dl Urine, 150 µg/L Hair, 120-300 mg/kg	Inorganic Pulmonary: corrosive pneumonitis GI tract: bloody diarrhea, necrosis Renal: proximal tubular dysfunction	Inorganic CNS: asthenic-vegetative syndrome (tremors, spasms, hyperexcitability, depression, hallucination), "Mad Hatter syndrome" GI tract: gingivitis, salivation Renal: immune glomerular disease Skin: acrodynia	Inorganic Binds cellular ligands with sulfhydryl groups Formation of immune complexes	Inorganic Hemodialysis and chelation Dimercaprol DMPS Penicillamine Calcium disodium edetate not useful
	Organic (methyl mercury) Industrial waste Shell fish Fungicide	Organic Blood, >30 µg/dl	—	Organic CNS: paresthesia, ataxia, dysarthria, deafness	Organic Degeneration of small nerve cells in cerebellum and visual cortex	Organic Chelation not helpful Interruption of enterohepatic cycling of mercury (biliary drainage, nonabsorbable thiol-resins)

Metal	Source	Diagnostic level	Acute toxicity	Chronic toxicity	Mechanism	Treatment
Nickel (Ni)	Cigarette smoke; Jewelry; Refining (mond process)	—	Systemic: fever, weakness; GI tract: emesis, diarrhea; Pulmonary: cough, respiratory failure; Hematopoietic: leukocytosis; CNS: cerebral edema	Skin: contact dermatitis; Pulmonary: carcinoma	—	Sodium diethyldithiocarbamate; Penicillamine; DMPS; Dimercaprol
Platinum (Pt)	Antineoplastic agents; Jewelry	—	—	Skin: allergic dermatitis; Renal: proximal and distal tubular dysfunction	Complex salts inhibit cell division; Bacterial mutagen	—
Selenium (Se)*	—	—	CNS: drowsiness, convulsions; GI tract: nausea, "garlic" breath; Hepatic: enzyme elevation; Hematopoietic: anemia	Musculoskeletal: discolored teeth; Skin: hair and nail loss, rash; Hepatic: necrosis, carcinoma; Endocrine: infertility	—	Dimercaprol contraindicated
Thallium (Tl)	By-product of iron, zinc, and cadmium refining; Rodenticides, insecticides; Depilatory; Production of halides (lens production)	Ingestion of 8-12 mg/kg	GI tract: irritation; CNS: ascending paralysis, psychic disturbances, dementia	Skin: alopecia; CNS: degeneration of peripheral nerves; Hepatic: necrosis; GI tract: gastroenteritis; Renal: nephritis; Pulmonary: edema	Competition with potassium in membrane transport system; Inhibition of mitochondrial oxidative phosphorylation; Disruption of protein synthesis	—
Tin (Sn)	Manufacture of solder, bronze, brass; Textile dyes; Fungicides, bacteriocides; Organic form most toxic (triethyl tin)	Urine, >24 µg/dl	—	Pulmonary: pneumonitis; CNS: encephalopathy, visual defects	Inhibition of ADP; Uncoupling of mitochondrial oxidative phosphorylation	—

*Denotes essential metal.

Continued.

Table 86-1 Heavy Metals Toxicity—cont'd

Metal	Source	Indicator of Toxicity	Target (acute)	Organs (chronic)	Mechanism of Action	Therapy (first agent listed is agent of choice)
Titanium (Ti)	Pigments used as whiteners (flour, cosmetics, confections) Manufacture of surgical implants	—	—	Pulmonary: fibrosis	—	—
Uranium (U) and radioactive elements	Nuclear fuel	—	Renal: failure Skin: burns GI tract: nausea, emesis	Renal: failure Musculoskeletal: bone abnormality Hematopoietic: marrow depression Carcinogenic Pulmonary: fibrosis Eye: cataracts	Bone deposition	DTPA Calcium disodium edetate
Vanadium (V)	By-product of petroleum refining Catalyst Manufacture of photography equipment, pigments, steel, insecticides	Serum, >50 μg/dl	Pulmonary: bronchitis GI tract: nausea, emesis, pain Cardiovascular: dysrhythmias CNS: depression	Pulmonary: interstitial fibrosis GI tract: tongue discoloration Renal: dysfunction	—	—
Zinc (Zn)*	Galvanizing process	—	Systemic: metal fume fever GI tract: diarrhea (ingestion of beverages in galvanized cans)	Pulmonary: interstitial fibrosis	Release of endogenous pyrogens Interstitial thickening	Penicillamine

*Denotes essential metal.

stances (e.g., arsenic) should be given maximum doses. Common chelation agents are discussed below and in Table 86-2.

Dimercaprol

Dimercaprol (BAL) is a dithiol compound with two sulfur atoms on adjacent carbon atoms that compete with critical ligand-binding sites. It forms a tightly bound nontoxic complex with inorganic mercury, antimony, bismuth, cadmium, cobalt, chromium, gold, and nickel. All dimercaprol-metal complexes can dissociate to some degree, with release of the metal in its active form. Dimercaprol's use is contraindicated in patients with cadmium, tellurium, and selenium toxicity because it enhances symptoms. It must be administered so that there is an excess of agent available to compete effectively with tissue ligands for complete metal binding. Dimercaprol is ineffective in the presence of large quantities of unbound metal; the degree of effectiveness in reversing signs of toxicity by reactivation of enzyme systems is proportional to the length of time the system has been exposed to the metal. Dimercaprol-metal complexes dissolve or become oxidized in acid media; thus alkalinization of the urine may increase excre-

tion and protect the kidney from tubular damage secondary to production and absorption of the metal.

Toxic reactions occur in 50% of patients receiving a dose of 5 mg/kg; symptoms can include headache, nausea, emesis, conjunctivitis, sweating, lacrimation, abdominal and perineal pain, tachycardia, hypertension, seizures, and coma. Cardiovascular effects are common, are dose related, and usually resolve within 30 to 60 minutes of injection. Children commonly experience drug-related fever, beginning with the second or third dose and persisting until completion of therapy.

Successful chelation may remove essential heavy metals normally found in enzyme systems such as catalases, carbonic anhydrase, peroxidases, and cytochromic enzymes. Dimercaprol must be given as a 10% solution by the deep IM route to avoid pain, local reaction, and formation of sterile abscesses. Hepatic insufficiency is a contraindication to its use.

Calcium Disodium Edetate

Calcium disodium edetate (calcium EDTA; ethylenediaminetetraacetic acid) forms a poorly dissociated ring complex with polyvalent metals that will displace calcium from the original molecule. Lead, zinc, cad-

Table 86-2 Chelating Agents

Agent	Dose Schedules	Toxicity	Comments

Dimercaprol	Severe intoxication:
	  3 mg/kg IM q 4 hr × 48 hr
	  2.5-3 mg/kg IM q 6 hr × 24 hr
	  2.5-3 mg/kg IM q 12 hr × 24 hr
	  2.5-3 mg/kg IM q 24 hr × 10 days
	Mild intoxication:
	  2.5 mg/kg IM q 4 hr × 48 hr
	  2.5 mg/kg IM q 12 hr × 24 hr
	  2.5 mg/kg IM q 24 hr × 4-12 days
	With calcium disodium edetate for lead poisoning:
	  4 mg/kg IM q 4 hr × 5 days
	5% ointment for treatment of skin lesions (arsenic, cadium) (not FDA-approved use)
		Hypertension, tachycardia
		Various GI effects
		Hemolytic anemia with G6PD deficiency
		Contraindicated with hepatic insufficiency except secondary to arsenic ingestion
		Dose not cumulative if given at 4 hr or greater intervals
		Increases toxicity from cadmium, tellurium, and selenium ingestion
			May go up to 4-5 mg/kg
			Modify dose schedule on basis of severity of symptoms
			Alkalinize urine to prevent dissociation of chelate-metal complex and to protect kidneys from direct metal toxicity
			Monitor urinary metal levels

Continued.

Table 86-2   Chelating Agents—cont'd

Agent	Dose Schedules	Toxicity	Comments
Calcium disodium edetate	Maximum safe dose: 1.5 g/m²/day in 2-3 doses Usual dose: 1 g/m² IV in 2-3 divided doses given over a minimum of 2 hr May be given as constant infusion over 12-24 hr	Hypocalcemic tetany with rapid IV administration Nephrotoxic T-wave abnormalities Histamine release reactions (hypotension, rash, sneezing, nausea, lacrimation) Contraindicated by anuria	Must establish good urinary output Poor GI absorption Obtain urinalysis daily; monitor electrolyte and creatinine values frequently, ECG continuously
DMPS	0.5 mg/kg IM or SC q 6-8 hr × 24 hr, then 0.5 mg q 8-12 hr × 24 hr; 0.5 mg/kg qd thereafter	Vertigo Nausea	Water soluble Effective through oral route
Deferoxamine	Usual dose: 20 mg/kg IM, followed by 10 mg/kg q 4 hr × 2, followed by 10 mg/kg IM q 4-12 hr prn Shock: Same dose by slow IV infusion, not to exceed 15 mg/kg/hr Maximum dose: 6 g or less	Histamine release reactions (hypotension with rapid IV administration, urticaria, abdominal discomfort) Cataracts: long-term use Contraindicated by anuria, pregnancy, renal disease	Poor GI absorption Urine discolored orange Monitor urinary iron levels
Dithiocarb	—	—	Investigational drug
DTPA	Usual dose: 25-50 mg/kg as a 25% solution by slow IV infusion qod × 3 or qd × 5 days May be repeated every 2 wk (at least 2 days of no therapy should precede institution of second dose schedule)	Hypocalcemic tetany with rapid IV administration Nausea, emesis, diarrhea Contraindicated with renal insufficiency	May be given IM
Penicillamine	Usual dose: 20 mg/kg/day PO for 14 doses given 3 hr after meals Maximum daily dose: 2 g or less Shock: Institute therapy with another agent	Proteinuria (usual) Immune complex membranous glomerulonephropathy Multiple diffuse dermatologic manifestations Contraindicated by penicillin sensitivity Bone marrow depression Hepatic dysfunction Hypoglycemia Concomitant iron Contraindicated in presence of immunosuppressants, gold salts, and phenylbutazone	Do not give PO iron with agent—decreases absorption Obtain urinalysis daily; monitor CBC with differential, hepatic enzymes frequently Frequent physical examination needed to assess peripheral nerve function and skin Iron spared in hemoglobin and cytochromes

mium, cobalt, copper, vanadium, and manganese are bound; thus it is the treatment of choice for patients with lead intoxication. The calcium salt instead of the sodium salt must be used so that excess calcium ions are available to replace calcium removed with chelation and to prevent an otherwise profound hypocalcemic tetany. The chelate half-life is 1 hour, with 50% urinary excretion of the complex in 1 hour. After 24 hours approximately 1% to 2% of the original dose remains in the body. The principal toxicity is a dose-related renal tubular dysfunction that includes proteinuria, glycosuria, hematuria, and eventually oliguria. If anuria occurs, the drug must be stopped. Minor side effects include histamine release (rash, nausea with IV administration, lacrimation, sneezing), ECG changes, and local reaction at injection sites. Calcium disodium edetate is poorly absorbed by the oral route and must be given parenterally as a 0.4% solution in 0.9% sodium chloride for IV use or as a 0.5% solution in procaine for IM use. Renal failure or failure to establish a brisk urinary output is a contraindication to the use of calcium disodium edetate. Increased renal excretion of potassium can occur, so electrolyte values must be monitored routinely, as must urine for the presence of protein or cellular elements.

2,3-Dimercapto-α-Propanesulfonic Acid

2,3-Dimercapto-α-propanesulfonic acid (DMPS) is a water-soluble derivative of dimercaprol, developed to reduce toxicity and unpleasant side effects. It effectively chelates inorganic and methyl mercury compounds, copper, nickel, and cadmium after a patient's recent, but not prolonged, exposure to them.

Deferoxamine

Deferoxamine (Desferal) is a hydroxylamine isolated from *Streptomyces pilosus* that has a specific affinity for ferric iron and competes successfully for iron in ferritin and hemosiderin but not in hemoglobin or heme-containing enzymes. Deferoxamine is poorly absorbed from the GI tract and must be given parenterally; in addition iron chelates in the GI tract can be reabsorbed, especially through damaged mucosa, and increase serum iron levels. Toxic effects include hypotension after rapid IV administration and occasional rashes and urticaria related to histamine release. Long-term therapy has been associated with cataract formation. The deep IM route is preferred, although the SC route has been shown to be effective

in the treatment of long-term iron overload. Deferoxamine is available in 250 to 500 mg ampules of lyophilized agent that must be reconstituted with sterile water. Administration will cause orangish discoloration of urine; loss of coloration indicates clearance of the iron-chelate complex. Urinary iron levels must be monitored, but very low levels may not be detected. In a patient with renal failure chelated iron compound can be removed by dialysis; the presence of severe renal disease and/or anuria generally contraindicates use of desferoxamine.

Dithiocarb

Dithiocarb (diethyldithiocarbamate) is the treatment of choice for acute nickel carbonyl poisoning. It may be administered orally for a patient with mild toxicity but must be administered parenterally for one with acute or severe symptoms.

Diethylenetriamine Pentaacetic Acid

Diethylenetriamine pentaacetic acid (DTPA) is a polyamino acid similar to calcium disodium edetate that generally has a greater affinity for metals. The calcium disodium salt must be used because of a high affinity of the drug for calcium; otherwise hypocalcemic tetany would occur. DTPA has been found useful for chelation of radioactive metals such as radium, strontium, and plutonium. Chelate-metal complexes appear rapidly in the urine, with 50% to 70% of a dose clearing within 4 hours. DTPA is poorly absorbed from the GI tract and must be given parenterally, usually by slow IV infusion. The patient must have intact renal function for excretion of DTPA.

Penicillamine

Penicillamine (Cuprimine) is a sulfhydryl amino acid that forms complexes with iron, copper, lead, arsenic, mercury, zinc, magnesium, manganese, and calcium that are subsequently excreted renally. It is the treatment of choice for copper toxicity. Since it is well absorbed from the GI tract, administration through the oral route is preferred. Hypersensitivity reactions characterized by fever, rashes of all types (urticarial, pemphigoid, morbilliform, papular, vesicular), pruritus, and lymphadenopathy can occur in up to one third of patients receiving the drug. Proteinuria commonly occurs with therapy and resolves spontaneously when penicillamine administration is stopped or the dose is reduced; hematuria or proteinuria >2 g/day may herald the development of an immune complex membranous glomerulonephropathy. Drug administration must be stopped if such severe hypersensitivity reactions occur. Iron deficiency anemia may occur in children receiving penicillamine therapy; if iron replacement therapy is needed, oral iron must be given several hours after penicillamine to avoid decreased absorption of the chelation agent. Since penicillamine has a similar derivation as penicillin, cross-reactivity occurs between the two drugs and sensitivity to penicillin is a contraindication to its use. Other toxic manifestations include bone marrow suppression, hepatic dysfunction with cholestasis, pancreatitis, hypogeusia, and peripheral neuropathies, including Guillain-Barré syndrome. Although the incidence of reactions is high, most symptoms resolve spontaneously with discontinuance of the drug.

Routine urinalysis to check for proteinuria must be done. A CBC with a differential count and frequent examination for skin and neurologic manifestation

are necessary as long as the patient receives penicillamine. Because of its effects on collagen and elastin, routine doses must be decreased before the patient has surgery and continued until wound healing is complete. Use of this agent is contraindicated in patients who receive drugs capable of bone marrow suppression (antimalarials, gold salts, immunosuppressants [particularly cancer chemotherapeutics], phenylbutazone) and who have renal insufficiency.

ADDITIONAL READING

American Hospital Formulary Service Drug Information 87. Bethesda, Md.: American Society of Hospital Pharmacists, 1987.

Goyer RA. Toxic effects of metals. In Klassen CD, Amdur MO, Dovll J, eds. Casarett and Doull's Toxicity: The Basic Science of Poisons, 3rd ed. New York: Macmillan, 1986, pp 582-635.

Klassen CD. Heavy metals and heavy metal antagonists. In Goodman and Gillman's The Pharmacological Basis of Therapeutics, 7th ed. New York: Macmillan, 1985, pp 1605-1627.

87 Street Drugs: Cocaine and PCP

W. Gary Reed · Ron J. Anderson

Many drugs fall into the category of "street drugs," and a detailed review of all of them is not possible in this text. Consequently, this chapter deals with two street drugs commonly encountered in critical care situations—cocaine and phencyclidine (PCP).

COCAINE
Background and Physiology
Cocaine is a powerful CNS stimulant that has been abused for decades in its pure form because of the intense euphoria it produces in the user. It is a white crystalline powder that has a short elimination half-life of approximately 40 minutes. It usually is taken intranasally ("snorting") by abusers, with an onset of action within minutes. Its short half-life usually results in repeated administration by the user to maintain the desired euphoria. A more rapid and intense euphoria can be obtained with IV injection or by smoking the free base form of the drug. Recently the smoking of this form of cocaine has increased dramatically with the emergence of an inexpensive crystalline form of the free base drug ("crack"). Oral use is rarely encountered except in persons trying to smuggle the drug by swallowing cocaine-filled condoms or balloons, which will occasionally rupture spontaneously.

The toxic manifestations of cocaine usually depend on its route of administration and the amount of drug used. With lower doses CNS stimulation results in euphoria, restlessness, and excitement, with occasional hyperpnea, diaphoresis, and vomiting. At higher blood levels tremor, hyperreflexia, respiratory depression, hyperthermia, hypertension, clonus, seizures, tachycardia, and ventricular dysrhythmias may occur. Rhabdomyolysis, which may be severe, is common in persons taking the drug in situations as-

sociated with intense muscle exertion. Chest pain with and without evidence of myocardial ischemia is common. Myocardial infarction caused by coronary artery vasospasm, premature atherosclerosis, or platelet plugging has also been reported. Occasionally patients die a sudden death ("caine reaction") after low doses of cocaine by any route of administration, probably because of a sensitization of the myocardium to circulating catecholamines, with subsequent ventricular dysrhythmias.

Monitoring and Laboratory Tests
Except for sudden death and with massive oral ingestion of cocaine, toxic effects of cocaine generally are short lived because of the short serum half-life of the drug. Consequently, measurement of serum levels of the drug is of little value.

Laboratory monitoring of patients is usually not necessary unless rhabdomyolysis is suspected, in which case serum muscle enzyme determinations (CPK) and creatinine, uric acid, electrolyte, and urinary myoglobin levels must be obtained.

The following must be carefully monitored in all patients with symptoms of intoxication from cocaine: vital signs to determine hypertension or hypotension, respiratory depression, hyperthermia, and tachycardia; neurologic status (for seizures); and continuous ECG (for ventricular dysrhythmias and myocardial infarction).

Treatment
The treatment of cocaine overdose is largely supportive, remembering that cocaine has a very short half-life and is frequently adulterated ("cut") with other toxic substances such as amphetamines, lidocaine, caffeine, or PCP.

1. With an intranasal or other mucous membrane application of cocaine any remaining drug must be removed by rinsing the mucous membrane with 0.9% sodium chloride solution.

2. With an oral ingestion of cocaine activated charcoal (1 g/kg) should be administered with a cathartic such as sorbitol (if patient is >1 year of age, 1 to 1.5 g/kg, maximum of 50 g per dose, as a 35% solution).

3. If the patient is comatose, is seizing, or has a depressed gag reflex, his airway must be protected with an endotracheal tube.

4. Hypotension can be treated with a 0.9% sodium chloride solution and Trendelenburg positioning. Vasopressors must be avoided if possible because of the susceptibility of the sensitized myocardium to serious ventricular dysrhythmias.

5. Systemic arterial hypertension is usually short lived and can be treated with a short-acting agent such as nitroprusside (1 μg/kg/min to start, then increase to achieve desired systemic arterial blood pressure) if no contraindication exists. Labetalol (0.25 mg/kg over 2 minutes) or propranolol (0.1 to 0.15 mg/kg IV in divided doses; maximum of 1 mg per dose over 1 minute) may also be used. Propranolol may also be used to treat the ventricular dysrhythmias associated with cocaine intoxication.

6. Hyperthermia must be treated aggressively with the use of cooling blankets or an ice water bath if condition is severe (≥104° F).

7. Seizures can be treated with a short-acting anticonvulsant such as diazepam (0.04 to 0.3 mg/kg IV; maximum dose should not exceed 0.6 mg/kg in 8-hour period) until seizures stop. Alternatively, lorazepam may be given at a dose of 0.05 to 0.15 mg/kg. Refractory seizures can be treated with conventional doses of phenytoin (15 mg/kg at 0.5 to 1.5 mg/kg/min, maximum of 50 mg/min) and/or phenobarbital (10 to 15 mg/kg at 25 to 50 mg/min).

PCP
Background and Physiology

PCP is a dissociative anesthetic that was discovered in the late 1950s while researchers were trying to synthesize nonnarcotic, nonbarbiturate anesthetics. Early trials with the drug resulted in distressing side effects that eventually led to the discontinuation of human studies in 1965. The street supply of PCP, however, was not curtailed even after veterinary use of the drug was stopped because the ingredients necessary for its synthesis are used extensively in industry, making it difficult to monitor sales of these ingredients.

PCP is self-administered, most commonly by smoking a drug-laced cigarette, usually marijuana, or by intranasal application ("snorting"). The drug can also be taken orally and, less commonly, by IV injection.

Within minutes PCP produces a "high" that lasts 4 to 6 hours. The drug also produces a sense of detachment from the environment and a tremendous sense of invulnerability that in some persons is pleasurable. Toxic manifestations of the drug depend on several factors, including the dose and route of administration, the premorbid emotional state of the user, and the presence of exteroceptive input.

Several psychiatric syndromes can result from the use of PCP, the most common of which is a schizophrenia-like illness that may appear at a time distant from the use of the drug and may be very difficult to treat. The occurrence of nonpsychotic violent behavior is very common, often resulting in severe self-mutilation and injury as well as acts of violence directed toward others.

The manifestations of PCP overdose generally fall into one of three stages, depending on the amount of drug ingested and the route of administration.

Stage 1. With this level of intoxication the patient is conscious and at extreme risk for violent behavior. The cardiovascular and respiratory systems are stable, although systemic arterial blood pressure, heart rate, and respiratory rate are increased. Usually the patient is ataxic, with a muscular rigidity. There is a decreased sensitivity to pain, although the patient is awake. The extreme muscular activity that occurs with this stage puts the patient at significant risk for rhabdomyolysis, volume depletion, and electrolyte abnormalities.

Stage 2. This stage represents a moderate overdose during which the patient is unconscious but has a competent airway. The pupils are usually at midpoint and reactive. There is a markedly decreased sensitivity to pain. Patients frequently have marked muscular rigidity and myoclonus, diaphoresis, hypersalivation, bronchorrhea, vomiting, and a propensity to develop laryngospasm. Seizures and rhabdomyolysis are common occurrences.

Stage 3. This stage represents a severe intoxication in which the patient is in coma and has a compromised airway. Brain stem reflexes are depressed, posturing is present, and patients are prone to seizures, systemic arterial hypertension, tachycardia, hypersalivation, and bronchorrhea. Hyperthermia and rhabdomyolysis commonly occur.

After ingestion of PCP patients are prone to develop a postingestion syndrome characterized by catecholamine excess, anxiety, depression, and violent behavior.

Monitoring and Laboratory Tests

Patients initially seen with PCP intoxication must have serum levels of the drug determined as well as arterial blood gas and pH, serum muscle enzyme, creatinine, uric acid, and electrolyte (especially potassium) values determined.

The patient's volume and hydration status must be followed carefully, as must his urinary output, systemic arterial blood pressure, neurologic status, and ECG. Generally patients do not need invasive hemodynamic monitoring or bladder catheterization unless hypotension or rhabdomyolysis are present.

Treatment

The treatment of PCP intoxication is primarily supportive, with special attention given to the behavioral problems exhibited by these patients.

1. "Talking down" to the patients is of no benefit. Patients need to be placed in a low sensory environment, and chemical restraint (diazepam, 0.1 to 0.3 mg/kg, maximum of 5 mg per dose, administered slowly by IV route) rather than physical restraint should be used whenever possible.
2. Phenothiazines must be avoided if possible because of their propensity to cause seizures.
3. If oral ingestion of the drug is suspected in patients with stage 2 or 3 intoxication, the stomach must be cleared by lavage, and activated charcoal (1 g/kg) can be administered with a cathartic such as sorbitol (if patient is >1 year of age, give 1 to 1.5 g/kg, maximum of 50 g per dose, as a 35% solution). Patients with stage 1 intoxication are generally too agitated to take oral medications.
4. Systemic arterial hypertensive crises can be treated with a short-acting drug such as nitroprusside (1 µg/kg/min to start, then increase until desired systemic arterial blood pressure is reached).
5. Tachycardia, ventricular dysrhythmias, and other signs of catecholamine excess can be treated with propranolol (0.01 to 0.1 mg/kg, maximum of 1 mg per dose over 1 minute).
6. Acidification of the urine increases the excretion of PCP, but using this procedure generally is not recommended because of the propensity of the drug to cause rhabdomyolysis.
7. Excretion of the drug can be enhanced by the induction of a 0.9% sodium chloride solution diuresis.
8. In patients with stage 1 intoxication all instrumentation must be avoided if possible. During stage 2 poisonings instrumentation precautions can be lifted except for oropharyngeal or tracheal suctioning because of the drug's tendency to cause laryngospasm. During stage 3 poisoning use of instrumentation is necessary because all patients must have endotracheal intubation.
9. All patients need psychiatric evaluation after detoxification for determining acute and chronic follow-up.
10. Patients must be followed closely for 1 week for the development of postingestion syndrome. During this time most patients will need treatment with propranolol.

ADDITIONAL READING

Allen RM, Young SJ. Phencyclidine-induced psychosis. Am J Psychiatry 135:1081-1084, 1978.

• Aronow R, Done AK. Phencyclidine overdose: An emerging concept of management. JACEP 7:56-59, 1978.

Balster RL, Chait LD. The behavioral pharmacology of phencyclidine. Clin Toxicol 9:513-528, 1976.

Barton CH, Sterling ML, Vaziri ND. Rhabdomyolysis and acute renal failure associated with phencyclidine intoxication. Arch Intern Med 140:568-569, 1980.

Benchinol A, Bartall H, Desser KB. Accelerated ventricular rhythm and cocaine abuse. Ann Intern Med 88:519-520, 1978.

• Burns RS, Lerner SE. Perspectives: Acute phencyclidine intoxication. Clin Toxicol 9:477-501, 1976.

Gay GR, Inaba DS, Sheppard CW, et al. Cocaine: History, epidemiology, human pharmacology and treatment. A perspective on a new debut for an old girl. Clin Toxicol 8:149-178, 1975.

• Miller SH. Cocaine toxicity. JAMA 239:2448-2449, 1978.

Noguchi TT, Nakamura GR. Phencyclidine-related deaths in Los Angeles County, 1976. J Forensic Sci 23:503-507, 1978.

Rappolt RT, Gay GR, Farris RD. Emergency management of acute phencyclidine intoxication. JACEP 8:68-76, 1979.

Rappolt RT, Gay GR, Inaba DS. Propranolol: Specific antagonist to cocaine. Clin Toxicol 10:265-271, 1977.

Rappolt RT, Gay GR, Inaba DS, et al. Use of inderal (propranolol-Ayerst) in 1a (early stimulative) and 1b (advanced stimulative) classification of cocaine and other sympathomimetic reactions. Clin Toxicol 13:325-332, 1978.

Russ C, Wong D. Diagnosis and treatment of the phencyclidine psychosis: Clinical considerations. J Psychedelic Drugs 11:277-282, 1979.

Shulgin AT, MacLean D. Illicit synthesis of phencyclidine (PCP) and several of its analogs. Clin Toxicol 9:553-560, 1976.

Siegel RK. Cocaine substitutes (letter). N Engl J Med 302:817, 1980.

Welch MJ, Correa GA. PCP intoxication in young children and infants. Clin Pediatr 19:510-514, 1980.

Wright HH, Sheth PA, Stasiowski MS. Phencyclidine-induced psychosis. South Med J 73:955-956, 1980.

88 Brown Recluse Spider Envenomation

Charles M. Ginsburg

BACKGROUND AND PHYSIOLOGY

Loxosceles reclusus (brown recluse spider), a member of the family Loxoscelidae, is indigenous to the southern and midwestern portions of the United States as well as to the temperate regions of Europe, South America, and Africa. Similar to other members of the genus *Loxosceles, L. reclusus* produces venom that causes localized dermatonecrosis at the envenomation site and occasionally systemic disease when it is injected into the skin and subcutaneous tissues of humans and animals.

The Spider

L. reclusus is a moderate-sized (2 to 5 cm), long-legged, fawn- to brown-colored spider that has a distinct violin-shaped area of pigmentation on its dorsal cephalothorax. Although highly mobile, the spider is reclusive, spending the majority of its time in remote dark locations (e.g., in woodpiles, under rocks and foundations, in basements). Attacks to humans are usually the result of provocation or when the nocturnally active spider encounters sleeping humans.

The Venom

The venom of the brown recluse spider is a complex mixture of low molecular weight protein and enzymes. After injection of crude venom into laboratory animals, dermatonecrosis, intravascular hemolysis, thrombocytopenia, hepatic and renal dysfunction, leukopenia, and death occur. The precise characterization and quantitation of the various venom components have not been completely elucidated; however, sphingomyelinase D, esterase, and hyaluronidase apparently are the major active enzyme components. Rees et al. have isolated a pure venom fraction that contains a protein containing sphingomyelinase D. Intraperitoneal injection of this extract into guinea pigs results in pulmonary edema, glomerulonephritis, leukopenia, thrombocytopenia, and death. Investigators have demonstrated that the venom fraction engages in a high-affinity interaction with sphingomyelin-containing cell membranes, and they have speculated that sphingomyelinase D incites perturbations of the cell membrane, resulting in the release of phospholipid-derived substances such as thromboxanes, prostaglandins, leukotrienes, and hydroxytetracosanic acid. These substances bind complement, resulting in platelet aggregation, leukocytic infiltration, vascular thrombosis, and ultimately tissue hypoxia and necrosis. Since sphingomyelin is ubiquitous in cell membranes, the effects of the venom are widespread.

The Bite

The activities of the individual at the time he encounters the spider generally determine the site of envenomation. The distal extremities, buttocks, and posterior thighs are the most common sites in diurnal envenomations. In contrast, the face and trunk, less common bite sites, are usually involved in nocturnal envenomations, during which the victim is generally unaware he has been bitten since there is little, if any, pain at the time of initial envenomation. Several hours after envenomation has occurred, pruritus, tingling, edema, erythema, and mild-to-moderate pain may occur at the local site. If sufficient toxin has been injected, the overlying skin becomes violaceous, and vesicles and blebs may appear at the envenomation site. Over the next 3 to 4 days the skin over the inoculation site becomes indurated and more tender, and a central area of necrosis and ulceration appears. Occasionally there may be a halo of pallid tissue surrounding the lesion; in some instances this area also becomes necrotic. During the next several days to weeks the area of necrosis may remain static or slowly enlarge, and the underlying dermis is destroyed, leaving an ulcerated, indurated necrotic crater. Healing of the lesions is protracted, taking weeks to months, and severe scarring is common.

Systemic reactions may occur in association with the local lesions. Although the precise incidence of these reactions is unknown, they are relatively uncommon, occurring in less than 10% of patients who have been envenomated. In general the onset of systemic signs and symptoms does not occur until 6 to 24 hours after envenomation, and it almost always antedates the appearance of necrosis in the local lesion. Fever, chills, tachycardia, asthenia, diarrhea, vomiting, arthralgia, and rash are the reactions most commonly reported. Seizures, paresthesias, alterations of the sensorium, hypotension, pulmonary edema, oliguria, and anuria are less frequent findings but, when present, bode an unfavorable prognosis.

The occurrence of fatal loxoscelism has been reported but is rare. The majority of deaths from patients in the United States has occurred in children younger than 5 years of age, and with few exceptions deaths have occurred only in patients who have developed disseminated intravascular coagulation (DIC) and renal failure after envenomation.

DIAGNOSIS

A myriad of laboratory abnormalities have been reported in patients with loxoscelism. Those most frequently reported are hemolytic anemia, thrombocytopenia, leukocytosis, DIC, biochemical evidence of hepatic and renal dysfunction, hypocomplementemia, and hypoglycemia. Since these abnormalities occur almost exclusively in patients with systemic reactions, it is unclear whether they are the result of the direct effect of the toxin or whether they occur secondary to acidosis and hypotension.

Diagnosis of envenomation by *L. reclusus* is made on clinical grounds. In many instances the diagnosis is often difficult since the bite may have been unnoticed and there is no routine diagnostic test available. In contrast to snake bite lesions the local lesion after brown recluse spider envenomation is generally not painful, and the envenomation site has little edema and discoloration until hours or days after envenomation has occurred. In rare instances vesicles or a bullae may form at the local site after Hymenoptera stings; however, these lesions rarely progress and generally resolve within 36 to 48 hours.

TREATMENT

Treatment of loxoscelism is directed at preventing or at least attenuating the amount of dermatonecrosis at the local site of envenomation as well as providing generalized supportive care for the small number of patients who develop systemic illness following envenomation. Over the years clinicians have used topical and intralesional corticosteroids, antimicrobials, antihistamines, vasodilators, and excisional therapy for prevention of dermatonecrosis and for acceleration of wound healing. Because of the paucity of controlled studies available in humans with necrotic arachnidism, there is no convincing evidence of the efficacy of any modality. In recent years investigators have evaluated the efficacy of the leukocyte inhibitor dapsone in animals and humans with local lesions. The results of the studies indicate this agent substantially reduces the need for early surgical intervention and also reduces the incidence of delayed wound healing and residual deformity. No data are available about its use in animals or in humans to indicate that dapsone attenuates or prevents systemic reactions.

Although a polyvalent antivenom has been used for treatment of a small number of patients in South America who have been envenomated by other members of the Loxoscelidae family, the antivenom is not commercially available in the United States, and, most important, there is no convincing evidence that this agent is efficacious in treating envenomation by *L. reclusus*.

ADDITIONAL READING

Babcock JL, Suber RL, Firth CH, Green CR. Systemic effect in mice of venom apparatus extract and toxin from the brown recluse spider. Toxin 19:463-471, 1981.

• Ginsburg CM, Weinberg A. Hemolytic anemia and multiorgan failure associated with a localized cutaneous lesion. J Pediatr 112:496-500, 1988.

Rees RS, Nanney LB, Yates RA, King LE. Interaction of brown recluse spider venom on cell membrane: The inciting mechanism? J Invest Dermatol 83:270-275, 1984.

• Rees RS, O'Leary JP, King LF. The pathogenesis of systemic loxoscelism following brown recluse spider bites. J Surg Res 35:1-10, 1983.

89 Trauma in Children

Dale Coln

BACKGROUND

Trauma is the major cause of death and disability in childhood. Ninety-five percent of injuries to children can be managed in the emergency department or on an outpatient basis. Injuries necessitating admission to the PICU are usually automobile related, frequently involve the head, and have a mortality rate of approximately 6%. Successful recovery requires the treating physician to have a compulsive sense of urgency in identifying and treating life-threatening injuries. The following points are key management factors:

1. Knowledge of the mechanism of injury helps in determining the type of injury.
2. The severity of head injury is the most important factor affecting recovery.
3. Hypotension is a late manifestation of blood loss.
4. The patient must be kept warm.
5. The findings from the abdominal examination can be unreliable.
6. Injury to the cervical spine can be occult.
7. All cases of hematuria must be investigated.
8. Relief of pain is important.

INITIAL ASSESSMENT AND TREATMENT
Mechanism of Injury

Important to the initial assessment is knowledge of the mechanism of injury. Children who fall from heights can incur head and upper extremity injuries but rarely intra-abdominal injuries. Compressive injuries to the upper abdomen and chest cause pulmonary contusions, myocardial contusions, disruption of the diaphragm, and injury to the renal pedicle. Children struck by cars frequently have multiple injuries involving the head, long bones, and intra-abdominal organs. Unrestrained automobile passengers sustain head and facial injuries.

Accidents when automobile lap belts are improperly positioned above the pelvis may cause disruption of the intestine or the abdominal muscles. An acute abdomen after trivial playground trauma suggests an injury to an *abnormal* intra-abdominal organ. Youngsters who are injured from overturned all-terrain vehicles sustain pulmonary contusions, fractures of the ribs and scapula, and major bronchopulmonary lacerations. A history inappropriate for the child's injury can alert the physician to the possibility of child abuse.

Airway

Establishing a satisfactory airway is the first priority in treating a patient who has sustained an injury. If immediate intubation is necessary, an effort must be made to keep the cervical spine in a neutral position to prevent injury or aggravation of an existing injury to the cervical cord from a cervical spine dislocation. Cricoid pressure must be used during the intubation to prevent aspiration of gastric contents on the assumption that every injured child has a full stomach.

Vascular Access and Treatment of Shock

The presence of shock mandates obtaining vascular access immediately, preferably in the upper extremities by venipuncture, although the lower extremity may be used if there is no evidence of intra-abdominal injury. In the hypotensive or comatose child the goal is to obtain vascular access in less than 2 minutes. If the initial venipuncture is not successful, a long-line Seldinger technique can be used to access the femoral or subclavian vein. Alternatives to venipuncture are cutdowns in the antecubital or saphenous veins. The early signs of shock are a rapid pulse and poor peripheral perfusion. Since hypotension occurs alarmingly late in children in shock (see Chapter 12), it is inappropriate to wait for the presence of hypotension to diagnose shock in pediatric patients. Hypovolemic shock is treated by the administration of lactated Ringer's solution at 10 ml/kg as a bolus. If the response is inadequate, a second 10 ml/kg bolus is given. The administration of packed red blood cells (10 ml/kg) is needed if there is not an adequate response to the second bolus. It is best to give no more than 40 ml/kg of crystalloid solution for acute resuscitation unless venous blood pressure and systemic arterial blood pressure are monitored. Frequent vital signs must be taken and recorded during volume resuscitation.

Continued Assessment

After the child's condition is stabilized, the priorities change. A complete examination, laboratory and roentgenographic studies, immobilization of fractures, maintenance of body heat, and administration of analgesics are in order. If the child is comatose or has evidence of intra-abdominal injury, a soft Anderson sump catheter is passed through the patient's nostril into the stomach. If the stomach is full, its contents must be washed out with 0.9% sodium chloride solution. A complete physical examination includes evaluation of mental status, CNS, chest, abdomen, and extremities. Notations are made of crepitus, tenderness, swelling, bruising, and limb deformity. Open wounds must be identified and accurately recorded. Extremity pulses are determined and recorded. Systemic arterial blood pressure, pulse rate, respiratory rate, and temperature are recorded. The child must be covered or an external heating lamp used to keep body temperature above 36° C.

Management of Pain

Analgesics and local anesthetics are administered to children after the initial assessment is complete. Meperidine (0.5 to 1.0 mg/kg IV) can safely be given unless there are severe respiratory or neurologic injuries. Midazolam (0.05 to 1.0 mg/kg IV) is useful if narcotics are contraindicated. Analgesics and local anesthetics are given before painful invasive procedures are performed in conscious children. Local skin anesthesia is provided with 1% lidocaine injected from a tuberculin syringe through a 30-gauge needle. To achieve longer anesthesia bupivacaine, 0.25%, is used for intercostal, axillary, and femoral nerve blocks.

Systemic Injuries

Central nervous system

Seventy percent of children who die from trauma do so because of a serious head injury. Most of these injuries occur because of acceleration and deceleration forces on the brain, frequently as a result of an auto-pedestrian accident that results in a shearing force starting immediately below the cortex and extending centrally. If the closed head injury is severe, decerebrate or decorticate posturing is present. Skull fractures usually produce local brain injuries of less severity. The Glasgow Coma Scale (Table 89-1) is essential in assessing the severity of neurologic damage in children. It is a satisfactory predictor of outcome for primary brain injury in children over the age of 1 year. In a child less than 1 year of age spontaneous motor movements frequently occur after a brain injury and will erroneously give the child a better neurologic score than his condition warrants. Glasgow Coma Scale scores of nine or less are an indication for neurosurgical consultation. Ventilation is indicated when scores are seven or less in a patient with a primary brain injury. Before intubation lateral roentgenograms of the spine must be done to exclude the presence of cervical injury.

A CT scan must be performed in a patient with a depressed level of consciousness, focal neurologic

Table 89-1   Glasgow Coma Scale

Eye Opening		Verbal Response		Motor Response	
Spontaneous	4	Oriented	5	Obeys	5
To voice	3	Confused	4	Localized pain	4
To pain	2	Inappropriate	3	Withdraws	3
None	1	Incomprehensible	2	Flexion	2
		None	1	None	1

signs, penetrating injuries, and depressed skull fractures. ICP monitoring must be started immediately in children with Glasgow Coma Scale scores of five or less. The ventricular catheter or dural monitor can easily be placed in the patient in the emergency department and does not interfere with the CT scan. Once the patient is intubated and has IV access established, blood can be drawn for determining arterial PO_2, PCO_2, and pH values. The child must be hyperventilated with sufficient FiO_2 to keep his arterial PO_2 >90 mm Hg. Ventilation is set at a rate that keeps the $PaCO_2$ at 25 to 30 mm Hg. Steroids, anticonvulsants, and antibiotics are not routinely administered. Surgery is rarely necessary in children with brain injuries and is reserved for patients with mass lesions and neurologic deterioration, open depressed fractures, and penetrating wounds.

If the brain-injured child is hemodynamically stable, initial fluid management is set at two thirds of the maintenance rate. Frequent measurements of electrolytes and osmolality are necessary because of the possibility of developing SIADH. Hourly urinary balance is recorded, and daily weights are monitored. Children whose level of consciousness deteriorates or in whom signs of cerebral herniation occur (pupillary dilation, abnormal motor responses) or in whom the ICP rises above 20 mm Hg are treated with immediate hyperventilation with hand ventilation. If this treatment does not lower the ICP, osmotic diuresis with mannitol (0.5 g/kg/IV) at a rate that does not decrease the systemic arterial blood pressure must be used. Mannitol necessitates insertion of a bladder catheter. For persistent ICP >20 mm Hg, the use of increased hyperventilation, continued osmotic diuresis, tubular diuretics, and IV thiopental (controversial) may be needed to control the intracranial hypertension. Death is most frequently correlated with elevated ICP, although mortality also depends on the extent of associated injuries and the primary neurologic injury.

Cervical spine injuries are not common in children but are easily overlooked because they frequently accompany a head injury and do not have associated cervical spine fractures.

Thoracic injuries

Hemothorax or pneumothorax is best treated by using tube thoracostomy. The preferred site is the seventh intercostal space in the midaxillary line. Incomplete expansion of the lung may necessitate insertion

of a second chest tube in the fourth intercostal space. Blood coming out of the chest tube at a rate >10 ml/kg/hr is an indication for thoracotomy. Most penetrating injuries of the chest can be successfully treated by tube thoracostomy. Exploration is necessary only in cases of continued bleeding or in the event that missiles have crossed the mediastinum.

Blunt trauma to the chest may cause pulmonary contusion, myocardial contusion, or rupture of the diaphragm. The more serious injuries to the chest are those that cause bronchial or tracheal disruption with massive air leaks. Multiple chest tubes may be necessary to control air leakage. Bronchoscopy is necessary for diagnosis of a bronchial tear, and it is followed by emergency thoracotomy. Myocardial contusion occurs rarely and is difficult to diagnose in children. Usually there are no ECG abnormalities or elevation of cardiac enzymes with these injuries. Low cardiac output, low systemic arterial blood pressure, and increased sensitivity to fluid administration are manifestations of myocardial injuries. If the mechanism of injury (i.e., a compressive force on the chest) leads one to suspect a myocardial contusion, echocardiography to look for abnormal ventricular wall motion is helpful. Monitoring the CVP and cardiac output is necessary to prevent fluid overload. Injuries to the diaphragm from blunt trauma are suspected if the chest roentgenograms show loops of bowel in the chest. However, this frequently is not the case, and the appearance is that of an "elevated diaphragm" or of a "hemothorax" that has not been evacuated by the chest tube drainage. Fluoroscopy and sonography of the diaphragm have been more helpful than CT scans in making the diagnosis.

Abdominal injuries

Most intra-abdominal injuries that occur in childhood are the result of blunt trauma. Although intra-abdominal injuries occur in only approximately 10% of children with blunt trauma, exsanguination from intra-abdominal injuries is the second leading cause of death from trauma in childhood. Disagreement surrounds the use of immediate surgery vs. observation with monitoring and blood replacement. The stated advantages of immediate surgery are that it provides earlier hemodynamic stability, shortens hospitalization, salvages more spleens, and has a greater margin of safety. The disadvantage is that surgery is not always necessary for treating injuries to solid intra-abdominal organs. The stated advantage of the nonoperative approach is that it avoids the risk and discomfort associated with an operation. The disadvantages of nonoperative treatment are the longer stay in the PICU, the longer hospitalization, the increased need for blood transfusion, the increased morbidity because of the delayed diagnosis of intestinal injuries, and the hazard of exsanguination from delayed bleeding from a liver injury.

Immediate surgery is performed on the basis of a positive peritoneal lavage, which detects 98% of intra-abdominal injuries. A negative perioneal lavage reliably predicts 100% survival after blunt abdominal trauma. The indications for peritoneal lavage are as follows: (1) an abdominal examination suggesting injury; (2) multiple trauma that occurred in an automobile accident; and (3) an altered state of consciousness if injury not known to have occurred exclusively to the head. The lavage is performed after the IV administration of midazolam and/or meperidine in the nonneurologically injured child. A bladder catheter is inserted before lavage. The lower portion of the abdomen is prepared with an iodine solution, and 1% lidocaine is used to produce anesthesia of the skin, subcutaneous tissue, fascia, and peritoneum. A commercially available peritoneal lavage kit is used, and a needle is inserted into the abdomen followed by a guidewire inserted through the needle. The peritoneal lavage catheter is inserted over the guidewire. Lactated Ringer's solution is instilled into the abdominal cavity in the following volumes for children: less than age 2 years, 250 ml; children 2 to 5 years of age, 500 ml; and children more than 5 years of age, 1000 ml. A positive peritoneal lavage is based on an aliquot of the 1000 ml of instilled fluid containing (1) a red blood count >100,000/mm³, (2) a white blood blood cell count >500/mm³, or (3) presence of bile, amylase, or bacteria. If the instilled amount of fluid was 250 ml, the red blood cell and white blood cell count on the aliquot must be divided by four. If 500 ml of fluid was instilled, the counts must be divided by two. This adjustment keeps the peritoneal lavage from being too sensitive in determining intra-abdominal injury. Experience in performing more than 800 peritoneal lavages for abdominal trauma indicates its use is safe, efficient, and reliable. It is the preferred test

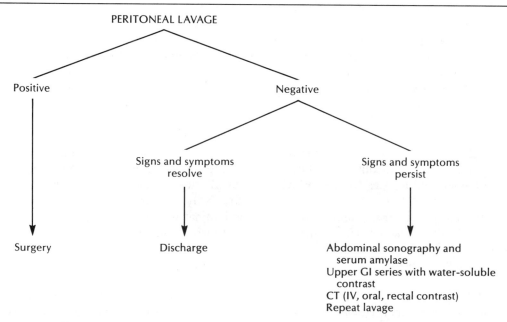

Fig. 89-1 Schema for determining the approach to treating abdominal trauma in the pediatric patient.

in determining the need for immediate surgery. A negative lavage does not exclude the presence of intra-abdominal injury, but the injury will not be a fatal one.

The selective use of the other diagnostic modalities is helpful in diagnosing stable patients. Studies comparing radionuclide scan, sonography, and CT scan for the detection of intra-abdominal injuries favor the use of a CT scan because a larger number of intra-abdominal injuries is detected. However, when compared with intraoperative findings, CT scans detect only 60% of intra-abdominal injuries in children and are unreliable for detecting pancreatic and small bowel injuries. Sonography is helpful in determining the presence of fluid in the abdomen and in evaluating injuries to the pancreas. Either an IVP or CT scan using IV contrast material is performed if microscopic hematuria is present; in a patient with gross hematuria a cystourethrogram is performed in addition to the IVP. A useful schema for managing blunt abdominal trauma in children is given in Fig. 89-1.

SPECIFIC ORGAN INJURIES FROM BLUNT TRAUMA

Spleen. The spleen is the most commonly injured intra-abdominal organ in childhood abdominal trauma. Ninety-eight percent of injured spleens can be salvaged by performing immediate surgery and repair. Nonoperative management is acceptable only for treating isolated splenic injuries in children with stable vital signs who do not need blood transfusions. Performing delayed exploration after failed nonoperative treatment frequently results in splenectomy.

Liver. The mortality for liver injuries from blunt trauma in children is approximately 20%. Exsanguination from liver injury is the second most common cause of traumatic death (after brain injury) in childhood. An alarmingly rapid deterioration from a liver injury can occur after several hours of apparent hemodynamic stability and is a significant risk factor to safe nonoperative management. Early exploration and control of hemorrhage is the preferred treatment for these injuries, which can extend into the hepatic veins.

Duodenum. A child with an intramural hematoma in the duodenum presents with vomiting resulting from obstruction several hours after an impaling injury to the right upper abdomen. Minimal upper abdominal tenderness usually is present. An upper GI series will demonstrate the obstruction in the second

portion of the duodenum. Resolution occurs within 4 to 5 days of using nasogastric suction, and surgery is usually not needed.

Pancreas. Impaling forces to the upper abdomen may injure the pancreas where it crosses the vertebral column and can result in complete disruption of the pancreatic duct or tearing of the pancreatic parenchyma. Some of these injuries are discovered during surgery after a positive peritoneal lavage. However, a number of pancreatic injuries in children are discovered because abdominal pain and elevated serum amylase suggest pancreatic injury. Sonography is helpful in detecting injury of the pancreas. If nasogastric suction and IV alimentation for 10 days does not result in complete resolution, an endoscopic retrograde pancreatogram is performed to determine whether or not the pancreatic duct is intact.

Small intestine. Injury to the small intestine occurs because the intestine is impaled against the spine. The child frequently does not have immediate symptoms but will develop signs and symptoms of peritonitis some hours after the injury.

Urinary tract. Renal injuries are common with blunt abdominal trauma in children. Most renal parenchymal injuries will heal without surgery. The serious urinary tract injuries are those that disrupt the renal vessels or the ureter at the ureteropelvic junction. An IVP must be performed in all injured children with hematuria, irrespective of the amount of blood. Extravasation of contrast material from a functioning kidney is not an indication for surgery. Bed rest is prescribed until hematuria clears, and the child is carefully monitored for continuing blood loss. However, extravasation of contrast from the medial side of the kidney and the failure to visualize the distal ureter suggest ureteropelvic disruption. Lack of kidney opacification on the pyelogram suggests renal vascular injury and is an indication for performing arteriography. Gross hematuria, especially after pelvic trauma, is investigated with a cystourethrogram. Disruption of the bladder usually necessitates operative intervention with suprapubic cystostomy.

PENETRATING INJURIES

Penetrating injuries are assessed according to their location, cause (gunshot, knife, foreign body), and local findings such as swelling, hemorrhage, tissue destruction, and functional deficit. Surgery is needed for penetrating wounds to the cranium, eye, neck, and abdomen. Selective operative management can be used for some knife wounds of the flanks and back. Most penetrating wounds of the chest respond well to tube thoracostomy, but surgery must be performed in patients with continued bleeding. Penetrating wounds of the extremities may need surgery for repair of vascular and neurologic injury.

Vascular injuries. Vascular injuries in children frequently go undetected because they do not produce obvious ischemia. Patients with vascular injuries caused by penetrating trauma are operated on for evidence of ischemia, absent distal pulses, severe bleeding, or arteriovenous fistulas. Preoperative arteriography is not often necessary. However, arteriography is helpful in patients with injuries to the base of the neck to determine the proper incision site for proximal vascular control. Orthopedic injuries that frequently cause major vascular problems are supracondylar fractures of the elbow and fracture-dislocations of the knee.

ADDITIONAL READING

• Bruce DA, Raphaley RC, Goldberg AJ, Zimmerman RA, Bilaniak LT, Schut L, Kuhl DE. The pathophysiology, treatment and outcome following severe head injury in children. Childs Brain 5:174-191, 1979.

Coln CD, Meyer DM, Thal ER, Weigelt JA, Redman HC. Comparison of computed tomography and diagnostic peritoneal lavage in the evaluation of children with blunt abdominal trauma. J Trauma (in press).

• Colombani PM, Buck JR, Dudgoon DL, Miller D, Haller JA. One-year experience in a regional pediatric trauma center. J Pediatr Surg 20:8-13, 1985.

Ramonofsky ML, Morse TS. Standards of care for the critically injured pediatric patient. J Trauma 22:921-933, 1982.

Sneed RC, Stover SL. Undiagnosed spinal cord injuries in brain-injured children. Am J Dis Child 142:965-967, 1988.

90 Lightning Injuries

Gary R. Turner

BACKGROUND AND PHYSIOLOGY

Lightning injuries are uncommon but dramatic; virtually every major organ system can be affected. Although lightning has a median current amplitude of approximately 25,000 amperes and involves potential differences of up to 1 billion volts and temperatures up to 50,000° F, approximately two thirds of the people struck by lightning survive. A short duration of exposure to the current (average of 0.2 second) and external flashover of the current to outside the body or to articles of clothing are among reasons given to explain how people can survive such an insult.

People are injured by lightning either directly, by a side flash, or by a step voltage. Victims of a direct strike often have evidence of current entry in the head or upper body. The current flows directly through the body to the ground, exposing the internal organs to injury unless an external flashover occurs. When people are carrying metal objects (e.g., golf clubs, umbrellas, fishing poles), the lightning can strike the object and be conducted through the hand into the body. Side-flash injuries occur when lightning strikes an object with a relatively high electrical resistance and then flashes over to a relatively better conductor nearby. People standing under a tree can be struck by a side flash when lightning hits the tree. Step-voltage injuries occur when lightning strikes the ground adjacent to where a person is standing and a potential difference is generated between the legs with current flowing through the legs and lower trunk. The victim often falls and suffers a temporary paralysis of the lower extremities. Fatalities can occur, especially if the victim was close to the point of impact; however, death is unusual in patients with this type of injury since the current does not traverse the heart or brain.

Thunder results from the rapid expansion of heated air adjacent to the lightning stroke. The resulting sound wave and blast effect also are capable of causing injury.

Lightning victims often suffer respiratory arrest, presumably secondary to the passage of current through the respiratory center. Although respirations may resume spontaneously, the duration of apnea may be prolonged. If effective basic life support is not given, the patient may suffer cardiac arrest secondary to hypoxia, with subsequent damage to the brain and other vital organs.

MONITORING AND LABORATORY TESTS

The most common and/or unusual manifestations of lightning injury in the major organ systems are listed in Table 90-1.

All patients struck by lightning must have an ECG. ECG changes after lightning injury are common and include nonspecific ST changes, T-wave inversion in the chest leads, and prolongation of the QT interval. The ECG usually returns to normal within a week, but it can remain abnormal for up to 1 year. Serial ECGs and cardiac isoenzyme studies are indicated in patients with ECG abnormalities.

A urinalysis must be done on all lightning victims. Although the occurrence of myoglobinuria is unusual compared to patients with other types of electrical injuries, it has been reported.

A hearing test and follow-up eye examination for cataracts are necessary for all survivors of acute injury. Other specific monitoring requirements will depend on the particular organ systems involved and the severity of illness. Neurologic assessment may be complicated by pupillary abnormalities (e.g., anisocoria, mydriasis) that have been reported to occur

Table 90-1   Manifestations of Lightning Injury in Major Organ Systems

Organ System	Complications	Comments
Respiratory	Apnea	May last up to 3 hr
	Lung contusion, ARDS	
Cardiovascular	Dysrhythmias	
	Asystole	
	Atrial or ventricular fibrillation	
	Frequent premature ventricular contractions	
	Myocardial injury, necrosis, infarction	
	Hypertension, tachycardia	Caused by increased endogenous catecholamines
	Congestive heart failure	Caused by myocardial damage
	Vasomotor spasm	Decreased pulses in extremities
Neurologic	Coma	
	Cerebral edema	
	Retrograde amnesia	
	Paresthesias	
	Paraplegia, hemiplegia	
	Seizures	
	Intracranial hemorrhage (subarachnoid, subdural, intracerebral)	
	Aphasia	
	Psychiatric problems (hysteria, depression)	
	Cerebellar ataxia	
Auditory	Tympanic membrane rupture	Most common ear injury
	Sensorineural hearing loss	May be permanent
Visual	Cataracts	1 mo to 2 yr afterward
	Corneal burns, retinal detachments	
	Optic atrophy	
	Abnormal pupillary response to light	
Renal	Myoglobinuria	
	Hemoglobinuria	
Gastrointestinal	Ileus	
	Stress ulcers	
Endocrine	SIADH	
Integumentary	Lichtenberg figures	Pathognomonic skin sign, dendritic macular rash that does not blanch
	Burns	Usually not severe
	Punctate entry and exit sites	
	Melting buckles, jewelry	
Musculoskeletal	Fractures	From falls and/or muscle contractions
	Compartmental syndromes	Rarely need fasciotomy
Hematologic	Positive direct and indirect antiglobulin (Coombs') test	Transient

secondary to lightning injury. Fixed and dilated pupils should not be immediately interpreted as a sign of cerebral death.

TREATMENT

Treatment of problems such as respiratory failure, dysrhythmias, hypertension, congestive heart failure, coma, cerebral edema, seizures, myoglobinuria, ileus, SIADH, and burns that can be associated with lightning injuries is nonspecific and supportive, as discussed elsewhere in this book. The "Lichtenberg figures" that may appear on the skin are not burns and tend to disappear spontaneously within 24 hours. Severe peripheral vasomotor spasm usually resolves without specific treatment; fasciotomies are needed only when soft tissue swelling compromises peripheral perfusion. Paresthesias and paralysis can resolve spontaneously within hours after the accident.

Effective cardiopulmonary resuscitation at the scene is extremely important for those victims who suffer a cardiopulmonary arrest as a consequence of lightning currents. The duration of apnea after a lightning injury often exceeds the duration of asystole; therefore in some cases artificial respiration alone may prevent recurrent asystole or ventricular fibrillation secondary to hypoxemia. There are numerous examples in the literature of victims who survived intact after receiving effective basic life support even though they first appeared dead at the scene of the accident.

ADDITIONAL READING

Abt JL. The pupillary responses after being struck by lightning. JAMA 254:3312, 1985.

Bartholome CW, Jacoby WD, Ramchand SC. Cutaneous manifestation of lightning injury. Arch Dermatol 111:1466-1468, 1975.

Chia BL. Electrocardiographic abnormalities and congestive cardiac failure due to lightning stroke. Cardiology 68:49-53, 1981.

Cwinn AA, Cantrill SV. Lightning injuries. J Emerg Med 2:379-388, 1985.

• Golde RH, Lee WR. Death by lightning. Proc Institution Elec Eng 123:1163-1180, 1976.

Hanson GC, McIlwraith GR. Lightning injury: Two case histories and a review of management. Br Med J 4:271-274, 1973.

• Kotagal S, Rawlings CA, Chen S. Neurologic, psychiatric and cardiovascular complications in children struck by lightning. Pediatrics 70:190-192, 1982.

Noel LP, Clarke WN, Addison D. Ocular complications of lightning. J Pediatr Ophthalmol Strabismus 17:245-246, 1981.

Stanley LD, Suss RA. Intracerebral hematoma secondary to lightning stroke: Case report and review of the literature. Neurosurgery 16:686-688, 1985.

Taussig HB. "Death" from lightning—and the possibility of living again. Ann Intern Med 68:1345-1353, 1968.

Yost JW, Holmes FF. Myoglobinuria following lightning stroke. JAMA 228:1147-1148, 1974.

91 Smoke Inhalation and Carbon Monoxide Poisoning

David A. Hicks · Nick G. Anas

BACKGROUND AND PHYSIOLOGY

Respiratory complications are responsible for much of the morbidity and mortality that result from fires; these pulmonary sequelae are caused by both smoke inhalation and carbon monoxide poisoning. Significant injury to the respiratory tract can occur even in the absence of surface burns. Because lung and respiratory tract damage due to smoke exposure most commonly occurs in persons trapped in confined places, the pediatric population represents a high-risk group.

Pulmonary injury from smoke inhalation may result from (1) heat exposure (thermal burn), (2) the inhalation of particulate matter, and (3) the effects of toxic fumes. In the clinical setting it is often difficult to determine which of these mechanisms has contributed to the pulmonary injury, since often they produce additive effects. Because the upper airway is an efficient heat exchanger, thermal injuries caused by direct flame exposure generally are limited to the area above the larynx. Since fully saturated air has 4000 times the heat capacity of dry air, steam injury may involve the entire tracheobronchial tree. Smoke tends to affect the larynx, trachea, and mainstem bronchi but does not often penetrate to the small airways and alveoli.

Toxic fumes are able to reach the pulmonary parenchyma and can cause more diffuse injury. Oxides of sulfur and nitrogen combine with water and form corrosive acids and alkalis that can irritate mucous membranes, induce bronchospasm, and denature proteins, resulting in widespread cellular destruction. The combustion of polyvinyl chloride produces at least 75 potentially toxic compounds, some of which damage type II pneumocytes, thereby interfering with surfactant production. Lipid-soluble toxic fumes dissolve within cellular membranes; in the tracheobronchial tree this may cause epithelial damage, sloughing of mucosa, and bronchiolar obstruction. Lipid-soluble toxins can directly injure the alveolar capillary membrane, leading to permeability pulmonary edema (adult respiratory distress syndrome). In turn, pulmonary macrophages are stimulated to release chemotactic mediators that sequester leukocytes and other cells of the circulation within the pulmonary capillary bed, causing further disruption of alveolar-capillary integrity. Thus the pulmonary effects of smoke inhalation can involve the entire tracheobronchial tree, alveoli, and pulmonary capillary bed. Gas-exchange abnormalities result from large and small airway obstruction, bronchospasm, pulmonary edema, surfactant deficiency, or obliteration of the pulmonary arterial bed.

Carbon monoxide (CO) is an odorless, colorless, and tasteless gas produced by incomplete combustion of organic fuels. Excessive exposure occurs in poorly ventilated areas in which wood or coal is being burned or, for example, in which a car engine remains running. CO causes toxicity because it avidly binds to hemoglobin; compared to oxygen it has 200 times the affinity for hemoglobin, resulting in a reduced oxygen-carrying capacity of the red blood cells. Carboxyhemoglobin (COHb) causes a leftward shift of the oxyhemoglobin curve, which increases the avidity of hemoglobin for oxygen; tissue oxygen tension must decrease to abnormally low levels before appreciable amounts of oxygen are released from the hemoglobin molecule (see Chapter 10). CO also binds to cytochrome oxidase a_3, interfering with cellular oxidation. Therefore CO induces hypoxia by reducing the oxygen-carrying capacity of hemoglobin, by inhibiting the release of oxygen from the hemoglobin molecule, and by interfering with cellular metabolism. The severity of tissue hypoxia is related to the COHb concentration in blood. The usual level of COHb is <1%. At levels of 20% to 30% headache, dyspnea, and mental confusion occur; at 30% to 40% nausea, irritability, visual impairment, chest pain, and tachycardia are common features; at 40% to 60% confusion, hallucinations, seizures, or coma predominate; at >60% cerebral edema, increased ICP, and death occur. The finding of cherry-colored skin, nail beds, and mucous membranes is unusual and does not appear until the level of COHb exceeds 40%.

Table 91-1 Physical and Laboratory Findings in Patients With CO Poisoning

System	Abnormalities
Central nervous system	Headache, mental confusion, hallucinations, seizures, coma
	CT scan of head
	Cerebral edema
	Cortical atrophy (late)
	Low-density areas in the globus pallidus (late)
	Increased ICP
	Increased cerebral blood flow
Cardiovascular	Increased heart rate and cardiac output
	ECG: ST depression, T-wave inversion, heart block, ectopy, atrial fibrillation
	Metabolic acidosis
Pulmonary	Comfortable respiratory rate and effort
	Normal Pao_2
	Reduced Sao_2 (measured)
Renal	Renal failure secondary to myoglobinuria
Skin	Cherry-red mucous membranes, nail beds, skin
	Blisters, erythema
Eye	Papilledema, retinal hemorrhages, blindness

Table 91-1 provides a list of physical and laboratory findings resulting from the organ system response to CO poisoning.

MONITORING AND LABORATORY TESTS

Information must be obtained about the type of fire (i.e., materials involved, presence of steam heat) that caused the injury, the length of the patient's exposure, and the location of the event (i.e., whether it was a closed or open space).

The patient is examined for external evidence of burns or smoke inhalation (e.g., burns of nose and lips, presence of singed nasal hairs). The degree of respiratory compromise is assessed through the patient's respiratory rate and effort, color, stridor, hoarseness, cough, and auscultatory findings of wheezing or crackles. The patient's level of consciousness must be determined.

Continuous cardiac (ECG) and respiratory monitoring, including continuous pulse oximetry, is started. However, one must recall that oxygen saturation (Sao_2) monitoring is less useful in cases of CO poisoning since it measures the percent saturation of hemoglobin-binding sites available for oxygen but not the sites bound by CO. In addition arterial blood gas tensions and pH are obtained. The Sao_2 must be measured directly (co-oximetry) and not extrapolated from the arterial oxygen tension (Pao_2) and body temperature.

The COHb level is most accurately determined by the spectrophotometric method; it must then be measured every hour until the value is <5%. A complete and differential blood count, as well as electrolyte and lactic acid levels are needed. The presence of lactic acidosis indicates significant tissue hypoxia.

A chest roentgenogram is obtained to determine the presence of aspiration pneumonitis, atelectasis, pulmonary edema, or hyperinflation. A 12-lead ECG will help determine the presence of rhythm disturbances or evidence of myocardial ischemia or infarction. Bronchoscopy or laryngoscopy may be used to determine the extent of laryngeal and upper airway injury and to remove debris. Placement of a central venous or pulmonary artery catheter may be considered if evidence of shock or severe hypoxia is present.

The use of CT scanning of the brain may be indicated to evaluate edema or concomitant trauma if the patient's level of consciousness is altered. In addition ICP monitoring may be indicated if there is physical or CT evidence of increased ICP.

TREATMENT

The goals of the management of a child with smoke inhalation and CO poisoning are (1) to reverse hypoxemia and tissue hypoxia, (2) to reduce COHb levels to a safe range, (3) to assure a patent airway and adequate alveolar ventilation, (4) to optimize fluid administration and cardiac output, and (5) to control seizure activity and increased ICP.

A tight-fitting, non-rebreathing mask should be used to administer 100% oxygen. Independent of its effect on oxygen saturation, 100% oxygen will increase the amount of dissolved oxygen in blood, increasing oxygen content while CO remains bound to hemoglobin. Hyperbaric oxygen administration (i.e., 100% oxygen at a pressure of 2 to 3 atm) has been recommended as a way to increase the amount of dissolved oxygen to 3 to 4 vol%, a figure sufficiently high to meet the body's oxygen demands. Administering 100% oxygen also accelerates the dissociation of CO from hemoglobin, reducing its half-life from 5 to 6 hours in room air to 1 to 2 hours. The 100% oxygen must be continued until the patient's COHb level is <5%; thereafter, it may be decreased slowly while maintaining SaO_2 >90%.

The patient's airway must be secured if there is evidence of symptomatic upper airway obstruction as determined by physical examination, arterial blood gas tension analysis, or bronchoscopy; the use of nasotracheal intubation (using either flexible fiberoptic bronchoscopy or inhalation anesthesia) is preferable to tracheostomy if visualization of the larynx is not obscured by burns or debris. If the damage proximal to the larynx is severe, an emergency tracheostomy may be necessary. Indications for airway support are as follows:

1. Symptomatic upper airway obstruction
2. Hypoventilation or apnea
3. Severe pulmonary edema necessitating use of PEEP therapy
4. Altered mental status and loss of airway reflexes
5. Evidence of increased ICP
6. Full-thickness facial burns, including those of the nose and lips
7. Facial burns associated with circumferential full-thickness burns of the neck

The airway or endotracheal tube is suctioned as indicated at a minimum of every 3 hours, and chest percussion therapy is given every 3 to 4 hours. If the patient is not intubated and has stridor or a crouplike cough, racemic epinephrine (2.25%) may be administered through a nebulizer every 2 to 4 hours at a dose of 0.2 to 0.3 ml in 2 ml 0.9% sodium chloride solution. Humidified gases must always be delivered to the patient's airway or endotracheal tube. Bronchospasm is treated with IV theophylline and nebulized β-adrenergic bronchodilators (see Chapters 34 and 133).

Assisted ventilation for hypercapnia ($PaCO_2$ >55 mm Hg) is begun. PEEP must be started to treat patients with hypoxemia unresponsive to supplemental oxygen therapy (PaO_2 <50 mm Hg in FiO_2 > 0.5) and with roentgenographic evidence of diffuse lung injury (e.g., pulmonary edema). Positive pressure ventilation must be avoided, if possible, in a patient with bronchospasm and a chest roentgenogram with evidence of gas trapping (i.e., hyperinflation) (see Chapters 10 and 128).

IV fluids can be administered at maintenance rates using D_5 0.45% sodium chloride solutions. If the blood volume status or the hemodynamic stability of the patient is uncertain, fluid therapy can be guided by measurement of cardiac filling pressures and output (see Chapter 12).

Antibiotics must not be used routinely. Their need must be determined by cultures, Gram-stain analysis of the sputum, and chest roentgenographic findings. Corticosteroids are not recommended routinely.

ICP monitoring is indicated if there is clinical or CT scan evidence of increased ICP (see Chapter 7).

ADDITIONAL READING
Smoke Inhalation

Crapo R. Smoke inhalation injuries. JAMA 246:1694, 1981.

Herndon D. Treatment of burns. In Herndon D, et al. Current Problems in Surgery. Chicago: Year Book, 1987.

Herndon D, Langner F, Thompson P, et al. Pulmonary injury in burned patients. Surg Clin North Am 67:31, 1987.

Herndon D, Thompson PB, Traber DL. Pulmonary injury in burned patients. Crit Care Clin 1:79, 1985.

Madden M, Finkelstein J, Goodwin C. Respiratory care of the burn patient. Clin Plast Surg 24:29, 1986.

Mellins R, Park S. Respiratory complications of smoke inhalation in victims of fires. J Pediatr 87:1, 1975.

Robinson L, Miler R. Smoke inhalation injuries. Am J Otolaryngol 7:375, 1986.

Schwartz D. Acute inhalation injury. Occup Med State Art Rev 2:297, 1987.

Shu C-S. New concepts of pulmonary burn injury. J Trauma 21:958, 1981.

Venus B, Matsuda T, Copiozo JB, et al. Prophylactic intubation and continuous positive airway pressure in the management of inhalation injury in burn victims. Crit Care Med 9:519, 1981.

Wiseman D, Grossman R. Hyperbaric oxygen in the treatment of burns. Crit Care Clin 1:129, 1985.

Carbon Monoxide Poisoning

Kirkpatrick J. Occult carbon monoxide poisoning. West J Med 1:52, 1987.

Marzella L, Myers R. Carbon monoxide poisoning. Am Fam Physician 39:186, 1986.

McMeekin J, Finegan B. Reversible myocardial dysfunction following carbon monoxide poisoning. Can J Cardiol 3:118, 1987.

Myers R, Snyder S, Emhoff T. Subacute sequelae of carbon monoxide poisoning. Ann Emerg Med 14:163, 1985.

Myers R, Snyder S, Limberg S, et al. Value of hyperbaric oxygen in suspected carbon monoxide poisoning. JAMA 246:2478, 1981.

Parish R. Smoke inhalation and carbon monoxide poisoning in children. Pediatr Emerg Care 2:36, 1986.

Wald P, Balmes J. Respiratory effects of short-term, high intensity toxic inhalations: Smoke, gases and fumes. J Intensive Care Med 2:260, 1987.

92 Drowning and Near-Drowning

Daniel L. Levin

BACKGROUND AND PHYSIOLOGY

Several different terms used in this discussion of near-drowning and drowning need to be defined initially to avoid later confusion.

drowning Death from asphyxia while submerged or within 24 hours of submersion.

near-drowning An episode of sufficient severity to warrant medical attention for the victim and that may eventually lead to morbidity and mortality.

drowning without aspiration of water Death from respiratory obstruction and asphyxia while submerged in water or within 24 hours of submersion.

drowning with aspiration of water Death within 24 hours from changes secondary to aspiration of water while submerged.

near-drowning without aspiration Survival of a victim, at least temporarily, after suffering asphyxia from submersion in water.

near-drowning with aspiration Survival of a victim, at least temporarily, after submersion in and aspiration of water.

secondary drowning Death following submersion from complications (e.g., ARDS, pneumonia, neurogenic pulmonary edema) more than 24 hours after the drowning but directly attributable to submersion.

immersion syndrome Sudden death, probably vagally mediated, due to cardiac arrest following contact with cold water (coincident use of drugs such as alcohol and/or sedatives may contribute to pathogenesis of this syndrome).

submersion injury Any submersion resulting in hospital admission or death (e.g., near-drowning, drowning, spinal cord injury).

save Water rescue or removal of victim from water by someone who perceived individual to be a potential victim of submersion injury.

Incidence and Epidemiology

The incidence and epidemiology of near-drowning and drowning in children less than 19 years of age is not specifically a PICU subject, but since these events are largely preventable they are worthy of discussion. Approximately 6000 non-boat drownings, 1200 boat-related drownings, 500 motor vehicle–related (submerged) drownings, and 1000 drownings of undetermined intent or suicide occur annually in the United States. When one realizes that near-drownings are three to five times as frequent as drownings and, it is estimated, there are 10 times as many saves as drownings, it is easy to understand why near-drowning and drowning are problems of epidemic proportions. The United States Consumer Product Safety Commission (USCPSC) estimates that in 1985, 3000 children less than 5 years old were treated in hospital emergency departments because of submersion accidents in residential pools. Approximately 235 children less than 5 years of age drowned in swimming pools in 1983. The number of pool drownings is roughly the same as the number of poisoning deaths (245) recorded for the same age group in 1969 before the enactment of the poison prevention packaging act. Approximately 85% of the deaths are in males, with a maximum incidence in the 10- to 19-year-old age group (Fig. 92-1). In the adolescent age group drowning represents the third most common cause of death overall and is second only to motor vehicle injuries as a cause of accidental death. The bimodal nature of the curve in Fig. 92-1 represents the peak risks for 1- to 2-year-olds and again for older male teenagers, but the complete absence of a second peak in females suggests a sex-related etiology among male victims.

In the PICU at Children's Medical Center, Dallas, Texas, from July 1, 1975, through July 31, 1989, 216 victims less than 19 years of age were seen (Table 92-1). Of them, 179 (83%) were 5 years of age or younger (Fig. 92-2). Overall, 34% died, and 11% suffered severe neurologic residua, many of them eventually dying. This experience is similar to that reported in most major centers in the United States, Canada, England, Australia, and New Zealand.

The USCPSC undertook a prospective analysis of near-drowning and drowning events in eight counties (5 in southern and northern California, 1 in Arizona, 2 in Florida) between May 1 and September 30, 1986. There were 142 near-drownings and drownings in children less than 5 years of age during this 5-month study, making it easy to accept that drowning is the number one leading cause of accidental death in children less than 5 years of age in California, Arizona, and Florida, the second leading cause in Texas, and the third overall in the United States. The incidents in young children mostly occur in private swimming pools (Table 92-2), regardless of geographical location. The leading identified cause for this astounding rate of accidents is the lack of an adequate barrier for small children between their own homes or yards and the pool. These children are not intruders; they are drowned in their own pools or in the pools of friends or relatives in whose homes they are invited guests. The accidents occur more frequently in warm weather but occur any month of the year (Fig. 92-3). There is a predominance of males over females even in younger victims, and females are almost missing from the later peak period because the later peak is related to water sports, boating, the daredevil syndrome, voluntary hyperventilation, and, most especially, alcohol. For victims brought to the hospital there is a high morbidity/mortality ratio compared to other forms of accidental injury requiring medical attention.

Pathophysiology

The drowning episode

Several pathogenic mechanisms of death can occur while a drowning victim is submerged. Brain death, the common final pathway, may be caused by cerebral hypoxia, carbon dioxide narcosis, laryngospasm, pulmonary reflexes, or vagally mediated cardiac arrest. Whereas drowning is technically death due to submersion in water and aspiration of water, the lat-

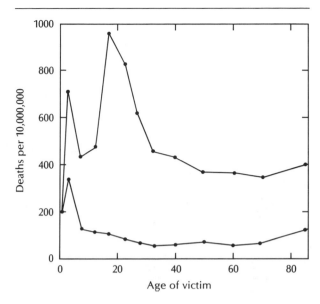

Fig. 92-1 Drowning rate in the United States, 1977-1979, for males (top line) and females (bottom line). (From Spyker DA. Submersion injury. Pediatr Clin North Am 32:113-125, 1985.)

Table 92-1 Near-Drowning Patients in Children's Medical Center PICU

Year	Near-Drownings	Expired	Severe Brain Damage
7/1/75-12/31/75	3	1	—
1976	8	4	—
1977	4	3	—
1978	11	4	—
1979	4	2	—
1980	11	4	1
1981	12	4	1
1982	14	4	1
1983	21	8	3
1984	20	6	3
1985	23	7	3
1986	26	7	6
1987	23	8	4
1988	25	9	2
1/1/89-7/31/89	11	3	—
	216	74 (34%)	24 (11%)

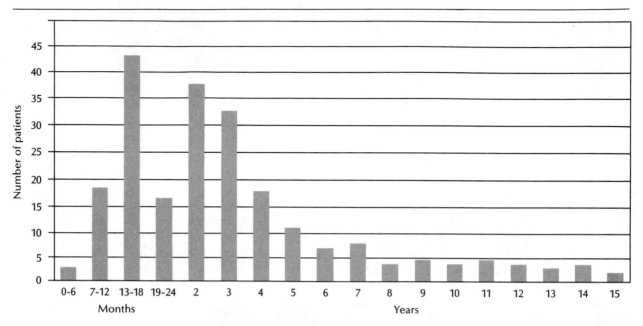

Fig. 92-2 Age of near-drowning victims, Children's Medical Center, Dallas, Texas (January 1, 1976–July 31, 1989).

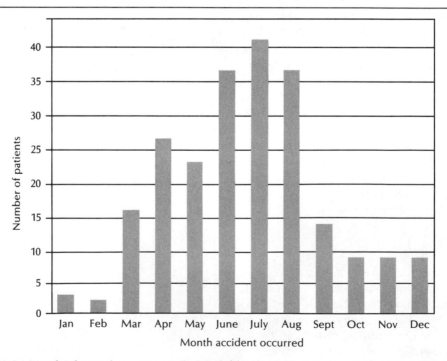

Fig. 92-3 Month of near-drowning accidents, Children's Medical Center, Dallas, Texas (1975-1989).

Table 92-2 Location of Near-Drowning
Accidents, July 1, 1975, to July 31, 1989,
Children's Medical Center PICU

Location	No. of Patients (%)
Pool	149 (69.7)
Lake	20 (9.3)
Bathtub	17 (7.9)
Bucket	5 (2.3)
Hot tub	9 (4.2)
Toilet	2 (0.9)
Miscellaneous	13 (6.0)
	216

ter three causes of death are due to submersion alone
without aspiration of water.

The volume of water aspirated or swallowed may
be large or small, and the depth of water may be
shallow. Laryngospasm may occur, and hypoxia may
follow without the active aspiration of water in as
many as 10% of victims. This is probably caused by
a small amount of water entering the larynx or trachea and eliciting a reflex causing spasm.

When a sober victim is first submerged, a period
of initial voluntary apnea occurs. There may not be
a struggle, but swimming movements occur. Younger
victims may simply sink to the bottom. In the younger
age group (less than 5 years) the diving reflex may
be stimulated and make a significant difference in
survival. Within seconds of the face's touching cold
water and before consciousness is lost, a reflex mediated by the trigeminal nerve sends sensory afferent
impulses to the CNS medullary respiratory center,
which causes bradycardia and shunting of blood from
cutaneous and splachnic vascular beds to the cerebral
and coronary circulations (i.e., the diving reflex). Systemic arterial blood pressure increases as well. These
reflex changes are independent of peripheral chemoreceptors and baroreceptors and are augmented
by progressively colder water temperatures and the
startle response. Infants who are taught to swim at a
very young age ("waterproofing") and who are not
afraid of the water may lack a startle response and
may be at greater risk for near-drowning. The victim
can hold his breath voluntarily until the break point
is reached, as determined by the oxygen and carbon

dioxide levels (peripheral and central chemoreceptors, respectively). The break point is when the individual will take an involuntary breath and occurs
at $PaCO_2$ levels of 51 mm Hg and PaO_2 of 73 mm Hg
after 87 seconds at rest in normal human volunteers.

After voluntary hyperventilation the break point
can be prolonged to 140 seconds ($PaCO_2$, 46 mm Hg,
and PaO_2, 58 mm Hg) at rest and 85 seconds ($PaCO_2$,
49 mm Hg, and PaO_2, 43 mm Hg) with exercise. The
break point may not occur while the victim is conscious if he has voluntarily hyperventilated to low
$PaCO_2$ values before submersion and hyperventilation
is followed by exercise (underwater swimming).
Hypoxia may cause loss of consciousness before activation of carbon dioxide receptors causes voluntary
breathing movements.

Within seconds of the first submerged breaths secondary apnea occurs and, if followed by involuntary
gasping under the water lasting for several minutes,
respiratory arrest follows. Dysrhythmias occur due
to hypoxia, and eventually cardiac arrest and brain
death occur. Once aspiration of fluid takes place,
metabolic acidosis and systemic arterial hypertension
persist even if the victim is saved or pulled from the
water.

How long hypoxia can be tolerated by an individual victim is a frequently asked question. It depends
on many factors, including the age of the victim, previous health, water temperature, and promptness and
effectiveness of the rescue effort. Young victims will
probably survive if submersion is <3 minutes and
up to 10 minutes in water 10° to 15° C. Survival after
longer submersions (15 to 20 minutes) is occasionally seen, and even longer times of up to 40 minutes
rarely are compatible with eventual recovery from
near-drowning in very cold water (0° to 15° C). Although the effect of surface cooling in young children
(large body surface area/mass ratio) and core cooling
due to aspiration and swallowing of very cold water
may play some role in patient survival after prolonged submersion by decreasing cerebral metabolic
rate, an active diving reflex with bradycardia and
shunting of the circulation to the cerebral and coronary circulations may be the most significant factor
in survival rather than a decrease in cerebral metabolic rate. In older victims very cold water may inhibit
effective swimming movements in even accomplished swimmers and induce vagally mediated cardiac dysrhythmias and coma in individuals with a
body temperature <34° C.

Aspirated fluid

Victims may aspirate fresh water or salt water and foreign matter either from the water itself or as stomach contents. Although the salinity of sea water varies, it usually has 34.48 g/kg (3.5%) of dissolved salts, of which 29.54 g/kg (2.9%) is sodium chloride. The Dead Sea in Israel is, for example, much different in both the quantity and nature of its salts. Fresh water also contains some salts and organic material. The contents of spas, bathtubs, cleaning pails, toilets, lakes, rivers, ponds, and stagnant water must be analyzed to know what the victim has aspirated.

After the victim inhales sea water, the hypertonic fluid pulls water from the circulation into the lungs,

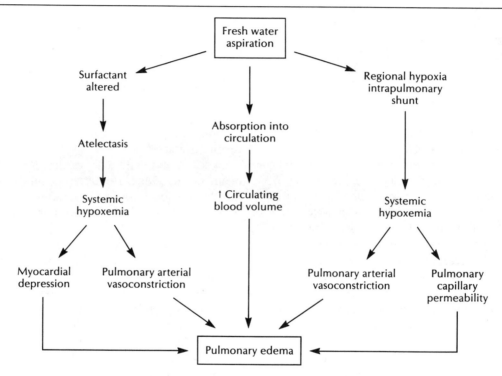

Fig. 92-4 Pathophysiology of pulmonary edema formation in near-drowning victims.

Table 92-3 Usual Laboratory Values After Near-Drowning*

	Sea Water		Fresh Water	
	Range	**Mean**	**Range**	**Mean**
Sodium	132-160	147 mEq/L	126-146	137 mEq/L
Potassium	3.2-5.4	4 mEq/L	2.4-6.3	4 mEq/L
Chlorine	96-127	106 mEq/L	88-116	98 mEq/L
Hemoglobin		14.8 g/dl		14.2 g/dl
Hematocrit		43%		44%

*Modified from Modell JH. Drowning. In Staub NC, Taylor AE, eds. Edema. New York: Raven, 1984, pp 679-693.

resulting in fluid-filled but perfused alveoli (pulmonary edema). Pulmonary surfactant is washed out. The victim becomes hypovolemic with greater amounts of sea water inhalation (>11 ml/kg), and blood volume can decrease to as little as 65% of the normal.

Aspiration of fresh water can cause an increase in blood volume because the hypotonic fluid is absorbed into the circulation when large amounts of fluid are aspirated. Surfactant is altered in a combination of regional hypoxia and intrapulmonary shunt, leading to systemic hypoxemia that causes reflex pulmonary arterial vasoconstriction, myocardial depression, and an alteration of pulmonary capillary permeability, all eventually leading to return of fluid to the lung and sudden pulmonary edema (Fig. 92-4).

Victims seen alive in hospitals rarely have aspirated enough fluid to cause life-threatening changes in blood volume, although pulmonary edema is common. For the same reason hospitalized victims of either sea water or fresh water accidents rarely have electrolyte disturbances (Table 92-3). Victims of sea water near-drowning would be expected to be hemoconcentrated and victims of fresh water near-drowning to be hemodiluted, but they are not. Fresh water near-drowning victims should have hemolysis with hyperkalemia and plasma free hemoglobin, although hyperkalemia is rare. An increased level of endogenous catecholamines even causes kaluresis, and serum potassium levels are usually decreased. Plasma free hemoglobin levels are usually <500 mg/dl and are not thought to cause renal dysfunction from plugging of tubules.

Pulmonary pathophysiology

The pulmonary pathologic events include:
Increased peripheral airway resistance
Variable degrees of laryngospasm
Reflex pulmonary vessel vasoconstriction, leading to pulmonary hypertension
Decreased lung compliance
Fall in ventilation-perfusion ratios
Fluid shifts across the alveolar membrane
Surfactant loss (salt water) or alteration in its properties (fresh water)
Foam and froth production
Anatomic changes in alveolar epithelial cells
When fluid is aspirated, a reflex via vagal efferents causes obstruction of the peripheral airways. The reflex is predominantly mediated through osmolality rather than volume of fluid; therefore its occurrence is more prominent with fresh water inhalation. Very small volumes of fresh water (1 ml/kg) can cause pulmonary vasoconstriction and result in pulmonary hypertension. Larger volumes of fluid (2.5 ml/kg) lead to vascular perfusion of nonventilated alveoli, and combined with loss or inactivation of surfactant, alveolar collapse and pulmonary hypertension result in decreased lung compliance. Within minutes of aspiration of small amounts of fresh water, an intrapulmonary shunt due to perfusion of nonventilated areas can increase from the normal of 5% to 18% to as much as 75%. Even though young victims may appear normal clinically within minutes or hours of the event, it may take days for the intrapulmonary shunt to return to pre-event levels.

As mentioned previously, fresh water moves across the endothelial and capillary membranes into the circulation, and plasma moves in the opposite direction, drawn by the hyperosmolality of sea water in alveoli. Surfactant is washed out by sea water and altered by fresh water. The airways may become obstructed by laryngospasm, bronchoconstriction, foam, mucus, inhaled foreign material, and stomach contents.

Neurologic pathophysiology

Metabolic acidosis and hypoxemia rapidly alter the blood-brain barrier, and even if the patient is saved at this point, cerebral edema occurs. Edema causes hemispheric swelling and shifts of brain across compartments (herniation). The edema probably does not cause brain cell injury but is an indication of the extent of the original and any subsequent hypoxic episodes. If the hypoxia is severe enough, brain death occurs.

Neurologic residua include prolonged unconsciousness with subsequent recovery (rare, but more likely when event occurred in very cold water), blindness, EEG changes, dilation of ventricles due to brain atrophy, and persistent coma, leading to death (more usual in patients with prolonged coma). I have treated two patients who developed cortical blindness after near-drowning but eventually recovered their vision.

Cardiovascular pathophysiology

The cardiovascular system in children is remarkably stable. Most victims have healthy hearts that can be resuscitated after prolonged periods of ischemia.

ECG changes, primarily bradycardia or asystole, can occur. Some victims may have ventricular fibrillation and need cardioversion during resuscitation. Systemic arterial blood pressure may be normal, high, or low, depending on oxygenation, acid-base balance, cardiac function, peripheral vascular resistance, the level of circulating endogenous and exogenous catecholamines, and elevated ICP.

Renal pathophysiology

Renal function is usually normal, but albuminuria, hemoglobinuria, oliguria, and anuria can occur. The dysfunction is probably due to ischemia rather than tubular damage from free hemoglobin.

Predictability of Outcome

When the victim is first seen, predicting the outcome is extremely difficult. No one finding (pulselessness, apnea, fixed and dilated pupils, duration of event, water temperature) reliably predicts outcome; therefore all victims who are submerged for an unknown length of time, except those with putrification, should receive CPR. When admitted to the emergency department, although certainty of outcome is still difficult to predict, those victims who are pulseless, apneic, and/or flaccid and comatose have a high likelihood of dying or surviving with extreme neurologic residua. Patients admitted to the PICU with apnea and signs of increased ICP have a high likelihood of death or survival with severe neurologic residua. Patients who are awake or have blunted awareness or responsiveness but who are not comatose have an excellent chance of survival with full recovery.

MONITORING AND LABORATORY TESTS

See also Chapter 4. Monitoring of the victim at the accident site includes checking for the presence of pulse, respirations, purposeful movement, and color. In the ambulance or emergency department, heart rate, ECG, respiratory rate, systemic arterial blood pressure, temperature, Glasgow Coma Scale score, serum electrolyte values, serum glucose and hematocrit values, and urinalysis must be checked. A chest roentgenogram must be taken, and for those with CNS or respiratory signs, arterial blood gas and pH values must be determined. The possibility of concomitant injuries, especially to the head and neck, must be considered.

In the PICU mild to moderately involved patients must be observed for signs of respiratory distress from aspiration of water and/or stomach contents and for signs of neurologic complications such as head trauma, seizures, or increased ICP. Severely involved victims will almost certainly need intubation and assisted ventilation. In addition they will need placement of a CVP catheter, arterial catheter, bladder catheter, nasogastric tube, and rarely a pulmonary artery catheter for treatment of severe persistent pulmonary edema and/or decreased cardiac output.

The need for ICP monitoring is quite controversial. Some authors believe that although ICP can be monitored and even treated, monitoring and treatment do not alter outcome and that all victims with elevated ICP have a poor outcome wth either death or severe neurologic residua. Others have noted that some victims with no measured increase in ICP also have a poor outcome and therefore ICP monitoring need not be done in any victims. Others believe that elevated ICP in combination with calculated cerebral perfusion pressure (CPP) is highly predictive of a poor outcome and that it should be monitored for that reason. Still other authors argue that even though those patients with an elevated ICP have a uniformly poor outcome, since the treatment of increased ICP necessitates interventions that may be harmful, especially for the brain, these interventions should not be used in the absence of a documented increase in ICP. Thus, according to this position, all patients who are severely involved must have ICP monitored. However, since none of these statements is based on a prospective, randomized clinical trial, I believe the subject is unresolved and still awaits such a study.

TREATMENT
In the Field

CPR must be given as quickly as possible. The one most devastating aspect of the drowning episode is hypoxemia, and mouth-to-mouth or mouth-to-nose ventilation must be given promptly, even in the water if necessary. All parents, child care personnel, and pool owners or supervisors should be certified in CPR. Supplemental oxygen must be given to all victims as soon as possible until it is proved that they no longer need it. Rescuers need to be cognizant of possible head and neck injuries and of the necessity for preventing aspiration of stomach contents. Once trained personnel arrive, bag and mask ventilation with proper positioning of the jaw and tongue, use of supplemental oxygen, and on occasion tracheal intubation may be needed. Inserting an IV catheter may be necessary for administration of fluids and medications (e.g., sodium bicarbonate, epinephrine) at the site, although epinephrine may be given intratracheally if the patient is intubated. Intraosseous infusion of fluids and medications is another route to consider. Rarely, cardioversion for defibrillation will be needed in the field.

In the Emergency Department

All patients must be given oxygen until it is proven they no longer need it by chest roentgenogram, arterial blood gas and pH determinations, and/or noninvasive pulse oximetry. All patients must have their stomach contents removed, particularly if they are not completely awake or lack intact protective airway reflexes. Because victims can swallow large amounts of fluid, they may vomit and aspirate the stomach contents even when they are neurologically intact; prolonged hospitalization for ventilatory care or even death can result from such an episode. All victims need to have their head and neck assessed for concomitant trauma. Severely affected patients may continue to need advanced cardiac life support, intubation and ventilatory assistance, and cardiac support with inotropic and vasoactive agents.

In the PICU
Pulmonary management

Pulmonary management is a primary factor early in the course of treatment. As mentioned previously, oxygen must be supplied at a rate sufficient to maintain SaO_2 ≥90% even to awake patients until it is proved they no longer need it. For severely involved patients PEEP is helpful in increasing lung volumes, decreasing oxygen requirements, and improving systemic oxygenation. Assisted mechanical ventilation will be necessary in patients with severe pulmonary edema and evidence of acute respiratory failure (see Chapter 10) and/or aspiration pneumonia and for patients with a pronounced CNS injury (e.g., Glasgow Coma Scale score <8) with seizures or neurologic depression.

Prophylactic use of broad-spectrum antibiotics for pneumonia is not indicated, although the high likelihood of aspiration of *Pseudomonas* in hot tub and spa victims makes use of antipseudomonal agents in these patients seem rational. Prophylactic use of corticosteroids for treatment of pulmonary complications has no support whatsoever according to properly performed studies.

Ongoing management of the pulmonary complications will depend on the patient's condition. In a few patients the pulmonary disease secondary to aspiration is a major problem, but in most children the lungs improve rapidly, and neurologic complications are the main problem.

Neurologic management

Neurologic complications can be devastating, with approximately 35% to 40% of young victims in most large pediatric centers dying with brain death and 10% surviving with severe neurologic residua. As indicated previously, monitoring and management of ICP is a major and controversial subject, specifically since no prospective randomly controlled studies exist about its efficacy. If one should choose to measure ICP and calculate CPP, progressive use of measures, including positioning, hyperventilation with mechanical ventilation, and osmotic and loop diuretics, is indicated to maintain an ICP <20 mm Hg and CPP >50 mm Hg (see Chapter 7). There is no evidence that barbiturate coma or steroids for treating a patient with an elevated ICP is of any benefit for improving outcome. Short-acting barbiturates interfere with white blood cell function and increase the risk of infection. Induced hypothermia not only lacks evidence for benefit in these patients, but its use may actually be harmful because it increases the risk for infection as a result of an alteration in white blood cell function. Seizures must be treated in a routine fashion (see Chapter 9). Hypovolemia can be corrected if the usual colloid/crystalloid considerations are kept in mind (see Chapter 12). Electrolyte abnormalities and renal failure rarely are specific problems.

Determination of brain death in these patients, as in most, may be difficult (see Chapter 24), but since they represent a growing and important source for human organ donation and transplantation, a specific and rigorous protocol for brain death must be available and followed from early in the course of treatment.

• • •

Prevention is more desirable than therapy, and this is particularly true in near-drowning and drowning in young children. Use of effective barriers with self-closing, self-latching doors and gates for residents, invited guests, and intruders will prevent 70% to 80% of these incidents in children under 5 years of age.

ADDITIONAL READING

Bohn DJ, Biggar WD, Smith CR, et al. Influence of hypothermia, barbiturate therapy, and intracranial pressure monitoring on morbidity and mortality after near-drowning. Crit Care Med 14:529-533, 1986.

Dean JM, McComb JG. Intracranial pressure monitoring in severe pediatric near-drowning. Neurosurgery 9:627-630, 1981.

Effmann EL, Merten DF, Kirks DR, et al. Adult respiratory distress syndrome in children. Radiology 157:69-74, 1985.

Fergusson DM, Horwood LJ. Risks of drowning in fenced and unfenced domestic swimming pools. N Z Med J 97:777-779, 1984.

Jacobsen JB, Nielsen H, Andersen PK. Resuscitation from drowning in cold water. N Engl J Med 305:580-581, 1981.

Jacobsen WK, Mason LJ, Briggs BA, et al. Correlation of spontaneous respiration and neurologic damage in near-drowning. Crit Care Med 11:487-489, 1983.

Levin DL. Near-drowning. Crit Care Med 8:590-595, 1980.

Lucking SE, Pollack MM, Fields AI. Shock following generalized hypoxic-ischemic injury in previously healthy infants and children. J Pediatr 108:359-364, 1986.

Modell JH. Treatment of near-drowning: Is there a role for H.Y.P.E.R. therapy? Crit Care Med 14:593-594, 1986.

• Modell JH. Drowning. In Staub NC, Taylor AE, eds. Edema. New York: Raven, 1984, pp 679-693.

Nussbaum E, Galant SP. Intracranial pressure monitoring as a guide to prognosis in the nearly drowned, severely comatose child. J Pediatr 102:215-218, 1983.

O'Rourke PP. Outcome of children who are apneic and pulseless in the emergency room. Crit Care Med 14:466-468, 1986.

Pearn JH. Current controversies in child accident prevention. An analysis of some areas of dispute in the prevention of child trauma. Aust N Z J Med 15:782-787, 1985.

Pearn JH. Pathophysiology of drowning. Med J Aust 142:586-588, 1985.

Pitt WR. Increasing incidence of childhood immersion injury in Brisbane. Med J Aust 144:683-685, 1986.

Rogers MC. Near-drowning: Cold water on a hot topic? J Pediatr 106:603-604, 1985.

Sarnaik AP, Preston G, Lieh-Lai M, et al. Intracranial pressure and cerebral perfusion pressure in near-drowning. Crit Care Med 13:224-227, 1985.

• Spyker DA. Submersion injury epidemiology, prevention, and management. Pediatr Clin North Am 32:113-125, 1985.

Taylor MJ, Houston BD, Lowry NJ. Recovery of auditory brain-stem responses after a severe hypoxic ischemic insult. Med Intelligence 309:1169-1170, 1983.

93 Aspiration Pneumonia

Paul Lubinsky · Nick G. Anas

BACKGROUND AND PHYSIOLOGY

Aspiration pneumonia is the entrance of either gastric or oropharyngeal contents into the tracheobronchial tree and is a common occurrence in PICU patients. Seventy percent of individuals with a depressed level of consciousness and 45% of normal individuals in deep sleep states have been shown to have evidence of aspiration pneumonia. In addition aspiration of gastric contents occurs in as many as 10% to 20% of patients during induction of anesthesia, the incidence being greatest with emergency induction. Aspiration episodes also occur frequently in association with head trauma, status epilepticus, and cardiopulmonary resuscitation. Aspiration pneumonia is frequently misdiagnosed and must be considered in the differential diagnosis of sudden, recurrent, or persistent pulmonary signs and symptoms. The conditions that predispose to aspiration pneumonia are presented on p. 694.

The initial phase of swallowing is voluntary and involves the movement of food from the mouth to the pharynx by the tongue. Once food is in the pharynx, the process is involuntary, and the individual protects himself from aspiration into the tracheobronchial tree by the following mechanisms: the soft palate guards the nares; the palatopharyngeal folds form a slit, retarding the passage of large food particles; the epiglottis covers the vocal cords, which close tightly; and the larynx moves upward and forward, pulling the esophagus open. Food enters the esophagus, and peristaltic waves move it to the stomach, where it is stored, mixed, and then propelled into the small intestine. The gastroesophageal sphincter prevents reflux of gastric contents into the esophagus. The integrity of this sphincter depends on (1) a mucosal valve formed by folds of gastric mucosa, (2) the gastroesophageal angle, and (3) the difference between thoracic and abdominal pressure (see Chapter 72).

The conditions predisposing to aspiration pneumonia result from alterations either in the integrity of the upper GI tract or airway or in the function of the swallowing mechanisms. Compromise of the esophageal sphincter may occur as the result of a number of factors. In the PICU the presence of a nasogastric tube represents a common situation in which the function of the esophageal sphincter is compromised. Alterations in thoracic or abdominal pressure (i.e., more negative pleural pressure or more positive abdominal pressure) favor the reflux of gastric food and juices. Children with upper airway obstruction generate large negative pressure swings within the thorax, making them vulnerable to aspiration episodes; this condition is particularly common in premature infants, in children with acute or chronic encephalopathies, and in children with enlarged tonsils and adenoids. Delayed gastric emptying occurs in association with stress or pain, secondary to hypoxic and ischemic insults, and after the administration of narcotic or anesthetic agents; delayed emptying increases the time during which the reflux of gastric contents can result in aspiration pneumonia. Increased gastric pressure (often in conjunction with delayed gastric emptying) may result from recent oral intake, intestinal obstruction, the presence of an abdominal mass or free fluid, or air forced into the stomach with mouth-to-mouth or bag-valve-mask ventilation. Also, lower esophageal sphincter pressure is decreased by certain drugs (e.g., morphine sulfate, diazepam, atropine) and an alkaline gastric pH. The emergency induction of anesthesia represents a situation in which the child is particularly vulnerable to an aspiration episode since the stomach may be full and emptying slowly; gas-

---

CONDITIONS PREDISPOSING TO ASPIRATION PNEUMONIA

Compromise of lower esophageal sphincter

Gastroesophageal reflux (i.e., incompetent sphincter)
Presence of nasogastric tube
Gastrostomy
Hiatal hernia
Tracheoesophageal fistula
Use of cardiopulmonary resuscitation (CPR)
Upper airway obstruction
Negative pressure ventilation
Muscular dystrophies
Scleroderma

Delayed gastric emptying

Anxiety or pain
Ileus or mechanical intestinal obstruction
Peptic or stress ulcers
Hypoxia or shock states
Use of narcotics or anesthetic agents

Increased gastric or abdominal pressure

Intestinal obstruction
Abdominal masses or fluid
Recent oral intake
Pregnancy or obesity
Depolarizing neuromuscular blockade (e.g., succinyl-
    choline)

Inability to protect upper airway

Hypoxic-ischemic encephalopathy (acute and
    chronic)
Severe head injury
Encephalitis or meningitis
Status epilepticus
Use of narcotic or anesthetic agents
Excessive alcohol intake
Suck-swallow incoordination
Rapid eye movement (REM) sleep

Anatomic or local factors

Vocal cord paralysis
Epiglottitis
Tracheal intubation
Tracheostomy
Decreased laryngeal sensation (e.g., after extubation
    or administration of topical anesthetics)
Tracheoesophageal fistula
Esophageal diverticulum
Pooling of pharyngeal secretions (e.g., with sinusitis,
    nasal hemorrhage, absent swallow reflex)
Nasogastric feeding (either continuous or by bolus)

---

troesophageal reflux may be promoted further by the use of depolarizing neuromuscular blockade (e.g., succinylcholine), during which gastric pressure increases with the onset of muscle fasciculations.

In addition to esophageal and gastric dysfunction a common problem in PICU patients is the inability to protect the upper airway. Children with acute and chronic encephalopathies (e.g., after head trauma, near-drowning, encephalitis, meningitis) often lose their cough and gag reflexes, which, in conjunction with the structural protection described previously, are responsible for preventing the aspiration of pharyngeal contents into the tracheobronchial tree. The loss of pharyngeal muscle tone also places the patient at greater risk for aspiration; pharyngeal hypotonia occurs during status epilepticus, after the administration of narcotic and anesthetic agents, and during rapid eye movement or deep sleep states.

Upper airway protection also is impaired by an endotracheal tube or decreased laryngeal sensation (e.g., after extubation of the trachea or the administration of topical anesthetics for bronchoscopy). The structure and function of the upper airway is altered in the presence of infectious processes (e.g., epiglottitis) or after trauma (e.g., vocal cord injury).

The clinical presentation of the child with aspiration pneumonia depends on the following factors: the volume of aspirated material, the type of aspirated material (e.g., particulate vs. nonparticulate, viscous vs. nonviscous), the pH of the stomach contents, the presence of bacteria in the aspirated material, and the state of host defense. The initial physiologic response to the entrance of foreign material into the tracheobronchial tree is designed to protect against further aspiration; cough and bronchospasm are the most common signs that aspiration has occurred. A volume of aspirated material >0.3 to 0.4 ml/kg appears to be sufficient to impair gas exchange by inducing either atelectasis or pneumonia. Hypoxemia (i.e., arterial oxygen tension [PaO_2] <70 mm Hg) is indicative of physiologically significant ventilation-perfusion imbalance.

The physiologic effect of particles within the aspirated material depends on their size. Large particles will obstruct either the trachea or mainstem and segmental bronchi and thus will impair alveolar ventilation most acutely and dramatically; small particles tend to distribute in more distal airways, resulting in either atelectasis or gas trapping. These disturbances lead to hypoxemia as the result of reduced ventilation relative to pulmonary perfusion. As a rule, particulate matter tends to cause greater destruction within the tracheobronchial tree and more extensive gas-exchange impairment than does nonparticulate or liquid material.

If the aspirated material has a pH <2.5, damage to the bronchial mucosa occurs, resulting in sloughing and bronchiolar obstruction with gas trapping. Wheezing is the predominant physical finding on chest auscultation, and alveolar ventilation is impaired because of the prolonged time needed for emptying of lung units. Airways resistance increases, and pulmonary compliance is reduced.

The less viscous the aspirated material (e.g., products containing hydrocarbons such as gasoline or kerosene), the more widespread is the destruction in the distal tracheobronchial tree. Disruption of alveolar-capillary membranes results in permeability pulmonary edema (i.e., ARDS); gas-exchange impairment in this disorder results from the development of both intrapulmonary shunting and dead space ventilation (see Chapter 35). If the inhaled material reaches the alveolar space, destruction of type II pneumocytes can occur, thereby interfering with surfactant production and resulting in atelectasis and reduced pulmonary compliance.

The spectrum of clinical problems after an aspiration episode is broadened by the possibility of aspirating infectious material. The mouth and oropharynx are colonized by many organisms; oropharyngeal secretions contain approximately 10^7 aerobic and 10^8 anaerobic organisms/ml. The distal airways and lung parenchyma are sterile under normal conditions. The risk of aspirating infected material is increased in patients with poor oral hygiene, with posterior nasal drainage due to sinusitis, and with

intestinal obstruction since the bacterial load of the gastric contents will be higher than under normal circumstances. The majority of community-acquired infections are due to anaerobic organisms: *Fusobacterium, Peptostreptococcus,* and *Bacteroides.* Hospitalized patients harbor additional organisms in the pharynx or stomach, including *Staphylococcus aureus, Escherichia coli, Streptococcus pneumoniae,* enterococcus, *Klebsiella pneumoniae, Serratia marcescens, Pseudomonas aeruginosa,* and *Citrobacter* species.

The sites within the lung most involved during an aspiration episode are the dependent areas, which are the bases in a standing person and the apices in a supine patient. However, hyperinflation may be widespread when bronchospasm occurs in reaction to the aspiration of foreign material. Additionally, ARDS can result in generalized pulmonary edema (see Chapter 35).

MONITORING AND LABORATORY TESTS

The goals of monitoring the patient with aspiration pneumonia are (1) to determine the extent of pulmonary involvement and gas-exchange impairment, (2) to ascertain the cause of the aspiration event, and (3) to identify other major organ system involvement (e.g., CNS or cardiovascular system).

The high-risk patient must be identified. Continuous respiratory and cardiac (ECG) monitoring as well as pulse oximetry, if available, is to be started.

Continuous assessment of the patient's respiratory status is necessary. Important physical signs include the presence of a cough, respiratory rate and effort, color, the presence of crackles or wheezing, and the adequacy of air movement by chest auscultation. The patient is observed for evidence of upper airway obstruction (i.e., stridor, noisy breathing, absent air entry during inspiration as judged by chest auscultation). Preferably the same person performs serial examinations of the patient during the course of the disease. Arterial blood gas tensions and pH are obtained to evaluate the adequacy of alveolar ventilation and systemic oxygenation.

The patient's neurologic status is assessed, particularly to determine level of consciousness and the presence of cough and gag reflexes.

Obtaining a chest roentgenogram will confirm the diagnosis of aspiration pneumonia and assess the degree of pulmonary involvement. The presence of parenchymal infiltrates, hyperinflation, pulmonary edema, or pneumothorax must be determined, as must the position of an endotracheal or nasogastric tube if present. An abdominal roentgenogram or ultrasound examination is indicated if there is physical evidence of gastric dilatation, intestinal obstruction, an abdominal mass, or ascites.

Tracheal specimens for Gram stain analysis and culture are needed from intubated patients. Tracheal and gastric aspirates must be analyzed for acid concentration (i.e., pH). Blood cultures must be obtained from a febrile patient (i.e., temperature >38.4° C).

Central venous or pulmonary artery blood pressure monitoring should be started in a patient with clinical and roentgenographic evidence of ARDS (see Chapter 35) or in a hemodynamically unstable patient.

Use of a barium contrast study of the upper GI tract may be considered for a patient suspected of having gastroesophageal reflux or anatomic abnormalities such as an esophageal diverticulum or hiatal hernia (see Chapter 72). When methylene blue dye is mixed in the formula or food of a patient suspected of aspiration pneumonia, the presence of the dye in tracheal secretions is diagnostic of aspiration events. Endoscopy of the esophagus and stomach may be used in patients suspected of having gastroesophageal reflux, ulcer disease, or anatomic abnormalities and bronchoscopy in patients suspected of inhaling particulate matter or of having anatomic abnormalities such as vocal cord paralysis or a tracheoesophageal fistula.

TREATMENT

The goals of treatment in patients with (or at risk for) aspiration pneumonia are (1) to prevent or reduce aspiration events by identification of high-risk pa-

---

TREATMENT OF ASPIRATION PNEUMONIA

Prevention

Identify the high-risk patient (see p. 694).

Place patients with emesis or impaired consciousness on right side with head down and suction oropharynx.

Elevate head of bed for patients with gastroesophageal reflux.

Administer metoclopromide, 0.1 mg/kg qid, to patients with gastroesophageal reflux.

Avoid administering a sedative or narcotics to patients with impaired airway reflexes.

Use small-bore nasointestinal tubes for tube feedings.

Intubate the trachea or perform tracheotomy in patients with loss of protective airway reflexes.

Acute aspiration episode

Suction the oropharynx.

Empty stomach and insert nasogastric tube.

Administer oxygen.

Administer D_5 0.25% sodium chloride solution at maintenance rate.

Administer aerosolized isoproterenol at 0.01 ml/kg in 2 ml 0.9% sodium chloride solution if patient is wheezing.

Administer aminophylline infusion if patient's response to aerosolized isoproterenol is inadequate.

Obtain a chest roentgenogram.

Determine arterial blood gas values and pH.

Provide intubation and suctioning to protect the patient's airway and/or provide assisted ventilation as necessary.

Preoperative treatment

Avoid enteral feeds 6 hours before surgery.

Administer ranitidine (1.5 mg/kg IVP q 6 hr) and/or Bicitra (0.5 ml/kg PO q 4 hr).

Suction the oropharynx and empty his stomach before induction of anesthesia or intubation.

Use Sellick's maneuver during intubation procedure.

Perform rigid bronchoscopy if particulate matter is present.

Antibiotics are not routinely indicated.

Steroids are not indicated.

Evaluate the patient for predisposing conditions; correct them when possible.

qid = four times a day; IVP = intravenous push; PO = by mouth.

tients and conditions, (2) to assure adequate alveolar ventilation and systemic oxygenation, and (3) to treat dysfunction in other major organ systems (e.g., CNS, cardiovascular system).

Placing the patient at high risk for an aspiration episode can be avoided by instituting the following policies:

1. Suction the oropharynx and empty the stomach before the induction of anesthesia and endotracheal intubation.
2. Intubate the trachea or perform tracheostomy in patients with lost airway reflexes (i.e., cough, gag, swallowing) and in those with upper airway obstruction that persists despite the use of conservative measures such as repositioning of the head and placement of an oropharyngeal airway.
3. Perform endotracheal intubation in high-risk patients using rapid-sequence induction (e.g., administering, in sequence, atropine at 0.02 mg/kg, thiopental sodium at 3 to 4 mg/kg, and succinylcholine at 1 mg/kg). Perform the Sellick maneuver (i.e., cricoid compression and esophageal obstruction) during the intubation procedure to minimize the possibility of reflux of gastric contents into the pharynx (especially when administering succinylcholine for neuromuscular blockade).
4. Increase gastric pH in high-risk patients by administering either histamine H_2-receptor antagonists (e.g., IV ranitidine at 1.5 mg/kg every 6 hours) and/or an actacid (e.g., Bicitra at 0.5 ml/kg every 4 hours). Avoid the use of particulate antacids in the high-risk situation.
5. Administer metoclopromide at 0.1 mg/kg to stimulate gastric emptying and to increase lower esophageal pressure in patients with evidence of gastroesophageal reflux.
6. Place the patient who is vomiting on his right side, with the head down to minimize the likelihood of an aspiration event. Place the patient with gastroesophageal reflux with the head of the bed elevated.
7. Place small-bore tubes past the pylorus and into the jejunum in patients who are receiving nasointestinal feeding.
8. Suction the stomach and assess the patient's level of consciousness as well as airway reflexes before performing tracheal extubation.

9. Avoid the use of sedative or narcotic agents in patients with impaired CNS function or with absent airway reflexes.
10. Avoid enteral feedings in a patient for 6 hours after anesthetizing his upper airway for bronchoscopy.

For the patient with aspiration pneumonia and respiratory compromise, the following policies must be instituted:

1. Suction the oropharynx and empty the stomach; consider using continuous nasogastric drainage until the patient is stabilized. Do not feed the patient.
2. Begin a continuous infusion of D_5 0.25% sodium chloride solution at a maintenance rate, and avoid IV administration of bicarbonate or acetate since recurrent vomiting results in metabolic alkalosis. Obtain serum electrolyte values and anticipate the presence of either hypokalemia or metabolic alkalosis or both. Administer oxygen at a concentration sufficient to maintain the arterial oxygen saturation (SaO_2 >90%.
3. Administer nebulized isoproterenol at 0.01 ml/kg in 2 ml 0.9% sodium chloride solution to a patient with wheezing and respiratory distress. Isoproterenol is the initial agent chosen because of its rapid onset of action; however, its use must be followed by administration of a β-sympathomimetic agent with more sustained action (e.g., albuterol) through a nebulizer if the wheezing persists (see Chapter 133).
4. Begin a continuous infusion of aminophylline if the wheezing and respiratory distress are not relieved by nebulized β-sympathomimetic drugs. See Chapter 34 for details about aminophylline administration and its potential side effects.
5. Perform endotracheal intubation, if necessary, for control of the upper airway or to reduce the risk of further episodes of inhalation. The latter goal is best accomplished by placing an endotracheal tube with an inflatable cuff (e.g., in children more than 8 years of age), which will allow for nearly complete protection of the tracheobronchial tree.
6. Begin providing assisted ventilation in patients with evidence of respiratory failure (i.e., arterial carbon dioxide tension >55 mm Hg) or with

respiratory muscle fatigue (see Chapter 10). Administer PEEP to the patient in whom hypoxemia persists despite the administration of 70% oxygen and in whom the pulmonary disorder is diffuse (e.g., permeability pulmonary edema) (see Chapter 128). Perform rigid bronchoscopy with the patient under general anesthesia if there is evidence of aspiration of particulate matter or if alveolar ventilation is significantly impaired.

7. Administer broad-spectrum antibiotic coverage (e.g., ceftriaxone at 100 mg/kg/day divided into two doses) if the patient is febrile or there is a suspicion or evidence that the inhaled material was contaminated with bacteria.

8. Do not routinely administer corticosteroids for episodes of aspiration pneumonia.

ADDITIONAL READING

• Bartlett JG, Gorbach SL. Triple threat of aspiration pneumonia. Chest 68:560, 1975.

Broeg PJ, Toung JK, Cameron JL. Aspiration pneumonia. Surg Clin North Am 60:1551, 1980.

• Gibbs CP, Modell JJ. Aspiration pneumonitis. In Miller RE, ed. Anesthesia. New York: Churchill-Livingstone, 1986, p 2023.

Johanson WG, Harris GD. Aspiration pneumonia, anaerobic lung infections and lung abscess. Med Clin North Am 64:385, 1980.

Metteny NA, Eisenberg P, Cameron JL. Aspiration pneumonia in patients fed through nasoenteral tubes. Heart Lung 15:256, 1986.

94 Near-Hanging and Choking Injury

Orval E. Brown · *Derek A. Bruce*

BACKGROUND AND PHYSIOLOGY

Hanging or strangulation injury occurs infrequently in childhood. The causes are accidents, attempted suicide, or nonaccidental injuries resulting from assaults or child abuse. The resulting defects are predominantly those of cerebral ischemia and/or hypoxia, depending on the type of injury. Cervical vertebral and cervical spinal cord injuries are extremely uncommon occurrences. Damage to the airway is always a concern in the early phase of resuscitation since laryngeal fractures occur and airway compromise is usually present to a greater or lesser degree.

Accidental injuries are usually the result of children getting their heads stuck in small spaces (e.g., between railings, out of car windows). In a child who attempts suicide, because there is usually a minimal drop of the body, fractures of the C2 laminae (hangman's fracture) and disruption of the vertebral arteries resulting in death rarely occur, and the injuries are usually the result of slow strangulation effects on the cerebrum. The nonaccidental, deliberate choking attempts also usually produce prolonged compression of the neck, resulting in laryngeal fractures and cerebral hypoxia followed by ischemia. Thus the management of this particular injury is based on the complex relationship between the airway damage and cerebral hypoxia and ischemia.

Pathophysiology
Nervous system

The external application of a tourniquet to the neck of animals results in severe reduction of cerebral blood flow but usually not complete cessation of flow. The initial effect is venous congestion followed immediately by arterial occlusion if the pressure is high enough. Thus the effects on the cerebral blood flow are those of severe oligemia. Past studies have stated that partial ischemia of the brain is more deleterious than complete ischemia because of the continued buildup of lactate acid levels in the former setting, resulting in a greater decrease in intracellular pH. Other studies have refuted this idea, suggesting that there is in fact no difference in effects between severe oligemia and ischemia. However, there is no question that the ultimate result of a near-hanging or near-strangulation injury is that of cerebral hypoxia and cerebral ischemia.

The initial effect of the neck compression is either occlusion of venous return from the brain resulting in venous engorgement or interference with ventilation as a result of airway compromise. In the latter case the response of the brain to systemic hypoxemia is vasodilation and an increase in cerebral blood flow in an effort (teleologically) to improve cerebral perfusion. Only when the hypoxia is sufficiently severe to result in systemic hypotension as a result of medullary ischemia or direct cardiac effects will vascular collapse occur, meaning that if the child has a cardiac arrest as a result of the systemic hypoxemia, the brain itself is likely to have sustained severe hypoxic injury before this event. Even if there is no cardiac arrest, severe injury to neurons may result despite the increase in cerebral blood flow, depending on the level of hypoxemia and the length of time over which it is present.

In addition to hypoxia systemic hypercarbia occurs, which causes further cerebral vascular vasodilatation. In the short run (for a few minutes) this vasodilatation may improve cerebral blood flow and thus serve some useful function. If the hypercarbia is prolonged, however, marked elevations of ICP will occur as a result of the vasodilatation. In addition the hypercarbia will result in further decreases in pH, both systemically and in the brain. If the hypoxic-hypercarbic insult continues long enough, severe brain swelling will result, and ultimately the ICP will equal the systemic arterial blood pressure, resulting in no cerebral blood flow and death.

When the compressive forces around the neck are sufficient to produce arterial occlusion, the insult to the brain primarily is one of ischemia. If, in addition, there is airway compromise, ischemia plus hypoxemia will occur, probably making any insult to the brain worse in a short period of time. Also, cerebral venous congestion will be present because of the occlusion of venous outflow from the brain. Thus the insult to the brain will be akin to that occurring with cardiac arrest, and lack of flow for more than 5 minutes will result in severe neuronal injury despite the absence of cardiac arrest.

The patency of the vertebral arteries is often preserved because they are encased in the bony canal from C1-6. Thus, if the compressing agent (e.g., hands or a thick rope) is quite wide, the vertebral arteries are protected unless the occlusive forces are very low in the neck. If the strangulation implement (e.g., a garrote) is thin, it can pass between the vertical body and lamina and compress the vertebral arteries also. In judicial hanging the cause of death is usually immediate and results from the weight of the body producing a hyperextension injury that fractures the lamina of C2. The weight of the body's continued fall then rotates it forward and tears the vertebral arteries, resulting in immediate death. This is rarely the case in near-hanging or hanging episodes in children because there is rarely a significant drop. The damage in these settings is due to either hypoxemia or hypercarbia, cerebral ischemia, or some combination of the two.

Neck and larynx

Near-hanging may cause laryngeal injury, ranging from minor endolaryngeal edema to massive laryngeal fracture with complete airway obstruction. These patients are initially seen with varied airway signs and symptoms in addition to neurologic and cervical spine injuries. All patients with a near-hanging injury must be evaluated for laryngeal fracture.

The patient can have either a stable airway with no stridor or respiratory obstruction or an unstable airway with stridor, respiratory obstruction, and possible hemoptysis. Patients with an unstable airway (i.e., with stridor or difficulty breathing) should be suspected of severe airway trauma and laryngeal fracture.

Patients with laryngeal injury can be categorized into three groups: minor, moderate, and massive injuries. Minor laryngeal trauma includes small endolaryngeal hematomas, edema, or small mucosal lacerations and no detectable laryngeal fracture. These patients have mobile true vocal cords and usually have a stable airway. Moderate laryngeal injuries include edema, hematoma, mucosal disruption, or laceration sufficient to cause upper airway obstruction that necessitates tracheotomy. These patients may have nondisplaced laryngeal fractures. Massive laryngeal injuries include displaced cartilage fractures, vocal cord immobility, cricoarytenoid joint dislocation, and severe endolaryngeal edema and mucosal tears. These patients usually need an immediate tracheotomy for airway support. Once it is done, the other systems may be evaluated and stabilized.

Clinical Findings

If the child's injuries were not deliberately produced, the history will be of a strangulation or a near-hanging event. When attempted murder or child abuse has been the cause, frequently no history can be obtained or the history is inappropriate to the injury (e.g., the child's being found hanging over the crib side) (see Chapter 95). The constellation of the history and the clinical findings makes the diagnosis clear in most cases.

When the child is examined, evidence of injury to the skin of the neck should be present (e.g., bruising, wheal formation, lacerations). If the injury has not caused immediate death, typically suffusion and swelling of the face and neck above the level of the occlusion are present. Petechial hemorrhages of the skin and conjunctiva are usually found. The tongue may be swollen, and retinal hemorrhages are frequently present. If the child is not in a coma, the severity of either the ischemia or hypoxia has been insufficient to produce immediate neuronal injury or severely increased ICP. Nonetheless, because of the pathology of the lesion, delayed cerebral swelling, brain edema, or delayed neuronal death can occur. In addition seizures superimposed on the initial injury may be detrimental. Thus careful observation for several days is necessary for the child who has had a near-hanging or strangulation injury but who is not comatose since the appearance of elevated ICP, seizures, or secondary leukoencepalopathy may be delayed during this time. In comatose children the outlook can be compared to that of children in other hypoxic-ischemic events (e.g., near-drowning). The deeper the coma and the longer it lasts, the worse are the chances for recovery. Indeed, if the Glasgow Coma Scale (GCS) score is not >6 with 3 to 4 hours after resuscitation, the child's chances of recovering to a normal state are close to zero.

One type of near-hanging occurs predominantly in adolescent males and is related to the onset of sexuality and masturbation. The adolescent frequently puts some kind of knotted implement around his neck to produce borderline hypoxia during masturbation. This is not infrequently done in the shower; if the child slips, the knot may tighten and result in a hanging episode, which may be fatal. Hanging is the most frequent method of teenage suicide.

MONITORING AND LABORATORY TESTS

Central nervous system. Frequent neurologic checks (see Chapter 4) must be done and documented, perhaps every 15 to 30 minutes during the first few hours, then every hour thereafter.

Airway. In addition to the usual monitoring of the airway (see Chapter 4) the following special procedures must be done. Patients with a stable airway are evaluated with the use of indirect laryngoscopy, if they are cooperative, or with fiberoptic nasolaryngoscopy. The condition of a patient with a stable airway may deteriorate either slowly or rapidly; thus intensive observation is indicated. If the patient's airway is unstable, a plan to provide an airway must be made, and immediate consultation with an experienced airway surgeon is essential. The larynx must be visualized by direct laryngoscopy to confirm the diagnosis.

After the airway is stabilized, which may require tracheotomy, a CT scan of the larynx is indicated. Injuries such as nondisplaced fractures and vocal fold hematomas will resolve spontaneously without operative intervention. CT permits rapid, accurate, noninvasive examination of the laryngeal cartilages, thus making operative intervention in these cases unnecessary. Severe edema of the endolarynx may obscure the diagnosis of displaced laryngeal fracture, but the diagnosis can be confirmed by CT. CT scanning of patients with massive laryngeal injury is not generally indicated since open exploration and repair of the

laryngeal fracture are necessary. However, if the patient is stable and undergoing CT of the CNS, the larynx may be scanned to provide further information to guide operative repair.

TREATMENT
Resuscitation

The first step in treating a child with a strangulation injury, as always, is to establish the A,B,Cs (*a*irway, *b*reathing, *c*irculation). All patients can be given a high concentration of oxygen, although bag and mask ventilation can be hazardous if there is disruption of the airway because it might make the obstruction worse. Maintaining the airway may be a major problem.

Intubation should only be attempted by an experienced physician and in the presence of an airway surgeon under optimal conditions, preferably in the PICU or operating room. Since the airway in these patients may be tenuous at best, under no circumstances should the patient be sedated or given a neuromuscular blocking agent until the airway has been evaluated by the airway surgeon. To do so could alter respiratory drive and function enough to convert a partial obstruction to a complete obstruction that cannot be relieved except by tracheostomy.

Patients with laryngeal fractures should never be intubated through the larynx since laryngeal fracture can disrupt the endolarynx and cause mucosal tears and cartilage fractures, making it difficult to pass an endotracheal tube into the lower airway. Asphyxiation and other severe laryngeal complications can ensue with attempts at intubation through the mouth. Patients needing airway support must undergo immediate tracheotomy while under local anesthesia. This procedure is done in the operating room. Management of minor laryngeal injury consists of close observation, elevation of the head of the bed, and humidification of inspired air. Patients with nondisplaced fractures are observed without performing open exploration. Patients with displaced fractures must undergo open surgical exploration with repair of the laryngeal fracture.

Patients with massive endolaryngeal injuries need primary laryngeal repair, which should be performed within 24 hours of the injury for the best results, as long as the patient is otherwise stable. The larynx is generally approached through a midline thyrotomy incision. Mucosal lacerations are repaired, and displaced thyroid and cricoid cartilage fractures are realigned and sutured. Dislocated arytenoids, if present, are repositioned. Laryngeal stents are avoided if possible but are indicated with severe disruption of the anterior commissure or with massive laryngeal injury resulting in an unstable cartilage framework despite the use of reduction and suturing. Stents are left in place for 3 to 4 weeks and then removed via a transoral endoscopic approach. Decannulation is performed as described in Chapter 135.

Only after the airway is patent can adequate breathing be established. The systemic arterial blood pressure may be difficult to reestablish in these children because of severe systemic acidosis, direct cardiac injury resulting from the hypoxemia, or medullary infarction with loss of vasomotor tone.

As noted previously, if the child has had a cardiac arrest or is in arrest in the emergency department, the injury to the brain will be severe and usually unsurvivable. The length of time allotted to resuscitative efforts must take into account the severity of the injury and the likelihood of recovery. If major difficulties are experienced in getting the cardiac function or systemic arterial blood pressure restored, the physician may question the value of continued resuscitative efforts in the presence of a likely dead brain.

Central Nervous System

Once the airway, ventilation, and systemic arterial blood pressure are reestablished, attention is directed to the CNS injury. In those children who have a GCS score of 8 or above, the concern about significant cerebral injury is small; however, a few of these children will develop delayed neurologic deterioration over the first few days. This deterioration may be due to either increased ICP, seizure, or delayed cerebral damage as a result of either neuronal or white matter dysfunction. An early CT scan, therefore, must be obtained to ascertain whether significant intracranial hemorrhage has occurred and to evaluate the density of the brain and the size of the CSF spaces. If delayed deterioration occurs, a repeat scan may show increased brain swelling.

The goals of management of these children with GCS scores of 8 or above are to maintain the serum osmolality at 280 to 300 mOsm, to limit IV fluids (generally 60% of maintenance), and to maintain normal systemic arterial blood pressure. Any systemic acidosis must be corrected slowly. Administering a bolus of sodium bicarbonate IV will result in an increase in alveolar carbon dioxide as the result of a sudden rise in arterial carbon dioxide and can produce vasodilatation in the brain and large increases in ICP, which in the presence of a tight (compressed) brain can conceivably produce herniation. There is no evidence that steroids or calcium blockers are helpful in preventing delayed deterioration or in affecting the acute injury. Administering prophylactic anticonvulsants to prevent seizures has not been shown beneficial.

Currently there are no specific drugs available to prevent the secondary damage. Research studies show that the delayed neural toxicity in this setting may be related to the release of glutamate, a putative neurotransmitter. The blockage of the glutamate uptake or release seems to result in preservation of neurons that would otherwise be damaged. If this experimental situation is applicable to humans, which seems likely, specific drugs that act at the site of glutamate action may become available for the treatment of the hypoxic-ischemic injury.

In those children who deteriorate late, elevated ICP is usually not the problem. But if the CT scan shows diffuse swelling, the use of ICP monitoring may be helpful in controlling and preventing secondary damage.

In comatose children with a GCS score of 7 or less, the problem is almost identical to that of the near-drowning or postcardiac arrest patient. Because of the venous congestion the occurrence of hemorrhage within the cerebrum is more likely. Thus CT scanning is indicated as soon as the patient is stabilized. The best that can be done is to establish normal vital signs as soon as possible. Although the ICP may be elevated, all the evidence suggests that the injury to the neurons has already occurred, and it has been our experience with a limited number of cases that if the ICP is elevated more than 20 torr, the outcome will be either death or vegetative survival, as is the case for children with near-drowning episodes. There is no evidence that aggressive efforts to control the ICP can alter outcome.

Routine administration of antibiotics is not indicated for treating the cerebral injury, although it may be indicated if damage to the larynx or trachea has occurred. The research work described previously suggests that the seizures that occur after ischemia and hypoxia may indeed be detrimental, causing further injury to the brain. Thus seizures, should they occur, must be aggressively treated with large enough doses of anticonvulsants to stop them. If necessary, EEG monitoring may be used to determine if seizures have been controlled. There is little evidence that the current anticonvulsant medications have much effect in those children with late onset of myoclonic seizures. These seizures frequently seem to arise within the reticular formation, and there is little or no evidence that they produce further cortical damage. They are, however, an indicator of severe brain injury with involvement of the less sensitive areas in the brain stem.

There is no evidence that prophylactic antiseizure medication is harmful; and if it is used, it must be given in large enough doses to achieve immediate blood levels sufficient to control seizures, and these blood levels must be monitored and maintained. Currently, however, there is no evidence that prophylactic antiseizure medication is beneficial.

• • •

In conclusion, the outcome from near-hanging or strangulation episodes in children correlates with the clinical examination on admission. The pathophysiologic process is similar to that associated with near-drowning episodes, and there currently is no evidence that any specific therapy directed toward the brain will alter the outcome. In those children in whom the ICP is elevated, death or vegetative survival is likely. In those children with a good GCS score on admission (i.e., 8 or above), recovery without significant neurologic or cognitive deficits can be expected.

ADDITIONAL READING

Allman FD, Nelson WB, Pacentine GA, et al. Outcome following cardiopulmonary resuscitation in severe pediatric near-drowning. Am J Dis Child 140:571-575, 1986.

Gisvold SE, Safar P, Hendrick HHL, et al. Thiopental treatment after global brain ischemia in pigtailed monkeys. Anesthesiology 60:88-96, 1984.

Kagstrom E, Smith ML, Siesjo BK. Local cerebral blood flow in the recovery period following complete cerebral ischemia in the rat. J Cereb Blood Flow Metab 3:170-176, 1983.

Kagstrom E, Smith ML, Siesjo BK. Recirculation in the rat brain following incomplete ischemia. J Cereb Blood Flow Metab 3:183-187, 1983.

Marshall LF, Durity F, Loundsbury R, et al. Experimental cerebral oligemia and ischemia produced by intracranial hypertension. Parts I and II. J Neurosurg 43:308-328, 1975.

Meldrum BS, Evans MC, Swan JH, et al. Protection against hypoxic/ischemic brain damage with excitatory amino acid antagonists. Med Biol 65:153-157, 1987.

Schaefer SD. Primary management of laryngeal trauma. Ann Otol Rhinol Laryngol 91:399-402, 1982.

• Schaefer SD, Brown OE. Selective application of CT in the management of laryngeal trauma. Laryngoscope 93:1473-1475, 1983.

Trone TH, Schaefer SD, Carder HM. Blunt and penetrating laryngeal trauma: A 13-year review. Otolaryngol Head Neck Surg 88:257-261, 1980.

95 Child Abuse and Shake Injuries

Paul R. Prescott · Derek A. Bruce

BACKGROUND

Child abuse has existed and exists today in all cultures. Historically, defining a given behavior as abusive or harmful varies both between and within cultures as well as over time. At various times in many cultures the father was the absolute head of the house, with the right to exercise life and death decisions over his property (i.e., his children). Given this right, children were deliberately exposed or killed if they were deformed, illegitimate, or simply not hardy enough to raise. Female infants were often considered a family burden and were similarly discarded. For centuries children were deliberately mutilated to increase their earnings as beggars; young boys were castrated for harem service or to preserve their high-pitched voices for choirs; and children were sacrificed to the gods for the greater good of the whole community. Passage of laws to make such abuse a crime did not necessarily bring it to a halt.

Some behaviors currently called abuse were once accepted as standard child-rearing methods. The culturally condoned neglect of infants given over to wet nurses for diverse reasons resulted in the death of many. At other times children were seen as inherently evil, justifying their severe beatings or confinement to instill proper behavior and to suppress their innate willfulness. Children were expected to show proper respect and complete obedience to their parents. Flogging was an acceptable disciplinary action in schools for children who were unruly or who did not learn their lessons. Several colonial states provided capital punishment for disobedient children. At the time parents and society viewed these behaviors as necessary to promote a proper familial and societal appearance.

During this and other countries' histories children as young as 5 or 6 years old were allowed to work long hours in substandard factories or were sold into indentured apprenticeships, a situation that was often precipitated by their parent's own severe poverty and in some ways is analogous to today's latchkey children.

Efforts to control abuse in the United States during the last half of the nineteenth century and first half of the twentieth century were directed toward enforcing the then-existing laws against child labor, slowly evolving to the concept of children's rights. Medically, many nonaccidental injuries were ascribed to accidents or unknown events. Between 1925 and 1946 Dr. John Caffey, a pediatrician by training and a leading pediatric radiologist, recognized that multiple fractures were due to trauma. His 1946 publication associating multiple fractures with subdural hematomas raised the question of parents causing the injuries, either covertly or overtly. Over the following years more articles in the medical literature drew the same conclusions, until Dr. C. Henry Kempe and colleagues, at a conference in 1961 and in an article in 1962, publicly coined the term "battered-child syndrome."

Definition and Etiology

What is ultimately defined as child abuse or neglect depends in large part on the society that sets the laws and how that society views and values children. Within the melting pot of the United States cultural differences must sometimes be taken into account. The parents' actions and their intent at the time in these cases should be viewed within the acceptable realm of behavior in their cultures. However, the effect on the child serves as a common denominator in defining abuse. The broadest possible definition for child abuse and neglect would include any behavior, whether overt or covert, on the part of a child's caregiver that interferes or might interfere with that child's normal growth and development physically, mentally, or emotionally. This definition allows for the potential of future injury based on past or present incidents and for a broader spectrum of harmful behaviors such as:

Physical abuse
Emotional abuse
Sexual abuse
Intentional drugging
Educational deprivation
Physical neglect
Nutritional neglect
Medical care neglect
Lack of supervision
Abandonment

An estimated one to two million cases of child abuse, with several thousand deaths, occur in the United States each year. In pediatric emergency departments, 10% of all trauma to children less than 3 years old and 25% of all fractures to children less than 2 years old are the result of abuse. In severe cases of abuse or neglect the long-term morbidity can be staggering. Learning and language deficiencies, developmental, mental, and growth retardation, blindness and deafness, psychosis, depression, suicide, juvenile and adult crime, prostitution, and drug abuse can all result.

Some of the causes of child abuse and neglect are rooted in the very fabric of society and its religious beliefs. "A man's home is his castle" and "spare the rod, spoil the child" are still commonly held beliefs that fail to teach child development and alternative disciplinary techniques. Often abusive parents were abused as children and repeat the cycle in their adult relationships and in relationships with their children, using the same parenting techniques that were used with them. Additionally, the demands placed on the child are unrealistic, from expecting less crying during infancy or complete control of elimination at too early an age to expecting the child to fulfill the parents' needs. To these parents their own needs are predominate. They often do not realize that the child has needs, or they misperceive those needs.

Factors frequently cited in the abusers are feelings of isolation, an inability to trust others, and low self-esteem. Environmental factors such as unemployment, poverty, and poor housing overstress an already stressed family. Child factors such as prematurity, developmental delay, disability, temperament, prolonged illness, and illegitimacy can mark the child as "different" and unable to fit into the parents' expected family picture.

Approximately 10% of abusive caregivers are psychotic or sociopathic. The remainder cannot reliably be separated from the nonabusive population by any known scale or test, a fact that must be remembered if nonaccidental injuries in families that do not fit the expected "profile" are to be recognized. Such instances of misdiagnosis occur in the Munchausen-by-proxy syndrome, in which parents are seen as doing the best they can while supporting the efforts of the medical staff. In other cases parents may fit the "sick-but-slick" syndrome, convincing everyone that they could not be responsible for their child's injury.

Legal Aspects

Before 1964 no effective or specific laws mandated the reporting of child abuse cases. The 1961 conference mentioned previously helped produce model child abuse laws that were enacted in one form or another by all the states. Reporting laws and providing relief for the child (such as temporary foster care placement) are parts of the civil code, with the purpose of protecting the child, not invoking criminal penalties against the abuser. Many states specifically require physicians and medical personnel to report abuse cases, others require all citizens to report them, and a few do both. No state requires absolute proof that a child has been abused or neglected or that a specific person be singled out as the abuser. Provided that a reasonable suspicion exists that a child has been or might be at risk, all states provide the informer immunity from civil and criminal responsibility if the report proves inaccurate. Penalties are generally provided for failing to report the abuse, and physicians may be held liable under malpractice laws for such failure. Each physician must become aware of the legal requirements in his own state.

Fifty percent of abused children sent back to the abusive environment without intervention will be reinjured, with one third of that group suffering permanent disability. All cases of significant injury involving a child must be investigated thoroughly. Even injuries consistent with a motor vehicle accident can actually be instances of abuse if no such accident occurred. Physicians and medical staff rarely have time to confirm the history, and this must be left to the reporting agency mandated by law to protect children.

DIAGNOSIS
History

The first step in diagnosing child abuse is to suspect it. Because very few injury patterns are pathognomonic for abuse, a complete medical history is vital. The physician must never directly accuse a person of child abuse or attempt to give legal advice.

The description of the events surrounding the injury must be as detailed as possible and include a complete developmental history and specific timing of symptoms and events leading to the admission. Some histories are diagnostic or at least highly suspect for nonaccidental injury (Table 95-1).

An inconsistent history is most frequent. Minor falls are blamed for causing complex skull or longbone fractures, multiple injuries, or closed head injury. In most falls of less than 36 inches little or no trauma occurs, and resulting fractures are simple and non-life threatening. The developmental level of the child must *always* be taken into account.

In abuse cases 30% of abusers delay seeking medical care for the child until the following morning; another 30% wait 1 to 4 days. In contrast there is no delay in seeking help after accidental injuries, or the delay is proportional to the child's age, the severity of the injury, and the time it takes for symptoms to become apparent to nonmedical personnel. Economic or transportation factors can be responsible for seeking delayed care although rarely in patients with severe injuries.

In an accidental injury, especially in toddlers, full details may not be known to the parent or caretaker if the accident happened out of his sight with no witnesses present. Either no explanation is offered or several explanations are offered over a period of days as minor past incidents are recalled. Unfortunately the same is often true in abuse cases. Nonaccidental injury is likely with all but the most minor injuries in pretoddlers and with severe or multiple injuries in all other children. The developmental history and the degree of trauma generally help to differentiate nonaccidental from accidental injuries. Any changes in the history made by the parents or discrepancies between different histories must be accurately documented.

Other diagnostic features include a recent family crisis or stress, a triggering event, unrealistic expectations for the child, a pattern of increasingly severe injury, abuse of parent as a child, and social isolation. The history must also include whether the birth was planned or unplanned, postnatal problems, and information about recent or chronic illness, crying, colic, toilet training, feeding and sleep problems, general behavior, and discipline. One or more of these frequently serve as the trigger that promotes the abusive incident. An understanding of the parents' knowledge of child development may show very unrealistic expectations of the child.

Past injuries, particularly a pattern of increasing severity, are common, although not often elicited initially. The social history may reveal a recent family

Table 95-1 Histories Offered in Abuse Cases

History	Comments
Child or parent accuses other parent or adult	Generally reliable if no custody disputes
No explanation given	Especially in pretoddler
Inconsistent with injury	Compare history with developmental level, severity of injury
Self-inflicted	Especially in pretoddler or if injuries are severe
Caused by sibling	Usually minor injury if true; if severe injury, referral to child protective services is still needed
Delay in seeking care	Especially in severe burns, fractures, closed head injury (see text)
Partial confession	Admits to some of trauma, usually not severest part
Varying or discrepant	Different histories at varying time or from different caretakers

crisis such as unemployment, eviction, separation, or divorce. Finally, when asked about his own childhood and disciplinary experiences, one or both parents may reveal a pattern seen through their eyes as appropriate, well-deserved dicipline.

Examination

All details of the physical examination must be thoroughly documented. CNS trauma, fractures, extensive bruising, and scalds in infants and toddlers and injuries to the buttocks, lower back, genitalia, inner thighs, earlobes, neck, and oral cavity at all ages should be considered nonaccidental until proved otherwise. However, the absence of marks, bruises, or fractures never rules out child abuse. Children with severe head and intra-abdominal injuries often have no visible external trauma.

Cutaneous lesions

External injuries are best documented on a body diagram. Estimating the age of external bruises and other injuries can document recurrent abuse. Although the rate of healing varies by age, body area, skin thickness, depth of injury, subcutaneous fat, blood supply, and other factors, bruises show specific color changes over time. Healing commences at the periphery and progresses centrally; therefore the color at the margin is used to approximate the age of the bruise (Table 95-2).

Bruises and burns are the two most common external signs of physical child abuse or neglect (Table 95-3). Patterned bruises do not usually occur accidentally and must be identified in the record as well as possible. Multiple or severe bruises, particularly on soft tissue areas, are always suspect. Even in tum-

---

Table 95-2 Dating of Bruises

Age of Bruise	Appearance
0-2 days	Swollen, tender
0-5 days	Red, blue, purple
5-7 days	Green
7-10 days	Yellow
10-14 days	Brown
2-4 weeks	Cleared

COMMON NONACCIDENTAL INJURIES

Cutaneous lesions

Bruises

Hand marks
    Pinch or grab
    Slap
    Choke
    Bilateral facial grab
Common object patterns
    Looped-cord
    Belt
    Buckle
    Switch
    Ankle or wrist ligature
    Wire coat hanger
Bite marks

Burns

Forced immersion
    Stocking or glove pattern
    Perineum or lower legs
Spill
Flame
Common contact patterns
    Cigarette
    Iron
    Curling iron
    Furnace grate
    Grill or griddle
    Stove burner

Head injuries

Traumatic alopecia
Skull fractures
Subarachnoid hemorrhage
Epidural hematoma
Parenchymal laceration
Subgaleal hematoma
Subdural hematoma
Intraventricular hemorrhage
Contusional hemorrhage
Focal or generalized cerebral edema

Abdominal injuries

Ruptured intestine, liver, spleen
Pancreatic pseudocyst
Duodenal or jejunal intramural hematoma
Renal trauma

Table 95-3   General Characteristics of Accidental vs. Nonaccidental Trauma

Trauma	Accidental	Nonaccidental
Bruises	Few other than on arms, shins in toddlers	Frequently multiple
	Rounded, nondescript	Often patterned or multishaped
	Over bony prominence	Same, plus soft tissue areas
	Location: shin, lower arms, iliac crest, chin, forehead	Location: trunk, upper anterior and inner thigh, back, buttocks, upper arms, chest, face, abdomen
Immersion burns	Asymmetric	Symmetric
	Often blurred	Clear, distinct margins
	Irregular splash marks	None or few
	Few spared areas	Patterned intertriginous sparing
	Partial thickness	Full thickness
	Location: random, consistent with history	Location: stocking or glove pattern, lower legs, buttocks, perineum
	Cause: consistent with pattern	Cause: unknown; self- or sibling-inflicted
Spill burns	Irregular margins	Same
	Face, arm, upper trunk, usually anterior	Same; multiple random areas if thrown
	Pattern: consistent with child's position	Pattern: inconsistent
Contact burns	Superficial or partial thickness	Deep or full thickness
	Small area of contact	Full contact area
	Blurred or no pattern	Clear pattern and margins
	Deeper at one edge	Uniform depth
	Exposed areas	Same but not limited
Skull fractures	Unilateral	Same or bilateral
	One bone	Same or multiple
	Single simple linear	Same or multiple, complex, depressed, diastatic
	Narrow (1-2 mm)	Same or wide, especially >5 mm
	Falls of 3-5 feet	Forceful blunt trauma
	No cerebral injury	Often associated with cerebral injury or hemorrhage

bling accidents such as falling down the stairs injuries tend to be minor and distally located.

The majority of deliberate burns are from scalding liquids, tend to occur in children less than age 3 years, and are deeper and more severe than accidental burns. In one recent series no full-thickness accidental scald burns were found. Classically there are no witnesses since the parent was "absent from the room at the time." Additional information such as the water temperature and the size of the container may be needed to make a certain diagnosis. Scald burns are time and temperature dependent, producing full-thickness burns to adult skin in 1 minute at 127° F,

in 30 seconds at 130° F, and in 2 seconds at 150° F. In contrast, 117° F on average is the threshold of pain for scalding liquids.

Bite marks, if clear and distinct, must be measured across the midcanine length. A width >3 cm generally means the attacker was more than age 8 years. If the marks are clear enough, a forensic dentist may be able to identify the person as accurately as fingerprints do.

Shake injuries

The results of nonaccidental trauma in the less than 2-year-old population of children are disastrous.

Table 95-4 Mortality After Admission to Hospital After Head Trauma in Children ≤2 Years (1981-1982)*

	All Causes	Child Abuse
No. of children†	73	7
No. of deaths	4 (5.5%)	3 (43%)
Deaths from child abuse	3	3

*Figures from the Children's Hospital of Philadelphia.
†Head injuries seen by the Pediatric Neurological Service.

Table 95-4 shows the results of one series of head-injured children less than 2 years of age seen at the Children's Hospital of Philadelphia. Nonaccidental trauma was responsible for approximately 10% of the injuries; yet child abuse resulted in 75% of the mortality, and similar figures have been reported by other authors. The other death in the series from this hospital was probably nonaccidental also, but this could not be fully ascertained. After severe CNS trauma in small children, 20% to 30% of the children will die, a similar number will be left with severe disability, and only 20% to 30% will make a reasonable recovery. Children that do recover have the problem of going back into the setting in which they were abused in the first place.

The uniqueness of the symptomatology of what has in the past, probably mistakenly, been called the shaken baby injury is the result of the age and developmental level of the children on whom this type of injury is perpetrated. This type of nonaccidental trauma in children frequently occurs as an isolated incident; therefore the absence of external signs is quite common. Rarely is there a suggestion of systematic child abuse. This type of injury usually occurs in a child less than 1 year of age, and the precipitating event is usually the child's uncontrollable crying. The adult response is usually one of frustration, and it appears quite likely that in the majority of cases the adult does not deliberately plan to injure the child. A sudden loss of control apparently is responsible for this type of trauma.

Recent studies strongly indicate that shaking alone cannot cause the life-threatening brain swelling, subdural hematoma, and brain injury that occur in these children. Chronic subdural hematomas in children

less than 1 year of age may result from repeated severe shaking injuries of sufficient degree to produce minor subarachnoid hemorrhage. This may result in clogging of the arachnoid villi, resulting in chronic extracerebral collections. These shaking events, however, are most unlikely to produce acute unconsciousness and severe brain damage. Some type of impact is probably required to develop the severe deceleration forces necessary to produce damage.

It seems reasonable to assume that after the shake injury has occurred the child must be discarded from the angry adult's arms. This is unlikely to be done gently, and frequently the child is tossed into the crib, onto a couch, or occasionally deliberately against a wall or floor. Shaking alone is unable to produce angular acceleration much greater than 9 or 10 *g*, which is well below the range needed to produce traumatic unconsciousness, let alone tearing of bridging of veins and subdural hematomas. However, with a single impact against even a soft mattress, angular accelerations in excess of 300 *g* are easily obtained. With a single impact against a hard surface the angular acceleration is as high as 400 or 500 *g*. If the head hits something solid (e.g., floor, wall), skull fractures are much more likely to occur than if the head hits something soft such as a mattress or couch.

In one study all the children who died had evidence of an impact injury as manifested by a skull fracture or galeal contusion. A common history that accompanies this injury is that the child fell from a couch. Simple falls from couches, changing tables, or beds do not produce this type of injury. However, the child may have bounced off the couch onto the floor after being discarded after the shaking event. We believe that there is usually an impact associated with the deceleration injury that produces the typical picture of "the shaken baby syndrome" and that this term should be changed to be "the shaken, impacted baby syndrome."

As emphasized previously, minor falls in children less than 1 year of age do not produce unconsciousness, very rarely produce brain damage, and essentially never produce retinal hemorrhages. Accidental skull fractures are very common occurrences in children less than 2 years of age, but these fractures are rarely associated with brain injury or disturbed consciousness and never with retinal hemorrhages. Thus in any sick baby seen in the emergency department or in a physician's office, if the history is not appropriate for the child's condition, an integral part of the physical examination, before any other intervention, is a retinal examination. This examination can be difficult to perform on an irritable baby, but severe degrees of retinal hemorrhage are easily seen.

The remainder of the physical examination can be misleading, especially in a child less than 6 months of age. The presence or absence of crying in response to painful stimuli is an important measure of consciousness. Conscious children cry, and unconscious children do not. Absence of crying in response to painful stimuli should put the physician on guard that a serious disturbance of brain function is present.

Infants can exhibit repeated involuntary eye opening in the absence of cortical function. This eye opening can be misinterpreted as spontaneous eye opening and the children assumed to be conscious. If carefully observed, this action will be seen to be rhythmic and not in response to any particular external stimuli. There are also no following responses of the eyes.

During the motor examination spontaneous bicycling types of movements of the arms and legs occur in small children despite almost absent cortical function. These movements are easily misinterpreted as voluntary motor function and again the child is believed to be better neurologically than he really is. Spinal cord reflex activity, which is often quite complicated in small children, is also easily misinterpreted as spontaneous motor function or withdrawal to pain and further clouds the neurologic examination. These are easy errors to make, especially if there is no history of head trauma. Examination of the fontanelle will usually reveal increased pulsations and some fullness, although significant elevations of ICP may not occur for some hours. Thus diagnosis is based on a high suspicion of nonaccidental trauma in all children less than 1 year of age who have disturbed consciousness and no reasonable history of severe trauma that might be a cause.

Because of the nonaccidental nature of the trauma, these children are frequently kept at home for 1 hour or more after the injury in the hope that they will recover consciousness. During this period a seizure or respiratory arrest may occur, precipitating a call to the ambulance service and resulting in the child's hospitalization. Retinal hemorrhages rarely if ever occur after cardiopulmonary resuscitation has been performed, although this is frequently given as an explanation. Trauma sufficient to produce coma, subarachnoid hemorrhage, acute subdural hematoma, and brain swelling or infarction will produce acute unconsciousness also. It is appropriate to assume that these injuries are acute and occurred close to the time the patient came to the hospital in a coma. Only if a large subdural or epidural hematoma is present is the history of slow deterioration over hours a possibility.

Therapy begins with diagnosis. Early care of the airway, control of seizures, and preservation of adequate ventilation come first. If the baby is flaccid or exhibits abnormal posturing, either extensor or flexor, and is exhibiting a full and tense fontanelle, emergency bilateral subdural taps are done. They often allow drainage of 5 to 15 ml of bloody CSF bilaterally, and this drainage may frequently result in improvement of the neurologic condition and breathing.

Once the baby is stable, a CT scan must be obtained. If the child is irritable, it is better to do the scan under general anesthesia with endotracheal intubation than to sedate him with oral or IV medication; the hypercarbia and hypoxemia that could accompany sedation with hypoventilation could cause further increases in ICP and a marked deterioration in the patient's condition. Rarely will the CT scan demonstrate any significant mass lesion. The most common pattern is that of a posterior triangular-shaped, interhemispheric collection of blood, although the incidence of small-to-large subdural hematomas varies from series to series. More extensive subdural hematomas can occur. Subarachnoid hemorrhage is frequently present. The most ominous and often overlooked of the CT findings is that of loss of the gray matter/white matter density difference, with or without brain swelling. This pattern is the result of transient or persistent cerebral ischemia and is usually followed by increases in ICP that may be immediate or delayed over 24 to 48 hours and frequently accompanied by seizures. Thus this pattern on the CT scan should warn the physician of the potential need for ICP monitoring and PICU care despite a neurologic examination that may appear fairly satisfactory. The second import of this finding of low density throughout the hemispheres is that there will almost certainly be a progessive loss of brain tissue, resulting in cerebral atrophy, which is the harbinger of a very poor prognosis for both survival and ultimate recovery.

Treatment. No specific therapies exist for shake injuries other than those for other children with increased ICP. Severely elevated ICP can occur in children with open fontanelles, and ICP monitoring is safe in this age group. Hyperventilation, strict control of seizures, osmotic agents, and barbiturates may all be necessary to control the ICP in this group of children. A great deal of the cerebral damage in children who are shaken and impacted apparently is caused by hypoxia and ischemia, and if the ICP is >20 mm Hg, the outlook for good recovery is very poor, an outcome similar to that for near-drowning patients. Because there is both traumatic and ischemic pathology, the efforts to control ICP are occasionally effective, and the outcome is better than expected, justifying the initial effort. In children with loss of gray matter/white matter density differential, the cerebellar or basal ganglia may appear to be of high density. They are, in fact, of normal density, the remainder of the brain being severely ischemic, and in this group of children the ICP and systemic arterial blood pressure are frequently equal when measured and confirm brain death.

•   •   •

The shaken-impact injury is the all-too-common cause of altered consciousness in children less than 1 year of age. In up to 50% of these children there is no history of trauma, and in the other 50% there is a history of only minor trauma. Minor trauma does not produce disturbed consciousness in young children, does not result in a full fontanelle, and essentially never produces retinal hemorrhages. It is critical that all physicians and nurses who deal with the pediatric patients, either in the emergency department or PICU, recognize this syndrome and maintain a high index of suspicion of such abuse in an unconscious child. The results of this injury are devastating: 30% die and 30% are left severely disabled. The only real cure is prevention; but early identification of the seriousness of the problem and early intensive intervention will result in a better outcome for some of the children.

Head injuries

The child's scalp must be palpated for soft tissue swelling and must be examined for bruises. However,

even after they receive a direct impact, skull fractures and externally visible scalp bruises are found in 50% or less. Blunt trauma from an open or closed hand, impact against the wall, floor, or other hard object, and rapid acceleration and deceleration cause the majority of nonaccidental injuries. Associated unilateral or generalized cerebral edema is the most life-threatening consequence of inflicted head injury.

Subdural hematomas originate from tearing of the bridging veins between the brain surface and the dural sinuses and are commonly associated with cerebral edema. In children less than 1 year of age the onset of symptoms is generally immediate or within minutes of nonaccidental trauma. Considerable force is needed to produce a subdural bleed in the normal child, making the usual history of falling out of bed or from a table untenable. A large percentage of the children develop obstructive hydrocephalus or cerebral atrophy with hydrocephalus ex vacuo.

Retinal hemorrhage often occurs in association with subdural hematomas or markedly increased ICP, yet it is uncommon in all but the most severe accidental head injuries. If it is noted, ophthalmologic consultation is warranted.

Despite the frequency of facial bruises and trauma in abused children, injury to the facial bones is rare. When present, the mandible or orbital regions are usually involved.

If traumatic alopecia has occurred recently, the child may have petechial hemorrhage at his hair roots, swelling, and tenderness. The remaining hair is not easily extracted, and the pattern of hair loss is diffuse, in contrast to that with alopecia areata.

Abdominal injuries

Severe intra-abdominal injuries can occur without obvious external injury or bruising. Nonaccidental injuries are frequently caused by blunt trauma from a punch or kick or by rapid deceleration from the child's being thrown. Plausible explanations are more frequent with these injuries, although simple falls and falls down stairs are inconsistent with the trauma. In many cases the history of abuse comes from the child's talking to hospital personnel when no family members are present.

Abdominal wall tenderness may mask more serious internal trauma or peritonitis. Symptoms may be vague and misleading, and the history rarely mentions direct trauma.

MONITORING, LABORATORY TESTS, AND RADIOLOGIC INVESTIGATION
(Table 95-5)

Coagulation studies are rarely needed in practice. Bruises caused by abuse are usually distinctive in shape, pattern, and location, whereas those of organic origin are nondescript and not limited to particular body areas.

Skeletal roentgenograms may reveal injuries that are unexpected or specific for nonaccidental trauma (Table 95-6). Such fractures in a child with other injuries or in a pretoddler or multiple fractures at different stages of healing are virtually pathognomonic for abuse provided metabolic diseases are ruled out. The relative age of skeletal injuries must be documented as accurately as possible (Table 95-7). This is especially important when multiple injuries at different stages of healing show a pattern of recurrent injury over time.

While the child is hospitalized, the abdomen must be reassessed every few hours at first for signs of distention, masses, and change in bowel sounds, which may reveal undetected trauma. The child's skin must be checked daily for a few days. Bruises present on the original examination may assume more distinctive shapes, and newly apparent, noniatrogenic bruises may be found.

Before the child's discharge vision, hearing, and developmental testing may be needed so that future caretakers will know the child's condition and disabilities. Follow-up physical therapy, ophthalmologic examination, and developmental training may be needed.

REPORTING

If, based on reasonable medical probability, a non-accidental injury is likely after full evaluation of the child, the appropriate state agency must be informed. Reports are usually required within a specified time. Most state laws define the means of doing this, whether by phone, written report, or both. Written reports must use common instead of medical terms (e.g., "jaw" instead of "mandible," "bruise" instead of "ecchymosis"). If a medical term is used, it must be briefly explained. The history or various histories can be summarized, followed by a brief interpretation of the pertinent positive and negative findings from the examination and laboratory and radiologic studies.

Table 95-5 Laboratory and Radiologic Studies

Test	Comments
Coagulation studies	Intracranial hemorrhage "Bruises easily" unless pattern-specific injury Widespread nonspecific bruises Family history of bleeding disorder Legal system requires testing
Urinalysis and amylase determination	Any abdominal signs or symptoms
Other chemical tests	History and examination specific
Skeletal roentgenogram	<2 yr: full skeletal survey 2-5 yr: examination guided; site specific >5 yr: rarely positive; site specific if history of fracture in prior 6 mo
Other roentgenograms and CT	History and examination specific

An opinion must be stated as to whether the injuries are nonaccidental.

The parents must be told that the report will be made in accordance with state law and that a child protective services worker or other person will want to interview them. This must be done before the agency personnel arrive unless it is highly probable the family will leave with the child.

If serious injuries have occurred to a child, the court may temporarily place custody of the child with the child protective agency. Depending on state law, this may mean that the caseworker or other professional assigned to the child, rather than the parents, has the legal right to give consent for specific medical procedures. Local law and custom prevail.

TESTIFYING IN COURT

Medical records are frequently subpoenaed for court hearings and must completely document the history, physical findings, and laboratory and radiologic findings.

If called to testify in court, the physician should

Table 95-6   Specificity of Radiologic Findings*

High Specificity	Moderate Specificity†	Common, but Low Specificity†
Metaphyseal lesions	Multiple fractures, especially bilateral	Clavicular fractures
Posterior rib fractures	Fractures of different ages	Long-bone shaft fractures
Scapular fractures	Epiphyseal separations	Linear skull fractures
Spinous process fractures	Vertebral body fractures and subluxations	
Sternal fractures	Digital fractures	
	Complex skull fractures	

*From Kleinman PK. Skeletal trauma: General considerations. In Kleinman P, ed. Diagnostic Imaging of Child Abuse. Baltimore: Williams & Wilkins, 1987, p 6.
†Moderate- and low-specificity lesions become high when history of trauma is absent or inconsistent with injuries.

Table 95-7   Timetable of Radiographic Changes in Children's Fractures*

Category†	Early	Peak	Late
1. Resolution of soft tissues	2-5 days	4-10 days	10-21 days
2. Periosteal new bone	4-10 days	10-14 days	14-21 days
3. Loss of fracture line definition	10-14 days	14-21 days	
4. Soft callus	10-14 days	14-21 days	
5. Hard callus	14-21 days	21-42 days	42-90 days
6. Remodeling	3 mo	1 yr	2 yr to epiphyseal closure

*From O'Conner JF, Cohen J. Dating fractures. In Kleinman P, ed. Diagnostic Imaging of Child Abuse. Baltimore: Williams & Wilkins, 1987, p 112.
†Repetitive injuries may prolong categories 1, 2, 5, and 6.

review the entire medical record, including roentgenograms and laboratory reports, and discuss the facts in advance with the prosecutor. The medical findings must be explained in lay terms, and those that are most pertinent must be pointed out. The physician is considered an expert witness, meaning that testimony can cover factual matters and an opinion about those facts is allowed based on reasonable medical probability. In court the physician must remain neutral. Testimony is meant to explain medical terms and facts to the court that would otherwise not be known or could be misinterpreted, not to make the case for the prosecuting attorney. Questions must be answered by the physician in a factual manner within his range of knowledge. If an answer is not known, he must say so, or if a question is not understood, he may ask to have it repeated or rephrased. Many times questions are asked in a "yes or no" fashion but cannot be answered that simply. If this is the case, an explanation should be given to the judge that the question cannot be answered yes or no and permission sought to explain; then the proceeding will continue according to the judge's ruling. No matter what, the physician must remain professional and calm; the best physician witness is one that, after hearing his testimony, the judge or jury members would feel confident in using for their own medical care.

ADDITIONAL READING

Allman FD, Nelson WB, McComb G. Outcome following cardiopulmonary resuscitation in severe pediatric near drowning. Am J Dis Child 140:571-575, 1986.

Aoki N, Masuzawa H. Subdural hematomas in abused children: Report of six cases from Japan. Neurosurgery 18:475-477, 1986.

Billmire ME, Myers PA. Serious head injury in infants: Accidental or abuse. Pediatrics 75:340-342, 1985.

Caffey J. Multiple fractures in long bones of infants suffering from subdural hematoma. Am J Radiol 56:163-173, 1946.

Cohen RA, Kaufman RA, Myers PA, et al. Cranial computed tomography in the abused child with head injury. Am J Nurs 146:97-102, 1986.

Duhaime AC, Gennarelli TA, Thibault LE, et al. The shaken baby syndrome. A clinical, pathological, and biomechanical study. J Neurosurg 66:409-415, 1987.

• Ellerstein N, ed. Child Abuse and Neglect: A Medical Reference. New York: John Wiley, 1981.

Hahn YS, Raimondi AS, McLone DC, et al. Traumatic mechanisms of head injury in child abuse. Childs Brain 10:229-241, 1983.

Helfer RE, Slovis TL, Black M. Injuries resulting when small children fall out of bed. Pediatrics 60:533-535, 1977.

Hobbs CJ. Skull fracture and the diagnosis of abuse. Arch Dis Child 59:246-252, 1984.

Joffe M, Ludwig S. Stairway injuries in children. Am J Dis Chil 141:383, 1987 (abstr).

Kempe R, Helfer R, eds. The Battered Child, 4th ed. Chicago: University of Chicago Press, 1987.

• Kleinman P, ed. Diagnostic Imaging of Child Abuse. Baltimore: Williams & Wilkins, 1987, pp 6, 112.

Krugman RD. Child abuse and neglect. Primary Care 11:527-534, 1984.

Lenoski EF, Hunter KA. Specific patterns of inflicted burn injuries. J Trauma 17:842-846, 1977.

Ludwig S, Warman M. Shaken baby syndrome: A review of 20 cases. Ann Emerg Med 13:104-107, 1984.

Moritz AR, Henriques FC. Studies of thermal injury: The relative importance of time and temperature in the causation of cutaneous burns. Am J Pathol 23:695-720, 1947.

Purdue GF, Hunt JL, Prescott PR. Child abuse by burning—An index of suspicion. J Trauma 28:221-224, 1988.

Rivera FP, Kamitsuka MD, Quan L. Injuries to children younger than 1 year of age. Pediatrics 81:93-97, 1988.

Wilson EF. Estimation of the age of cutaneous injuries in child abuse. Pediatrics 60:750-752, 1977.

Zimmerman RA, Bilaniuk LT, Bruce DA, et al. Computed tomography of craniocerebral injury in the abused child. Radiology 130:687-690, 1979.

96 Psychosocial Aspects of Pediatric Intensive Care: The Parents

Lenetta G. Hogue

BACKGROUND

The implementation of innovative medical practices in the care of critically ill children has fostered a greater understanding of parents' psychosocial needs relating to pediatric critical care.

The hospitalization of a sick child is very stressful to a family. This stress is magnified when the child must be admitted to the PICU. Parents often must relinquish their previously held status and familiar roles as they enter a foreign environment in which they have very little influence and even less control. Admission of a child to a PICU often places the child's family in a situation that it is ill prepared to handle. Parents may experience feelings of helplessness and hopelessness since the patient's outcome is not always readily known.

Admitting a child to a PICU can hurl the family into a state of crisis. Family members may experience a grief reaction characterized by shock, disbelief, disorganization, and anxiety. The family must rely on a variety of coping mechanisms to maintain equilibrium in the family unit and to adapt to the crisis. In addition it is difficult for many parents to comprehend the nature of their child's health problems and treatment plan because they lack medical training. This can add confusion and concern to an already taxing family situation. A child's hospitalization can also add enormous financial and environmental strain on the family. In addition the location of the PICU may remove the parents from family and other social support networks.

Research has shown that information is essential to help parents cope with the stress of their child's illness. Thus PICU personnel, particularly medical, nursing, and social work staff, have a responsibility to act as a team in providing information to parents and in fostering better communication with them. Health care professionals need to anticipate parents' questions rather than wait for them to be voiced. Many health care professionals forget that parents can be overwhelmed and unwilling to voice questions or concerns because they are intimidated by the PICU setting and the medical regimen. Appropriate intervention by members of all disciplines can address the parents' emotional concerns and help reinforce their coping mechanisms to achieve successful crisis resolution.

EVALUATION

An unresolved family crisis may drastically affect the outcome of the patient's illness. To provide support to the family the PICU personnel must continuously assess and reassess the family dynamics and the parents' coping abilities.

Research supports the significance of including families in developing a plan of care for patients, especially in times of crisis. Parents may use the gathering of information as a strategy to help them anticipate what to expect and what to do next. The information that health care professionals share with the parents must be presented in a clear, concise, and timely fashion. Parents often require repeated explanations because their high anxiety level makes it difficult for them to retain information. As the family's stress decreases, the parents will be able to provide more support to the patient.

Evaluating the emotional adjustment of the patient's parents to the PICU is also of vital importance. Parents will almost certainly experience a great deal of distress when their child is hospitalized. Many parents exhibit bizarre signs of emotional stress, whereas others show no such behavior. Parental emotional responses must be closely monitored to ensure that the child's hospitalization does not disrupt the parent-child relationship. Parents who experience extreme overreaction or underreaction may need closer monitoring and provision of additional intervention and support. Research has shown that single-parent families, parents with preexisting psychiatric problems, and parents experiencing grief from previous losses are more likely to be at greater emotional risk during a crisis. How family members cope with their concerns and fears is largely determined by their intellectual capacities, cultural orientation, individual philosophies, and life experiences.

Some parents display a hopeful, optimistic attitude toward their child's hospitalization. Others may exhibit a negative or pessimistic attitude no matter how grave or hopeful their child's condition may be. Many parents experience the stages of anticipatory grief that are similar to those described by Kübler-Ross regarding object loss: (1) initial shock and denial characterized by refusal or inability to accept the existing situation; (2) feelings of anger, rage, and envy; (3) bargaining or an attempt to postpone the inevitable; (4) depression, in which previous anger is replaced by a feeling of sadness and a sense of great loss; and (5) eventual acceptance, involving a decrease in previous agitation and the onset of a degree of quiet expectation. These stages become very real to the parents as they deal with an anticipated or actual death of a child. Not all parents will experience each of these stages or have the ability to work through them during the course of the child's stay in the PICU. The PICU team members must be alert to and familiar with these stages and accept them as a normal part of the parents' emotional adjustment.

The patient's family must also be evaluated in terms of what social support systems are available to them. Support can be obtained from a variety of sources, including other family members; social, religious, or work affiliations; hospital personnel; other families with a child in the PICU; and community social agencies. Many parents will suffer additional emotional stress because their support systems are inadequate. It is important to assess what support systems are available and whether they are adequate to provide the parents with positive assistance and reinforcement.

INTERVENTION STRATEGIES

Parental stress can be greatly diminished through appropriate interventions on the part of the PICU health care team members, who can intervene in a variety of areas to offer support to a patient's family.

A universal need for all parents with a hospitalized child has been identified as the need for hope. All parents must be allowed to hope that their child may recover, no matter how grave the child's condition.

Parents must also be acquainted with the PICU unit and the waiting room. Thus the PICU personnel must take an active role in providing a tour of the unit itself and the waiting room. It is not unusual to see families keeping an anxious vigil in PICU waiting rooms. A major task for the social worker involves acclimating the patient's family to the hospital environment. Most PICUs must adhere to strict visiting policies, and frequent power struggles may evolve between staff and parents. Parents often feel the need to remain close to their child. Because parents will be bombarded with an array of important decisions to make, they need to feel comfortable in the waiting room as well as in the PICU itself.

Research indicates that parents' ability to cope can be improved when they know who is responsible for the care of their child and know they can communicate with involved staff as often as necessary. Parents are not always aware of who is caring for their child. PICU health care members must introduce themselves every time they speak with patient's parents. During the patient's PICU stay parents are often unable to remember names from one visit to the next. Therefore it is useful to give parents the names and titles of those individuals caring for their child in written form.

The literature emphasizes the need to ensure that the parental role is maintained despite the child's hospitalization. Parents are often forced to deal with deprivation of their normal parenting role. Hospital personnel must work together to ensure that this interruption in parental responsibility is minimized. Parents may be encouraged to assist with the patient's daily care if medically possible, providing them with an opportunity to reduce feelings of helplessness. When possible, parents may even be encouraged to carry out routine patterns of discipline.

Parents need to be encouraged to express their feelings about the patient's hospitalization. Parents will experience a barrage of different feelings. If they are not able to vent these feelings successfully, communication between the parent and the health care team can be impeded. A PICU parent support group can provide a prime opportunity for parents to discuss their feelings. The leader of the group can gather a great deal of information about the parents' coping mechanisms. Information may be shared with other health care professionals to reduce not only the parent's stress, but that of the medical staff.

Referral to outside agencies may also benefit patient families. A child's hospitalization can often be financially, psychologically, and socially taxing. At times community resources can best address specific family needs.

Parents may become concerned about the patient's siblings and their reactions to the patient's hospitalization. Parents often experience lengthy separations from the siblings who remain at home, creating additional parental stress. Parents may need some guidance in dealing with the siblings' potential feelings of abandonment and isolation and with their own guilt feelings related to decreased time and attention available for their nonhospitalized children.

Parents also need to be able to express their grief openly. The PICU health care team may try to facilitate the expression of grief whenever possible. Parents need to feel it is acceptable to experience feelings of anger and sadness. When a patient is critically ill or dying, the family must be afforded longer periods of time to spend with the patient. If a patient does die, it is imperative that the family be provided an opportunity to be alone with the patient's body.

One of the most important interventions the health care team can provide is follow-up contact with the family. This is essential not only for those families who have lost a child but also for families of children who may transfer to a ward or be discharged home. Families can benefit greatly from follow-up in those instances in which an autopsy must be performed. It not only provides the patient's parents an opportunity to ask questions and gain better understanding but also affords the health care team an opportunity to observe how the family is coping

after the child's death. Ongoing contact with the PICU social worker can be very important to the patient's family in ensuring that the family is appropriately referred to outside community resources that are best suited to meet their needs.

With consistent effort on the part of the PICU health care team, parental stress can be greatly diminished. If the team members are open, honest, and available throughout all aspects of the patient's care, recovery, not only for the patient but for the family as well, will be better.

ADDITIONAL READING

Caroff P, Mailick MD. The patient has a family: Reaffirming social work's domain. Soc Work Health Care 10(4):17-34, 1985.

Cataldo MF, Jacobs HE, Rogers MC. Behavioral/environmental considerations in pediatric inpatient care. In Russo DC, Varni JW, eds. Behavioral Pediatrics: Research and Practice. New York: Plenum, 1982.

Epperson M. Families in sudden crisis: Process and intervention in a critical care center. Soc Work Health Care 2(3):265-273, 1977.

Fiser DH, Stanford G, Dorman DJ. Services for parental stress reduction in a pediatric ICU. Crit Care Med 12:504-507, 1984.

• Gowan NJ. The perceptual world of the intensive care unit: An overview of some environmental considerations in the helping relationship. Heart Lung 8:340-344, 1979.

• Hansen M, Young DA, Carden MPH, Carden FE. Psychological evaluation and support in the pediatric intensive care unit. Pediatr Ann 15:61-69, 1986.

Korblum H, Marshall R. A clinical social worker's function as consultant in the neonatal intensive care unit. Soc Work Health Care 7(1):57-64, 1981.

Kübler-Ross E. On Death and Dying. New York: Macmillan, 1980.

Lust BL. The patient in the ICU. A family experience. Crit Care Q 6:49-57, 1984.

Mahan CK, Krueger JC, Schreiner RL. The family and neonatal intensive care. Soc Work Health Care 7(4):67-78, 1982.

Miles MS. Impact of the intensive care unit on parents. Issues Compr Pediatr Nurs 3(7):72-90, 1979.

Molter NC. Needs of relatives of critically ill patients: A descriptive study. Heart Lung 8:332-339, 1979.

Murdach AD. Skills and tactics in hospital practice. Soc Work 28(4):279-284, 1983.

Rodgers CD. Needs of relatives of cardiac surgery patients during the critical care phase. Focus Crit Care 10:50-55, 1983.

Schilling RF II, Schilling RF. Social work and medicine: Shared interests. Soc Work 31(3):231-234, 1987.

Sheridan MS, Johnson DR. Social work services in a high-risk nursery. Health Soc Work 1(2):87-103, 1976.

Silverman E. The social worker's role in shock—trauma units. Soc Work 31(4):311-313, 1986.

Spatt L, Ganas E, Hying S, Kirsch ER, Koch M. Informational needs of families of intensive care unit patients. QRB January, 16-21, 1986.

Videka-Sherman L. Research on the effect of parental bereavement: Implications for social work intervention. Soc Serv Rev 61(1):102-116, 1987.

Waldron JA, Asayama VH. Stress, adaptation, and coping in a maternal-fetal intensive care unit. Soc Work Health Care 10(3):75-89, 1985.

York GY. Religious-based denial in the NICU: Implications for social work. Soc Work Health Care 12(4):31-45, 1987.

97 Psychosocial Aspects of Pediatric Intensive Care: The Patient

Vicki D. Kelley

BACKGROUND

The PICU presents many challenges to a child's ability to cope with unfamiliar, painful, and distressing hospital experiences. The child who does not cope successfully may exhibit psychosocial upset during and after a hospital stay. Some children are more vulnerable, but all children need support and planned interventions to meet the unique threats posed by hospitalization. Careful assessment and planned interventions can help children face the challenges of a PICU admission.

Responses to PICU Hospitalization: Guidelines for Assessment

The ways children respond to hospitalization are determined by many factors. Children most likely to have posthospital psychological upset are those 6 months to 4 years of age who have had repeated hospitalizations and/or a hospital stay longer than 1 week. Other factors have been identified as increasing a child's vulnerability to psychological upset, including developmental considerations, environmental influences, medical diagnosis, and idiosyncratic (personal) influences.

Developmental considerations

Children at different ages have diverse cognitive and behavioral skills. The developmental stage of the child has implications for both the child's coping ability and the planning of interventions to support the child.

Infants and toddlers. Infants are in the sensorimotor stage of development; that is, they deal with the environment through their senses and cope with experiences through motor activity. The environment in the PICU can be overstimulating to the senses and restrictive motorically. Work with infants emphasizes that unusual physical inactivity is frequently a characteristic of the psychologically vulnerable child and that therapy that enables the child to be active on his own behalf can reduce symptomatic behavior, enhance developmental competencies, increase coping behavior, and lead to decreased vulnerability.

Toddlers are in the developmental stage of autonomy vs. shame or doubt, which assumes that a child's positive self-worth and feeling of self-control lead to a sense of autonomy. Newly acquired and mastered personal and environmental control may be removed from a child in the PICU because of his medical condition and necessary treatment. These limitations may lead the infant to use various adaptive or maladaptive coping mechanisms as he attempts to regain control.

Some typical coping behaviors seen in infants and toddlers in the PICU are regression; clinging; changes in physical and/or play activity; decreased exploration; social, physical, or emotional withdrawal; and protest. These coping behaviors represent the individual child's attempts to deal effectively with the PICU experience and need not necessarily be perceived as negative.

Preschoolers. Children approximately 2 through 6 years of age are in the preoperational stage of thinking. These children are egocentric in their thought processes and believe that the world revolves around them. They are unable to process the abstract concepts of illness and disease. Magical thinking is common during these years. Thinking in this way can cause children to believe that hospitalization is a punishment for something they did.

Coping behaviors of preschoolers vary from child to child. Some typical behaviors occurring in reponse to a PICU stay include physical and verbal aggression, regression, withdrawal, and protest. Many children may verbalize their frustration, confusion, and fear. These behaviors, although often difficult for staff members to understand, signal the child's coping efforts and need for acceptance and support.

School-age children. Children approximately 7 to 11 years of age have developed the cognitive capability to reason inductively. Inductive reasoning allows the child to understand a concept better if he has had active experience with it. School-age children who have the opportunity to ask questions, actively manipulate equipment, and visit the unit before admission may display greater understanding of the PICU experience and, as a result, may cope better.

School-age children need to feel industrious and productive. Children develop more positive self-concepts with successful accomplishments. School-age children who experience a PICU stay are usually limited in opportunities to be productive and to feel in control.

Coping behaviors of school-age children may manifest as regression, aggression, withdrawal, protest, and denial. These behaviors may be situationally appropriate when the child is faced with a PICU admission. Efforts to direct the child's feelings into activities that provide choices and feelings of control may be initiated to successfully counteract less effective coping behavior.

Adolescents. Formal operations, a stage of cognitive development, may begin with individuals 12 years of age and older. Adolescents have attained the ability to use deductive reasoning. They can conceptualize ideas and occurrences that they themselves have never experienced or seen. Although tours of the PICU are valuable in preparation for admission, adolescents are better able to imagine the PICU environment without the concrete experience. They are capable of abstract thinking and can use questions, intellectualization, rationalization, and analysis to cognitively master the PICU environment and related experiences.

Identity vs. role confusion is the developmental crisis adolescents experience. They are striving to-

ward independence yet are faced with losing this independence during a PICU stay. Allowing adolescents to make independent choices when possible, respecting their privacy, and recognizing their skills encourage positive identity and coping throughout a PICU stay.

Environmental considerations

Being aware of the child's environment is important. The primary environment of the child is the family: its composition, attitudes, experiences, culture, cohesiveness, and values. Also, has the child been in the PICU previously? Has the child had previous experiences with hospitals? A child who has experienced a grandparent's hospitalization and death, for example, may egocentrically conclude that he will also die or be separated from his family forever, as was his grandparent.

Medical diagnosis

Medical diagnosis is a key factor in influencing how a child responds to the PICU. What limitations are placed on the child as a result of his illness or treatment? What fears are related to the diagnosis and resulting treatment? What feelings of loss result from conditions that alter the child's body image?

Idiosyncratic (personal) characteristics

Idiosyncratic characteristics are those character traits that make a child unique. Each child displays a different temperament and personality. The following are considered dimensions of temperament: activity level, rhythmicity, approach, adaptability, threshold, intensity, mood, distractibility, and persistence. Recognizing a child's temperament and personality can help tailor supportive interventions for each child in the PICU. If the child is shy, has a low intensity level, and adapts slowly to change, he may be labeled incorrectly as depressed; this is particularly true if he is compared to a child of high intensity who is social, outgoing, and persistent. Idiosyncratic characteristics make each child unique. Plans for each child must reflect this uniqueness.

A child's response to a PICU hospitalization is related to many factors, and compiling information about a child's response to a PICU stay is a constant process. Methods of gathering this information include direct observation and interactions with the child, observations of family interactions, discussions with family members, and staff communication. Understanding the child's developmental level, environmental influence, and unique personality assist the PICU staff in understanding a child's behavior and in planning specific interventions to support the child.

INTERVENTIONS

Interventions can be developed that encourage positive coping within the PICU environment. These interventions, frequently carried out by child life specialists, involve the child's family as well as the PICU staff. Two general categories of interventions are developmental and environmental.

Developmental Interventions

Developmental interventions are provided based on understanding of each child's age and unique temperament. These interventions promote emotional attachment, preparation, control and mastery, and play.

Emotional attachment

Separation from parents and other primary support persons is a major factor in psychological upset for a child hospitalized in the PICU. Methods to provide emotional support and attachment and visitation can be encouraged to assist the child in knowing he has not been abandoned. Visitation policy may limit the amount of time the family can be with its child, so placing pictures of family members near the bed provides the child with a concrete reminder that his family continues to be supportive and is near. Tape recordings of familiar sounds such as his mother's voice can provide a sense of security. The sense of smell can be used to provide sensory connection of the infant's emotional attachment (e.g., a father's T-shirt can be placed in the crib). For older children and adolescents emotional attachments may expand beyond the family circle. Visitation and contact with peers through letters, cassette tapes, or photographs provide emotional support.

Family involvement is not the only intervention that can be kept consistent. Primary staff members are an important part of a child's sense of predictability, trust, and routine. When a primary staff member provides a child with truthful and well-thought-out information and answers, the child's PICU experience can be less ambiguous and therefore less stressful. Building a trusting staff relationship with an adolescent is important in helping him feel comfortable when expressing his feelings and asking questions.

Preparation

Preparation can decrease stress and anxiety in the hospitalized child by providing him with information and experiences that promote understanding and mastery of an upcoming event. The event could be a surgery, a procedure, and/or an admission to the PICU. What a child fantasizes or imagines about the PICU can be more upsetting than the actual experience or environment. Preparation allows the child to experience the PICU environment before the time he might feel most vulnerable (e.g., after surgery). Useful preparation activities include tours, sensory experiences, play, and modeling. Unfortunately many children who experience the PICU are those who are admitted on an emergency basis and for whom extensive preparation is not possible.

Tours offer the child the opportunity to visit the unit, meet staff members he will encounter later, ask questions, and manipulate objects in the environment. Children learn through active experimentation. Manipulating objects such as oxygen tubing, cardiac leads, catheters, and IV lines helps the child know what to expect as a patient in the PICU. When parents are involved in preparation tours, the child feels their support in what will become his new environment. Such preparation can also decrease the parent's stress, which, in turn, can decrease the child's stress.

Sensory preparation is a crucial aspect in preparing children for upcoming events, including surgery and PICU admission. Children's concerns revolve around what will be felt and experienced. Preparation can deal with what children will see, hear, feel, smell, and taste. For example, preparing a child for surgery could include seeing and touring the recovery room, feeling and smelling the oxygen with which he will awaken, manipulating the gauze bandage, and feeling where the bandage will be placed.

Play is one way a child learns about the world. Play is educational and expressive and can be a valuable method to prepare the child for coping with the PICU experience. Dolls, stories, puppets, and actual medical equipment can be used as preparation methods to teach the child why procedures are performed and how equipment is used.

Modeling is learning by imitation. Filmed modeling in which the child watches another child encounter a stressful situation, feel scared, receive support, and then adapt to the situation has been a successful modeling technique. Older children have shown more positive reactions to this preparation method than younger children since younger children tend to respond best to sensory preparation.

To determine the most effective method of preparation the individual child must be assessed. Factors to consider when providing preparation interventions are age, developmental level, cognitive capabilities, medical information, timing between preparation and the procedure or surgery (e.g., too much time gives the younger child opportunities to fantasize and may actually increase stress), and anxiety level of parents. Children are sensitive to parental anxiety, and decreasing parents' stress can lead to decreased stress in the child. PICU social work staff members can be particularly helpful in this regard.

Control and mastery

The PICU environment provides few opportunities for the child to feel autonomous. Because of medical necessity, the child in the PICU is given little control over what happens. When possible, it is extremely important to offer the child choices. The choices may be simple but must always be realistic (e.g., does the child want to take medicine from a cup or a syringe?). The child who is allowed these choices believes that he has some control over what happens to him, and having control leads to a sense of mastery. If the child believes he has mastered experiences and the environment, his feelings of vulnerability will decrease, and a positive sense of coping can emerge.

Methods to encourage control and mastery vary with the individual child and by developmental level. For the school-age and adolescent child predictable experiences can be encouraged by posting a daily schedule on the child's bed. The child thus gains a sense of mastery over the experiences because he knows what to expect. This scheduling and predictability allows the child to increase trust in the staff and his environment.

Involvement in familiar, goal-oriented activities gives the young child a sense of mastery. Providing a child with a crib toy similar to the one he has at home is more comforting than presenting a toy he has never seen. Continuation of activities that adolescents find valuable may include hobbies, music, art, literature, sports, and mobile video games. Such an attempt at facilitating the adolescent's adjustment

to the PICU setting may help him develop a positive self-concept.

Play

The importance of play for the hospitalized child has been well documented. Play increases cognitive mastery and can be an expressive tool that allows the child a cathartic experience. In addition play can be diversional, allowing the child the opportunity to experience pleasure in an environment that is potentially overwhelming and unfamiliar. Play can enhance a child's sense of control and normalization.

Medical play provided by a well-trained professional (e.g., a child life specialist) is a valuable intertervention. Medical play enables the staff to understand better the child's perception of the PICU experience. Such play can be nondirective or directive. Nondirective medical play allows the child to manipulate and explore medical equipment independently while the staff member closely observes the child's expression of feelings, understanding, misconceptions, or fears. Directive medical play is more goal directed in that it can be educational for the child. Staff members can clarify misunderstandings, explain what the child is experiencing, and help define what is expected of the child during procedures.

Environmental Interventions

PICU staff members have responsibility to provide interventions that encourage positive patient coping. The following examples are environmental interventions specific to the child experiencing the PICU.

Controlling the factors that cause environmental overload (noise, lighting, crowding, painful or disturbing touch and odors) of the PICU can be a challenge. Constant noise in the environment can be muted with tape recordings and soothing music. Taped messages from friends help to provide continuity for the school-age child. An effective way to decrease the extreme, possibly stressful auditory stimulation of the PICU is to have the patient wear headphones while listening to tapes.

Complex care in the environment necessitates constant lighting. It may be beneficial to place children near windows where a day/night cycle can be observed. Infants often keep their eyes closed or fixated on a bright light. Appropriate visual stimulation that is positioned at angles to shade the eyes but allows enough light for viewing the patient can increase the child's visual exploration.

Many PICUs are crowded. A conscious effort must be made by every staff member to control the negative effect of crowding. If a child is awake and alert, he will probably feel less vulnerable if groups of staff members discuss issues away from the bedside. Locating equipment as far from the bed as safely possible allows the child a larger area that he may perceive as his own space.

Painful and disturbing touch and odors are part of the critical care environment. The issue facing staff members is how to provide positive, soothing touch and pleasant smells. One obvious intervention may be to allow time to provide stroking or massage; however, some children need a verbal cue before even gentle touch is initiated until they learn that not all touch in the PICU is painful. Disturbing odors from alcohol, tape, and plastic may be sensory factors that are easily overlooked because staff members have learned to shut them out. Olfactory stimulation that is pleasant and/or familiar can be provided to counteract the unpleasant smells. A parent's article of clothing or pillows and blankets from home have scents that are familiar and comforting to the child.

CONCLUSION

A multidisciplinary approach to programming for the child in the PICU can effectively meet the child's needs. Assessments by and communication between all disciplines will result in an effective approach to helping the PICU patient and family. With appropriate assessment, support, and planned intervention, the child patient in the PICU can maintain psychological well-being while physical well-being is strengthened.

ADDITIONAL READING

• Baker CF. Sensory overload and noise in the ICU: Source of environmental stress. Crit Care Q 6(4):66-80, 1984.

Bates TA, Broome M. Preparation of children for hospitalization and surgery: A review of the literature. J Pediatr Nurs 1:230-239, 1986.

Bellack JP, Fore CV. The young child in the critical care unit. In Fore C, Poster EC, eds. Meeting Psychosocial Needs of Children and Families in Health Care. Washington, D.C.: Association for the Care of Children's Health, 1985, pp 43-51.

Betz CL, Poster EC. Incorporating play into the care of the hospitalized child. Issues Compr Pediatr Nurs 7:343-355, 1984.

Douglas JWB. Early hospital admissions and later disturbances of behavior and learning. Dev Med Child Neurol 17:456-480, 1975.

Ferguson F. Childhood coping: Adaptive behavior during intensive care hospitalization. Crit Care Q 6(4):81-93, 1984.

• Jones L. Pediatric Intensive Care Units: Strategies for Emotional and Developmental Support. Dallas: Children's Medical Center of Dallas, 1986.

Liakapoulou M, Patterson A, Samaraweera S, Finnegan L. Developmental interventions in infancy during lengthy hospitalizations. J Dev Behav Pediatr 4:213-217, 1983.

McCue K. Medical play: An expanded perspective. J Assoc Care Child Health 16(3):157-161, 1988.

Nagera H. Children's reactions to hospitalization and illness. Child Psychiatry Hum Dev 9:3-19, 1978.

Piaget J. The Language and Thought of the Child. New York: Meridian Books, 1953.

Provence S. Some relationships between activity and vulnerability in the early years. In Anthony EJ, Koupernik C, eds. The Child in His Family: Children at Psychiatric Risk. New York: John Wiley & Sons, 1974, pp 157-166.

Ruddy-Wallace M. Temperament: Assessing individual differences in hospitalized children. J Pediatr Nurs 2:30-36, 1987.

Thomas R. Comparing Theories of Child Development. Belmont, Calif.: Wadsworth, 1979.

98 Psychosocial Aspects of Pediatric Intensive Care: The Staff

Katherine Lipsky

BACKGROUND

The crisis orientation of the PICU that envelops pediatric patients and their families also affects PICU staff members. This focus on crisis creates certain environmental conditions and work expectations that place unique stresses and challenges on PICU personnel. The purpose of this chapter is twofold: to identify the particular stresses intrinsic to the PICU milieu and to delineate specific organizational interventions that can attenuate such stresses, thus, hopefully, improving job performance, enhancing staff satisfaction, and reducing unit turnover.

In the PICU setting emergency is routine. What is considered normal work in a PICU would be considered an emergency necessitating maximal attention in many other areas of hospital life. PICU staff members must become accustomed to this intensity if they are to avoid working in a state of chronic fear and exhaustion. At the same time, however, they must remain alert so that at any given moment they can make an immediate distinction between what is serious and what is not. The frenetic PICU environment exposes staff to a massive array of sensory stimuli; space is often limited, and the noise level is often high. Patient acuity demands constant vigilance. Highly complex technologic procedures and equipment must be mastered. Distraught parents must be informed and supported. In an environment in which every procedure is potentially lifesaving, any mistake in judgment or execution could prove catastrophic. Finally, death is an ever-present possibility in the PICU, an unrelenting reminder to the staff of their

own vulnerability. It is, then, in this highly charged, fast-paced, overstimulating environment that PICU physicians and nurses go about the daily business of trying to save the lives of the critically ill children entrusted to their care.

The detrimental effects that a PICU admission can have on patients and their families are more thoroughly researched and documented than are the potential repercussions of those same environmental influences on the PICU medical staff. Medical and surgical attending physicians bear the ultimate responsibility for patient management decisions. Rotating house officers are forced to respond quickly and accurately to emergency situations in an unfamiliar setting. Many interns and residents are scheduled to work long, consecutive hours during their PICU rotations. Often their nursing colleagues have more PICU experience and may question their authority and judgment.

Although the literature related to physician stress and coping in the critical care setting is still quite limited, certain trends in terms of shared stresses and common coping strategies have emerged. The most common stressor described by both house staff and faculty attending physicians is providing prolonged care to patients with multisystem failure and a poor prognosis. Other commonly reported stresses included the frequent deaths of pediatric patients and a sense of loss over the children's untapped potential, constant emergencies calling for quick and difficult decision making, and ethical dilemmas in patient care. The physical setting of the unit itself frequently was named as a significant stressor, specifically the close quarters and high noise level. Sleep deprivation also was cited repeatedly as a PICU-associated stressor. Several studies examined the relationship between sleep deprivation and progressive deterioration in the ability to perform tasks related to patient care in terms of vigilance, motivation, and emotional stability.

The most frequently reported mechanisms for coping with the demands of the PICU environment include the following behaviors: strong and consistent leadership by the attending physician; good communication among physicians, both within the house staff ranks and between house officers and faculty attending physicians; open communication between physicians and PICU nursing staff; opportunity for adequate sleep recovery; availability of psychosocial support personnel such as a full-time social worker assigned to the unit; the use of humor; and involvement in out-of-work activities such as hobbies or exercise.

These physician coping mechanisms underscore the importance of providing both formal and informal settings in which communication can take place across health care disciplines and within the physician hierarchy. The goal of these communication opportunities is to turn the potential for indifferent or competitive relationships among physician/physician and physician/nurse coworkers into supportive or collegial relationships.

Nurses form the core of the patient care team, and they have to function in the hectic PICU environment week after week. Physically the nurse is the staff member who spends the most time in the PICU. Psychologically it is the nurse who must interact with family members and with the numerous medical, technical, and support personnel who make transient appearances. Studies that examine the effects of PICU work exposure on nursing staff are reported in the literature more extensively than are similar studies performed on physicians. Much of the research in the area of nursing focuses on three major themes: stressors inherent in PICU nursing and the relationship of such stressors to nurse burnout and to job satisfaction.

The literature on stressors inherent to the PICU divides nursing responses into three major categories: (1) the physical environment of the PICU; (2) direct patient care variables; and (3) professional and interpersonal issues. Although certain problems

and concerns span all three categories, use of these general divisions helps to focus on specific nursing reactions to the PICU milieu.

The physical environment of the PICU presents its nursing staff with many challenges. PICUs frequently are separated physically from other nursing units. Critical care nurses may be required to wear distinctive uniforms that mark them as different from their nursing colleagues. The highly specialized PICU nurses often are viewed with considerable ambivalence by other nursing personnel, adding psychological separation to geographic distance. Space is often limited; noise volume is often high; the environment is overcrowded and overstimulating; the physical demands of the job can be considerable; and complex technical equipment, intricate monitoring devices, and precise and delicate procedures must all be mastered.

Direct patient care stressors most frequently described in the nursing literature center around the demanding acuity level of PICU patients and around the issues of death and dying. Nurses report feeling the pressure of making critical decisions about life and death issues and struggling over the ethical dilemmas that are associated with the provision of critical care. The demands of distraught relatives can drain emotions and consume nursing time. The fear of making mistakes may become chronic and paralyzing since it is realized that margins for error can be small and that a clinical misjudgment could prove catastrophic. Paradoxically, in the midst of this emergency-oriented atmosphere of the PICU patient care requires that the nurses carry out incessant repetitive routines. Nurses are often so involved in collecting and charting data that they have frustratingly little time to interpret the information obtained. Finally, death is imminent in the PICU, serving as a constant reminder of the nurses' own mortality.

The professional and interpersonal issues most frequently described as PICU nursing stressors are divided equally between knowledge preparation inadequate for task demand and unsatisfactory work relationships. Feelings of inadequate preparation can interfere with decision-making ability and increase fear of failure, which in turn can contribute to suboptimal performance. Dissatisfaction with work relationships includes those with fellow staff nurses, with physicians, and with nursing administration. Competitive or indifferent relationships with nursing coworkers were repeatedly reported as high sources of stress. Relations with physicians tended to be characterized by two negative aspects: overzealousness and lack of experience. Physicians were viewed as either inappropriately encroaching on nursing authority and responsibility or as lacking in specific PICU knowledge and shirking their responsibility. The most frequently reported stressor related to nursing administration was a rigid policy-setting framework that was out of touch with and therefore unresponsive toward the daily demands of a PICU's harried pace.

Certainly the number and variety of nursing stressors just reviewed offer ample evidence that the PICU setting provides significant environmental, patient care, intrapsychic, and interpersonal challenges. However, although early nursing studies tended to suggest that PICU nurses were under more stress and thus in geater danger of burnout than were their non-critical care colleagues, the better designed, later studies comparing PICU nurses to non-unit-based nurses failed to support that premise. Indeed, several recent studies have revealed that nursing job satisfaction was comparable in PICU and non-PICU areas, that nursing turnover rates in both areas were virtually identical, and that the level of subjective distress reported by nursing staff in PICU areas was no greater than that reported in non-critical care areas. Thus, although stressors intrinsic to the PICU environment may be high and may have certain unique characteristics, they are not necessarily perceived by critical care nursing staff as more negative than the stressors described by floor nursing staff as intrinsic to their own work environment.

Still, burnout and job dissatisfaction are evident among all nursing ranks today. Accordingly, it is important to recognize the signs and symptoms of burnout and to delineate strategies of intervention designed to diminish the potential for professional burnout and enhance job satisfaction, quality, and productivity. Burnout is characterized by physical and emotional exhaustion and a loss of compassion and respect for patients. It is the behavioral manifestation of an individual's inability to cope with constant emotional stress. Characteristic behavioral signs and symptoms include irritability, rigidity, suspiciousness, emotional distancing, inappropriate or cruel use of humor, loss of concern, and decreased ability to make plans or decisions. Absenteeism, serious on-the-job errors, and patient neglect can be the tangible results of a nurse experiencing burnout. Burnout also can occur as a group phenomenon, with a whole unit getting swept into its negative and paralyzing spiral. Signs and symptoms that can typify a unit undergoing burnout include the following group behaviors: scapegoating, expressions of helplessness and hopelessness, lack of cooperation or initiative, and a critical attitude toward coworkers.

INTERVENTIONS

Because job demands and job fatigue are both very real, it is valuable to investigate intervention strategies designed to help nurses cope with stresses inherent in working in a PICU. In general such interventions fall into two broad categories: knowledge enhancement and facilitation of group cohesion. Knowledge enhancement can be achieved through carefully planned orientation, training, and ongoing in-service education programs. Group cohesion can be facilitated through opportunities to participate in group social activities and through provision of formal nursing support groups. Before examining the potential effectiveness of each of these alternatives, it is important to emphasize that no organizational intervention designed to increase job satisfaction or reduce job turnover is a substitute for a full and balanced life away from the hospital setting.

The PICU nurse must possess a broad knowledge base, quick recall, and the ability to apply knowledge with speed and accuracy to be able to deal with the complexity and variety of diseases, treatment regimens, and equipment she encounters in the PICU. A thorough initial period of orientation and training is essential. This training must focus on work characteristics specific to the PICU and must include both technical and psychosocial aspects of patient care. The nursing literature identifies knowledge as a major mechanism for coping successfully with stress. Studies reveal an inverse relationship between the two variables; as knowledge increases, the critical care nurse's perception of stress tends to decrease. The indication that knowledge about stressors apparently reduces the severity of a stress reaction underscores the utility of comprehensive orientation and training for newly hired PICU nursing staff. Regularly scheduled, compulsory ongoing education sessions also must be provided. PICU nurses must be given the tools they need to keep abreast of the ever-expanding therapeutic and technologic interventions available to them. In addition to such physiologic and technologic topics, ongoing in-service education subjects must include conflict resolution and philosophic, ethical, psychological, cultural, interpersonal, and grief issues related to pediatric critical care.

One useful forum for ongoing education in which the preceding topics can be addressed is the health team staff meeting. Weekly meetings can be held that are attended by PICU medical, nursing, respiratory therapy, and psychosocial staff. Each meeting could proceed as follows: one complex patient is presented. Problems are identified and a treatment plan is devised and agreed on that includes individual staff responsibilities for follow-up care. Medical, nursing, and psychosocial aspects of the case are examined. Staff issues related to the particular patient and his family are raised and discussed. The nursing care plan devised as the result of such a staff meeting is shared with personnel on all work shifts. In this way nurses who were unable to attend the conference are recognized as potential contributors to the patient's overall health care planning.

A growing body of nursing literature indicates that the encouragement and facilitation of a feeling of group belonging and commitment offers the best basis for cooperative resolution of the many practical and emotional problems inherent in working in a PICU.

One supportive measure that can be taken to develop staff cohesion involves planned social activities. Spontaneous informal socializing often occurs among PICU nurses. Such activities can enhance morale and promote a sense of group identity. In addition several large planned annual events can be scheduled that are aimed at increasing feelings of solidarity and esprit de corps. For example, a yearly holiday party for patient graduates from the unit can provide PICU nurses with rewarding tangible testimony to their own competence and caring.

Another supportive measure is to ensure the delivery of appropriate positive feedback. Too often mistakes are pointed out, whereas good work is not recognized or rewarded. Establishing systems to provide encouragement and positive reinforcement can help improve staff morale and heighten staff members' feelings of belonging to an elite and motivated group. The PICU social worker often is in an ideal position to pass on words of praise from patient families and work colleagues that might otherwise remain unknown to PICU nursing staff.

The creation of ongoing nursing support groups for unit nurses is yet another supportive measure

that can be taken to enhance a sense of group cohesion and commitment. The support groups can be designed to explore both the positive and negative aspects of the PICU work experience. An important distinction must be made between the support group and a therapy group. A therapy group consists of identified patients seeking to make changes in their personal behaviors and lives. In contrast, a support group serves to enhance job performance and satisfaction. Support groups deal with intrapsychic issues only when they are interfering with the workplace. Care must be taken to ensure that group communication focuses on the PICU situation rather than expanding into more general self-exploration. Verbal interchange must not be allowed to interfere with comfortable working relationships between group sessions.

Support group meetings can provide an opportunity for the following: an avenue for expressing and resolving intragroup concerns; recognition that uncertainty and anxiety are acceptable feelings shared by all PICU nurses; a safe forum in which doubts and errors can be discussed without hostility amid the realization that minor mistakes are inevitable and need not be a paralyzing source of guilt or shame; a sharing of knowledge, both technical and interpersonal, that individual nurses have found useful in dealing with problems arising on the job; and an arena for developing constructive collective solutions to problems and exchanging effective group suggestions for improved unit communication.

There is a growing trend to use support groups for nurses in critical care settings. However, the literature makes it clear that not all support groups succeed. Indeed, many fail to achieve group attendance and cohesion. Certain factors that have been identified as positive indicators for group success include groups that were initiated in response to staff nurse requests and were supported, but not mandated, by nursing administration; groups that were kept highly structured and did not allow early expression of intense negative feelings; groups in which the leader was not an actual nursing staff member but was known and respected by the group (e.g., a psychosocial professional working in the hospital); and groups in which problems discussed were chiefly interpersonal and could be dealt with inside the group rather than the group's focusing primarily on environmental or administrative issues beyond its control.

Recent research comparing support groups that succeed with those that fail stresses the importance of a highly structured format. Groups must be time limited, with an option for renewable time expansion. Short-term support groups, if properly led, apparently are as constructive as long-term ones.

A practical starting point for initial nursing support group sessions is the discussion of a problem patient or patient family. This early focus on patient-related, rather than intrastaff, concerns accomplishes two objectives: first, it allows the leader time to gain the group's trust, including trust about confidentiality issues; second, it demonstrates to group members that the group will not be overwhelmed by its own aggression, a common concern for individuals newly embarked on a group experience.

Another format structure that is common to successful groups is for the leader to provide closure at the end of each group session. This closure process must include three components: (1) a brief summary of the discussion content, (2) restatement of the positive actions or solutions suggested by the group, and (3) setting of an agenda for the next session that is built on the current session.

The major goals of support groups for PICU nurses include enhanced morale, improved communication, and reduced turnover, with the hope that these changes will ultimately result in better patient care. Research studies that measure these specific outcome variables must be carefully conducted to evaluate objectively the success of nursing support groups and to determine whether the growing use of this modality is justified in the PICU setting.

In contrast to the staff nurses, the nursing leader of the PICU is in a lonely and difficult position in terms of job stresses and coping options available to deal with those stresses. The nurse leader often must handle conflicting needs and expectations. At times she literally is enmeshed in incompatible roles since she must perform administrative policy and, at the same time, protect staff nurses from undue negative stressors, some of which are created by the very administrative management that she serves.

The position of nurse supervisor is a pivotal one. Research shows that her leaderhip style strongly affects the attitudes and behavior of the PICU staff nurses. Effectiveness of critical care nursing leadership style has been studied along two major variables: consideration and structure. Consideration emphasizes concern for group members' needs and stresses mutual trust, respect, and two-way communication. Alternatively, structured leadership emphasizes the achievement of organizational goals and pushes for production. Studies have shown that high-consideration leadership is associated with increased job satisfaction and decreased staff burnout. Staff nurse job satisfaction scores have been found to be lower in critical care units with head nurses whose leadership style is perceived as low consideration and high structure.

The nurse director of a PICU, therefore, must seek to strike an appropriate balance between considering staff needs and ensuring unit productivity. This is often a difficult balance to maintain with staff nurses, nursing administration, and PICU medical faculty potentially setting differing directions and priorities. Unfortunately group support and social activities open to staff nurses to help them cope with stress reduction may not be appropriate or available for leaders' participation. Fortunately stress relief can be available from working with a fair and consistent PICU medical director, having a nursing administrator as a supervisor who herself ranks high in consideration leadership style, or gaining support from nursing directors of other care areas in the hospital who understand the sense of wearying isolation that can play a significant part in any nursing leadership role.

• • •

In summary, the PICU setting places demands and stresses on its medical and nursing staff as well as on its patients and their waiting families. Selye's classic work on stress promotes the following description: stress is defined as the nonspecific response of the body to demands made on it that can have both negative *and positive* valences. Staffing a PICU, as physician or nurse, presents continuous and complex challenges and pressures. It also presents powerful and unique chances for life-saving interventions and for feelings of mastery and worth. Perhaps no concept captures the essence of the challenge before PICU staff as vividly or succinctly as the ancient Chinese symbol for crisis. This symbol is comprised of the juxtaposition of two separate characters—one is danger; the other, opportunity.

ADDITIONAL READING

Bryson RW, Anderman M, Sampiere JM, et al. Intensive care nurse: Job tension and satisfaction as a function of experience level. Crit Care Med 13:767-769, 1985.

Chiriboga DA, Bailey J. Stress and burnout among critical care and medical surgical nurses: A comparative study. Crit Care Q 9(3):84-92, 1986.

Cronin-Stubbs D, Rooks CA. The stress, social support and burnout of critical care nurses: The results of research. Heart Lung 14:31-39, 1985.

Duxburg ML, Armstrong GD, Drew DJ, et al. Head nurse leadership style with staff burnout and job satisfaction in neonatal intensive care units. Nurs Res 33(2):97-101, 1984.

• Eisendrath SJ, Link N, Matthay M. Intensive care unit: How stressful for physician? Crit Care Med 14:95-98, 1986.

Esteban AN, Ballesteros P, Caballero J. Psychological evaluation of intensive care nurses. Crit Care Med 11:616-620, 1983.

Finn A, Speidel BD. Shift system for senior house officer on call duties on a neonatal intensive care unit. Br Med J 296:343-344, 1988.

Fiser DH, Stanford G, Dorman D. Services for parental stress reduction in a pediatric ICU. Crit Care Med 12:504-507, 1984.

Goldman LS, Chase PK. Depression in intensive care units. Int J Psychiatry Med 17(3):201-211, 1987.

• Hay D, Oken D. The psychological stresses of intensive care unit nursing. Psychosom Med 34(2):109-118, 1972.

Huckabay LMD, Jagla B. Nurses' stress factors in the intensive care unit. J Nurs Adm 9(2):21-26, 1979.

Keane A, Ducette H, Adler DC. Stress in ICU and non ICU nurses. Nurs Res 34(4):231-236, 1985.

Lewis DJ, Robinson JA. Assessment of coping strategies of ICU nurses in response to stress. Crit Care Nurs 6(1):38-43, 1986.

MacNeil JM, Weisz GM. Critical care nursing stress: Another look. Heart Lung 16:274-277, 1987.

Mann EE, Kunkan JJ. Retaining staff: Using turnover indices and surveys. J Nurs Adm 18(7/8):17-23, 1988.

Norbeck JS. Types and services of social support for managing job stress in critical care nursing. Nurs Res 34(4):225-230, 1985.

Selye H. The Stress of Life. New York: McGraw-Hill, 1971.

Spoth R, Konewko P. Intensive care staff stressors and life event changes across multiple settings and work units. Heart Lung 16:278-284, 1987.

Stratton H. Managing stress in the ICU. Nurs Mirror 161(14):15, 1985.

Vincent P, Coleman WF. Comparison of major stressors perceived by ICU and non ICU nurses. Crit Care Nurs 6(1):64-69, 1986.

Weiner MF, Caldwell T, Tyson J. Stresses and coping in ICU nursing: Why support groups fail. Gen Hosp Psychiatry 5:179-183, 1983.

• Weiner MF, Caldwell T. The process and impact of an ICU nurse support group. Int J Psychiatry Med 13(1):47-54, 1983.

99   The PICU Experience: The Parents' Point of View

Bill Hare · Cathy Hare

The following presents two parents' views of the PICU experience. Because we are distinct individuals we often react to situations in somewhat different manners. Bill tends to remain calm in emergencies; Cath relies on emotion. For that reason our memories of events must be balanced. What we had in common during this ordeal was our beautiful 14-year-old daughter Laura. As her parents, we submit the following narrative.

Bill: I remember very clearly going to our family physician's office with Cath and Laura as we often did with our kids—another cold or flu . . . quick visit . . . go fill the prescription . . . have them home for a few days. I was a little concerned when the doctor said to go to the hospital for a few tests.

Cathy: We settled Laura into a room, and nurses came in to try to take a blood sample. Laura was not cooperating, and I remember being embarrassed by her hostility. I couldn't understand why she didn't seem to hear me talking to her or to the doctors and nurses. People seemed anxious about her. I wanted them to give her something, to *do* something, then let us take her home. It soon became apparent that this was serious. Bill had not come back yet, and the doctor was talking about transferring her to Children's Medical Center by *ambulance*. She may have Reye's syndrome. This cannot be happening; dear God, let me wake up!

Bill: When I returned from the airport, I went to find Cath and Laura, expecting to find them in the outpatient area, but they weren't there. I stepped off the elevator; two doctors approached me and said that Laura was very sick and needed to be transported to Children's Medical Center immediately. There was a lot of commotion going on—nurses and aides

trying to get Laura ready to move—all very efficient and professional but with very little time for explanations. Reye's syndrome was mentioned, along with some equally bad possibilities, but none of them meant anything to me. It all seemed to be going so fast, and it was so unexpected. I walked out of that elevator into a crazy world that seemed to be going 100 miles an hour. I felt confused, helpless, uncertain of exactly what was goint on; yet everyone wanted decisons—now!—but decisons about what? Were these choices, or were they just trying to be nice? No choice really, based on what they said. Sure, I agree; we'll transfer her to Children's. Cath and I didn't have more than a minute to talk. I remember we did decide that Cath would go in the ambulance, and I'd follow her. The impact still hadn't hit me.

Cathy: I had never even been in an ambulance before. I kept thinking to myself, "Why Children's? We don't know any doctors who practice there." The ambulance attendants were wonderfully kind. I could hear Laura yelling in the back. They didn't use the siren because they said it might frighten her.

Bill: Thirty minutes later I was in another hospital trying to find Cath and Laura. I was directed to the third floor intensive care unit, which was to become our home for the next 10 days. But we couldn't go in; so we just sat there for several hours.

Cathy: We sat for awhile; our friend and priest joined us, and we started the incredible waiting. We called Michael, Laura's older brother, to let him know where we were. He kept asking us how she was, but we didn't have any answers.

Bill: We tried to kill time by going down to the coffee shop and walking around the halls, but even that was distracting. There were young kids everywhere, all of them obviously very sick; some were in wheelchairs, others in little wagons pulled by their brothers or sisters, some by themselves with IV's stuck in their arms and hung from poles that they pushed along the corridors. This was obviously a place for kids who were very, very sick. So what was Laura doing here? When they finally let us in to see Laura, she didn't seem to recognize us. She was like a crazy woman, beating and screaming at people, yelling and even trying to *bite* nurses. Our priest went in with us.

Cathy: Although I was angry that we had had to wait several hours to see Laura, I realized when we walked into the unit that we would have been in the way. There were four or five other children in surrounding beds, all hooked up to machines. It was like walking into a movie set filming a disaster scene. We had to put on protective, sterilized gowns and masks. As we walked back down the hallway, I began to cry and told Bill we had to call my mother and sister. I needed to make those phone calls and yet didn't know what to tell them except to get to Dallas as soon as possible. That was the first time the seriousness of the situation hit home for me. I was afraid Laura was not going to make it.

Sometime in that first night we were told that Reye's syndrome can be brought on by taking aspirin if the child has the flu or chickenpox. I had given her aspirin. I simply cannot describe the sense of guilt I felt. I had caused her to be in this condition! Probably many parents of children in PICU incorrectly blame themselves for their child's being there. The one you love most in the world, for whom you would lay down your life, is there, and you are somehow to blame.

Bill: We had to wait again for several hours. Then we began a parade that lasted all through the night, with various doctors and surgeons and nurses inviting us to sit in a little room, the family waiting room, explaining all the details, none of which we really understood, and asking us to sign various releases and forms. It went on like that all night, each time requiring progressively more dramatic action.

Cathy: Out of a fog we found ourselves discussing the chances of our baby's survival. I remember being told that she might be "salvageable." I do not know how you can move from terror to feeling more terrified, but it happened. It was like the sound of a swiftly moving river turning into a flood. It simply increased in volume and speed until I thought my mind and heart would explode.

The doctor in charge was very professional and extremely honest about Laura's condition. She told us the hospital policy was to give parents all the pertinent facts and to explain our child's condition clearly. I remember wishing she were not so blunt. As the night progressed and our nerves became raw, I became rigid, resented the doctor's professionalism, and began thinking she was somehow responsible for all this. How irrational parents can become in this situation. We have no choice but to trust in the expertise of doctors, but it is not easy to let someone else take charge of a child to whom you have given birth and raised. There is almost a sense of outrage.

I also remember seeing all the people in the waiting area and wondering, "What is wrong with their children? How long have they been here?" They were a roomful of strangers with whom we were somehow intimately connected, and the connecting link was seriously ill children. I wondered why they were there; but during the entire time we were there, I never entered into a meaningful conversation with any of them. I think it was out of fear. Somehow the fear of death is so pervasive. It took all the emotional strength I could muster to hang on myself, let alone try to be brave or consoling to someone else. As I write this, the words seem so selfish; but they were true, at least for me.

Bill: At some point we were told that they would have to drill a hole in Laura's skull to determine the amount of pressure on the brain.

Cathy: When they asked our permission to insert the catheter, I thought, "My God, her brain! Even though this is a fine hospital, shouldn't we consider having her transferred to New York or somewhere else? She's so young; what if they slip and she is brain damaged? Can I deal with that?" We were told Laura was being put into a drug-induced coma. Words become ominous. "Coma—people go into comas and never come out of them! Don't do that to our baby!" But you come down to only one choice—trust.

Bill: They wanted to tell us about all these choices and have us make decisions; and we were practically going crazy, hardly able to understand what they were saying, much less make some decisions. I knew in the back of my mind that they knew what they were doing. But after a while we told them we wouldn't go back in that little room for any more conferences. Just do what they had to do and tell us about it as soon as they could. I have always felt that

I have been a person who could look at any situation, digest the facts, and, like a computer, spit out the answer almost instantaneously. But in this case it was as though they were talking to me in Chinese. I could hardly figure out what they were talking about, much less make decisions. All I wanted them to do was make Laura well. I was getting angry with them. They were like some sort of bureaucratic paper mill that kept pushing these forms at us to sign. What good were they anyway? I was tired of forms and of doctors. Above all, however, I didn't want to upset them or do anything that would cause Laura to be in any jeopardy. So we signed the forms and tried to keep our sanity through the night.

Cathy: I suppose looking back on it, the family conference room became the symbol of awful decisions. Like Bill, I also eventually refused to go back in there. We made several more phone calls to friends, relatives, and priests, including one to Laura's high school, and we spoke to the dean. What would have been a routine call to report her absence was instead a tearful conversation that ended as did all our other calls—please pray for her.

Bill: By morning they told us Laura might stay in a coma for 5 to 7 days, that it was better for her and gave her a better chance of survival—great choice of words. All night the doctors and nurses could see how upset we were, and they tried to keep us as calm as possible, but words like "coma" and "survival" tend to make you a little crazy and not too logical or organized.

I remember going in to see Laura early the next morning, and my first reaction was, "God, I've never seen so many machines hooked up to a person before." There were tubes everywhere—in her mouth, in her nose, a catheterization tube, IVs in her arms, a monitor in her skull, ECGs bleeping across the screens, digital readouts of blood pressure and heart rate. It was an incredible array of equipment. It reminded me of something out of a science fiction movie; I was actually fascinated about how all of it really worked. It distracted me from the reality of what was going on. I know I bugged the nurses and the doctors for days every time that I was in there about what each one meant, what the normal ranges were, and how the numbers were going. It became important to me that I wasn't just standing idly by. I grew to understand what numbers they were looking for. It took away some of that helplessness and gave me something to concentrate on.

Cathy: I remember the first time I saw Laura hooked up to those intimidating machines. Some had numbers; some had blips. The staff had carefully and patiently explained the importance of each. Bill said he was able to understand and "decode" them and in that way had a sense of participation. All I could think was, "What if they are not connected properly? What if there is a power failure? What if the people who clean around her bed should accidentally unplug one? What kind of grades did these nurses and doctors get in medical training?" I didn't ask these questions, but they all revolved around and around in my brain like horses on a carousel.

My mother and sister arrived early that morning. We followed the rules, mostly because the nurses at the station asked us to and because they were simply so wonderful to us and to my mother, letting us visit as often as we liked as long as we were not in the way of other patients and parents.

During the next few days we answered endless questions about her past medical history. Had she ever taken drugs? Parents of a teenager today have to respond honestly, "We do not know." Dear God, I thought, please do not let her have a drug problem. The days became times for waiting for test results, for signing a release for a liver biopsy. To the average person the word *biopsy* is terrifying. Waiting for those results, waiting and praying, became a way of life.

Bill: We waited there for hours and days for Laura to make a comeback. I'd go in to see Laura during the day. Even though she was in a coma, I'd talk to her about all the equipment and what good treatment she was getting and tell her how her numbers were going—and how she should hang in there. There were times when I would see something change, and I would call the doctor or nurse and feel particularly good if they did something or adjusted something that would bring that number back down or settle it more. It was as though I were part of the team, helping to make her better. I was determined to know as much about that equipment as any doctor or nurse in that hospital.

Cathy: How did I fill the spaces of time between going in to see Laura? Bill and I never left the hospital at the same time except at night when my sister slept on the floor of the waiting room. We felt someone had to be present in case the situation changed. Like the other families we ate most of our meals in the hospital dining room. We had so many wonderful friends who came to be with us. We would try to catch some naps sitting up in chairs, but tension and strain made that nearly impossible. As long as we had each other to talk to or our family and friends were there, I was distracted. But then something would grab my heart, and I would feel the fear creep back to the surface. I spent a lot of time praying my rosary or reading the Bible.

Bill: Checking in and out of the nurses' station became our regular routine. We always wanted them to know where we were. We spent a lot of time walking around the courtyard visiting with friends. It was difficult seeing those kids in the hallways pushing their portable IV units. We could never totally relax during those days Laura was in the coma. I appreciated the distraction when people would come by to see us. It made the time go faster.

Cathy: Some of our friends brought their children when they came, and many of Laura's friends from school came by. It helped me to see normal kids horsing around and to put my arms around them. One day our son Michael came. He was having such a difficult time with all of this. His high school graduation was just a week away, and we were having to spend all our time at the hospital. I remember telling him not to jump from one bench to the other because he might fall and hurt himself. He looked at me like I'd lost my mind. I wondered if I had.

Bill: There were an awful lot of ups and downs during those 10 days. I felt very confident about the treatment Laura was getting. The staff in the hospital was fantastic. I really admired their dedication and had a lot confidence in what they were doing. Yet we were both very anxious about what was going to happen.

Cathy: Our family has always had a strange yet wonderful sense of humor. I consider the ability to laugh in the face of trauma a gift from God. Somehow there was comic relief there. I began to do imitations of the various doctors.

It also had occurred to me that our insurance company was not going to pick up the entire tab for this stay. I refused to worry about it because we had no choice, and it was all up to God anyway.

One day Bill disappeared, then returned to tell me he had gone to the Psychiatric Unit of Parkland to see if they had any empty rooms. He was halfway serious, and it broke me up because I knew he was close to the edge and the pressure was getting to him. My normally in-control Bill was feeling desperately out of control.

Bill: I remember the morning of the fifth or sixth day. Early in the morning they told me that Laura had been doing much better and that they were going to try to bring her out of the coma. Cath was in the motel getting some sleep; when she arrived, I told her that things were looking good. We were both very optimistic for a few hours, but then they came and said it didn't work. It was a really crushing blow. They tried to assure us that they were going to try it again, but I remember wondering to myself, "If it doesn't work, how many times can you try it?" It was a very tough setback. Doubts began to creep back into my mind. We'd been there for 6 days and didn't seem to be making any progress. How long was this going to last?

Cathy: That day, when we were told she was not yet strong enough to be brought out of the coma, was probably one of the lowest points of the entire stay. One of the nurses let me see Laura as they were increasing the drugs. I stood there next to Laura and could see tears in her eyes. Up to now I had convinced myself that she was in no pain, was not aware of where she was. The sight of those tears made me frantic. I simply sat down on the floor and sobbed. A lovely, young nurse came over to me, helped me up, and reminded me in the most gentle voice that tears are a sign of life, they don't necessarily mean pain, they are just a natural, physical reaction to the lights. She probably saved my sanity with those words. I could again concentrate on the positive fact; she was still alive.

Later that same day a baby in the bed next to Laura died. I was asked to leave the unit and saw the parents coming down the hall toward me. I couldn't look at them. Two years later I dreamed of that moment and realized that I felt not only sadness for them, but a sense of relief that it was not my child who had died.

Bill: On the first day the nurses had suggested that we bring Laura's portable tape player and favorite tapes to the hospital. They told us that people in comas may be able to hear or at least are possibly aware of the surrounding noises. They thought familiar voices and songs would help keep her calm. In a matter of hours we had tapes of her favorite rock groups, her school classmates, her riding group, and some soothing music. No matter when we went in, she had music playing. The doctors and nurses would change the tapes and vary what she heard. I wondered if she could really hear it or if they were just telling us that so that we would feel better. Much later, Laura would tell us that she thought she remembered some of those tapes.

On the eighth or ninth day they tried to bring Laura around again; this time she reacted positively. Cath left the hospital to get some lunch. As they took away different pieces of equipment, they would come tell me. I was impatient for it to be over with, but they said it would take a long time. I wanted to go in there and unhook all that stuff myself and take her home. During that day they let me in more frequently, and each time I was more encouraged as one by one the pieces of equipment could be unhooked. At one point when I went into the unit, she still had a tube down her throat, and she couldn't say anything. She opened her eyes every once in a while, and when I held her hand, she could squeeze my finger a little. By now I was emotionally drained. Cath and I had spent a lot of time crying by ourselves, but I didn't want Laura to see me crying. I was so glad she could squeeze my finger, but I had to get up and go out of the room. She needed her strength to keep coming back and didn't need to worry about me or Cath.

Cathy: When I returned to the hospital that evening, some friends of ours were waiting out in front of the hospital for me. They whisked me upstairs where I found Bill. He told me she had squeezed his fingers. I couldn't believe she was going to be all right! We simply stood and held each other for a few minutes. I know my mother and sister were there, and everyone seemed to be crying. I quickly went in to see her; but then they asked us to go back to our motel and get some sleep, and they would call us during the night.

Some time early the next morning the phone rang, and I talked to a nurse. But then I fell asleep. An hour later I woke up in a panic and told Bill the hospital had called, but I couldn't remember what they said. We called back and with relief heard our nurse say, "Laura is doing great, and you can come and see her." They had told her where she was and what had happened, including why part of her head had been shaved. We raced to the unit, hurriedly donned our sterile duds, and ran down the hall. There she was, sitting up in her bed, drinking a Coke! Did she look thin! But the atmosphere in that room was one of sheer joy. Everyone from the nurses' station people to the doctors and nurses to the other children's parents were rejoicing with us.

Bill: Her mouth was very sore, and we could give her little pieces of ice. She couldn't talk, but she knew we were there. All the fear and anxiety we had had for her seemed to disappear. I felt excited and optimistic for the first time—as I had felt when she had been born. It had been a horrible 10 days, but now she was going to make it. Later that day she was moved to the fourth floor. Our nurse told us that her first question was "Has Mike graduated yet?" We asked if she would be able to attend his graduation 2 days later and were told, "Let's see how she does tonight."

Cathy: Although I was elated at her recovery, I was reluctant to have her moved out of the unit. I had become totally dependent on all the staff there and quite frankly didn't want to trust her to someone else. Later that day Laura told me she had a migraine headache, and I panicked. I ran downstairs to the unit, found her doctors, and begged them to come and see her. Although they did call and request some medication for her, they gently explained that she would be all right, and I needed to deal with the staff on the floor. It was like breaking the unbilical cord. For so long I had relied on each of them; now it was as though we were on our own. Of course I soon realized how wonderful everyone at Children's is.

We had asked all our friends to send her balloons when she came out of the coma. You forget how many people you talk to. Within hours her room was a sea of color. A few of her best friends were allowed to visit her. They sat on the bed with her and teased her about missing her exams, related the inevitable rumors circulating around school, and generally acted like teenagers. It was a joy to see!

We were told she could go home the next day. It was her *fifteenth birthday*. The nurses on the fourth floor had a cake and a present for her. She did attend her brother's high school graduation in a wheelchair. Bill and I cried all the way through it.

Laura's recovery was a miracle—a miracle of technology. Although we prayed constantly along with literally hundreds of others, our prayers were words, thoughts, and pleadings. The staff's very actions were a prayer, and for them we are deeply grateful. So many people were involved with her: our family doctor, the entire hospital staff, our priests, family, and friends. We simply do not know, even nearly 3 years later, how to thank all of them.

Today Laura is a normal, healthy, happy teenager who frequently drives us crazy as she tries to decide where to go to college next year. Those days at Children's seem like a distant, foggy memory. They were terrible, awful days, but they made an impression on us personally and influenced the value we now place on things. Our family motto has become, "As long as we are all healthy, it just doesn't matter."

We were sometimes unreasonable to deal with, often demanding, and even rude. Yet the staff was consistently empathetic. They obviously cared a great deal about their patients and the patients' families. They realized that under terrible stress even nice people can become unreasonable. For that kindness—God bless them. Laura may be just one of their successes; she is our "baby."

100 Delivering Culturally Sensitive Care

Mary Elaine Jones

BACKGROUND

Hospital health professionals working in PICUs are part of a cultural scene. A cultural scene has a shared body of knowledge and values, a specific language, codes of behavior, and rules for dress that all its members share and understand.

Each member of the health team brings his own individual cultural heritage, beliefs, and values to the cultural scene. Superimposed on these beliefs is his socialization as a professional into the hospital subculture. The family and patient also bring to the patient-professional encounter their own individual beliefs about cause and cure of illness, their socialization experiences within their cultural or ethnic heritage, and any additional past experiences with health care or hospitalization.

The crisis nature of a family's encounter with the PICU brings into strong relief each participant's differences in world view, values, and beliefs. The patient and family may come with a different definition of what constitutes illness, its cause and cure. How the patient and family behave during the illness episode depends in large part on their beliefs and values and on their socialization experiences within their cultural or ethnic traditions.

A second factor in the behavioral response of the patient and family is the encounter with the hospital bureaucracy and with scientific technology, which results in "culture shock." The family members enter a foreign territory in which familiar cues for behaving are missing and in which they lack knowledge of the language and rules. Hospital efficiency takes control of a child from the family, and hospital routine risks depersonalizing both the child and family. Culture shock may initially manifest itself in disorientation and disorganization, undefined anger, fears, anxiety, and feelings of helplessness and hopelessness.

Because the hospital cultural scene is powerful and families are less powerful in this confrontation of cultures, adaptation must occur for effective communication to result. A form of *acculturation,* or what Oberg calls the beginning resolution phase of culture shock, takes place on the part of the patient and family. Acculturation is the process of a subordinate group borrowing cultural elements and traits from a dominant culture. In this period the individual seeks to learn new patterns of behavior that are appropriate to the new setting. This is best seen in the PICU when parents adopt the language of the cultural scene or become involved with the machinery used to care for their child. Parents' ability to adjust depends on subjective characteristics such as age, previous experience with adapting to new situations, and overall coping style. Adjustment also depends on how responsive and sensitive hospital professionals are to parents' needs.

Health professionals have a unique opportunity to provide culturally sensitive care in the PICU setting. For the professional two potential natural barriers to providing culturally sensitive care are ethnocentrism and stereotyping. Both are attitudinal and judgmental processes.

Ethnocentrism is judging another's culture in relation to one's own culture. It is the opposite of cultural relativity, an attitude that customs, beliefs, and behaviors should be viewed within the context of other person's culture. An example of ethnocentrism is the failure to acknowledge the patient's (or the patient's parents') view of the illness episode. The very act of asking the patient's view sanctions his cultural tradition.

To *stereotype* is to generalize rather than to individualize. Numerous studies have documented that health professionals often label patients as good or bad according to subjective characteristics such as cooperativeness, emotional responsibility, or complaining vs. noncomplaining. Another form of stereotyping relates specifically to cultural traits, with the generalization that persons of a particular culture *all* think, believe, and behave in a certain, specific way (e.g., "Black people believe in contagious magic"; "Hispanics believe in the evil eye"). Stereotyping in this way eliminates variation in beliefs and practices; it is in direct contrast to individualization and humanization of care.

ASSESSMENT

Patients and families come to the hospital with varying degrees of adherence to traditional explanations of the cause of illness and beliefs about treatment. In addition the behavioral response to hospitalization and resulting acculturation will vary, depending on these beliefs and on past experiences with health care providers and hospitals. The task of providing culturally sensitive care requires the PICU staff to make two kinds of cultural assessment: self-assessment and assessment of the patient and his family. Self-assessment by the health professional should cover two areas. First, what are the health professional's own beliefs about family support during crises, pain relief for children, modesty, self-control, cleanliness, eating and sleeping schedules, time, success, failure, mothering, parenting? Health professionals should be cognizant of their own cultural behavior as a means of sensitizing themselves to other cultural behaviors.

Second, how much general knowledge, both formal and informal, does the health professional have about the beliefs and values of the cultural populations served? Each person has a responsibility to acquire a basic knowledge about individual cultural groups. Important beginning areas of comparison for the health professional include the following:

Traditional illness beliefs and curing practices; definition of causation
Family structure and organization styles
    Role of family during illness
    Attitudes toward children
    Decision-making roles

Time and work orientations; labor divisions within the family
Religious beliefs and practices; role of religion in illness
Basic value system and world view
Language
Nutritional practices; role of food during illness

The second assessment involves a cultural assessment of the patient and family. A number of guides are available and are listed in the reference section. Two strategies are important. The first strategy is to determine whether a family or patient is adhering to traditional beliefs and explanations about illness and cure. Harwood summarizes important predictors of adherence to traditional medical practices, which can be adapted for use as a triage tool to assess all patients. They include the following:

Recent immigration
Immigration from rural rather than urban setting
Immigration at an older age
Maintenance of close ties to ethnic networks
Frequent migration back and forth to mother country
Little to no experience with illness or medical services
Low formal education

The older, recent immigrant from a rural part of his country may not have had experience with scientific explanations of cause and cure of illness and may adhere to traditional explanations. However, it should be noted that all patients/families under stress may rely on nonscientific, nonmainstream explanations for illness.

The second strategy of patient assessment is to determine the patient's explanation of the illness episode. Families come to the health encounter with a health tradition that includes beliefs about causation and cure. Why does the patient/family behave the way it does? What are the patient's cultural values that give meaning and provide a rationale for behaving?

Kleinman proposes that patient-professional communication can only progress if the clinical encounter includes an assessment of cultural factors to identify the discrepancies between the health professional's beliefs and the patient's beliefs about the illness episode. His clinical assessment includes three basic steps.

The first step in this process is to determine the patient's perception of the cause of the illness or event, including how it occurred, the pathophysiology, the expected course and prognosis, and the treatment that should be administered. This step involves asking the patient what he thinks caused the illness and why. The professional thus seeks to understand the meaning of the illness episode to the patient and his family.

The second step is to compare the patient's explanation with the professional's own explanation of the cause and cure. It is here that the cultural gap becomes evident. The distance between the professional's beliefs and those of the patient/family can impede communication and compliance with health regimens.

The third step is to negotiate the differences between what the patient believes and what the professional believes. Eliciting a patient's explanatory model of illness requires sensitivity and listening to cues to understand how the patient's views may differ from those of the professional who is in a position of power and authority.

MANAGEMENT

The goal of a health professional committed to providing culturally sensitive care is to become a culture broker for the patient and family. In a sense the patient needs a bridge of understanding to make a healthy transition into the cultural scene of the PICU. For the professional it requires self-study and a desire to accumulate knowledge about cultural differences. It requires an openness to differences among human beings in order to search for the universals of human experience. Additional considerations in assuring that such care is delivered should include the following.

Staff education. Delivering culturally sensitive care requires that each member of the health team understands the cultural beliefs, values, and health behaviors of the populations served. To be effective the concepts detailed must be systematized and reflected in plans of care for patients.

Language barriers. To speak another's language is to understand the nuances of meaning and the emotional context. Communication is enhanced by knowing the language of the patients/families served. However, if staff members are not fluent in the patient's language, the staff should have access to interpreters. The professional should direct his conversation to the patient/family rather than to the interpreter. Specific areas in which differences in styles of communicating may exist are in the use of handshake, the meaning of eye contact in conversation,

and how much time is used in social preliminaries before the actual content of the interaction.

Time differences. Concepts of time are embedded in the socialization process of each culture. Time has specific meaning for an efficient professional working in a hospital. Prompt action during an emergency and adherence to medication and treatment schedules are important in saving lives and are necessary for an efficiently run unit. Some families' times schedules, depending on their cultural heritage, may not conform to the professional's concept of time. Learning a particular family's orientation to time is a necessary part of the communication and intervention interaction.

Biologic variations. A number of biologic variations occur in different ethnic and racial groups, including skin color variations and susceptibility to disease. A number of these variations such as care of the skin and hair have specific implications for bedside care. Learning these variations ensures not only accurate and safe nursing/medical intervention but also considerate care.

Adaptation of care. The central goal of culturally sensitive care is to negotiate the differences between patient and professional in the definition and meaning of the illness and to assure communication about the treatment regimen. This requires acculturation on the part of the patient/family and can be facilitated by adapting medical/nursing care at the bedside to meet the individual needs of the patient. For example, care may need modification to ensure modesty beliefs are preserved and care of body functions conforms to patient beliefs about sex roles. Differences in pain tolerance and expression may require specific changes in routines. Dietary beliefs about specific foods or food preparation or foods that are believed to cause illness or enhance healing comprise another area in which routines may be modified. Adjustment of standard policies regarding numbers of visitors and the role of the clergy and lay healers during illness and crisis is another area that can enhance patient/family comfort.

Therapeutic negotiation. The steps outlined in the "Assessment" section for negotiating differences in beliefs about cause and cure may need to be ongoing. Continuous monitoring of the patient/family's understanding of new procedures as changes in the patient's condition occur must be considered. The ultimate goal is to establish and maintain bicultural communication in a setting that allows for multicultural diversity.

ADDITIONAL READING

Bloch B. Bloch's assessment guide for ethnic/cultural variations in ethnic nursing care. In Orque MS, Block B, Monrroy LSA. Ethnic Nursing Care. St. Louis: CV Mosby, 1983, pp 49-75.

Bogdan R, Brown MA, Foster SB. Be honest but not cruel: Staff/parent communication on a neonatal unit. Hum Org 41:6-16, 1982.

Brink PJ, Saunders JM. Culture shock: Theoretical and applied. In Brink PJ, ed. Transcultural Nursing: A Book of Readings. Englewood Cliffs, N.J.: Prentice-Hall, 1976, pp 126-138.

• Foster G, Anderson BG. Medical Anthropology. New York: John Wiley, 1978.

• Harwood A, ed. Ethnicity and Medical Care. Cambridge, Mass.: Harvard University Press, 1981.

Kleinman A. Clinical relevance of anthropological and cross-cultural research: Concepts and strategies. Am J Psychiatry 135:427-431, 1978.

Lorber J. Good patients and problem patients: Conformity and deviance in a general hospital. J Health Soc Behav 16:213-225, 1975.

Lynch LR, ed. The Cross-Cultural Approach to Health Behavior. Rutherford, N.J.: Fairleigh Dickinson University Press, 1969.

Mead M. Understanding cultural patterns. In Lynch LR, ed. The Cross-Cultural Approach to Health Behavior. Rutherford, N.J.: Fairleigh Dickinson University Press, 1969, pp 445-451.

Oberg K. Culture Shock. Indianapolis: Bobbs-Merrill, 1954.

Paul B. Anthropological perspectives on medicine and public health. In Lynch LR, ed. The Cross-Cultural Approach to Health Behavior. Rutherford, N.J.: Fairleigh Dickinson University Press, 1969, pp 26-42.

Taylor C. In Horizontal Orbit: Hospitals and the Cult of Efficiency. New York: Holt, Rinehart & Winston, 1970.

101 Suicide

David A. Waller · Graham J. Emslie

BACKGROUND

The purpose of this chapter is to provide guidelines for the psychological assessment and management of children and adolescents who have made suicide attempts that result in hospitalization in a PICU. Children and adolescents admitted to a PICU with injuries, poisonings, or unexplained metabolic imbalance may be suffering from a recognized or unrecognized suicide attempt. This is true for all ages. Although completed suicides are rare in children, 25% of depressed children as young as 5 years of age verbalize suicidal ideation or death wishes. If they act on these feelings, these younger children will more often present as "accident victims" (e.g., from running into traffic, jumping from heights, ingestions). Substance abuse or alcohol abuse often complicate the management of adolescent suicide attempts.

Fifty percent to eighty percent of suicides are associated with depression; therefore direct or indirect evidence of depression is a warning sign that the current situation may be a result of suicidal or self-destructive behavior. Warning signs of depression include a recent change in the individual with social withdrawal, change in peer group, recent drop in grades, changes in appetite or weight, decreased energy or fatigue, substance or alcohol abuse, and non-specific somatic complaints.

MONITORING

An interview with the patient's parents will elicit any recent changes in behavior possibly associated with depression. Most children and adolescents will admit to suicidal behavior if asked directly. Even very young children (i.e., preschoolers) who may not understand the permanence of death can think about ending one's life as a way to get out of feeling bad. Children will usually confide these feelings if they sense that the interviewer understands how unhappy and hope-less children (and adults) can feel sometimes. The child may be asked whether he has been feeling lately that it might be better to have never been born or not to be alive any longer. Further guidelines for interviewing are provided later in this chapter.

TREATMENT

Once the situation is identified as a suicide attempt, the most important idea to convey to both children and parents, assuming the patient survives, is that survival represents an *opportunity,* a second chance on which to capitalize. Psychiatric consultation can help ensure that the opportunity is not wasted.

The opportunity alluded to is in reality twofold: an opportunity to *understand* the nature of the distress that led to the attempt and an opportunity to begin a process of *change* so that distress of suicidal proportions hopefully does not recur. By the time the child or adolescent is transferred or discharged from the PICU, clear-cut progress in each of these areas, as described below, should have occurred.

Understanding the Distress

Once the child or adolescent is feeling well enough and thinking clearly enough to be interviewed about the suicide attempt, efforts must be made to establish the kind of atmosphere in which the patient will feel comfortable sharing feelings. Often he will feel guilty about what has happened, correctly surmising that from the family's (or possibly even some of the staff's) point of view such behavior is simply "wrong" or uncalled for and should never be repeated. There may be a sense that the patient "did it for attention" and a feeling that such "manipulative" behavior should not be rewarded. Yet the key to gaining access to the child's distress is somehow to create a non-judgmental climate for the sake of discussion of the child's feelings and in spite of countervailing personal emotions and reactions.

Asking children straight-out why they did it usually evokes a simple shrug of the shoulders or an "I don't know" defensive response. More helpful is to get to know the child a bit (e.g., how old he is, his place of residence, likes and dislikes, grade in school). "Everyone feels unhappy at times; tell me about the kinds of things that you have felt unhappy about" is a good lead-in to discussing the events and feelings that prompted the suicide attempt.

It is important to assess the child's present feelings about suicide. Is there a sense of disappointment (even personal failure) that the attempt failed? Children with active suicidal ideation must be monitored at all times. More often children, like adults, do not feel suicidal immediately after an attempt. The tensions that led up to the event have been temporarily discharged. The real danger is that the distress that was present will be minimized or denied, with assurances given by the child and his parents that they are certain it will never happen again. In this situation attention must be redirected toward achieving an understanding of the distress that led up to the attempt.

Family members may also experience an array of distressing feelings (e.g., guilt over having contributed in some way to the problem or for not recognizing it sooner, even anger at the patient for subjecting them to an experience like this). Relatives or neighbors may contribute to the parents' sense of failure by accusations, stated or implied, which may be quite unjustified. Support must be provided as indicated and attention gently redirected to the issue of change.

Change

Suicidal thinking and behavior are often based on a premise of hopelessness and helplessness. There is a sense not only of distress, but that nothing can be done to make things better. The seeds of this perception may be biologic or psychosocial (or both). Thus an adolescent with "affective illness" (depressive disease) may respond differently from other adolescents to the usual stresses and upsets of this time of life. Sleep difficulty, inappropriate guilt, feelings of low self-esteem, hopelessness about the future, and suicidal thinking and behavior may all constitute parts of an episode of depression, which, if identified, may respond to psychotherapy and antidepressant medication. In contrast, another child may feel hopeless because of literally being caught in a destructve family environment that he can do nothing to change.

It is crucial, however, that no child or adolescent hospitalized because of a suicide attempt leave the PICU setting until there are the *beginnings* of a plan that will result in a favorable change of whatever factors, biologic or psychosocial, that have contributed to the attempt. Policies and procedures for management of suicidal patients in a PICU must be established. Often patients are transferred to a medical floor for further care. Until continued suicidal risk has been evaluated (preferably by a trained child and adolescent psychiatrist), it may be necessary to provide one-to-one observation by either staff or family members. The psychiatric consultant will assist in developing an appropriate plan for further care, which may necessitate transfer to a psychiatric unit for a more thorough evaluation.

Patients (and families) may sometimes resist such plans, citing the familiar "stigma" associated with psychiatric hospitalization and expressing concerns for "how it will look on the school records" (remind them that completed suicide means there are no further school records). In some instances outpatient follow-up may be satisfactory, especially if one senses a real commitment from both patient and parents to follow through and if an appointment can be scheduled (before discharge) for an outpatient evaluation to take place within a day or two of discharge from the hospital. But if the child or adolescent remains very depressed during the course of hospitalization, if there is still suicidal thinking, or if there is a problematic family situation that cannot easily be changed, psychiatric hospitalization is warranted.

•   •   •

To summarize, child and adolescent suicide attempts represent an opportunity to begin to understand distress and to begin to make a favorable change in a child's or adolescent's life. Such beginnings can take place in the PICU. Although a certain degree of shock and dismay (and even denial) is to be anticipated, the opportunity for initiating understanding and change must not be allowed to slip away.

ADDITIONAL READING

Looney JG, Oldham DG, Claman L, Crumley FE, Waller DA. Suicide by adolescents. Tex Med 81:45-49, 1985.

Weinberg WA, Emslie GJ. Depression and suicide in adolescents. Int Pediatr 2:154-159, 1987.

102 Legal Aspects of Pediatric Intensive Care

Patricia T. Driscoll

The provision of health services is heavily regulated by law, especially when the health care of minors is concerned. Health care providers often tend to resent the "intrusion," as they perceive it, of law into medicine. This is hardly a defensible position since legal rules, however imperfectly constructed, reflect societal values, which must and should be considered in medical decision making. The dilemma for health care professionals is to recognize the appropriate relationship between law and medicine in everyday practice. A fundamental knowledge of legal issues is essential.

SOURCES OF LAW

The laws applicable to the issues surrounding the delivery of health services stem from many different sources, including the United States Constitution and the constitutions of individual states, federal and state court decisions, federal and state statutes and regulations, and various local laws and ordinances. Some of these laws have nationwide impact, whereas some have only local applicability. Some laws impose criminal liability for violations, whereas others provide only a civil remedy such as an action for damages. Moreover, the law is not static. At its most basic level law is an expression of public policy. It is the expression of the way society views a given matter at a particular time. Consequently, laws change when underlying public policy changes. The evolution of laws governing the relative rights and responsibilities of parents and their minor offspring is an example of this process. The movement from nearly complete parental autonomy to the contemporary children's rights perspective largely reflects societal perceptions regarding minority.

CONSENT FOR MINORS

The treatment of minors gives rise to several questions in connection with obtaining sufficient consent. There are differences in the facts of each situation and in individual state law via case or statute, which render the answering of these questions with legal certainty difficult. On occasion, therefore, a physician and the hospital must rely on their best judgment in a particular case.

Parents are vested with custody and control over their minor children; therefore they may consent to nearly every form of health care for a minor child. The consent of only one parent is sufficient. If the health professional knows that the other parent would object, although not legally required to do so, he should seek to mediate the dispute in a manner that addresses the best interest of the child. When parents are separated or divorced, the parent who has actual control of the minor child at the time the health care need arises, even if he or she is not the legal custodian, generally may give effective consent. The treating professional may proceed in good-faith reliance on the representation of the presenting parent and need not insist on proof of custodial status. If, however, there is reason to believe that an absent custodial parent would object to the treatment, the professional may want to seek judicial guidance unless the delay would jeopardize the welfare of the child. This will ensure that the physician does not become embroiled in a custody dispute, which is ancillary to the health need of the minor.

The question of whether any adult besides a parent may consent to medical treatment for a minor child frequently arises in situations in which a parent is unavailable. Historically the answer has been that except in emergency situations, no one other than parents is authorized to consent. A few states have enacted statutes that provide for persons other than parents to consent to treatment of children. Generally these laws permit any adult who is caring for the child at the time health care is needed to act in place of the parents if parents are absent and/or cannot be reached. Often this is within the context of emergency or emergent care. Even in states that have no such statutes, there are cases in which the health care professional has been found blameless for treating a minor on the consent of another adult. These cases are few and were based on what seemed reasonable at the time in view of the type of treatment needed and the age of the child. Therefore, to treat with consent of an adult other than a parent, a provider must ascertain whether a statute allows this action in the jurisdiction; if not, he should proceed only when an emergency exists or if the facts of the situation are very compelling.

Children admitted to the PICU from a foster home present special considerations for consent, depending on the nature of the foster placement. Morrissey, Hoffman, and Thorpe offer the following helpful summary:

1. Foster parents or representatives of custodial institutions generally may consent to routine or necessary care of the minor they are responsible for on a day-to-day basis.
2. If the proposed treatment is elective, major, or bears significant risks, and placement has occurred as a result of voluntary action on the part of the natural parents, the consent of the natural parents should be obtained. If their whereabouts are unknown, the supervising social agency should be contacted.
3. If the proposed treatment is elective, major, or bears significant risks, and placement was initiated by a government entity, and parental rights have been terminated, or the minor surrendered for adoption, the supervising social agency may consent.
4. If the health need is an emergency, general emergency principles govern.*

The Minor's Consent

Generally the consent of a minor need not be obtained before initiating medical treatment if parental or other authorized adult consent is present. There

*From Morrissey J, Hoffman A, Thorpe JC. Consent and Confidentiality in Health Care of Children and Adolescents. New York: Free Press, 1986.

are circumstances, however, in which the consent of the minor is sufficient or when the consent of the minor is necessary.

Emancipated minors may consent to their own medical care. Minors are generally considered emancipated when they are married or otherwise no longer subject to parental control and are not supported by their parents. The specific factors necessary to establish emancipation are usually set forth by statute and vary from state to state. Some states require that the parent and child agree on the emancipation, so a minor cannot achieve that state by running away from home. In some states emancipation is established by the courts, and no statutory definition exists. Confusion about the criteria by which emancipation is determined, concern about possible liability if an incorrect determination is made, and doubts about who is financially responsible have made health care providers understandably reluctant to accept the doctrine of emancipation. However, the emerging concept of minors' rights and an underlying policy judgment that endorses the benefit of teenage minors' independent access to obtaining timely medical treatment make it incumbent on hospitals to establish an appropriate policy to help guide practitioners confronted with the issue.

Mature minors (although not emancipated) may consent to some medical care. Some states have enacted statutes that authorize older minors to consent to any medical treatment or minors of any age to consent to treatment for specific conditions such as venereal disease or drug abuse. The age limits and scope of treatment to which minors can consent vary from state to state. In states that do not have applicable consent statutes the risk of liability for treating a mature minor on his own consent is negligible if the criteria suggested by Morrissey, Hoffman, and Thorpe are met:

1. The minor is 15 years of age or over.
2. The minor is able to give an informed consent; that is, in the judgment of the treating physician, the minor appears to understand and appreciate the benefits and risks of the proposed treatment and to make a reasoned decision based on such knowledge.
3. The proposed treatment is for the minor's benefit and not for the benefit of another.
4. The proposed treatment is deemed necessary according to best professional judgment.
5. The treatment does not involve complex, high-risk medical procedures or complex, high-risk surgery.

Consent in Emergency Situations

Situations may arise in the PICU in which emergency, urgent, or necessary procedures are deemed by the physician to be needed and the parent or legal guardian is unavailable to consent. In an emergency no consent is required. The law presumes or implies consent from the facts; that is, given the urgency of the health need, any reasonable parent would want his child to be treated promptly. Most states have also enacted specific statutes addressing the treatment of minors in emergency situations. Many health care professionals believe that a minor must be in clear and imminent danger of death before emergency care may be given in the absence of parental consent. In fact, the cases do not support this definition of emergency. The term "emergency" is usually defined by the courts as including not only situations in which the patient is in danger of death, but also situations in which a delay in treatment would increase the risk to the patient's health or in which treatment is necessary to alleviate pain. The vast majority of the statutes dealing with emergency care of minors and parental consent also define emergency in broad terms and afford physicians latitude in exercising their professional judgment about when an emergency exists and parental consent need not be obtained.

With few exceptions there is no legal requirement that a physician obtain a concurring medical opinion that an emergency exists before providing care or initiating a procedure for a minor. At this time only South Carolina, North Carolina, and Oklahoma have second-physician rules and only if surgery is contemplated. These states also waive the requirement when another opinion is not readily available under the circumstances. The "two-physician rule" has grown out of medical practice and may have sound clinical basis; however, with the exception of the states listed above, there is no legal requirement for it by legislative mandate or judicial opinion.

It is difficult to formulate absolute rules to assure that the health professional's decision will be deemed appropriate in an emergency. However, the following guidelines will help practitioners:

1. If sound clinical judgment is exercised, courts will rarely question a professional's decision, especially in an emergency in which clinical decisions must be made quickly.
2. When the minor is very young, an emergency should be defined somewhat more narrowly.
3. Procedures that are irreversible (e.g., removal of body part or sterilization) should not be performed in the absence of parental consent unless there is no other alternative and attempts to obtain parental consent are not possible or have proved fruitless.
4. Parents should always be consulted when it is possible to do so, both for the initial treatment and any extensions of treatment.

Refusal of Consent for Treatment

If the parent or guardian consents to treatment but the minor patient possesses both maturity and understanding and refuses, the provider should in most instances recognize the minor's rights as paramount and not proceed with the treatment. If a mature and understanding minor consents to treatment and the parent or guardian refuses, the same approach is advisable; that is, rely on the minor's consent.

What happens when parents of a minor who lacks maturity and understanding affirmatively refuse consent for treatment that a physician deems necessary for the child? This conflict generally arises in three types of situations. First, parents may withhold consent for religious reasons. Second, parents may not wish to impose procedures they deem extraordinary in an attempt to prolong their child's severely compromised life. Third, standard medical treatments may be rejected in favor of forms that are less traditional and more questionable in nature. There are obvious ethical dilemmas involved in these situations that are beyond the scope of this chapter. However, it is important to keep in mind that not all instances of parental refusal are incompatible with good health care or inconsistent with best medical judgment.

If the health provider is confronted with parental refusal and believes the decision is not compatible with appropriate medical care and will place the child's health in jeopardy, he has two options. The physician or hospital can seek a court order to override the parents' refusal, or the matter can be reported to the local child protective agency as medical neglect. In all states the law considers the withholding of necessary medical treatment from a child to constitute abuse and/or neglect and mandates the reporting of such cases. It is the role of the designated agency to investigate and take protective action, including court proceedings when necessary. Once the proper notifications are made, it is the court's function, not the physician's, to decide when a child shall be treated against the parent's will. There need be no concern about liability for making a report of neglect that is later determined to be unfounded. Every state grants immunity to reporting individuals as long as they acted in good faith.

INFORMED CONSENT

Consent, technically, is a simple yes or no on the part of the individual authorized to consent. However, the law concerning consent in health care mandates that the individual giving consent be provided with sufficient information to make an informed decision. The issue of informed consent and minors can be confusing because of the overlap of the rights of minors to give legal consent in some situations and the developmental ability of an individual minor to give informed consent. In most cases encountered in the PICU the minor is not legally entitled to give consent, and in these situations the physician looks to the parents or guardian for informed consent on behalf of the minor child. Consent alone protects the health care provider from liability for battery, whereas informed consent is necessary to protect the provider from liability for negligence.

The courts have struggled to outline general principles to facilitate meaningful informed consent and have developed two standards for determining the adequacy of information given to obtain consent: (1) the professional or reasonable physician standard and (2) the materiality or reasonable patient standard. The states are almost equally divided on which standard to apply. In states using the first standard the physician has a duty to provide the information that a reasonable practitioner would provide under the same or similar circumstances. Under the second standard the extent of the physician's duty to provide information is determined by the patient rather than by professional practice. Information that is material to the decision must be disclosed (i.e., what a reasonable person would want to know before reaching a decision). Courts recognize that it is not feasible to inform the decision maker of all risks associated with a procedure. However, the practitioner should consider disclosure of the following factors:

1. Diagnosis. This includes the medical steps preceding diagnosis, including tests and their alternatives. The right of informed refusal requires disclosure of the risks of foregoing a diagnostic procedure.
2. The nature and purpose of the proposed treatment.
3. The risks of the treatment. The threshold of disclosure varies with the product of the probability and the severity of the risk.
4. The probability of success.
5. Treatment alternatives. Practitioners should disclose those alternatives that are generally acknowledged within the medical community as feasible.
6. The prognosis if the treatment is not given.

More than half of the states have enacted legislation dealing with informed consent, largely in response to the perceived malpractice crisis. The statutes take a variety of forms, but they all share the common thread of moving the informed consent standard toward greater deference to medical judgment. At least 12 states have enacted statutes that make a signed consent form presumptively valid consent. It is therefore imperative for the practitioner to become familiar with individual state law in formulating appropriate procedures for obtaining valid informed consent.

The physician is responsible for providing the necessary information to obtain informed consent before proceeding with diagnostic or therapeutic procedures. Other independent practitioners who order procedures have a similar responsibility concerning those procedures. The hospital is generally not liable for failure of the physician to secure informed consent unless the physician is an employee or otherwise acting on behalf of the hospital. Some physicians rely on hospital personnel (nurses in particular) to obtain consent. This can be a dangerous practice since the physician remains responsible and cannot ensure the adequacy of the process if done by another.

TERMINATION OF LIFE-SUPPORT SYSTEMS FOR MINORS

The termination of artificial life-support systems and the withholding of conventional treatment from handicapped infants present a special set of issues in the PICU. There are no clear-cut legal criteria at this time to guide parents and doctors in resolving these decisions. However, the decisional law of the last decade and, to some extent, recently enacted "living will" statutes provide some guidance in this developing area of jurisprudence. Apparently parents or other surrogates may assert a minor's constitutional right of privacy to refuse artificial life support if the minor is terminally ill or in an irreversible comatose state. The doctrine of substituted judgment accords great weight to parental decisions when the parents are fully informed about the medical prognosis and treatment alternatives. However, the question of whether a less compelling diagnosis and prognosis justify the discontinuance of life support or withholding of treatment is less clear, especially in light of current federal regulatory activity in the area of child abuse. The 1985 amendments and accompanying regulations require that medically indicated treatment not be withheld from a handicapped infant unless (1) the infant is chronically and irreversibly comatose; (2) the treatment would merely prolong dying and not be effective in ameliorating or correcting all the infant's life-threatening conditions or would be futile in terms of the survival of the infant; or (3) the treatment would be virtually futile in terms of survival of the infant and the treatment itself under such circumstances would be inhumane. Courts, parents, and medical professionals are currently also being faced with the problem of whether artificial means of furnishing nourishment and hydration may be withheld or withdrawn based on the same standards governing other mechanical life-support systems.

Hospital ethics committees, although not a panacea for these dilemmas, may play a useful role in generating discussions of the difficult medical, moral, and legal problems involving treatment of critically ill minors. Examination of these cases by a multidisciplinary committee increases the probability that such treatment decisions are informed and consistent with the broadest moral values of society. Providers, confronted with questions in this complex and unsettled area, should consult with appropriate hospital administrative or legal personnel to ascertain what legal obligations, if any, must be met.

MALPRACTICE

Health care providers and the public frequently interchange the terms "malpractice" and "negligence." Although the distinction is technical, there is a difference. Negligence is a general term that denotes conduct lacking in due care. Anyone can be liable for negligence. Malpractice is a more specific term and examines a professional standard of care as well as the professional status of the caregiver. Malpractice is the failure of a professional person to act in accordance with the prevailing professional standards or failure to foresee consequences that a professional person, having the necessary skills and education,

should foresee. To be successful in a malpractice cause of action the injured party-plaintiff must prove the following:

1. Duty owed to the patient (i.e., a doctor/patient or nurse/patient relationship exists).
2. Breach of the duty owed the patient (i.e., failure to conform to the standard of care as established by expert testimony).
3. Injury (i.e., breach of standard is not enough; the patient must suffer injury or damages as a result).
4. Proximate cause (i.e., the injury must have been incurred directly because of the breach of duty owed the patient).

The presence of all the required elements of a cause of action for malpractice does not necessarily mean that a lawsuit will be filed. The fifth element that is required is a willing plaintiff. Whether or not an injured party becomes a willing plaintiff is usually based on patient (family) expectation. As a rule patients and their families lack the technical sophistication to recognize whether a bad outcome is an unavoidable complication or an iatrogenic injury. Lacking this knowledge, the care is judged on the basis of two criteria: (1) Was the outcome consistent with the perceived seriousness of the original medical condition? (2) Was the care delivered in a professional manner (i.e., did the PICU staff appear competent, and were the providers responsive to the patient's needs)? Although the families of PICU patients perceive the condition of the patient as serious and are usually more prepared for a bad outcome, it is important to keep the parents apprised of all facets of treatment and prognosis to reduce the likelihood of a lawsuit. Remember, it is people, not the action or event that triggered a bad outcome, who sue.

Liability for negligence or malpractice in an institutional setting involves essentially the same issues discussed previously. The major difference in determining liability in the hospital or PICU setting is the complications that derive from the multiplicity of potential defendants. When a patient injury results in a medical malpractice lawsuit, the patient's attorney will usually sue the hospital and all the persons involved in the patient's care. The court will ultimately sort out the tangle of overlapping responsibility in finding liability (if it in fact exists). However, the court's view of the responsibility for the patient's care may differ from that of the PICU team. This viewpoint could result in individuals being held legally responsible for actions taken by persons they were not supervising. For example, under some states' medical practice acts members of the medical staff committees who approve PICU "standing orders" could be found liable for patient injuries caused by inappropriate application of those protocols. Therefore, both legally and medically, it is obviously advantageous to delineate responsibility clearly and, if possible, to have one physician in charge of the patient's care. There should also be one specific nurse in charge of coordinating all nonphysician personnel involved in the patient's care. This nurse should possess appropriate PICU clinical skills and should ensure that the patient receives proper nursing care, that ordered tests are done and results reported, and that ancillary personnel are properly integrated into the PICU routine. The determination of proper nurse staffing levels in PICUs is becoming a major issue in hospital cost-containment efforts. Although it is tempting to save money by reducing nursing staff, this decision should be considered with caution. A nursing shortage can, in itself, be determined to be a breach of proper care sufficient to create liability for patient injuries.

The PICU deals in state-of-the-art medical care involving the latest therapies and equipment. Therefore it is essential that all personnel be sufficiently trained in the use of the technology to avoid the risk of liability for breach of the standard of care. The PICU should have a formal training program for all personnel in the use of new equipment or procedures. There should also be a mechanism for ensuring that all personnel maintain proficiency in the tasks in which they are involved. Requirements for use of specific equipment should include knowing how to use all the offered features of the equipment and recognition of equipment malfunction as well as the physiologic and therapeutic events that the equipment monitors or supports. Similarly, certification in a new procedure should include demonstration of the ability to perform the procedure properly, recognition and treatment of the possible complications, and knowledge of when to use the procedure. There are situations when modifications may be needed to correct equipment defects or to change equipment capabilities to improve patient care. However, it is important to appreciate the magnitude of the legal risks involved in this type of modification. If a patient suffers injury, the manufacturer will claim the injury was due to the modification rather than to an intrinsic defect. Modification of equipment, therefore, should be undertaken with great caution.

The "malpractice crisis" and proposed reforms of the tort system have been discussed a great deal. It is unlikely, however, that either the substantive law defining negligence/malpractice or the process for determining liability will be substantially altered in most jurisdictions. There is not an apparent consensus about either the nature of the problem or of the solution. To limit potential liability the health care provider should be aware of relevant legal doctrines but, more important, be cognizant of prevailing professional standards and incorporate this knowledge and sound professional judgment into everyday practice.

MEDICAL RECORDS

Complex medical problems, along with the multiplicity of personnel involved in the care of patients in the PICU, demand that an accurate, effective, and up-to-the-minute medical record that coordinates and documents patient care activities be kept. Unfortunately the focus on the medical record as a legal document has reduced both its legal and medical effectiveness. Medical professionals, repeatedly told that the best defense is a good medical record, often forget that a medical record is valuable only to the extent that it documents the actual rendering of good medical care. A poor record may prevent providers from establishing the good care that was given to the patient, but a good record is not a substitute for good care. The misunderstanding of the purpose of the medical record as a legal tool has led to the inclusion of so much data in the record that it is sometimes impossible to retrieve necessary information in a timely manner.

The primary purposes of the medical record are to ensure continuity of care, to provide rapid access to recent information about the patient's condition, and to serve as an audit tool for evaluation of the care rendered. The PICU record must be structured to accomplish these objectives. If this is done, the record will automatically provide legal protection. Personnel in the PICU must be wary of creating off-the-chart record-keeping systems, especially if the information they contain is not recorded in the medical record. Simple narrative charting does not usually meet the recording needs of the PICU, nor should this method of charting be retained if outmoded.

Flow sheets and other methods of abbreviating information have developed for ease of understanding and transmission. It is important that these documents be used consistently and that blank spaces be avoided. A simple "NA" or like designation will alert the reviewer (attorney or court) that proper consideration was given to the subject and that it was not simply overlooked.

For the medical record to accomplish its medical purposes it must be legible, complete, and accurate. As a legal tool, the same applies. A record that cannot be interpreted because of illegible entries, the use of abbreviations that have no standard means of interpretation, or obvious lapses of time with no recording casts doubt not only on the record, but on the credibility of those providing the care embodied in the record. All entries in the medical record should be relevant, concise, objective, and factual. The record should be a representation of the actual care the patient received. No attempt should be made to obscure incidents or the planned approach to the patient by omitting this information from the record. For example, if it is determined that a patient is not a candidate for CPR, the appropriate order should be written. Similarly, if an incident occurs in the PICU that involves a patient, the filing of an incident report, which should not become a part of the chart, does not preclude the need to document the facts relative to the patient's diagnosis, care, or treatment in the medical record.

The medical record is often the single most important document available to a practitioner in the defense of a negligence/malpractice action and ordinarily is admissible as evidence of what happened in the care of the patient. An ambiguous or illegible record is often worse than no record since it documents a failure of the involved professional staff to communicate clearly and thus reflects on the care the patient received. The professional is well advised to treat the record as an important aspect of the overall service provided the patient and to handle it with the same skill and diligence as other phases of diagnosis and treatment.

Confidentiality

The hospital owns the physical medical record, subject to the patient's interest in the information in it. The medical record and information contained therein are considered confidential, as are all private communications made to a professional within the professional relationship. Release of information that has not been authorized by the patient (parents) or is not made pursuant to statutory, regulatory, or other legal authority may subject the hospital and staff to liability. The rise of consumer-rights activism, growing concepts of a right to privacy, and increasing concern over the compilation of expansive dossiers made possible by computer technology without the knowledge or consent of the individual concerned have prompted increased judicial and legislative activity. Health care providers should be aware of relevant federal and state statutes and regulations that create a positive duty not to disclose medical information except as specified.

The law provides little guidance concerning who may have access to or authorize the release of information contained in the record of minors. In the absence of statutory or common law authority the generally accepted rule is that the information may be released only on authorization of one of the parents or a guardian and that the parent or guardian may be allowed access to the record on behalf of the patient. This approach does not address potential conflicts of interest, the invasion of the minor's own confidences, or possible future discriminatory consequences of such disclosure. For example, many potentially compromising diagnoses made in childhood may be conjectural and either subsequently disproved or confirmed but resolved before adulthood. Yet this information commonly remains in the health medical record or third-party data banks indefinitely as fact. Too few parents and providers give sufficient thought to the possible long-term consequences and take corrective or preventive steps.

The dilemma about how to preserve the confidentiality of minors represents a major health record privacy problem. Protection against inappropriate disclosures of confidential information requires diligence on the part of providers. The less confidential the information that is recorded in the record, the fewer will be the opportunities for unintentional and/or harmful disclosure. Health providers have a tendency to record far more than is needed for either documentation or the provision of care. Only necessary data should be recorded and should be done in a manner that is specific to the degree necessary for documentation and therapeutic purposes. Professionals should clearly distinguish between those diagnoses that are conjectural hypotheses or academic exercises, and hence eliminated, and those that are borne out. This is especially relevant in an environment in which clerical coding is done pursuant to diagnosis-related groups (DRGs). The health record is a permanent document that often is reposited outside the control of either the patient or provider, particularly when the patient is a minor. Confidentiality and privacy can best be assured by careful discrimination on the part of health care providers themselves in determining what is written and the manner in which it is stated.

CHILD ABUSE AND NEGLECT

In every American jurisdiction it is the legal obligation of the examining health care provider to report suspected cases of child abuse to authorities designated by statute. Significantly, all of the statutes provide immunity from civil liability for reporting in good faith, and in at least 31 states failure to report child abuse can result in criminal prosecution. When the physician assesses a child to determine whether reasonable cause exists to believe the child is abused or neglected, careful notations must be made in the medical record. Specifically, a detailed and objective documentation and description of all pertinent physical findings should be noted as should information pertinent to time sequences and parental explanations. The diagnosis of child abuse is not always clear. When in doubt, it is suggested that the physician should always report its possibility. Morrissey, Hoffman, and Thorpe suggest the following constructive approach toward possible abusing parents to ease the difficult position in which health care providers are placed in these situations:

1. The parent accompanying the child should be advised relatively promptly of the physician's concerns (and why), but not in adversarial terms.
2. The physician should explain that he or she is not making a legal finding that a child is abused, but that the law requires the reporting of any suspected case. There is no option. (Let the law be the scapegoat.)
3. The subsequent process should be explained. (Child abuse protocols already exist in most acute pediatric care facilities.) Most importantly, the parent should be helped to understand that even if the suspicion of abuse is confirmed, the primary objective is to rehabilitate, not punish.

4. Ample opportunity should be given for the parents to express their side of the matter and to be heard, even if their account is posed in angry terms. Even if not at fault, it is difficult for anyone to be so accused and not respond defensively. But the provision of "equal time" will be the best method of opening up parents' concern over loss of control and problems encountered in raising the child, and of motivating them for treatment.

Regardless of other factors, providers should remember that the ultimate disposition of the case is up to the agents of the state. Reporting must take place before the child is allowed to leave the facility unless there is no possibility of further harm if discharged home. Parents should not be allowed to sign the child out, and authorities should be contacted if they do so. The most important issues are following the best interest of the child and preventing further harm.

CONCLUSION

The PICU presents many complex medical and legal issues for which there is little case or statutory law to provide direction. However, analysis of the various issues involved and application of sound principles can offer a reasonable course. Points to consider include the following:

1. The courts have always been reluctant to invalidate the physician's best judgment when it is invoked on the behalf of a minor and intended to benefit the minor and when the minor's best interests have been given all due consideration.
2. A well-documented record is the best defense against any legal challenge.
3. Advance planning and negotiation from a therapeutic rather than legal or adversarial position will avoid many unnecessary adversarial situations. Policies must be developed to deal with troublesome situations.
4. The capacity to deal empathetically with the differential concerns, fears, and anxieties of both parents and minors will avoid many legal actions.
5. At least a basic knowledge of the law and its principles will provide some clarity in murky circumstances.
6. When in doubt, consult an attorney.

ADDITIONAL READING

Brennan JA. Do not resuscitate orders for the incompetent patient in the absence of family consent. Law Med Health Care 14:13-19, 1986.

Guidelines on the termination of life-sustaining treatment and care of the dying. A Report by the Hastings Center. New York: Hastings Center, 1987.

Guido GW. Legal issues in nursing. Norwalk, Conn.: Appleton & Lange, 1988.

Hegland K. Should hospitals be responsible for informed consent? Law Med Health Care 11:860-877, 1983.

Holder A. Parents, courts and refusal of treatment. J Pediatr 104:516-524, 1983.

Jackson CC. Severely disabled newborns. J Leg Med 8:135-177, 1987.

• McMenamin JP. Children as patients. In American College of Legal Medicine. Legal Medicine. St. Louis: CV Mosby, 1988, pp 251-284.

• Morrissey J, Hoffmann A, Thorpe JC. Consent and Confidentiality in Health Care of Children and Adolescents. New York: Free Press, 1986.

Pozgar GD. Legal Aspects of Health Care Administration, 3rd ed. Rockville, Md.: Aspen, 1987.

President's commission for the study of ethical problems in medicine and behavioral research. Washington, D.C.: U.S. Government Printing Office, 1983.

Richards EP, Rathbun DC. Risk management in the intensive care unit. In Benesch K, Abramason N, Grenvik A, Meisel A, eds. Medicolegal Aspects of Critical Care. Rockville, Md.: Aspen, 1986, pp 11-29.

Roach WH, Chernoff SN, Easley CL. Medical Records and the Law. Rockville, Md.: Aspen, 1985.

Scheb JM. Termination of life support systems for minor children: Evolving legal responses. Tenn Law Rev 54:1-30, 1986.

• Shapiro RS, Frader JE. Critically ill infants. In Benesch K, Abramason N, Grenvik A, Meisel A, eds. Medicolegal Aspects of Critical Care. Rockville, Md.: Aspen, 1986, pp 61-84.

Smith RS. Disabled newborns and the federal child abuse amendments: Tenuous protection. Hastings Law J 37:32-63, 1986.

Southwick AF. The law of hospital and health care administration, 2nd ed. Ann Arbor: Health Administration Press, 1988.

Wlody GS, Smith S. Ethical dilemmas in critical care: A proposal for hospital ethics advisory committees. Focus Crit Care 12(5):41-46, 1985.

103 Role of the Clergy in the PICU

Ron Somers-Clark

To understand the role of the clergy in a PICU, one must not simply regard the clergy as persons who offer religious support to families. Such a statement is not meant to negate the importance of religious traditions with all their meaning and importance to families encountering life, illness, pain, and suffering. Religious traditions and beliefs are expressions of a person's faith, which is that inner, more personal orientation to life and living that defines a person's way of being. The threat that illness poses to the life of the patient, his family, and persons working in a PICU is a threat that by its very nature raises the deepest faith concerns. Rarely, if ever, would anyone working in a PICU encounter a family whose basic faith system is not challenged as its members are confronted with a threat to their child's health. Therefore the clergy's role is to support persons as they act according to their faith during their interactions in the PICU.

The clergy has a unique leadership role among families in this society. The role of the patient's visiting clergy and the role of the clinically trained hospital chaplain may be similar but different in scope in a PICU. There are powerful emotional family systems with which clergy interact. The visiting clergy may not only be involved with both the patient and his family but may also be the leader of the congregational family from which the patient gains support. The scope broadens for the hospital chaplain whose role and leadership result from his representing the larger faith community in an ecumenical ministry. In addition the hospital chaplain gains entrée to the family as a member of the health care (family) team. Often the chaplain is accepted by the patient and family or visiting clergy and is seen by them as their liaison and spokesperson to the PICU team. These varying relationships of both the visiting clergy and the hospital chaplain place the clergy/chaplain in an excellent position to offer support directly to the patient or to foster such support to the patient through the family.

It is the clergy/chaplain's role to recognize and assist the patient and family to draw on their unique faith system, including appropriate religious rites and rituals such as prayer, emergency baptism, and worship. These more traditional forms of ministry may be offered by the visiting clergy or the hospital chaplain as needed.

The hospital should have a chaplain available in the PICU or on call with a quick response time 24 hours a day. In the majority of cases the nonthreatening chaplain will be a ready friend and ally to an anxious family. The skilled hospital chaplain can encourage positive attitudes through which families accept the chaplain's ministry while dispelling negative stereotypes that families may possess.

Serious and critical illnesses of children often throw families either into actual grief or into a process similar to the stages of grief. The clergy/chaplain must be available quickly after the child is admitted to the PICU since the child's family may be in a stage of *shock and disbelief*. Often the situation seems like a bad dream, and the family members believe it cannot be happening to their child and family. Quickly they move to a stage of *anger*. The anger may be felt toward God for the injustice of their innocent child's suffering and illness, expressed toward family members or staff, or quietly turned inwardly on themselves. Most parents feel responsible for their children and express guilt and regret to varying degrees. Some family members may begin to move into a stage of *bargaining* with God or in subtle ways with staff.

751

As reality sets in, many move to varying forms of *acceptance* of what is occurring.

In all stages of the PICU process families hope for their child's recovery and relief from suffering. Regardless of the child's condition, the clergy/chaplain is in a position to assist the family with realistic hope.

In addition to being sensitive to the family's coping with faith, the clergy/chaplain may enable staff members to be sensitive to the developmental stage of the patient. Many younger children or very ill children are not able to communicate much. However, siblings may need care when the adult's expression of faith is not as helpful to them. The chaplain may assist the family or staff in caring for the needs of these siblings.

In addition to the pastoral support offered during initial phases of family care, the chaplain must be one of the primary caregivers for families during crisis or death of the child. Assisting physicians with caring for the family before, during, and after important discussions about the child's condition, the decision to cease aggressive support, or death news is an appropriate role for the PICU chaplain. The clergy/chaplain may assist the parents and relatives in their grief work as they hold their child and say good-bye. The chaplain may also assist other staff members with the request for organ donation or autopsy or as other important matters are discussed.

Through care, understanding, and assessment of the patient's family and faith community, the chaplain may offer one of many perspectives to the medical staff as decisions are made about the child's care and treatment. The chaplain or the Clinical Pastoral Education chaplain resident may make rounds with the medical staff to discuss family concerns or offer an additional perspective to medical ethical discussions that often accompany PICU care.

The PICU chaplain must also be available as a caregiver to staff members and to provide assistance with the overall concerns of the unit itself. Such friendly support in times of staff grief and work stress would be akin to the care the clergy would give to his congregation. The element of spiritual care is difficult to measure. The hope and energy needed for healing and relief of pain and suffering certainly entails faith and a spiritual dimension. It is important to honor the power of such energy, not only for healing of the patient's family, but for supporting the PICU caregivers as well.

ADDITIONAL READING

Fowler J. Stages of Faith: The Psychology of Human Development and the Quest for Meaning. New York: Harper & Row, 1981, pp 9-15, 120-213.

Friedman EH. Generation to generation: Family process in church and synagogue. In Gurman AS, ed. The Guilford Family Therapy Series. New York: The Guilford Press, 1985, pp 1-8.

Kübler-Ross E. On Death and Dying. New York: Macmillan, 1973, pp 38-156.

104 Ethical Issues in Intensive Care: Autonomy, Utility, Justice, and Truthfulness

William M. Longworth

Many decisions in the intensive care unit are relatively free of agony (e.g., when satisfactory protocol meets the needs of a presenting problem). It is amid conflicts and imponderables that quandries and dilemmas arise: conflicts among claims pulling in different directions with competing weights and imponderables of outcome that in the most difficult cases cannot be clearly seen, much less weighed. Judgments are made in response to crisis. When there is time, they often reflect a consensus among physicians, health care personnel, and family. Just as often, perhaps, difficult judgments are made in the midst of conflict: conflict with different sides of one's own judgment or conflict with other participants. Application of the ordinary principles of ethics (autonomy, utility, justice, truthfulness), although their use alone cannot resolve dilemmas, can help to sift the issues and clarify critical points of decision.

Apart from these principles' limitations in all medical contexts, they are further qualified in two important respects by circumstances special to the PICU. First, the *autonomy* of the child is severely restricted. Even in the most difficult circumstances, however, self-determination is not totally nonexistent, for individual aspects of temperament and character are manifested in physiologic responses to crises. But the minimal information gained from such inferences does not begin to provide the needed assistance available from either the stated preferences or known values of established adult relationships. It is only this information that helps to "tilt" a decision when outcomes are closely balanced. Since the child has diminished self-determination, physicians and par-

ents must decide in terms of the child's best interest. With parents or their designates playing an increasingly important role in these decisions, it is important that physicians not unduly restrict the full expression of their informed judgment. Even with sensitivity to pluralism of family values and with attention, care, and openness to informed judgments of health care personnel, it is still physicians who have responsibility both for treatment decisions and for guiding the decision-making process.

The principle of *utility* seeks a favorable balance of good over harm, benefits over burdens. Difficulties enough accompany balancing decisions of this sort in any intensive care setting. The special circumstances of pediatrics entail duration of outcome. If the child responds to treatment and his quality of life is gravely impaired, the burdens to the child and to those entrusted with care can be considerable, and they persist. Amid the imponderables of these decisions, judgments about outcome must still be ventured, and in many cases bad news cannot be forever postponed. Quality-of-life questions must be honestly and realistically faced. Financial costs of treatment and cost to family and society become more relevant the more quality of life is projected as severely impaired. It is better to speak of "obligatory" instead of "heroic" treatment. Efforts are to be expended commensurate with outcome. When medical factors indicate that continued treatment causes suffering to the child and only prolongs dying, obligation to treat becomes an obligation to discontinue treatment. When this situation exists, the physician must guide the parents toward this decision and help them accept the death of the child. In these situations one is not always absolutely certain of what is right. But applying sensitivity and openness to the range of factors, combined with a rigorous and thoughtful honesty brought to critical reflection in conversation with others, allows a sense of what is right most often to emerge.

The principle of utility seeks balance of benefits over burdens. The principle of *justice* seeks fairness in their distribution. On the large scale in our society difficult choices are forthcoming between performing miracle procedures at the high end of medical care and making standard treatment available to all. The challenge of new frontiers is the life force of medicine. Applying honesty and rigor toward prospects and using restraint in performing costly procedures postpone the day when social and legislative pressure will arbitrarily restrict both research and treatment choices in individual cases. At present pressure for access to intensive care treatment should not cause the withdrawal of treatment in situations in which that treatment is obligatory.

Truthfulness is the principle that guards both the integrity of the other principles and the process of their application. Truthfulness must be understood, not in the narrow or technical sense of verbal veracity, but in the broadest sense of truth about the total situation. This means that physicians, health care personnel, and families not only have an obligation to speak truth to one another, they also have a deeper and more profound obligation to listen for the truth. The capacity for denying bad news is enormous. To keep this capacity from causing harm, everyone has to listen: to the responses of the child, to expressions of hope, and also to information about the prolonged drain on resources of all by the severely damaged child. Enhanced technical capacities and the entire drive of medicine is to fix problems. But displaying courage and honesty is also necessary in accepting tragedy when it cannot be avoided.

Truthfulness is the guardian both of the process and of the outcome. Competence, sensitivity, openness, and rigorous honesty; listening to the responses of the child, to health care personnel, to family, and to reports of strains on resources; humility in judging as best one can . . . if these principles are practiced by all, a sense of what is right emerges, and in most cases the right thing is done.

ADDITIONAL READING

Abram MB, Dunlop GR, Jacobson BK. Deciding to Forego Life-Sustaining Treatment. President's Commission for the Study of Ethical Problems in Medicine and Biomedical and Behavioral Research. Washington, D.C.: U.S. Government Printing Office, 1983.

Beauchamp TL, Childress JF. Principles of Biomedical Ethics, 3rd ed. Oxford: Oxford University Press, 1989.

105 Denial or Termination of Treatment in a PICU

Angela R. Holder

BACKGROUND

Issues of denial or termination of curative therapies in a PICU may involve a number of situations. First, parents may initiate a request to allow a child to die in a situation in which the physicians believe that the child should be treated. Second, parents and physicians may agree that further treatment is futile and that the child should be allowed to "die in peace." Third, the physicians may believe that further treatment is futile, and the parents may wish "everything done." Fourth, in any of the above situations there may be a disagreement between the parents, the parents may not be able to understand the situation no matter how carefully it is explained to them, or the physicians may be trying to deal with an adolescent single mother and her extended family. The primary issue is who can agree to what. Any of these situations creates a different legal problem.

THE PARENT WHO REFUSES TO CONSENT TO TREATMENT
Child Abuse and Neglect

Parental refusal to obtain adequate medical care for a child is, by definition, child neglect under the child abuse statutes in each state. Courts are willing to intervene in most circumstances in which physicians ask them to do so and will order the child treated over parental objections. Parents also may be criminally prosecuted under child neglect statutes.

Religious Objections to Treatment

The most frequent situation in which parents wish to refuse treatment for a child is one in which their objections are based on religious conviction. For example, Jehovah's Witnesses refuse to consent to blood transfusions but will consent to other forms of medical intervention; some members of faith-healing sects refuse to permit any forms of medical care. Courts have uniformly held that parental rights to freedom of religion under the First Amendment do not extend to allowing their children to die or become disabled. There is clear law that a competent adult has the right to refuse any treatment for himself even if death will result; the same autonomy does not extend to one's child's well-being.

A few cases within the recent past have dealt with the right of an adolescent member of such a sect to refuse chemotherapy. Although these cases occur much too infrequently to allow drawing generalized conclusions about "the state of the law" on the issue, it seems that once judges determine that the adolescent's refusal of treatment is not the result of parental coercion but is an independently held conviction, a 16- or 17-year-old youth may be permitted to make this decision. Courts seem, however, to disallow the wishes of children younger than 16 years old and order them treated over their objections and the wishes of their parents.

Courts will order treatment of these children even if the issue is not the child's death but concerns a prognosis of substantial disability. For example, court orders to treat children of faith-healing sect members have been granted to allow treatment of children with epilepsy, severely infected tonsils and adenoids (conditions that were predicted to cause deafness), congenital facial deformities severe enough to preclude the child's possibilities for a normal life, and significant speech problems.

Nonreligious Objections to Treatment

Some parents who are perfectly willing to consent to most forms of medical intervention for their children are opposed to particular interventions deemed necessary by physicians. These situations are, in general, treated in legal terms in the same way that religious objections are handled; namely, most, if not all, courts will rule in favor of the therapy if the physicians ask for such an order and the situation is urgent. In fact, however, courts are much more likely to consider the parents' reasons as significant. Judges tend to be mainline, middle-class people (they have been through college and law school); members of nonmainline religious groups tend in many cases to be less than well-educated or articulate and may find themselves dismissed as members of "nut groups." Alternatively, well-educated parents who refuse to consent to blood transfusions because they are afraid their child might get AIDS or refuse chemotherapy because they would rather have their child die than be subjected to the side effects of the drugs are, in fact, much more likely to be taken seriously at a judicial hearing than those whose objections to identical interventions are based on religious beliefs.

Transfer of Care

If the objecting parent is able to find a licensed physician who is willing to assume responsibility for the care of the child within the parent's desired limitations (e.g., a physician who is willing to give a child laetrile instead of chemotherapy), in most circumstances a court will allow transfer of the child to the new physician even though his philosophy is not that of mainstream medicine. The theory is that once a parent takes a child to a physician and agrees with that physician on a course of treatment, the parent has met the requirements of the law of child neglect. If the nonmainstream physician's theories are dangerous to the child's health, it should be up to the state's medical licensing board to deal with the situation instead of asking a judge to choose between alternative schools of medical thought. The right to pursue alternatives, incidentally, involves only a parent's right to take the child to another physician. A court will not grant a parent's request to transfer care of a child to a chiropractor, naturopath, or other nonmedical healer.

Permissible Limits of Refusal

Courts take seriously parents' refusal to consent to treatment when the risks of treatment are great and benefits may not be as obvious. For example, a judge may be confronted with a child whose heart defect is grave but who is not likely to die immediately and parents who are refusing permission for performing high-risk heart surgery on the child. Since the cardiac surgeon who is asking for the court order to operate cannot assure the parents or the court that the child will survive the surgery and the immediate postoperative period, the parents' statement that "it's just too dangerous" is likely to prevail. This, of course, is not a situation in which desperate measures are being attempted to save the life of a child whose death is both imminent and inevitable unless "something" is done and no less-risky procedure can be expected to achieve the same result.

Any parent has the right to refuse to allow his child to participate in a clinical investigation, even, for example, when the drug being tested is much more likely to be successful in curing the child than any available approved drug. Federal research regulations specifically provide that any research subject or his duly authorized representative must be told that participation is voluntary and that refusal to participate will involve no penalty or loss of benefits to which the subject is otherwise entitled.

Criminal Prosecution of Parents

Criminal prosecution of parents for medical neglect of their children almost entirely occurs in instances in which the parents, for reasons involving religion, inertia, or some other factor, do not take an obviously sick child to a physician at all. Disagreement with physicians' recommendations and consequent refusal to consent to treatment, however irrational, may well result in court-ordered care, but it will not result in criminal prosecution of the parent.

• • •

Physicians who are taking care of a child who is sufficiently ill or injured to be a patient in the PICU are almost certain to prevail if they ask a judge to issue an order for life-saving or disability-preventing treatment that parents are refusing. If the parents have a physician who uses an alternative therapy that they do find acceptable and who is willing to care for the child, however, the PICU physician must be prepared to convince the judge that the proposed alternative therapy will clearly be ineffective, not just less effective than the treatment for which the order is being sought. The proposed course of treatment must also be within the broadest realm of mainstream medicine.

AGREEMENT NOT TO PURSUE FURTHER THERAPY

When a physician caring for a child whose parents are refusing treatment requests a court order to allow performance of the treatment under the state's child neglect statutes, it is extremely unusual for the order not to be granted. When, however, parents and physicians agree that providing further treatment is inappropriate and some third party—welfare agencies, police, or school personnel—attempts to intervene, courts invariably follow the judgment of the treating physicians and allow the refusal to stand.

One important point about the cases in which physicians have requested court orders to treat children is that in all of them it is clear that the treatment, if given, would either cure the child or allow him to lead a much more normal life than otherwise would be possible. There are *no* cases in which the treatment sought to save a child's life would result in long-term serious disabilities as opposed to death (e.g., saving a child's life by removing a brain tumor, but leaving the child blind but with a normal life expectancy).

A mentally competent adult has the right on his own behalf to refuse lifesaving treatment that will prolong a miserable or painful existence; this is the principle behind the increasing insistence in this country on "death with dignity." Parents should be allowed to make the same decision for their children. In the few cases in which courts have been asked to rule on the parents' right to order a respirator disconnected for a child who is in a persistent vegetative state, as long as the judge is satisfied that the diagnosis and prognosis are correct, parents are permitted to make that decision.

Decisions to forego surgery, to disconnect a respirator, or to omit some other form of treatment must be based on correct diagnoses. To allow a child to die and then discover at autopsy that the prognosis actually was much better than had been predicted is not only a tragedy, but it is likely to result in a successful malpractice suit. For this reason many departments of pediatrics have policies requiring all such situations to be presented to the institution's Pediatric Ethics Committee. Review by such a committee will also serve to establish that the decision was a reasonable one in the light of current pediatric knowledge and practice.

Decisions to forego lifesaving treatment must be made solely on the basis of the child's condition.

Factors such as economics (the family may have difficulties affording therapy after the hospitalization) or social concerns (the family may not be bright enough to meet the child's needs) are entirely out of place in this calculation. Any decision to allow a child to die because his family is poor or ignorant and, in the physician's estimation, could not care for the child if he recovered from his illness or injury is not only arrogant paternalism in its worst form, but it is quite clearly actionable malpractice.

Criminal prosecution of either the parents or the physician after making a decision to forego treatment is almost unprecedented in U.S. medical history, and fear of criminal charges should not control medical decision making in these cases. As long as the decision was reasonable (which approval by a pediatrics ethics committee would certainly indicate) and the child was kept comfortable and "allowed to die," no prosecutor would be interested in taking action. However, active euthanasia, otherwise known as "mercy killing," is murder and is likely to be prosecuted as such.

PARENTAL REFUSAL TO AGREE TO NONTREATMENT

On occasion physicians realize that a child is unlikely to awaken from a coma or is brain dead or that whatever treatment is available will only prolong the dying process for a child; but when the situation is explained to the parents, they "want everything done."

If a child is brain dead, as determined by standard medical criteria, parental permission to disconnect a respirator or other life-support machinery is not legally required. Although removing life supports against the wishes of a parent is not usually permitted in most PICUs, the brain-dead child is legally dead, and the situation can be dealt with as is any death. The death certificate may be signed and the life-support system disconnected. The parents should never be asked for permission; they need only be told their child is dead. Particularly in the case of a sudden death, such as a child who is perfectly healthy and happy one moment and in a horrible accident the next, it may be humane pediatric practice to keep the child on the respirator for a few days until the family members can come to grips with their loss, but it is not legally required.

If the child's condition is the result of child abuse, parents may object vehemently to disconnection of the respirator. As soon as the child is pronounced dead, they may be arrested for murder instead of assault, so it is entirely in their interests to postpone a declaration of death as long as possible. Particularly in these cases and frequently in others in which parents simply cannot accept their child's death, prudence may dictate that a court order be obtained before the child's life-support system is disconnected. In several cases involving children who were brain dead as the result of abuse, courts have ruled that the physician may declare the child dead and disconnect the respirator over parental objection, but it is extremely unlikely that the court would allow a physician to disconnect life-support machinery if the child did not meet all criteria for brain death and was in a chronic vegetative state.

If the child is not brain dead but is clearly in a permanent state of coma, parental refusal to disconnect a life-support system must be respected. Counseling may change the parent's mind, but as long as the parent refuses, that decision must be respected.

SPECIAL PROBLEMS IN CONSENT
Consent of One Parent

In an urgent situation, if one parent is willing to agree to therapy but the other refuses, consent may be obtained from the one and treatment begun. In a situation of less urgency, however, if negotiation does not bring agreement and the treatment carries significant risk (e.g., any surgery performed with the child under general anesthesia), it is probably prudent to ask a judge for a court order to treat the child. If one parent wants the child treated and the other is not making positive objections or is away or so detached that he is not actually involved, the consent of one parent is sufficient, and no court order is required.

If parents are divorced, although the one with legal custody does ultimately have the paramount right to give consent, noncustodial parents remain parents and certainly have the right to be involved in their children's medical care. If the child is brought to the hospital by one parent and the other is not available, the parent who is present has the right to make all necessary decisions, even if he is not the custodial parent.

Uncomprehending Parents

As all pediatricians know, giving an explanation to parents sometimes fails. The parents simply cannot comprehend the situation, treatment cannot be further delayed, the risks may be great, and an impasse is reached. In some cases of sudden-onset critical illness or an accident, the parents may be perfectly capable of understanding things and are just shocked. In those cases normal ability to reason will return, and emergency care may be given in the meantime. Non-physician members of the health care team, particularly nurses in the PICU and the unit's social workers and clergy, may, in fact, be more adept at communicating with parents in this situation than the child's physicians, since the parents may perceive the physician as a more threatening figure.

If lack of comprehension is the result of a language barrier, the obvious solution is to obtain an interpreter. Most medical centers have lists of interpreters who can translate for non-English-speaking patients and their families, and critical care units in particular need to have access to interpreters on very short notice. Assuming that the parents' language is one expected within the community (e.g., French, Spanish), it would be absolutely no defense to an informed-consent suit later that the physician could not speak the parents' language, no interpreter was on duty, and no explanation could be made. The hospital (as opposed to the physician) would no doubt be liable for its negligence in failing to have the interpreter available. When the language is not one expected to be found within the community, however, and if reasonable effort is made to find an interpreter, but no one can be located, presumably there would be no liability. "Reasonable effort," incidentally, would presumably include trying to find a nonmedical faculty member or graduate student who speaks the language if the hospital is located in a community with a university offering instruction in the language in question.

In some situations the parents speak English, they are not in shock, and they simply cannot understand what they are told. If persistent efforts by physicians, nurses, chaplains, and social workers do not result in understanding and no members of the more extended family are available to assist, it is certainly possible to initiate a proceeding for a court order for treatment. This step, however, should be reserved for interventions carrying substantial risk for the child.

Many infants and small children are the children of minor parents. A minor mother, who may legally surrender her child for adoption without the approval of her family, may also make medical decisions for her child in spite of the fact that she is under age. Minor fathers who are married to the child's mother also have the same rights to consent to treatment as an adult parent would, but if the couple is not married and the father is not present, his opinion does not have to be sought, and his consent is not required. Although many adolescent mothers and their babies live with the mothers' families, the mother, not her parents (the child's grandparents), is the appropriate party from whom to obtain consent. This does not preclude discussion with the extended family if they are present and involved, but the young mother herself must consent.

In many cases the parents may not be present. In particular, an adolescent mother may have left her child with her own mother and gone away to begin a new life, but the grandmother has never been appointed legal guardian of the child. In situations in which there is guardianship resulting from lack of the presence of the mother, the grandparent should be treated as if he were the child's parent and allowed to make decisions about the child's medical care.

ADDITIONAL READING

Ewald LS. Medical decision-making for children: An analysis of competing interests. St Louis Law J 25:689, 1982.
• Holder AR. Parents, courts and refusal of treatment. J Pediatr 103:515, 1983.
• Sher EJ. Choosing for children: Adjudicating medical care disputes between parents and the state. NYU Law Rev 58:157, 1983.

Cases

In re B., 92 Cal App 3d 796, cert den 445 U.S. 949, 1980 (refusal of heart surgery for child with Down's syndrome).

In re Barry, 445 So 2d 365, FL 1984 (parents and physicians may decide to disconnect life support systems for a permanently comatose child).

In the Matter of the Appeal in Cochise County Juvenile Action, 650 p 2d 459, AZ 1982 (refusal to obtain any medical care for children after one died of peritonitis; mother believed in faith healing).

In re Custody of a Minor, 379 N.E. 2d 1053, 393 N.E. 2d 836, 1979 (refusal to consent to chemotherapy; parents wished to give the child laetrile; this is the famous case about Chad Green).

In re D.L.E., 645 P 2d 271, CO 1982 (mother who believed in faith healing refused to allow child to be medicated for epilepsy).

In re Hamilton, 657 SW 2d 425, TN 1983 (religious objections to use of chemotherapy).

In re P.V.W., 424 So 2d 1015, LA 1982 (parents and physicians have the right to decide together to remove respirator from a child in a persistent vegetative state).

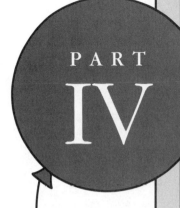

PART

IV

Equipment and
Techniques

106 The Physical Setting: Conceptual Considerations

Maureen Zipkin · Daniel L. Levin

BACKGROUND

The role that the actual physical environment plays in the successful management of critically ill children must not be underestimated. A well-designed unit facilitates the work of the entire health care team and supports both the child's and family's needs for privacy, quiet, and comfort. It is critical that the design of the unit addresses the needs of all these people.

Even in the most ideal of circumstances, designers of PICUs inevitably face numerous constraints, including financial, geographic, personnel, and political issues. The challenge to the designers and planners is to identify and prioritize the major functions and requirements of the unit and choose among the many options to meet these objectives. Without careful ordering of objectives, decisions about unit design cannot be made optimally.

It is also critical that the design team adopt a long-range perspective of the unit's functions and requirements. This futuristic perspective must be based on a comprehensive strategic planning process and reflect a unit mission that has evolved from careful analysis of both internal and external factors. In today's rapidly changing health care environment, it is unwise to assume that patient populations, team composition and function, treatment modalities, and resources currently available will remain as they are in the future. Major changes in any one of these variables can drastically change the physical requirements of the unit. Therefore a unit designed for the future must be adaptable and expandable and must maximize the resources of space, time, equipment, communication, and personnel.

ALLOCATION OF SPACE

One of the first decisions to make is about division and allocation of a limited amount of space. This is perhaps the most difficult decision and one that is essential to the effective and efficient functioning of the unit (Fig. 106-1).

Patient Care Areas

Before decisions about allocation of space can be made, the number of bed spaces to comprise the unit must be determined. The number of beds can be determined by analyzing the following data. Historical PICU occupancy statistics provide the starting point. In addition to looking at average daily census, it is important to look at the maximum daily census. If adequate systems are not in place to ensure efficient patient flow out of the unit, it is highly likely that the maximum census will greatly exceed average daily census. The number of beds available in the unit must accommodate this increased patient load, even if only for 6 hours out of the day. It is also important to consider other variables that will affect future bed use such as the competitive health care environment in the city, the planned addition or deletion of programs that involve a PICU stay, and demographic trend projections for the area. Finally, the number of beds in the unit may in part be determined by comparing space per patient required and desired with actual space available.

State codes govern the amount of space required per patient and the minimum distance required between patients. For example, in Texas the Hospital Licensing Standards stipulate that neonatal intensive care areas must have a minimum area of 100 square

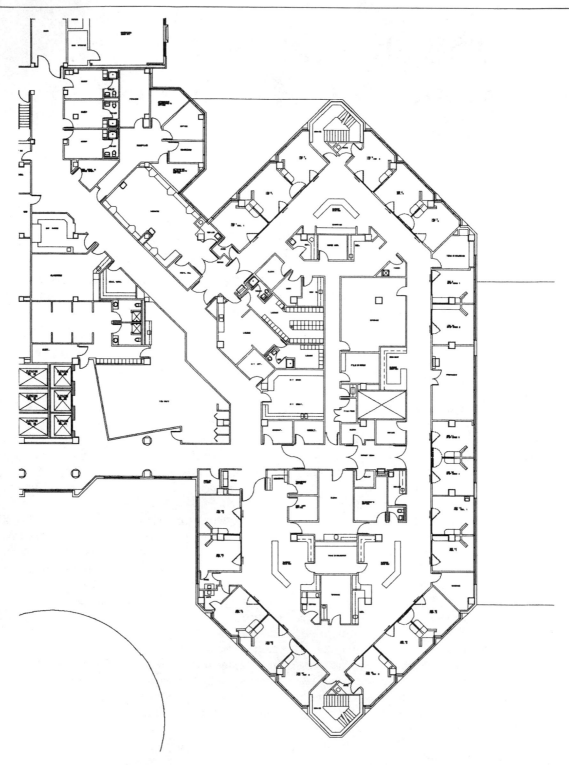

Fig. 106-1   Overall unit design. (Courtesy HKS, Inc., Dallas, Tex.)

feet per bed and that the distance between beds must be at least 6 feet. Pediatric intensive care areas require a minimum square footage of 120 feet. Clearance between beds must be at least 4½ feet. The amount of space required by code may be much less than the amount of space desired. Technologically sophisticated units may require as much as 200 square feet per bed to accommodate routine (numerous IV poles and pumps, ventilator) and special patient care needs (hemodialysis, extracorporeal membrane oxygenation, portable nuclear scans) (Fig. 106-2). Individual bed space requirements may limit the overall bed capacity of the unit.

Minimum requirements for isolation are also gov-erned by state codes. In Texas one private room to be used for seclusion and/or isolation must be provided for each 10 beds or one for each unit if the overall bed capacity is less than 10 beds. It is also necessary for planners to consider the isolation requirements or preferences for anticipated patient populations. For example, although their use is not a universal practice, individual transplant surgeons may desire isolation rooms for their patients. Also to be considered are the recommendations of the Centers for Disease Control for replacing traditional forms of isolation with body substance isolation, thereby decreasing the number of isolation rooms required.

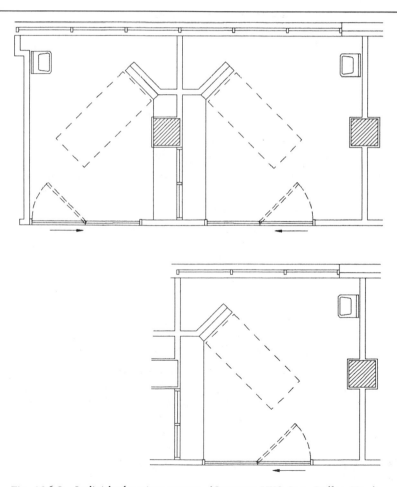

Fig. 106-2   Individual patient rooms. (Courtesy HKS, Inc., Dallas, Tex.)

Support Services

State codes also govern the minimum requirements for kinds of support areas. For example, in Texas the Hospital Licensing Standards stipulate that a storage space of not less than 20 square feet be provided in neonatal intensive care areas. Other requirements include having a workroom, examination and treatment room, formula room, janitor closet, and soiled workroom.

In addition to allocating space for support areas as required by state codes, planners must consult with all members of the PICU multidisciplinary team to discuss their individual space requirements before making a final decision about allocation of space for support services. A systematic analysis of needed support areas can address the topics of equipment, services, communication, and personnel.

Regardless of what the codes suggest, a storage space of only 20 square feet is inadequate for a large, technologically sophisticated unit. The only way to determine how much storage space is needed is to measure equipment and carts, multiply by the exact quantities, add the totals, and include additional square footage to accommodate new equipment.

The following services' space needs must be considered: respiratory therapy, surgery, pharmacy, radiology, dietary, social service, child life, pastoral care, materials management, education, biomedical engineering, and clerical support. A unit with an automated patient data management system will also need space allocated for that system.

Every unit must have space(s) allocated for electronic and human communications. This may be the central nursing station in a small unit or a separate communications center in addition to multiple nursing stations in a large unit. The central communications center will house the master telephone and intercom systems, contain computer and pneumatic tube terminals, and serve as the coordinating center for the entry and exit of staff, visitors, equipment, and supplies. It is also necessary to provide space away from the patient areas for staff communication with each other and for staff communication with families.

Allocating space for unit personnel for both work-related activities and relaxation is essential. An adequate number of classrooms and conference rooms must be provided so that multiple functions can occur at once. It is also important that staff members have a comfortable and private lounge in which to relax and socialize. Locker facilities must be provided

in or adjacent to the unit. Finally, office space should be located on the unit for all members of the multidisciplinary team.

It is also important to provide support areas such as on-call rooms, office space, small library facilities, and desk space for physicians who use the PICU.

Family Support Areas

In Texas the Hospital Licensing Standards require that PICUs provide sleeping space for parents who must be under the control of and in communication with the PICU staff. Space should also be allocated for other parent-support facilities such as a lounge, grieving rooms, quiet rooms, shower and lavatories, locker facilities, kitchenette, and vending areas, and the facilities should be near local and long-distance telephone facilities.

DESIGN OF SPACE

Although Hospital Licensing Standards and other accreditation organizations have certain requirements that guide the design of space, numerous options confront the planners as they enter the process of spatial design. Prioritization of unit objectives will guide the decision process.

Patient Care Areas

When designing the patient care areas, planners must consider the current trend of providing care with fewer people, a result of both personnel shortages and cost-containment reasons. The acuity level of the patients as well as the technologic sophistication of the unit also must be considered. A fast-paced, technologically sophisticated unit with a lean staffing component dictates that resources needed for the care of patients be in close proximity to those patients and that access to and visualization of patients be unimpeded by physical barriers and inefficient traffic patterns.

The above considerations will guide the choice between an open bay arrangement or enclosed cubicles in the patient areas. If the general population of the unit is comprised of critically ill children needing extensive technology and personnel on a continuous basis, providing an open bay or cubicles with sliding walls is desirable. This design allows expansion of the space around the patient and its adaptation to accommodate a sudden and/or sustained influx of equipment and personnel (Fig. 106-2). The nature and quantity of invasive monitoring devices also help establish the requirements for the spacial layout. All children who are invasively monitored or who are aided by life-support equipment need constant observation and monitoring. This is more easily accomplished in an open bay arrangement than in an area with an enclosed cubicle design. When working with critically ill, unstable, or potentially unstable children, it is likely that the prioritized list of unit requirements places patient safety and quick access to patients ahead of patient privacy or infection control. Although individual cubicles are superior to the open bay arrangement for provision of privacy and quiet and for minimizing cross-contamination, supporting concerns that have a higher priority (e.g., ready access) require that the open bay or cubicles with sliding walls be chosen. If affordable, the cubicle with sliding walls appears to be the best solution since multiple objectives can be met with this design.

If space and finances allow, one additional patient area that is desirable is a special procedures room. The functions of this room can be multiple, including initial placement of catheters and tubes, performance of minor and/or major surgical procedures, and provision of a holding area for a patient whose own room is not yet ready. To accommodate these multiple functions this room must contain the same design as the individual bed spaces in the rest of the unit but also must contain equipment and features needed in an operating room. This includes a surgical table that can accommodate fluoroscopy equipment (a portable C-arm), multiparameter monitoring capabilities, an anesthesia machine and electrosurgical unit, an overhead surgical light, a scrub sink, and blanket and solution warmers. The general lighting system can be zoned so that certain areas of the room can be illuminated while fluoroscopy is in progress. The headwall system must contain several more vacuum outlets and access to additional medical gases such as nitrous oxide and nitrogen. C-lockers at one end of the room can house supplies and small pieces of equipment.

In the design of the individual bed spaces the overall patient population of the unit as well as the long-term plans for the unit must be considered. It is also imperative that designers consider the trends in current and future monitoring capabilities. A large technologically sophisticated PICU in a tertiary care facility has significantly different bedside requirements from those of a small PICU in a community hospital. Additionally, a unit committed to purchasing new monitors that provide modules to replace numerous stand-alone monitoring devices actually may have decreased electrical and space requirements at the bedsides. Automated patient data management systems create specific requirements for each bedside.

Numerous vendors manufacture custom-made headwalls or columns that are capable of providing virtually every physical resource needed at the bedside. Numbers and location of electrical outlets, grounding inlets, vacuum and oxygen and air outlets, alarm buttons, communications systems, lighting controls, equipment brackets, and storage capabilities can all be individually tailored (Fig. 106-3). Achieving the optimum arrangement of these systems necessitates collaboration of a multidisciplinary team comprised of physicians, nurses, respiratory therapists, biomedical engineers, and architects.

Key issues to address in the design of the bed space include provision of adequate access both to patients and to the resources at the bedside, unimpeded visualization of both the patient and the monitoring devices, expandability of space, and privacy. It is essential that electrical, vacuum, oxygen, and air outlets are positioned so that cables and tubings attached to them do not impede patient contact or visualization. Also, it is essential that the patient's position does not impede access to all of these outlets. Additionally, the layout of the bed space must accommodate health care providers of varying heights. This becomes particularly important when choosing the height of cardiac monitors and computer screens, since they are typically placed at a height that allows visualization from other more distant positions. The large number of cables going from the patient to the monitors must feed into a central transmission system rather than drape individually across the patient and his space.

Support Services

Storage space must be near the patient areas to facilitate efficiency. Movable furniture such as C-lockers on adjustable tracts will provide needed flexibility as storage needs change over time. Storage areas also must have numerous electrical outlets at both floor height and counter height so that chargeable equipment can remain plugged in.

Support service areas can function as work areas or office areas. Services such as respiratory therapy, pharmacy, radiology, dietary, and clerical support

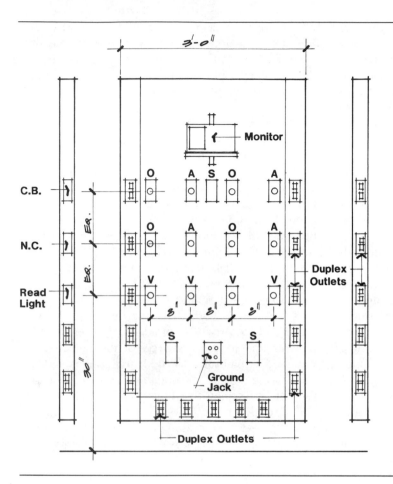

Fig. 106-3 Headwall for the patient's bed. (Courtesy HKS, Inc., Dallas, Tex.)

need actual work areas designed for them. The capabilities of the pharmacy and radiology satellite areas must mimic those provided in the central pharmacy and the radiology department. Other services such as social services, pastoral care, and child life will need offices of a standard design.

The communications areas must be designed to provide adequate space and seating for a variety of team members. If space allows, it is desirable to provide a separate area in which physicians can review charts, write orders, and talk on the phone. Nursing stations must be located and designed to facilitate visualization of numerous patients in the event that nurses must leave the bedside to perform functions at the nursing station. The design of the family con-

ference rooms must accommodate four to five family members and several health care team members in a comfortable manner and must provide privacy.

Staff conference rooms and classrooms must be designed to accommodate a variety of functions. It is desirable for each of these rooms to have blackboards and projection screens. Storage space for in-service videotapes, equipment, procedure manuals, and reference materials must either be provided in a small library in the unit or be incorporated into a conference room or classroom. The staff lounge needs to include comfortable sofas and chairs for use during relaxation. A small area of the lounge should be designed as a kitchenette with a refrigerator and microwave.

Family Support Areas

The parent sleeping area is preferably separate from the general visitors' lounge. The furniture in the lounge needs to be arranged so that the room is divided into numerous small sections to provide as much privacy as possible. If space allows, a game table can be provided at one end of the lounge. Providing a message board will facilitate family and visitor communication with each other. Shower and lavatory facilities need to be accessible from both the sleeping and lounge areas. Grieving and quiet rooms need to be located away from the general family area so that privacy is maximized for particularly distraught family members.

ADDITIONAL READING

Fein IA, Strosberg MA. Managing the Critical Care Unit. Rockville, Md.: Aspen, 1987, pp 113-125.

Texas Department of Health. Hospital Licensing Standards. Hospital and Professional Licensure Division, sections 7-3 and 7-4. May 1986.

107 Electrocardiographic and Respiratory Monitors

Stephanie M. Ford · Frances C. Morriss

BACKGROUND AND INDICATIONS

The use of bedside ECG and respiratory monitors is a mainstay of monitoring in the PICU. The ECG provides information about the electrical conduction system of the heart, the absolute heart rate, and relative changes in the heart rate. Each waveform represents one myocardial contraction and the electrical activity generated by it. It is not, however, representative of the contractility of the heart. The respiratory component of the monitor records respiratory effort through measurement of thoracic impedance.

All patients admitted to the PICU are immediately placed on ECG and respiratory monitors. These monitors generally allow visualization of an ECG and a respiratory tracing on an oscilloscope and give a numeric readout of heart and respiratory rates per minute. The instrumentation on the monitors includes the following controls:

1. On-off switch
2. Oscilloscope
3. Brightness control
4. Heart rate digital display
5. Rate alarms
6. Position control
7. Size control
8. Gain control
9. mm/sec control
10. Run/hold/record control
11. Calibration control
12. Mode control
13. Lead control

ELECTROCARDIOGRAPHIC MONITORING
Technique

The rate alarms must be set for each patient. A safe range is 10 to 15 beats above and below the patient's normal heart rate range. The position control knob allows determination of the position of the ECG tracing on the oscilloscope. The entire complex (high and low points) must be visible on the screen. The size control knob allows adjustment of the size of the complex for better visualization. The gain control (also known as sensitivity) knob allows adjustment of the height of the ECG complexes and alters the internal sensing mechanism of the monitor. This mechanism counts the R waves, and if the ECG complexes are too high or too low, the monitor will count them incorrectly. The millimeters per second (mm/sec) control determines the speed at which the ECG complexes will move across the screen. The common practice is to leave this control at the 25 mm/sec position. Increasing the speed to 50 mm/sec causes the complexes to spread, and decreasing the speed results in their being closer together. The 50 mm/sec speed is useful in making a diagnosis such as determining the presence or absence of P waves. The run/hold/record control allows continuous monitoring in the *run* mode; freezing the waveform on the oscilloscope in the *hold* mode; and recording the pattern on the central monitor on the *record* mode. The calibration control allows calibration of the monitor against a consistent standard so that abnormalities in the tracing can be measured. Most monitors are calibrated to a 1 mm standard. The mode control determines whether the monitor is on continuously or is on standby. Since different leads provide different electrical images of the heart, the lead control allows selection of a lead for cardiac monitoring. All monitors have leads I, II, and III; some have additional settings.

Proper ECG lead placement is critical in obtaining clear ECG tracings that are easily interpreted. Typical lead placement involves chest leads I, II, and III. The negative electrode (may be labeled "RA") is placed on the right midclavicular line at the second intercostal space. The positive electrode (may be labeled "LA" or "LL") is placed on the left midclavicular line at the second intercostal space; and the ground electrode may be placed on the lower abdomen or on either leg.

Modified chest lead (MCL) placement may be required for some PICU patients because of the presence of large dressings and/or small available skin surface area. The negative electrode (or RA) is placed on the outer section of the left clavicle, and the ground is placed on the right shoulder. The positive electrode (or LA or LL) is placed at the fourth intercostal space on the left sternal border. Specific monitor guidelines listed in the manufacturer's manual should be noted. The nurse must be aware of the initial lead monitored by the equipment.

The use of either of these lead systems provides sufficient information about the conduction system to be useful on a long-term basis. Finding ideal lead placement in the pediatric patient is often difficult; therefore it is imperative that changes in the ECG tracing be interpreted over time rather than as an isolated event. Before the ECG electrode is placed on the skin, the area must be defatted with an alcohol swab and scrubbed dry with a gauze pad to remove the dry layer of epithelium.

The central station provides continuous monitoring of the ECG via telemetry, which transmits the patient's ECG by an antenna system. A central station consists of a memory bank, an oscillosope, a recorder, and an alarm system. The memory bank stores specific information and allows retrieval. The recorder permits the printing of hard copy of rhythm strips, which may be initiated from either the central station or the patient's bedside. The oscilloscope can provide constant tracings of ECGs and invasive pressure tracings.

Risks and Complications

As with any piece of equipment, the ECG monitor is only as reliable as its operator. It is the responsibility of the doctors, nurses, and respiratory therapists to become familiar with the workings of the monitor and to be able to troubleshoot it. The monitor is a machine and therefore capable of malfunctioning, so it is necessary always to examine the patient when an alarm sounds. Once it is established that the patient is stable, the equipment can be checked for problems. The patient (or the parent at the bedside) needs to be reassured that the problem is mechanical and that it will be resolved shortly.

When troubleshooting the problem, the electrodes must be checked for the presence of adequate gel. If applying pressure over the center of an electrode corrects the problem, the electrodes are probably dry and need changing. Electrodes placed over a skin fold or a large muscle mass can transmit electromyographic (EMG) signals. Next, the lead wires and patient's monitor cable must be checked for poor connections or exposed wiring. If still no solution is found, it may be necessary to remove the monitor and send it for inspection by biomedical engineers.

The gel on the electrodes may be irritating to the skin, and placement sites must be changed every 24 to 48 hours. On very small infants the site may need changing more frequently because of the hypertonicity of the gel, which may cause skin ulceration. Karaya ECG pads are available for use on infants and may be less irritating to the skin than the conventional pads.

RESPIRATORY MONITORING
Technique

Most respiratory monitors have a digital readout and a corresponding oscilloscopic waveform. The amplitude of the waveform reflects the depth of the respiration. Therefore mechanically ventilated patients may have waveforms of varying sizes, one representing the ventilator breath and one representing the patient's spontaneous respiration. Respiratory monitors must include an alarm system with high and low alarm limits that are set for each patient. They must also include an option for an apnea alarm with 10-, 15-, or 20-second intervals.

The most commonly used form of respiratory monitoring involves impedance pneumography. This method records the changes in resistance of an electrical field that result from changes in tidal volume caused by respiratory effort. The changes in resistance (impedance) are measured as the distance changes between a pair of electrodes placed on either side of the chest. With proper electrode placement and the use of filters in the system, the same two electrodes used for ECG monitoring may be used for respiratory monitoring.

Another method of monitoring a patient's respiratory effort uses a mattress containing a layer of wire mesh that measures change in thoracic capacitance. The mattress is placed in an Isolette or, if a larger bed is used, under the child's thoracic cavity. When motion is not detected within a preset time interval, an alarm will sound.

Several methods of determining respiratory airflow in the neonate have been recently developed. Quantitative measurement of respiratory airflow requires the use of a pneumotachograph, which is a device that provides a uniformly low resistance to airflow, with measurement of pressures on each side of the resistance. Change in pressure with uniform resistance is proportional to change in airflow. The pneumotachograph is used at the proximal end of the endotracheal tube in an intubated patient or through a face mask in the spontaneously breathing infant.

Qualitative assessment of airflow can be performed with instruments that determine temperature, respiratory noise, and carbon dioxide level. Changes in temperature during inspiration and expiration are detected using a thermistor, a device that varies electrical resistance in relation to temperature. Acoustic detection of respiratory effort has been tried using a microphone encapsulated in silicone and placed at the end of a 5 F, mushroom-tipped suction catheter placed at the nostril. A filter was also included in the device to help determine actual expiratory noise from background noise. A microphone equipped with a filter has also been attached to the chest wall to determine airflow by monitoring expiratory sounds. Detection of carbon dioxide in expired air is accomplished through a device that attaches inside a small conical face mask, which has Velcro straps that attach it to a hat on the infant's head. The apnea alarm system is set to go off at appropriate preset intervals.

Risks and Complications

False positive apnea alarms will occur, and the nurse must make every attempt to change electrode placement, adjust the monitor sensitivity, or reposition the patient (when possible) in an effort to minimize their happening. Repeated false alarms are irritating and/ or frightening to the patient and/or parent. Also they

may cause the PICU staff members to become nonchalant in their response (cry wolf!) and not to respond quickly to a true emergency.

Impedance pneumography transmits all chest wall movement, whether it is related to respiratory effort or not. It does not distinguish effective respiratory efforts from noneffective respiratory effort such as occurs with upper airway obstructions. Patients with unstable respiratory status need additional respiratory monitoring such as transcutaneous devices or pulse oximeters (see Chapters 120 to 122). As with all monitoring devices, it is imperative that the caregiver examine and assess the patient on an ongoing basis for signs and symptoms of distress and correlate this information with the monitor's data.

The apnea mattress is less prone to ECG interference but may pick up more artifact because of the patient's movement. The qualitative monitors need close supervision of the device actually used to measure respiratory effort to ensure their proper placement. However, they do measure direct airflow rather than chest wall movement and may be more helpful in monitoring the respiratory status of infants.

ADDITIONAL READING

Decker S. Continuous EKG monitoring systems. Nurs Clin North Am 22(1):1-11, 1987.

Dransfield DA, Philip AGS. Respiratory airflow measurement in the neonate. Clin Perinatol 12(1):21-30, 1985.

McIntosh N. The monitoring of critically ill neonates. J Med Eng Technol 7(3):121-129, 1983.

Pomerance JJ, Duncan RG. Basic equipment needs for neonatal monitoring. Clin Perinatol 10(1):189-203, 1983.

Rolfe P. Neonatal critical care monitoring. J Med Eng Technol 10(3):115-120, 1986.

Scordo KA. Taming the cardiac monitor. Part I. Nursing 82 12(8):58-63, 1982.

Scordo KA. Taming the cardiac monitor. Part II. Nursing 82 12(9):60-67, 1982.

Webster HW. Bioinstrumentation: Principles and techniques. In Hazinski MF, ed. Nursing Care of the Critically Ill Child. St. Louis: CV Mosby, 1984.

Werthammer J, Kasner J, DiBenedetto J, Start AR. Apnea monitoring by acoustic detection of airflow. Pediatrics 71:53-55, 1983.

108 Pressure Transducers

Kyoo H. Rhee · Pam Holbrook

INDICATIONS

The mercury manometer, although excellent for recording steady pressure, cannot respond to pressure changes that occur more rapidly than approximately one cycle every 2 to 3 seconds. When it is necessary to have accurate and constant information because of rapidly changing pressures in the PICU patient, a high-fidelity type of recording system using a mechanoelectrical pressure transducer is needed. More important in the PICU patient is the accurate measurement of the constant direct pressures when the indirect measures are difficult to obtain because of the small size and/or deformity of the extremity or are impossible to obtain noninvasively because of the location (CVP, LAP, PAP, ICP). In addition indirect monitoring can often be misleading (e.g., in a patient with peripheral vasoconstriction, shock, or limb damage), making direct invasive monitoring a necessity.

TECHNIQUE
The Transducer

An electronic pressure transducer is a device that converts the mechanical motion of fluid in the tubing connected to the pressure source into electrical signals. A typical transducer comprises a very thin and highly stretched metal membrane (diaphragm), which forms the base of a fluid-filled, clear plastic dome. The dome is connected through pressurized tubing to a catheter within the vessel or chamber to be monitored.

Sensing elements connected to the diaphragm convert its movement by the pressure change into an electrical signal. There are several types of sensing devices (Fig. 108-1):

1. Strain gauge: Wires or semiconductor elements change their electric resistance when distorted.
2. Inductance gauge: The diaphragm is connected to a dust-iron core, the movement of which changes the inductance of the coil.
3. Capacitance gauge: The diaphragm is connected to one plate of a variable capacitor; the changes in capacitance between the plate and diaphragm can be recorded electronically.

The electrical output (signal) produced by the sensing device is both small and noisy (full of irregularities). Therefore the signal must pass through a preamplifier for filtering and then through an amplifier for enlargement. After amplification the signal passes to a recording or display device, which may be a digital or metered readout, an oscilloscope, and/or paper (Fig. 108-1).

The pressure transducer must be zeroed to atmospheric pressure before calibration. The transducer must be properly attached to the patient's catheter and to the pressure module and must be properly positioned. For example, transducers for measuring arterial and venous blood pressures must be placed at the level of the right atrium or midchest. Transducers for measuring ICP must be placed at the level of the third ventricle or external auditory canal (any unusual or different placement for a specific purpose must be noted by the physician in the orders). The stopcock must then be turned off to the patient and the transducer opened to air. The pressure module is then adjusted until it reads a consistent zero, according to the manufacturer's instructions.

Most pressure monitoring systems use an electronic calibration system, making calibration with a mercury manometer obsolete. High-pressure catheters (i.e., arterial) are calibrated to 200 mm Hg and low-pressure catheters (i.e., right atrium, left atrium, pulmonary artery, ICP) to 40 mm Hg. Some of the newer monitors calibrate all catheters (high and low pressure) to 100 mm Hg.

To calibrate the system the stopcock must be first turned off to the patient and then the transducer opened to air. The calibration device is adjusted to

200 or 40 mm Hg or to manufacturer's specification. The level of the transducer must be checked for improper placement, or it will result in incorrect pressure readings. If the transducer level is too low, the fluid pressure in the tubing will weigh on the transducer and produce a falsely high reading. The reverse is also true; if the transducer is too high, the lack of fluid pressure will create an artificially low reading. Transducers must be recalibrated frequently; generally low-pressure catheters are calibrated at least

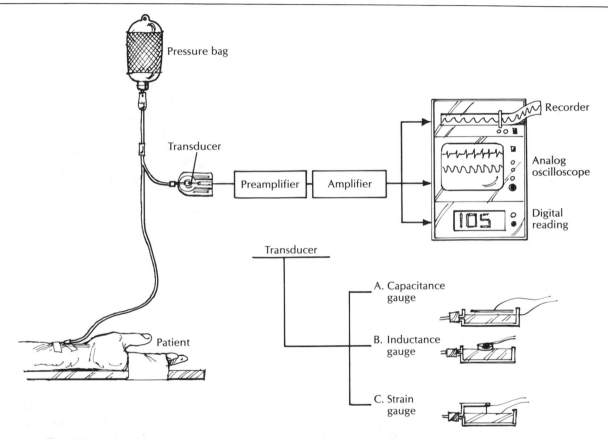

Fig. 108-1   Components of a continuous pressure measuring system and types of electric pressure transducer.

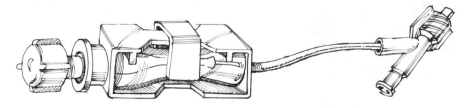

Fig. 108-2   The Intraflow device.

every 4 hours and high-pressure catheters every 8 hours. Performing recalibration must be considered for patients with changes in pressure readings after extensive catheter manipulation (e.g., multiple blood draws, weighing).

Air

Air bubbles present within the system will dampen waveforms and produce inaccurate readings, since air will compress at a ratio different from that of the fluid.

Continuous vs. Intermittent Readings

Continuous pressure readings are preferable to intermittent readings, and they are made possible with the use of the Intraflow device. The Intraflow (Fig. 108-2) is a disposable plastic device that fits between the transducer, the fluid source, and the patient and allows continuous pressure reading concurrent with continuous fluid infusion to the patient. It comes in either a 3 or 30 ml/hr size. Generally a pressure bag, inflated to 300 mm Hg, is used with a 3 ml/hr Intraflow. An infusion pump with a rate of up to 30 ml/hr may be used with the 30 ml/hr Intraflow device. This device cannot accept a flow rate greater than its maximum capacity even if the infusion pump is set a greater rate (e.g., 35 ml/hr).

Manifolds

In patients needing monitoring of multiple pressure catheters a manifold that allows reading of multiple pressure catheters off a limited number of transducers may be used (Fig. 108-3). Care must be taken to label all catheters appropriately to avoid medication or fluid errors.

TPN and Intraflow Devices

Recently, we have noted that TPN and/or intralipid infusions given through CVP catheters with Intraflow devices in place have resulted in abnormally high

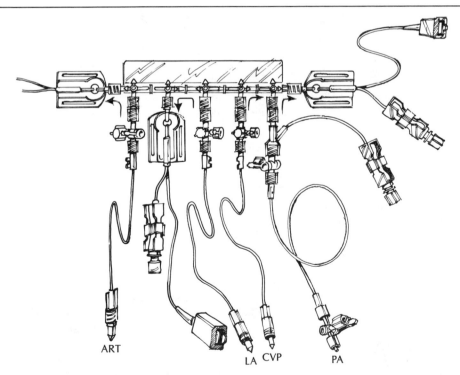

Fig. 108-3 This manifold allows reading of four pressure lines off the three transducers. Although three catheters give continuous readouts, a fourth may be read intermittently by turning the stopcock to the transducer. Note that all catheters are labeled to avoid confusion.

readings. It is possible that the density of the TPN and/or lipids may interfere with the Intraflow device's ability to regulate pressure from the infusion pump. Therefore, when the CVP is read during TPN and lipid infusions, the fluid source must be temporarily turned off to obtain the reading.

Disposable Transducers

Many PICUs are currently using the completely disposable transducers. Many of the contaminants found in transducers come from the hands of personnel during manipulation or from breaks in technique during some change. Therefore the invention of the

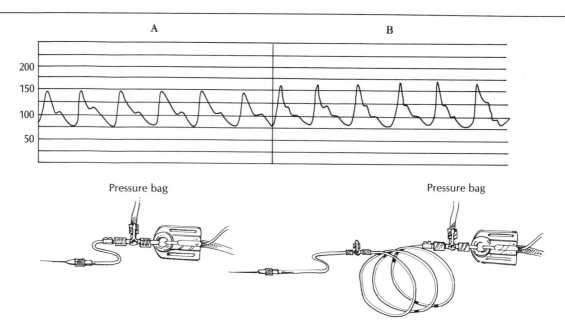

Fig. 108-4 **A,** Pressure recording from short extension tubing. **B,** Pressure recording from long extension tubing. Note approximately 20 mm Hg difference in systolic pressure caused by overshooting by *B* system.

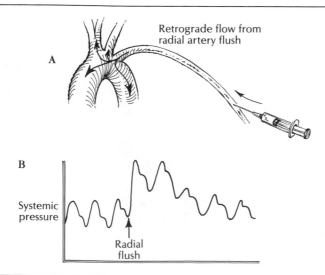

Fig. 108-5 **A,** Schematic drawing of retrograde blood flow caused by vigorous radial flush. **B,** Acutely elevated systemic arterial blood pressure during radial flush with high-pressure bag.

one-piece, single-use transducer can result in a reduction in the risk of infection. Cost effectiveness, always an issue, is currently being evaluated. One particular advantage of using the disposable transducer is the elimination of the frequent repair that is necessary for the permanent transducer. If the permanent transducer is used constantly, wear and tear are great, and greater range of inaccuracy occurs with the transducer (i.e., more drift in the reading). Many newer monitoring systems reject the transducers with unacceptable drift (i.e., will not zero). Zeroing and calibration of disposable transducers is the same as for permanent ones.

RISKS AND COMPLICATIONS

Most of the risks associated in pressure monitoring occur with the indwelling catheter and not the transducer. The risks of infection, emboli, bleeding, and electrocution from an indwelling catheter may be reduced when the catheters are removed as soon as the patient is stabilized. The risk of infection may be reduced by using strict sterile technique when placing the catheter, when setting up the transducer, and whenever it is necessary to break into the tubing system. Disposable systems may reduce the incidence of infection from the tubing system as discussed previously.

Erroneous reading may be prevented by using stiff, noncompliant extension tubing of the shortest possible length (Fig. 108-4). Avoiding the use of more than one stopcock between catheter and transducer will also reduce the chance of error.

Retrograde flow caused by vigorous flush while using a high-pressure bag may cause embolism to vital organs such as the brain (Fig. 108-5). The use of high-pressure bags for flushing pressure lines must be avoided. Instead a small syringe may be used for gentle flushing with 0.5 to 1.0 ml of flush solution.

As with all electronic devices, the electrical system must be grounded and constantly monitored for excessive leakage (>10 μA).

ADDITIONAL READING

American Heart Association. Invasive Monitoring Technique. Textbook of Advanced Cardiac Life Support. Dallas: The Association, 1987, pp 155-157.

Butt WW, Gow R, Whyte H, et al. Complications resulting from use of arterial catheters: Retrograde flow and rapid elevation in blood pressure. Pediatrics 76:250-254, 1985.

Geddes LA. The significance of a reference in direct measurement of blood pressure. Med Instrum 20:331-332, 1986.

• Gravenstein JS, Paulus DA. Invasive monitoring. In Gravenstein JS, Paulus DA, eds. Clinical Monitoring Practice, 2nd ed. Philadelphia: JB Lippincott, 1987, p 106-139.

Grossman W. Pressure measurement. In Grossman W, ed. Cardiac Catheterization and Angiography, 3rd ed. Philadelphia: Lea & Febiger, 1986, pp 118-134.

Guyton AC. Physics of blood, blood flow, and pressure: Hemodynamics. In Guyton AC, ed. The Textbook of Medical Physiology, 7th ed. Philadelphia: WB Saunders, 1986, pp 210-211.

• Lough ME. Introduction to hemodynamic monitoring. Nurs Clin North Am 1:89-110, 1987.

Luskin RL, Weinstein RA, Nathan C, et al. Extended use of disposable pressure transducers: A bacteriologic evaluation. JAMA 7:916-920, 1986.

Prys-Roberts C. Invasive monitoring of the circulation. In Saidman LJ, Smith NT, ed. Monitoring in Anesthesia, 2nd ed. New York: John Wiley, 1984, pp 79-93.

109 Infusion Pumps

Carolanne Capron · Gretta Liljeberg · Frances C. Morriss

BACKGROUND AND INDICATIONS

Infusion pumps are a necessity in the modern PICU. A variety of available models for both constant and intermittent infusions can be used to ensure the constant rate of infusion necessary to administer potent medications with short half-lives (i.e., catecholamines, lidocaine, insulin, thiopental), the constancy of volume administration per unit of time, and the patency of the vessel. Conditions for which infusion pumps are most useful include (1) maintenance of line patency of intra-arterial or central venous catheters; (2) infusion of hypertonic solutions centrally (e.g., parenteral hyperalimentation); (3) infusion of vasoactive substances (e.g., epinephrine, dopamine, nitroprusside); and (4) assurance of accurate volumes in small patients.

TECHNIQUE
Equipment
Intermittent infusion pumps

Intermittent infusion pumps have gained popularity in the PICU setting. Most are easy to use, portable, and battery operated. They allow infusion of low fluid volumes at a constant rate over a preset time interval, providing greater patient safety than with the old unregulated hand-push method. The procedure for the pump's use varies according to the manufacturer, and the equipment manual must be reviewed to learn specifications. The majority of intermittent infusion pumps use 1 to 50 ml syringes connected to microbore extension tubing for delivery of low volumes. They are used primarily to administer timed, intermittent doses of medications such as antibiotics and anticonvulsants.

It is important to maintain these pumps carefully, especially since they are portable and at increased risk for damage due to mishandling and dropping. Care must also be taken to prevent any fluids from entering the pump mechanism. The drugs that are used must be carefully placed in a disposable syringe, with none administered that might undergo pharmacologic changes (e.g., nitroglycerin, pentobarbital). Before the infusion device is connected to the patient, air must be purged through the tubing, eliminating the possibility of an air embolism.

A residual amount of fluid will remain in the tubing and cannot be infused. This residual amount must be calculated as extra volume to be added when the syringe is initially filled, or the residual medication must be flushed from the tubing with 0.9% sodium chloride solution at the end of the infusion. Secure access must be established to the continuous infusion line or heparin-locked device. New needle-locking devices are available that prevent needle dislodgment from an infusion port. In all cases it is important to establish set procedures within the PICU for the use of intermittent infusion pumps.

Continuous infusion pumps

There are three types of constant infusion devices. The first uses a peristaltic action in propulsion of liquid through tubing sequentially compressed by rollers. A second uses constant pressure on the plunger of a syringe, and a third uses sequential low-volume filling from a volumetrically regulated cassette. In general constancy and accuracy of rate and volume are best provided by the cassette pump.

Each of the pump types allows battery-powered operation and allows the rate of infusion to be changed. Battery operation may be essential in maintaining accurate infusion rates during transport within or between hospitals. Many pumps are available that will work up to 8 hours on battery power and recharge within 20 to 30 minutes. Available infusion rates range from 0.1 to 999 ml/hr. These rates have been established as accurate when infused through catheters in comparison with winged-needle devices of a comparable diameter.

Setting Up the Pump

Fluid sources containing only 2 to 3 hours of fluid must be connected via a burette chamber to the pump, thereby decreasing any possibility of fluid overload caused by pump malfunction. Pump rates and infusion volumes must be established according to manufacturer's guidelines. Pump alarm systems may be activated by obstruction of the line, presence of air, pump malfunction, low battery states, and infusion completion. New pumps that detect infiltration are being tested. The fluid system and pump function must be checked routinely at the beginning of each shift for proper fluid amount and rate of flow and to ensure that alarms are turned on.

RISKS AND COMPLICATIONS

Infiltration remains the main complication associated with use of the infusion pump. Since the majority of pumps do not sense infiltration, they will continue to deliver fluid and/or medication despite catheter dislodgment. Therefore the patency of the catheter must be frequently assessed at the insertion site. Extravasation of medicine and/or hypertonic solution into the skin can result in severe tissue damage. The use of clear IV catheter dressings (Tigoderm, Venoguard) allows more complete visual assessment of the catheter insertion site.

110 Radiant Warming Devices

Gene A. Basham

BACKGROUND AND INDICATIONS

The use of incubators and radiant warmers is standard practice in the maintenance of body temperature in the neonate. Incubators operate by convection, circulating heated, humidified air around the infant. The use of double-walled units is preferred in the clinical setting. These units reduce the amount of radiant heat loss, thereby providing greater protection against changes in room temperature and minimizing oxygen and caloric consumption by the infant. Air temperature may be controlled by either a servomechanism or manual adjustment. Incubators are not generally used during the infant's acute phase of illness because of the lack of accessibility to the infant for performing procedures and because they provide a less stable thermal environment when ports or access panels are open for frequent interventions.

Conversely, radiant warmers provide easy access to the infant, with minimal effect on temperature control. They consist of electrically heated elements positioned overhead that emit infrared rays downward to the infant. The heat source may be either an infrared lamp or a quartz heating tube or coil. The rays must be in the far infrared range plus invisible to the eye at 3 to 12 μm. Visible light does not provide a good heat source since much of this light is reflected off the skin, and it may interfere with assessment of the patient's color. In comparison, far infrared radiation is absorbed by the skin to a depth of less than 1 mm and is completely absorbed by the cornea to prevent penetration through the eyes. Heating of the skin causes vasodilation, which allows the transfer of heat to deeper tissues through conduction and blood circulation. Another advantage of the radiant warmer over the incubator is the former's ability to provide greater heat output for the extremely premature infant.

Standard criteria for the design specifications in evaluating a radiant warmer include (1) high and low patient temperature alarms, (2) defective probe or heater alarms, (3) power indicator, (4) constant infant temperature indicator, (5) visible control point setting, (6) manual and automatic servomechanism capabilities, and (7) minimal radiation of visible light. Electrical safety features must include low leakage (<100 μA), the inability of line voltage variation to affect heater output, radio frequency compatibility, and overcurrent protection. Additional features needed include (1) resistance to tipping, (2) mobility, (3) secure side panels, (4) storage space, (5) a tilting mattress, (6) ample space for performing radiographic procedures and using phototherapy lights, (7) ease in cleaning, and (8) protection for the infant and caretaker from hot surfaces.

TECHNIQUE

The radiant warmer should be prewarmed before use if at all possible, for it may take up to 30 minutes for the mattress to warm sufficiently. The use of white linen increases the warming efficiency. When the infant is positioned in the warmer, the skin probe must be attached to him immediately. The probe must have a foam-backed, self-adhesive, reflective shield. The temperature probe can never be placed beneath the infant since it will result in ineffective warming of the infant as the result of its sensing both the infant's body heat and the mattress temperature. Conversely, a loose probe could cause hyperthermia. Skin probes are designed by manufacturers for specific units and are calibrated for the unit accordingly. The interchanging of manufacturers' probes can interfere with warming capabilities. The skin probe site must be monitored frequently and changed routinely, depending on the infant's skin integrity. The set point for the skin temperature is usually 36.5° C for the term infant and 37.0° to 37.5° C for the preterm infant.

Initially the infant's axillary temperature must be checked at least every 30 minutes to determine the ideal set point. After thermal stability is achieved, the temperature may be checked routinely every 2 to 4 hours.

Changes in skin temperature may be the first sign of cold stress since core temperature drops only after the infant's compensatory response to cold stress is no longer successful. For this reason the bedside nurse may wish to monitor the power output trends of the warmer. The servomechanism mode of the warmer may mask temperature instability in the infant. Objects such as phototherapy lights, surgical drapes, blankets, and clothes can also affect the amount of heat the infant receives, leading to hypothermia or hyperthermia. Sudden temperature changes must be corrected and the cause investigated. During radiographic procedures the film must never be allowed to come into contact with the infant's skin.

RISKS AND COMPLICATIONS

Assessment of the infant for normothermia is essential. It is difficult to protect the infant in the radiant warmer from drafts; therefore the location of the radiant warmer must be considered in relation to heating or cooling vents. Shields can be made and placed over vents to redirect airflow and to assist in maintaining a normothermic environment.

One of the primary problems associated with the use of radiant warmers is hyperthermia, typically caused by a loose skin probe. Hyperthermia in the infant may be manifested by tachycardia, flushing, and lethargy with an increase in metabolism and oxygen consumption. The servomechanism probe status can be checked through the infant's vital signs (at least every 2 hours). Any fluctuations in power output must be investigated and monitored closely. Temperature probe accuracy must be checked periodically as part of a regular maintenance program for the radiant warmer as a whole. The concomitant use of phototherapy light increases the risk of hyperthermia and may necessitate adjustment of the heater set point.

Increased insensible water loss (IWL) is another area needing special attention, with the infant more vulnerable to convective and evaporative heat loss than the older child. This problem is magnified in the preterm infant because of the increased ratio of body surface area to body mass. Along with IWL, the basal metabolic rate and oxygen consumption are higher for the infant in a radiant warmer. Daily weight, strict intake and output, and serum sodium and urinary specific gravity must be monitored closely. Maintenance fluid requirements will increase from 20% to 50% and vary from infant to infant. A heat shield made of plastic food wrapping material stretched across the warmer will decrease IWL to some extent by reducing air turbulence around the infant and decreasing convective and evaporative heat loss. The infant may be weaned to an incubator or open crib as his condition stabilizes.

An additional problem is that of skin damage. Infants with poor peripheral circulation are at a greater risk for skin damage if placed too close to the heat source. Skin damage may also occur in the preterm infant with a delicate skin condition due to excessive drying. These patients must be monitored closely for areas of breakdown over pressure points such as the buttocks, elbows, and heels. Other adverse effects stemming from infrared radiation include cataracts, flash burns of the skin, and heat stress.

ADDITIONAL READING

Baumgart S, Engle WD, Fox WW, Polin RA. Effects of heat shielding on convective and evaporative heat losses and on radiant heat transfer in the premature infant. J Pediatr 99:948-956, 1981.

• Bell EF. Infant incubators and radiant warmers. Early Hum Dev 8:351-375, 1983.

Bell EF, Gray JC, Weinstein MR, Oh W. The effects of thermal environment on heat balance and insensible water loss in low-birth-weight infants. J Pediatr 96:452-459, 1980.

Committee on Environmental Hazards. Infant radiant warmers. Pediatrics 61:113-114, 1978.

Committee on Environmental Hazards. Infant radiant warmers, evaluation. Health Devices 3:4-23, 1973.

• Dodman N. Newborn temperature control. Neonatal Network 5:25-28, 1987.

Ducker DA, Lyon AJ, Russell RR, Bass CA, McIntosh N. Incubator temperature control: Effects on the very low birth weight infant. Arch Dis Child 60:902-907, 1985.

Fitch CW, Korones SB. Heat shield reduces water loss. Arch Dis Child 59:886-888, 1984.

Hull D, Sheldon A. Open or closed incubators. Arch Dis Child 61:108-109, 1986.

LeBlanc MH. Relative efficacy of radiant and convective heat in incubators in producing thermoneutrality for the premature. Pediatr Res 18:425-428, 1984.

LeBlanc MH. Relative efficacy of an incubator and an open warmer in producing thermoneutrality for the small premature infant. Pediatrics 69:439-445, 1982.

• Malin SW, Baumgart S. Optimal thermal management for LBW infants nursed under high-powered radiant warmer. Pediatrics 79:47-54, 1987.

Marks KH. Energy metabolism and substrate utilization in LBW neonates under radiant warmers. Pediatrics 78:465-472, 1986.

Marks KH, Gunther RC, Rossi JA, Maisels MJ. Oxygen consumption and insensible water loss in premature infants under radiant heaters. Pediatrics 66:228-232, 1980.

Sauer PJJ, Dane MJ, Visser HKA. New standards for neutral thermal environments of healthy very low birthweight infants in week one of life. Arch Dis Child 59:18-22, 1984.

Thompson MH, Stothers JK, McLellan NJ. Weight and water loss in the neonate in natural and forced convection. Arch Dis Child 59:951-956, 1984.

Whiteside D. Proper use of radiant warmers. Am J Nurs 78:1694-1696, 1978.

111 Temperature-Sensing Devices

Kathy Thomas · Frances C. Morriss

BACKGROUND AND INDICATIONS

Monitoring body temperature and maintaining a normal range of body temperature are of extreme importance in the pediatric patient. The pediatric patient's body surface area is large in relation to body mass; therefore body heat may be lost quickly, causing cold stress and increased oxygen consumption, especially in the infant population.

Temperature may be defined as the degree of heat in a body or substance generated by the movement of the molecules within it. Temperature, measured in terms of degrees, has two fixed points from which the rest of the scale is determined: the temperature at which water boils (boiling point) and the temperature at which water freezes (freezing point). Body temperature is most commonly measured on either the Fahrenheit (F) or centigrade (C) scale. The boiling point on the Fahrenheit scale is 212°, with a freezing point of 32°. On the centigrade scale the boiling point is 100° and the freezing point 0°. To convert a Fahrenheit or centigrade temperature to the opposite scale, the following equations may be used:

$$°C = (°F - 32) \times 5/9$$
$$°F = (°C \times 9/5) + 32$$

The cells of the human body operate most efficiently within a narrow range of temperatures, 97.5° to 99° F or 36.4° to 37.2° C.

Changes in temperature are measured by using other physical properties of the substance that change relative to but in a direct linear fashion with the temperature change of that substance. The two major types of temperature-sensing devices measure either expansion changes caused by changing temperature or changes in electrical resistance corresponding to temperature changes.

Thermoexpansive Thermometers

The mercury thermometer, a thermoexpansive thermometer, uses the element's ability to expand or contract with small changes in temperature. Mercury has several other useful properties: it is a liquid at the range of temperature likely to be measured; rapid heat conduction allows uniform expansion of the medium with any rise or fall in temperature; it is opaque for easy visibility; and it is cohesive when in contact with glass. A thin-walled reservoir bulb containing mercury is placed in direct contact with the skin or mucous membrane. The temperature of mercury within the bulb reaches equilibrium with the temperature of the skin or mucous membrane. The volume of the mercury expands in the small capillary tube in direct proportion to the increase in temperature. It is amplified for easy visualization, and the level of the mercury is compared to the temperature calibration etched on the glass stem.

Most mercury thermometers have a scale from 94° to 106° F and are most often used in monitoring the temperature of patients with contagious diseases. However, a "hypothermic" mercury thermometer with a temperature scale to below 94° F can determine profound hypothermia. It is necessary when an exact admission body temperature is needed to document hypothermia in patients (e.g., with near-drowning or environmental cold exposure).

Thermoresistive Thermometers

Thermoresistive thermometers are the thermistor and the thermocouple. The thermistor is reusable and consists of a metal oxide semiconductor located at the tip of the temperature probe. Nickel and manganese are usually used as the metal oxide because of their wide sensing range, −60° to 100° C. The thermistor is attached to an insulated wire that leads to a digital monitor. Since the resistance of a conductor changes with its temperature, a measure of electrical resistance of a specific conductor can be used to express degrees of temperature. When the probe is placed on the patient's skin or is inserted rectally, a change (measured by a Wheatstone bridge) in electrical resistance occurs in the probe. Current flowing through a meter, calibrated for temperature, is proportional to the resistance in the bridge's measuring limb. The resistance, in turn, is proportional to the temperature of the transducer probe.

The thermocouple is disposable and operates on the principle that current in a circuit constructed of two unlike metal elements will be directly proportional to the difference of the temperatures of the two junctions of the metals. If one of the junctions is maintained at a standard temperature, the current between the two metal junctions will reflect the difference of the two temperatures.

Thermistor and thermocouple probes are flexible, lightweight, small, inexpensive, and extremely sensitive to slight temperature variances. They are frequently used in continual monitoring of servomechanism infant warmers, incubators, heating and cooling blankets, continuous temperature monitoring devices (including indwelling probe on vascular catheters), and intermittent measurement sensors (electronic thermometers).

In addition to thermistors and thermocouple devices the liquid crystal temperature strips are sensitive to change in skin temperature. The temperature is read from the adhesive strip as the color of the liquid crystal changes with changes in skin temperature. Since studies have shown that liquid crystal temperatures may inaccurately reflect core temperatures, the use of this device must be correlated with a more accurate temperature-sensing device.

RISKS AND COMPLICATIONS

Safety, accuracy, convenience, and speed of measurement are considerations that are important in selection of a temperature-sensing device for use in the PICU. Selection of a probe and its placement should take into account the patient's age, his level of activity, the reason the temperature must be monitored, and any health conditions that might affect probe placement or accuracy (e.g., skin conditions, nares patency, recent rectal or esophageal surgery). For active children with routine health problems obtaining intermittent axillary temperatures is the most

appropriate method; intermittent oral, rectal, and all continuous methods are either impractical, uncomfortable, or relatively inaccurate. An alternative choice may be the use of a digital probe, which measures core temperature from tympanic membrane radiant heat. The use of rectal probes, both intermittent and continuous, is specifically inappropriate for neonates less than 1 month of age or weighing <2500 g because of the danger of bowel perforation and the high rate of associated morbidity; skin probes are inappropriate for use in patients with extensive skin damage or breakdown. In addition any condition that causes vasoconstriction and decreased skin blood flow (shock, low temperature, use of α-adrenergic agonists) will cause inaccurate skin and axillary measurements, and an alternate monitoring site must be considered. All glass devices used for determining intermittent temperatures can break and cause tissue damage. These probes are particularly inadvisable for active children. With the advent of disposable probes and probe covers, the likelihood of spreading infection from one patient to another has been minimized.

Situations that must be continuously monitored include (1) patient with potentially unstable low temperature needing use of a servomechanism warming device (e.g., neonate, patient with diminished subcutaneous tissue); (2) unstable or cold environmental conditions (e.g., operating room, transport conditions); (3) patient with preexisting or induced hyper- or hypothermia (e.g., cardiopulmonary bypass); and (4) patient with unstable temperature or the potential for instability (e.g., malignant hyperpyrexia, thyroid storm, extensive burns). If large differences between surface and core temperature such as may occur with rapid warming and cooling are anticipated, more than one site of temperature monitoring may be useful. In this situation at least one probe should measure core temperature. Core temperature is best reflected in most patients by nasopharyngeal or tympanic membrane probes. In patients with pulmonary artery catheters containing thermistors, blood temperature may be measured directly. Continuous tympanic membrane monitoring with an indwelling probe is associated with an unacceptable incidence of tympanic membrane perforation. All indwelling probes, particularly thermistors within vascular catheters, provide a path for direct electrical access to body cavities. All such devices must have isolated circuitry to prevent accidental defibrillation. For any

Table 111-1   Technique for Probe Use

Type of Thermometer	Site	Technique	Problems or Complications
Thermoexpansive			
Glass mercury	Axilla	Hold in place 3-7 min before reading	Slow
	Rectum	Insert 3 cm	Uncomfortable; perforation; not recommended in neonates
	Mouth	Insert beneath tongue (postero-lateral aspect) for 2-4 min	Breakage with trauma to mouth; not recommended for uncooperative patients; slow
Thermoresistive			
Digital, intermittent Continuous probes*	All sites	See individual manuals	See individual manuals
	Skin	Avoid bony prominences; shield from exogenous heat sources; must have good blood flow in skin	Falsely low reading over areas of low blood flow; skin breakdown or reaction to adhesive
	Rectum	Insert 3 cm	Skin breakdown; false elevation from presence of feces; uncomfortable
	Nasopharynx or esophagus	Estimate distance from nares to angle of jaw (nasopharynx) or mouth to midchest level (esophagus; behind right atrium)	False high reading if used in conjunction with endotracheal tube through which patient is receiving warmed gases; nosebleed and mucosal ulceration
Indwelling vascular probes*	Via catheter	Calibration; checked electronically before calculations by cardiac output monitor	See Chapter 116

*For all indwelling probes, a path for direct electrical access to body cavities is present; isolated circuitry must be present.

patient with an indwelling probe, skin or tissue breakdown remains a problem, and the insertion site must be checked routinely for tissue integrity.

To ensure accurate temperature readings, proper placement of temperature probes and proper technique of taking temperatures manually must be followed (Table 111-1).

To ensure the accuracy of indwelling and continuous probes, they must be in contact with tissue having appropriately high blood flow and not be exposed to other sources of heating and cooling. Skin probes should make full skin contact in areas in which bony prominences will not interfere and must be insulated from radiant warming devices. Feces in the rectum can prevent thermal contact. Warm gases in an endotracheal tube or cool lavage solutions in a nasogastric tube can affect the accuracy of an esophageal probe. All digital devices must be used according to the manufacturer's specifications; when using the more conventional techniques, the most common problem of accuracy results from allowing insufficient time for equilibration between the patient and the temperature-sensing device.

ADDITIONAL READING

• Blitt CD. Monitoring in Anesthesia and Critical Care Medicine. New York: Churchill Livingstone, 1985, pp 450-455.

Dornette WHL. Instrumentation and Anesthesia, 2nd ed. Philadelphia: FA Davis, 1964, pp 5-7.

• Merenstein GB, Gardner SL. Handbook of Neonatal Intensive Care. St. Louis: CV Mosby, 1985, pp 88-89.

Rogers MC. Textbook of Pediatric Intensive Care, 2nd ed. Los Angeles: Williams & Wilkins, 1987, pp 1440-1441.

112 Transport

Lela W. Brink · Beth Clark

BACKGROUND

Specialized pediatric transport systems have evolved in parallel with the growth and development of PICUs. As a relative newcomer in the transport field, pediatric systems have the opportunity to use the adult and neonatal experience to achieve the goal of rapidly delivering expert pediatric care to any critically ill child.

Early civilian transport programs developed during the 1970s. Adult programs grew along two avenues: (1) rapid transport of ill or injured patients from a nonhospital environment to a medical facility and (2) interhospital transport of critically ill patients to specialized medical facilities. Scene responses began with minimally trained ambulance personnel responding to injury calls and progressed to the use of sophisticated mobile ICUs staffed by personnel skilled in advanced life support and capable of delivering sophisticated medical care on the scene. Helicopters were incorporated into civilian transport programs because of their ability to respond in multiple environments and *rapidly* transport the patient to an appropriate facility. Well proven on the battlefields of Korea and Vietnam, helicopters have become sophisticated intensive care transport vehicles that can be outfitted to any need. Fixed-wing transport, widely used in the military for long-distance transport during the war, is becoming a more significant element of civilian transport systems.

As ICUs have become more specialized, so have transport systems. The emergency medical system's response to accident or injury is significantly different from that of specialized hospital-based providers who target specific populations. With the attempts at regionalization of neonatal care and the development of a three-tiered system to categorize the level of care offered at a facility, transport of critically ill neonates has become an essential component of the delivery of perinatal care. To assure the proper triage of critically ill neonates, perinatal networks have evolved, interrelating minimal care facilities (level I) with facilities with more sophisticated capabilities for neonatal intensive care (level II or III). Tertiary centers (level III) respond to the needs of their referral centers by providing comprehensive transport teams trained to respond promptly to the delivery (or potential delivery) of a critically ill neonate by bringing appropriate equipment and personnel to the scene to stabilize the child and prepare him for transport. This has been coupled with extensive outreach education programs based in the tertiary care facilities and has markedly improved the level of care for premature infants.

As pediatric intensive care evolves as a specialty, several factors distinguish it from its neonatal and adult counterparts. To take care of a wide range of patients varying in age and size from neonates to adolescents requires specialized equipment, an appreciation for the physiologic changes that accompany growth and development (see Chapter 2), and an appreciation of the wide variety of illnesses and injuries that affect this population. A knowledge of the medical needs of each age child and the appropriate use of the equipment in each age group defines the specialized role of personnel involved with pediatric transport and pediatric intensive care.

TECHNICAL CONSIDERATIONS
Development of a Pediatric Transport Program

As early as 1980 sophisticated emergency transport networks were evolving. The Denver model of a pediatric emergency transport network described in that year suggests the use of a regionalized network centered in a PICU with an excellent communication system allowing any physician access to the expert consultation he needs to care for an ill child. Such consultation may or may not result in a transport or referral to the center but can always improve the level of pediatric care.

To initiate the formation of a pediatric transport system, an assessment must be made of the needs of the referral region. This can be done through retrospective review of referral patterns, inquiries to referring hospitals, or a combination of these. Once the extent of the referral region has been determined and the expected number of transports assessed, basic determinations can be made concerning the type and amount of equipment, the number and type of vehicles, and the number of personnel and their level of skill and training.

The general equipment for pediatric transport has been well described in a number of sources. The list of medications needed for transport generally parallels that used in the specific PICUs. Although they may vary with the program or with a specific transport, suggested basic equipment and supplies are listed on pp. 788-789. Special equipment needs reflect the interests of the consultants available at the transport center and may include supplies for techniques such as extracorporeal membrane oxygenation (ECMO), continuous arteriovenous hemofiltration (CAVH), or specialized ventilatory techniques.

Personnel needs may be met by a combination of administrators, physicians, nurses, respiratory therapists, and allied medical personnel (e.g., EMTs, paramedics, physician assistants, perfusionists), depending on the needs and mission of the individual program. The training requirements for each category of personnel and their job descriptions must be defined early in the development of the program.

The acuity of the patients; the size, geography, and weather of the referral area; and the crew requirements must be considered in determining the mode of transportation and types of vehicles to use. The specific equipment needed to outfit each vehicle must be specified, and the need for backup or supplemental vehicles must be defined before contracting with a vehicle operator.

Specific equipment must be evaluated and obtained. All equipment must meet the specifications for hospital use plus specifications applied by the regulatory agencies involved in transport (state and local Emergency Medical Services [EMS], Federal Aviation Agency [FAA], Department of Transportation [DOT].

The management of interhospital communication and crew and vehicle dispatch must be evaluated and specific protocols established. A mechanism for interfacing with hospital disaster planning as well as dealing with a transport system disaster must be established.

Selection of Personnel

All personnel involved in transport must have excellent medical skills, extensive pediatric critical care experience, and clinical experience within the base hospital, and they must have the ability to deal with physicians and staff from diverse backgrounds in unfamiliar settings. The close quarters of the transport environment make team cooperation essential, and all members must be able to relate well.

The members of the pediatric transport team will vary with the goals of the system, the number of personnel involved, the support services available, and the needs of the particular patient and transport.

Administrative personnel may include any of the following, depending on program requirements.

Medical director. The medical director should be a specialist in pediatric critical care medicine and transport. He is responsible for all medical aspects of the transport, including initial and follow-up consultation and patient status evaluation. The director must be able to interact with all administrative personnel to ensure the smooth functioning of all aspects of the transport program. Having experience or interest in public relations and marketing is helpful, especially if he is initiating a program. If a flight program is active, having training in flight physiology and/or flight medicine is necessary.

Nursing coordinator. The nursing coordinator should be a registered nurse with experience in transport and critical care. This person is responsible for supervision of personnel and all educational aspects of the program, including the medical aspects of transport, safety, and transport physiology. He is responsible for outreach education and follow-up with referring centers and is also responsible for establishing and supervising the quality assurance program, supervising the development of a policy and procedure manual governing transport, and ensuring that it is current. PICU, transport, and management experience are necessary.

Administrative coordinator. This person is responsible for the financial and support aspects of the program, including equipment acquisition and maintenance, vehicle acquisition and maintenance, and contractual interactions with the vehicle operators to ensure cooperation with the quality assurance program and programs established in compliance with the requirements of the regulatory agencies. In smaller programs these responsibilities may be assumed by the medical director and nursing coordinator.

Director of communication. This position is necessary if a program is going to operate its own dispatch center. The director of communication is responsible for the maintenance of the communications center, the communications equipment in the center, and the transport vehicles as applicable; for establishing dispatch protocols in cooperation with

the other members of the administrative team; and for conducting the quality assurance and safety programs essential to the operation of the dispatch center. He must be aware of all Federal Communications Commission (FCC) and other regulatory agency policies that affect dispatch and must ensure compliance with these regulations.

• • •

Transport team crew members must include a core of personnel selected according to the specific needs of a transport. Resource personnel include the following.

Emergency medical technicians. Certified by the state regulatory agency, trained in basic life support

---

EQUIPMENT

Nursing supply bag

Syringes	Foley catheters	Tape measure
60 cc (5) Luer-Lok	No. 6 (2)	Dextrostix
60 cc (3) catheter tip	No. 8 (2)	K-Y jelly
20 cc (5)	No. 10 (1)	Povidone-iodine (Betadine) pads (10)
10 cc (5)	No. 12 (1)	Alcohol pads (10)
5 cc (5)	No. 14 (1)	Cotton balls
3 cc (5)	Feeding tubes	Safety pins
1 cc (10)	No. 5 (2)	Band-Aids
IV catheters*	No. 8 (3)	Scissors
24 g (10)	NG tubes	Hemostats
22 g (4)	No. 10 (1)	Adhesive tape
20 g (3)	No. 12 (1)	Miscellaneous trays
18 g (3)	No. 14 (1)	Thoracostomy tube tray
Butterfly needles	Intraosseous needles	Thoracostomy tubes (10, 12, 16, 20)
25 g (3)	Large (1)	Venesection tray
23 g (3)	Small (1)	Pleuro-Vac (1)
T-connectors (5)	Heimlich valve (2)	Foley drainage bag (urimeter)
Extension tubing (3)	Chest tube clamp (1)	Stethoscope
Wrist restraints (4)	Needles	Calculator
Armboards	20 g 1 inch (5)	Monitor
Child (2)	22 g 1 inch (5)	ECG pads
Infant (2)	22 g 1½ inches (5)	ECG lead wires (6)
BP cuffs	18 g 1½ inches (5)	Infusion pumps
Adult (1)		
Child (1)		
Infant (1)		
Neonatal No. 4 (1)		

*g = gauge.

with supplemental training in pediatrics, EMTs assist in patient preparation and operate the ground transport vehicles. They are responsible for all aspects of operation and maintenance of the vehicles and must ensure compliance with a preventive maintenance program.

Respiratory therapists. Respiratory therapists must be registered or registry eligible and licensed by the state regulatory agency. They must receive training in advanced life support and specific training in advanced airway skills, including intubation. They must be proficient in ventilator management and blood gas sampling and interpretation.

Paramedics. Certified and/or licensed by the state regulatory agency, paramedics have received training in advanced life support techniques and are able to assist in the stabilization and preparation of the patient for transport. Additional experience and/or training in pediatrics at the base institution is needed.

Transport nurse. The transport nurse is a registered nurse with a minimum of 6 months' experience in pediatric critical care and with training in transport medicine. If this person is acting as a team leader, he may need extensive additional experience in critical care as well as training in specialized techniques for stabilization and transport of the pediatric patient.

Transport physician. All transport physicians must be experienced in the management and stabilization of the critically ill pediatric patient, must be trained in transport medicine, and must have received an

---

Respiratory therapy equipment list

ET tubes: 2.5-9.0 mm (2)
Stylets: small, large (2)
Magill forceps: small, large (1)
Laryngoscope handles (2)
Miller blades 0, 1, 2, 3 (1)
MacIntosh blades 2, 3 (1)
Light bulbs (2)
AA batteries (2)
Resuscitation bags (Laerdal) (1)
    Infant, pediatric, adult
Oral airways (graduated sizes) (1)
Resuscitation masks: 0, 1, 2, 3, 4, 5, adult (1)
Suction catheters: sizes 6, 8, 10, 12, 14 g (2)
DeLee suction (1)
Yankauer suction (1)
Portable suction apparatus (1)
O_2 supplies
    Infant O_2 cannula (2)
    Pediatric O_2 cannula (2)
    O_2 tubing (2)
    Infant O_2 mask (1)
    Pediatric O_2 mask (1)
    Adult O_2 mask (1)
    Ventilation mask: adult, pediatric, infant (1)

Aerosol delivery
    Nebulizers (2)
    Albuterol (Ventolin) (1)
    Isoproterenol (Isuprel) (1)
    Isoetharine (Bronkosol) (1)
    Metaproterenol (Alupent) (1)
    Terbutaline (5 vials)
Flashlight
TB syringes (3)
Normal saline vials (3)
Pediatric ventilator circuit (1)
ABG kit (2)
Adapters for in-line nebulization
Tracheostomy adapters
Pulse oximeter
    Neonatal probe (2)
    Adult probe (2)
Capnograph (optional)
    Sensors
Anesthesia bag setup (1 and 2 L bags, PEEP value)
O_2 tubing connectors (1)
E cylinder regulator (1)

orientation to communication protocols. A minimum of 3 years of pediatric training is needed.

Consulting physicians. Resource physicians within the transport network must be easily accessible to referring physicians. These physicians must receive an orientation to communication procedures and work closely with the transport physician or medical director.

• • •

Because of the emotional and physical stresses of transport, crew fitness is essential. An initial assessment before employment and a routine program of annual reevaluation must be established. A comprehensive medical history must be completed by all crew members and reviewed by the medical director. All crew members must be aware of any physical fitness requirements, including height and weight restrictions. The individual programs must determine any physical limitations (e.g., ability to lift a specified load) and must establish policies for dealing with disabilities (temporary or permanent) that preclude participation in transport. Vehicle size, payload requirements, and patient care specifications will help determine the crew fitness requirements for an individual program.

Personnel Training

Specific training requirements are determined by the needs of the individual program. At each level personnel must have the appropriate state, local, or national certification or licensure. All team members must have documented experience in pediatric critical care and must receive extensive orientation to the policies and procedures of the base hospital. Certification in base life support (adult and pediatric) must be current. Personnel certified in advanced life support procedures must be available on every transport.

If an air transport program is in place, the training requirements proposed by the Department of Transportation and the American Society of Hospital Based Emergency Air Medical Services (ASHBEAMS) in 1988 must be met. All regulatory agency policies at the local, state, and national levels must be investigated to ensure that the program remains in compliance with these requirements.

Training in specialized skills such as airway management, vascular access, ventilatory management,

ECMO, or other procedures needed within the specific transport program must be incorporated into the educational program. Initial skills training and skills maintenance records must be fully documented and maintained in the personnel files.

Well-delineated protocols must be developed in an attempt to provide uniform care within the transport environment. All personnel must receive orientation to these protocols, and any deviation from a routine protocol must be documented. Protocols must be available in the base facility, at the dispatch center, and when applicable, in the transport vehicles.

Selection of Pediatric Transport Equipment

The selection of equipment reflects the needs of the individual program. Major equipment purchases such as the Isolette, transport stretchers, monitors, and ventilators must be usable in any of the transport vehicles. If the program has the capabilities for simultaneous transport, having duplicate equipment may be necessary.

Each crew member should be responsible for stocking and transporting his own equipment. Having individual medication, nursing supply, and respiratory therapy bags allows for practical separation of equipment. Sample equipment lists and transport information record (Fig. 112-1) need to be modified to reflect the program's needs. Ready transport bags of durable material with sufficient compartments must be systematically stocked and maintained with the necessary equipment.

The pharmacist needs to monitor all medications, assuring that all drugs included in transport are current. To facilitate accounting for narcotics and controlled drugs, these medications must be maintained as a separate unit and signed for at the time of a transport, and an accurate accounting of all medications must be given on return from transport.

The respiratory therapist must ensure that all airway equipment, oxygen delivery systems, and ventilators are maintained. Transport ventilators, oximeters, capnography equipment, and the appropriate sensors must be ready for use at all times.

The EMT is responsible for maintaining the ambulance and seeing that the appropriate supplies and equipment are stocked. Regular inventories and equipment checks must be documented as part of the quality assurance program.

Call taken by _____ Date _____ Time _____
Patient name _____ Date of birth _____ Wt. _____
Referring physician _____ Phone _____
Referring hospital _____ Phone _____
Referred to Dr. _____
Provisional diagnosis (1) _____ (2) _____
Patient destination _____ Phone _____

Present illness:

Onset:

Progression:

Physical examination (within last hour)   Ht. _____ Wt. _____
Vital signs   T _____ P _____ RR _____ (pattern) BP _____
☐ HEENT   ☐ WNL _____
☐ Lungs   ☐ WNL _____
☐ Heart   ☐ WNL _____
☐ Abdomen   ☐ WNL _____
☐ Extremities   ☐ WNL _____
☐ GU   ☐ WNL _____
☐ Neuro   ☐ WNL _____
(LOC, pupils, cough, gag, motor, posturing, flaccid, etc.)

Laboratory data

CBC: Metabolic: Renal:
   Hb _____   Na _____   BUN _____
   Hct _____   K _____   Cr _____
   WBC _____   Cl _____   UA _____
   Platelets _____ HCO_3 _____
PT _____   Ca _____
PTT _____   Glu _____

ABG: Time: _____   Other: Liver: CSF:
   pH _____   pH _____   AST _____   Cell ct. _____
   Pco_2 _____ Pco_2 _____   ALT _____   _____
   Po_2 _____ Po_2 _____   Bili _____   Glucose _____
   BE _____   BE _____   Ammonia _____   Protein _____
   Fio_2 _____ Fio_2 _____   Gram's stain _____
                                                                          CIE _____

Fig. 112-1   PICU transport information record.

Continued.

Interventions

Antibiotics _____

Medications _____

X-rays _____

Other _____
_____

Intubated	☐ Yes	☐ No
Trach	☐ Yes	☐ No
IV:	☐ Yes	☐ No
Fluid _____	Rate _____	
Fluid _____	Rate _____	
Arterial line	☐ Yes	☐ No
NG	☐ Yes	☐ No
Foley	☐ Yes	☐ No

Requested studies/procedures prior to arrival of team

Lab _____

X-ray _____ Fluid change _____

Management _____
_____

Disposition

☐ Accept   ☐ Refuse _____

Team Composition: ☐ MD   ☐ RN   ☐ RT _____

Vehicle: ☐ Ambulance   ☐ Helicopter   ☐ Plane

Special needs: (1) Isolette _____ (2) _____ (3) _____

Airport/landing specifications _____

Response time

Initial phone call out of hospital _____

Team dispatch _____

Team arrival _____

Problems encountered

_____
_____
_____
_____
_____
_____
_____
_____
_____

Fig. 112-1, cont'd   PICU transport information record.

PHARMACY SUPPLY LIST

Normal saline (NS) solution (10 ml) (10)
Sterile water (10 ml) (5)
IV fluids
    D_5W, 250 ml
    $D_5\frac{1}{4}NS$, 250 ml
    $D_5\frac{1}{2}NS$, 250 ml
    NS, 500 ml
    $D_{10}W$, 250 ml
Albumin, 25%
Albumin, 5%, or Plasmanate
Resuscitation medications
    Atropine, 1 mg/10 ml (2)
    Epinephrine, 0.1 mg/ml 10 ml (2)
    $NaHCO_3$, 8.4% (50 ml) (1)
    $NaHCO_3$, 8.4% (10 ml) (1)
    CaCl, 10% (10 ml) (1)
    Dextrose, 50% (50 ml) (1)
    Naloxone, 0.4 mg/ml (1)
Vasoactive drugs
    Dopamine, 200 mg/5 ml (2)
    Dobutamine, 250 mg/20 ml (1)
    Epinephrine, 30 mg/30 ml (1)
    Nitroprusside, (50 mg vial) (2)
    Prostaglandin E_1, 500 µg/ml (1) (as needed)
    Isoproterenol, 1 mg/5 ml (5)
    Propranolol, 1 mg/ml (1)
    Hydralazine, 20 mg/ml (2)
Controlled drug box
    Sodium thiopental, 500 mg vial (1)
    Phenobarbital, 65 mg/ml 2 ml vials (2)

Pentobarbital, 100 mg/2 ml (1)
Morphine, 10 mg/ml (2)
Fentanyl, 100 µg/2 ml (4)
Lorazepam, 2 mg/ml (2)
Midazolam, 5 mg/ml (1)
Miscellaneous
    Acetaminophen suppository, 650 mg (1)
    Acetaminophen suppository, 120 mg (1)
    Aminophylline, 250 mg/10 ml (3)
    Ampicillin, 1 g vial (1)
    Cefuroxime, 750 mg vial (2)
    Diphenhydramine, 50 mg/ml (2)
    Diazoxide (Hyperstat), 300 mg (1)
    Furosemide, 20 mg/2 ml (2)
    Gentamicin, 80 mg/2 ml (1)
    Glucagon, 1 mg vial (1)
    Heparin, 10000 U/10 ml (1)
    Insulin, human, regular, 100 U/ml
    Lidocaine, 100 mg/5 ml (1)
    Lidocaine, 1% 10 ml (1)
    Phenytoin, 100 mg/2 ml (2)
    Potassium chloride (2)
    Sodium polystyrene sulfonate (Kayexalate), pre-mixed (1)
    Methyprednisolone sodium succinate (Solu-Medrol), 125 mg (1)
    Succinylcholine, 20 mg/ml (1)
    Vecuronium, 10 mg vial (2)
    Mannitol, 12.5 mg/50 ml (2)

Vehicle Selection

The selection and configuration of the transport vehicle must meet the needs of the program. Consideration must be given to the modes of transport to be used (ground, fixed wing, rotorcraft), distance traveled, time in the vehicle, number of patients to be handled, equipment, and crew weight and bulk.

Ground ambulances vary in size, capability, and optional equipment available. Once a needs assessment has been made, the configuration of the vehicle can be proposed. The vehicle chosen must be large enough to carry the patient, crew members, and equipment safely. Appropriate storage space must be available, and patient care must be delivered with relative ease. Monitoring equipment must be restrained during transport yet easily visible to the medical personnel. On-board air, oxygen, suction, and power must be adequate for the distance designated for ground transport.

Rotorcraft (helicopters) come in an assortment of configurations and must fulfill the needs of the program, patient, and crew. Cost and availability will affect the choice of vehicle and its configuration.

Single- and dual-engine vehicles are available. The benefits attributed to single-rotor vehicles include rapid start-up time, lower fuel costs, and lower main-

---

ROTORCRAFT AVAILABLE FOR AIR TRANSPORT

Single-engine craft

Bell 206 BIII Jet Ranger
Bell 206 LII Long Ranger
Aerospatiale Astar AS350
Aerospatiale Alouette III SA 316

Twin-engine craft

MBB BK 117
MBB BK 105
Aerospatiale Twinstar AS355F
Aerospatiale Dauphin SA 365N
Bell 222
Bell 412
Augusta 109A
Sikorsky S76

---

tenance costs. The major disadvantages are cabin size, limited access to the patient, and significant limitations placed on the number of crew that may accompany the transport. Dual-engine vehicles have a greater safety margin but have slower start-up time and higher fuel and maintenance costs. The larger cabin allows more access to the patient, greater flexibility in choosing the on-board equipment, and an overall larger payload. The advantages of the larger craft may include a longer transport distance, thereby widening the area that can be serviced by helicopter. No matter how helicopter transport programs are evaluated, the extensive vehicle maintenance costs and preventive maintenance requirements are the primary limitations on their expansion.

Landing and takeoff requirements, vehicle operating conditions, and general weather considerations greatly affect the selection of vehicle.

Fixed-wing craft come in a variety of sizes and cabin configurations. The use of fixed-wing craft for longer distances is well documented, but recent experience demonstrates the benefits of fixed-wing craft for shorter transports in some parts of the country. The size and weather characteristics of the region and landing strip configuration and availability must be evaluated to determine the type and size of craft

required. New FAA regulations for fixed-wing air ambulance operations are expected in late 1988 or 1989.

Once the program's vehicular needs and specifications have been determined, negotiations must begin with an operator. Several types of operating arrangements are possible. Careful review of the operator's records concerning safety, maintenance, and compliance with regulatory agencies must be undertaken. His availability, responsibility, and financial stability must be assessed. If possible a visit to a program operated by the vendor should be undertaken before final contract discussions. Involving the appropriate administrative personnel early in these discussions is beneficial.

ORGANIZATION OF A COMMUNICATIONS CENTER

The communications center may be as simple as a designated phone line and a protocol for triage. Optimally, such a center would be physically separate, quiet, and private. Phone information from the referring hospital, the information given, and consultations must be recorded for verification and documentation purposes (Fig. 112-1). Personnel answering the telephones must be knowledgeable about the transport program and its procedures and protocols.

If vehicle dispatch is to be managed by the same communications center, appropriate telephone, radio, and recording equipment must be available. The communications personnel must be well trained in the medical aspects of transport, in radio communication with ground and air vehicles, and in government regulations that govern such communication at the local, state, and federal levels. A fully operational communications center acting as dispatch for a transport program with fully operational ground and air capability must be able to provide ground-to-air communication and ground-to-ground communication and be able to communicate with the air traffic control and weather facilities involved.

For each program the communications center provides the major contact with the nonhospital public. The role and functioning of the communications center must be the professional interface for the hospital-based transport program with the emergency medical, fire, police, and ambulance systems in the area. The complexities of the communication center will mirror its role within the transport program, and its growth will reflect the growth of the program.

DISASTER PLANNING

Two components of disaster planning must be considered. The first is determining how the transport program will interface with the hospital disaster plan and also determining what role, if any, it is expected to play in local and statewide disaster planning. The level of response in each circumstance must be delineated, and the impact on the program's services must be noted. These policies must be placed in the programs policy and procedure manual and be reviewed regularly.

The second major aspect of disaster planning is the formal construction of a protocol to deal with the occurrence of a vehicle accident involving transport vehicles and personnel. This plan must ensure prompt communication with all team members and appropriate family members. A mechanism for delivering accurate information to media representatives in a timely fashion must cxist. The hospital public relations department, pastoral care, and social service departments must determine how they will interface with this aspect of the disaster plan. If pos-

sible a separate area in which crew members and families can gather to receive information and support is designated. A single phone line needs to be dedicated to handling calls related to the accident and must be answered by a well-prepared spokesman. When possible and appropriate, personnel must attempt to keep the system functioning. If not, an alternative backup system must be activated to respond to referral calls.

ADDITIONAL READING

American Academy of Pediatrics Committee on Hospital Care. Guidelines for air and ground transport of pediatric patients. Pediatrics 78:943-950, 1986.

American Society of Hospital Based Emergency Air Medical Services. Air Medical Crew National Standard Curriculum. Samaritan AirEvac and Department of Transportation. 1988.

Dobrin RS, Block BA, Gilman JI, Massaro TA. The development of a pediatric emergency transport system. Pediatr Clin North Am 27:633-645, 1980.

113 ICU Computerization

John E. Brimm · Lorene S. Nolan

BACKGROUND AND INDICATIONS

Computers are playing an increasingly important role in the management of ICU patients. Bedside instruments such as patient monitors and infusion pumps incorporate computers to improve their capabilities for performing patient care such as measuring blood pressure, interpreting cardiac rhythms, and regulating IV infusions. The scope of ICU computerization, however, goes beyond its uses in instrumentation. Currently, the major emphasis is on automation of the manual tasks involved in patient care documentation.

Two decades ago a few pioneering institutions began using computers to automate the collection of vital signs. Today's systems, called clinical information management systems (CIMS), automate many of the traditional medical records, including flowsheets, physician's orders, nursing care plans, assessments, and progress notes. Nurses and physicians are beginning to use electronic versions of the flowsheet and chart for recording and reviewing information. Hospitals are placing computer displays and keyboards at patient bedsides as well as at nursing stations to replace the use of paper and pencil.

OBJECTIVES OF ICU COMPUTERIZATION

The broad objectives of ICU computerization are to improve the quality of patient care and to reduce hospital operating costs. Five specific objectives follow:

- To be the official version of the medical record for all of the clinical staff: nurses, physicians, respiratory therapists, and others. To achieve this objective the system must be accessible at all appropriate locations such as the patient bedside and nursing station, and it must be highly reliable.

- To automate all the steps in creating the chart, from physicians' orders to the Kardex to the flowsheet. The system cannot offer a partial solution such as automating half the flowsheet nor can it require double charting such as recording an entry both on paper and again into the computer.

- To collect data once from the person who is responsible for it and then automatically transcribe it into all appropriate parts of the chart. Computers eliminate time-consuming and error-prone transcription steps such as copying a medication order onto both the Kardex and the medication administration record.

- To collect information automatically. As computers are used in more bedside instruments and hospital ancillary departments, the CIMS can acquire information automatically from them.

- To extend users' abilities. For example, computers can check ordered medications for drug-drug interactions and for inappropriate dosages; notify users when medications are overdue or new laboratory results are available; calculate doses of drugs based on a patient's weight; and provide on-line reference information.

As these objectives are increasingly met, computers will revolutionize the way that information is managed in the critical care unit because paper and pencil cannot extend users' abilities, but computers can. A new generation of ICU computer systems, based on the availability of high-performance bedside workstations, is enabling this revolution.

TECHNIQUE
Equipment

The computer equipment used in ICUs can vary in cost and complexity from the use of a simple personal computer placed at a nursing station to an interconnected network of high-performance workstations placed at every bedside. Regardless of the specific configuration or the manufacturer, however, all systems have most of the following components.

Equipment	Use
Processor	The hardware that executes the software (computer programs) that control the system's operation.
Display	The TV-like monitor that presents text and graphics generated by the processor. The display is the primary output device for presenting information to users.
Disk	The floppy or hard drive that is used for storing computer programs and data.
Keyboard	The input device that is used as a major method for controlling the system and for entering data.
Mouse	The small "pointing device," placed next to the keyboard, that contains one to three buttons for selecting items on the computer display. Other pointing devices include touch screen, light pen, and track ball.
Printer	The output device that generates paper reports for backup and the permanent medical record. Printers are generally placed at the nursing station.

A workstation consists of a processor, disk, display, keyboard, and mouse. Workstations are interconnected by a local area network, or LAN, so that the individual workstations function together as one system. The LAN enables users to review any patient's data from any bedside or nursing station.

Applications

The applications provided by a CIMS have improved over the last decade as a result of advances in underlying computer technology and a better understanding of clinical requirements. ICU computer applications are extremely varied; the remainder of this chapter gives an overview of some of the major ones.

Vital signs flowsheet. Computers acquire data automatically from patient monitors for documenting vital signs. The documentation process entails verifying that the monitored values are correct or modifying them if they are not before storing them. Data from other bedside instruments such as noninvasive blood pressure devices and oximeters can also be captured automatically. Some observations or measurements such as a Glasgow Coma Scale score must be assessed by the nurse and entered manually. An example of a computerized flowsheet is shown in Fig. 113-1.

Graphs and trends. Manual flowsheets use either a tabular or graphic format for recording data; if another presentation is needed, the data must be recopied into the new format. Data entered into a computer can be presented in either tabular or graphic format without double entry. Trends of vital signs can be plotted automatically over various time intervals. These graphs can be presented on the computer display or printed on paper.

Respiratory flowsheet. Manual charting of ventilator settings and respiratory measurements is time consuming, particularly if detailed changes are tracked. Computers can acquire ventilator data directly from the ventilators and blood gas results from the laboratory. Derived respiratory variables such as oxygen saturation or shunt fraction can be calculated automatically. Thus a respiratory flowsheet can be generated effectively without manual intervention.

Hemodynamic and other calculations. Early ICU systems provided the capability to calculate derived cardiorespiratory variables such as vascular resistance and shunt fraction to gain valuable physiologic insight from this knowledge. Entry of data into calculators, with subsequent copying onto the flowsheet, is no longer needed; ICU systems provide these calculations as a by-product of the charting process, and both the primary and derived data are included in the electronic record.

Intake and output. Critically ill patients often receive five or more IV infusions and have a comparable number of tubes, drains, and other output categories. Recording this information is difficult, and calculation of totals at the end of the shift is notoriously inaccurate. With a CIMS this process is almost totally automated. IV labels are transferred directly onto the flowsheet after entry of the physician's orders. Hourly volumes from infusion pumps and drainage devices can be acquired automatically, and, from them, the systems can calculate running, shift, and daily totals of various IV fluids and outputs and even compute nutritional intakes such as daily caloric and protein intake. Thus maintaining the intake/output flowsheet can be almost entirely automated.

Medications. Nurses must spend effort ensuring that medications are administered correctly as scheduled; infusions of vasoactive drugs may be changed and documented as frequently as every 5 minutes. When the physician's orders are entered into a computer, however, the system can present a chronologic list of medications to be administered and alert nurses when they are due. Systems are also commonly used to calculate patient-specific dosages and infusion rates for drugs based on the patient's weight. Further, systems can calculate the dosage for drugs such as gentamicin based on pharmacokinetic mod-

els. Many systems incorporate checks for drug-drug interactions, allergies, and inappropriate dosages. All of these warnings and notifications result in a decrease in medication errors.

Ancillary department communications. Whereas information used in the ICU is mainly generated there, ICU orders and requisitions go to ancillary departments such as the laboratory and pharmacy, and results from those departments are returned to

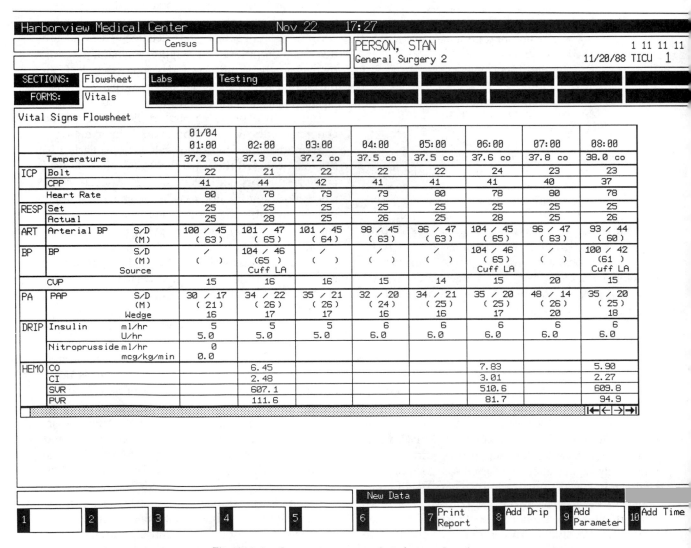

Fig. 113-1   Computer-generated vital signs flowsheet.

and charted in the ICU. Currently, laboratory results are reported either by telephone or by printed result slip; then the nurse transcribes them to the flowsheet. In addition much time is spent in telephoning the laboratory to check on a test's status and to obtain results.

When the laboratory and other ancillary departments are computerized, the ICU system must interface with those departmental computer systems. With such interfaces results can be directly transferred and made immediately available at the bedside in a clinically useful format such as a flowsheet. Messages alert users to the availability of new results, particularly critical values.

Physician's orders. Physician's orders pose the greatest challenge in the documentation process because they drive most diagnostic and therapeutic interventions. After trying either to decipher illegible handwriting or to interpret incomplete orders, nurses or clerks must transcribe these orders to requisitions forms, the Kardex, and the flowsheet, at times to five or more documents, with an associated risk of error.

Computers can enhance the creation of orders and ease the associated burden of documentation by doing the following:

- Providing standard order sets according to physician, unit, and problem such as a sepsis workup, which can be entered quickly
- Transcribing orders to the appropriate departments and forms
- Requiring the complete entry of the order so that assumptions by the nurse are reduced
- Checking for the appropriateness of repetitive laboratory tests or medication doses
- Generating derivative orders for the nurse such as invoking nursing protocols when a patient is to be placed on a ventilator

Perhaps the greatest benefit provided by computer systems is called "closing the order loop," implying that for every order, a CIMS drives the documentation process so that there is verification of whether or not the order was executed. For example, when a medication is ordered, the system ensures that all appropriate administration of the medication is accounted for. Closing the order loop has profound implications for improving the quality assurance process as com-

pared to the current manual system, in which no guarantees exist that a patient will receive an ordered treatment.

Reference information. A CIMS is much more than an automated version of the medical record. It is an information utility that offers capabilities well beyond the manual charting system. For example, systems are programmed with edit checks to reduce the possibility of erroneous entries. They can provide a drug formulary with dosage and administration information, which can be used as a reference when writing orders. They can contain reference information such as a hospital's policies and procedures (e.g., a procedure for calibrating a transducer or for inserting a catheter), which can be displayed on a workstation at the bedside whenever a nurse or physician needs this information. Using a CIMS as an information utility, a kind of on-line electronic library, promises ultimately to replace traditional textbooks.

Quality assurance. The medical record serves as the major legal reference for the care given to a patient. Maintaining accurate records is critically important, both for assisting with the ongoing care of patients and for protecting personnel against malpractice claims. Computers can provide many checks to ensure that care is given as ordered and according to policy; further, the systems ensure that this care is easily and clearly documented. Moreover, as this care is documented, the electronic medical record can be systematically audited. Unlike manual records in which chart reviews are difficult at best, the electronic record is a database that can be queried to study the efficacy of a particular procedure or to document outcomes.

SUMMARY

The examples cited in this chapter only hint at the transformation of information management that computerization promises. The benefits of computerization of the ICU chart are compelling. The quality of the chart can clearly be improved; a computerized record is more accurate, timely, complete, legible, auditable, and accessible. The past decade has seen tremendous improvement in bedside instrumentation as a result of the introduction of computers. The next decade will see corresponding improvements in the capabilities of CIMS, and they will effectively replace current manual charting methods.

114 Venous Access

Luis O. Toro-Figueroa · Katherine A. Hammond

BACKGROUND

Peripheral and central venous catheterization is indispensable in the care of critically ill children. Over the past decade various procedures and catheter technologies have evolved. All these changes give the pediatrician a more versatile armamentarium that he can tailor to meet the needs of his patients.

PERIPHERAL VENOUS CANNULATION

Peripheral venous catheterization is indicated in all patients who need IV medications or fluids, in patients who are at risk for cardiopulmonary arrest, and in some patients for blood sampling and occasionally for exchange transfusions.

Peripheral venous access may be obtained through two techniques: percutaneous insertion or cutdown insertion. The percutaneous approach has the following advantages: (1) safety, (2) ease of personnel training, (3) low rate of complications, (4) numerous access sites, and (5) no disfiguring scars. The disadvantages of percutaneous venous catheterization include the following: (1) inserting the cannula may be difficult in patients with poor peripheral perfusion (i.e., in shock or cardiopulmonary arrest) or in chronic patients with poor peripheral access because of previous venous cannulations; (2) it provides an indirect route for administration of resuscitation drugs to the central circulation; and (3) in some cases it limits the amount of fluid that can be delivered rapidly

The primary advantage of peripheral cutdown is direct visualization and cannulation of the desired vessel in patients with poor peripheral perfusion or in those with no access because of numerous prior percutaneous catheterizations. The disadvantages of the cutdown technique include (1) the need for more

specialized training, (2) a higher complication rate, (3) wound scarring, (4) indirect route for administration of resuscitation drugs to the central circulation, and (5) in some cases limitation of the amount of fluid that can be delivered rapidly.

Technique
Access sites (Fig. 114-1)
Preferred sites for percutaneous peripheral venous catheterization, in order of preference, are (1) the back of the hand (dorsal metacarpal and dorsal venous network), (2) the foot (dorsal venous arch, venous plexus of the dorsum, median, and marginal vessels), (3) the forearm (median antebrachial and accessory cephalic veins), (4) the ankle (greater and lesser saphenous veins), (5) the antecubital fossa (median cephalic and basilic veins), (6) the arm (cephalic, basilic, and axillary veins), (7) the scalp in newborns and infants (superficial temporal, occipital, posterior auricular, frontal, and supraorbital veins), (8) the neck (external jugular vein), and (9) the thigh (greater saphenous and femoral veins).

The preferred sites for peripheral venous cutdown insertion are (1) the lesser saphenous vein (ankle), (2) the antecubital fossa (median cephalic and basilic veins), (3) the external jugular vein, and (4) the greater saphenous vein (thigh).

Equipment
All necessary equipment for the procedure must be set up before attempting cannulation to decrease the chances of causing accidental decannulation while attempting to locate equipment after catheterization of a vessel. The equipment necessary for percutaneous cannulation and a venous cutdown are as follows:

Peripheral venous cannulation equipment

Armboards appropriate for patient's size (hand and foot
   immobilization)
Benzoin sticks
Infusion pump
IV fluid
IV tubing with a microdrip chamber
Needles or catheters
   Butterfly needle, 19, 21, 23, 25 gauge
   Over-the-needle catheters, 14, 16, 18, 20, 22, 24 gauge
Povidone-iodine ointment
Povidone-iodine pads
Protective goggles (universal precaution)
Rubber bands
Small paper cup (protect scalp cannula)

Sodium chloride flush solution, 10 ml vial
Surgical gloves and mask (universal precautions)
Surgical tape, 1/2 and 1 inch
Syringes
   3 ml syringe with 3/8-inch needle
   10 ml syringe
T-connector (optimal)
Tourniquet

Venous cutdown cannulation equipment

Catheters (short or long), 18, 25 gauge (see also above)
Lidocaine, 1%
Plastic catheter introducer
Surgical procedure lamp
Vascular access tray (see below)
Other equipment (same as above)

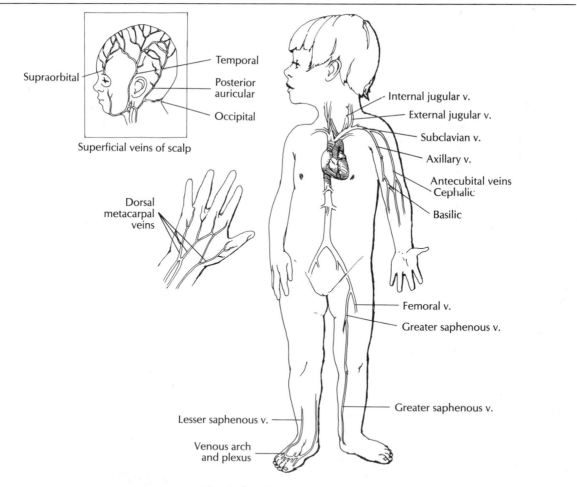

Fig. 114-1 Venous sites.

Vascular access tray (sterile)

Syringe for flush solution, 10 ml
Clear dermal tape
Draping towels
Five 4 × 4 inch gauze sponges
Four-inch curved eye-dressing forceps
Four-inch straight eye-dressing forceps
Needle holder
Scalpel blades, Nos. 11 and 15
Scalpel handle
Smooth forceps
Small scissors
Suture on needle, 4-0 silk or nylon
Toothed forceps
Two 5-inch curved mosquito hemostats
Umbilical tape

Insertion

Percutaneous insertion. Using aseptic technique prepare the area in which the cannula will be inserted with povidone-iodine solution. Apply a tourniquet proximal to the insertion site. Anchoring a rubber band around the patient's head above the eyebrows to avoid any ocular damage may be useful for scalp venipunctures in infants. Allow the povidone-iodine solution to dry for 30 seconds. Visualize and palpate an appropriate vein. Straight vessels provide better insertion sites. Approach the vessel in the direction of blood flow. The use of nitroglycerin ointment (0.4 mg for infants <1 year old; 0.8 mg for children >1 year old) aids in performing venous cannulation in children without causing systemic effects.

When using a butterfly needle, flush it with 0.9% sodium chloride solution before insertion to ensure that the needle and tubing are free of air and bubbles. Grab the needle by the butterfly wings with the bevel up. Stretch the skin over the vessel with your free hand to anchor the vessel. Puncture the skin with the needle 0.5 to 1.0 cm distal to the desired vessel puncture site. Advance the needle along the vein's axis until vessel puncture is accomplished. At this point there should be blood return into the stylet's hub; proceed to advance the catheter into the vessel. After inserting the cannula, attach a 3 ml syringe filled with 0.9% sodium chloride solution to the needle and aspirate gently to corroborate blood return. After blood return is obtained, release the tourniquet and flush the tubing and needle. Fluid must flow freely. Tissue swelling and/or discoloration is an indication of extravasation. If the line has good blood return

and flushes properly, secure it with adhesive tape, avoiding the skin insertion site. Connect it to the rest of the infusion system at this point. A small self-adhesive dressing can be applied to the skin insertion site, protecting the site from ambient contamination but allowing easy inspection.

The approach with the over-the-needle catheter is similar except that there is no need to flush the catheter before insertion and the insertion technique for the Teflon cannula is different. Once the vessel is pierced with the needle and blood returns into the hub, advance the needle slightly into the lumen of the vein until the Teflon catheter is within the vessel. At this point hold the needle in a stationary position while the catheter is slowly advanced over the needle. Some personnel prefer to advance the catheter while rotating it over the needle. Once the catheter is advanced, carefully remove the needle and allow blood to return through the catheter. Remove the tourniquet at this point and flush the catheter. If the catheter flushes without signs of extravasation, secure it with adhesive tape, connect it to the infusion system, and cover it with a sterile dressing.

Cutdown insertion. The lesser saphenous venous cutdown is the only cutdown site discussed in this section (Fig. 114-2). All other sites are described in the literature listed in Additional Reading. The techniques vary only in anatomic location of the vessel.

The saphenous vein at the ankle should be located superior and anterior to the medial malleolus (Fig. 114-2, *A*). Aseptically apply povidone-iodine to the surgical site three times and let dry. Infiltrate the area with lidocaine. Drape the surgical site and set up the necessary equipment (i.e., mount scalpel blade, draw flush solution, paint the T-connector). Cut a cardboard wedge in a triangular shape with a base 1 cm from the cardboard that holds the surgical suture material. Recheck the patient for analgesia. Make a 1 cm incision at the upper limit of the medial malleolus, starting at the most anterior quarter of the malleolus and extending anteriorly. Find the saphenous vein by scraping the tibia from anterior to posterior with the hemostat closed and the curve down to pick up the tissue bundle that contains the saphenous vein and nerve. Open the hemostat wide to separate the nerve and the vein from the connective tissue. Use the two eye-dressing forceps, alternating them in an opening and closing fashion, to dissect the saphenous vein. The vein is round, pink, and elastic; the nerve is flat, white, and stringlike.

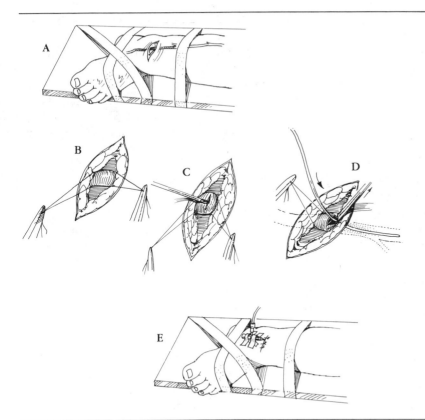

Fig. 114-2   Saphenous vein cutdown.

After dissecting the vein place a stay suture (6 cm long) distally and another proximally. Do not tie the vessel. Place a hemostat, holding the ends of each stay suture together (Fig. 114-2, *B*). Slip the triangular-shaped cardboard under the vessel. While exerting gentle traction on the distal stay suture, cannulate the vein using the same technique as for percutaneous insertion of over-the-needle catheters. For inserting long catheters make a puncture incision with an 18- or 20-gauge needle in the middle of the vessel (Fig. 114-2, *C*). Introduce the plastic catheter introducer into the vessel's lumen, opening the puncture incision. Pick up the tip of the long catheter with the eye-dressing forceps and introduce it gently into the vessel. Advance the catheter gently until the length desired is introduced (Fig. 114-2, *D*).

After the catheter has been placed, check for blood return; then flush the catheter with a 0.9% sodium chloride solution, observing the patient for signs of extravasation. Close the surgical wound with single stitches. Suture the catheter to the skin and the T-connector (Fig. 114-2, *E*). Cleanse the wound of blood with 0.9% sodium chloride solution or povidone-iodine solution. Apply adhesive tape to the catheter and T-connector for more stability without covering the wound. Finally, secure the stay sutures with tape distally and proximally. These sutures are helpful in stopping bleeding around the catheter. If such an event happens, gently pull the stay sutures to enhance hemostasis.

Maintenance

The dressing must be changed every 48 hours. The skin insertion site dressing must be minimal in size to allow inspection for signs of infiltration and infection (i.e., cellulitis, phlebitis) every hour and 8 hours, respectively. A transparent self-adhesive dressing can be used and must be changed when it no longer is occlusive. IV fluids must be changed every 24 hours and IV tubing every 72 hours.

Catheter removal

The Centers for Disease Control recommend that the insertion site be changed every 72 hours, but availability of other sites must be taken into account. The risk of catheter-induced septicemia or suspected septicemia from peripheral Teflon catheters is very small in general pediatric patients. In patients admitted to the general pediatric ward the risk of colonization and catheter-related septicemia is apparently not adequate reason for removing IV catheters at 72 hours when local or systemic signs of inflammation or infection are absent. Our policy states that in patients with minimal vascular access and no signs of local or systemic infection the catheter may be left longer than 72 hours. This requires documentation by the physician in the progress notes.

Risks and Complications

Peripheral venous cannulations have a low rate of complications, which can be separated into two categories: infectious and noninfectious. The infectious complications are local cellulitis, phlebitis, colonization, and septicemia. The noninfectious complications are arterial cannulation, chemical or mechanical phlebitis, extravasation, thrombosis, and embolus formation.

Extravasation of some drugs may cause skin and deep tissue necrosis. The use of hyaluronidase decreases and in some cases prevents tissue injury by temporarily destroying the interstitial cement and increasing diffusion of extravasated fluid through the tissues. Investigators have used 15 units of hyaluronidase in infants and 300 units of hyaluronidase in rabbits without secondary effects. As many as 750,000 units has been used in animals with virtually no adverse effects. For optimal effect hyaluronidase must be administered within 1 hour of extravasation.

CENTRAL VENOUS CATHETERIZATION

Central venous catheterization (CVC) is used for (1) CVP measurement, (2) CVP waveform analysis, (3) secure delivery of drugs to the central circulation, (4) administration of high-concentration parenteral alimentation, (5) rapid infusion of large volumes of fluids or blood products, (6) exchange transfusion, or (7) an alternate route for parenteral fluids or drugs for patients in whom peripheral venous cannulation is no longer possible.

Rapid delivery of drugs to the central circulation during resuscitation can best be achieved through CVC.

CVC can be accomplished in two ways: percutaneously or cutdown. The advantages of the percutaneous technique over the cutdown technique are (1) no remaining disfiguring scar, (2) more quickly performed, and (3) simpler to learn. The advantage of the cutdown technique over the percutaneous technique is direct visualization of vessels in those patients who are in shock or who are difficult to cannulate percutaneously.

Technique

Access sites (Fig. 114-1)

Any peripheral vessel (see "Access Sites" in section on peripheral venous catheterization) can be used to access a central vein if a long enough catheter is used to reach the central circulation. Usually the more peripheral the site is, the smaller the catheter that may be used. Peripheral sites such as the scalp, hands, and feet generally do not lend themselves to cutdowns. In addition to the list of percutaneous peripheral insertion sites, the following deep veins are available for CVC placement (in order of preference): (1) external jugular vein, (2) internal jugular vein, (3) femoral vein, and (4) subclavian vein.

The internal jugular vein should not be catheterized in patients with increased ICP since the catheter may impede venous return from the head and elevate ICP. In patients with high intrathoracic pressure and in small infants the subclavian approach should be avoided when possible because of the high incidence of pneumothorax.

Equipment

The variety of CVCs available has increased over the past few years, giving the physician the advantage of tailoring the catheter to the patient's needs.

CVCs are classified into two categories: (1) short vs. long term and (2) single vs. multiple lumen. Most short-term catheters (up to 3 weeks of use) are constructed from polyethylene or polyurethane. Polyurethane is preferred over polyethylene because of its elasticity and lesser thrombogenicity. Silicone is the preferred material for long-term catheters since it is less thrombogenic and more pliable than polyurethane. Polyurethane catheters coated with hydromer (isocyanate prepolymer, hydrogel interpolymer of polyvinylpyrrolidone) have been reported to be less thrombogenic than silicone, polyvinylchloride, and noncoated polyurethane.

Multiple-lumen catheters have made simultaneous drug administration and monitoring possible. Cath-

Table 114-1   Generic Central Venous Catheter Guidelines

No. of Lumina	Size (F) (max)	Length (cm) (min)	Age (weight)	Site
Single	3	10	Newborn (3 kg) to 6 mo (8 kg)	Neck/subclavian
Single	3	30	Newborn (3 kg) to 6 mo (8 kg)	Basilic/femoral
Single	4	15	6 mo (8 kg) to 2 yr (13 kg)	Neck/subclavian
Single	4	45	6 mo (8 kg) to 2 yr (13 kg)	Basilic/femoral
Single	5	20	2 yr (13 kg) to adult	Neck/subclavian
Single	5	60	2 yr (13 kg) to adult	Basilic/femoral
Double	4	10	Newborn (3 kg) to 6 mo (8 kg)	Neck/subclavian
Double	4	30	Newborn (3 kg) to 6 mo (8 kg)	Basilic/femoral
Double	5	15	6 mo (8 kg) to 2 yr (13 kg)	Neck/subclavian
Double	5	45	6 mo (8 kg) to 2 yr (13 kg)	Basilic/femoral
Double	7	20	2 yr (13 kg) to adult	Neck/subclavian
Double	7	60	2 yr (13 kg) to adult	Basilic/femoral
Triple	5	15	6 mo (8 kg) to 2 yr (13 kg)	Neck/subclavian
Triple	5	45	6 mo (8 kg) to 2 yr (13 kg)	Basilic/femoral
Triple	7	20	2 yr (13 kg) to adult	Neck/subclavian
Triple	7	60	2 yr (13 kg) to adult	Basilic/femoral

eters with up to three noncommunicating lumens are presently available in a single catheter body. Exit ports are usually separated to facilitate simultaneous use. Sizes vary from as small as less than 1 F to as large as 14 F. Combining different materials and single- or multiple-lumen designs with the wide range of sizes that are available offers a large number of catheters for use in pediatric patients. At least 18 catheter manufacturers are in the market; some make customized catheters, and others have a standardized product line. Table 114-1 lists generic catheters that provide a wide range of options, taking into account the patient's age, the insertion site, the catheter size, and the length and number of lumina.

Insertion

Percutaneous insertion. There are three percutaneous techniques: (1) the Seldinger technique, (2) the through-the-needle technique, and (3) the combined technique.

The Seldinger technique consists of locating the desired vessel percutaneously with a small-gauge search needle mounted on a syringe. The syringe is removed from the needle when blood is returned (Fig. 114-3, *A*), and a thin-walled needle is introduced following the same trajectory of the search needle until entry into the vessel is gained (Fig. 114-3, *B*). A guidewire is passed through the needle into

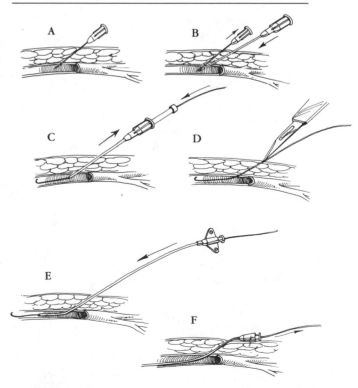

Fig. 114-3   Percutaneous venous access. Seldinger technique.

the vessel, advancing one fourth to one third of the wire (Fig. 114-3, *C*). The thin-walled needle is removed, leaving the guidewire in place (the search needle is also removed at this point) (Fig. 114-3, *D*). A catheter is inserted over the wire, making certain the guidewire is visible through the proximal end of the catheter before advancing it into the vessel (Fig. 114-3, *E*). A twisting motion is used to advance the catheter (slight enlargement of the entry site with a scalpel may be necessary). After the catheter is introduced into proper position, the guidewire is removed gently (Fig. 114-3, *F*).

The through-the-needle technique of catheterization consists of venous cannulation with a needle or catheter large enough to accommodate a catheter once a vessel is cannulated (Fig. 114-4, *A*). The catheter is then advanced into the vessel, and the introducing needle or catheter is removed (Fig. 114-4, *B*). Usually these setups have some kind of protective device to cover the sharp end of the needle to protect

the catheter or have a needle that can be broken in half longitudinally and removed. This technique is useful for placing small, long Silastic catheters into small vessels and advancing them to the central circulation (especially useful in premature infants). This technique of insertion does not allow pulling back the catheter because of the possibility of shearing it with the needle.

The third technique is a combination of the Seldinger technique and the through-the-needle technique. Vascular access is obtained using the same guidewire approach (Fig. 114-5, *A*). A peel-away sheath is introduced over the wire into the vessel, and the wire is removed (Fig. 114-5, *B* and *C*). A catheter of smaller diameter than the peel-away sheath is introduced into the vessel, and after the catheter is positioned as desired, the sheath is pulled and peeled, leaving the catheter in place (Fig. 114-5, *D-F*). This technique is useful for placement of soft large-diameter catheters (i.e., Broviac or Hickman

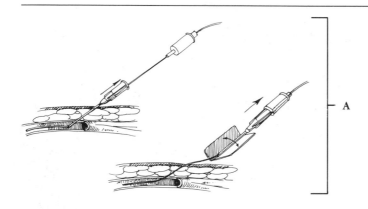

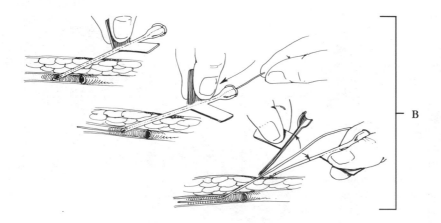

Fig. 114-4   Percutaneous venous access. Through-the-needle technique.

typc) because it allows the use of vessel dilators and the sheath offers little resistance to the advancement of a floppy catheter.

The percutaneous cannulation techniques for use in the external and internal jugular vein, femoral vein, and subclavian veins are discussed in detail in this section. The percutaneous catheterization of the basilic vein is omitted since the technique is similar to that used with a peripheral IV catheter. The only modifications would be the application of the Seldinger, through-the-needle, or combined technique.

External jugular vein cannulation (Fig. 114-6). Restrain the child's arms and legs and turn his head to the side opposite to the catheterization site (right side preferred). Place the child in a 20- to 30-degree Trendelenburg position and identify the external jug-

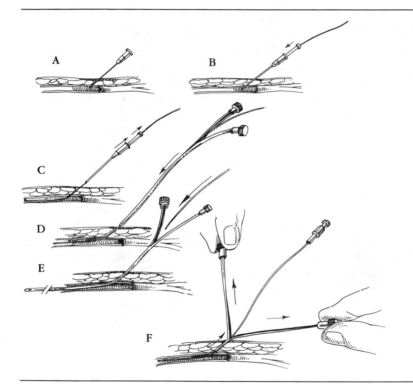

Fig. 114-5 Percutaneous venous access. Combination technique.

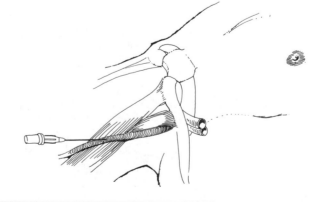

Fig. 114-6 Technique for external jugular vein catheterization.

ular vein (it is helpful to occlude it distally with a finger at the base of the neck). Use complete aseptic technique and give a local anesthetic. Cannulate the vessel using the Seldinger technique or through-the-needle technique, depending on the catheter desired (difficulty may arise passing the catheter centrally since it may go into the subclavian vein following the trajectory into the arm or in some instances may not

advance past the bifurcation). Check for proper catheter placement (Fig. 114-7) and suture the catheter in place.

Internal jugular vein cannulation. The four different approaches to the catheterization of the internal jugular vein are anterior, central, posterior, and low. Only the central approach is discussed in this chapter since the anterior and posterior approaches are modifications of the same technique. The low approach is also omitted since it is believed to have a higher incidence of pneumothorax than the other three approaches.

Immobilize the patient in the Trendelenburg position (Fig. 114-8); place a diaper roll between his shoulders and hyperextend his neck. The right side approach is preferred because of the lower position of the lung's apical pleura, less likelihood of injuring the thoracic duct, and a straighter route to the right atrium. Identify the landmarks as described previously. Cleanse the area surgically using sterile technique, including the use of cap, mask, and gloves. Anesthetize the area with lidocaine.

When using the central approach to the internal jugular vein cannulation (Fig. 114-9), identify the sternocleidomastoid muscle and the carotid artery. The two lower heads of the sternocleidomastoid muscle form a triangle, with the apex cephalad and the base caudad. Locate the apex of the triangle and introduce the search needle at a 30-degree angle to the coronal plane, diverting caudally parallel to the sagittal plane or slightly down the ipsilateral nipple. Do not advance the needle past the clavicular level to avoid pleural puncture. Redirecting the needle 5 to 10 de-

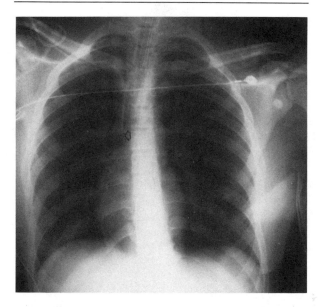

Fig. 114-7   Chest roentgenogram to confirm CVP placement.

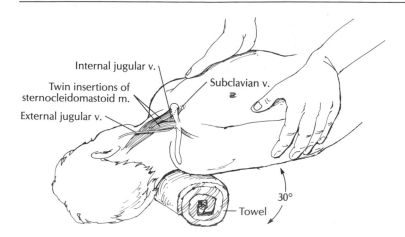

Internal jugular v.

Twin insertions of sternocleidomastoid m.

External jugular v.

Subclavian v.

30°

Towel

Fig. 114-8   Central venous catheterization. Trendelenburg position.

grees laterally may be needed to achieve cannulation.

When venous blood is freely obtained with the search needle, leave the needle in place and remove the syringe. Introduce a thin-walled needle and complete the procedure, following the instructions as described for the Seldinger technique. Caution must be taken not to let any port or needle open to air since negative intrathoracic pressure can pull air through the needle into the vein, resulting in air embolism. Once the catheter is in place, secure it

with several stitches. After securing the catheter, check for proper catheter placement as described below.

Femoral vein cannulation (Fig. 114-10). Immobilize the patient in a frog position. Identify the femoral pulse and surgically cleanse the area using sterile technique. Administer a local anesthetic to the area. Insert the search needle medial to the femoral pulse, 1 to 2 cm below the inguinal ligament, advancing it cephalad at a 45-degree angle until blood flow is obtained (do not go past the inguinal ligament to avoid intra-abdominal puncture of a femoral vessel). After achieving cannulation with the search needle, complete the Seldinger technique. Confirm catheter position and secure the catheter as previously described.

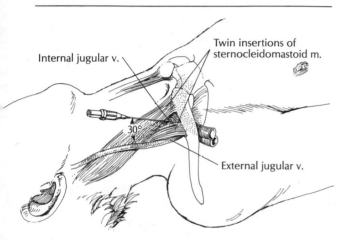

Fig. 114-9   Technique for internal jugular vein catheterization.

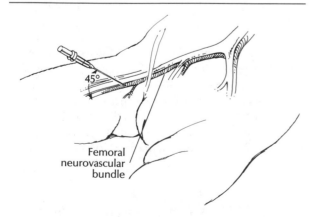

Fig. 114-10   Technique for femoral vein catheterization.

GUIDELINES FOR CONFIRMATION OF PROPER CVC PLACEMENT

1. External surface measurement: The distance from the point of the insertion site to the point between the second and third rib at the costochondral junction.
2. Waveform analysis: A central venous pressure waveform with its characteristic A, C, and V waves with the presence of respiratory cycle fluctuation ensures intrathoracic placement (pressure lower during spontaneous inspiration).
3. Chest roentgenogram: An anteroposterior chest roentgenogram should confirm the presence of the tip of the catheter at the superior vena caval–atrial junction (Fig. 114-7). The lateral chest roentgenogram may be helpful when catheter malposition is suspected from the anteroposterior roentgenogram.
4. IV dye contrast study: May be helpful when anatomic variations are suspected or in confirming malposition.
5. Sonography: Advocated by some authors as a noninvasive, nonradiating procedure but lacks prospective clinical studies to support its accuracy.
6. Electrocardiographic (ECG) confirmation: ECG of catheter placement has been attempted using two techniques: ECG signal through a guidewire and ECG signal through a saline solution–filled catheter with an ECG sensor attached at the outside port. This method also lacks prospective clinical confirmation.

Subclavian vein cannulation (Fig. 114-11). The infraclavicular approach in small infants is recommended only when no other routes are available. The proper technique must be followed carefully to avoid causing a pneumothorax and injury to the subclavian artery or internal thoracic artery.

Immobilize the child in a 30-degree Trendelenburg position (Figs. 114-6 and 114-7) with his head turned to the side opposite the area being cannulated. Identify the following landmarks: suprasternal notch, junction of the middle and medial thirds of the clavicle, and the pectoral shoulder groove (Fig. 114-11, *A*). Surgically scrub the area and apply a local anesthetic. Introduce a thin-walled needle at the junction of the middle and medial thirds of the clavicle, directing it toward a finger placed in the suprasternal notch. The syringe should be parallel to the frontal plane, lying in the pectoral shoulder groove. Advance the needle, applying gentle negative pressure under the clavicle toward the clavicular sternal junction at the level of the fingertip in the suprasternal notch. When free flow of blood is obtained, rotate the needle 90 degrees so the bevel faces caudad to facilitate the passage of the guidewire into the superior vena cava (Fig. 114-11, *B* and *C*). Remove the syringe carefully, occluding the needle to prevent air embolism; then complete the Seldinger technique for catheter placement. Secure the catheter and confirm catheter position as previously described.

Cutdown insertion. The cutdown technique for performing CVC placement is similar to that for performing peripheral venous cutdowns. The preferred site is the basilic vein. The greater saphenous vein at the groin, the internal and external jugular veins, and the femoral vein may also be used but are not discussed in this chapter (see Additional Reading for further information). Only the anatomic considerations for the basilic vein cannulation are discussed here. The rest of the technique combines the peripheral venous cutdown and percutaneous CVC placement techniques. The anatomic landmarks for the basilic vein are the brachial pulse, the humerus' medial epicondyle, and the groove between the biceps and triceps muscles. A 1 cm incision transverse to the vessels should be made approximately 1 cm above the antecubital fold medial to the brachial pulse and lateral to the epicondyle transversing the biceps/triceps groove. Blunt dissection should reveal the basilic vein, the median nerve, and the brachial artery. The basilic vein lies deep within the groove and occasionally may be found behind the brachial

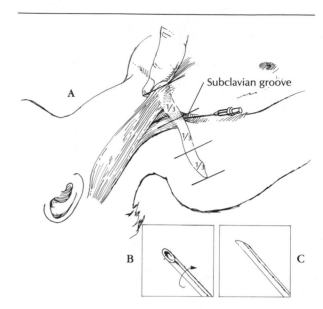

Fig. 114-11 Infraclavicular approach to subclavian vein cannulation.

artery or the median nerve. Cannulation of the vein may be done using the Seldinger technique or going directly into the vessel as previously described.

CVP interpretation

CVP directly correlates with right atrial pressure (RAP), which reflects right ventricular end-diastolic pressure (RVEDP) when the physiologic and anatomic conditions of the right heart are normal. Clinically, CVP is used as an indicator of preload, although right ventricular end-diastolic volume (RVEDV) is a better indicator of preload.

Ventricular compliance and transmural ventricular distending pressure are the major components of RVEDV. The transmural distending pressure is the intracavitary pressure (RVEDP) minus the juxtacardiac pressure (i.e., intrathoracic pressure). Therefore RVEDP is only one of the variables that determine RVEDV. Clinically, two-dimensional echocardiography provides right ventricular end-diastolic dimensions that are better correlates of RVEDV.

Waveform analysis

A normal CVP waveform is composed of five components (Fig. 114-12): (1) the A wave, which represents atrial contraction; (2) the X descent, which rep-

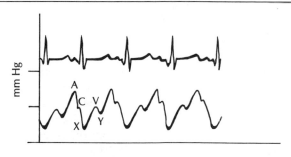

Fig. 114-12   CVP waveform.

resents atrial relaxation; (3) the C wave, which represents the closing and bulging of the tricuspid valve at the onset of ventricular systole; (4) the V wave, which represents passive venous filling of the right atrium during ventricular systole; and (5) the Y descent, which represents rapid atrial emptying after opening of the tricuspid valve.

The A wave follows the ECG's P wave by 80 msec in adults. The distance between the A wave and the P wave is equal to the PR interval. When the PR interval is prolonged, the C wave becomes more accentuated. The V wave occurs near the ECG's T wave. The CVP waveform's relationship with the ECG is helpful in distinguishing it from other pressure tracings.

CVP waveform analysis can be divided into four categories: (1) elevated A wave, (2) elevated V wave, (3) elevated A and V waves, and (4) abnormalities related to dysrhythmias. An elevated A wave may be caused by tricuspid stenosis, pulmonary stenosis, pulmonary hypertension, and right ventricular failure. Tricuspid insufficiency causes elevation of the V wave. The causes of elevation of the A and V waves are volume overload, cardiac tamponade, constrictive pericardial disease, and left ventricular failure. The abnormalities associated with dysrhythmias are no A waveform during atrial fibrillation, the summation of the A and V waveforms (cannon A waves) during junctional rhythm, and no A waves during ventricular pacing.

Maintenance

To maintain the patency of venous catheters, fluids must be administered by constant infusion through an infusion pump. Since this is a low-pressure line, CVP lines can be satisfactorily maintained with infu-

sion rates as low as 2 to 3 ml/hr. In addition 1 unit of sodium heparin per 1 ml of fluid in the solution may be used to maintain patency.

CVC blood sampling is useful except that it may not be considered representative of mixed venous blood gas since there are three major venous contributors into the atrium: the sinus venosum (lowest oxygen content), the superior vena cava (intermediate oxygen content), and the inferior vena cava (highest oxygen content). Depending on the area in which the CVC lies, the blood gas values will reflect different contributions to the right atrial blood volume.

When CVP readings are desired, attach the catheter to a transducer system with a 30 ml/hr flow-directed device. If the fluid administration rate exceeds 30 ml/hr, the continuous display of pressure by the 30 ml/hr flow-directed device cannot be used. However, by deleting the flow-directed device, pressures may be obtained by turning the stopcock off to the fluid source to obtain intermittent CVP readings. Since the CVP is a low-pressure line, recalibration of the transducer every 4 hours is necessary. The administration of lipids through CVCs in line with the continuous flow-directed device renders the CVP unreliable unless the fluid source is occluded momentarily.

Strict adherence to aseptic technique (use of mask included) during catheter manipulation and care should be maintained. To aid in the prevention of local and systemic infections, the following CVC care must be provided: (1) fluid changed every 24 hours, (2) central dressing changed at least three times weekly (M, W, F) or when dressing is nonocclusive, (3) site observed for erythema, swelling, and/or drainage, (4) dressing checked for any leakage of fluid, and (5) delivery system connections cleansed for 30 seconds with iodine solution before opening them.

CVC dressing changes include removal of the old dressing using aseptic technique including wearing mask and sterile gloves; cleansing around the catheter insertion site with acetone-alcohol without touching the catheter itself, followed by application of povidone-iodine at the catheter site and along the catheter for 3 to 5 cm; placing a drop of iodine ointment on the insertion site; topping with two split pieces of sterile 2 × 2 gauze, each facing the opposite way over the catheter; covering the area with nonporous tape to form an occlusive dressing; and coiling the catheter on top of the 2 × 2 gauze before the application of the occlusive tape to prevent direct tension on the catheter. When skin breakdown is noted, the frequency of dressing changes must be decreased. Other antimicrobial cleansing agents are available for use in patients allergic to povidone-iodine solutions.

Catheter removal

Removal of venous catheters is indicated when the patient's condition no longer necessitates their use. Catheter removal is also indicated when catheter clotting is suspected. Before removal of a clotted catheter, use of the streptokinase or urokinase protocol to dissolve central line clots (see Chapter 149) should be considered. Other indications for catheter removal include any signs of local infection, phlebitis, sepsis, and/or positive blood cultures obtained through the catheter (catheter colonization).

After removal of the catheter continuous pressure must be applied to the catheter insertion site for 5 to 10 minutes until no bleeding is noted. The catheter must be inspected to confirm that the entire catheter has been removed and the tip sent for culture. The site must be topped with providone-iodine ointment, dressed with a small self-adhesive bandage or gauze pad, and inspected daily until healing occurs.

Risks and Complications

CVC complications can be classified as infectious, thrombotic, mechanical, cardiopulmonary, and others.

Infectious complications. Infectious complication rates as high as 11% have been reported. They may be classified as local (site or wound cellulitis and phlebitis), systemic (sepsis), and catheter colonization. Systemic infection and catheter colonization can be differentiated by comparing semiquantitative blood cultures (peripheral and through the catheter). A negative peripheral blood culture with a positive catheter culture indicates catheter colonization, and when both cultures are positive, with a semiquantitative catheter blood culture fivefold greater than the peripheral, catheter-related sepsis is indicated. When the difference between semiquantitative cultures is less than fivefold, the presence of noncatheter-related sepsis or bacteremia is most likely. Catheter-related sepsis or colonization in a hemodynamically stable patient may be eradicated with the catheter in place when antibiotics are infused through the catheter. Persistent positive blood cultures or a hemodynam-

ically unstable patient is an indication for catheter removal.

Thrombotic complications. Thrombotic complications have been reported in association with low blood flow states, extended catheter life, sepsis, high glucose concentrations, and catheter material (in decreasing order of prevalence: polyvinyl, polyethylene, polyurethane, silicone). When thrombus formation is suspected, it may be confirmed by a sonogram or dye-contrast study. If the presence of a thrombus is confirmed, the catheter should be removed, and/or treatment with heparin, urokinase, and/or thrombectomy should be considered. In many partial occlusion situations conservative management with catheter removal and observation usually leads to clot reabsorption.

Mechanical complications. Mechanical complication rates as high as 25% have been reported. These complications include occlusions, fractures, and dislodgments. Occlusion is the most common complication, clotting being the leading cause. Clotted catheters may be recannulized using urokinase to dissolve the clot. Catheter occlusions secondary to medication precipitation do not resolve with the administration of urokinase. Catheter fractures may be repaired using a blunt needle, suture, and glue technique. Catheter dislodgment can be prevented by securing the suture, minimizing patient movement, and confirming catheter placement using roentgenograms or sonography and waveform analysis.

Cardiopulmonary complications. The cardiopulmonary complications associated with CVC placement include pneumothorax, hydrothorax, hemothorax, dysrhythmias, embolism, and cardiac tamponade. These complications are responsible for the great majority of deaths associated with CVC placement. Pneumothorax, hydrothorax, and hemothorax are more often associated with subclavian and internal jugular (low more frequently than high insertion) approaches, with the subclavian approach having the higher complication rate.

Dysrhythmias most frequently occur during catheter insertion, atrial placement, the catheter's lying against the tricuspid valve, or dislodgment into the right ventricle. They are prevented by maintaining the catheter at the superior vena cava–right atrium (SVC-RA) junction. When catheter dislodgment causes dysrhythmias, the catheter must be pulled back to the SVC-RA junction.

Embolism may be caused by air leaking into the system or a thrombus being dislodged. Air embolism most commonly occurs when the catheter is open to air, especially when the patient is spontaneously breathing. Embolism secondary to thrombus dislodgment is most frequently seen when catheters are removed. A thromboembolic phenomenon should be suspected in any patient with a CVC or after its removal when a patient has sudden onset of hypoxia and/or respiratory distress.

Cardiac tamponade is the most serious catheter-related complication and the most difficult to diagnose (see Chapter 40). A mortality rate of 50% to 100% has been reported and is caused by the difficulty in identifying the insidious onset of signs and symptoms that usually lead to a rapid drop in cardiac output and cardiac arrest. The clinical picture of cardiac tamponade includes sudden neck vein distention, increased CVP, sudden onset of duskiness or cyanosis, apnea, grunting, bradycardia, tachycardia, paradoxical pulse, increasing hypotension, decreasing pulse pressure, distant heart sounds, restlessness, confusion, nausea, epigastric discomfort, respiratory distress, loss of CVP waveform, and inability to draw blood back from the catheter. Although some cases of tamponade occur during catheter insertion, the most frequent presentation has a delayed onset. Cardiac tamponade must be suspected in any patient who suffers a cardiac arrest with a central line in place or who has a history of CVC removal close to the event. Any patient with the above-mentioned clinical picture must be evaluated for the possibility of cardiac tamponade secondary to perforation. The same preventive measures mentioned under pneumothorax apply to cardiac perforation. The risk of perforation is greater with (1) atrial placement of the CVC, (2) a left-sided venous approach, (3) a subclavian approach, (4) stiff catheters, and (5) beveled catheters. Cardiac tamponade must be immediately treated with administration of a volume expander through another route and with inotropic agents, cessation of infusions through the suspected catheter, aspiration through the suspected CVC, pericardiocentesis, and in some cases pericardial window or pericardial tube placement (see Chapter 143).

Others. Additional complications of CVCs include arterial puncture during insertion, fluid extravasation, Horner's syndrome, subdural collection of fat emulsion (neonates), superior vena cava syndrome, thoracic duct injury, and venostasis. In general most CVC-related complications are recognizable; therefore mortality and morbidity may be preventable. Usually there is a higher incidence of morbidity and mortality in infants because of their smaller anatomy and vague symptomatology.

UMBILICAL VEIN CATHETERIZATION

Umbilical vein catheterization (UVC) into the central circulation of newborn infants is possible up to 7 days of age. The advantages of this procedure are easy access, simplicity of procedure, and accommodation of large-diameter catheters. Disadvantages of the procedure are listed in Chapter 115. UVC is only for short-term use. The principal indications for its use are exchange transfusion, route of administration for resuscitation drugs in the delivery room, CVP monitoring, and administration of high-concentration glucose.

Technique
Access site

The umbilical stump contains a single large, thin-walled vein usually located cephalad of the umbilical arteries.

Equipment

See Chapter 115.

Insertion

Immobilize the patient, surgically scrub the umbilical stump, and place a fenestrated sterile drape around it. Prepare the equipment while the providone-iodine solution dries (i.e., flush catheter, mount scalpel blade, connect catheter to transducer and fluid source). Place a curved hemostat at the distal end of the umbilical stump; pull gently and turn it cephalad over the instrument. With the scalpel blade slowly cut the cord superficially 2 cm above the skin margin. Advance toward the center of the cord until the vein is partially transected. Ideally no more than half the vein's circumference must be cut. Remove any visible clots within the vein. Introduce the catheter gently until a CVP waveform with respiratory fluctuations can be observed (Fig. 114-13, *A*). Be careful not to allow air into the fluid system since it can cause air embolism during inspiration. Secure the catheter with Dermick tape and suture to the umbilical stump (Fig. 114-13, *B*). An H-type adhesive tape bridge can be used to further secure the catheter to the abdominal wall (Fig. 114-13, *C*). An anteroposterior roentgenogram of the chest and abdomen must be taken to confirm a properly positioned catheter at the SVC-RA junction (Fig. 114-14).

Maintenance

Refer to "Maintenance" in section on central venous catheterization.

Catheter removal

The UVC should be removed when the indications for insertion are resolved or when there is evidence of omphalitis, catheter colonization, or sepsis. The catheter must be removed slowly and inspected for integrity. After removal of the catheter, pressure must be applied around the umbilical stump for 5 to 10 minutes to obtain hemostasis.

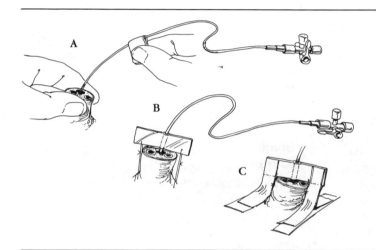

Fig. 114-13   Umbilical vein catheterization and securing the catheter.

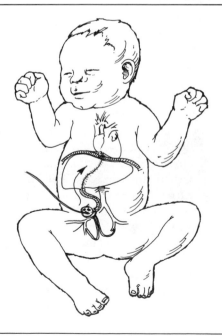

Fig. 114-14   UVC placement confirmation.

Risks and Complications

In addition to the complications listed in Chapter 115, the following complications are common: necrotizing enterocolitis, hepatic infarction, hepatic abscesses, and bowel perforation during exchange transfusion.

ADDITIONAL READING

Aaronson IA. Letter to the Editor. J Pediatr Surg 18:657, 1983.

Agarwal KC, Ali Khan MA, Falla A, Amato JJ. Cardiac perforation from central venous catheters: Survival after cardiac tamponade in an infant. Pediatrics 73:333-338, 1984.

Aldridge HE, Jay AWL. Central venous catheters and heart perforation. Can Med Assoc J 135:1082-1084, 1986.

Asaadi M, Seltzer MH. Subclavian intravenous catheterization for hyperalimentation. Resident & Staff Physician, August 1980, pp 53-58.

Balagtas RC, Bell CE, Edwards LD, Levin S. Risk of local and systemic infections associated with umbilical vein catheterization: A prospective study in 86 newborn patients. Pediatrics 48:359-367, 1971.

Birman H, Haq A, Hew E, Aberman A. Continuous monitoring of mixed venous oxygen saturation in hemodynamically unstable patients. Chest 86:753-756, 1984.

Borow M, Crowley JG. Prevention of thrombosis of central venous catheters. J Cardiovasc Surg 27:571-574, 1986.

Brahos GJ. Central venous catheterization via the supraclavicular approach. J Trauma 17:872-877, 1977.

Cameron GS. Central venous catheters for children with malignant disease: Surgical issues. J Pediatr Surg 22:702-704, 1987.

Cobb LM, Vinocur CD, Wagner CW, Weintraub WH. The central venous anatomy in infants. Surg Gynecol Obstet 165:230-234, 1987.

Colley PS, Artru AA. ECG-guided placement of Sorenson CVP catheters via arm veins. Anesth Analg 63:953-956, 1984.

• Cote CJ, Jobes DR, Schwartz AJ, Ellison N. Two approaches to cannulation of a child's internal jugular vein. Anesthesiology 50:371-373, 1979.

DeFalqie RJ. Percutaneous catheterization of the internal jugular vein. Anesth Analg 53:116-121, 1974.

Demey HE, Colemont LJ, Hartoko TJ, Roodhooft AMI, Ysebaert DK, Bossaert LL. Venopulmonary fistula: A rare complication of central venous catheterization. JPEN 11:580-582, 1987.

Diemer A. Central venous Silastic catheters in newborns: Localization by sonography and radiology. Pediatr Radiol 17:15-17, 1987.

• Dronen SC, Yee AS, Tomlanovich MC. Proximal saphenous vein cutdown. Ann Emerg Med 10:328-330, 1981.

Durand M, Ramananathan R, Martinelli B, Tolentino M. Prospective evaluation of percutaneous central venous Silastic catheters in newborn infants with birth weights of 510 to 3920 grams. Pediatrics 78:245-250, 1986.

• Filston HC, Grant JP. A safer system for percutaneous subclavian venous catheterization in newborn infants. J Pediatr Surg 14:564-570, 1979.

• Filston HC, Johnson DG. Percutaneous venous cannulation in neonates and infants: A method for catheter insertion without "cut-down." Pediatrics 48:896-901, 1971.

Flynn PM, Shenep JL, Stokes DC, Barrett FF. In situ management of confirmed central venous catheter-related bacteremia. Pediatr Infect Dis 6:729-734, 1987.

Fraschini G, Jadeja J, Lawson M, Holmes FA, Carrasco HC, Wallace S. Local infusion of urokinase for the lysis of thrombosis associated with permanent central venous catheters in cancer patients. J Clin Oncol 5:672-678, 1987.

Garland JS, Nelson DB, Cheah TE, Hennes HH, Johnson TM. Infectious complications during peripheral intravenous therapy with Teflon catheters: A prospective study. Pediatr Infect Dis 6:918-921, 1987.

Gilhooly J, Lindenberg J, Reynolds JW. Central venous silicone elastomer catheter placement by basilic vein cutdown in neonates. Pediatrics 78:636-639, 1986.

Greenspoon JS, Terrasi J. Central venous catheterization: Are complications related to the route? Am J Obstet Gynecol 155:1143, 1986.

• Groff DB, Ahmed N. Subclavian vein catheterization in the infant. J Pediatr Surg 9:171-174, 1974.

• Hall DMB, Geefhuysen J. Percutaneous catheterization of the internal jugular vein in infants and children. J Pediatr Surg 122:719-722, 1977.

Henderson AM, Sumner E. Late perforation by central venous cannulae. Arch Dis Child 59:776-789, 1984.

Hodge D, Delgado-Paredes C, Fleisher G. Central and peripheral catheter flow rates in "pediatric" dogs. Ann Emerg Med 15:1151-1154, 1986.

Holt RW, Heres EK. Creation of subcutaneous tunnel for Broviac and Hickman catheters. JPEN 9:225-226, 1985.

Hughes WT, Buescher ES. Pediatric Procedures, 2nd ed. Philadelphia: WB Saunders, 1980, pp 87-121.

Iberti TJ, Katz LB, Reiner MA, Brownie T, Kwun KB. Hydrothorax as a late complication of central venous indwelling catheters. Surgery 94:842-846, 1983.

Ikeda S, Schweiss JF. Maximum infusion rates and CVP accuracy during high-flow delivery through multilumen catheters. Crit Care Med 13:586-588, 1985.

• Kanter RK, Zimmerman JJ, Strauss RH, Stoeckel KA. Central venous catheter insertion by femoral vein: Safety and effectiveness for the pediatric patient. Pediatrics 77:842-847, 1986.

Kitterman JA, Phibbs RH, Tooley WH. Catheterization of umbilical vessels in newborn infants. Pediatr Clin North Am 17:895-912, 1970.

Knox WF, Hooton VN, Barson AJ. Pulmonary vascular candidiasis and use of central venous catheters in neonates. J Clin Pathol 40:559-565, 1987.

• Krausz MM, Berlatsky Y, Ayalon A, Freund H, Schiller M. Percutaneous cannulation of the internal jugular vein in infants and children. Surg Gynecol Obstet 148:591-594, 1979.

Laurie SWS, Wilson KL, Kernahan DA, Bauer BS, Vistnes LM. Intravenous extravasation injuries. The effectiveness of hyaluronidase in their treatment. Ann Plast Surg 13:191-194, 1984.

Lemmer JH, Zwischenberger JB, Bove EL, Dick M. Lymph leak from a femoral cutdown site in a neonate: Repair with fibrin glue. J Pediatr Surg 22:827-828, 1987.

Levy JH, Nagle DM, Curling PE, Waller JL, Kopel M, Tobia V. Contamination reduction during central venous catheterization. Crit Care Med 16:165-167, 1988.

Linder LE, Curelaru I, Gustavsson B, Hansson HA, Stenqvist O, Wojciechoiski J. Material thrombogenicity in central venous catheterization: A comparison between soft, antebrachial catheters of silicone elastomer and polyurethane. JPEN 8:399-406, 1984.

Mactier H, Alroomi LG, Young DG, Raine PAM. Central venous catheterisation in very low birthweight infants. Arch Dis Child 61:449-453, 1986.

Maki DG, Cobb L, Garman JK, Shapiro J, Ringer M. Multicenter trial of an attachable silver-impregnated subcutaneous cuff for prevention of infection with central venous catheters. Abstract of the 1987 Interscience Conference on Antimicrobial Agents in Chemotherapy.

Malatack JJ, Wiener ES, Gartner JC, Zitelli BJ, Brunetti E. Munchausen syndrome by proxy: A new complication of central venous catheterization. Pediatrics 75:523-525, 1985.

Marx JA, Rosen P, Jorden RC, Moore EE. Proximal saphenous vein cutdown: When and why? Ann Emerg Med 11:167, 1982.

Maschke SP, Rogove HJ. Cardiac tamponade associated with a multilumen central venous catheter. Crit Care Med 12:611-613, 1984.

Meland NB, Wilson W, Soontharotoke CY, Koucky CJ. Saphenofemoral venous cutdowns in the premature infant. J Pediatr Surg 21:341-343, 1986.

• Morgan WW, Harkins GA. Percutaneous introduction of long-term indwelling venous catheters in infants. J Pediatr Surg 7:538-541, 1972.

Motte S, Wautrecht JC, Delcour C, Bellens B, Vincent G, Dereume JP. Verbal arteriovenous fistula following central venous cannulation: A case report. J Vasc Dis 37:731-734, 1986.

Mulvihill SJ, Fonkalsrud EW. Complications of superior vs. inferior vena cava occlusion in infants receiving central total parenteral nutrition. J Pediatr Surg 19:752-757, 1984.

Nicolson SC, Sweeney MF, Moore RA, Jobes DR. Comparison of internal and external jugular cannulation of the central circulation in the pediatric patient. Crit Care Med 13:747-749, 1985.

Pegelow CH, Narvaez M, Toledano SR, Davis J, Oiticica C, Buckner D. Experience with a totally implantable venous device in children. Am J Dis Child 149:69-71, 1986.

Pietsch JB, Nagaraj HS, Groff DB. Simplified insertion of central venous catheter in infants. Surg Gynecol Obstet 158:91-92, 1984.

• Prince SR, Sullivan RL, Hackel A. Percutaneous catheterization of the internal jugular vein in infants and children. Anesthesiology 44:170-174, 1976.

Puntis JWL. Percutaneous insertion of central venous feeding catheters. Arch Dis Child 61:1138-1140, 1986.

Quan SF. Mixed venous oxygen. Am Fam Physician 27:211-215, 1983.

• Ramanathan R, Durand M. Blood cultures in neonates with percutaneous central venous catheters. Arch Dis Child 62:621-623, 1987.

• Rao TLK, Wong AY, Salem MR. A new approach to percutaneous catheterization of the internal jugular vein. Anesthesiology 46:362-364, 1977.

Schug CB, Culhane DE, Knopp RK. Subclavian vein catheterization in the emergency department. A comparison of guidewire and nonguidewire techniques. Ann Emerg Med 15:769-773, 1986.

• Seldinger SI. Catheter replacement of the needle in percutaneous arteriography. Acta Radiol 39:368-376, 1953.

Sharkey SW. Beyond the wedge: Clinical physiology and the Swan-Ganz catheter. Am J Med 83:111-122, 1987.

Sherman MP, Vitale DE, McLaughlin GW, Goetzman BW. Percutaneous and surgical placement of fine silicone elastomer central catheters in high-risk newborns. JPEN 7:75-78, 1982.

Shiu MH. A method for conservation of veins in the surgical cutdown. Surg Gynecol Obstet 134:315-316, 1972.

Shulman RJ, Pokorny WJ, Martin CG, Petitt R, Baldaia L, Roney D. Comparison of percutaneous and surgical placement of central venous catheters in neonates. J Pediatr Surg 21:348-350, 1986.

Simon RR, Hoffman JR, Smith M. Modified new approaches for rapid intravenous access. Ann Emerg Med 16:44-49, 1987.

• Smith-Wright DL, Green TP, Lock JE, Egar MI, Fuhrman BP. Complications of vascular catheterization in critically ill children. Crit Care Med 12:1015-1017, 1984.

Snydman DR. Letter to the Editor. Ann Surg 200:101, 1974.

Stark DD, Brasch RC, Gooding CA. Radiographic assessment of venous catheter position in children: Value of the lateral view. Pediatr Radiol 14:76-80, 1984.

Starr DS. Letter to the Editor. Ann Surg 206:683, 1987.

Starr DS, Cornicelli S. EKG-guided placement of subclavian CVP catheters using J-wire. Ann Surg 204:673-676, 1986.

Sterner S, Plummer DW, Clinton J, Ruiz E. A comparison of the supraclavicular approach and the infraclavicular approach for subclavian vein catheterization. Ann Emerg Med 15:421-424, 1986.

Stine MJ, Harris H. Subdural collection of intravenous fat emulsion in a neonate. Clin Pediatr 24:40-41, 1985.

Sullivan CA, Knoefal SH. Cardiac tamponade in a newborn: A complication of hyperalimentation. JPEN 11:319-321, 1987.

Symchych PS, Krauss AN, Winchester P. Endocarditis following intracardiac placement of umbilical venous catheters in neonates. J Pediatr 90:287-289, 1977.

Teplick RS. Measuring central vascular pressures: A surprisingly complex problem. Anesthesiology 67:289-291, 1987.

Tocino IM, Watanabe A. Impending catheter perforation of superior vena cava: Radiographic recognition. Am J Roentgenol 146:487-490, 1986.

Vaksmann G, Rey C, Breviere GM, Smadja D, Dupuis C. Nitroglycerine ointment as aid to venous cannulation in children. J Pediatr 111:89-92, 1987.

Verweij J, Kester A, Stroes W, Thijs LG. Comparison of three methods for measuring central venous pressure. Crit Care Med 14:288-290, 1986.

Wachs T, Watkins S, Hickman RO. "No more pokes": A review of parenteral access devices. Nutr Support Services 7:12-18, 1987.

Warner BW, Gorgone P, Schilling S, Farrell M, Ghory MJ. Multiple purpose central venous access in infants less than 1000 g. J Pediatr Surg 22:820-822, 1987.

Watson AR, Bahoric A, Wesson D. A central venous (W-B-W) catheter for multipurpose vascular access in children. Artif Organs 10:59-61, 1986.

Wechsler RJ, Byrne KJ, Steiner RM. The misplaced thoracic venous catheter detailed anatomical consideration. CRC Crit Rev Diagn Imaging 21:289-305, 1982.

• Woo-Sup A, Joong-Shin K. An easy technique for long-term central venous catheterization and subcutaneous tunneling of the Silastic catheter in neonates and infants. J Pediatr Surg 21:344-347, 1986.

Zenk KE, Dungy CI, Greene GR. Nafcillin extravasation injury. J Dis Child 135:1113-1114, 1981.

115 Arterial Catheters

Luis O. Toro-Figueroa · Kim Yeakel

BACKGROUND

Continuous arterial catheterization was first introduced into pediatric practice in the middle of the 1960s with the use of umbilical artery catheterization in neonates. Peripheral artery catheterization came into use in the early 1970s, providing pediatricians with intra-arterial access for monitoring older children. Both systemic arterial approaches have evolved into safer techniques with increased familiarity and improvements in equipment. Peripheral and umbilical catheterization offer different alternatives in vascular monitoring of the neonate. The clinician must try to individualize his patient's needs and match them with the procedure that offers fewer risks.

PERIPHERAL ARTERY CATHETERIZATION

Arterial cannulation is indicated in critically ill children who may need continuous systemic arterial blood pressure and pulse monitoring and waveform display; frequent determination of arterial blood gas and pH_a, which can be obtained with the patient in a steady-state condition; indocyanine green cardiac output determinations; exchange transfusions; or frequent or large-volume blood sampling (relative indication) for laboratory analysis and/or crossmatching of blood.

Some of the advantages of peripheral arterial cannulation are (1) low incidence of complications, (2) multiplicity of available sites, (3) applicability to any size or age patient, (4) preductal blood sampling, (5) precoarctation systemic arterial blood pressure monitoring, and (6) rapid and easy access (especially with the percutaneous methods).

Peripheral arterial catheters have the following disadvantages: (1) amplification of systolic blood pressure readings the more distal the catheter is placed along the arterial system (i.e., pedal arterial blood pressures have been reported as much as 25.1 ± 12.3 mm Hg greater than radial arterial blood pressures); (2) scarring after catheter removal (especially with cutdowns); (3) unreliability for pressure monitoring in patients with high systemic vascular resistance; and (4) inability to accommodate indwelling electrodes for continuous monitoring of pH_a or Pao_2.

Peripheral artery cannulation of neonates has gained popularity over the past decade. At least three studies demonstrate a lower incidence of major and minor complications in neonates with peripheral arterial catheters, similar to that in older children.

Technique
Access sites

Preferred sites for cannulation in order of preference are radial, posterior tibialis, dorsalis pedis, ulnar, femoral, brachial, axillary, and temporal arteries (Fig. 115-1). Temporal artery catheterization has been associated with middle cerebral artery infarction secondary to retrograde embolization through the carotid artery. Femoral or brachial artery cannulation is discouraged except in extreme situations because of lack of collateral circulation and the large area to which they supply blood.

Although the axillary artery has better collateral circulation, it is more difficult to cannulate. In addition, since there is little experience or published data in pediatric patients supporting its safety, we use this site infrequently.

Equipment

Equipment needed for both percutaneous and cutdown arterial catheterization is as follows:

Percutaneous arterial catheterization equipment

Adhesive tape, ½ and 1 inch
Appropriate size catheter
    Adolescent to adult, 18-20 gauge
    School-age children, 20-22 gauge
    Toddlers to infants, 22 gauge
    Premature infants, 24 gauge
Armboard
Benzoin sticks
Iodine solution and ointment
Continuous flush device, 3 ml/hr
Gloves (universal precautions)
Heparin, 1000 U/ml; add 1 U/ml of arterial line fluid
Lidocaine, 1%
Monitor with pressure module

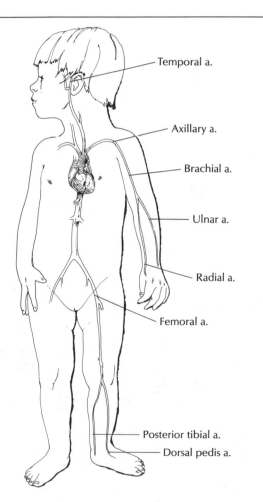

Fig. 115-1   Arterial sites.

Papaverine, 60 mg/ml; add 60 mg/500 ml of arterial
    line fluid
Protective goggles (universal precautions)
Pressure infuser (inflate to 300 mm Hg)
Pressure transducer
0.225%, 0.45%, and 0.9% sodium chloride solution, 500
    ml
Suture, 4-0 nylon or silk, with straight-cutting needle
Syringes
    3 ml syringe with ⅜-inch, 25-gauge needle
    10 ml syringe
T-connector

Arterial cutdown catheterization equipment

Sterile surgical gown and gloves
Surgical mask
Surgical procedure lamp
Vascular access tray (see below)
Other equipment (see above)

Vascular access tray (sterile)*

Syringe with a 20-gauge needle for flush solution, 10
    ml
Clear dermal tape
Draping towels
Five 4 × 4 inch gauze sponges
Four-inch curved eye-dressing forceps
Four-inch straight eye-dressing forceps
Needle holder
Scalpel blades, Nos. 11 and 15
Scalpel handle
Smooth forceps
Small scissors
Suture on needle, 4-0 silk or nylon
Toothed forceps
Two 5-inch curved mosquito hemostats
Umbilical tape

Insertion

A modified Allen test must be performed before placing an arterial catheter in the radial, ulnar, pedal, or
tibial arteries. In the upper extremity the modified
Allen test consists of having the patient clench and
compress his hand and then occluding his ulnar and
radial arteries. Release the ulnar artery; if the hand
flushes in less than 5 seconds, the flow is adequate
from the ulnar collaterals. The test must be repeated
to assess the radial circulation.

---

*Items needed for skin infiltration and solution withdrawing may
be added aseptically to the tray by the assistant.

Before cannulating the artery, place the patient's hand, wrist, and distal third of forearm in a supine position on an armboard of a size appropriate for the patient's age. Use 4 × 4 inch gauze pads under the wrist and proceed to secure the extremity with adhesive tape while maintaining the wrist in an extension angle of 30 degrees. Care must be taken to leave the fingertips free for visual inspection. Apply tape securely but gently to prevent pressure sores or occlusion of collateral circulation and venous drainage. To immobilize the ankle place a well-padded board on the external aspect of the extremity, placing the ankle in an anatomic position. Extra padding may be added to prevent pressure sores around the external maleolus. The toes must always be visible for further inspection. The only other area that may need immobilization is the elbow on the rare occasion when brachial artery catheterization is performed in infants and children. For this purpose the elbow must be immobilized in an anatomic position.

Sterile technique must be maintained at all times. The site must be surgically cleansed three times with an iodine solution for 3 minutes. The iodine must be dry before proceeding to obtain maximum bactericidal effect.

With a small-gauge needle infiltrate the skin and deep tissue with lidocaine. Take care not to infuse lidocaine directly into a vessel (aspirate for blood before injecting the lidocaine). Infiltration must be gentle and the quantity sufficient to produce local analgesia but not so much as to impede palpation of the arterial pulse. After 5 minutes test for local analgesia before proceeding. Before attempting cannulation, ensure that all necessary equipment is readily available and the tubing and catheters are flushed with solution.

Cannulation of a peripheral artery may be performed via percutaneous catheterization or cutdown insertion.

Percutaneous technique. The two preferred methods of percutaneous peripheral artery catheter insertion are direct and transfixation (Fig. 115-2). The direct method is similar to the technique used to start a peripheral IV catheter. Palpate for the arterial pulse; then approach the area with the catheter at a 30-degree angle, penetrating the anterior wall of the artery. When blood flushes back into the catheter, advance the catheter.

In the transfixation method approach the artery at a 45-degree angle and penetrate both walls. After achieving transfixation remove the catheter's inner needle and pull the catheter back slowly until blood returns into the catheter reservoir. When blood return is observed, advance the catheter into the vessel.

Connect a T-connector and a 10 ml syringe with flush solution free of air bubbles to the catheter to prevent unnecessary blood loss and to test for patency. Patency can be documented by the free flow of blood into the syringe and by observing the arterial waveform once the catheter and tubing are connected to the transducer-monitor system (Fig. 115-3).

The catheter must be sutured to the skin and further secured using tincture of benzoin and adhesive tape. Apply two ½-inch adhesive tape strips in butterfly fashion and cover them with a short strip of 1-inch adhesive tape. Take care to leave the skin insertion site visible for inspection. A small amount of iodine ointment may be applied to the skin insertion site. A small self-adhesive bandage may be used to dress the skin insertion site area since it is easily removable and therefore permits frequent examination of the skin site (Fig. 115-4).

Cutdown technique. The radial artery cutdown method is the only one discussed in detail in this section. The technique for cutdown of other sites is similar with the exception of the anatomic landmarks.

First, identify the anatomic landmarks. The radial artery is medial to the brachioradialis tendon and proximal to the lower radial epiphysis on the volar side of the wrist. Palpation is best achieved proximal to the palmar branch. The flexor carpi radialis tendon lies medial to the radial artery followed by the median nerve on the palmaris longus tendon as one moves more medially (Fig. 115-5).

Drape the surgical site and set up the necessary equipment (i.e., mount scalpel blade, draw flush solution, prime the T-connector). Cut a cardboard wedge with a base of approximately 1 cm from the cardboard that holds the suture material to use later during the procedure. Recheck the skin site for local analgesia.

Make a 1 cm incision transverse to the artery's path. Use a single stroke to expose the subcutaneous tissue. With both mosquito hemostats gently dissect parallel to the vessel using a blunt technique. Do not tear or cut any tissue within the operative site. Identify the structures using the aforementioned landmarks. In general arteries are round, pulsating, elastic, and bright red (except in hypoxic patients). Veins are flat,

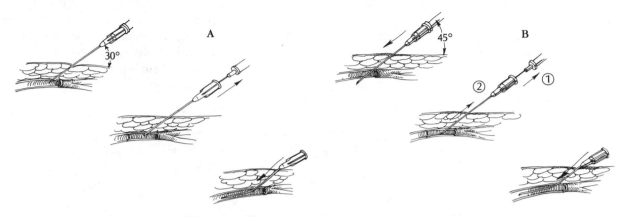

Fig. 115-2   Percutaneous techniques. **A**, Direct. **B**, Transfixation.

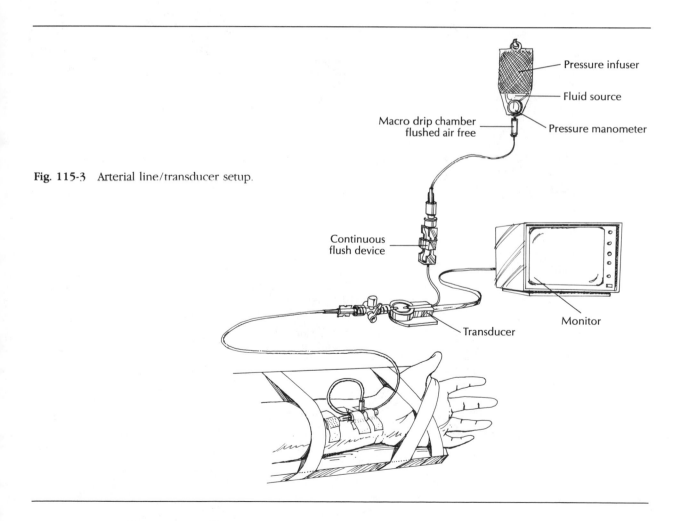

Fig. 115-3   Arterial line/transducer setup.

very pliable, and darker than arteries. Nerves are flat, pale, and stringlike. Tendons are white, round, and ropelike. Muscle tends to be beefy and friable. Finally, bone tends to be solid and white.

After identifying the artery elevate it gently using a curved hemostat. Place a 4-0 stay suture (6 cm long) distally and another proximally. *Do not* tie the vessel. Place a hemostat holding the ends of each stay suture together (Fig. 115-6, *A*). Proceed gently to remove from the vessel all connective tissue that may lead to

"false channeling" when inserting the catheter. The best way to accomplish this is to stretch the artery carefully by opening the forceps in an alternating fashion from the underside of the vessel. Do not attempt to pick, pull, or cut any tissue off the artery since doing so may lead to arterial rupture (Fig. 115-6, *B* and *C*).

After removing all undesired tissue pull on the distal stay suture and slip the cardboard wedge under the vessel (Fig. 115-6, *D*). Exert gentle traction on the

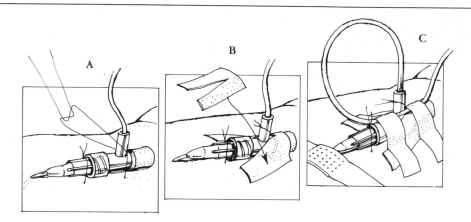

Fig. 115-4 **A,** Suture-secured arterial line. **B,** Adhesive tape–secured arterial line. **C,** Self-adhesive small bandage protecting the insertion site.

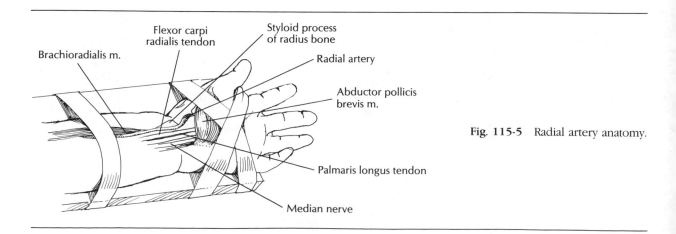

Fig. 115-5 Radial artery anatomy.

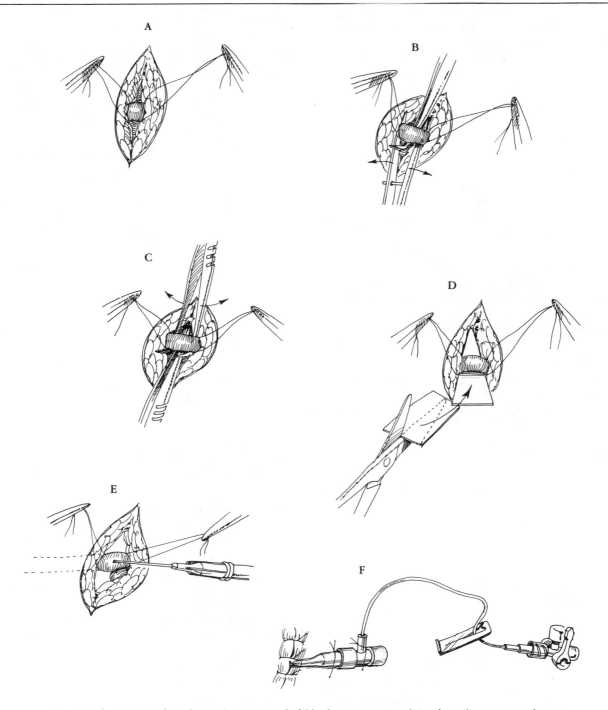

Fig. 115-6 A, Arterial cutdown. Stay sutures held by hemostats. **B** and **C,** Blunt dissection with eye-dressing forceps. **D,** Cardboard wedge in position. **E,** Pulling on the stay suture and advancing the catheter. **F,** Closing of surgical wound and securing of arterial catheter.

distal stay suture, and cannulate the vessel using the same direct technique described in the percutaneous insertion method (Fig. 115-6, *E*).

Advance the catheter slowly, thus decreasing the likelihood of vasospasm. Attach the flushed T-connector and syringe and check for patency in a fashion similar to that used in the percutaneous technique. Do not connect the T-connector to the transducer until the surgical wound is sutured and the catheter is secured in place since doing so may lead to decannulation if the tubing is accidentally pulled.

Close the surgical wound with single stitches and suture the catheter hub securely to skin as well as the T-connector (Fig. 115-6, *F*), thus giving the unit more stability. Clean the wound of blood with 0.9% sodium chloride solution and/or iodine solution. Apply adhesive tape in a fashion similar to that used in the percutaneous technique. Wound and dressing care is also similar to that of percutaneous catheters. Finally, secure the stay sutures by taping them to the skin both distal and proximal to the incision. If bleeding occurs around the catheter, pull the stay sutures gently to enhance hemostasis. The stay sutures must never be tied around the catheter. After 24 hours or when a bleeding diathesis has been corrected, the sutures may be removed by pulling them out through the wound.

Pressure waveform

A continuous pressure waveform tracing must be displayed on the monitor screen at all times, and ideally a printout of the waveform with a simultaneous ECG tracing is available. An arterial waveform consists of a systolic phase, a dicrotic notch, and a diastolic phase. There are some differences between peripheral and aortic artery pressure waveforms. The aortic waveform tends to be flatter and have a more marked dicrotic notch (Fig. 115-7). The dicrotic notch of an arterial waveform coincides with ECG T waves, which represent ventricular repolarization.

Arterial waveforms also may be helpful in diagnosing the severity of cardiac dysrhythmias since the waveform will vary when the cardiac output is altered by the dysrhythmia. Pulsus alternans, caused by diminished ventricular performance, and pulsus paradoxus, caused by high intrapleural pressure, can be noted in the continual waveform tracing. In the spontaneously breathing patient with pulsus paradoxus the arterial pressure tracing will decrease during inspiration and will rise during expiration. In the me-

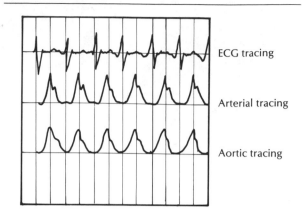

Fig. 115-7 Pressure waveform: aortic vs. peripheral artery.

chanically ventilated patient with pulsus paradoxus the arterial pressure tracing will increase during inspiration and will decrease during expiration. Hypovolemia may be diagnosed by a very narrow waveform or by the evidence of respiratory cycle–associated waveform arterial depression.

Maintenance

To obtain blood for sampling from the peripheral arterial catheter, clamp the fluid source at the T-connector. Clean the injection site with iodine and let it dry before inserting a 25-gauge needle. After inserting the needle let five drops of fluid and blood drip onto a gauze pad to displace heparinized fluid from the catheter and T-connector. Attach a 1 or 3 ml syringe and draw the desired amount of blood. The use of a larger syringe can cause arterial spasm. After drawing blood unclamp the T-connector; the volume of pressurized fluid that accumulated during the time the connector was clamped will be enough to flush the catheter adequately. If the catheter is on an infusion pump (recommended when infusion rates <3 ml/hr are needed) or fails to clear with the back-pressure, gently flush the system with 1 to 2 ml of heparinized fluid. *Do not* use the continuous flow device to flush the catheter, for it delivers large amounts of fluid rapidly. In addition the flow generated by this device when released will cause arterial retrograde flow, which can reach the arch vessels and possibly cause CNS embolization or an acute increase of ICP (see Fig. 108-5). Once the T-connector is unclamped, observe the monitor for the return of the arterial waveform.

No fluids other than 0.225%, 0.45%, or 0.9% sodium chloride solution may be infused through an arterial line. No medications except heparin (1 to 5 units/ml) and papaverine (60 mg/500 ml) may be infused through any arterial catheter. Heparin may prevent clot formation, and papaverine may prevent arterial spasm. Papaverine is contraindicated in patients with ICP precautions since it will cause cerebral vessels to dilate, increasing cerebral blood flow and worsening ICP. Heparin may not be infused in those patients with severe bleeding diathesis or in anhepatic patients.

Tubing and fluids must be changed every 24 hours, and the catheter insertion site must be inspected daily. If any signs of cellulitis are present, the catheter must be removed and the catheter tip and blood cultured. A wound culture is also indicated in the case of inflammation at the cutdown site. The area distal and proximal to the catheterization must be inspected for blanching, redness, cyanosis, and changes in temperature and/or capillary refill time. In febrile patients blood must be obtained for culture from the arterial catheter and at a peripheral site to help to distinguish bacteremia or sepsis from catheter colonization (see Chapter 114).

Catheter removal

The indications for catheter removal are the following: (1) stabilization or resolution of the indications for cannulation of the artery; (2) catheter-related infection (local or systemic) or colonization by microorganisms; (3) evidence of clot formation (i.e., dampened tracing or sluggish blood flow; and (4) any evidence of thrombosis or mechanical occlusion of the artery (i.e., edema, discoloration, cold extremity).

To remove a peripheral arterial catheter cut the securing stitch, pull the catheter gently, and hold pressure on the area for 5 to 10 minutes. The fluid source need not be clamped before removal of the catheter, hopefully preventing the formation of clots within the arterial circulation. In patients with bleeding disorders correcting the deficiencies and applying pressure hemostasis for longer periods may be necessary.

Risks and Complications

The reported incidence of complications from peripheral artery catheterization varies from 0.3% to 51%.

Complications of peripheral arterial catheterization

Arteriovenous fistula formation
Arterial-intimal flaps
Arteriospasm
Arteritis
Bacteremia or sepsis
Bleeding
Cellulitis
Cerebrovascular accidents (especially with use of temporal site)
Colonization with a microorganism
Electrocution
Embolization
Hematoma
Necrosis of an extremity
Peripheral nerve damage
Skin sloughing (ischemia)
Thrombosis

The most commonly reported complication is arterial thrombosis. Factors that increase the incidence of thrombosis are low cardiac output states, lack of use of heparin, lack of use of the continuous flush method, small wrist circumference, length of catheterization (>4 to 7 days), lack of collateral circulation (modified Allen's test >5 seconds), longer catheter diameter relative to arterial diameter, tapered catheters, lack of experience with the procedure, size of hematoma before insertion, and age of patient (<5 years). Arterial recanalization has been reported in up to 100% of occluded radial arteries up to 75 days after decannulation. If thrombosis is suspected, the catheter must be removed and the extremity checked hourly for pulses, warmth, and discoloration. Application of heat to the opposite extremity may cause reflex vasodilation and increase flow through an incomplete obstruction. Thrombolytic therapy with streptokinase or urokinase (see Chapter 149) and early consultation with a vascular surgeon should be considered.

There are at least three reports of cerebral thromboembolic events related to the use of temporal artery catheterization. Retrograde embolization through the carotid artery is thought to play a role as the mechanism of injury. The use of temporal arterial catheters is discouraged for this reason.

Infection-related complications have been reported at a rate ranging from 1.27% to 25%. One study reported a colonization rate of 18% and a 4% incidence of septicemia. Factors associated with increased risk of infection were insertion by surgical cutdown, cannulation longer than 4 days, and presence of local inflammation. Another study reported a colonization rate of 25%, with an incidence of septicemia of only 0.6% in pediatric patients. When catheter-related infection is suspected, cultures must be obtained as outlined in Chapter 114, use of the arterial catheter must be discontinued, and broad-spectrum antibiotics must be administered for both gram-negative and gram-positive (*Staphylococcus epidermidis* included) organisms. Antifungal therapy must be used when fungal disease is suspected clinically.

Bleeding at the site of insertion is another common complication. When bleeding occurs, one must make certain that all tubing connectors are tightly sealed and that there are no cracks or defective materials. Interlocking tubing connectors are available, and their use decreases the potential for bleeding secondary to loose tubing connections. Bleeding abnormalities must be corrrected if possible. Applying local pressure for a limited time can help achieve hemostasis and prevent excessive blood loss. The distal extremity must be carefully inspected during the application of local pressure to prevent too great a pressure resulting in tissue ischemia. Circular bandages are not recommended since they may lead to ischemia. When an arterial cutdown is bleeding, the stay sutures may be pulled gently to achieve hemostasis. *Do not* tie these sutures. If bleeding persists, use of the catheter may have to be discontinued.

Vascular spasm is another complication that may lead to the discontinuation of use of an arterial catheter and even to tissue necrosis. Papaverine may be used as a continuous infusion, as previously described, to prevent vasospasm. Diluted lidocaine, 0.1 ml of 1% lidocaine in 0.9 ml of 0.9% sodium chloride solution, infused slowly may dilate the constricted artery. Warming the opposite extremity may also be helpful. If arteriospasm does not resolve, the arterial catheter must be removed.

In patients with pacemakers the display of the arterial waveform is paramount to monitoring cardiac function since an ECG tracing or the pacemaker artifact will continue to appear in the monitor screen and can be counted as heart rate by the electronic sensing device without any corresponding cardiac output being generated. An asystolic patient will not have a low heart rate alarm initiated in these circumstances. A decrease in pressure or a flat-line waveform may be the first sign of trouble since the heart rate will be fixed at the preset pacing rate.

Pressure waveform changes will also alert the health care team to mechanical problems with the system. Underdamping may be caused by an inappropriately sensitive monitor or transducer, high-compliance tubing, air bubbles in the system, tube kinking, lipid deposition in the transducer dome, clot formation, tubing being too long (>7 feet), compliant injection sites (T-connectors), leakage (e.g., in tubing, connections, stopcocks, injection sites), or vasospasm. Overdamping may occur when the monitor-transducer system is too sensitive or there is a faulty flush device and/or air bubbles within the system. When a waveform is underdamped, one must make certain the patient is stable first and that a change in hemodynamic status is not responsible for the waveform change. Another patient-related event that may cause waveform underdamping and is life threatening is exsanguination from leakage or disconnection of the arterial catheter system. The whole system must be readily visible and the waveform constantly displayed to prevent a leak in the system from resulting in a fatal hemorrhage.

The use of very small catheters in and of itself does not account for overdamping since significant differences have not been found in pressures recorded using 22- and 24-gauge catheters.

UMBILICAL ARTERY CATHETERIZATION

Arterial cannulation is indicated in critically ill neonates who may need continuous systemic arterial blood pressure and pulse monitoring and waveform display; frequent determination of arterial blood gases and pH_a, which can be obtained with the patient in steady-state condition; continuous Pao_2 and pH_a determinations through indwelling electrodes; exchange transfusions; or frequent or large-volume blood sampling (relative indication) for laboratory analysis and/or crossmatching of blood.

The advantages of umbilical artery catheters are rapid and easy access, less skill needed to perform than a peripheral arterial cutdown; the insertion of larger sized catheters, making the use of indwelling electrodes possible; decreased scarring after the removal of the catheter; and the ability to monitor aortic pressure, which in certain cases (i.e., high peripheral vascular resistance) may be more indicative of organ perfusion pressures than those pressure measurements obtained from a peripheral arterial catheter under similar circumstances.

The disadvantages of umbilical artery catheters include a higher incidence of minor and serious complications when compared with peripheral arterial catheters (see "Risks and Complications"); a postductal sampling site, which may lead to erroneous interpretation of arterial blood gas values in some neonates; the potential for inappropriate treatment of hypotension in a patient with coarctation of the aorta; and an inaccessible route after approximately 10 days of life.

Technique
Access sites

The umbilical cord usually contains two small, round, thin-walled arteries located caudally. The umbilical vein is usually larger, flat, and located centrally or cephalad. Cords with single arteries are more difficult to cannulate.

Equipment

Equipment necessary for these techniques is listed below.

Umbilical artery catheterization equipment

Blunt needle, 18 gauge
Catheters (polyvinylchloride with single end hole)
    No. 5 F for infants >1500 g body weight
    No. 3.5 F for infants <1500 g body weight
Continuous flush device, 30 ml/hr
Continuous infusion pump
IV fluid; add sodium heparin (1 U/ml)
Low compliance pressure tubing, 4 feet long
Monitor with pressure module
Pressure transducer setup
Pressure transducer dome
Sterile measuring tape
Sterile surgical gown and gloves
Surgical mask, goggles, and cap
Surgical procedure lamp
Three-way interlocking stopcock (three)
Vascular access tray (see p. 819)

Insertion

An indwelling umbilical artery catheter may be placed by either of two methods: direct placement or cutdown. Strict sterile technique must be used. Although no local analgesia is needed for direct umbilical catheterization, for the cutdown method of anesthetic infiltration technique similar to that for the

peripheral artery cutdown method must be used. The infant must be monitored throughout the whole procedure, ideally with a cardiorespiratory monitor and pulse oximeter.

Direct technique. Set up the equipment and flush all tubing and the catheter. Immobilize the infant with arm and leg restraints and clean the umbilical site as previously described for peripheral artery catheterization. Tie an umbilical tape loosely at the base of the cord without including skin. The tape may be tightened if bleeding occurs.

Measure the distance between the umbilicus and the acromioclavicular junction. Sixty-five percent of this measurement plus the length of the umbilical stump should be the distance from the insertion site to the third or fourth lumbar vertebra. Mark this distance on the catheter with the sterile transparent dermal tape in a butterfly fashion.

Place a curved hemostat at the distal end of the stump, pull gently, and turn the stump cephalad over the instrument (Fig. 115-8, *A*). With the scalpel blade, slowly cut the cord superficially 2 cm above skin level. Advance toward the center of the cord gently until an artery is partially transected. Ideally no more than half the artery's circumference must be cut.

Dilate the artery with the curved eye-dressing forceps. The curved forceps allows better control and visualization. Dilation must be gentle and progressive to minimize arterial rupture or spasm.

After flushing the catheter free of air and all bubbles insert it into the artery using the pincer or an eye-dressing forceps to grasp it (Fig. 115-8, *B* and *C*). Advance the catheter in a smooth fashion using gentle pressure to overcome the resistance met when passing from the hypogastric artery to the femoral artery (Fig. 115-8, *D*). Confirm placement by aspirating blood and observing the waveform when connected to the transducer-monitor system. Secure the catheter by placing sutures from the butterfly tape to the umbilical skin. An H-type tape bridge is recommended to secure the catheter to the abdominal wall as an extra safety measure (Fig. 11-8, *E* and *F*).

Finally, the catheter tip position must be confirmed. An anteroposterior abdominal roentgenogram will show the catheter tip at the level of the third or fourth vertebra (Fig. 115-9).

Cutdown technique. Equipment setup, infant immobilization, skin preparation, and umbilical tie can be done as in the direct technique. Catheter length

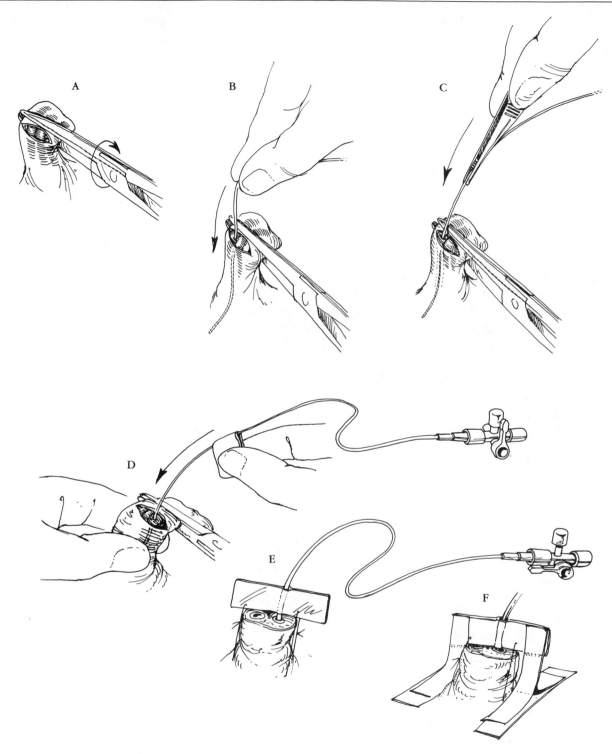

Fig. 115-8 Umbilical artery placement. **A,** Umbilical artery catheterization. Pulling stump gently and turning it cephalad over hemostat. **B,** Introducing and advancing catheter. **C-F,** Inserting and securing catheter.

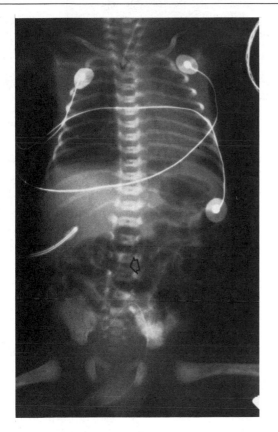

Fig. 115-9 Proper position of umbilical artery catheter as seen on thoracoabdominal roentgenogram.

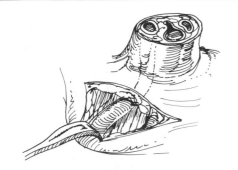

Fig. 115-10 Umbilical artery cutdown.

is determined in a fashion similar to the direct method with the exception of eliminating the stump distance.

A 1 cm skin incision is made 1 to 2 mm below the umbilicus. The fascia is identified, and a transverse incision is made to either side of the midline, medial to the rectus muscle (Fig. 115-10). The artery must be distinguished from the urachus; the urachus will widen into the dome of the bladder by pulling the suspected structure superiorly. In addition the umbilical artery may have pulsations.

After the artery is identified it can be isolated with stay sutures in a fashion similar to that used for a peripheral arterial cutdown. A cardboard wedge under the artery may be helpful with immobilization, arteriotomy, and cannulation. Cannulation and confirmation can be done as in the direct technique. The surgical wound may be closed and dressed as stated in the peripheral cutdown method. The catheter must be secured as mentioned previously.

Pressure waveform

See the section "Pressure Waveform" for peripheral artery catheterization.

Maintenance

To draw blood from the umbilical arterial catheter, attach a 1 ml syringe to the stopcock and turn the stopcock off to the fluid source (Fig. 115-11). Gently aspirate 0.5 to 1.0 ml of fluid (depending on the length of catheter to stopcock) to clear the catheter of the heparinized fluid and turn the stopcock off to all ports (quarter turn). Remove the syringe and attach the sampling syringe. Turn the stopcock off to the fluid source and aspirate the desired amount of blood. After drawing the blood turn the stopcock a quarter of a turn, remove the sampling syringe, and attach a syringe with flush solution. Flush the catheter with 1 to 2 ml of heparinized saline solution, turn the stopcock off to the sampling port, remove the flush syringe, and place a sterile injection cap on the sampling port. Observe the monitor for the return of the arterial waveform. With small infants it is necessary to monitor closely the amount of discarded blood as blood loss. If it is necessary to return blood to the infant, it must be given only through a venous catheter.

D_5W or $D_{10}W$ solution, in addition to sodium chloride solutions, may be infused through umbilical artery catheters. No medications except for heparin may be infused through an umbilical artery catheter. A small amount of heparin (1 to 5 units/ml) may help prevent clot formation, although heparin may not be infused in those patients with a severe bleeding diathesis or in anhepatic patients.

Tubing and fluid changes and catheter insertion site inspection must be done following the same guidelines as for peripheral arterial catheters. If any signs of cellulitis are present, the catheter must be removed and the catheter tip and blood cultured. An

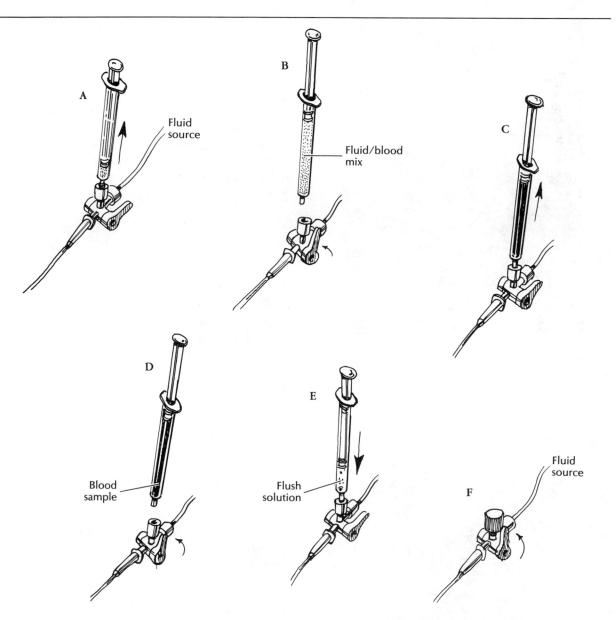

Fig. 115-11 Umbilical artery catheter. Blood sampling. **A,** Stopcock off to fluid source. **B,** Stopcock off to all ports. **C,** Drawing sample. **D,** Stopcock off to all ports; remove sample syringe. **E,** Flush catheter. **F,** Stopcock off to sampling port.

umbilical stump culture is also indicated for a patient with cellulitis at the umbilical site. The lower extremities must be inspected for blanching, redness, cyanosis, and changes in temperature and/or capillary refill time. In febrile patients blood must be drawn for culture from the arterial catheter as well as at a peripheral site to help to distinguish bacteremia or sepsis from colonization.

Catheter removal

The umbilical artery catheter must be removed over a 20- to 30-minute period to allow the umbilical artery to constrict to prevent free bleeding on removal of the catheter. All catheters must be inspected for thrombus formation and for integrity on removal.

Risks and Complications

The reported incidence of complications from umbilical artery catheterization ranges from 8.6% to 95%.

Complications of umbilical artery catheterization

Bleeding
Cellulitis
Congestive heart failure (secondary to aortic thrombosis)
Electrocution
Embolization
False abdominal aortic aneurysm
Infectious arthritis
Ischemia to intra-abdominal organs (secondary to thrombosis and/or embolism)
Lower extremity ischemia
Necrotizing enterocolitis
Osteomyelitis
Pelvic exsanguination
Refractory hypoglycemia
Sepsis or bacteremia
Thrombosis
Vascular perforation

Thrombus formation is the most common and probably the least diagnosed complication. It may occur in as many as 95% of patients when thrombus formation is diagnosed by aortography in infants with umbilical artery catheters. The incidence of clinically significant thrombosis formation secondary to use of umbilical artery catheters is 3.3% to 6%. As in patients with peripheral arterial catheters, these thrombi reabsorb with time, or there may be pericatheter fibrin formation. The concern is that when an organ distal to the occlusion is affected, the outcome is usually dismal since there is no collateral circulation to abdominal aorta. Reported complications include the loss of an extremity, transverse myelitis, renovascular hypertension (renal artery thrombus), intestinal necrosis, gluteal muscle necrosis, and skin necrosis. Whenever thrombus formation is suspected, use of the umbilical catheter must be discontinued. Abdominal ultrasonography, CT, or aortography as well as early medical treatment with streptokinase or urokinase can be considered, and early consultation with a vascular surgeon is encouraged.

The incidence of umbilical artery catheter colonization has been reported to be as high as 62%. The incidence of septicemia is similar to that for peripheral arterial catheters, 2.6% in one series. Colonized or infected umbilical arterial catheters must be managed in a similar fashion to peripheral arterial catheters.

Bleeding around the catheter can be successfully stopped by gently tightening the umbilical tape around the stump. Once the bleeding has stopped, do not leave the tape tied permanently since doing so may lead to tissue necrosis. Bleeding from faulty or untightened tubing or connectors can be managed in a fashion similar to that for peripheral arterial catheters.

Administration of any medication, including antibiotics, and direct mechanical trauma secondary to catheter insertion may lead to arterial intimal damage. Any of these causes may lead to internal flap formation, which in time serves as a site for thrombus formation.

Spasm of the iliac artery may be stopped by warming the opposite extremity when the spasm is unilateral. If blanching persists, use of the catheter must be discontinued.

ADDITIONAL READING

Abramowsky CR, Chrenka B, Fanaroff A. Wharton jelly embolism: An unusual complication of umbilical catheterization. J Pediatr 96:739-741, 1980.

Adams JM, Speer ME, Rudolph AJ. Bacterial colonization of radial artery catheters. Pediatrics 65:94-97, 1980.

Anagnostakis D, Kamba A, Petrochilou V, Arseni A, Matsaniotis N. Risk of infection associated with umbilical vein catheterization. J Pediatr 86:759-765, 1975.

Bedford RF. Wrist circumference predicts the risk of radial-arterial occlusion after cannulation. Am Soc Anesthesiol 48:377-378, 1978.

• Bedford RF, Wallman H. Complications of percutaneous radial-artery cannulation: An objective prospective study in man. Anesthesiology 38:228-236, 1973.

Boros SJ, Nystrom JF, Thompson TR, Reynolds JW, Williams HJ. Leg growth following umbilical artery catheter–associated thrombus formation: A 4-year follow-up. J Pediatr 87:973-976, 1975.

• Briassoulis G. Arterial pressure measurement in preterm infants. Crit Care Med 14:735-738, 1986.

Bull MJ, Schreiner RL, Garg BP, Hutton NM, Lemons JA, Gresham EL. Neurologic complications following temporal artery catheterization. J Pediatr 96:1071-1073, 1980.

• Butt W, Whyte H. Blood pressure monitoring in neonates: Comparison of umbilical and peripheral artery catheter measurements. J Pediatr 105:630-632, 1984.

Butt W, Shann F, McDonnell G, Hudson I. Effect of heparin concentration and infusion rate on the patency of arterial catheters. Crit Care Med 15:230-232, 1987.

• Caeton AJ, Goetzman BW. Risky business: Umbilical arterial catheterization. Am J Dis Child 139:120-121, 1985.

Casalino MB, Lipsitz PJ. Contamination of umbilical catheters. J Pediatr 78:1077, 1971.

• Cochran WD, Davis HT, Smith CA. Advantages and complications of umbilical artery catheterization in the newborn. Pediatrics 42:769-777, 1968.

Cohen A, Reyes R, Kirk M, Fulks RM. Osler's nodes, pseudoaneurysm formation, and sepsis complicating percutaneous radial artery cannulation. Crit Care Med 12:1078-1079, 1984.

• Cole FS, Todres ID, Shannon DC. Technique for percutaneous cannulation of the radial artery in the newborn infant. J Pediatr 92:105-107, 1978.

• Downs JB, Chapman RL, Hawkins IF. Prolonged radial-artery catheterization. Arch Surg 108:671-673, 1974.

Downs JB, Rackstein AD, Klein EF, Hawkins IF. Hazards of radial-artery catheterization. Anesthesiology 38:283-286, 1973.

• Fiser DH, Graves SA, van der AA J. Catheters for arterial pressure monitoring in pediatrics. Crit Care Med 13:580-583, 1985.

Gardner RM. Direct blood pressure measurement–dynamic response requirements. Anesthesiology 54:227-236, 1981.

Gardner RM, Schwartz R, Wong HC, Burke JP. Percutaneous indwelling radial-artery catheters for monitoring cardiovascular function. N Engl J Med 290:1227-1231, 1974.

• Gupta JM, Robertson NRC, Wigglesworth JS. Umbilical artery catheterization in the newborn. Arch Dis Child 43:382-387, 1968.

• Harris MS. Umbilical artery catheters: High, low, or no. J Perinat Med 6:15-21, 1978.

Hecker JF. Thrombogenicity of tips of umbilical catheters. Pediatrics 67:467-471, 1981.

• Henry CG, Gutierrez F, Lee JT, Hartmann AF, Bell MJ, Bower RJ, Strauss AW. Aortic thrombosis presenting as congestive heart failure: An umbilical artery catheter complication. J Pediatr 98:820-822, 1981.

Johnson FE, Sumner DS, Strandness DE. Extremity necrosis caused by indwelling arterial catheters. Am J Surg 131:375-379, 1976.

• Johnstone RE, Greenhow DE. Catheterization of the dorsalis pedis artery. Anesthesiology 39:654-655, 1973.

Kaye W. Invasive monitoring techniques: Arterial cannulation, bedside pulmonary artery catheterization, and arterial puncture. Heart Lung 12:395-427, 1983.

Kirkpatrick DMBV, Kodroff M, Ehrlich FE, Salzberg AM. Pelvic exsanguination following umbilical artery catheterization in neonates. J Pediatr Surg 14:264-269, 1979.

Krauss AN, Albert RF, Kannan MM. Contamination of umbilical catheters in the newborn infant. J Pediatr 77:965-969, 1970.

Lehmiller DJ, Kanto WP. Relationships of mesenteric thromboembolism, oral feeding, and necrotizing enterocolitis. J Pediatr 92:96-100, 1978.

Lim MO, Gresham EL, Franken EA, Leake RD. Osteomyelitis as a complication of umbilical artery catheterization. Am J Dis Child 131:142-144, 1977.

Lowenstein E, Little JW, Lo HH. Prevention of cerebral embolization from flushing radial-artery cannulas. N Engl J Med 285:1414-1415, 1971.

Malloy MH, Nichols MM. False abdominal aortic aneurysm: An unusual complication of umbilical arterial catheterization for exchange transfusion. J Pediatr 90:285-286, 1977.

Marsh JL, King W, Barrett C, Fonkalsrud EW. Serious complications after umbilical artery catheterization for neonatal monitoring. Arch Surg 110:1203-1208, 1975.

Mathieu A, Dalton B, Fischer JF, Kumar A. Expanding aneurysm of the radial artery after frequent puncture. Anesthesiology 38:401-403, 1973.

Mayer T, Matlak ME, Thompson JA. Necrosis of the forearm following radial artery catheterization in a patient with Reye's syndrome. Pediatrics 65:141-143, 1980.

McGregor M. Pulsus paradoxus. N Engl J Med 301:480-482, 1979.

Miyasaka K, Edmonds JF, Conn AW. Complications of radial artery lines in the paediatric patient. Can Anaesth Soc J 23:9-14, 1976.

Morris T, Bouhoutsos J. The dangers of femoral artery puncture and catheterization. Am Heart J 89:260-261, 1975.

Mozersky DJ, Buckley CJ, Hagood CO, Capps WF, Dannemiller FJ. Ultrasonic evaluation of the palmar circulation: A useful adjunct to radial artery cannulation. Am J Surg 126:810-812, 1973.

Nagel JW, Sims JS, Aplin CE, Westmark ER. Refractory hypoglycemia associated with a malpositioned umbilical artery catheter. Pediatrics 64:315-317, 1979.

Pape KE, Armstrong DL, Fitzhardinge PM. Peripheral median nerve damage secondary to brachial arterial blood gas sampling. J Pediatr 93:852-856, 1978.

Park MK, Robotham JI, German VF. Systolic pressure amplification in pedal arteries in children. Crit Care Med 11:286-289, 1983.

Peter G, Lloyd-Still JD, Lovejoy FH. Local infection and bacteremia from scalp vein needles and polyethylene catheters in children. J Pediatr 80:78-83, 1972.

Prian GW, Wright GB, Rumack CM, O'Meara OP. Apparent cerebral embolization after temporal artery catheterization. J Pediatr 93:115-118, 1978.

Rajani K, Goetzman BW, Wennberg RP, Turner E, Abildgaard C. Effect of heparinization of fluids infused through an umbilical artery catheter on catheter patency and frequency of complications. Pediatrics 63:552-556, 1979.

• Randel SN, Tsang BHL, Wung JT, Driscoll JM, James LS. Experience with percutaneous indwelling peripheral arterial catheterization in neonates. Am J Dis Child 141:848-851, 1987.

Ryan JF, Raines J, Dalton BC, Mathieu A. Arterial dynamics of radial artery cannulation. Anesth Analg 52:1017-1025, 1973.

• Sellden H, Nilsson K, Larsson LE, Ekstrom-Jodal B. Radial arterial catheters in children and neonates: A prospective study. Crit Care Med 15:1106-1109, 1987.

Shapiro GG, Krovetz LJ. Damped and undamped frequency responses of underdamped catheter manometer systems. Am Heart J 80:226-236, 1970.

Shinozaki T, Deane RS, Mazuzan JE. The dynamic responses of liquid-filled catheter systems for direct measurement of blood pressure. Anesthesiology 53:498-504, 1980.

• Spahr RC, MacDonald HM, Holzman IR. Catheterization of the posterior tibial artery in the neonate. Am J Dis Child 133:945-946, 1979.

• Todres ID, Rogers MC, Shannon DC, Moylan FMB, Ryan JF. Percutaneous catheterization of the radial artery in the critically ill neonate. J Pediatr 87:273-275, 1975.

Tooley WH, Myerberg DZ. Should we put catheters in the umbilical artery? Pediatrics 62:853-854, 1978.

Tyson JE, deSa DJ, Moore S. Thromboatheromatous complications of umbilical arterial catheterization in the newborn period. Arch Dis Child 52:744-754, 1976.

Wessel DL, Keane JF, Fellows KE, Robichaud H, Lock JE. Fibrinolytic therapy for femoral arterial thrombosis after cardiac catheterization in infants and children. Am J Cardiol 58:347-351, 1986.

• Wiedemann HP, Matthay MA, Matthay RA. Cardiovascular-pulmonary monitoring in the intensive care unit (Part 1). Chest 85:537-549, 1984.

• Wigger HJ, Bransilver BR, Blanc WA. Thromboses due to catheterization in infants and children. J Pediatr 76:1-11, 1970.

• Youngberg JA, Miller ED. Evaluation of percutaneous cannulations of the dorsalis pedis artery. Anesthesiology 44:80-83, 1976.

• Zerella JT, Trump DS, Dorman GW. Access for neonatal arterial monitoring. J Pediatr Surg 14:270-275, 1979.

116 Swan-Ganz Pulmonary Artery Catheters and Left Atrial Catheters

Luis O. Toro-Figueroa · Marjorie Craft ·
Michelle Morris-Copeland · David E. Fixler

SWAN-GANZ PULMONARY ARTERY CATHETERS
Background

The first clinical application for catheterization of the right heart with a flow-directed, balloon-tipped catheter was described by Swan and associates in 1970. The Swan-Ganz catheter has been modified over the years, adding functions that help obtain more accurate physiologic information. Presently the catheter can provide information on intracardiac pressures and cardiac output, ventricular pacemaker therapy, and continuous monitoring of mixed venous oxygen saturation. Each of these functions requires a separate channel within the catheter. The most commonly used configuration is a four-channel catheter, which is available in both No. 5 and 7 F sizes for pediatric and adult patients. A thermistor (for the thermodilution technique for the measurement of cardiac output), a balloon lumen (for flotation and occlusion), a distal lumen (for measurement of pulmonary arterial blood pressure and pulmonary arterial occlusion pressure), and a proximal lumen (for measurement of right atrial blood pressure) are the most common components of the four-channel Swan-Ganz catheter. A fifth channel is currently used in adults for a right ventricular (middle) port or a distally placed fiberoptic line for continuous measurement of mixed venous oxygen saturation. The right ventricular port may be used to monitor pressures within the ventricle or as an access to the ventricular muscle mass for placement of cardiac pacing wires when needed for emergency pacing. The mixed venous oxygen saturation can be continuously monitored, giving a "real-time" estimate of cardiac output provided that hemoglobin concentration, arterial oxygen saturation, and oxygen consumption remain constant. No studies are available that provide data about the efficacy or safety of either of these new applications of the Swan-Ganz catheter in pediatric patients.

A variety of distances between the proximal and distal lumens is available; 10, 15, 20, and 30 cm distances are standard. Special-order Swan-Ganz catheters with shorter distances between distal and proximal ports are available for pediatric use. A two-dimensional plot (Fig. 116-1) using the square root of age compared to the middle right atrium to right pulmonary artery distance is available to predict proximal to distal port distances. The clinical validity of these equations is still being studied, but the graph may be helpful to clinicians whose patients may need special-order catheters.

Cardiac pressure monitoring

Catheterization of the pulmonary artery through the right side of the heart provides the following direct pressure measurements: (1) right atrial blood pressure (RAP) or central venous blood pressure (CVP) (see Chapter 114), (2) right ventricular blood pressure (RVP) using single measurements during insertion or withdrawal, (3) pulmonary arterial blood pressure (PAP), and (4) pulmonary arterial occlusion pressure (PAoP) (see Fig. 116-2 for normal pressures).

PAoP provides indirect information about pulmonary hydrostatic pressure and left ventricular end-diastolic pressure (LVEDP). PAoP is not equivalent to pulmonary hydrostatic pressure, especially in patients who have increased pulmonary vascular resistance. Clinicians have used PAoP as a reflection of the LVEDP. During ventricular diastole the mitral valve is open and the left ventricle is directly connected with the left atrium and the pulmonary veins, which are in continuity with the pulmonary capillaries (wedge pressure) and the occluded pulmonary artery (PAoP). This continuous closed circuit allows the clinician to use PAoP as a reflection of the LVEDP only under certain conditions.

Criteria for proper PAoP measurement are as follows: (1) a and v waves must be present in the PAoP waveform (Fig. 116-3, *A*), they must appear and disappear quickly with inflation and deflation of the balloon, and PAoP must have the least respiratory variability; (2) catheter patency must be documented by free flow of blood with the balloon inflated; (3) the occlusion blood sample oxygen tension must be 10 mm Hg greater than the pulmonary arterial blood oxygen tension, although this criterion may not hold true when the catheter tip is in a low $\dot{V}/\dot{Q}$ zone (e.g., in a patient with pneumonia); (4) PAoP must be less than or equal to pulmonary artery diastolic blood pressure (PADP) (when large v waves are present [e.g., with mitral valve disease], the area between the a and v wave must be used to determine the PAoP); and (5) the catheter tip must be below the left atrium on the lateral chest roentgenogram.

Even if the above criteria are met and the aforementioned clinical situations are not present one cannot necessarily assume that LVEDP reflects left heart preload. Preload correlates better with left ventricular end-diastolic volume (LVEDV). LVEDP is a major component of LVEDV but is not its only determinant (Fig. 116-4). Juxtacardiac pressure and ventricular compliance also have a significant effect on the LVEDV. Changes in any of these components may shift the ventricular pressure-volume curve to the right or the left with or without any changes in the LVEDP. There is not a good correlation between PAoP and LVEDV. Two-dimensional echocardiography provides left ventricular end-diastolic dimensions that correlate with LVEDV.

Pulmonary arterial blood pressures and waveforms must be monitored continuously to determine catheter migration and accidental wedging. A normal

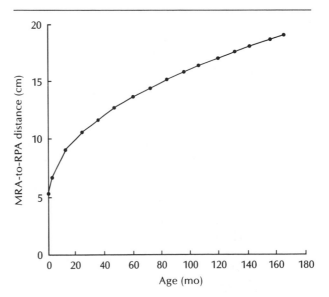

Fig. 116-1 MRA-to-RPA distance = 1.504 + 0.156 × Length − 0.117 × SSSP. (MRA = middle right atrium; RPA = right pulmonary artery; SSSP = distance from suprasternal notch to suprapubis.) (From Borland LM. Allometric determination of the distance from the central venous port to the wedge position of the balloon-tip catheter in pediatric patients. Crit Care Med 14:974-976, 1986.)

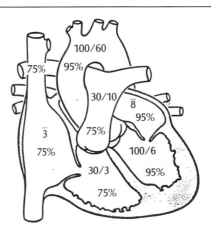

Fig. 116-2 Catheterization data in the normal pediatric heart with pressure (torr) and oxygen saturation (%). (From Ream AK, Fogdall RP. Acute Cardiovascular Management: Anesthesia and Intensive Care. Philadelphia: JB Lippincott, 1982.)

RELATION OF PAoP TO LVEDP IN DIFFERENT CLINICAL SITUATIONS

Decreased left ventricular compliance (PAoP = LVEDP/LVEDV)

Two physiologic causes

With decrease in volume there is a left shift along a single Frank-Starling curve.

With increased intrinsic stiffness there is a left shift along the family of Frank-Starling curves.

Intrinsic causes of decreased ventricular compliance

Principal causes
  Ventricular hypertrophy
  Ventricular ischemia
  Ventricular fibrosis
  Ventricular tumors
  Ventricular infiltrative processes (e.g., amyloidosis)
  Pericardial disease
Other causes
  Increased temperature
  Increased osmolality
  Increased heart rate

Eccentric balloon occlusion (PAoP > LVEDP)

Balloon occludes the distal port directly or through placement against the vessel wall.

Incorrect transducer placement

Correct position: see "Technique of Catheter Insertion."

Increased pulmonary vascular resistance (PAoP > LVEDP)

Causes
  Alveolar hypoxia
  Chronic obstructive pulmonary disease
  Hypercarbic states
  Open heart surgery
  Pulmonary embolism

Overwedging (overocclusion) (PAoP > LVEDP)

Condition results from distention of pulmonary vasculature and/or from occlusion of tip of catheter.

Pulmonary venous obstruction (PAoP > LVEDP)

Causes
  Atrial myxomas
  Increased intrathoracic pressures
  Mediastinal fibrosis
  Pulmonary venous thrombosis
  Thoracic tumors

Respiratory effects (PAoP ≥ LVEDP)

Record PAoP and respiratory cycle on paper simultaneously.
  Spontaneous breathing: Read PAoP at end-inspiration. If using digital readout, use *systolic PAoP*.
  Mechanical ventilation: Read PAoP at end-expiration. If using digital readout, use *diastolic PAoP*.
West's zones
  Zone I: $P_A > P_a > P_v$; PAoP > LVEDP
  Zone II: $P_a > P_A > P_v$; PAoP > LVEDP
  Zone III: $P_a > P_v > P_A$; PAoP = LVEDP
PEEP
  West's zone III may convert into a zone II or I; PAoP is > LVEDP (usually PEEP 15 or lower if hypovolemia is present).
  When PAoP increases by more than 50% of the change in applied PEEP, a non-zone III placement should be suspected.
  PEEP will increase pericardial pressure (PP), and PP will be transmitted to the LV, elevating LVEDP and decreasing LVEDV (left shift of Frank-Starling curve).
  Effects of PEEP on pleural pressure decrease in low-compliance lungs.
  PEEP's effect on pleural pressure may be assessed by direct measurement of pleural pressure or midesophageal pressure in lateral decubitus position.

Valvular heart disease

Mitral valve disease: (PAoP > LVEDP)
  Mitral stenosis (large a wave)
  Mitral insufficiency (large v wave)
Aortic regurgitation (PAoP = LAP > LVEDP)

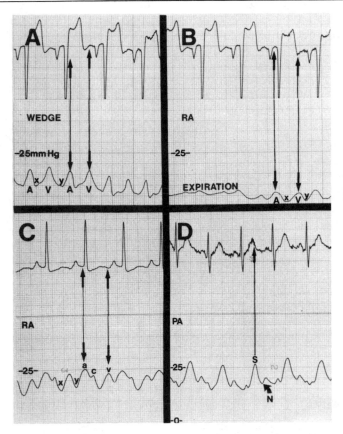

Fig. 116-3 **A,** Normal wedge pressure waveform. The peak of the A wave follows the peak of the ECG P wave by 240 msec, whereas the peak of the V wave occurs after the ECG T wave. **B,** Normal RAP waveform. The peak of the A wave follows the peak of the ECG P wave by 80 msec, whereas the peak of the V wave occurs at the end of the ECG T wave. During inspiration the RAP falls and the A and V waves become more prominent. **C,** RAP waveform from a patient with first-degree atrioventricular block. The c wave is clearly visible. The RAP is elevated because of right ventricular infarction. **D,** Normal PAP waveform. The peak systolic pressure (*S*) occurs within the ECG T wave. The dicrotic notch (*N*) is present. (From Sharkey SW. Beyond the wedge: Clinical physiology and the Swan-Ganz catheter. Am J Med 83:111-122, 1987.)

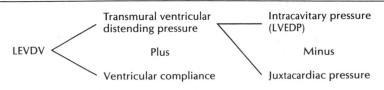

Fig. 116-4   Relation of LVEDV to LVEDP.

PAP waveform is composed of a systolic phase, dicrotic notch, and diastolic phase (Fig. 116-3, *D*). An ECG and PAP waveform must be simultaneously available for interpretation.

Pulmonary systolic blood pressure normally would reflect right ventricular systolic blood pressure. In the absence of most of the factors mentioned on p. 836, PADP would reflect left atrial pressure (LAP) within 4 mm Hg (Fig. 116-2). When the PAP and PAoP are within 4 mm Hg, there is no need to occlude the pulmonary artery by inflating the balloon. PADP may be elevated by any clinical disorder or therapeutic intervention that increases pulmonary vascular resistance (e.g., open heart surgery, chronic obstructive pulmonary disease, alveolar hypoxia, hypercarbic states, pulmonary embolism), pulmonary venous blood pressure (e.g., pulmonary venous obstruction, mitral valve disease, left ventricular failure), and pulmonary blood flow (e.g., left-to-right intracardiac shunt, some aortopulmonary shunts).

In clinical practice misinterpretation of Swan-Ganz data may be minimized through careful evaluation of the patient's clinical status, knowledge of the disease process, meticulous use of PAoP criteria for measurement, and frequent reevaluation of the patient and pulmonary arterial catheter data after therapeutic interventions.

Indications

Indications for placement of a Swan-Ganz catheter are (1) shock unresponsive to fluid resuscitation; (2) any low cardiac output state in which inotropy and/or vasodilatory therapy must be used and the effectiveness of therapy assessed; (3) pulmonary arterial hypertension surveillance and management; (4) any pulmonary process in which high PEEP (usually >10 cm H_2O) or high peak inflating pressures may increase juxtacardiac pressures and thereby depress myocardial function (e.g., ARDS); and (5) preoperative placement in patients in whom the need for this monitoring postoperatively is anticipated such as patients undergoing liver transplantation and patients in whom a complex congenital heart defect is being corrected.

Thermodilution Technique for Cardiac Output Measurement

Measurement of cardiac output is often important in treating a child in shock or with low-output state. Changes in cardiac output are useful in estimating the effect of inotropic and vasoactive agents and assisted ventilation. Thermodilution indicators have proved satisfactory since the indicator (cold) is easily detectable and nontoxic and produces no cardiorespiratory changes. In this method a known volume of liquid, either at room temperature or at 0° to 4° C, is introduced at one point in the circulation (right atrium), and the change in intravascular blood temperature is measured distally (at the catheter tip). Currently available instruments electronically integrate the area under the thermodilution curve and display the cardiac output in liters per minute. This value is divided by the body surface area of the child to give the cardiac index.

The thermodilution technique can provide accurate reproducible values if several conditions are met: (1) the duration of the injection must be <2 seconds; (2) the volume and temperature of the solution must be accurately determined; (3) the temperature of the injectate must be preserved; (4) the temperature of the pulmonary artery blood must be determined; (5) the injection site and thermistor recording site must be located in areas where the injectate is completely mixed with the blood (this is best accomplished with a central venous or right atrial injection site and a thermistor site in the main pulmonary artery or a proximal branch); and (6) the subject must be in a relatively steady state as reflected by the heart rate and systemic arterial blood pressure. Abrupt changes of these variables during the injection may result in an invalid determination. The thermodilution technique is not an accurate measurement of cardiac output when tricuspid insufficiency or intracardiac mixing occurs.

It is important to measure the temperature of the injectate accurately. When injecting room temperature solutions, two vials of the injectate must be available, one as a reservoir from which the injectate is withdrawn and the other for monitoring the temperature of the injectate with an external thermistor probe. When an iced injectate is used, several vials of injectate solution are placed in an ice bath. One of the vials serves as a site to monitor the injectate temperature. Just before injection the fluid is rapidly drawn into the syringe with minimal handling of the syringe barrel. Injectate-filled syringes are not placed directly into the ice bath because of possible contaminant seepage into the syringe. A period of approximately 40 minutes is needed to cool the vials to 0° C.

The syringe is attached to the proximal port and is injected as quickly (<2 seconds) and evenly as possible. The injection catheter must not contain any medications. An alternative system is the American Edward's CO-Set closed injectate system in which the cardiac output may be determined without entering the tubing system and a more consistent injectate temperature is maintained.

When using different volumes and temperatures for injectates, computation constants are supplied by the manufacturer according to the catheter size.These constants are fed into the cardiac output computer to compensate for the stated variables. We place these catheter sizes and calibrator numbers on a card labeled *Swan-Ganz* and post it on the patient's bed where it is clearly visible.

The reproducibility of the cardiac output measurements is checked by performing triplicate determinations. These replications must be done within a few minutes of one another and must yield values within 10% to 15% of each other. The first determination of the triplicate may be off by more than 15% because of temperature changes within the catheter; therefore it may be eliminated and the subsequent two determinations averaged.

Insertion

Vascular access for Swan-Ganz catheter placement can be attained using either the percutaneous or cutdown method. Preferred insertion sites are the internal or external jugular, basilic (most commonly used in adolescent patients), femoral, subclavian, or axillary veins. The use of the jugular and subclavian veins must be avoided in patients with increased ICP since the catheter may impede venous return from the head and raise ICP. In patients with high intrathoracic pressures and in small infants the subclavian approach must be avoided because of the high incidence of pneumothorax.

Percutaneous vascular access using the Seldinger technique provides a rapid and safe method for catheter placement. Other advantages of this method are better hemostasis, more aesthetically pleasing appearance after removal, more available vascular sites, and a lower incidence of infections (according to some authors).

A Teflon vascular sheath with a T-connector for fluid administration and an airtight valve that allows introduction, repositioning, removal, and replacement of the catheter is recommended. Before inser-

tion of the Swan-Ganz catheter the balloon patency must be tested by attaching a syringe and injecting the prescribed volume of air. This can be done by the person inserting the catheter since it is a sterile procedure.

Pulmonary arterial blood pressures are monitored using a transducer with a 30 ml flush device and low-compliance tubing. The flush device may be omitted if the flow rate is >30 ml/hr, but the infusion pump pressure will introduce an artifact and increase pressure readings. Standard fluids may be used to prime the tubing, and heparin may be added to them. One to five units of heparin per milliliter of fluid may be used. The lower the flow rate, the higher the concentration of heparin needed to prevent clotting. Care must be used in priming the tubing and all stopcocks since any air in the system is a potential embolus and/or may dampen pressure readings.

The transducer must be placed at the intersection of the midaxillary line and the intermammary line (left atrial level). Zeroing and calibration of the transducer must be performed according to the monitor's specifications. Once the catheter has been properly set up and tested, a sterile sleeve can be placed over it to maintain catheter sterility and allow repositioning of the catheter without the introduction of bacteria into the vascular space.

Placement of the tip of the catheter into the pulmonary artery may be accomplished at the bedside using the flotation method, with or without the help of fluoroscopy. Continuous ECG and pressure monitoring is required. The flotation method uses the flow of blood to move the catheter through the right side of the heart. The clinician must follow waveform changes closely to determine catheter position. The catheter can be advanced with the balloon deflated into the superior or inferior vena cava and then advanced further until respiratory fluctuations are observed in the venous pressure tracing. These fluctuations indicate intrathoracic position of the catheter tip. While mean pressure is monitored, the balloon should be inflated with sterile carbon dioxide (0.5 ml/5 F and 1.5 ml/7 F) and floated into the right ventricle. A ventricular waveform and an increase in the mean blood pressure will be detected. After the monitor has been changed to diastolic pressure readings, flotation into the pulmonary artery should be continued while the waveform change and increase in blood pressure are observed. Flotation of the catheter should continue until a PAoP tracing is observed.

(See Fig. 116-2 for intracardiac blood pressures and Fig. 116-5 for a pressure tracing of right heart catheterization.)

Once the catheter is in position, the balloon is deflated and the sterile sleeve extended over the catheter and secured to the T-connector of the sheath. The catheter is then secured with surgical tape or with a commercially available clamp. Once the catheter is secured, the list of criteria for proper PAoP measurement must be rechecked. Anteroposterior and lateral chest roentgenograms must also be obtained to determine if there is a redundant catheter loop in the right ventricle and if the catheter tip is below the left atrium (West's lung zone III in which Pa > Pv > PA).

Careful monitoring is required to observe for changes in the pulmonary artery waveform. The pulmonary artery line must be calibrated every 8 hours, with any change in the patient's position, and/or with sudden changes in the PAP. Any air bubbles or clot formation may dampen the pulmonary artery waveform. Air bubbles in the catheter must be aspirated via the stopcock and the catheter flushed. If the air is aspirated, heparinized 0.9% sodium chloride solution may be used to flush the catheter to clear any blood from the tubing. If a wedged waveform persists, the catheter must be repositioned since a catheter lodged against the vessel wall can result in a wedged waveform.

The insertion site must be inspected at least every 48 hours and the sterile dressing changed, with any redness, edema, or leakage from the site noted. Skin site and blood cultures are recommended whenever the patient is febrile or has suspected sepsis or signs of insertion site cellulitis.

PAoPs are obtained by slowly inflating the balloon

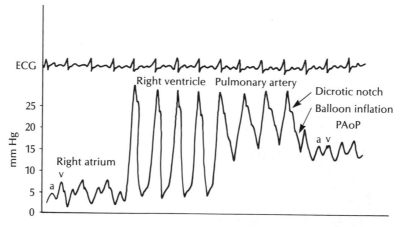

Fig. 116-5 Representative recording of pressures as a Swan-Ganz catheter is inserted through the right side of the heart into the pulmonary artery. The first waveform is a right atrial tracing with characteristic a and v waves. The right ventricular, pulmonary artery, and pulmonary artery wedge tracings follow in sequence. The pressures and waveforms shown here are normal. Note that the wedge tracing shows a and v waves transmitted from the left atrium. In addition the wedge pressure (mean) is less than pulmonary artery diastolic pressure. The wedge tracing is not always this distinct, but a very damped tracing or a mean wedge pressure greater than pulmonary artery diastolic pressure usually indicates some mechanical problem in the system (e.g., air bubble in the connecting tubing, catheter tip "overwedged," balloon inflated over distal orifice, catheter tip in zone 1 or zone 2). In a patient with severe mitral regurgitation the large transmitted left atrial v waves occasionally may cause the wedge tracing to resemble a pulmonary artery tracing. In such a case careful analysis of the waveforms and attention to where peak pressure occurs in relation to the ECG complex usually will avoid misinterpretation. (Redrawn from Matthay MA. Invasive hemodynamic monitoring in critically ill patients. Clin Chest Med 4:233-49, 1983.)

port while observing the pulmonary artery waveform for a wedge tracing (Fig. 116-3, *A* and *B*). The balloon is inflated only until the waveform changes to a wedged waveform. Overinflation can result in balloon rupture, pulmonary artery rupture, or pulmonary infarction and falsely high PAoP readings. A normal resistance will be felt while the balloon is inflated. To deflate the balloon the syringe is removed from the lumen and the balloon is allowed to deflate spontaneously; the air must not be aspirated since this may lead to balloon rupture. When blood is noted in the balloon lumen, the balloon has ruptured. This port must not be used again. When removed, the catheter must be inspected to determine if any part of the ruptured balloon has been embolized.

Indications for removal of the catheter are as follows: (1) when the reasons for its placement have been resolved or are static; (2) evidence of fibrin sheath or clot formation (i.e., damped tracing after ruling out wedging and air bubble in the system or echocardiographic evidence); (3) pulmonary embolism that can be traced to the Swan-Ganz catheter; (4) intractable dysrhythmias; and (5) colonization of the catheter by microorganisms.

When removing a Swan-Ganz catheter one must be sure the balloon is deflated. Pressure recordings and waveform inspection can be performed as the catheter tip is withdrawn into the different cardiac chambers. Blood gas values may also be obtained to rule out left-to-right intracardiac shunts in patients after open heart surgery. The balloon must always be inspected for rupture once it is removed.

Risks and Complications

The safety vs. the risks of placement of 22 Swan-Ganz catheters has been demonstrated in a study of catheterization performed at the patients' bedside in 19 pediatric-age patients. The following complications were reported: catheter malposition (4), balloon rupture (3), dislodgment (2), pneumothorax during vascular access attempted into an internal jugular vein (1), femoral cutdown site bleeding (1), hypotension with balloon inflation (1), transient premature ventricular contractions (14), and failure to "wedge" balloon (9).

In another study of 774 vascular catheterizations (of which 47 were pulmonary artery catheters) in 467 children, 4.1% of patient's experienced bleeding, arterial obstruction, and/or sepsis. A knot in one pulmonary artery catheter was reported with no impact in the patient's outcome. No other specific mention of significant complications related to Swan-Ganz catheters was made. A composite of complications has been reported in both pediatric and adult patients.

LEFT ATRIAL CATHETERS
Background and Indications

Left atrial blood pressure reflects LVEDP when there is no mitral valve disease or aortic regurgitation. Open heart surgery increases peripheral vascular resistance, rendering PAoP inaccurate in relation to LAP. In addition mitral valve disease (regurgitation or stenosis) renders PAoP inaccurate. Many thoracic surgeons prefer direct placement of a left atrial catheter to obtain a more reliable reflection of LVEDP.

COMPLICATIONS OF SWAN-GANZ CATHETERIZATION

Access site bleeding
Arch vessel injury
Balloon rupture
Cardiac perforation with or without tamponade
Catheter dislodgment
Catheter-related sepsis
Cellulitis of insertion site
Central vascular puncture during access
Coronary sinus occlusion
Dysrhythmias
Entanglement with other central venous catheters
Failure to wedge balloon
False pulmonary artery aneurysm
Hypotension during balloon inflation
Knotting of the catheter
Luminal obstruction
Myocardial laceration
Pneumothorax
Pulmonary artery rupture
Pulmonary embolization
Pulmonary infarction
Superior vena cava syndrome
Thermistor malfunction
Thrombocytopenia
Thrombus formation
Triscuspid and/or pulmonic valve damage
$\dot{V}/\dot{Q}$ mismatch during wedging

Technique

A polyurethane 16-gauge Sentinel catheter is inserted through the chest or abdominal wall left of the midline. An incision is then made in the tip of the left atrial appendage. After insertion the catheter is secured with a purse-string suture.

Extreme care must be taken to keep the catheter free of air bubbles. Any air embolism will go to the systemic circulation and has great potential for causing catastrophic complications.

Left atrial lines are always set up using a 3 ml flush device with low-compliance tubing and a pressure infuser for fluid delivery. Placing this system on a pump involves a much higher risk of air entering the system. A 0.9% sodium chloride solution or 0.45% sodium chloride solution is infused through the catheter's lines with heparin (1 unit/ml) added as an anticoagulant.

Risks and Complications

Medication administration and blood sampling are not done through the left atrial catheter since this increases the incidence of air embolism and clotting, which are the two most common complications.

The third complication is bleeding at the atrial incision on removal. The mediastinal chest tube must not be removed until all surgically placed atrial catheters have been removed. If bleeding occurs at a rate of more than 3 ml/kg/hr, thoracotomy and insertion site repair must be considered.

Inability to remove the left atrial catheter is the fourth known complication. It may result from the catheter's being trapped by the suture at the atrial appendage or from sectioning or breaking of the catheter below the skin level. In either case a thoracotomy may be necessary to remove the catheter.

ADDITIONAL READING

- Bellamy PE, Mercurio P. An alternative method for coordinating pulmonary capillary wedge pressure measurements with the respiratory cycle. Crit Care Med 14:733-734, 1986.

Birman H, Haq A, Hew E, Aberman A. Continuous monitoring of mixed venous oxygen saturation in hemodynamically unstable patients. Chest 86:753-755, 1984.

Bouchard RJ, Gault JH, Ross J Jr. Evaluation of pulmonary arterial end-diastolic pressure as an estimate of left ventricular end-diastolic pressure in patients with normal and abnormal left ventricular performance. Circulation 44:1072-1079, 1971.

- Bourland LM. Allometric determination of the distance from the central venous pressure port to wedge position of balloon-tip catheters in pediatric patients. Crit Care Med 14:974-976, 1986.

Buchbinder N, Ganz W. Hemodynamic monitoring: Invasive techniques. Anesthesiology 45:146-154, 1976.

Colardyn F, Vandenbogaerde J, De Niel C, Jordaens L. Ventricular pacing via a Swan-Ganz catheter: A new mode of pacemaker therapy. Acta Cardiol 41:23-29, 1986.

- Colgan FJ, Stewart S. An assessment of cardiac output by thermodilution in infants and children following cardiac surgery. Crit Care Med 5:220-225, 1977.

Daily EK, Shoreder JS. Techniques in Bedside Hemodynamic Monitoring, 3rd ed. St. Louis: CV Mosby, 1986.

Damen J, Bolton D. A prospective analysis of 1400 pulmonary artery catheterizations in patients undergoing cardiac surgery. Acta Anaesthesiol Scand 30:386-392, 1986.

Damen J, Verhoef J, Bolton DT, Middleton NG, Van Der Tweel I, De Jonge K, Wever J, Nijsen-Karelse M. Microbiologic risk of invasive hemodynamic monitoring in patients undergoing open-heart operations. Crit Care Med 13:548-555, 1985.

Eisenberg PR, Jaffe AS, Shuster DP. Clinical evaluation compared to pulmonary artery catheterization in the hemodynamic assessment of critically ill patients. Crit Care Med 12:549-553, 1984.

Elliott CG, Zimmerman GA, Clemmer TP. Complications of pulmonary artery catheterization in the care of critically ill patients. Chest 76:647-652, 1979.

Fairfax WR, Thomas F, Orme JF. Pulmonary artery catheter occlusion as an indication of pulmonary embolus. Chest 86:270-271, 1984.

Fein AM, Goldberg SK, Walkenstein MD, Dershaw B, Braitman L, Lippmann ML. Is pulmonary artery catheterization necessary for the diagnosis of pulmonary edema? Am Rev Respir Dis 129:1006-1009, 1984.

Feinberg BI, LaMantia KR, Addonizio P, Geer RT. Pulmonary artery catheter–associated thrombocytopenia: Effect of heparin coating. Mt Sinai J Med 54:147-149, 1987.

- Freed MD, Keane JF. Cardiac output measured by thermodilution in infants and children. J Pediatr 92:39-42, 1978.

Ganz WW, Forrester JS, Chonette D, Donoso R, Swan J. A new flow-directed catheter technique for measurement of pulmonary artery and capillary wedge pressure without fluoroscopy. Am J Cardiol 25:96, 1970.

Goodman DJ, Rider AK, Billingham ME, Schroeder JS. Thromboembolic complications with the indwelling balloon-tipped pulmonary arterial catheter. N Engl J Med 291:777, 1974.

Hasan FM, Weiss WB, Braman SS, Hoppin FG. Influence of lung injury on pulmonary wedge–left atrial pressure correlation during positive end-expiratory pressure ventilation. Am Rev Respir Dis 131:246-250, 1985.

Hasan FM, Malanga AL, Braman SS, Corrao WM, Most AS. Lateral position improves wedge–left atrial pressure correlation during positive-pressure ventilation. Crit Care Med 12:960-964, 1984.

Heard SO, Davis RF, Sherertz RJ, Mikhail MS, Gallagher RC, Layon J, Gallagher TJ. Influence of sterile protective sleeves on the sterility of pulmonary artery catheters. Crit Care Med 15:499-502, 1987.

Hoar PF, Wilson RM, Mangano DT, Avery GJ, Szarnicki RJ, Hill JD. Heparin bonding reduces thrombogenicity of pulmonary-artery catheters. N Engl J Med 305:993-995, 1981.

Johnston WE, Royster RL, Vinten-Johansen J, Gravlee GP, Howard G, Mills SA, Tucker WY. Influence of balloon inflation and deflation on location of pulmonary artery catheter tip. Anesthesiology 67:110-115, 1987.

Kaplan JA. Hemodynamic monitoring. In Kaplan JA, ed. Cardiac Anesthesia. New York: Grune & Stratton, 1987, pp 202-206.

Kron IL, Joob AW, Lake CL, Nolan SP. Arch vessel injury during pulmonary artery catheter placement. Ann Thorac Surg 39:223-224, 1985.

Lange HW, Galliani CA, Edwards JE. Local complications associated with indwelling Swan-Ganz catheters: Autopsy study of 36 cases. Am J Cardiol 52:1108-1111, 1983.

Martin C, Auffray JP, Saux P, Albanese J, Gouin F. The axillary vein: An alternative approach for percutaneous pulmonary artery catheterization. Chest 90:694-697, 1986.

McMichan JC, Baele PL, Wignes MW. Insertion of pulmonary artery catheters—a comparison of fiberoptic and non-fiberoptic catheters. Crit Care Med 12:517-519, 1984.

• Moore RA, McNicholas K, Gallagher JD, Niguidula F. Migration of pediatric pulmonary artery catheters. Anesthesiology 58:102-104, 1983.

Morris AH, Chapman RH, Gardner RM. Frequency of wedge pressure errors in the ICU. Crit Care Med 13:705-708, 1985.

Moser KM, Spragg RG. Use of the balloon-tipped pulmonary artery catheter in pulmonary disease. Ann Intern Med 98:53-58, 1983.

Myers ML, Austin TW, Sibbald WJ. Pulmonary artery catheter infections. A prospective study. Ann Surg 201:237-241, 1985.

Nadeau S, Noble WH. Misinterpretation of pressure measurements from the pulmonary artery catheter. Can Anaesth Soc J 33:352-362, 1986.

Nelson LD, Martinez OV, Anderson HB. Incidence of microbial colonization in open versus closed delivery systems for thermodilution injectate. Crit Care Med 14:291-293, 1986.

Perkins N, Cail WS, Bedford RF, Elinger JH, Buschi AJ. Internal jugular vein function after Swan-Ganz catheterization. Anesthesiology 61:456-459, 1984.

• Pollack MM, Reed TP, Holbrook PR, Fields AI. Bedside pulmonary artery catheterization in pediatrics. J Pediatr 96:274-276, 1980.

Quan SF. Mixed venous oxygen. Am Fam Physician 27:211-215, 1983.

Quintana E, Sanchez JM, Serra C, Net A. Erroneous interpretation of pulmonary capillary wedge pressure in massive pulmonary embolism. Crit Care Med 11:933-935, 1983.

Raper R, Sibbald WJ. Misled by the wedge? The Swan-Ganz catheter and left ventricular preload. Chest 89:427-434, 1986.

Ream AK, Fogdall RP. Acute cardiovascular management: Anesthesia and intensive care. Philadelphia: JB Lippincott, 1982, p 576.

Robin ED. The cult of the Swan-Ganz catheter. Ann Intern Med 103:445-449, 1985.

Rosenbaum L, Rosenbaum SH, Askanazi J, Hyman AI. Small amounts of hemoptysis as an early warning sign of pulmonary artery rupture by a pulmonary arterial catheter. Crit Care Med 9:319-320, 1981.

Ross RM. Bedside calibration of pulmonary artery catheters. Chest 84:506-507, 1983.

Samsoondar W, Freeman JB, Coultish I, Oxley C. Colonization of intravascular catheters in the intensive care unit. Am J Surg 149:730-731, 1985.

Settergren G. The calculation of left ventricular stroke work index. Acta Anaesthesiol Scand 30:450-452, 1986.

Shah KB, Rao T, Laughlin S, El-Etr AA. A review of pulmonary artery catheterization in 6245 patients. Anesthesiology 61:271-275, 1984.

• Sharkey SW. Beyond the wedge: Clinical physiology and the Swan-Ganz catheter. Am J Med 83:111-122, 1987.

Sibald WJ, Driedger AA, Myers ML, Short AIK, Wells GA. Biventricular function in the adult respiratory distress syndrome: Hemodynamic and radionuclide assessment, with special emphasis on right ventricular function. Chest 84:126-134, 1983.

Sise MJ, Hollingsworth P, Brimm JE, Peters RM, Virgilio RW, Shackford SR. Complications of the flow-directed pulmonary-artery catheter: A prospective analysis in 219 patients. Crit Care Med 9:315-318, 1981.

Smith-Wright DL, Green TP, Lock JE, Egar MI, Fuhrman BP. Complications of vascular catheterization in critically ill children. Crit Care Med 12:1015-1017, 1984.

• Swan HJC, Ganz W. Use of balloon flotation catheters in critically ill patients. Surg Clin North Am 55:501-520, 1975.

• Swan HJC, Ganz W, Forrester J, Marcus H, Diamond G, Chonette D. Catheterization of the heart in man with use of a flow-directed balloon-tipped catheter. New Engl J Med 283:447-451, 1970.

Thomson IR, Dalton BC, Lappas DG, Lowenstein E. Right bundle-branch block and complete heart block caused by the Swan-Ganz catheter. Anesthesiology 51:359-362, 1979.

Traeger SM. "Failure to wedge" and pulmonary hypertension during pulmonary artery catheterization: A sign of totally occlusive pulmonary embolism. Crit Care Med 13:544-547, 1985.

Whalley DG. Correlation of central venous and pulmonary capillary wedge pressures. Can Anaesth Soc J 31:203-204, 1984.

• Wiedemann HP, Matthay MA, Matthay RA. Cardiovascular-pulmonary monitoring in the intensive care unit (Part 1). Chest 85:537-549, 1984.

Wilkerson DK, Rosen AL, Gould SA, Sehgal LR, Sehgal HL, Moss GS. Oxygen extraction ratio: A valid indicator of myocardial metabolism in anemia. J Surg Res 42:629-634, 1987.

Zidulka, Hakim TS. Wedge pressure in large vs. small pulmonary arteries to detect pulmonary venoconstriction. J Appl Physiol 59:1329-1332, 1985.

117 Intraosseous Infusions

Michael L. Ponaman · Linda White

BACKGROUND AND INDICATIONS

The quest for rapid, safe, and effective intravascular access in infants and small children remains a challenge for those involved in pediatric resuscitation and emergency and intensive care. Recently there has been a renewal of enthusiasm for intraosseous infusions. Drinker, Drinker, and Lund first described the technique in 1920 in animal studies and proposed it as a possible route for blood transfusions in small children. The technique was popularized clinically by Tocantins in the 1940s. During this period large studies were published, some with over 1000 infusions, that demonstrated high rates of success (i.e., >94%) and a low incidence of serious complications. Substances mentioned in these reports as being infused included lactated Ringer's solution, 0.9% sodium chloride solution, whole blood, plasma, sodium bicarbonate, glucose solutions, and contrast material. With the greater availability of disposable IV catheters and better surgical technique, the use of intraosseous infusions fell into obscurity in the 1950s and 1960s.

Despite these technical advances instances continued to occur in which percutaneous IV access was not possible and a surgical approach unacceptably delayed lifesaving treatment. These problems, combined with the growing number of individuals with specific interests and expertise in pediatric resuscitation, rekindled interest in intraosseous infusions in the early 1980s. It is believed that substances pass from the marrow cavity into the central circulation through noncollapsible sinusoids and medullary venous channels, with absorption times and drug effectiveness equivalent to those achieved through the IV route. This may explain the effectiveness of this route of administration even during CPR when it is generally thought that blood flow is preferentially shifted away from the lower extremities toward the head and upper extremities. Recent case reports and studies have documented the successful administration of the following substances: epinephrine, atropine, insulin, morphine, lidocaine, calcium gluconate, dopamine, dobutamine, and isoproterenol.

Although newer studies may expand the role of intraosseous infusions even further, we currently recommend reserving their use for life-threatening situations in which other methods of intravascular access are not quickly available and endotracheal administration is not recommended. In addition it is advisable to establish the more conventional intravascular route as soon as possible. In any event the infusion must be discontinued within 12 hours, even if this means starting a second intraosseous infusion at an alternate location since the incidence of osteomyelitis apparently increases significantly when intraosseous infusions are allowed to remain in place for longer periods of time (see "Risks and Complications"). Specific instances in which intraosseous lines may be beneficial include:

1. Fluid resuscitation in hypovolemic shock (crystalloid or isotonic colloid solution)
2. Initial correction of metabolic acidosis with bicarbonate
3. Administration of anticonvulsants in patient with status epilepticus
4. Initiation of vasopressor therapy with epinephrine, dopamine, dobutamine, or isoproterenol

TECHNIQUE

The procedure is relatively simple and easy to learn. Early proponents recommended gaining experience and familiarity with the landmarks by practicing on cadavers. The preferred sites in children 0 to 5 years of age are the proximal tibia approximately one fingerbreadth (2 to 3 cm) below the tubercle on the anterior medial surface (rather than the anterior surface) and the distal femur 2 to 3 cm above the external condyles in the midline (Fig. 117-1).

The equipment needed for the procedure is as follows:

Intraosseous infusion equipment

For children <18 months old, 18- to 20-gauge spinal or intraosseous needle

For older children, 13- to 16-gauge bone marrow or intraosseous needle

Lidocaine, 1% (three syringes and 25-gauge needle)

Povidone-iodine swabs

T-connector

10 ml syringes (2)

Sterile saline solution

Mask, gown, and sterile gloves

¼-inch tape

1-inch tape

Padded board

IV tubing setup

Hemostats

New commercially prepared intraosseous needles with guards to prevent too deep penetration and mechanisms that provide ease in stabilizing and securing the needle are available. In their absence an 18-gauge spinal needle or a large-bore short bone marrow needle is an excellent alternative.

Strict aseptic technique must be used throughout the procedure. The skin is first cleansed with povidone-iodine solution and infiltrated with 1% lidocaine to the periosteum. The needle is inserted almost perpendicular to the skin and angled slightly away from the growth plate (i.e., caudal for the tibial site and cephalad for the femur). The needle is advanced until the periosteum is palpated, and the bone is penetrated with a boring or screwing motion. Entrance into the bone marrow cavity is signified by a loss of resistance. The stylet is then removed, and a 10 ml syringe, filled halfway with 0.9% sodium chloride solution and connected to a T-connector, is attached to the needle.

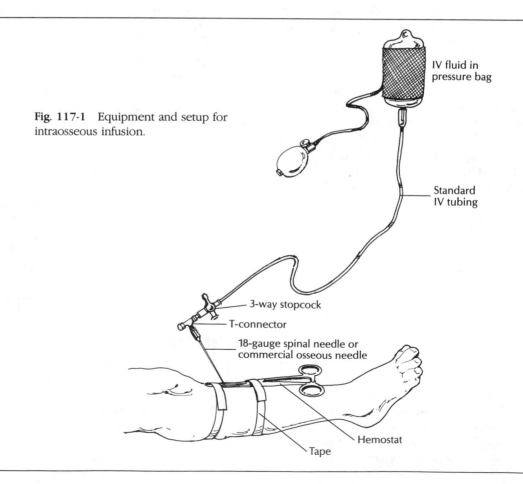

Fig. 117-1 Equipment and setup for intraosseous infusion.

IV fluid in pressure bag

Standard IV tubing

3-way stopcock

T-connector

18-gauge spinal needle or commercial osseous needle

Hemostat

Tape

Aspiration of bone marrow may be used as a second confirmation of proper position, even though the bone marrow may clot the needle. (Some authors recommend that no infusion be attempted unless bone marrow is first aspirated.) A final test for proper position is flushing 5 to 10 ml of 0.9% sodium chloride solution through the syringe using only a slight amount of pressure and observing for extravasation as the fluid is infused. This maneuver also clears the syringe of any clot. Conventional IV tubing is then attached to the needle. Fluid can then be allowed to flow by gravity or be placed in a pressure bag for rapid infusions (up to 41 ml/min with pressure of 300 mm Hg).

The method selected for stabilizing the needle depends on the type of device used. The newly designed intraosseous needles with protective guards may be adequately secured with tape. However, securing the bone marrow or spinal needle may be more challenging. A hemostat or clamp may be attached across the needle at the level of the skin and then secured to the leg with tape. The limb must be secured to a padded board, immobilizing the extremity.

RISKS AND COMPLICATIONS

No recent prospective or retrospective studies review the complications from intraosseous infusions. The majority of information was reported in large series published in the 1940s or in anecdotal reports. Most complications apparently result from failure to place the needle properly, infusions of hyperosmolar fluids, and less commonly infection. If the needle is left superficial to the marrow cavity, either intramuscular or subperiosteal injection can occur. There is at least one report in the literature of pressure necrosis resulting in bone reabsorption from a subperiosteal injection. Superficial placement of the needle in the distal femur can result in deposition of infused material in the knee joint via the upper extension of that joint's synovial cavity beneath the quadriceps tendon.

Deep placement of the needle through both the anterior and posterior cortex is possible, which would result in deposition of fluid in the popliteal space. This space is enclosed by fascia, and a compartment syndrome could ensue (particularly if fluid is infused through a pressure bag), compromising flow through the tibial vessels with resulting damage to the tibial nerve.

If two attempts at an intraosseous infusion are made in close proximity, fluid infused through the needle may leak from the hole left in the bone by the first attempt. Leakage of fluid from around the entry site of the needle can occur when the needle is left in place for protracted periods of time and small movement and jarring of the needle slowly enlarges the entry hole. Signs of extravasation include redness, blanching, and edema.

Although minor superficial infections and cellulitis have been described, more serious deep infections such as osteomyelitis and arthritis are rare. In one series of 944 infusions of isotonic bicarbonate, blood, and serum, no cases of osteomyelitis were found. The series with the highest incidence reported three cases out of 35 patients; however, all these patients had been given continuous infusions for more than 12 hours. Osteomyelitis can occur even though the needle is no longer in place. Health care providers must observe for heat, redness, and swelling at the site.

Anecdotal reports of gas gangrene and ischemic or thrombolic events distal to the infusion site exist but are extremely rare. It is probably accurate to compare the complications listed above with complications known to have occurred with other types of parenteral therapy during their period of development. The frequency of most complications is similar to that of other procedures involving placement of a hollow tube or needle in the body, plus the additional complication of osteomyelitis, which occurs rarely when placement is reserved for patients with the indications mentioned previously. In addition it would be valuable to know the complication rate of intraosseous infusions vs. that of more traditional routes of infusions attempted during life-threatening situations.

ADDITIONAL READING

Berg RA. Emergency infusions of catecholamines into bone marrow. Am J Dis Child 138:810-811, 1984.

Brickman KR, Rega P, Guinness M. A comparative study of intraosseous versus peripheral intravenous infusion of diazepam and phenobarbital in dogs. Ann Emerg Med 16:1141, 1987.

Drinker CK, Drinker KR, Lund CC. The circulation in the mammalian bone marrow. Am J Physiol 62:1-93, 1922.

Heinild S, Sondergaard T, Tudvad F. Bone marrow infusion in childhood. Experiences from a thousand infusions. J Pediatr 30:400-412, 1947.

Hodges D, Delgado-Pardes C, Fleisher G. Intraosseous infusion flow rate in hypovolemic pediatric dogs. Ann Emerg Med 16:305-307, 1984.

Manley L, Haley K, Dick M. Intraosseous infusion: Rapid vascular access for critically ill or injured infants and children. J Emerg Nurs 14:63-69, 1988.

Spivey WH, Lathers CM, Malone DR, et al. Comparison of intraosseous, central and peripheral routes of sodium bicarbonate administration during CPR in pigs. Ann Emerg Med 14:2235-2239, 1985.

Rosetti VA, Thompson BM, Miller J, et al. Intraosseous infusion: An alternative route of pediatric intravascular access. Ann Emerg Med 14:885-888, 1985.

Tocantins LM, O'Neil JF. Complications of intraosseous therapy. Ann Surg 122:266-277, 1945.

Tocantins LM, O'Neil JF, Jones HW. Infusions of blood and other fluids via the bone marrow, applications in pediatrics. JAMA 117:1220-1234, 1941.

Tocantins LM, O'Neil JF, Price AH. Infusions of blood and other fluids via the bone marrow in traumatic shock and other forms of peripheral circulatory failure. Ann Surg 114:1085-1992, 1941.

118 Intracranial Pressure Monitoring

Cole A. Giller · Frederick H. Sklar · Mary Grandy Baker

Detection and treatment in the PICU of patients with intracranial hypertension requires an understanding of the methods of monitoring intracranial pressure (ICP). A variety of ICP monitoring systems are available to the clinician. Some are reliable; most are invasive; and none is perfect. Noninvasive techniques are also used, and they range from palpating the fontanelle to sophisticated Doppler evaluations. This chapter discusses techniques and problems related to the most commonly used ICP monitoring devices.

INDICATIONS

ICP monitoring may be important in the PICU care of children with presumed intracranial hypertension as a result of head trauma, hydrocephalus, cerebral tumors, and metabolic disorders. For instance, marked elevation of ICP can occur after head trauma, and the use of pressure monitoring guides ICP-reduction therapy. Changes in the pressure measurements may suggest the development of an expanding hematoma. For treatment of patients with trauma a rule of thumb is to monitor those patients whose mental status is less than purposeful and those who need intubation. Since cerebral edema and ventricular effacement are frequent CT findings after trauma, ventricular puncture may be difficult.

Hydrocephalus occasionally produces rapid and potentially life-threatening elevations of ICP. Monitoring by ventriculostomy can document pressure changes; CSF drainage will bring pressures back into safe ranges. Similarly, monitoring patients with intracranial tumors can provide warnings of increasing edema, hemorrhage, or hydrocephalus. Disorders such as metabolic disturbances, Reye's syndrome, and lead intoxication can result in cerebral edema, and ICP monitoring can guide intensive pressure-reduction therapy.

VENTRICULOSTOMY

The standard technique for monitoring ICP is ventriculostomy. A fluid-filled catheter is positioned within a ventricle, and pressure is monitored with a transducer.

Procedure (Fig. 118-1)

The patient is sedated if necessary and placed supine with his head in neutral position. The nondominant right side is usually chosen for insertion. The scalp is shaved, prepared, and draped with sterile towels. The skin is generously infiltrated with lidocaine in the midpupillary line at the coronal suture.

In infants it is sometimes easier and safer to make the twist drill hole just anterior to the coronal suture

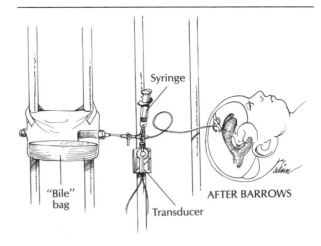

Fig. 118-1 Standard apparatus for ICP monitoring and CSF drainage from a ventriculostomy.

VENTRICULAR TAP TRAY

1 Children's Hospital hand drill
1 Burton-Blacker hand drill
1 Adson forceps *with* teeth
1 sponge forceps
1 suture scissors
1 needle holder
1 No. 11 and 1 No. 15 knife blade
1 custard cup
1 18-gauge 1½-inch spinal needle (metal)
1 18-gauge 3½-inch spinal needle (metal)
1 18-gauge 3½-inch Cone needle
1 20-gauge 3½-inch Cone needle
4 green surgical towels
20 4 × 4 inch sponges
1 Weitlaner retractor
1 Lampert rongeur
1 knife handle
1 3½-inch Gelpi retractor

1 16-gauge 3½-inch Cone needle (new)
30-inch extension set
Povidone-iodine ointment and Tegaderm
1 three-way stopcock
1 18-gauge needle disp
1 22-gauge needle disp
1 25-gauge needle disp
1 10 cc Luer-Lok syringe disp
1 package bone wax
1 straight ventricular catheter
1 bile bag
1 package 3-0 Ethilon suture (31663)
1 package 4-0 Ethilon suture (699)
1 T-connector
1 vial 1% lidocaine
1 No. 5 pediatric feeding tube
1 10 ml vial 0.9% sodium chloride solution (without preservative)

---

or fontanelle rather than to attempt to pass a catheter through the suture or fibrous fontanelle. In this way the rigid skull stabilizes the ventriculostomy catheter.

A 4 mm transverse skin incision is made. In older children the incision is continued through the periosteum, and a twist drill hole is made while the drill is firmly supported to avoid accidental penetration of the dura and brain. Some twist drill devices have adjustable safety stops. In infants the skull may be very thin so that gentle rotatory pressure with a hand-held drill bit may suffice to create a hole.

The dura is penetrated several times with an 18-gauge needle, and the subdural space is checked for fluid. A ventriculostomy catheter fitted with a stylet is then introduced through the twist drill hole and directed toward the medial canthus of the ipsilateral eye while the catheter is held perpendicular to the skull. A gentle "pop" is often felt as the catheter punctures the ependymal surface of the ventricle. These landmarks are meant only as estimates for the surgeon to use while guiding the catheter into the frontal horn. It may be more appropriate to visualize in one's mind a picture of the ventricular system in relation to the coronal suture and to aim appropriately. A CT scan is helpful in case of ventricular shift or effacement.

Alternative procedure

In an alternative technique a No. 14 or No. 16 Cone needle is introduced into the frontal horn. The needle is then removed and replaced with a No. 5 pediatric feeding tube filled with 0.9% sodium chloride solution. The tube is slowly threaded into the frontal horn along the needle tract. Tapping the ventricle first with a Cone needle is sometimes easier, especially when the ventricles are small.

CSF will flow from the catheter if the ventricle has been successfully cannulated, although flow may be nearly absent if the ventricles are small or the pressure is low. Nevertheless, the fluid in the catheter should pulsate and flow freely into the ventricle when the distal end of the catheter is elevated. A stopcock is attached, with ports connecting to a pressure transducer and drainage bag. The catheter is secured to the scalp with sutures, and a sterile occlusive dressing is applied (Fig. 118-1).

Use

ICP may be monitored with the transducer at the level of the foramen of Monro. The stopcock can be used to drain CSF intermittently. Alternatively, CSF can be drained continuously; pressure can be regulated by the height of the drainage bag or that of the inline valve to the bag available in some systems. The bag must be drained when full and sampled for cell counts when clinically indicated. CSF drainage may not be possible if the ventricles are small, since the ventricular walls may collapse around the tube and occlude the catheter. Pressure readings are not accurate if fluid is draining at the same time that the readings are made.

Technical difficulties

Small ventricles may be difficult to cannulate. Visible CSF pulsations within the catheter or a pulsatile waveform may be the only evidence of successful puncture.

The ICP waveform may dampen at any time, and flow of CSF may decrease, indicating either a decrease in ICP or an obstructed system. Applying light pressure over a jugular vein should increase the ICP in the former circumstance and may help to distinguish the two situations. Small volumes of 0.9% sodium chloride solution (without preservative) (0.1 to 0.2 ml) may be used to flush the catheter. An improved waveform that rapidly dampens indicates intraparenchymal position of the catheter tip or a collapsed ventricular system. Finally, a CT scan can confirm catheter position. All tubing must be checked for patency and kinking. The proper position of the drainage bag must be determined at the time of catheter insertion to ensure consistency when draining the system.

When replacing ventriculostomies, removing the old catheter before introducing the new one permits untoward CSF leakage, possibly making retapping the ventricle difficult or impossible. Accordingly, the new catheter must be placed before the old one is removed.

Risks and complications

The infection rate for intraventricular catheters is 3% to 5% and remains low as long as the catheter is replaced every 4 or 5 days. The most common infection is ventriculitis. The new catheter is generally positioned on the opposite side. Some surgeons tunnel the catheter under the scalp a considerable distance from the twist drill hole and insist that this procedure protects against infection and decreases the urgency to change ventriculostomy catheters. Prophylactic antibiotics are not used. Scalp IV catheters are contraindicated because of increased risk of local infection.

The risk of intracranial hemorrhage during insertion is less than 2%. Anticoagulation and untreated coagulopathies are contraindications to invasive ICP monitoring. The occasional CSF leak is easily stopped with either a suture or a collodion-soaked cotton ball.

OTHER TECHNIQUES
Ventricular Taps

Occasionally it is desirable simply to tap the ventricle to obtain samples of CSF for the laboratory or for emergency CSF drainage and ICP reduction. For older children the procedure is the same as for performing ventriculostomy with a Cone needle. For infants an 18-gauge spinal needle can be used to puncture the ventricle percutaneously through the fontanelle or coronal suture. Gentle twisting of the needle may be needed to pass through the coronal suture. A suture and collodion-soaked cotton ball may be placed after the procedure for managing CSF leakage.

Shunts

A ventricular shunt with a reservoir or pumping device can be tapped to measure ICP, to obtain CSF for laboratory samples, or to drain CSF in an emergency. The scalp over the shunt is shaved, prepared, and draped. A 23-gauge butterfly needle is introduced into the shunt. In the case of sudden neurologic or cardiopulmonary deterioration due to shunt malfunction, tapping the shunt may not yield fluid. A spinal needle can be introduced through the shunt directly into the ventricle as a lifesaving procedure.

Subdural Recordings

If the ventricles are small and difficult to tap, a subdural catheter may be used to measure pressure. This technique works well only for patients with thin skulls and may soon be replaced entirely by intraparenchymal monitors.

Procedure

The insertion site for the subdural catheter is chosen in the midpupillary line directly over bone at or near the coronal suture. A twist drill hole is made as with a ventriculostomy, and a small rongeur is used to enlarge the hole. A small skin retractor and some bone wax are useful for maintaining hemostasis. The dura is sharply incised, and a No. 5 feeding tube filled with 0.9% sodium chloride solution is slipped beneath the dura with the aid of a venous catheter introducer. The tube is directed anteriorly and advanced several centimeters. In practice the subdural catheter is introduced after attempts at tapping the ventricle have failed.

Use

The catheter usually needs to be flushed with 0.1 to 0.2 ml 0.9% sodium chloride solution (without preservative). Dampening of the pressure tracing may indicate partial occlusion of the catheter and inaccurate pressure measurements. The subarachnoid space is frequently entered, permitting slow CSF drainage in approximately one third of cases. The catheter is attached to the collection system as indicated previously for intraventricular catheters in cases in which CSF drainage is possible.

Risks and complications

Complications are the same as for ventriculostomy except for a lower incidence of ventriculitis.

Intraparenchymal Recordings

Fiberoptic ICP monitoring systems are currently available that are not fluid filled. They are positioned directly within the brain parenchyma. Since use of these catheters does not require ventricular puncture, they are not prone to the problems of obstruction or ventricular collapse. These systems are technically easier to insert and maintain than ventricular catheters but may be associated with significant signal or baseline drift over several days. CSF drainage is not possible with these fiberoptic devices.

Procedure

A twist drill hole is made with a bit supplied in the kit. The drill allows adjustment for pediatric skull thickness. A hollow metal connector is screwed firmly into the hole, and a probe is used to pierce the dura. The fiberoptic tube is calibrated and passed through the connector into the brain tissue to a depth of 2 to 3 cm and withdrawn 1 mm. A connection hub connects over the catheter to seat it into place. An ICP waveform should be apparent on the monitor.

Use

Flushing and recalibration are not necessary. Care must be taken not to bend or break the fiberoptic catheter.

Risks and complications

Complications are the same as for ventriculostomy except for a lower incidence of ventriculitis.

Subarachnoid Bolt

Although some institutions use subarachnoid bolts as ICP monitors, we believe that readings from these devices are frequently unreliable. Moreover, the previously described systems offer compelling advantages. However, a discussion of subarachnoid bolts is included for sake of completeness.

Procedure

After a twist drill hole is made, a No. 11 knife blade is used to incise the dura in a cruciate fashion. A small curette is useful to scrape the dura against the bone edge to widen the opening. A hollow stainless steel bolt is screwed into the skull until the tip of the bolt is presumably in the subarachnoid space and the bolt is secure. The bolt is flushed with 0.9% sodium chloride solution (without preservatives) using a 20-gauge needle and connected to a pressure transducer. A waveform should be apparent on the monitor. The skull must be thick enough to support the bolt; some bolts with wider threads have been adapted for use in the thin skulls of infants.

Use

Dampening of the waveform is a persistent problem and may indicate obstruction of the bolt. Flushing with 0.1 to 0.2 ml of 0.9% sodium chloride solution (without preservatives) or gentle probing of the bolt with a lumbar puncture needle may clear the obstruction. If the bolt is partially obstructed, recorded pressures may be entirely erroneous. Screwing the device further into the skull may also restore the waveform.

Risks and complications

The complications are the same as for ventriculostomy except for decreased risk of ventriculitis.

•   •   •

A proper working knowledge of the equipment is needed to ensure accuracy of the readings obtained from the above-mentioned monitoring devices. Orders must be specific about positioning the patient's head; keeping it either elevated or flat must be determined so that consistency in care is observed.

ADDITIONAL READING

Allen R. Intracranial pressure: A review of clinical problems, measurement techniques and monitoring methods. J Med Eng Technol 10:299-320, 1986.

Jenkins JG, Glasgow JFT, Black CW, et al. Reye's syndrome: Assessment of intracranial monitoring. Br Med J 294:337-338, 1987.

Kaiser AM, Whitelow AGL. Intracranial pressure estimation by palpation of the anterior fontanelle. Arch Dis Child 62:516-517, 1987.

Kaktis JV. An introduction to monitoring intracranial pressure in critically ill children. Crit Care Q 3:1-8, 1980.

• Lundberg N, Kjallquist A, Kullberg G, et al. Non-operative management of intracranial hypertension. In Kuayenbuhl H, ed. Advances and Technical Standards in Neurosurgery, vol 1. Berlin: Springer-Verlag, 1974.

• McGraw CP. Continuous intracranial pressure monitoring: Review of techniques and presentation of method. Surg Neurol 6:149-155, 1976.

McGraw CS, Alexander E Jr. Durometer for measurement of intracranial pressure. Surg Neurol 7:293-295, 1977.

Mitchell P. Intracranial hypertension: Implications of research for nursing care. J Neurosurg Nurs 12:145-154, 1980.

Mollman HD, Rockswald GC, Ford SE. A clinical comparison of subarachnoid catheters to ventriculostomy and subarachnoid bolts: A prospective study. J Neurosurg 68:737-741, 1988.

Ostrop RC, Luerssen TG, Marshall LF, et al. Continuous monitoring of intracranial pressure with a miniaturized fiberoptic device. J Neurosurg 67:206-209, 1987.

Raju TWK, Vidysager D, Papazafiraton C. Intracranial pressure monitoring in the neonatal ICU. Crit Care Med 8:575-581, 1980.

Robinson RO, Rolfe P, Sutton P. Non-invasive method for measuring intracranial pressure in normal newborn infants. Dev Med Child Neurol 19:305-308, 1977.

Sundbärg G, Nordström CH, Messeter K, et al. A comparison of intraparenchymal and intraventricular pressure recording in clinical practice. J Neurosurg 67:841-845, 1987.

Vries JK, Becker DP, Young HF. A subarachnoid screw for monitoring intracranial pressure: Technical note. J Neurosurg 39:416-419, 1973.

Zeideiman C. Increased intracranial pressure in the pediatric patient: Nursing assessment and intervention. J Neurosurg Nurs 12:7-10, 1980.

119 Echocardiography

Nancy A. Ayres

BACKGROUND AND INDICATIONS

Recent advances in diagnostic ultrasound technology have dramatically changed the clinician's ability to provide accurate, noninvasive evaluations of intracardiac anatomy and cardiac function and to characterize blood flow within the heart. The three modalities of echocardiography are motion-mode (M-mode) or single-plane imaging, two-dimensional (2-D) real-time imaging, and Doppler echocardiography.

M-mode and 2-D imaging use short pulses of ultrahigh-frequency sound waves. A transducer transmits the ultrasonic wave into the body and a portion of the sound wave is reflected back to the transducer from each tissue interface. The transducer is calibrated to convert elapsed time from transmission of the sound wave to reception into a measurement of distance. Thus the spatial relationship of the reflected echoes with different acoustic densities is processed by the computer to create an image. The 2-D images provide tomographic sections of the heart and great vessels. With real-time 2-D echocardiography rapid image updating produces remarkably detailed images of intracardiac structures, valves, and myocardium in motion.

The Doppler shift of the frequency of ultrasound is a noninvasive modality used to measure the direction and velocity of blood flow within the heart and great vessels. The clinical application of 2-D and Doppler echocardiography allows accurate diagnosis of many congenital cardiac lesions, obviating the need for invasive catheterization before surgical intervention. In addition many neonates and infants coming to the PICU with symptoms of cardiogenic shock can be quickly evaluated by using 2-D echocardiography, allowing the clinician to establish or exclude cardiac disease as the cause of the shock. Several applications of M-mode, 2-D, and Doppler echocardiography are discussed.

TECHNIQUE
M-Mode Echocardiography

M-mode echocardiography is useful in determining quantitative measurements of cardiac chamber size, wall thickness, and left ventricular function. Myocardial contractility or left ventricular function is frequently expressed as a shortening fraction:

$$\frac{\text{LV end-diastolic dimension} - \text{LV end-systolic dimension}}{\text{LV end-diastolic dimension}} \times 100$$

The normal mean shortening fraction is 30% to 36%, with a range of 28% to 45%. An increased shortening fraction is found in patients with large left-to-right shunts, increased cardiac output, and volume overload. A diminished shortening fraction is found in patients with myocarditis, cardiomyopathies of various etiologies, hypoxic myocardium, cardiovascular shock, and end-stage cardiac or renal disease. By measuring sequential left ventricular shortening fractions, the myocardial response to therapeutic interventions can be periodically and noninvasively monitored.

Two-Dimensional Echocardiography

To visualize cardiac structures in the neonate or premature infant ultra-high-frequency transducers (i.e., 5.0, 7.5, 10 mHz) are necessary. Since high-frequency transducers provide poor penetration, lower frequency 3.5 to 2.25 mHz transducers are used for older children.

The tomographic cardiac images obtained from different positions along the long and short axis of the heart and great arteries allow evaluation of the size and shape of both normal and abnormal cardiac structures. The precise anatomic information revealed by 2-D ultrasonic images has revolutionized the diagnosis of complex congenital heart disease. Infants and children with septicemia, hypoglycemia, hypoxemia, pneumonia, CNS disorders, and cardiac disease frequently present with similar clinical symptoms. The neonate presenting with cardiovascular shock may have sepsis, hypoplastic left heart syndrome, critical valvar aortic stenosis, an interrupted aortic arch, severe coarctation of the aorta, myocarditis, or cardiomyopathy. Alternatively, in the cyanotic newborn, transposition of the great vessels, pulmonary valve atresia, tricuspid atresia, tetralogy of Fallot, truncus arteriosus, and total anomalous pulmonary venous return must be differentiated from pulmonary artery hypertension or pneumonia. A complete 2-D echocardiogram rapidly assists in distinguishing the structural intracardiac lesions from myocardial dysfunction.

Complications associated with prolonged use of central catheters such as intracardiac thrombi and mycotic or bacterial vegetations can be identified by 2-D imaging. In addition perforation of the atrium or the ventricle resulting in pericardial effusion is most readily recognized by 2-D imaging.

Pericardial effusions are easily identified and quantitated by using M-mode or 2-D echocardiograms. However, 2-D imaging, with its recently improved visualization of the right heart, has enabled the clinician to identify two signs of pericardial tamponade: right atrial and right ventricular diastolic collapse. These signs indicate significant hemodynamic compromise. Since the right atrial wall is thinner than the right ventricular free wall, an early sign of impending pericardial tamponade is loss of the normal convexity of the right atrial free wall. Right atrial collapse during atrial relaxation is the most sensitive and reliable sign of pericardial tamponade (Fig. 119-1).

In the cyanotic neonate who needs an atrial balloon septostomy to improve systemic oxygenation, the procedure can be safely performed with 2-D echo visualization in the PICU. The 2-D echocardiogram allows the cardiologist to position and observe the atrial septostomy catheter as it is pulled across the atrial septum and to assess the size of the atrial septal defect created. 2-D echocardiography may also be used to assist the cardiologist in placing a central catheter and in performing a pericardiocentesis.

Intracardiac shunting can be detected in patients with pulmonary hypertension or residual cardiac defects after cardiac surgery. Intracardiac shunting can be visualized using 2 D imaging of the heart while several milliliters of agitated 0.9% sodium chloride solution or the patient's blood are rapidly injected. The injection creates microcavitations that are detected by ultrasound and that opacify the various cardiac chambers as the injectate progresses through

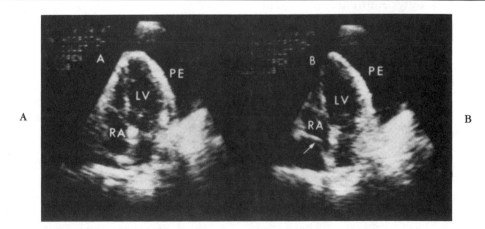

Fig. 119-1 These apical four-chamber 2-D echocardiograms demonstrate a patient with a large pericardial effusion *(PE)*. The right atrial *(RA)* free wall has a normal orientation in **A**; however, a diastolic frame (**B**) demonstrates collapse (arrow) of the right atrial free wall. *LV,* Left ventricle. (From Feigenbaum H. Echocardiography, 4th ed. Philadelphia: Lea & Febiger, 1986.)

the heart. The microcavitations are cleared from the blood by passing through the lungs. Thus right-to-left shunting is detected by opacification of the left heart by the microcavitations injected into the right heart. In most cases the site of shunting is detected by visualizing the microcavitations passing across a defect in the atrial or ventricular septum. To demonstrate left-to-right shunting agitated saline solution or blood must be infused into the left ventricle or atrium. However, the use of Doppler echocardiography is rapidly replacing this method of detecting intracardiac shunting.

Doppler Echocardiography

The most recent advancement in ultrasound is Doppler echocardiography, which provides noninvasive determination of the direction and velocity of blood flow, pressure differences, valvular regurgitation, intracardiac and valvular stenoses, and intracardiac shunting.

To measure the velocity of blood two Doppler techniques are used: continuous wave (CW) and pulsed wave (PW) ultrasound. The CW Doppler technique has no limit on the maximum velocity for measurement; thus higher flow velocities are most accurately determined using the CW mode. With the PW mode the time needed to receive the echoed signal is a function of depth of the reflecting surface; thus depth is defined, but the maximum velocity is limited. Therefore CW and PW Doppler complement each other by respectively determining the maximum velocity and position of flow.

The most common application of Doppler echocardiography is to predict a pressure difference across an obstruction by using the modified Bernoulli equation, which states the pressure difference (mm Hg) $= 4V^2$, where V is the peak velocity of flow across an area. Thus the difference across a stenotic valve, pulmonary artery band, intracardiac membrane, or a ventricular septal defect is estimated by using the Doppler technique. In addition the pulmonary artery blood pressure may be estimated from pulmonary or tricuspid regurgitation if no pulmonary obstruction is present. To estimate the peak systolic pulmonary artery blood pressure, the mean right atrial blood pressure (which may be assumed to be 5 mm Hg) is added to the peak pressure difference predicted from the regurgitant jet across the tricuspid valve or to the diastolic pulmonary artery blood pressure predicted from regurgitant jet across the pulmonary valve. The noninvasive estimation of the systolic pulmonary artery blood pressure may be useful in the patient with pulmonary hypertension or chronic lung disease.

Doppler evaluations of pulmonary blood flow in the cyanotic neonate with pulmonary atresia, pulmonary stenosis, or severe tetralogy of Fallot enables one to determine whether these infants depend on ductal blood flow for pulmonary perfusion or have antegrade blood flow into the pulmonary artery. In addition, for the neonate with critical pulmonary or aortic valve stenosis, Doppler-predicted pressure gradients allow the cardiologist to make necessary decisions about surgical interventions without performing cardiac catheterization. Moreover, Doppler evaluation of the ill premature infant has markedly improved the sensitivity and specificity of diagnosing the presence of a patent ductus arteriosus (PDA). When a PDA is present, the left-to-right shunting is displayed by the Doppler technique as a continuous or bidirectional flow pattern in the pulmonary artery and descending aorta. In addition the relative degree of shunting through the PDA may be defined by an echocardiographic Doppler study. The accuracy of a Doppler study in conjunction with a 2-D echocardiogram has alleviated the need for invasive diagnostic catheterizations in many critically ill newborns.

Doppler echocardiography is used to define the source of a new or residual murmur in the critically ill child or in the child after cardiac surgery. AV valve insufficiency frequently occurs in patients with left ventricular dysfunction. The degree of valvar insufficiency can be quantitated and mapped by performing a complete Doppler study. Cardiac output can also be estimated by a Doppler study. However, the measurements necessary to calculate cardiac output are tedious to obtain, and the results are variable. Thus at this time the Doppler technique has not replaced thermodilution determinations of cardiac output in most PICUs.

The most recent addition to Doppler ultrasound technology is color flow. With color Doppler technology the blood flow patterns are superimposed on the 2-D echo image. The Doppler signal is assigned a color based on computer analysis of the velocity, turbulence, and direction of blood flow. Flow toward the transducer is usually coded red, whereas blood flow from the transducer is coded blue. Greater intensities of color indicate higher flow velocities. Thus color Doppler imaging provides direct visualization of the anatomy in conjunction with display of intra-cardiac flow by rapidly updating color images. Because of their thin chest wall, color Doppler images are sharper in children than in adults and provide more information for diagnosis. Color Doppler imaging has improved the accuracy of detecting lesions such as septal defects, valvular regurgitation, and peak flow velocities across stenotic areas.

The tremendous advancements of 2-D, Doppler, and color Doppler echocardiography over the past few years could fill several books. The purpose of this chapter is to introduce the field of echocardiography and allow better understanding of the uses and limitations of echocardiography since the abilities of skilled technologists and echocardiographers are needed to assist in the interpretation of most studies.

RISKS AND COMPLICATIONS

There are no known risks or complications associated with these techniques.

ADDITIONAL READING

Feigenbaum H. Echocardiography, 4th ed. Philadelphia: Lea & Febiger, 1986.

Goldberg SJ, Allen HD, Marx GR, Flinn CJ. Doppler Echocardiography. Philadelphia: Lea & Febiger, 1985.

Goldberg SJ, Allen HD, Sahn DJ. Pediatric and Adolescent Echocardiography, 2nd ed. Chicago: Year Book, 1980.

120 Transcutaneous Oxygen Monitoring

David A. Hicks · Nick G. Anas

BACKGROUND AND INDICATIONS

The development of noninvasive monitoring of blood gas tensions has evolved from the need to assess continuously the critically ill patient's pulmonary (gas exchange) function and to evaluate rapidly the response to therapeutic intervention. The measurement of blood gas tensions at the surface of the skin is made possible by a technology that is simple to use and painless for the patient. In contrast with PaO_2 and $PaCO_2$ determinations in which the values reflect the partial pressure of the gases in blood, the transcutaneous oxygen tension ($PtcO_2$) and carbon dioxide tension ($PtcCO_2$) values reflect both gas exchange (i.e., PaO_2 and $PaCO_2$) and skin perfusion (i.e, cardiac output).

Gas exchange occurs at the surface of the skin, and the epidermis is provided with microcirculation far in excess of its metabolic requirements. Oxygen diffuses from the upper portion (dome) of the epidermal capillary loops to the skin surface at a rate that is determined by (1) the PO_2 gradient between the blood and skin surface, (2) the diffusion properties of the multiple layers of the skin, and (3) the oxygen delivery to and oxygen consumption of the skin. Therefore the $PtcO_2$ value is a measure of tissue PO_2 and is determined by the following factors: the arterial oxygen tension (PaO_2), cardiac output, systemic vascular resistance (SVR), capillary density, mitochondrial oxygen use, and skin thickness. Therefore $PtcO_2$ monitoring cannot be used independently to measure either the PaO_2 or cardiac output. The $PtcO_2$ value approximates the PaO_2 only under conditions of hemodynamic and metabolic stability. The ratio of $PtcO_2$ to PaO_2 is referred to as the $PtcO_2$ index and provides a means for interpreting the $PtcO_2$ value. As the index approaches unity, $PtcO_2$ monitoring be-

comes a means of following the patient's PaO_2 and therefore pulmonary (gas exchange) function. During shock states the index approaches zero, and $PtcO_2$ monitoring becomes a marker of the adequacy of cardiac output and peripheral (tissue) perfusion. In other words, the $PtcO_2$ index reflects the extent to which the $PtcO_2$ values are either PaO_2 dependent or flow dependent.

To determine whether a change in the $PtcO_2$ is primarily related to a respiratory or to a circulatory derangement, a simultaneous PaO_2 measurement must be obtained, and an assessment of cardiac output must be performed (either directly by thermodilution techniques or indirectly by the physical examination and laboratory findings described in Chapter 12). Studies have demonstrated that in patients with a cardiac index >2.2 L/min/m^2, the $PtcO_2$ correlates well with the PaO_2. When the cardiac index is <1.5 L/min/m^2, there is poor correlation between the $PtcO_2$ and PaO_2 (a reduced $PtcO_2$ index) but close correlation between the $PtcO_2$ and the cardiac index. Table 120-1 summarizes the use of $PtcO_2$ as a marker of the PaO_2 or cardiac output.

Other physiologic principles must be understood when using $PtcO_2$ monitoring. Because the $PtcO_2$ value is blood flow dependent, the presence of a stable systemic arterial blood pressure (BP) does not guarantee good correlation between the $PtcO_2$ and PaO_2. Systemic arterial blood pressure may be maintained in the presence of reduced cardiac output by a concomitant increase in SVR (BP = CO × SVR), and this phenomenon is particularly common in pediatric patients. For example, studies have demonstrated that during hypovolemic shock, the patient's systemic arterial blood pressure does not decrease until the cardiac output is reduced to 75% of its baseline value and yet peripheral perfusion may be significantly compromised.

The effect of cardiac output on $Ptco_2$ monitoring is demonstrated further in animal studies of the use of positive end-expiratory pressure (PEEP) in an ARDS model. As PEEP was progressively increased, the $Ptco_2$ followed the improving Pao_2 only until the cardiac output became adversely affected (see Chapter 128). When the cardiac index declined, the $Ptco_2$ decreased and correlated with oxygen delivery. The maximum $Ptco_2$ values corresponded to the maximum mixed venous tension ($P\bar{v}o_2$) or the minimal arteriovenous oxygen content difference ($a\text{-}vDo_2$).

Other factors that reduce the correlation between the $Ptco_2$ and Pao_2 include the finding that the $Ptco_2$ index falls as the Pao_2 becomes more abnormal (e.g., <70 mm Hg). The linearity of this relationship is lost as the patient becomes more hypoxemic, even in the presence of adequate peripheral perfusion. Finally, conditions of deep hypothermia (which reduces cutaneous circulation), excessive edema, and extreme obesity limit the use of tco_2 monitoring.

The clinical circumstances in which tco_2 monitoring has proved most valuable include:

1. Assessment of neonates and infants with respiratory distress syndrome, shock states, and ductus arteriosus right-to-left shunting
2. Intraoperative monitoring of gas exchange and cardiac output
3. Fetal and maternal oxygen tension monitoring
4. Continuous assessment of patients during transport
5. Initial stabilization of patients needing either mechanical ventilation or inotropic support or both
6. Assessment of the adequacy of tissue oxygen delivery to skin flaps and to patients with burns

Monitoring of the neonate and infant with respiratory distress and/or shock syndromes has been improved by the use of transcutaneous techniques. Monitoring of tco_2 allows better control of the Pao_2, thereby avoiding the extremes of hypoxemia and hyperoxemia, and allows rapid detection of hypoxemia, which could result in life-threatening bradycardia or apnea if undetected and untreated. The effect of procedures during which patients are moved and disturbed, such as weighing and feeding, can be more accurately determined; smoother, safer weaning from supplemental oxygen can be accomplished; and sleep hypoxemia can be more easily documented. Simultaneous measurement of $Ptco_2$ at pre- and postductal sites (e.g., right arm and abdomen, respectively) may provide evidence of right-to-left shunting at the level of the ductus arteriosus caused by pulmonary artery hypertension. Furthermore, $Ptco_2$ monitoring can detect a reduction in oxygenation more rapidly than can noninvasive oxygen saturation (Sao_2) monitoring when the Pao_2 values exceed 90 to 100 mm Hg. With reduced cardiac output the $Ptco_2$ will fall as peripheral perfusion worsens; simultaneously, the heat output of the sensor will increase to compensate for the loss of cutaneous blood flow (see below). The $Ptco_2$ value then becomes a gauge of peripheral oxygen delivery.

TECHNIQUE

The tco_2 sensor uses a standard Clark polarographic electrode that is modified so that it can be heated and mounted on the skin (Fig. 120-1). The basic principle of the polarographic O_2 electrode involves the reaction of oxygen with a metal surface. A silver chloride cathode and a platinum anode are placed in a buffered solution that is retained by a semipermeable membrane. Oxygen diffuses across the membrane

Table 120-1 $Ptco_2$ as a Guide to Pao_2 and Cardiac Output

$Ptco_2$	Pao_2	Cardiac Output	Interpretation
Reduced	Reduced	Unchanged	Hypoxemia
Reduced	Unchanged	Reduced	Shock
Reduced	Reduced	Reduced	Reduced oxygen delivery
No change	Unknown	Unknown	Uninterpretable
Increased	Increased	Unchanged	Hyperoxia
Increased	Unchanged	Increased	Improved perfusion

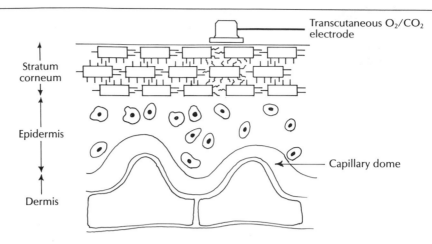

Fig. 120-1   Placement of a dual O_2/CO_2 sensor and a cross-sectional display of the skin layers and capillary bed through which gas exchange occurs at the skin surface.

and is reduced on contact with the platinum, yielding electrons that generate a current that is proportional to the Po_2. Under usual conditions oxygen flow through the skin is relatively low, and the measured $Ptco_2$ is much less than the Pao_2. This problem is minimized by heating the skin surface, thus increasing oxygen diffusion, causing a rightward shift of the oxyhemoglobin dissociation curve, and inducing hyperemia. The polarographic electrode is capable of varying the heat output to maintain the skin surface at a fixed temperature.

Calibration of the sensor is performed at two points. The zero point is checked with a null solution (sodium bisulfate), and room air is used as the high point. The electrode is then fixed to the skin by placing a drop of electrolyte solution between the semipermeable membrane and skin to facilitate oxygen diffusion. The heating coil is then energized, and the electrode temperature is maintained at 43° to 45° C. The warm-up time for the tco_2 monitor at the skin surface is approximately 10 to 15 minutes.

RISKS AND COMPLICATIONS

Pitfalls in tco_2 monitoring are related to misunderstanding the physiologic principles described previously. To reiterate, the $Ptco_2$ value is both Pao_2 and flow dependent. Accurate interpretation of changes in the $Ptco_2$ value necessitates obtaining a simultaneous determination of the Pao_2 and cardiac output

(or other physical examination and laboratory indicators of the adequacy of peripheral perfusion). Thus the $Ptco_2$ value most accurately reflects tissue oxygen delivery.

Practical clinical considerations include the presence of skin burns and calibration errors. There is always a potential for causing an electrode-size skin burn with the heated $Ptco_2$ electrode (*burn* is defined as a blister or second-degree injury). The incidence of burns is a function of the electrode temperature and the length of time the electrode remains in the same location. Studies have shown that burns are prevented by adhering to the following rules regarding temperature and duration of monitoring at a single site: for premature babies, 43° C for 2 hours; for newborn babies, 43.5° C for 4 hours; and for children, 44° C for 6 hours. Even with proper use, a hyperemic spot that fades in 24 to 48 hours remains on the skin after each use.

As with any type of electrical equipment, proper calibration with minimal drift is important to maintain accurate monitoring. In practice most drift is at the high calibration point (room air). Therefore this point must be checked before each use. The low (zero) calibration point is usually more stable and only needs checking after a membrane is changed. The electrode membrane must be changed when the drift exceeds 1% per hour; if properly treated, the membrane lasts for 1 week or more.

ADDITIONAL READING

• Brown M, Vender JS. Noninvasive oxygen monitoring. Crit Care Clin 4:499, 1988.

Hansen T, Tooley W. Skin surface carbon dioxide tension in sick infants. Pediatrics 64:942, 1979.

Herrell N, Martin RJ, Pultusker M, et al. Optimal temperature for the measurement of transcutaneous carbon dioxide tension in the neonate. J Pediatr 97:114, 1980.

Merritt T, Liyamasawd S, Boettrich C, et al. Skin surface CO_2 measurements in sick preterm and term infants. J Pediatr 99:782, 1981.

• Stock MC. Noninvasive carbon dioxide monitoring. Crit Care Clin 4:522, 1988.

Tabata BK, Kirsch JR, Rogers MC. Transcutaneous blood gas measurements. In Rogers MC, ed. Textbook of Pediatric Intensive Care. Baltimore: Williams & Wilkins, 1987, p 1423.

Tremper KK, Mentelos RA, Shoemaker WC. Effect of hypercarbia and shock on transcutaneous carbon dioxide at different electrode temperatures. Crit Care Med 8:608, 1980.

Tremper KK, Shoemaker WC. Transcutaneous oxygen monitoring of critically ill adults with and without low flow shock. Crit Care Med 9:706, 1981.

Tremper KK, Shoemaker WC, Shippy CR, et al. Transcutaneous P_{CO_2} monitoring on adult patients in the ICU and the operating room. Crit Care Med 9:752, 1981.

121 Transcutaneous Carbon Dioxide Monitoring

David A. Hicks · Nick G. Anas

BACKGROUND AND INDICATIONS
(see also Chapter 120)

The transcutaneous CO_2 tension ($PtcCO_2$) must exceed the capillary and arterial PCO_2 to provide the gradient necessary to transport carbon dioxide out of the tissue beds and into the venous circulation. The $PtcCO_2$ exceeds the $PaCO_2$ in neonates by a mean of 15 to 20 mm Hg and in adults by 10 to 35 mm Hg. If the gradient between $PtcCO_2$ and $PaCO_2$ remains constant, the $PtcCO_2$ becomes an accurate monitor of the $PaCO_2$. The correlation between the $PtcCO_2$ and $PaCO_2$ is greater than for $PtcO_2$ and PaO_2; the linear correlation coefficient approximates 0.8 to 0.9 in patients with adequate cardiovascular function. A reduction in cardiac output increases the $PtcCO_2$ value but has a minimal effect on the $PaCO_2$. In adults, when the cardiac index falls to <1.5 L/min/m^2, the $PtcCO_2$ is inversely related to the cardiac index, and quantitatively the $PtcCO_2$ and $PaCO_2$ changes correlate poorly. As in $PtcO_2$ monitoring, the degree of shock can be assessed by measuring the $PtcCO_2$-$PaCO_2$ gradient; a larger gradient reflects poor peripheral perfusion. Acidosis and hypoxemia will also increase the $PtcCO_2$ value out of proportion to an increase in $PaCO_2$.

The $PtcCO_2$ response to changes in $PaCO_2$ is slow at 3 to 4 minutes. Nonetheless, in the presence of stable hemodynamic and metabolic function, $tcCO_2$ monitoring provides a useful gauge of alveolar ventilation. Clinical circumstances in which $tcCO_2$ monitoring has been shown to be valuable include ventilator management of the patient with respiratory distress and/or shock, transport of the critically ill neonate or infant, and performance of invasive procedures such as bronchoscopy and cardiac catheterization. Newborns and young infants with respiratory distress and shock syndromes have benefited most from $PtcCO_2$ monitoring, since these populations represent the groups in whom the correlation between $PtcCO_2$ and $PaCO_2$ is greatest and in whom invasive blood gas monitoring is often more difficult and tedious to attain. Monitoring of $tcCO_2$ also is useful in the operating room to monitor gas exchange in the hemodynamically stable child.

TECHNIQUE

The $tcCO_2$ probe that is applied to the patient's skin contains a heater, an electrode, and a thermistor. Similar to the tcO_2 system, warming softens the skin, thereby making the physical barrier to diffusion more permeable; it also results in capillary dilatation and augments carbon dioxide production locally. Warming the skin to 44° C increases the response time to $PaCO_2$ changes and is necessary to obtain clinically useful $PtcCO_2$ values. The electrode is an outgrowth of Severinghaus' modification of Stowe's electrochemical sensor that is commonly used in blood gas analyzers. The typical $tcCO_2$ sensor consists of a pH-sensitive glass electrode, a silver chloride reference electrode, a membrane permeable to carbon dioxide, and a bicarbonate electrolyte solution. After the skin is warmed, carbon dioxide diffuses through the Teflon membrane into the bicarbonate solution. The CO_2 reacts with H_2O to form H_2CO_3, which dissociates into H^+ and HCO_3^-. The H^+ production alters the pH of the solution, increasing the electrical potential between the glass electrode and the reference electrode. This change in electrical potential is converted to millimeters of mercury and is displayed as the $PtcCO_2$ value.

A new probe necessitates a warm-up period of approximately 1 hour to allow the electrolyte solution to distribute evenly over the glass electrode, which is fragile and expensive.

Calibration of the equipment generally is performed in vitro at high and low carbon dioxide concentrations (e.g., 5%, 10%) and in vivo by comparing the $Ptcco_2$ value with a simultaneously obtained $Paco_2$ value.

RISKS AND COMPLICATIONS

As with $Ptco_2$ monitoring, $Ptcco_2$ monitoring is inaccurate or invalid if the observer is unaware of the physiologic determinants of its value. Therefore changes in the $Ptcco_2$ must be compared to the $Paco_2$ and to the state of peripheral perfusion.

Burns of the skin surface occur if the site is not changed every 2 to 4 hours, if the thermostat that controls skin temperature fails, or if hypotension reduces peripheral perfusion, resulting in poor dissipation of heat.

• • •

In summary, both $Ptco_2$ and $Ptcco_2$ monitoring offer noninvasive means of following blood gas exchange and tissue perfusion in critically ill children.

Electrodes that simultaneously monitor both $Ptco_2$ and $Ptcco_2$ are available, but warming of the skin, scrupulous attention to details such as calibration, frequent changing of the monitoring site to prevent burns, and a comparison with arterial blood gas tensions and tissue perfusion are necessary. These techniques provide a way to rapidly assess the gas-exchange status of the patients and their response to therapeutic intervention and allow increased safety for the patient during such procedures as transport, bronchoscopy, cardiac catheterization, and surgery.

ADDITIONAL READING

Hansen T, Tooley W. Skin surface carbon dioxide tension in sick infants. Pediatrics 64:942, 1979.

Herrell N, Martin RJ, Pultusker M, et al. Optimal temperature for the measurement of transcutaneous carbon dioxide tension in the neonate. J Pediatr 97:114, 1980.

Stock MC. Noninvasive carbon dioxide monitoring. Crit Care Clin 4:522, 1988.

Tremper KK, Mentelos RA, Shoemaker WC. Effect of hypercarbia and shock on transcutaneous carbon dioxide at different electrode temperatures. Crit Care Med 8:608, 1980.

122 Oxygen Saturation Monitoring

David A. Hicks · Nick G. Anas

BACKGROUND AND INDICATIONS

The measurements of arterial oxygen saturation (SaO_2) and tension (PaO_2) are used in the management of PICU patients with cardiopulmonary disorders to assess the adequacy of systemic oxygenation. In conjunction with cardiac output and hemoglobin concentration the SaO_2 determines oxygen availability or delivery to the vital organs; the PaO_2 represents the maximal tension driving oxygen to its mitochondrial sites of use. Hypoxemia (PaO_2 <50 mm Hg or SaO_2 <90%) is the result of a reduced alveolar oxygen (PAO_2) concentration, alterations of ventilation-perfusion ($\dot{V}/\dot{Q}$) matching, disruption of diffusion of oxygen across the alveolar-capillary membrane, or depression of cardiac output (see Chapter 10).

The relationship of SaO_2 to PaO_2 is expressed by the oxyhemoglobin dissociation curve (Fig. 122-1). The dissociation curve is sigmoidal in shape. At PaO_2 values >60 mm Hg the curve flattens and demonstrates that hemoglobin is maximally saturated; therefore hemoglobin molecules exposed to the high concentration of oxygen within the alveoli will be transported to peripheral vascular beds nearly 100% saturated. At PaO_2 values <60 mm Hg the curve is steep and demonstrates that small changes in oxygen tension result in large changes in hemoglobin saturation. Therefore a small reduction in PaO_2 results in greater unloading of oxygen from hemoglobin and increases the gradient for oxygen delivery to tissue vascular beds.

The position of the oxyhemoglobin dissociation curve may shift to the right or left, reflecting changes in the affinity of hemoglobin for oxygen. The quaternary structure of the hemoglobin molecule regulates its affinity for oxygen and is altered by several factors: arterial carbon dioxide tension ($PaCO_2$), hy-

drogen ion concentration (pH), body temperature, the hemoglobin concentration of 2,3-diphosphoglycerate (2,3-DPG), and the type of hemoglobin. The PaO_2 value at which the hemoglobin molecule is 50% saturated (P_{50}) is used as an index of the relative position of the oxyhemoglobin dissociation curve. The "normal" P_{50} is 27 mm Hg (i.e., assuming normal body temperature, pH, $PaCO_2$, and red blood cell 2,3-DPG content, hemoglobin is 50% saturated when the PaO_2 value is 27 mm Hg). A shift to the right of the

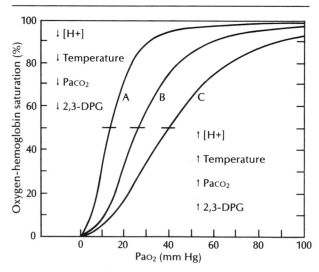

Fig. 122-1 Oxyhemoglobin saturation curve. *B*, Normal. Abnormalities that result in an increased, *A*, or a decreased, *C*, affinity of the hemoglobin molecule for oxygen are shown beside the outer curves. The P_{50} value for each curve is represented by a horizontal dash at the 50% saturation level.

curve (i.e., increased P_{50}) implies a lowered affinity of oxygen for hemoglobin. Conversely, a shift to the left (i.e., decreased P_{50}) means that oxygen is bound more avidly to hemoglobin.

Acidosis, hypercapnia, and hyperthermia (variables that reflect stress or disease) shift the curve to the right (Fig. 122-1) so that SaO_2 is reduced at any given PaO_2. This shift allows oxygen unloading to tissues under stress to occur more readily. Alkalosis, hypocapnia, and hypothermia increase the affinity of oxygen for hemoglobin, thereby reducing the P_{50}. This results in a reduced PaO_2 relative to SaO_2 and limits the delivery of oxygen to cellular mitochondria. For example, when alkalosis is induced to reduce pulmonary arterial blood pressure or when hypocapnia is used to treat intracranial hypertension, oxygen delivery and use may be impaired by the leftward shift of the oxyhemoglobin dissociation curve.

2,3-DPG also regulates oxygen affinity for hemoglobin. It lowers hemoglobin affinity by binding to beta chains of hemoglobin A or to gamma chains of hemoglobin F (fetal hemoglobin). For example, anemia leads to increased 2,3-DPG levels (increases the P_{50}), whereas storage of bank blood with acid-citrate-dextrose (ACD) preservation results in depletion of 2,3-DPG (reduces the P_{50}).

The type of hemoglobin may determine oxygen binding. For example, fetal and sickle cell hemoglobins more avidly bind oxygen than does hemoglobin A. Methemoglobin is a hemoglobin molecule in which iron is oxidized; therefore it cannot bind oxygen (see Chapter 49). Tissue hypoxia and acidosis occur when methemoglobin levels exceed 30%. Finally, oxygen binding may be inhibited by substances with greater affinity for hemoglobin such as carbon monoxide (therefore the SaO_2 is reduced). Carbon monoxide also limits oxygen delivery by reducing the P_{50} (i.e., shifting the oxyhemoglobin dissociation curve to the left).

Indications for using continuous pulse oximetry are as follows:

1. Management of critically ill patients in the PICU
2. During transport of patients both within and between hospitals
3. Pre- and postoperative assessment of systemic oxygenation
4. Perioperative manipulations to improve systemic oxygenation
5. Polysomnography (sleep) studies
6. Radiographic or invasive monitoring procedures that place the patient in a high-risk situation
7. Home care of oxygen-dependent children
8. Heavy sedation of the patient

TECHNIQUE

SaO_2 monitoring (in conjunction with the assessment of cardiac output, hemoglobin concentration, pH, urinary output, and mental status) is invaluable in determining the adequacy of systemic oxygenation. If SaO_2 monitoring is used along with mixed venous saturation ($S\bar{v}O_2$) measurements, the relationship of oxygen consumption to oxygen delivery can be used to follow and dictate therapeutic interventions (see Chapter 124). In the absence of technology capable of measuring the PaO_2 and oxygen consumption in specific tissue beds (e.g., brain, myocardium, kidney), continuous systemic oxygen measurements provide the most reliable description of the cardiorespiratory state of the patient and responses to therapy. As a generalization, SaO_2 monitoring provides a gauge of pulmonary function by demonstrating trends that reflect the adequacy of gas exchange.

An ideal monitoring system must include the following capabilities. (1) It must be continuous; intermittently obtained information from critically ill patients may not accurately reflect the trend and is less useful than continuous data in assessing the response to a therapeutic intervention. (2) Monitoring must be as noninvasive as possible, must not be painful to the patient, and must depend on minimal patient cooperation. Invasive procedures are often painful and increase the risk of complications such as infection. (3) Finally, the data that are collected must be valuable to the medical staff in terms of management. Continuous pulse oximetry meets these criteria, explaining its widespread acceptance in the care of PICU patients. In addition the numerical readout of oxygen saturation is easily interpreted by all members of the health care team. Over the last 5 years noninvasive continuous SaO_2 monitoring has replaced intermittent intra-arterial sampling as the optimal method for determining the adequacy and trend of systemic oxygenation in critically ill patients.

The technique of continuous pulse oximetry is based on the following principles: (1) the color of blood is a function of SaO_2; (2) the optical properties of hemoglobin determine the color of blood at var-

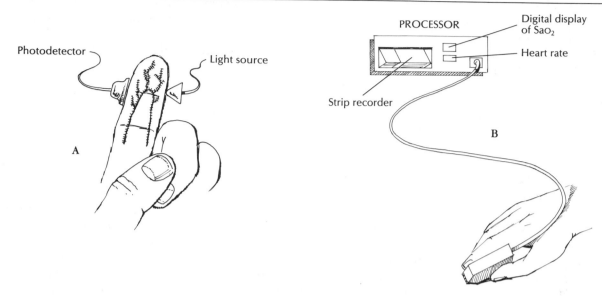

Fig. 122-2   A, Oximeter probe-detector and light source. **B,** Finger pickup and oximeter. The strip chart can be useful for a permanent record.

ious SaO$_2$ levels; and (3) the total absorption of a system of absorbers is the sum of their individual absorbances (Beer-Lambert law). In most of the commercially available pulse oximeters two wavelengths of light (red and infrared) are used to determine the ratio of oxygenated hemoglobin to deoxygenated hemoglobin. Visible red light (660 nm) is absorbed more by deoxygenated hemoglobin than by oxyhemoglobin; infrared light (940 nm) is absorbed more by oxyhemoglobin than deoxygenated hemoglobin. These two wavelengths of light (red and infrared) are passed through the chosen arterial bed (e.g., finger, heel, earlobe), and the percent oxyhemoglobin and deoxygenated hemoglobin are determined by measuring the ratio of infrared and red light transmitted to the photodetector (Fig. 122-2). This type of analysis excludes the measurement of other hemoglobin molecules that may be present, such as methemoglobin or carboxyhemoglobin (two conditions, for example, in which continuous pulse oximetry provides misleading or inaccurate information).

Continuous pulse oximetry also provides measurement of heart rate independent from that obtained from impedance chest wall leads. The pulsating vascular bed in the site chosen for monitoring creates a change in the light path length that modifies the amount of the light detected. The oximeter determines the pulse rate from the change in the amount of light that is absorbed from systole to diastole. The SaO$_2$ value is accurate only if the heart rate as measured by the pulse oximeter correlates with the heart rate as determined either by chest wall impedance or by palpation.

The application of the continuous pulse oximeter is simple. The use of digits (or the heel in a newborn) provides easy access and multiple sites. No heat pretreatment to "arterialize" the bed is necessary, as is the case with transcutaneous oxygen and carbon dioxide monitoring systems. A microprocessor performs the calibration, measurements, and readout functions, making it easy to use. The initial reading occurs within 10 to 15 seconds of application of the probe. The probes available are small, relatively inexpensive, disposable, and durable (Fig. 122-2).

Continuous pulse oximetry has obviated the need for intra-arterial monitoring in most circumstances. The use of arterial blood samples for SaO$_2$ measurements is indicated in those instances in which noninvasive measurement is not possible or is inaccurate (see below).

RISKS AND COMPLICATIONS

For the purposes of this discussion, risks and complications of continuous, noninvasive SaO_2 monitoring are defined as those situations in which this technique provides inaccurate, misleading, or insufficient information.

Inaccurate measurements occur in situations in which there is significant reduction in vascular pulsation, which is detected by a discrepancy between the oximeter heart rate measurement as compared to that obtained by chest wall impedance, palpation, or auscultation. These situations include hypotension, hypothermia, peripheral vasoconstriction, and motion artifact. Motion artifact limits the use of oximetry in circumstances in which the patient and monitor are unobserved and a hard copy readout of SaO_2 values is obtained (e.g., home sleep studies). Newer technologies will soon be available that measure heart rate independent of vascular pulsation, allowing the detection of motion artifact as a cause of a reduced SaO_2. An additional source of error is introduced by extraneous light sources consisting of wavelengths near the measured frequencies (e.g., infrared radiation heaters and ultraviolet phototherapy for treating hyperbilirubinemia). Injection of dyes such as methylene blue, indigo carmine, indocyanine green, and fluorescein also interferes with SaO_2 measurements. Finally, the present technology does not provide accurate data when SaO_2 falls below 50%.

Misleading information is obtained in the following situations. Because only oxyhemoglobin and reduced hemoglobin are detected by pulse oximetry, the presence of abnormal hemoglobin types such as carboxyhemoglobin or methemoglobin can lead generally to an overestimation of the true SaO_2. In these circumstances intra-arterial sampling and measurement of SaO_2 by co-oximetry is necessary for accurate determinations. Several problems are related to the shape of the oxyhemoglobin dissociation curve (i.e., the fact that SaO_2 and PaO_2 are not linearly related throughout the wide range of possible PaO_2 values). A significant reduction in PaO_2 (e.g., from 300 to 90 mm Hg) may occur without a change in SaO_2 (i.e., SaO_2 will remain at 98% to 100%). In this situation a physiologically significant event is not detected by the pulse oximeter. More commonly, a reduction in SaO_2 from 98% to 92% will not be appreciated as significant, even though it reflects a decrease in PaO_2 (e.g., from 100 to 70 mm Hg) and represents a position much closer to the steep portion of the oxy-

hemoglobin dissociation curve. Another situation in which the shape of the curve may be responsible for misleading information is that in which hypoxemia occurs as a result of hypoventilation. As a rule the reduction in PaO_2 that results from hypoventilation is inversely proportional to the increase in $PaCO_2$ (see Chapter 10). For example, in a patient breathing room air an increase in $PaCO_2$ from 40 to 60 mm Hg will result in a reduction in PaO_2 from 100 to 80 mm Hg, with little if any change in the SaO_2 value. This phenomenon will be further masked by the administration of supplemental oxygen, which may allow a reduction of PaO_2 from 150 to 130 mm Hg but no change in SaO_2 when hypoventilation has resulted in a 20 mm Hg increase in the $PaCO_2$ value.

Misleading information also occurs because of changes in the position of the oxyhemoglobin dissociation curve. A reduced P_{50} indicates that oxygen is bound to hemoglobin more avidly; therefore, for any given PaO_2 value, the SaO_2 will be higher than if the curve were in the normal position. A patient in whom alkalosis or hypocapnia has been induced will demonstrate a greater SaO_2 value relative to the PaO_2, and the degree of intrapulmonary shunt will not be appreciated (or accurately calculated) using SaO_2 measurements as a guide.

Conditions exist in which insufficient information is provided by noninvasive pulse oximetry. This may result in misapplication of the data. Specifically, oxygen delivery depends on cardiac output and hemoglobin concentration as well as on SaO_2. A reduction in SaO_2 may be accompanied by an increase in cardiac output that is sufficient to maintain adequate oxygen delivery. Additionally, oxygen delivery and oxygen consumption are not consistently related in all circumstances (e.g., oxygen consumption is reduced relative to delivery in patients with ARDS); thus simultaneous determination of the $S\bar{v}O_2$ values may be necessary to evaluate the adequacy of SaO_2 (see Chapter 124).

• • •

The availability of continuous pulse oximetry has improved the early detection of changes in systemic oxygenation and has resulted in a more rapid response to adverse alterations in gas exchange. The technology is safe, accurate, and easy to use, and the data displayed are useful, particularly if the user is aware of the potential for obtaining misleading or insufficient information.

ADDITIONAL READING

• Barker SJ, Tremper KK. Advances in oxygen monitoring: Pulse oximetry: Applications and limitations. Int Anesthesiol Clin 15:3, 1987.

Boyson PG, Broome JA. Noninvasive monitoring of lung function during mechanical ventilation. Crit Care Clin 4:527, 1988.

Brown M, Vender JS. Noninvasive oxygen monitoring. Crit Care Clin 4:493, 1988.

Bryan-Brown CW, Baek SM, Makebali G, et al. Consumable oxygen: Availability in relation to oxyhemoglobin dissociation. Crit Care Med 1:17, 1973.

Cohen DE, Downes JJ, Raphaely RC. What difference does pulse oximetry make? Anesthesiology 68:181, 1988.

Fanconi S, Doherty P, Edmonds J, et al. Pulse oximetry in pediatric intensive care: Comparison with measured saturations and transcutaneous oxygen tension. J Pediatr 107:362, 1985.

Marin JJ. Monitoring during mechanical ventilation. Clin Chest Med 9:73, 1988.

• Nichols DG, Rogers MC. Developmental physiology of the respiratory system. In Rogers MC, ed. Textbook of Pediatric Intensive Care. Baltimore: Williams & Wilkins, 1987, p 100.

123 End-Tidal Carbon Dioxide Monitoring (Capnography)

Nick G. Anas

BACKGROUND AND INDICATIONS

End-tidal carbon dioxide ($etCO_2$) monitoring, or capnography, is the measurement and display in waveform of carbon dioxide concentration in exhaled gases. The value of noninvasive monitoring of blood gas tensions is the ability to follow continuously the patient's pulmonary (i.e., gas-exchange) function and to assess immediately the response to therapeutic intervention. The $etCO_2$ concentration is a function of the following factors: (1) the arterial carbon dioxide tension ($Paco_2$), (2) the cardiac output, (3) the percent dead space ventilation (V_D/V_T), and (4) airway time constants. Thus $etCO_2$ monitoring can be used to follow the adequacy of alveolar ventilation, to estimate changes in the patient's metabolic status (i.e., production of carbon dioxide), to evaluate the adequacy of cardiac output, and to assess pulmonary perfusion relative to alveolar ventilation (i.e., the percent dead space ventilation). The limitations of capnography are related to the fact that there are multiple determinants of the $etCO_2$ value (see Chapter 10).

As a method for assessing alveolar ventilation, capnography is valid when the $Paco_2$ is equal to the end-tidal carbon dioxide tension ($Petco_2$). The $Paco_2$ value is determined by the Pco_2 of perfused alveoli (whether or not they are ventilated), whereas the $Petco_2$ value represents the Pco_2 of all ventilated alveoli (whether or not they are perfused). Any condition that reduces pulmonary perfusion of ventilated alveoli (i.e., increases dead space ventilation) will increase the disparity between the $Paco_2$ and $Petco_2$. This fact is the basis for the calculation of dead space ventilation using the following equation:

$$V_D/V_T = \frac{Paco_2 - Petco_2}{Paco_2}$$

Therefore, as dead space increases, the $Petco_2$ underestimates $Paco_2$.

Conditions that increase dead space ventilation and therefore reduce $Petco_2$ can be categorized into those that reduce cardiac output (hypovolemia, depressed myocardial contractility, cardiac arrest, increased systemic afterload), those that increase pulmonary vascular resistance (pulmonary vasospasm, excessive positive end-expiratory pressure [PEEP]), those that reduce the cross-sectional area of the pulmonary vascular bed (ARDS, multiple pulmonary emboli), and those that obstruct blood flow in large pulmonary arteries (air and thrombotic emboli). In all of these situations the $Paco_2$-$Petco_2$ gradient will increase, making capnography not a measurement of alveolar ventilation but a marker of pulmonary perfusion. Alternatively, conditions that increase the $Paco_2$ (either reduced alveolar ventilation or increased carbon dioxide production) will be reflected by an increased $Petco_2$, provided that pulmonary perfusion remains constant.

In the PICU $Petco_2$ monitoring of critically ill children can be used in the following fashion. A change in the $Petco_2$ value is an indication for measurement of the $Paco_2$ and reevaluation of the patient's pulmonary and hemodynamic status. A reduction in $Petco_2$ with a concomitant reduction in $Paco_2$ (i.e., a constant gradient) is consistent with either improved alveolar ventilation (V_A) or reduced carbon dioxide production ($\dot{V}co_2$). A reduction in $Petco_2$ in the presence of unchanged or increased $Paco_2$ reflects an increase in dead space ventilation. If simultaneously obtained mixed venous (pulmonary artery) blood gas tensions demonstrate increased carbon dioxide ($P\bar{v}co_2$) and reduced oxygen ($P\bar{v}o_2$), such a critical reduction in cardiac output has occurred that alveolar

Table 123-1   Comparison of $Petco_2$ and $Paco_2$ Values in Critically Ill PICU Patients

$Petco_2$	$Paco_2$	Differential Diagnosis
Reduced	Reduced	Improved alveolar ventilation
		Reduced CO_2 production
Reduced	Unchanged or increased	Reduced cardiac output or cardiac arrest
		Increased pulmonary vascular resistance
		Reduced cross-sectional area of pulmonary vascular bed
		Pulmonary embolus
Increased	Increased	Reduced alveolar ventilation
		Increased CO_2 production
Increased	Unchanged	Increased airway resistance
		Excessive alveolar compliance
Unchanged	Unknown	No guarantee of cardiopulmonary stability

blood flow is reduced and cannot keep pace with carbon dioxide production, and oxygen extraction has increased, resulting in a widened arterial-venous oxygen difference ($a\text{-}vDo_2$). An increase in $Petco_2$ with a concomitant increase in $Paco_2$ is consistent with either reduced $\dot{V}a$ or increased $\dot{V}co_2$ (e.g., associated with malignant hyperthermia syndrome). An increase in $Petco_2$ with an unchanged $Paco_2$ (i.e., a reduced gradient) is an unusual circumstance that occurs when dead space ventilation is minimal and the time constants of the airway (either resistance or compliance) are increased. In the pediatric population this situation is present in patients with severe small airways obstruction (e.g., bronchiolitis) in whom the slowest emptying lung units may have $Petco_2$ values that exceed the $Paco_2$ as a result of the pendelluft effect (see Chapter 10). Table 123-1 summarizes the clinical use of simultaneous measurements of $Petco_2$ and $Paco_2$.

TECHNIQUE

For all practical purposes $etco_2$ monitoring in critically ill patients can be performed only in those with either an endotracheal tube or tracheostomy in place.

The carbon dioxide tension in an exhaled gas mixture may be determined either by infrared absorption analysis or by mass spectrometry. This discussion focuses on the use of the infrared technique since mass spectrometry has limited use in the PICU because of its expense, slow response time, bulkiness, and the requirement for labor-intensive repair.

The molecules that define the structure of a gas exhibit characteristic absorption spectra determined by their composition and configuration. Infrared energy reacts with these molecules, and the degree of absorption depends on the reactivity and the number of molecules present. Carbon dioxide strongly absorbs infrared light at a wavelength of 4.28 nm; thus this wavelength is used to measure gaseous carbon dioxide. The infrared energy is passed through a chamber that contains a sample of exhaled carbon dioxide, and a lens directs the unabsorbed radiation onto a detector. The higher the carbon dioxide tension in the exhaled gas mixture, the more the radiation is absorbed and the less it is directed to the detector. The detector creates an electrical signal proportional to the intensity of incidental radiation and thus the $Petco_2$ of the sample. The signal is processed to display a continuous waveform of the $Petco_2$ values. Fig. 123-1 demonstrates a normal pattern of exhaled Pco_2 over time.

The gas to be analyzed can reach the sample chamber in one to two ways (Fig. 123-2). *Sidestream* analyzers pump the exhaled gas sample from the trachea through small-bore tubing to a remote analyzer. This method adds little weight or dead space to the breathing circuit. However, the narrow lumen of the sample tube often becomes obstructed by airway secretions. The response time is slow compared to that of mainstream analyzers. *Mainstream* analyzers are attached directly to the endotracheal tube or tracheostomy. Because the analyzer is part of the breathing circuit, the response time is very rapid. However, the analyzer is heavy and must be supported to prevent endotracheal tube kinking or dislodgment.

As described in the previous section, changes in $Petco_2$ must be compared to the $Paco_2$ value to determine the cause of the gas-exchange derangement. Assuming that they correlate (i.e., dead space ventilation is constant), hypoventilation can be diagnosed by an increase in the height of the capnogram (Fig. 123-3) and hyperventilation by a reduction in the height of the capnogram (Fig. 123-4). Apnea, disconnection from a ventilator circuit, or esophageal in-

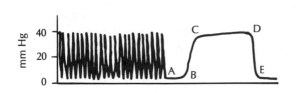

Fig. 123-1 Normal Petco$_2$ pattern. Left side of the tracing of exhaled carbon dioxide tension is obtained with a reduced paper speed; the Petco$_2$ value of 40 mm Hg is demonstrated with each breath. The right side demonstrates four sections of an entire cycle marked by the letters *A, B, C, D, E*. Segment *AB* is the initiation of the expiratory phase of the respiratory cycle during which gas is removed from the anatomic deadspace. As perfused alveoli empty, the Petco$_2$ increases rapidly to a peak (*BC*). A plateau (*CD*) is achieved and must be evident to assure an accurate Petco$_2$ determination. The segment marked *DE* represents the initiation of the inspiration phase of the respiratory cycle.

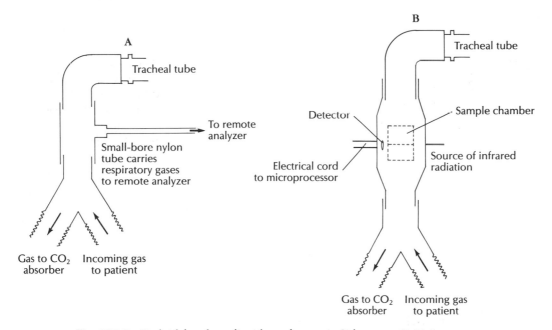

Fig. 123-2 End-tidal carbon dioxide analyzers. **A,** Sidestream. **B,** Mainstream.

Fig. 123-3 Increase in Petco$_2$ is consistent with hypoventilation; this diagnosis is confirmed by demonstrating an increase in arterial carbon dioxide tension (Paco$_2$).

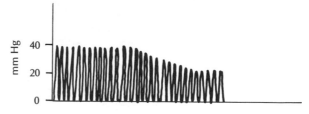

Fig. 123-4 Reduction in Petco$_2$ is consistent with hyperventilation.

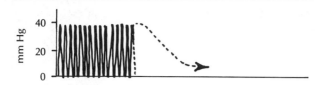

Fig. 123-5   Reduction in Petco₂ from 40 to 0 mm Hg is consistent with situations in which no alveolar ventilation is occurring (apnea) or those in which malfunction or improper placement of the endotracheal tube has occurred.

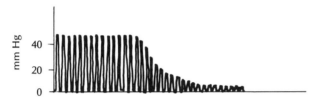

Fig. 123-6   Petco₂ tracing demonstrates progressive reduction as cardiac arrest occurs, resulting in decreased pulmonary perfusion.

Fig. 123-7   Petco₂ tracing is consistent with compromised pulmonary perfusion by hypovolemia, increased pulmonary vascular resistance, or the administration of excessive positive end-expiratory pressure (PEEP).

tubation results in reduction of Petco₂ toward zero (Fig. 123-5). If reduction in Petco₂ occurs in the presence of an unchanged or increasing Paco₂, an increase in dead space ventilation can be inferred. Fig. 123-6 demonstrates the capnogram typical of cardiac arrest in which the Petco₂ value progressively falls and ends in small waves that result from carbon dioxide production by the lungs. Fig. 123-7 demonstrates a more subtle reduction in Petco₂ caused by reduced pulmonary perfusion.

RISKS AND COMPLICATIONS

For the purposes of this discussion, complications of etCO₂ monitoring are defined as misinterpretation of the displayed data, which can occur because of misunderstanding of the physiologic principles or as a result of mechanical dysfunction of either the monitoring or ventilating apparatus. The first situation occurs when the changing Petco₂ value is not compared to a simultaneously obtained Paco₂; it cannot be assumed that pulmonary perfusion and carbon dioxide production have remained constant. The second category includes situations in which a change in the Petco₂ value is the result of mechanical and not patient malfunction.

A sudden reduction in Petco₂ to zero may indicate one or more of the following mechanical defects: obstructed endotracheal tube, defective carbon dioxide analyzer, ventilator malfunction, or endotracheal tube malposition. A sudden increase in the Petco₂ baseline may be the result of a saturated carbon dioxide absorber, the presence of water in the analyzer, or a calibration error.

•   •   •

In summary, etCO₂ monitoring for the intubated patient may provide a means for following alveolar ventilation or carbon dioxide production or pulmonary perfusion provided that a changing Petco₂ value is compared to a simultaneously obtained Paco₂ value. Additionally, it is valuable in assessing the patency or proper placement of an endotracheal tube, perhaps in adjusting PEEP by determining adverse effects on dead space ventilation, and for following the effectiveness of cardiopulmonary resuscitation.

ADDITIONAL READING

Baudendistel L, Goudsouzion N, Cote C, et al. End-tidal CO_2 monitoring: Its use in the diagnosis and management of malignant hyperthermia. Anaesthesia 39:1000, 1984.

• Falk JL, Rackow EC, Weil MH. End-tidal carbon dioxide concentration during cardiopulmonary resuscitation. N Engl J Med 318:607, 1988.

May WS. Respiratory monitoring. Int Anesthesiol Clin 163:159, 1986.

Murray JP, Modell JM. Early detection of endotracheal tube accidents by monitoring carbon dioxide concentration in respiratory gas. Anesthesiology 59:344, 1983.

• Nunn JF, Hill DW. Respiratory dead space and arterial to end-tidal CO_2 tension differences in anesthetized man. J Appl Physiol 15:383, 1960.

Raemer DB, Francis D, Philip JH, et al. Variation in P_{CO_2} between arterial blood and peak expired gas during anesthesia. Anesthesiol Analg 62:1065, 1983.

• Stock MC. Noninvasive carbon dioxide monitoring. Crit Care Clin 4:511, 1988.

Weil MH, Bitera J, Trevino RP, et al. Cardiac output and end-tidal carbon dioxide. Crit Care Med 13:907, 1985.

124 Oxygen Consumption Measurements

Gary Goodman

BACKGROUND AND INDICATIONS

The goal of supportive care of the critically ill patient is to sustain adequate transport of oxygen relative to need. The adequacy of tissue oxygenation depends on the volume of oxygen delivered to the tissues (oxygen transport) and the volume consumed by the tissues (oxygen consumption). Arterial oxygen content (CaO_2) is the sum of oxygen chemically bound by hemoglobin (Hb) and the oxygen physically dissolved in the plasma. The amount of chemically bound oxygen is directly related to the concentration of hemoglobin and to the degree to which hemoglobin is saturated with oxygen (SaO_2). Arterial oxygen content is calculated by the following equation:

$$CaO_2 = (Hb \times 1.34 \times SaO_2) + (PaO_2 \times 0.003)$$

where 1.34 is the estimate of the mean volume of oxygen that can be bound by 1 g of normal hemoglobin when it is fully saturated, PaO_2 is the arterial oxygen tension, and 0.003 is the solubility coefficient of oxygen in plasma. $C\bar{v}O_2$ is calculated by the same formula using $P\bar{v}O_2$.

Oxygen transport or delivery (DO_2) is the volume of oxygen delivered to systemic vascular beds per minute and is the product of CaO_2 and cardiac index (CI) (cardiac output corrected for body surface area or indexed):

$$DO_2 = CaO_2 \times CI$$

Oxygen uptake is the amount of oxygen that diffuses from the capillaries into the tissues. Oxygen uptake can be inferred from the arterial-venous content difference ($a\text{-}vDO_2$), which is determined by using a mixed venous blood gas value obtained from a pulmonary artery catheter:

$$a\text{-}vDO_2 = CaO_2 - C\bar{v}O_2$$

where $C\bar{v}O_2$ is the mixed venous oxygen content.

Oxygen consumption may then be estimated using the Fick equation, which relates oxygen consumption to cardiac output and arterial-venous oxygen content difference:

$$O_2 \text{ consumption} = VO_2 = CI \times a\text{-}vDO_2 \times 10$$

where 10 is a correction factor. Oxygen delivery normally exceeds oxygen uptake by threefold. In certain disease states, however (most notably ARDS and septic shock), the normal relationship between oxygen delivery and consumption is altered such that oxygen use depends on oxygen delivery, a phenomenon known as supply dependency of oxygen uptake. This apparently is caused by both increased oxygen use and impaired oxygen extraction (see Chapters 12 and 35).

TECHNIQUE

Assessment of oxygen delivery and consumption may be made both by physical examination and by calculation of hemodynamic variables. Clinical indicators measure end-organ function and reflect adequacy of tissue oxygenation (Table 124-1).

Specific hemodynamic calculations can be determined with data collected from invasive monitoring (Table 124-2). Intermittent measurement of hemodynamic variables and calculation of oxygen transport variables can be used to follow trends and to document the response to therapeutic manipulations such as positive end-expiratory pressure (PEEP) and inotropic support. Continuous monitoring with transcutaneous devices, pulse oximetry, and mixed ve-

874

nous fiberoptic oximetry can detect early changes in the patient's oxygen status.

Continuous pulse oximetry is extremely useful clinically since it can accurately determine Sao_2, which is linearly related to Cao_2 (see Chapter 122). Invasive oxygen saturation monitoring can measure

continuously mixed venous oxygen saturation ($S\bar{v}o_2$), which reflects $C\bar{v}o_2$. Mixed venous oxygen saturation and content values estimate the average oxygen consumption in all tissues, and changes in $S\bar{v}o_2$ infer a change in the overall oxygen delivery-extraction process. By rearranging the Fick equation relating oxygen consumption to cardiac output and arteriovenous oxygen content difference, the determinants of mixed venous oxygen content are more obvious:

$$C\bar{v}o_2 = Cao_2 - (\dot{V}o_2/CI \times 10)$$

Thus a reduction in mixed venous oxygen content (and thus saturation) may be caused by (1) decreased arterial oxygen saturation, (2) decreased cardiac output, (3) decreased hemoglobin concentration, or (4) increased oxygen consumption.

However, neither the oxygen delivered to nor the oxygen returned from the tissue is a complete measure of tissue oxygen use because both fail to measure the tissue function of specific vital organs. It is essential to monitor end-organ function simultaneously, especially the brain, kidneys, and metabolic indices, using the clinical indicators outlined in Table 124-1.

Table 124-3 reviews the pathophysiology of different disease states that may affect oxygen content, delivery, or use. Optimizing oxygen consumption involves treating the underlying disease process and augmenting compensatory mechanisms that balance the pathophysiologic derangement. For example, decreased oxygen content due to pulmonary edema can be compensated for by increasing cardiac output,

Table 124-1 Clinical Assessment of Tissue Oxygenation

Organ System	Clinical Sign or Laboratory Measurement	Alteration
Metabolic	Core temperature	Hypothermia
	pH	Acidosis
	Serum lactate	Elevation
Central nervous system	Mental status	Confusion or depression
Cardiac	Perfusion	Delayed capillary refill
	Systemic arterial blood pressure	Hypotension
Pulmonary	Arterial blood gas tensions	Hypoxemia, hypercapnia
	Respiratory muscle function	Hyperpnea, apnea
Renal	Urinary output	Decreased

Table 124-2 Clinical Measurement and Calculation of Oxygen Variables

Variable	Measurement or Calculation	Normal Range
Arterial blood gas	Pao_2	80-100 mm Hg
	Sao_2	90%-100%
Hemoglobin	Oxygen *content* = Cao_2 = $(Sao_2 \times Hb \times 1.34) + (0.003 \times Pao_2)$	17-20 ml/dl
Cardiac index	Oxygen *delivery* = Do_2 = $Cao_2 \times CI \times 10$	570-670 ml/min/m²
Mixed venous blood gas	$P\bar{v}o_2$	37-43 mm Hg
	$S\bar{v}o_2$	70%-76%
Arterial-venous oxygen difference	a-vDo_2 = $Cao_2 - C\bar{v}o_2$	4-5 ml/dl
Oxygen *consumption*	$\dot{V}o_2$ = $CI \times$ a-v$Do_2 \times 10$	120-200 ml/min/m²
Oxygen *extraction* ratio	$\dot{V}o_2/Do_2$	20%-30%

Table 124-3   Derangements of Oxygen Transport

Mechanism	Pathophysiology	Clinical Examples
Decreased oxygen	Hypoxemia	Pneumonia
	Anemia	Hemorrhage
	Reduced hemoglobin-binding sites	Sickle cell hemoglobin, methemoglobin, carbon monoxide poisoning
Decreased oxygen delivery	Decreased cardiac output	
	Inadequate preload	Hypovolemia
	Diminished contractility	Cardiomyopathy, heart surgery, congenital heart disease
	Excessive systemic afterload	Systemic hypertension
	Excessive pulmonary afterload	Pulmonary hypertension
	Reduced regional blood flow	Elevated intracranial pressure
	Increased Hb affinity for oxygen	Alkalosis, hypothermia, carbon monoxide poisoning
Altered oxygen use	Increased tissue oxygen requirements	Burns, hyperpyrexia, hyperthyroidism
	Inability of tissues to use oxygen	Septic shock

Table 124-4   Manipulation of Oxygen Parameters

Goal	Method
Oxygen content	
Increase oxygen-carrying capacity	Transfusion of packed red blood cells: hematocrit 35%-45%
	Maintenance of normal pH
	Maintenance of normothermia
Increase hemoglobin saturation	Administration of supplemental oxygen
	Continuous positive airway pressure
	Positive end-expiratory pressure
	Positive pressure ventilation
Increase dissolved oxygen	Hyperbaric oxygen
Oxygen delivery	
Optimize cardiac output	
Heart rate	
Low	Administration of atropine, isoproterenol; placement of cardiac pacemaker
High	Provision of sedation, volume, pharmacologic therapy
Preload	Maintenance of optimum cardiac filling pressures
Contractility	Administration of glucose, calcium, oxygen, inotropic agents
Afterload	
Pulmonary	Maintenance of increased alveolar oxygen, hyperventilation, alkalosis; administration of pharmacologic vasodilators
Systemic	Administration of pharmacologic vasodilators
Oxygen uptake	
Optimize unloading of oxygen	Maintenance of normothermia, acid-base balance Sao_2 >85%
Optimize regional blood flow	
Renal	Administration of low-dose dopamine (3-5 μg/kg/min)
Cerebral	Decrease intracranial pressure
	Maintenance of cerebral perfusion pressure
Cardiac	Support of diastolic blood pressure
Decrease oxygen use	Administration of sedatives, muscle relaxants, paralysis
	Mechanical ventilation (to decrease work of breathing)
	Maintenance of normothermia

thereby increasing oxygen delivery to tissue beds. In disease states such as ARDS or septic shock in which there is supply dependency of oxygen uptake, increasing oxygen delivery may be lifesaving. With determination of oxygen delivery a minimally acceptable value can be maintained by manipulating the various components of the oxygen delivery system in a specific manner rather than adjusting for Pao_2 or Sao_2 endpoints, which may overshoot or undershoot the desired oxygen delivery objective. Table 124-4 illustrates the various manipulations that favorably affect oxygen delivery and consumption. It is important not only to improve oxygen content, delivery, and uptake, but also to reduce oxygen use by lowering the metabolic requirements of the body. Monitoring clinical signs of end-organ function in addition to invasive determination of hemodynamic and oxygen variables allows the clinician to document the response to therapy. Altered mental status, diminished urinary output, metabolic acidosis, and accumulation of lactic acid are ominous signs of tissue hypoxia.

RISKS AND COMPLICATIONS

Therapeutic manipulations based on the measurement of cardiopulmonary variables can be instituted safely in a PICU in which the nursing and medical staffs are knowledgeable about their significance as well as the limitations of the technology. Noninvasive bedside monitoring of heart rate, respiratory rate, and temperature; Doppler measurement of systemic arterial blood pressure; and continuous pulse oximetry can be accomplished with few risks and complications. Invasive measurement of arterial blood pressure with indwelling vascular catheters may be complicated by infection, bleeding, vasospasm, or emboli. Pulmonary artery catheters pose many potential risks, including bleeding, infection, dysrhythmias, and emboli. See appropriate chapters for details on these procedures.

ADDITIONAL READING

• Cain SM. Assessment of tissue oxygenation. Crit Care Clin 2:537-550, 1986.

Dantzker DR, Gutierrez G. The assessment of tissue oxygenation. Respir Care 30:456-462, 1985.

Katz RW, Pollack MM, Weibley RE. Pulmonary artery catheterization in pediatric intensive care. In Barness LA, ed. Advances in Pediatrics. Chicago: Year Book, 1983, pp 169-190.

Shapiro BA, Harrison RA, Walton JR. Pulmonary artery blood gases. In Harrison RA, Walton JR. Clinical Application of Blood Gases. Chicago: Year Book, 1977, pp 227-235.

• Snyder JV, Pinsky MR, eds. Oxygen Transport in the Critically Ill. Chicago: Year Book, 1987.

• Swedlow DB, Cohen DE. Invasive assessment of the failing circulation. In Swedlow DB, Raphaely RC, eds. Cardiovascular Problems in Pediatric Critical Care. New York: Churchill Livingstone, 1986, pp 129-168.

125 Bedside Pulmonary Function Testing of Infants

M. Douglas Cunningham

BACKGROUND AND INDICATIONS

Methods for determining the dynamics of newborn and infant lungs have been available for several decades, but bedside applications for critically ill infants undergoing mechanical ventilation have only recently been developed. The various methods have included body plethysmography, spirometry, and pneumotachography. Of these, only pneumotachography has been adapted for rapid bedside measurement of airflow, tidal volume, and transpulmonary pressure. Most recent developments have included computer-assisted systems for recording the basics of infant lung mechanics and calculating dynamic lung compliance and respiratory system resistance.

The pneumotachograph is an open capillary mesh resistor that provides a slight, but constant resistance to respiratory airflow. The change in pressure across the resistive element is proportional to flow. Most available systems use the Fleisch 00 or 0 pneumotachograph (OEM Medical Inc., Richmond, Va.) for establishing the change in pressure across the flow-resistive mesh and a Validyne MP45 differential pressure transducer (Validyne Engineering Corp., Northridge, Calif.) for detecting the pressurer change and to establish the flow signal. Volume is electronically integrated from flow and recorded as tidal volume. Standard pressure transducers and a recorder complete the necessary instrumentation for determining airway pressure, esophageal pressure, and transpulmonary pressure. An approved clinical device for bedside testing of lung mechanics for infants is currently available as the PeDS unit (pulmonary evaluation and diagnostic system, Medical Associated Services, Inc., Philadelphia, Pa.). It is an assembly of pneumotachograph, transducers, and a computer with a software program designed for producing a specific set of pulmonary functions, which are currently limited to dynamic compliance (C_{dyn}), total respiratory system resistance (R_{trs}), inspiratory resistance, expiratory resistance, respiratory time constants (K_t), and work of breathing. Each of these functions is calculated from the measured values of airflow, tidal volume, and transpulmonary pressure. Methods for determining other recognized pulmonary functions such as thoracic gas volume, vital capacity, functional residual capacity, and forced expiratory volume are being developed for infants, but applications for an intensive care setting are not yet available.

The management of three clinical situations involving sick neonates and infants (infants with chronic lung disease of infancy, infants with respiratory distress syndrome, and infants undergoing extracorporeal membrane oxygenation) have been facilitated by bedside pulmonary function testing during intensive care, recovery, and convalescence. Mechanical changes in the progression of chronic lung disease of infancy (bronchopulmonary dysplasia) are well recognized, as are the responses of those infants to pharmacologic agents (diuretics, bronchodilators, steroids). Documentation of increasing dynamic compliance has been noted to be an indicator of lung recovery during extracorporeal membrane oxygenation (ECMO). Finally, bedside pulmonary function testing offers an assessment that may assist in deciding to change ventilator settings during mechanical ventilation of infants with respiratory distress syndrome and other acute respiratory diseases.

TECHNIQUE
Airflow

For the determination of flow ($\dot{V}$) of respiratory gases a pneumotachograph (00 Fleisch for infants 5 kg or less, 0 Fleisch for larger infants) is inserted between the endotracheal tube and the ventilator circuit. The airflow waveform reveals inspiratory and expiratory flow and the point of zero flow at midinspiration and midexpiration (Fig. 125-1). The airflow waveforms differentiate between spontaneously generated breaths of infants breathing with continuous positive airway pressure (CPAP), breathing freely through a face mask, or breathing during intermittent mandatory ventilation in contrast to mechanical breaths generated through an endotracheal tube by a pressure-limited, time-cycled ventilator.

Transpulmonary Pressure

Transpulmonary pressure (P_{tp}) is the airway pressure (Paw) taken at the mouth or at the junction of the endotracheal tube and ventilator circuit; the esophageal pressure (P_{es}) is the airway pressure taken by balloon in the lower third of the esophagus. In the case of spontaneous breaths the airway pressure (generated as the diaphragm descends) and esophageal pressure (a reflection of intrathoracic pressure) are recorded as negative values. Transpulmonary pressure waveforms are displayed for both mechanically and spontaneous generated breaths in Fig. 125-1.

Volume

Breath volume corresponds to the points of zero flow between end-inspiratory flow and end-expiratory flow. Since volume is an integral of flow, it is proportional to the area beneath the inspiratory flow waveform (Fig. 125-1). The Fleisch 00 pneumotachograph indicates flow from as little as 5 ml/sec to nearly 100 ml/sec, with most pneumotachographs being linear in response between 15 and 80 ml/sec. Normal values for infant tidal volume (V_T) are 2.5 to 10 ml/kg, depending on birthweight, maturity, respiratory disease, and whether or not the infant is receiving mechanical ventilation (Table 125-1).

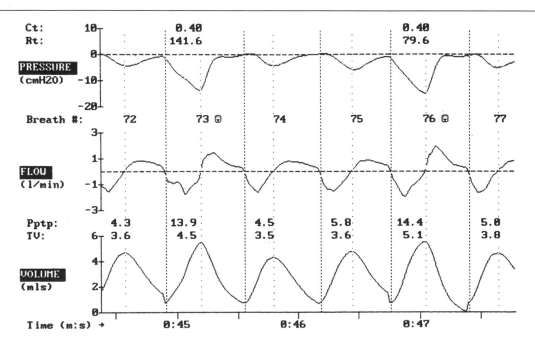

Fig. 125-1 Waveforms of scalar output of the PeDS pulmonary function testing system from an infant undergoing intermittent mechanical ventilation. Note that breaths 73 and 76 were mechanically generated, in contrast to breaths 72, 74, and 75, which were taken spontaneously.

Table 125-1   Examples of Pulmonary Function Measurements of Infants

Patients	$\dot{V}$	P_{tp}	V_T	C_{dyn}	R_{trs}	R_{exp}	Comments
A. One-week-old, 1050 g infant with respiratory distress syndrome							
Spontaneous breaths taken during mechanical ventilation	37.80	3.74	4.47	1.83	48.00	41.00	Normal values. Discontinuance of mechanical ventilation would depend on respiratory drive.
Data for mechanically generated breaths	55.70	6.67	8.87	1.84	63.00	109.00	Somewhat higher resistance values are occasionally seen with mechanical breaths.
B. Five-day-old, 1080 g infant with respiratory distress syndrome							
Spontaneous breaths	37	10.40	7.13	0.76	126.00	271.00	Poor compliance is evident, with striking increase of resistance values in spontaneous breaths.
Mechanical breaths	58	9.10	6.74	0.73	112.00	123.00	
Same infant, 28 days of age, receiving oxygen and continued ventilator support; moderate bronchopulmonary dysplasia on chest roentgenogram							
Spontaneous breaths	45	8.6	6.97	1.16	145.00	179.00	Despite modest improvement of C_{dyn}, spontaneous R_{exp} remains high, consistent with chronic lung disease of infancy (bronchopulmonary dysplasia).
Mechanical breaths	49	9.8	5.75	1.05	185.00	154.00	
C. Four-day-old, 1370 g infant with respiratory distress syndrome							
Spontaneous breaths	31	3.37	5.54	1.84	24.00	29.00	Infant was removed from ventilator support on day 6, with uneventful recovery thereafter. Spontaneous breath values are consistent with clinical course, mechanical breath data to the contrary.
Mechanical breaths	46	13.1	11.73	0.74	26.00	159.00	
D. One-month-old, 2160 g infant with bronchopulmonary dysplasia	24.1	9.00	5.2	0.72	166.42	253.75	Moderate improvement of C_{dyn} and resistance values has occurred.
Same infant, 3 months old	66.6	20.00	12.3	1.59	95.02	138.09	
E. Newborn with normal lungs; birthweight, 3590 g	57	3.6	6.3	5.17	60	63	—

Another instrument, solely for monitoring neo-natal and infant tidal volume, is available as a ther-mocalibrated nonresistive anemometer (NVM1; Bear Medical Inc., Riverside, Calif.). As a bidirectional flow detection device, it also electronically integrates vol-ume from airflow. Advantages of the anemometer over the pneumotachograph include not being af-fected by humidification of respiratory gases, being lightweight, having only 1.5 ml dead space, and con-tinuously recording for longer periods of time. It does not provide a scalar display, and like the PeDS unit, it does not distinguish between mechanical and spontaneous tidal volumes.

Compliance

Lung compliance may be expressed as static or dy-namic. Static compliance is determined when flow is interrupted at peak inspiration and maximal volume and change of intrathoracic pressure is observed. In contrast, dynamic compliance is a measure of chang-ing transpulmonary pressure at points of no flow between peak inspiration and peak expiration, and corresponding changes in volume are observed:

$$C_{dyn} = \frac{\Delta V_T}{\Delta P_{tp}}$$

Although static compliance determinations are con-sidered more accurate, an interrupted system for ob-serving flow, pressure, and volume relationships is preferable in a critical care situation. Dynamic com-pliance depends on accurate esophageal measure-ment of intrathoracic pressure. The unstable chest wall of infants and unequal ventilation may introduce a source of error into esophageal pressure changes. Normal compliance values for newborn infants are estimated to be 2.00 to 3.00 ml/cm H_2O/kg. Very low birthweight infants with dynamic compliance values of 1.00 to 1.2 ml/cm H_2O/kg (Table 125-1) may re-cover from respiratory distress syndrome and be weaned from mechanical ventilation.

Changes in lung compliance can be illustrated as pressure-volume loops (Fig. 125-2). The more com-pliant lungs need less pressure for inflation, achieve greater volume, and result in more vertical loops. Lungs with poor compliance need greater pressure for inflation, achieve less volume, and result in more protracted and horizonal-appearing pressure-volume loops.

Resistance

Respiratory system resistance is a reflection of the volume, velocity, and density of gases. The respiratory system has inherent resistance to gas flow, largely because of the diameter and length of the conducting system (trachea and bronchi), the bronchial subdi-visions, and the viscosity of the lung tissues. Taken together, the resistance as measured with the avail-able instrumentations is a measure of total respiratory system resistance. Resistance is calculated from the measured change in transpulmonary pressure and change in airflow.

$$R_{trs} = \frac{\Delta P_{tp}}{\dot{V}}$$

Normal newborn and infant respiratory system re-sistance values are expected to be 15 to 60 cm H_2O/L/sec (Table 125-1); however, determinations of re-sistance have proved to vary considerably. For infants studied with an endotracheal tube in place, the length, diameter, and curvature of the tube influence the resulting resistance. The position of the tube within the trachea or its proximity to the carina can result in higher than expected resistance values. The condition of the infant can directly affect resistance values. For example, accumulating secretions, exces-sive hydration, and an infant attempting to over-breathe or resist the ventilator can create widely dif-ferent resistance values.

Increased resistance has been found to be a hall-mark of chronic lung disease of infancy. Resistance values >100 cm H_2O/L/sec early in the first week of life have been associated with a protracted clinical course of oxygen dependence and mechanical ven-tilatory assistance. More specifically, differentiation between inspiratory and expiratory resistance has re-vealed marked increases of resistance in expiration. Further demonstration of increased resistance is il-lustrated by flow-volume loops (Fig. 125-2). Slight narrowing of the airways is normal during expiration, but in many patients with bronchopulmonary dys-plasia it appears to be accentuated and is recordable as limited expiratory flow. Deformation of the flow-volume loop corresponds with markedly increased expiratory resistance in contrast to inspiratory resis-tance.

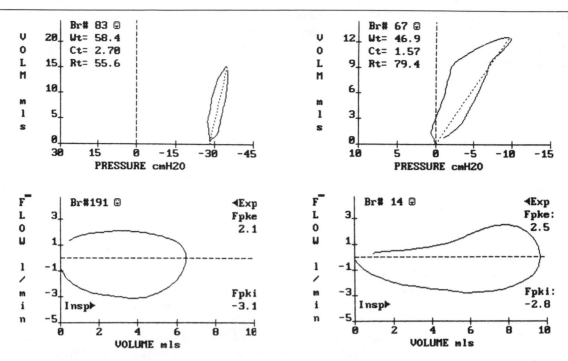

Fig. 125-2 Flow-volume and pressure-volume loops. Loops on the left represent normal breaths of an infant breathing spontaneously through an endotracheal tube with continuous positive airway pressure (2 cm H₂O) just before extubation. The loops on the right represent breaths generated spontaneously during intermittent mandatory ventilation and represent poor lung compliance (pressure-volume) and increased expiratory resistance (flow-volume).

Time Constant

The product of compliance and resistance is the time constant (K_t). It is the time (in fractions of a second) required for proximal and alveolar airway pressure to reach equilibrium. As pressure in the airways changes, so will the volume of respiratory gases. It is the time, either during inspiration or expiration, in which 63% of the respired gases can be exchanged. Three time constants (3 K_t) is the time needed for 95% exchange of gases. Because airways normally narrow during expiration, any exaggeration of expiratory time becomes important in the ventilator management of obstructive diseases such as meconium aspiration and chronic lung disease of infancy. For example:

$$K_t = \text{Compliance} \times \text{Resistance}$$

$$K_t = 0.005 \text{ L/cm H}_2\text{O} \times 30 \text{ cm H}_2\text{O/L/sec}$$

$$(K_t \text{ of normal newborn} = 0.15 \text{ sec})$$

$$3 \times K_t = \text{Time for 95\% exhalation of tidal volume}$$

$$3 \times K_t = 0.45 \text{ sec as minimal expiratory time}$$

But, if an infant has respiratory distress syndrome with poor compliance and increased expiratory resistance, K_t is prolonged:

$$K_t = 0.0008 \text{ L/cm H}_2\text{O} \times 200 \text{ cm H}_2\text{O/L/sec}$$

$$K_t = 0.16 \text{ sec}$$

$$3 K_t = 0.48 \text{ sec}$$

Given these pulmonary functions, and if the ventilator rate is 80 breaths per minute with an inspiratory to expiratory ratio of 1:1, the expiratory time is reduced to 0.375 second. It can be assumed that the ventilator rate setting is inconsistent with the sick infant's time constant of 0.48 second and sets the stage for air trapping and air leakage.

RISKS AND COMPLICATIONS

The procedures and instrumentation used in studying lung mechanics at the bedside of infants in intensive care cause minimal risk. Care must be taken not to alter ongoing nursing and respiratory care. The benefit of using bedside studies for infants resides mostly in not having to disturb the stable temperature environment and cardiovascular and respiratory monitoring that is in progress.

Potential but unreported risks include overheating of airway gases by the pneumotachograph heater and a slight increase of PEEP (1 to 2 cm H_2O) because of the resistance of the pneumotachograph, with a slight increase of Pao_2 (2 to 5 torr). On occasion the 1.7 ml of added dead space of the pneumotachograph has been accompanied by an increase of $Paco_2$ (4 to 8 torr). Continuous testing is not recommended in a patient with an esophageal balloon in place and without suctioning and control of oral and pharyneal secretions.

Routine calibration of the system is always required, including recalibration of individual pneumotachographs.

Interpretation of data dictates that users of any pulmonary function testing system establish a database with clinical correlates for the patient population. Normal and abnormal values for newborn and infant pulmonary functions have varied considerably in published reports.

ADDITIONAL READING

Bancalari E. Pulmonary function testing and other diagnostic laboratory procedures. In Thibeault DW, Gregory GA, eds. Neonatal Pulmonary Care. Norwalk, Conn.: Appleton-Century-Crofts, 1986, pp 195-233.

Cunningham MD, Desai NS. Methods of assessment and findings regarding pulmonary function in infants less an 1000 grams. Clin Perinatol 13:299-313, 1986.

Engelhardt B, Elliott S, Hazinski TA. Short-term and long-term effects of furosemide on lung function in infants with bronchopulmonary dysplasia. J Pediatr 109:1034-1039, 1986.

Gerhardt T, Hehre D, Feller R, Reifenbergh L, Bancalari E. Serial determination of pulmonary function in infants with chronic lung disease. J Pediatr 110:448-456, 1987.

• McCann EM, Goldman SL, Brady JP. Pulmonary function in the sick newborn infant. Pediatr Res 21:313-325, 1987.

Mortola JP, Saetta M. Measurements of respiratory mechanics in the newborn: A simple approach. Pediatr Pulmonol 3:123-130, 1987.

• Sly PD, Brown KA, Bates JHJ, Spier S, Milic-Emilli J. Non-invasive determination of respiratory mechanics during mechanical ventilation of neonates: A review of current and future techniques. Pediatr Pulmonol 4:39-47, 1988.

126 Oxygen Administration

Becky Wade · Gary Elmore

INDICATIONS

The use of supplemental concentrations of oxygen is common in patients with various disorders. Four primary indications for oxygen therapy are (1) hypoxemia, (2) increased work of breathing, (3) increased myocardial work, and (4) pulmonary hypertension.

Hypoxemia results from a variety of pathophysiologic mechanisms (see Chapter 10), and increased demands of both the ventilatory and cardiovascular systems are common responses of the patient to hypoxemia. All children with symptomatic pulmonary hypertension need an increase in inspired oxygen concentration to reduce pulmonary vascular tone.

Many devices that supply varying concentrations of oxygen are available for use in infants and children. Despite the type of delivery device chosen, patient cooperation is essential for maximum effectiveness. In most cases a little extra attention and reassurance are all that may be needed to gain the cooperation of an infant or child.

TECHNIQUE

Incubators. Closed incubators, like most incubators, may be used to provide supplemental oxygen and can provide a stable thermal environment for the newborn infant. Most incubator units are designed with air-entrainment devices, which restrict the maximum FiO_2 within the unit to 0.40, depending on the liter flow of oxygen used. Higher concentrations of oxygen can be obtained by closing the air-entrainment port, allowing only oxygen to enter the incubator. In some cases an FiO_2 up to 0.85 may be achieved with the proper liter flow of oxygen. A red flag is used with most incubators to indicate whether the FiO_2 being used is above or below 0.40; in the vertical position the red flag indicates an FiO_2 >0.40; in the horizontal position, an FiO_2 of 0.40 or less is being achieved.

The desired FiO_2 in an incubator is often not obtained because of leaks. For example, the FiO_2 drops rapidly when the portholes are opened; when maintaining a stable FiO_2 is important, an oxygen hood may be used inside the incubator. Saline and bicarbonate solutions must never be used for humidification in an incubator since they will cause salt deposits to build up on the fan and motor, damaging the unit. Instead, only distilled water may be used.

Hoods. Oxygen hood devices are the most effective delivery device when precise concentrations are essential for infants and small children who are not intubated. Hoods must be made of clear Plexiglas for optimum visibility of the infant. An FiO_2 of up to 1.0, or 100% oxygen, is attainable with adequate oxygen flow rates. The flow rate into the hood must be high enough to maintain the desired oxygen concentration without allowing carbon dioxide to accumulate. Generally, a flow rate of 8 to 12 L/min is adequate to flush the system.

Hoods come in varying sizes and designs. Some hoods such as the Oxyhood are designed with the large-bore connection perpendicular to and several inches above the base, thus generating a more turbulent flow of gas and making it difficult to maintain a stable FiO_2. With this design the top of the hood must remain enclosed to aid in stabilizing the FiO_2 being delivered. However, if the infant is in a radiant-heating system, much of the heat may be absorbed by the lid of the Oxyhood. In this type of design the area surrounding the infant's neck must remain open to allow the escape of carbon dioxide. In contrast to the Oxyhood, the halo type of design provides more vortex flow because the large-bore tubing is connected to a T-adaptor that is parallel to the base of the halo (Fig. 126-1). This provides a more stable oxygen concentration, and carbon dioxide is allowed to escape through the open top of the halo. Since the top of the halo is always open, a pad or cloth diaper may be placed around the neck opening to protect the infant's skin.

Tents. Mist tents were once popular devices for the administration of supplemental oxygen concentrations of up to 50% for infants and small children. One of their major advantages was increased mobility of the patient since they may cover the entire body or just the head and upper chest. However, tents are used less and less frequently because they are cumbersome, access to the patient is limited, they are difficult to maintain, they must be sealed tightly around the patient, and some patients find them frightening. Stable oxygen concentrations are difficult to maintain due to leaks in the system. Also, when the tent is opened for access to the patient, the oxygen concentration drops rapidly. Most tents must be equipped with a refrigeration system to maintain adequate temperature control. Open-top tents do not need a refrigeration system since heat is allowed to escape through the top. A temperature 5° to 7° C lower than room temperature must be maintained for maximum patient comfort.

Masks. Several different mask types that deliver varying concentrations of oxygen are manufactured (Fig. 126-2). Most masks are manufactured in infant, pediatric, and adult sizes. All masks must be made of soft, pliable plastic and must be transparent so that the patient's face is visible. The simple oxygen mask delivers a low to moderate oxygen concentration, depending on the liter flow. The simple mask is not the mask of choice if a stable Fio_2 is desired, since the concentration is directly affected by the oxygen flow rate and patient's inspiratory flow rate. Aerosol masks may deliver up to 100% oxygen, provided that the flow is adequate to meet inspiratory demand. Nonrebreathing masks are designed with one-way leaf valves and a reservoir bag that partially collapses during inspiration. The nonrebreathing masks deliver moderate to high concentrations of oxygen. Partial-rebreathing masks are similar in design to a simple oxygen mask but, like the nonrebreathing mask, are equipped with a reservoir bag. This particular mask is capable of delivering up to 60% oxygen. Venturi masks deliver precise concentrations that vary from 24% to 50%. Masks allow easy accessibility to the patient but are not usually tolerated for extended periods.

Face tents. Face tents are loose fitting and are generally accepted well by children. With adequate flow rates, a stable oxygen concentration can usually

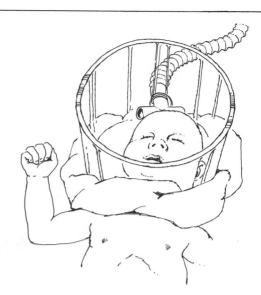

Fig. 126-1   Infant halo type of hood.

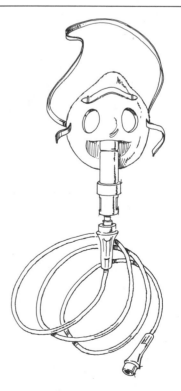

Fig. 126-2   Oxygen mask.

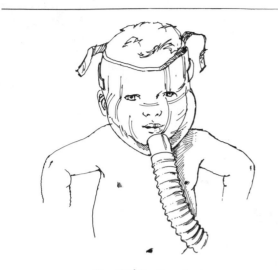

Fig. 126-3 Face tent.

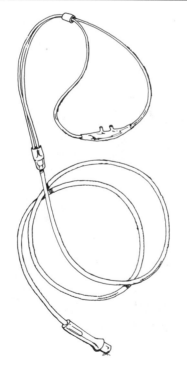

Fig. 126-4 Nasal cannulas.

be provided. When properly set, the oxygen concentration provided should be equal to that of the source gas. Because face tents are only manufactured in adult sizes, they are usually inverted for use in smaller patients (Fig. 126-3), creating a smaller reservoir and a better fit for the pediatric patient.

Nasal cannulas and catheters. Nasal cannulas and catheters are used to deliver low flows and low concentrations of oxygen. The oxygen concentration delivered by the nasal cannula and catheter varies with changes in the patient's inspiratory flow rate. In addition care must be taken to ensure that the cannula or catheter does not fit too snugly, occluding the infant's nares, since infants are obligate nose breathers. Most nasal cannulas and catheters manufactured currently are distributed in neonatal, pediatric, and adult sizes, providing a more precise fit and increased tolerance by smaller patients. With these devices the patient is easily accessible, and oxygen therapy need not be circumvented for feedings. Oxygen flows of <1 to 6 L/min are needed with these devices. Nasal catheters are usually not well tolerated since they are inserted nasally to the level of the uvula in most patients. Cannulas are generally tolerated well and are often used for patients who need chronic oxygen therapy because of the low flows and low concentrations they deliver (Fig. 126-4).

T-bars and tracheostomy masks. The most direct method of delivering oxygen is through either an endotracheal tube or a tracheostomy tube. These devices can deliver precise oxygen concentrations when an adequate flow is used. The flow must be high enough to meet the patient's inspiratory flow demands and not allow room air entrainment. In some instances a short reservoir tube placed on the expiratory side of a T-bar can be used to stabilize the FiO_2 instead of increasing the flow rate. Achieving concentrations of up to 100% oxygen is possible with both devices. When either device is used, it must be monitored closely to ensure that unnecessary tension is avoided since this tension may cause inadvertent extubation.

RISKS AND COMPLICATIONS

Because of its potential toxicity, oxygen must be considered a drug and must be closely monitored. The risk of toxicity can be decreased by following certain guidelines. The patient's PaO_2 must be closely monitored by obtaining arterial blood gas values and by using transcutaneous oxygen monitors and oxygen saturation monitors (pulse oximeters) (see Chapters 120 and 122). The FiO_2 must also be closely monitored and must be analyzed by the respiratory therapist at least every 4 hours and with each change in FiO_2.

Probably the most common form of oxygen toxicity in the neonate or infant is retrolental fibroplasia, a form of systemic oxygen toxicity resulting partly from delivery of excessive PaO_2 to the retinal arteries. Pulmonary oxygen toxicity is characterized by a decrease or cessation in mucociliary activity, a decrease in surfactant production, absorption atelectasis, and $\dot{V}/\dot{Q}$ abnormalities. Both pulmonary and systemic oxygen toxicity depends on both the oxygen concentration and the duration of administration of oxygen and varies from one individual to the next. Generally a PaO_2 of 60 to 80 mm Hg is considered reasonable in most patients to decrease the possibility of pulmonary or systemic oxygen toxicity. As the patient's condition begins to improve, the weaning process also starts. In a patient who has had long-term oxygen therapy, the FiO_2 must be decreased in decrements of no more than 0.10.

ADDITIONAL READING

Burgess WR, Chernick V. Respiratory Therapy in Newborn Infants and Children. New York: Thieme, 1986.

Burton, GC, Hodgkin JE. Respiratory Care, A Guide to Clinical Practice, 2nd ed. Philadelphia: JB Lippincott, 1984, pp 700-702.

127 Intubation

Frances C. Morriss · Jean Stone · Lynn M. Butler

INDICATIONS

Despite the often emergency nature of airway problems in children, placement of an endotracheal tube must be approached in a deliberate and calm manner if trauma to the airway and patient instability are to be avoided. Regardless of the indications for intubation, airway control must be established immediately with the use of bag and mask ventilation while equipment, personnel, and supplies are being readied. Intubation will proceed more safely in an oxygenated and physiologically stable patient. Although establishing a patent airway and adequate ventilation is not synonymous with intubation, intubation provides a closed system for ventilation while ensuring patency and protecting the airway. Specific indications for intubation are listed below:

Apnea
Acute respiratory failure (Pao_2 <50 mm Hg in patient with Fio_2 >0.5 and $Paco_2$ >55 mm Hg acutely; see Chapter 10)
Need to control oxygen delivery (e.g., institution of PEEP, accurate delivery of Fio_2 >0.5)
Need to control ventilation (e.g., to decrease work of breathing, to control $Paco_2$, to provide muscle relaxation)
Inadequate chest wall function (e.g., in patient with Guillain-Barré syndrome, poliomyelitis, flail chest)
Upper airway obstruction
Need to protect the airway of a patient whose protective reflexes are absent

TECHNIQUE

The process of intubation involves placement of a flexible tube into the opening of the upper airway, the larynx, from the oropharyngeal or nasopharyngeal route using a lighted blade to assist visualization. The soft tissues of the oral cavity (tongue, tonsils,

uvula) must be displaced and the axis of the pharyngeal airway aligned with the axis of the larynx to accomplish tube placement (Fig. 127-1). Laryngoscopy and intubation elicit a number of physiologic responses and reflexes that must be recognized and managed appropriately:

Airway protective reflexes (neurologically mediated via glossopharyngeal and vagal nerves)
Glottic closure (laryngospasm)
Cough
Gag and retch
Sneeze
Cardiovascular responses
Sinus bradycardia (direct vagal stimulation)
Tachycardia and hypertension (neuroendocrine mediation via sympathetic efferents)
Dysrhythmias, especially if patient becomes hypoxic

Equipment

All necessary equipment for airway support including intubation must be available and functional before attempting intubation. The equipment may be placed in a portable cart or tool box since this is helpful for emergency situations in which speed may be essential. Minimal equipment needs are listed below:

Intubation equipment

Laryngoscope handles and blades of various sizes and types
Oral endotracheal tubes of various sizes with standard 6 mm connectors
Suction equipment (source of vacuum, tonsil suction, catheters)
Nasogastric or large-bore, soft red-rubber catheters
Bag, mask, and oxygen
Atropine
Supplies for securing endotracheal tube
Oral and nasal airways of various sizes
Gloves and goggles

Optional equipment
    Nasotracheal tubes
    Magill forceps
    Stylets
    Specialized tubes
    Manometer
    Lubricant
    Afrin nasal spray
    Intubation pillow

Straight laryngoscope blades (Miller, Phillips, Seward) are more useful in neonates and infants because the rigidity of the infantile epiglottis hampers the use of a curved blade (MacIntosh), which is usually placed in the vallecula behind the epiglottis. Miller blade sizes from 0 to 3 are needed; the 0 blade (used for premature infants) is only shorter than the 1 blade and is not scaled down in size in any other way. A short, stubby handle can be particularly useful for intubation of a patient with a short neck and/or a prominent chest. Batteries and light bulbs must be checked regularly for proper function.

Uncut *oral* endotracheal tubes should range in size from 2.0 to 6.0 mm uncuffed and 5.5 to 8.0 mm cuffed. Although cuffed tubes of sizes smaller than 5.5 mm are available, they are not recommended because the addition of a cuff to an endotracheal tube decreases the tube's internal diameter; since the resistance for laminar flow is related inversely to the fourth power of the tube's radius, a small decrease in the internal diameter results in a large increase in resistance. Cuffs, if used, must be the low-pressure,

high-volume type to minimize circumferential tracheal mucosal trauma. Appropriately sized standard 6 mm connectors need to be packaged with each tube. The composition of the tube must be compatible with human tissue; polyvinylchloride tubes have low tissue toxicity and suitable malleability without being rigid. Tubes with a shoulder (Cole) are not recommended because of trauma to the glottis. Desirable characteristics of tube design include sequential centimeter indicators along the length, identification of tube size on the connector or cuff pilot tube, and a radiopaque marking to assess position.

The tonsil suction is the most effective device for removing blood and thick mucus from the airway. Catheters are more effective for removing secretions from the endotracheal tube. As with other procedures that expose the operator to body secretions, gloves and glasses or goggles should be worn during intubation.

Technique

Assemble all the necessary equipment and obtain the aid of other health care personnel to assist with patient positioning, monitoring, and airway management. Continuous cardiorespiratory monitoring (ECG, systemic arterial blood pressure, heart rate, oxygen saturation) is desirable throughout the procedure; if such monitoring is unavailable, one assistant must be responsible for monitoring pulse and oxygenation by visual assessment. If it is practical, secure an IV line for drug administration.

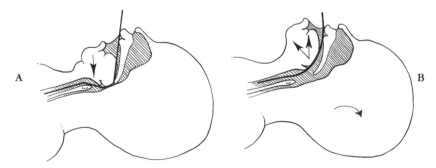

Fig. 127-1 Alignment of the axis of the larynx with that of the oropharynx. **A,** Airway obstructed by oropharyngeal soft tissue; the laryngeal opening cannot be visualized. **B,** Obstructing soft tissue has been lifted out of airway by positioning head, pulling jaw forward, and lifting tongue to allow alignment of oropharynx with the larynx and adequate visualization.

Empty the stomach with a large-bore NG tube, soft, oral red rubber catheter, or suction catheter and remove the tube. This step is particularly important if the patient has been fed recently or has gastric distention.

Oxygenate the patient with 100% oxygen for several minutes to replace alveolar air with oxygen and thus provide an added source of oxygen should the patient become apneic. Optimal saturation for intubation is 100% or whatever the patient's normal saturation is. If the patient is a premature infant, optimal saturation is 96% to 97%.

While the patient receives oxygen, check the laryngoscope function and select the appropriate type and size tube. Proper tube diameter for children more than 2 years of age may be estimated by the formula:

$$\text{Tube size} = \frac{\text{Age in years}}{4} + 4.5$$

The diameter of the patient's fifth finger correlates well with airway size. In children more than 8 to 10 years of age cuffed tubes are appropriate, especially if sealing the airway is desirable. Most children this age need a 6.0 to 6.5 mm tube; often the presence of a cuff is sufficient to prevent an air leak around the tube. Also select a tube one size larger and one size smaller than the expected size. *For emergency situations oral tube placement is technically easier to perform and therefore safer and faster.* If a cuffed tube is selected, test the cuff for patency and absence of leaks. Consider the use of atropine (0.2 mg/kg IV) to block the vagus nerve, especially in neonates and infants in whom bradycardia is common.

Position the child with the intubator at his head, removing the head of the bed if necessary. The patient's head must be in the sniffing position (i.e., head slightly extended with the jaw thrust forward) (Fig. 127-2). The normal occipital prominence of a neonate will maintain a sniffing position. Hyperextension of the head will obstruct the airway and interfere with visualization of the larynx (the axis of the laryngeal and oropharyngeal airways diverges with hyperextension). An assistant must gently restrain the patient's arms, shoulders, and head and direct a flow of oxygen over his face. Open the patient's mouth wide and insert the laryngoscope blade (grasped firmly in the left hand) in the right side of the mouth. Move the blade to the midline, keeping the tongue trapped to the left of the blade. Place a curved blade in the vallecula behind the epiglottis and a straight

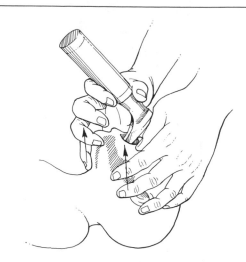

Fig. 127-2 Sniffing position: correct head position for intubation. Head is slightly extended, jaw elevated and pulled forward, and laryngoscope inserted on right side of mouth.

blade in front of the epiglottis. Lift superiorly with a motion from the shoulder. Do not bend the wrist since this forces the blade against the teeth and gums and raises the blade tip, pushing the larynx out of the line of vision (Fig. 127-3). As the blade is lifted and withdrawn slightly, the larynx should drop into view.

From the right side of the mouth insert the endotracheal tube under direct vision several centimeters through the vocal cords. Insertion of the tube down the blade may entrap the tube in the blade groove, preventing easy placement. Gentle posterior or downward pressure over the cricoid cartilage may be helpful in visualizing a larynx that appears to be displaced anteriorly (only the arytenoid cartilages are seen in Fig. 127-4). In a neonate this can be done by the intubator with the fifth finger; however, in older infants and children an assistant must apply the pressure. Since the infantile larynx is funnel shaped, the tube tends to abut anteriorly as it is advanced; this may be corrected by flexing the patient's head slightly or by twisting the tube in a corkscrew motion.

If at any time the patient becomes desaturated or bradycardic, institute bag and mask ventilation with 100% oxygen immediately. The smallest diameter of the infant airway is at the cricoid cartilage; thus a tube may pass through the vocal cords and then meet resistance. Do not force the tube if this occurs; rein-

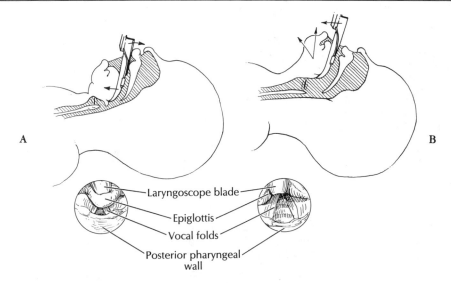

Laryngoscope blade
Epiglottis
Vocal folds
Posterior pharyngeal
wall

Fig. 127-3   Proper and improper use of laryngoscope blade. **A,** Tip of blade is in the vallecula and is being levered against the superior alveolar ridge. Note that the epiglottis is pushed down (inset), obscuring the laryngeal opening. **B,** Tip of blade has picked up the epiglottis, and blade is being lifted, not levered. Note that airway soft tissue is trapped behind blade and view of larynx is improved (inset).

tubate with a smaller sized tube. Inflate the cuff (if present) with a small amount of air only if necessary to eliminate an air leak around the tube. Should the patient regurgitate stomach contents, quickly place him in the lateral head-down position and suction the pharynx with the tonsil sucker.

Once the patient's trachea is intubated, ventilate him with a breathing bag and check for bilaterally equal breath sounds. Use a rapid rate of bag compressions so the person listening can easily distinguish this respiratory pattern from air movement in a spontaneously breathing but esophageally intubated patient. Louder or absent breath sounds on one side indicate that the tube lies in a mainstem bronchus and must be withdrawn until the breath sounds become equal. Breath sounds should be absent over the stomach; with esophageal intubation, transmitted breath sounds can be heard over the chest but will be louder over the stomach. In addition the child will be able to phonate. The chest wall will move with pressure on the breathing bag; absent movement suggests an obstructed tube or esophageal intubation. If the child is breathing spontaneously, look for corresponding movement of the bag. If any doubt exists about tube position, use the laryngoscope to

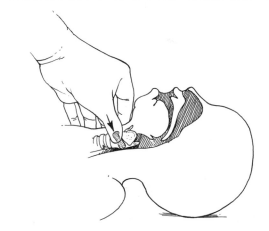

Fig. 127-4   Application of cricoid pressure. Gentle pressure applied perpendicularly over the cricoid cartilage will occlude the esophagus, protecting against passive regurgitation, and will push the larynx inferiorly.

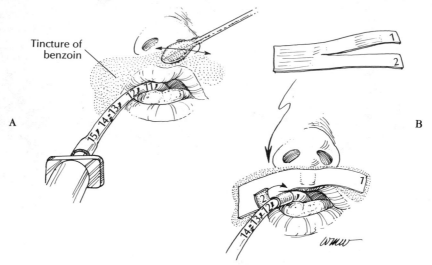

Fig. 127-5 Securing an oral tube. **A,** Tube position (length) is checked and tincture of benzoin applied to upper lip. **B,** Tape is torn in half for approximately half of its length. Upper portion of tape is applied to upper lip and lower portion is wrapped securely around the tube.

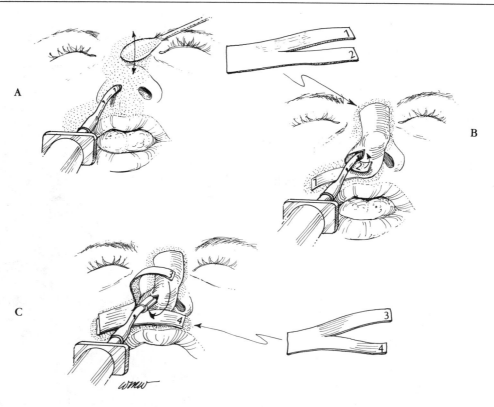

Fig. 127-6 Securing a nasotracheal tube. **A,** Tube position is noted in centimeters along tube, and tincture of benzoin is applied to the bridge of nose and upper lip. **B,** Tape is prepared in same manner as for oral tube and is applied to the bridge of nose. One end *(1)* is applied to the upper lip and the second *(2)* to the shaft of the tube. **C,** A second piece of tape is prepared since most nasotracheal tubes are used for long-term problems and must be very secure. The untorn end is applied to the cheek with the lower piece *(4)* laid securely along the upper lip; the other is wrapped around the tube with the first piece of tape underlying the wrap. Note that the area where the tube and its connector meet is left unobscured for observation.

visualize the patient's vocal cords and check tube position visually. If the patient's condition deteriorates, remove the tube, reestablish bag and mask ventilation, and check for plugging or other mechanical problems.

Check the tube for appropriate size by assessing the amount of air leakage present when graded positive pressure (using a manometer in the circuit) is applied. A leak of air that occurs around the tube at 15 to 25 cm H_2O pressure indicates proper tube diameter. With leaks occurring at >25 cm H_2O pressure, tracheal mucosal damage is more likely. With leaks noted at <15 cm H_2O pressure, mechanical ventilation may be difficult because of the large leak. The leak is best heard by auscultation, placing a stethoscope over the larynx or the open mouth.

Stabilize the tube with adhesive tape and tincture of benzoin (Figs. 127-5 and 127-6). Do not release the tube until it is secure and the patient is restrained. Obtain a chest roentgenogram to check tube position; the tip should lie in the trachea, midway between the carina and the clavicles. Accidental extubation is much more likely when the tip is above the clavicles. Check for pneumothorax as well. Once correct position is established, cut the tube to an appropriate length to minimize dead space.

Special Considerations

Conditions in which special considerations exist that modify intubation are as follows:
    Upper airway obstruction
    Abnormal airway anatomy
    Increased intracranial pressure
    Abnormalities of the cervical spine
    Full stomach
    Need to change an existing endotracheal tube in an unstable patient
    Asthma (see Chapter 34)

Upper airway obstruction

Patients with upper airway obstruction, particularly if it is life threatening, must be handled by the most experienced intubator available. A protocol for management of this type of emergency must be established (see Chapter 33). Such intubations are preferably done in the operating room with a surgical team on standby for performing emergency tracheostomy. If intubation is attempted in the PICU, a bronchoscopist must be available to secure the airway in an alternate fashion. Should standard tube placement

be impossible, under no circumstances can a neuromuscular blocking agent be administered until it is absolutely established that the patient either can be ventilated satisfactorily or can be intubated. Paralysis under any other condition is fatal because relaxation of muscles and soft tissues will obstruct the airway.

Abnormal airway anatomy

A number of anatomic features can increase the difficulty of intubation.
    Normal neonatal anatomy
    Inability to open mouth fully
    Inability to extend neck
    Dental curtain (missing or broken teeth) or intraoral appliance
    Short, thick neck
    Hypoplastic mandible
    Macroglossia
    Midfacial or palatal abnormalities
    Active bleeding in the mouth, nose, or lower airway
    Airway masses
    "Anterior larynx"
If possible, a cursory assessment of the airway must be done before the intubation attempt, including visual inspection of the face and intraoral cavity, estimation of the range of motion of the neck and jaw, and measurement of the anteroposterior distance from the mentum of the mandible to the hyoid bone (Schwartz hyoid maneuver). In adults this distance is at least 3 cm (two fingerbreadths) and in infants, 1.5 cm. Reduction of this distance implies that the potential space for displacement of oral soft tissues (the space encompassed posteriorly by the hyoid, laterally by the mandibular rami, and anteriorly by the mandibular mentum) is limited and laryngoscopic visualization of the airway may be impossible. This condition is sometimes referred to as an "anterior larynx." Identification of a potentially difficult intubation will introduce more caution into the instrumentation process. It must be ascertained whether an experienced intubator is available to assist with the procedure; special techniques such as blind intubation, tongue traction by suture, or fiberoptic laryngoscopy may be needed. The laryngoscope must be used initially to assess the airway anatomy and to remove secretions without attempting to place a tube. Use of a styleted tube with a hockey-stick configuration may be helpful (Fig. 127-7). This type

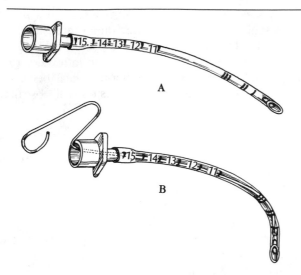

Fig. 127-7 A, Usual curvature of endotracheal tube. **B,** Styleted oral endotracheal tube with tip directed anteriorly.

of patient must not be paralyzed until the ability to ventilate him adequately by bag and mask has been demonstrated.

Increased intracranial pressure

The patient with increased ICP may not tolerate airway instrumentation under the usual circumstances. With impairment of cerebral autoregulation, ICP becomes directly related to cerebral perfusion pressure, and any event that increases heart rate and systemic arterial blood pressure or causes increased blood flow to the CNS (vasodilators, hypercapnea) can cause a symptomatic increase in ICP. For preservation of cerebral function, intubation must be accomplished in a way that eliminates the expected cardiovascular responses. This is done by anesthetizing the patient before intubation.

Begin by assuring that ventilation can be supported in the usual fashion. Administer a sleep dose of thiopental sodium (4 mg/kg/IV), which is thought to decrease ICP, and follow with a nondepolarizing neuromuscular blocking agent; vecuronium (0.1 to 0.2 mg/kg/IV), which does not release histamine and does not stimulate sympathetic afferents, is the agent of choice. Hyperventilate the patient (end-tidal or transcutaneous carbon dioxide monitoring is helpful); the carbon dioxide level must be 20 to 25 mm Hg. Assess the neuromuscular blockade with a nerve

stimulator; all twitches should be absent (see Chapter 130). At this point the patient is incapable of a Valsalva maneuver and has a $Paco_2$ level that is associated with vasoconstriction. If twitches are present, continue to hyperventilate the patient until they disappear. At this point administer a small dose of thiopental (1 mg/kg/IV) or lidocaine (1.5 mg/kg/IV) to blunt any cardiovascular reflexes that might be activated with intubation. Intubate the patient 30 to 60 seconds after this injection and perform continuous ECG, heart rate, and systemic arterial blood pressure monitoring. No change in the monitored cardiovascular variables or in the pupil size indicates achievement of a level of sedation that will probably successfully protect the CNS. Should the patient exhibit symptoms (hypertension, bradycardia, pupillary dilation) suggestive of ICP decompensation, institute measures to decrease ICP. Should the patient need immediate intubation because of cardiorespiratory arrest, the primary goal is to reestablish oxygenation; the above procedure should be aborted.

Cervical trauma or abnormalities

Compromise of the function of the cervical spine secondary to trauma (fractured cervical vertebrae) or congenital subluxation (trisomy 21, achondroplasia) mandates handling intubation in such a way that the neck remains in a neutral position (no flexion or extension). The neck may be stabilized before intubation with axial traction; if not, someone, preferably a neurosurgeon in the case of traumatic injury, can manually stabilize the neck during the procedure. The presence of traction, particularly when combined with other types of head and neck trauma, may make conventional intubation difficult. Fiberoptic or blind awake intubation may be necessary to place a tube without moving the neck.

Intubation of a patient with a full stomach

Emergency intubation undertaken on an unprepared patient who may have a full stomach necessitates special consideration. A recent meal, trauma, shock, narcotics, bleeding into the airway, pregnancy, gastroesophageal reflux, and any type of intestinal obstruction can cause retention of liquid, particulate matter, and acid in the stomach. Such a patient must be intubated while awake so that protective airway reflexes are intact should regurgitation of stomach contents occur. If this type of intubation is inadvisable, a rapid-sequence IV technique that reduces the period of time the patient is without protective airway reflexes and without airway support can be used. Administer 100% oxygen for at least 3 minutes to replace air in the lung and thus increase the period of time the patient can be apneic without concomitant hypoxia. Atropine (0.02 mg/kg/IV) may be given to block the vagus nerve. Administer a nonparticulate antacid such as sodium citrate and citric acid to neutralize stomach pH, and empty the stomach with a NG tube, although the use of an NG tube does not preclude the possibility of aspiration of gastric contents.

Give by IV push in rapid sequence an agent to produce unconsciousness rapidly (thiopental, 4 to 5 mg/kg, or ketamine, 2 mg/kg) and a rapidly acting muscle relaxant (succinylcholine, 2 mg/kg). Paralysis ensues in 30 seconds, allowing the intubation to be done almost immediately. As soon as the patient loses consciousness, apply manual pressure perpendicularly over the cricoid cartilage (Sellick maneuver; Fig. 127-4). Since the cricoid is the only complete tracheal ring, perpendicularly applied pressure will displace the cartilage, occlude the esophagus, and prevent passive regurgitation at a time when the patient does not have protective reflexes. Maintain cricoid pressure until successful intubation and ventilation have been accomplished. Avoid the use of positive pressure ventilation once the patient is areflexic and until the airway is protected with a tube. Positive pressure ventilation can cause gastric distention and increases the likelihood of regurgitation. If, however, the intubation attempt fails or the child cannot tolerate even very short periods of apnea, bag and mask ventilation is permissible if inflation pressures are kept <15 cm H_2O pressure and effective cricoid pressure is maintained throughout the procedure. Children 10 years of age or older are usually intubated with cuffed endotracheal tubes to provide more complete sealing of the airway. Since this is a very rapid technique involving intentional apnea, the intubator must be absolutely certain he can place a tube. Since little time elapses from administration of succinylcholine to placement of the tube, the full range of cardiovascular responses (tachycardia, hypertension, increased intracranial and intraocular pressure) will be seen. Because succinylcholine is a drug with many contraindications and side effects, this technique is best used or supervised by an anesthesiologist. Younger children, particularly neonates, should be intubated while awake because of the expected difficulties related to their normal anatomy.

Changing an Endotracheal Tube

The need to change the existing endotracheal tube to another site or another size is best done on the unstable patient by an experienced intubator. The goal is to replace one tube with another without losing control of the airway (i.e., one tube is placed at the same time the original tube is removed). After placing the patient on 100% oxygen, untape the existing tube and move it to the left side of the mouth (if it is placed orally) still connected to the patient's ventilatory support system. Have an assistant hold it in place. Insert a nasal tube or use the laryngoscope and insert an oral tube. Trap the original tube behind

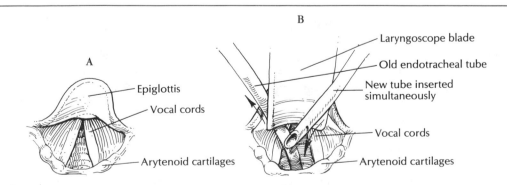

Fig. 127-8 Replacement of an endotracheal tube without removing the original tube. **A,** Normal anatomy of larynx as seen by the intubator. **B,** View seen with the original endotracheal tube in the airway and the new tube placed adjacent to it for insertion under direct vision.

the blade and move the second tube into place beside the first (Fig. 127-8). At this point two endotracheal tubes can be visualized, with the one on the left traversing the vocal cords and the one on the right wedged closely beside the first. Have the assistant slowly remove the first tube and advance the second tube either manually or with Magill forceps. Do not remove the first tube until both tubes are in direct vision. Although it may take several attempts to accomplish this procedure, it is safer and preferable to removing the artificial airway in a patient who is unstable and difficult to intubate. Use of a nondepolarizing neuromuscular blocking agent such as atracurium or vecuronium can facilitate this process. Ventilate the patient throughout the procedure to avoid hypoxia.

RISKS AND COMPLICATIONS

The risks of endotracheal intubation are related to the skill of the intubator and the conditions under which the intubation is done. In a series of 100 consecutive patients needing intubation in a PICU, one series described four cardiopulmonary arrests, two cases of anoxic cerebral injury, and one death. Even intubations performed in a deliberate manner with proper equipment and assistance may carry a significant risk in PICU population.

The most common and potentially most severe problem arising during intubation is hypoxia accompanied by bradycardia or other dysrhythmias. Patients must be monitored closely during intubation attempts, and should signs of instability occur, adequate ventilation must be restored.

Inability to place an endotracheal tube is always a possibility, and failure to do so in a patient with a life-threatening airway obstruction can result in death. Experienced assistance must be sought for patients whose anatomy or condition suggests difficulty. Under no circumstances should the inexperienced intubator resort to the use of sedatives or neuromuscular blocking agents without adequate and skilled support. Failure to ventilate the apneic or paralyzed patient can cause rapid death.

Long-term complications of intubation are discussed elsewhere (see Chapter 36). Early complications occur during the procedure and are traumatic in nature. They include damage to the teeth, gums, and oropharynx; epistaxis; creation of an air leak or perforation, particularly in a struggling, hypoxic child; and direct trauma to laryngeal structures. Re-

peated attempts at tube placement may exacerbate existing airway obstruction by increasing edema in the upper airway. Aspiration pneumonitis secondary to inhalation of stomach contents into the airway can be a severe and life-threatening complication. For a patient with reduced cardiovascular reserve (especially in a patient with pulmonary arterial hypertension), increased ICP, or increased intraocular pressure, the normal response to airway manipulation may cause additional instability or deterioration. Since many of these complications are more likely to occur in the awake, struggling child, a case can be made for the routine use of sedation for intubation of these patients when they are relatively stable, are well oxygenated, and have no anatomic airway problems.

ADDITIONAL READING

• Applebaum B. Tracheal Intubation. Philadelphia: WB Saunders, 1976.
• Bishop MJ, ed. Physiology and consequences of tracheal intubation. Probl Anesth 2(2):entire issue, 1988.
Blanc VR, Tremblay NAG. The complications of tracheal intubation. Anesth Analg 53:203-210, 1974.
Eckenhoff JE. Some anatomic considerations of the infant larynx influencing endotracheal anesthesia. Anesthesiology 12:401-410, 1951.
Fassoulaki A, Eforakopoulou M, Vassiliou M. Metabolic responses (Vo_2, Vco_2 and energy expenditure) associated with nasal intubation of the trachea. Anesth Analg 68:112-115, 1989.
Lee KWT, Downs JJ. Pulmonary edema secondary to laryngospasm in children. Anesthesiology 59:347-349, 1983.
Manchikauti L, Colliver JA, Marrero TE, et al. Assessment of age-related acid aspiration risk factors in pediatric, adult and geriatric patients. Anesth Analg 64:11-17, 1985.
Marshall TA, Deeder R, Par S, et al. Physiologic changes associated with endotracheal intubation in preterm infants. Crit Care Med 12:501-503, 1984.
• Orlowski JP, Ellis NG, Amin NP, et al. Complications of airway intrusion on 100 consecutive cases in pediatric ICU. Crit Care Med 8:324-331, 1980.
Salem MR, Mathrubhuthan M, Bennett EJ. Difficult intubation. N Engl J Med 295:879-881, 1976.
Salem MR, Wong AY, Collins VJ. The pediatric patient with a full stomach. Anesthesiology 39:435-440, 1973.
• Stahling LC, Zander HL, eds. Anesthetic Implications of Congenital Anomalies in Children. New York: Appleton-Century-Crofts, 1980.
White A, Kauder PL. Anatomical factors in difficult direct laryngoscopy. Br J Anaesth 47:468-472, 1975.

128 Continuous Distending Pressure and Assisted Ventilation

David M. Habib · Ronald M. Perkin

BACKGROUND AND INDICATIONS

Assisted ventilation may be defined as the movement of gas into and out of the lung provided by an external device connected directly to the patient. The device may be a resuscitation bag, a continuous distending pressure apparatus, or a mechanical ventilator. It may be attached to the patient by way of a face mask, endotracheal tube, tracheostomy, or the chest (i.e., negative pressure mechanisms).

Assisted ventilation is a supportive technique; it is not curative. It can accomplish no more than maintain blood gas tension homeostasis within acceptable physiologic limits for a period of time. Its purposes are to provide alveolar ventilation (i.e., carbon dioxide removal), optimal systemic oxygenation, and a reduction in the work of breathing.

Children may need assisted ventilation for a variety of conditions, which may or may not have a primary pulmonary etiology. It is difficult to categorize indications for assisted ventilation by disease entity. Not only would this create an endless list, but with each disease the degree of involvement at which point assisted ventilation is needed would have to be defined. The clinical indications for commitment to assisted ventilation are best stated in terms of categories based on neurologic and cardiopulmonary pathophysiology.

Indications for assisted ventilation

Central nervous system dysfunction
    Head and spinal cord injuries
    Mass lesions
    Abnormalities in breathing control
    Infection
    Status epilepticus
    Drug effect
Respiratory pump failure
    Neuromuscular failure
    Loss of mechanical integrity of the respiratory apparatus
    Nutritional debilitation
    Respiratory muscle fatigue
Respiratory failure caused by intrinsic pulmonary disease
    Alveolar disorders
    Interstitial disorders
    Airway diseases
Circulatory problems
    Cardiac arrest
    Shock syndrome
    Pulmonary arterial hypertension
Surgical indications
    After cardiac surgery
    Intraoperative trauma to lung or airway
    Extensive abdominal surgery
    Need for high-dose analgesics
    Trauma

In addition in some instances instituting assisted ventilation only to reduce the oxygen cost of breathing may improve a patient's ability to overcome a major physiologic insult.

Pulmonary Compliance

Compliance of the lung is defined as the change in volume per unit change in distending airway pressure ($\Delta V/\Delta P$) and is determined by elastic forces within the lung as well as the surface tension generated by the air-tissue interface within the alveoli. Pulmonary compliance therefore is a measure of "stiffness" and is described by a sigmoid curve that has a diminishing slope at either end where large and small lung volumes exist. Chest wall compliance is determined by the integrity of its supporting structure (i.e., rib cage) and by the volumes of the lung and abdominal cavity. Since a greater negative intrapleural pressure must be generated to inflate a less compliant lung, the patient's work of breathing increases, and gas exchange in general becomes less efficient. Disease states associated with reduced lung or chest wall compliance are as follows:

Conditions associated with decreased lung or chest wall compliance

Increased elastic recoil forces
 Hyaline membrane disease
 Severe bronchiolar-alveolar pneumonia (bacterial, viral, fungal, aspiration, opportunistic organisms)
 Severe diffuse pulmonary edema (cardiogenic, hydrostatic, neurogenic)
 Adult respiratory distress syndrome (permeability pulmonary edema)
 Diffuse atelectasis
 Interstitial inflammation; fluid or fibrotic process
 Radiation pneumonitis and chronic changes
Reduced chest wall, lung, and diaphragmatic excursion
 Thoracic trauma and abdominal surgery
 Pleural effusions (blood, chyle, exudates, transudates)
 Pneumothorax
 Reduced diaphragmatic excursion caused by abdominal distention (ascites, gastric or intestinal gas, peritoneal dialysis, after gastroschisis repair)
 Paralysis of diaphragm
 Thoracic bone deformities (severe kyphoscoliosis)
Alveolar overdistention
 Asthma
 Bronchiolitis
 Severe meconium aspiration
 Severe bronchopulmonary dysplasia
 Severe laryngotracheobronchomalacia
 Excessive PEEP or CPAP
 Inadequate assisted ventilator expiratory time

Calculation of the static and dynamic lung compliance when a child is on a mechanical ventilator is useful both to identify causes of acute respiratory distress and to provide a trend value to monitor the course of the patient's pulmonary function (see "Problem Management"). Static compliance is obtained by dividing the tidal volume by the static (plateau) inflation pressure, which can be obtained by occluding the exhalation port just before exhalation. This measurement estimates actual pulmonary compliance. Dynamic compliance is obtained by dividing the tidal volume by the peak inspiratory pressure. Dynamic compliance is always lower (i.e., the pressure requirement for the same change in volume is greater) than static compliance, and the difference is a reflection of resistance to airflow.

Functional Residual Capacity

Functional residual capacity (FRC) is that volume of gas retained in the lung at the end of the expiratory phase of the respiratory cycle. It is decreased in patients with respiratory failure resulting from alveolar or interstitial disease. With atelectasis the FRC falls, and the number of alveolar units that participate in gas exchange decreases. Acute functional loss of alveoli leads to systemic arterial hypoxemia. A major goal of assisted ventilation is to return FRC toward normal and therefore improve systemic oxygenation.

Airway Resistance

Airway resistance is the pressure difference (between mouth and alveoli) or driving pressure needed to move respiratory gases through the airways at a constant flow rate. Airway resistance is determined by (1) the flow rate or velocity of airflow, (2) the length of the airways, (3) the physical properties (viscosity and density) of the gas breathed, and (4) the radius of the airways. The most important determinant of airway resistance is the airway radius. Therefore even minor degrees of constriction from bronchospasm, collapse from interstitial edema or emphysema, narrowing from swelling, or obstruction from mucous accumulation can cause a significant increase in airway resistance (i.e., resistance is inversely related to the fourth power of the radius as defined by Poiseuille's law).

Time Constants

The time constant of a patient's respiratory system is a measure of how quickly the lungs can inhale or exhale or how long it takes for alveolar and proximal airway pressures to equilibrate. The product of airway resistance and pulmonary compliance defines the time constant. A knowledge of time constants aids greatly in choosing the safest and most effective ventilator settings for an individual patient.

Various diseases can alter the time constant, depending on the pathologic site. In addition different segments of the lung may have different time constants. In diseases that cause increased airway resistance, such as asthma or bronchopulmonary dysplasia (BPD), the time constants of alveolar units will increase, causing slower filling and emptying of the diseased alveolar unit. In diseases that result in decreased compliance (e.g., ARDS), the time constant will decrease, causing the alveolar unit to have a faster filling and emptying time. Three to five time constants are required to allow complete filling or emptying of an alveolar unit. In a normal infant one time constant equals approximately 0.15 second, and three time constants equal 0.45 second.

Inadequate expiratory time in mechanically ventilated patients can lead to air trapping and occult end-expiratory pressure (auto-PEEP, inadvertent PEEP, or intrinsic PEEP). Auto-PEEP is a relatively common but seldom appreciated occurrence. The patient with high (increased) compliance (e.g., with alveolar destruction or emphysema) or increased resistance is at risk for gas trapping, and the appropriate ventilator settings must be selected to prolong the duration of the expiration phase as much as possible. Signs of gas trapping include overexpansion of the chest, decreased chest wall movement and carbon dioxide retention, increased arterial oxygen tension (PaO_2) in infants with pulmonary shunts or decreased PaO_2 in infants with extrapulmonary right-to-left shunting, and signs of deterioration of cardiovascular function (i.e., reduced cardiac output). A simple method for detecting auto-PEEP is to occlude the endotracheal tube at end-expiration and to measure the equilibration pressure distal to the occlusion. In the presence of gas trapping the pressure distal to the airway occlusion will remain higher than the measured PEEP unless there are leaks around the endotracheal tube or the patient makes spontaneous respiratory efforts during the occlusion.

A large portion of the airway resistance in an infant or child receiving assisted ventilation may be secondary to use of an endotracheal tube or its connectors. This becomes exaggerated if the tube is partially kinked or obstructed by secretions and may be responsible for gas trapping and auto-PEEP.

TECHNIQUE

Mechanical ventilatory assistance can be provided by a variety of methods and devices. This discussion is limited to negative pressure ventilators, continuous distending pressure (CDP), and intermittent positive airway pressure devices.

Negative Pressure Ventilators

Negative pressure ventilators generate a pressure differential between mouth pressure and alveolar pressure (and hence provide gas movement) by decreasing alveolar pressure. Negative pressure ventilators range from tank ventilators, or "iron lungs," to abdominal and thoracic cuirasses. These devices, however, are cumbersome, prevent access to the patient, and provide varying alveolar ventilation.

Although negative pressure ventilators are not extensively used, they still maintain a role in the management of children with neuromuscular disorders who have normal pulmonary function but reduced alveolar ventilation.

Continuous Distending Pressure

Ineffective oxygenation of patients with acute respiratory failure, despite the use of a high-concentration supplemental oxygen, led to the application of PEEP and CPAP. PEEP is defined as a residual pressure above atmospheric pressure maintained at the airway opening at the end of expiration. Although it may be used during spontaneous ventilation, it is most commonly used in conjunction with mechanical ventilation. CPAP is usually defined as a pressure above atmospheric pressure maintained at the airway opening throughout the respiratory cycle during spontaneous breathing. Thus pressure in the airway is always positive when CPAP is used.

Technical consideration

Many devices and systems have been developed to deliver CPAP. All work on the same principle, using continuous gas flow, a reservoir bag, a valve to produce above ambient expiratory pressure, and a humidification device (Fig. 128-1). The system needs gas flow rates sufficient to provide two to three times the patient's minute volume to avoid rebreathing of exhaled gases.

CPAP is most commonly applied to the patient's airways via an endotracheal tube. Other modes of application include face mask or nasal prongs.

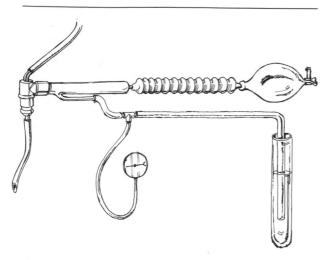

Fig. 128-1 A ventilator device capable of generating positive end-expiratory pressure.

Physiologic effects of PEEP and CPAP

Pulmonary effects. Improvement in arterial oxygenation that occurs with PEEP or CPAP has been recognized since its earliest use. The mechanisms believed to be important in improving oxygenation include (1) increasing FRC by alveolar distention and recruitment of collapsed units, (2) redistributing lung water from the gas-exchanging alveolar spaces to the interstitial compartment, and (3) altering the ventilation-perfusion relationship.

The increase in FRC that results from use of PEEP or CPAP depends not only on the compliance of the lung but also on the compliance of the chest wall. Thus the efficacy of PEEP and CPAP is influenced by factors such as position, pleural effusion, abdominal distention, and muscular tone as well as by the inflation characteristics of the lung. When FRC is increased, ventilation to poorly ventilated or collapsed alveoli improves, lung compliance improves, intrapulmonary shunt decreases, and PaO_2 increases. However, lung compliance may decrease when PEEP or CPAP is applied, probably as a result of overdistention of alveoli. If alveolar overdistention occurs, dead space ventilation will increase (see Chapter 10).

Redistribution of blood flow in relation to ventilation may cause a decrease in PaO_2 in a patient with unilateral lung disease. Application of PEEP or CPAP to the normal lung may cause overdistention of alveoli and an increase in pulmonary vascular resistance, diverting blood flow to the sick lung, which does not have the same increase in volume and pulmonary vascular resistance with PEEP or CPAP is applied. Increased blood flow to the diseased lung may increase intrapulmonary shunting and decrease PaO_2.

A beneficial effect often attributed to PEEP and CPAP is the redistribution of alveolar liquid, both within the alveolus itself and through actual transfer of liquid from the alveolus to the interstitial compartment. Removal of alveolar liquid shortens the diffusion distance for gases into the bloodstream, thereby improving oxygenation. However, the total volume of water contained in the lung is not reduced.

Cardiovascular effects. PEEP and CPAP therapy has long been known to reduce cardiac output. Considerable work has been done to investigate the mechanism of this reduction. Two separate mechanisms have been identified: an increase in intrapleural pressure that decreases venous return and an increase in lung volume that, through an unknown mechanism not related to reduction in venous return, causes ventricular dysfunction. Several mechanisms have been suggested to account for the ventricular dysfunction, including changes in coronary blood flow, an increase in right ventricular afterload caused by increased pulmonary vascular resistance, a reflex change in contractility, changes in the compliance of the left ventricle, compression of the heart by the distended lungs, and a humorally mediated depression of the heart. A reduction in cardiac output can be severe enough to offset the benefits of increased arterial oxygen content and can result in an actual decrease in systemic oxygen transport (see Chapters 12 and 35).

Renal effects. Significant water retention (manifested as weight gain), a positive water balance, hyponatremia, a decrease in the hematocrit, and pulmonary edema without signs of cardiac failure are frequently seen when positive pressure is applied to the airway. The effects on renal function are complex and may involve one or a combination of the following factors: (1) elevation in antidiuretic hormone level, (2) activation of the renin-angiotension-aldosterone axis, (3) redistribution of intrarenal blood flow to juxtamedullary nephrons, and (4) a reduction in atrial natriuretic peptides.

Central nervous system effects. The use of PEEP or CPAP may result in or intensify intracranial hypertension, cerebral ischemia, or both. These effects are directly related to the amount of CPAP or PEEP applied and vary inversely with lung compliance. Changes in ICP correlate with changes in CVP and pleural pressure. Decreased cerebral perfusion pressure may be related to a decrease in cardiac output and mean systemic arterial blood pressure as well as an increase in ICP.

Indications and applications of PEEP and CPAP

PEEP and CPAP are commonly used in the treatment of the ARDS and hyaline membrane disease (HMD). However, other uses of expiratory pressure have emerged.

Uses of PEEP or CPAP

Acute lung injury
  Adult respiratory distress syndrome
  Hyaline membrane disease
  Diffuse pneumonia
  Aspiration syndromes
Others
  Apnea
  Asthma and bronchiolitis
  Tracheobronchomalacia
  Chronic lung diseases
  Postoperative care
  Pulmonary edema
  Artificial airways
  Intracardiac left-to-right shunts
  Weaning from mechanical ventilation

For many of these the therapeutic goals of PEEP and CPAP are quite different from those for patients with ARDS and HMD, and in some of them PEEP or CPAP is used to treat airway rather than alveolar disease. PEEP or CPAP is most likely to benefit patients with acute or diffuse lung disease associated with reduced FRC. If hypoxemia persists despite supplemental oxygen administration (e.g., >50%), a trial of PEEP or CPAP is indicated.

PEEP or CPAP is generally increased in small increments (2 to 3 cm H_2O); oxygenation and hemodynamic performance must be monitored during these changes. As arterial oxygen tension (i.e., PaO_2) improves, the fraction of inspired oxygen (FiO_2) can be reduced. A PaO_2 >60 mm Hg results in a hemoglobin saturation >90% and is adequate in most pa-

tients. A "safe" FiO_2 level has not determined; however, a value below 0.5 is well tolerated by most patients for an extended period. The optimal level of PEEP or CPAP remains controversial. The amount of PEEP or CPAP administered must be guided by the ability to reduce FiO_2 while maintaining adequate tissue perfusion (i.e., cardiac output) and oxygenation. Although positive airway pressure improves oxygenation and allows a reduction in FiO_2, it may impair cardiac performance and expose a patient to pulmonary barotrauma (e.g., pneumothorax). Thus continuous monitoring is necessary to gain the benefit of PEEP or CPAP and to avoid or minimize its adverse effects and complications.

After the patient's condition has improved, PEEP or CPAP must be reduced in a carefully controlled fashion (i.e., in 2 cm H_2O increments). Premature withdrawal or sudden discontinuation of PEEP or CPAP may lead to a precipitous fall in PaO_2 and FRC. Procedures such as tracheal suctioning that temporarily result in the removal of PEEP must be kept to a minimum whenever possible.

Positive Pressure Ventilators

Before positive pressure ventilation can be instituted, a stable airway must be established usually by placing an endotracheal tube. Like the normal upper airway, endotracheal tubes have nonlinear pressure-flow characteristics; therefore resistance increases progressively with increasing flow rates. In addition, at any given flow rate, the pressure loss across the endotracheal tube depends primarily on its internal radius. As the size of the tube decreases, therefore, resistance increases exponentially. Most of the time the effect of increased resistance may be overcome during positive pressure ventilation, but it may present difficulties as minute ventilation is decreased when the patient is weaned from the ventilator.

The anatomy of the infant's and small child's airway is such that uncuffed endotrachal tubes must be used. Ideally, to minimize laryngeal damage, there must be a small air leak during positive pressure ventilation. The presence of air leaks, however, may cause difficulties in adequately ventilating a child, especially when pulmonary compliance is decreased.

Small plugs of mucus may decrease the radius of an already small tube, greatly increasing tube resistance. Frequent suctioning of the endotracheal tube (e.g., every 4 hours) and proper humidification of inspired gases are essential; when a patient's condition deteriorates, the possibility of an obstructed endotracheal tube must be considered.

Respiratory failure may be defined as either a reduction in arterial oxygen tension (i.e., Pao_2 <50 mm Hg) or an increase in arterial carbon dioxide tension (i.e., $Paco_2$ >55 mm Hg). The two types of respiratory failure have different pathophysiologic mechanisms; thus the mode of ventilatory support required to correct the abnormality differs (see Chapter 10).

Ventilation

Patients in whom ventilatory failure is characterized by increased $Paco_2$ and respiratory acidemia require mechanical ventilation (see Chapter 10). The ventilatory cycle may be considered in terms of the inspiratory and expiratory phases. The inspiratory phase of mechanical ventilation pertains to the positive pressure breath and may be divided into the following phases: initiation, gas flow during inspiration, and termination of the inspiratory phase.

Initiation. Several modes of positive pressure mechanical ventilation have been developed. Most ventilators available in intensive care units can provide several of these different modes, alone or in combination with CPAP or PEEP.

Controlled mechanical ventilation (CMV) delivers mechanical breaths at a predetermined interval; no gas flow is available for spontaneous ventilation. Therefore, if the patient attempts to breathe, he will decrease his airway pressure, but no gas will flow into his lungs. Additionally, the patient's spontaneous effort to breathe may interfere with the mandatory breaths delivered by the mechanical ventilator (i.e., the patient may be "fighting the ventilator").

To prevent this struggle the patient's spontaneous breaths must be eliminated, which can be accomplished by inducing alveolar hyperventilation and respiratory alkalemia, by administering either respiratory depressant drugs, or by inducing neuromuscular blockage (Table 128-1). Sedation facilitates the patient's breathing in phase with the ventilator so that the minimum peak airway pressure can be determined without the child's coughing and straining. Muscle relaxants increase chest wall compliance, reduce oxygen consumption, and maximize patient cooperation. These drugs must always be used in combination with sedation, since they have no sedative properties. Ventilation with the help of muscle relaxants and/or sedatives must be limited to the following situations:

1. Requirement for very high airway pressures such as in a patient with asthma
2. Critically inadequate oxygenation such as in ARDS
3. Ventilator intolerance such as in an anxious infant
4. Nonpulmonary indications such as head injury

Assisted mechanical ventilation (AMV) was developed to permit the patient to control the rate at which mechanically assisted breaths are delivered. When a patient attempts to take a breath during AMV, the machine senses the decrease in airway pressure, and a positive pressure breath is delivered with a predetermined tidal volume.

Although this mode does reduce the sensation of suffocation, alveolar hyperventilation and respiratory alkalemia may occur, particularly in the anxious infant.

Intermittent mandatory ventilation (IMV) was initially developed as a technique of weaning. It was, however, soon adopted as a mode of mechanical ventilatory support with distinct advantages over assist and control modes. IMV allows the patients to breathe spontaneously and yet provides a certain preselected number of mechanically delivered breaths in contrast to the method of controlled or assisted ventilation in which all of the minute ventilation is mechanically provided. With IMV both spontaneous and mechanical breaths have identical inspired oxygen concentrations, using a second circuit with low-resistance, one-way valves and continuous gas flow to prevent rebreathing of expired gases. Some of the advantages of IMV over conventional ventilation include (1) ventilation with lower mean airway pressures, leading to less cardiovascular depression and less barotrauma; (2) reduced need for sedation or paralysis in patients requiring mechanical ventilation; (3) less tendency for alveolar hyperventilation or hypoventilation; (4) maintenance of spontaneous respiratory activity, which results in the continuous exercise of respiratory muscles; and (5) more even distribution of ventilation and pulmonary blood flow.

With IMV the mechanical volume is delivered at a specific predetermined interval at any time during the patient's respiratory cycle. Thus the mechanical volume could be delivered while the patient is exhaling or at the peak of his spontaneous respiration.

Table 128-1   Commonly Used Drugs to Facilitate Mechanical Ventilation

Trade Name	Generic Name	Route	Dose	Side Effects	Comments
Chloral hydrate	Chloral hydrate	PO, PR	20-40 mg/kg	CNS depression Vomiting GI irritation	Do not exceed 2 g/24 hr Hepatic metabolism
Versed	Midazolam	IM, IV	0.05-0.15 mg/kg	Respiratory depression	Hepatic metabolism
Ativan	Lorezepam	PO, IM, IV	0.05 mg/kg	Respiratory depression	Hepatic metabolism
Morphine	Morphine	PO, IM, IV, PR	0.05-0.2 mg/kg 20-100 µg/kg/hr as continuous infusion	CNS depression Hypotension Histamine release Constipation and delayed gastric emptying	Hepatic metabolism Half-life: 2-2½ hr
Sublimaze	Fentanyl	IM, IV	2 µg/kg—low dose 2-20 µg/kg—moderate dose 20-75 µg/kg—anesthesia induction 1-10 µg/kg/hr as continuous infusion	Respiratory depression Muscle rigidity in chest wall	Hepatic metabolism: may be used by continuous infusion
Pavulon	Pancuronium	IM, IV	0.1-0.15 mg/kg	Tachycardia Hypertension	Renal metabolism (55%-70%) Hepatic metabolism (30%-45%)
Metubine	Metocurine	IM, IV	0.3-0.5 mg/kg	Hypotension Histamine release	Renal metabolism
Tracrium	Atracurium	IM, IV	0.4-0.6 mg/kg—intubation 0.1 mg/kg—maintenance	Histamine release at high doses or with rapid administration	Nonenzymatic Hoffmann elimination May be used as a constant infusion
Norcuron	Vecuronium	IM, IV	0.75-0.1 mg/kg—intubation dose 0.1-0.15 mg/kg—repeated dose	No histamine release No circulatory effects	Metabolism: renal, 15%; biliary, 30%-50% May be used as a continuous infusion

Although this possibility has not been shown to be of clinical importance, some new ventilators incorporate a synchronized intermittent mandatory ventilation (SIMV) circuitry. This incorporation of SIMV into the ventilator apparatus is an expensive addition, and its value has been questioned.

New methods of ventilatory support, designed for specific problems and made possible by new mechanical ventilators, have recently been developed. These newer methods of mechanical ventilation include pressure support ventilation, high-frequency ventilation, mandatory minute ventilation, differential lung ventilation, inverse ratio ventilation, and airway pressure release ventilation. Most of these ventilatory modes are currently available, even though there are few critical studies that assess their clinical value. They claim to benefit one or more aspects of ventilatory assistance, specifically to improve ventilation-perfusion imbalance, to minimize positive pressure–related cardiovascular compromise, to decrease the work of breathing, or to facilitate the weaning process. However, a considerable gap exists between the rapidly increasing ventilatory options and knowledge of how best to ventilate a patient with a particular disease at a certain time.

Gas flow during inspiration. The only function of the ventilator during the inspiratory phase is to force gas into the lungs. For a gas to move from one area to another, a pressure difference must exist between two points of a conducting system. In mechanical ventilation this pressure difference is found between the generated pressure of the ventilator and alveolar pressure. Based on the magnitude of the generated pressure, a ventilator can be classified as either a pressure generator or a flow generator. Flow generators are used most often.

Ending the inspiratory phase. The inspiratory phase may be ended when a certain pressure, volume, time, or flow is achieved. Ventilators may thus be classified according to what limits the gas flow and what factor ends the ventilator cycle. Most neonatal and infant ventilators are pressure-limited, time-cycled ventilators, whereas those used in children and adults are volume limited and either volume or time cycled.

For each type of ventilator the variables remain the same: flow ($\dot{V}$), volume (V), pressure (P), respiratory frequency (f), and ratio of inspiration to expiration (I:E). The difference between the types of

Table 128-2 Ventilator Types: Controlled vs. Determined Variables

Variable	Ventilator Type (cycle)		
	Pressure	Volume	Time
Flow	Controlled	Controlled	Controlled
Volume	Determined	Controlled	Determined
Pressure	Controlled	Determined	Determined
Frequency	Controlled	Controlled	Controlled
I:E	Determined	Determined	Controlled
Fio₂	Controlled	Controlled	Controlled

ventilators relates to which of the variables the operator can manipulate or to which variables the operator can control or set and which become determined variables as a result of the settings (Table 128-2).

Pressure-cycled ventilators terminate the inspiratory phase when a preselected airway pressure is achieved. Once this pressure is attained, an exhalation valve opens, initiating the expiratory phase. The volume delivered to the patient and the time or duration of inspiration will vary according to airway resistance, pulmonary compliance, and integrity of the ventilator circuit. Significant changes in the duration of inspiration may signal a problem either in the patient or in the machine. A short inspiratory time can result from decreased pulmonary compliance, a restriction or obstruction in the endotracheal tube or the ventilator circuit, or an increase in the patient's airway resistance. Regardless of cause, a smaller tidal volume will be delivered because the cycling pressure is reached prematurely. When a pure decrease in lung compliance has taken place, tidal volume cannot be restored by adjusting flow rate. The corrective procedure is with the cycling pressure, which must be increased. However, with increases in airways resistance adjusting the flow rate alone may be of some value in restoring volume because of the relationship that exists between flow rate and step rise in the initial mouth pressure.

In the event of an airway leak or ventilator disconnection, cycling pressure cannot be achieved, and inspiration will be prolonged indefinitely.

In contrast to pressure-cycled ventilators, many

ventilators (e.g., volume, time, or mixed) may incorporate a pressure-limiting feature as a safety device. These ventilators vent any excess pressure (and therefore volume) to the atmosphere.

There is no simple way to predict the initial requirements of the pressure-cycling mechanism because the extent of the patient's pulmonary dysfunction is not established. Clinical judgment dictates the cycling pressure selected and is customarily in the range of 10 to 20 cm H_2O. The exact setting for flow rate is also impossible to establish but is initially adjusted to provide an adequate inspiratory time (e.g., 0.3 to 0.6 second).

Once the preliminary settings are made, the patient is connected to the ventilator. The optimal tidal volume and minute ventilation of infants and children are then assessed by listening for air entry and exit, observing chest expansion, measuring exhaled volume, and obtaining arterial blood samples for blood gas tension and pH analysis.

A ventilator is *volume cycled* when the inspiratory phase is ended at the moment a predetermined volume has been delivered into the patient circuit. Compared to the pressure-cycled ventilator, the initial regulation of the volume-cycled ventilator is straightforward. The operator determines the volume to deliver. As a starting point, the setting for tidal volume is 10 to 15 ml/kg of body weight. Once the desired tidal volume is established, provisions must be made to assure that the volume is delivered within a reasonable time. With most volume-cycled ventilators a flow rate control is present and provides the necessary means of regulating the length of the inspiratory phase.

As soon as the patient is connected to the ventilator, the volume delivered to the patient must be verified with a volume-measuring device (e.g., spirometers). Not all of the volume selected at the ventilator will reach the patient. Some will be lost in the ventilator circuit as a consequence of the system's compliance. Volume may also be lost because of a leak (uncuffed tubes) or if the patient is disconnected from the circuit. The usual method of correcting for lost volume is by slowly increasing delivered volume until the desired return volume is achieved. The flow rate may then need further adjustment to maintain inspiratory time.

With changes in lung conditions the pressure developed by the ventilator to deliver the set volume will change. For example, if the patient's lung compliance decreases, more pressure is needed to deliver the same tidal volume. Conversely, if the patient's compliance improves, less pressure must be developed by the ventilator to deliver the same tidal volume. Other factors that may produce increased pressure readings in volume-cycled ventilators include kinked ventilator tubing, a malpositioned or obstructed endotracheal tube, water condensate in ventilator tubing, increased airway resistance caused by secretions or bronchospasm, and changes in the patient's position.

Ventilators that are *time cycled* change from the inspiratory phase of the breathing cycle to the expiratory phase only after a predetermined time has elapsed. In time-cycled ventilators the cycling is independent of the volume delivered to the patient and the pressure required to deliver the volume. If the pressure increases to deliver a set flow rate in a given time, this increase in pressure may be caused by the same factors as seen for pressure increases in volume-cycled ventilators (e.g., decreased pulmonary compliance, increased airway resistance, occluded endotracheal tube). The same rationale applies to a decreased pressure reading when tidal volume is delivered with a time-cycled ventilator (e.g., leaks in the ventilator-patient circuit, change in patient position).

Time-cycled ventilators do not control volume directly but deliver a volume proportional to the product of flow rate and inspiratory time. Therefore the volume delivered will remain constant as long as the flow rate remains constant. Thus the ideal time-cycled ventilator is one that operates as a flow generator.

In time-cycled ventilators the frequency of ventilation is determined by the inspiratory and expiratory controls. If tidal volume is increased by prolonging the inspiratory time, respiratory rate decreases unless expiration time is decreased. Conversely, if the inspiratory time is decreased to reduce the tidal volume, the ventilatory rate will increase unless expiratory time is increased. If one plans to manipulate the tidal volume without changing inspiratory time, the flow rate can be manipulated.

Expiratory phase. This phase begins when the ventilator's exhalation valve opens. Expiration may proceed in several ways: (1) passively until atmospheric pressure is attained, (2) against an expiratory resistance, or (3) against a positive end-expiratory pressure.

The expiratory time usually is not set but results from the set inspiratory time, flow rate, and ventilator rate. Because the airways tend to collapse during expiratory time, expiratory time constants normally are longer than inspiratory time constants. In diseases such as asthma this difference is accentuated. If the expiratory time is not adequate, the alveoli will not completely empty, resulting in auto-PEEP (see "Time Constants").

Some ventilator circuits, especially when applied to small children with rapid ventilator rates, may have a flow resistance in exhalation valves that causes a functional expiratory retard. It may result in higher expiratory pressures, impairment in ventilation, and difficulty when the patient is in the weaning phase.

Oxygenation

Physiologic mechanisms that give rise to inadequate pulmonary capillary oxygen uptake and hypoxemia include ventilation-perfusion mismatching, shunting, hypoventilation, low inspired oxygen concentration, and diffusion abnormalities (see Chapter 10).

Hypoxemia can be corrected (i.e., increase PaO_2) by several methods. The appropriate choice is based on the specific pathophysiologic process causing the hypoxemia (see "Problem Management" section of this chapter). Increasing the oxygen concentration of the delivered gas will increase the PaO_2 whenever the cause of the hypoxemia is hypoventilation, a diffusion impairment, or ventilation-perfusion mismatching. However, when severe shunt (>20%) is the cause of hypoxemia, increasing the inspired oxygen concentration will not be effective.

PEEP or CPAP is the cornerstone of treatment for patients with acute lung injuries characterized by diffuse alveolar infiltration, decreased FRC, reduced pulmonary compliance, increased intrapulmonary shunt, and arterial hypoxemia refractory to high concentrations of oxygen (see previous section).

Although PEEP is the most commonly used therapy, numerous studies have documented a relationship between oxygenation and mean airway pressure (MAP). MAP is defined as the area under the pressure curve of one ventilatory cycle. Any ventilatory variable that alters the area under the pressure curve translates into a change in MAP. The value of MAP therefore is that it considers not only PEEP, but also peak inspiratory pressure, inspiratory time, ventilator rate, and the pressure waveform created by the ventilator.

The main ventilator manipulations used to improve oxygenation with volume-limited ventilation are tidal volume, inspiratory time, and PEEP. If a pressure-cycled ventilator is used, the manipulations used for improved oxygenation are peak inspiratory pressure, inspiratory time, and PEEP. The optimal level of PEEP (or MAP) is controversial. Different levels of PEEP may be considered best, depending on whether lung compliance, PaO_2, oxygen delivery, intrapulmonary shunt, or dead space ventilation is used to make this determination.

Weaning

Weaning ("liberating" is another and possibly more accurate descriptive term) from mechanical ventilation is determined by clinical trial. Criteria for the initiation of weaning rest on rather ill-defined clinical factors and are not absolute. Generally, weaning from respiratory support is not instituted until hemodynamic stabilization is achieved, the patient is alert and responsive, and all metabolic abnormalities have been corrected. Hypoglycemia, hypophosphatemia, hypomagnesemia, hypocalcemia, hypokalemia, and hypochloremic metabolic alkalemia may all prevent successful weaning. The chest wall and diaphragm must be intact and capable of generating at least -20 cm H_2O pressure at the airway (inspiratory force), and the child must be able to generate a volume of 10 cc/kg body weight of gas with maximal effort (vital capacity). Arterial blood gas and pH values must be stable, and the FiO_2 should be <0.5. The weaning process can begin only after the PaO_2 is acceptable (e.g., $PaO_2 \geq 60$ mm Hg), with a PEEP of <10 cm H_2O.

Nutrition is important in guaranteeing successful weaning from mechanical ventilation. Malnourished children have diminished respiratory drive and low energy stores, which are rapidly depleted. In addition malnutrition decreases the diaphragm's muscle fiber cross-sectional area, resulting in decreased diaphragmatic contractility and enhanced fatigability.

Just as too few calories can have important consequences on a patient's ability to wean from mechanical ventilation, too many calories can also result in respiratory failure. Excessive carbohydrate intake, for example, increases carbon dioxide production, which necessitates increased minute ventilation to facilitate carbon dioxide excretion.

Finally, weaning can be inhibited by multiple other factors, including fever, infection, sedation, psychological status, pain, and structural neurologic damage. Pharmacologic stimulation of respiratory centers with doxapram or medroxyprogesterone is beneficial only in patients with hypoventilation syndromes (e.g., congenital alveolar hypoventilation).

The goal of weaning is to minimize the number of assisted breaths and to have the patient breathe spontaneously during the ventilator's expiratory phase. The two main methods of decreasing ventilatory support currently used are IMV (or SIMV) and T-tube or CPAP trials.

When weaning with IMV, the ventilator rate is gradually decreased over a period of hours to days. Weaning can continue as long as the arterial blood gas tensions and pH remain within an acceptable range and as long as hemodynamic and metabolic stability is maintained. As the amount of spontaneous ventilation increases, the increased work of breathing may cause the child's overall condition to change before blood gas and pH values deteriorate. Tachycardia, hypertension or hypotension, and anxiety are signs of instability. Paradoxic chest wall–abdominal motion, alternating use of intercostal muscles and the diaphragm, and apnea are signs of respiratory muscle fatigue (see Chapter 10). Frequent assessment of the arterial blood gas and pH values (e.g., every 4 hours) and observation of the child's clinical condition are essential throughout the weaning process. Loss of previously gained weight may occur with prolonged increase in work of breathing.

Fortunately most patients who require mechanical ventilation can be easily weaned from ventilator support by using the IMV technique. Difficult-to-wean patients typically have underlying pulmonary disease, neurologic disease, severe systemic disease, malnutrition, or multiple organ failure. For these patients a carefully planned weaning process using alternative methods such as brief CPAP trials, pressure support ventilation, or mandatory minute ventilation may be initiated.

Certain medications may be helpful in the weaning process. Bronchodilators, either inhaled or IV, may help weaning by relieving bronchospasm, improving diaphragmatic muscular strength, and facilitating mucous clearance. The ability of the patient to generate a strong cough is important to a successful extubation and must be assessed. Meticulous attention must also be paid to fluid balance, hematocrit values, and the detection of infection.

Before extubation is considered, careful assessment of the quality and volume of endotracheal secretions is essential. Large, thick secretions may cause extubation to fail if the child cannot cough and clear them adequately. Additionally, extubation should not be attempted in a child without intact airway reflexes (i.e., cough, gag, swallowing).

MONITORING AND LABORATORY TESTS

The goals of monitoring of the mechanically ventilated patient are to assess the adequacy of alveolar ventilation and systemic oxygenation and to check for the multiple possible complications.

The initial assessment of adequate alveolar ventilation and systemic oxygenation is made by clinical observation (see Chapter 10). The observations include vital signs, detection of respiratory distress, assessment of respiratory muscle performance, auscultation of the chest, and assessment of circulation and of the quality and quantity of pulmonary secretions.

Assessment of gas exchange includes use of arterial or capillary blood gas analysis, continuous pulse oximetry, transcutaneous gas analysis (carbon dioxide and oxygen), end-tidal carbon dioxide, mixed venous oxygen saturation, respiratory dead space, and intrapulmonary shunt.

Cardiovascular performance is assessed by determining cardiac output (pulse, systemic arterial blood pressure, urinary output, arterial blood pH, capillary refill), calculated oxygen delivery and consumption, renal and fluid-electrolyte balance, and central venous and pulmonary artery blood pressures.

Lung and chest wall mechanics are evaluated by determining static pressure volume relationships, airway resistance, airway pressure, tidal volume delivered, dynamic compliance, and esophageal pressure. Strength and muscle reserve can be monitored by determining vital capacity and maximal inspiratory pressure and using electromyography. The ventilator performance itself must be monitored continuously and documented in the chart every hour. Variables to monitor include respiratory rate, tidal volume delivered, airway pressure, percentage of inspired oxygen, and temperature of gas delivered.

RISKS AND COMPLICATIONS

Positive pressure ventilation is associated with numerous physiologic and mechanical complications.

Complications of positive pressure ventilation

Positive mean airway pressure
    Decreased cardiac filling and output
    Altered distribution of ventilation and pulmonary
       blood flow
    Extravascular water accumulation
    Pulmonary parenchymal damage
    Gastrointestinal malfunction
    Cerebral ischemia and/or intracranial hypertension
       (decreased central venous return)
    Alveolar hypoventilation or hyperventilation
    Alveolar rupture with extra-alveolar free air
Endotracheal or tracheostomy tubes
    Mucosal damage
    Accidental malposition or extubation
    Partial or complete tube obstruction
    Pneumonia
Operation of ventilator
    Mechanical failure
    Alarm failure
    Inadequate nebulization or humidification

To prevent these complications, it is imperative to comprehend not only how and when to apply airway pressure therapy, but also how and when the therapy may be detrimental or contraindicated. The clinical goal of positive pressure ventilation is to optimize ventilatory mechanics and gas exchange while minimizing impairment of the central and peripheral circulations.

Most adverse physiologic responses to positive pressure ventilation result from inappropriately high MAP (see previous discussion on PEEP). Elevation of the MAP may detrimentally affect cardiac filling and output. Depressed cardiac output and changes in peripheral vascular resistance and blood flow can lead to hypotension, oliguria, and fluid retention, all of which tend to aggravate pulmonary pathology and decrease systemic oxygen transport. Hemodynamic monitoring, IV fluid therapy, and cardiovascular pharmacologic therapy are inseparable from positive airway pressure therapy (see Chapter 12).

Positive pressure ventilation may also adversely affect the distribution of ventilation and pulmonary perfusion. Inappropriately high levels of MAP can lead to overinflation of alveoli, increased dead space ventilation, decreased pulmonary compliance, fluid accumulation in the lungs, and increased intrapulmonary shunt. The beneficial effects and optimal level of positive MAP depend on the underlying pulmonary pathology.

Alveolar rupture and its sequelae constitute the most frequent life-threatening complication of ventilatory assistance (Fig. 128-2). The capacity for instant recognition, evaluation, and relief of these disorders is a primary requisite for PICU personnel.

The occurrence of mechanical failure is more often due to personnel errors than defective equipment. The common mechanical misadventures such as disconnected tubes, extubation, endotracheal tube obstruction, and apparatus malfunction are largely preventable and underscore the need for continuous electrical and human monitoring of both the machine and the patient.

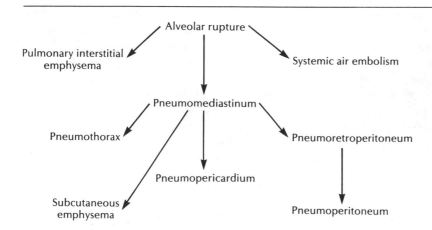

Fig. 128-2 Barotrauma complicating mechanical ventilation.

Problem Management

Acute respiratory distress occurring in the patient on ventilatory support may be caused by the patient or by ventilator malfunction. Common ventilatory dilemmas and their possible causes are listed in Table 128-3.

Table 128-3   Ventilator Dilemmas

Problem	Possible Causes

High peak airway pressure and normal plateau pressure	High peak inspiratory flow rate
	High resistance in endotracheal tube or ventilator connector
	  Small endotracheal tube
	  Kinking
	  Obstruction
	  Secretions
	High airway resistance
	  Secretions
	  Bronchospasm
	  Edema
	  Foreign body
	  Tracheobronchomalacia or stenosis

High plateau and peak pressure	Alveolar overdistention Pulmonary edema Consolidation Atelectasis Mainstem bronchus intubation Pneumothorax Chest wall constriction Abdominal distention Agitation, seizures
Auto-PEEP	Obstructed expiratory circuit Insufficient expiratory time
Low exhaled volumes	Leak from circuit Cuff leak Insufficient delivery Bronchopleural fistula
Increased respiratory rate	Change in clinical status Low tidal volume Insufficient flow rate
No spontaneous breaths	Respiratory alkalosis Sedation CNS problems

Acute hypoxemia. Hypoxemia or worsening systemic oxygenation is a common problem in the PICU patient. Ventilator-related problems, patient-related problems (including progression of the underlying disease), superimposed disorders, interventions, procedures, and medications can all adversely affect the patient's oxygenation. Impaired oxygenation however, is not always due to worsening lung problems. In fact, *sudden* changes in PaO_2 are usually circulatory (e.g., pulmonary arterial hypertension, decreased cardiac output) or metabolic (e.g., increased oxygen demand) in origin if gross ventilatory changes have been excluded (e.g., pneumothorax, bronchial intubation, change in FiO_2, ventilator malfunction).

CAUSES OF IMPAIRED OXYGENATION IN MECHANICALLY VENTILATED PATIENTS

Ventilator-related problems

Endotracheal tube obstruction or malposition
Improper ventilator settings
Ventilator or breathing circuit malfunctions

Progression of underlying disease process
Onset of a new problem

Pneumothorax
Atelectasis
Aspiration
Bronchospasm
Retained secretions
Pulmonary edema
Nosocomial pneumonia
Decreased cardiac output
Increased oxygen demand

Interventions and procedures

Suctioning
Position change
Chest physiotherapy
Thoracentesis
Dialysis
Medications
    Bronchodilators
    Vasodilators

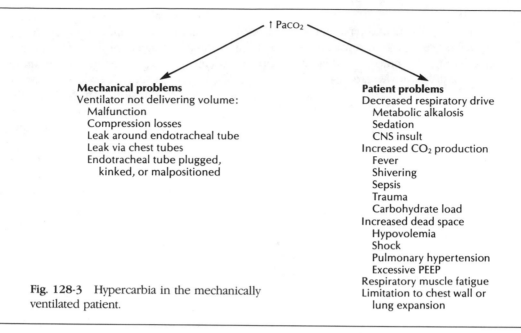

Fig. 128-3 Hypercarbia in the mechanically ventilated patient.

Acute hypercarbia. The adequacy of ventilation of the patient is assessed by the arterial partial pressure of carbon dioxide ($Paco_2$). A frequent problem that develops in patients on mechanical ventilation is hypercarbia (i.e., $Paco_2$ >55 mm Hg in acute conditions). Fig. 128-3 provides an algorithm to aid in differential diagnosis.

An increase in the production of carbon dioxide will necessitate an increase in ventilation to avoid hypercarbia. Occasionally excessive carbohydrate administration results in hypercarbia in compromised patients. Although the administration of adequate calories is essential, excessive calories administered as carbohydrates leads to the formation of fat and the liberation of carbon dioxide. The process is readily reversed by decreasing the carbohydrate load. A few conditions, as part of their abnormal physiology, cause an increase in carbon dioxide as part of their abnormal physiology, cause an increase in carbon dioxide production; they include hyperthyroidism, malignant hyperpyrexia, and drug withdrawal syndrome.

ADDITIONAL READING

Bancalari E. Inadvertent positive end-expiratory pressure during mechanical ventilation. J Pediatr 108:567-569, 1986.

Cane RD, Shapiro BA. Mechanical ventilatory support. JAMA 254:87-92, 1985.

Craig RC, Pierson DJ, Carrico CJ. The clinical application of positive end-expiratory pressure (PEEP) in the adult respiratory distress syndrome (ARDS). Respir Care 30:184-201, 1985.

Dupuis YG. Ventilators: Theory and Clinical Applications. St. Louis: CV Mosby, 1986.

• Marin JJ. Monitoring during mechanical ventilation. Clin Chest Med 9:73-100, 1988.

• McWilliams BC. Mechanical ventilation in pediatric patients. Clin Chest Med 8:597-609, 1987.

Perkin RM, Levin DL. Adverse effects of positive-pressure ventilation in children. In Gregory GA, ed. Respiratory Failures in the Child. New York: Churchill Livingstone, 1981, pp 163-187.

Pierson DJ. Alveolar rupture during mechanical ventilation: Role of PEEP, peak airway pressure, and distending volume. Respir Care 33:472-486, 1988.

Tyler DC. Positive end-expiratory pressure: A review. Crit Care Med 11:300-308, 1983.

129 Analgesia and Sedation

Michael L. Ponaman · Elizabeth Farrington · Frances C. Morriss

INDICATIONS

A reluctance to prescribe analgesic drugs to alleviate postoperative and other pain in neonates and children has existed for years. Such reluctance has been attributed to questions about whether or not neonates and infants perceive pain and to concerns about potential harmful effects of opioid analgesics, such as respiratory depression. Studies conducted in the 1940s on neurologic development concluded that neonatal responses to painful stimuli were decorticate in nature and that neonates lacked perception of localized pain. Recently this conclusion has been reevaluated in light of new observations of patient responses to painful stimuli.

In the recent studies neonates' reactions in response to repeated heel lancing and to circumcision included increased heart rate, respiratory rate, and systemic arterial blood pressure; movement of upper and lower limbs; facial grimacing; palmar sweating; changes in skin conductivity; increased transcutaneous carbon dioxide readings, and decreased arterial oxygen partial pressure. In neonates undergoing circumcision these responses were blunted by opiate-induced analgesia or penile nerve block. In addition recent work has demonstrated a significant neonatal endocrine response to surgical stress; the response was more marked when an analgesic was not given. When evaluating infants undergoing circumcision with and without penile block, researchers reported the autonomic nervous system response observed in both newborns and adults is similar. Studies on neonates who have been circumcised have shown that behavioral changes may persist for more than 22 hours postoperatively in those who did not receive analgesics. Conclusions from these studies support the hypothesis that neonates are capable of feeling and reacting to painful stimuli, and as a result, analgesia is indicated as part of their medical management.

Pain and anxiety increase the heart rate, respiratory rate, and muscle activity, which all contribute to increases in metabolic rate and oxygen consumption. If oxygen delivery cannot be increased sufficiently to meet the greater demand, anaerobic metabolism resulting in metabolic acidosis can ensue. Hormonal studies conducted in infants and children who underwent surgery under minimal anesthesia reported a marked release of catecholamines, growth hormone, glucagon, cortisol, aldosterone, and other corticosteroids as well as suppression of insulin secretion. These changes led to severe and prolonged hyperglycemia caused by a breakdown of carbohydrate and fat stores. Marked increases in blood lactate, pyruvate, total ketone bodies, and nonesterified fatty acids were also noted. Increased protein breakdown was documented after surgery by changes in plasma amino acids, elevated nitrogen excretion, and increased 3-methylhistidine:creatinine ratios in the urine. In a randomized, controlled trial using adequate or minimal anesthesia the stress responses were inhibited in the adequate anesthesia group. Use of appropriate analgesics and anxiolytics in the PICU could prevent some unnecessary metabolic abnormalities and ameliorate a preexisting catabolic state.

In addition to causing exhaustion of carbohydrate reserves the severe and prolonged hyperglycemia associated with stress and pain may have important clinical implications because of its effect on plasma osmolality. In preterm neonates the association of hyperlactatemia and a rapid increase in plasma osmolality may have a deleterious effect on the renal cortex and cerebral substance and may lead to intraventricular hemorrhage.

Since cardiorespiratory, hormonal, and metabolic changes have been reported in infants and children in response to pain and anxiety, proper use of analgesic and anxiolytic medications may result in additional physiologic benefits to the patient. The medications can be as beneficial to the patient as assisted ventilation or inotropic support.

Tracheal intubation and often ventilation in both preterm and full-term neonates while they are awake causes a significant decrease in tco$_2$ together with increases in systemic arterial blood pressure and ICP. The rise in ICP may be associated with an increased incidence of intraventricular hemorrhage. The increases in ICP with intubation were, however, abolished in preterm neonates who were anesthetized. In addition infants' cardiovascular responses to tracheal suctioning were abolished by using opiate analgesia.

Sedation can sometimes be beneficial for patients with airway obstruction (both upper airway and reactive airways disease) if agitation is creating unnecessary effort and energy expenditure. Treatment of such a patient who does not have an artificial airway, however, must be contingent on several prerequisites: (1) that the agitation is not a sign of hypoxia, (2) that the increased effort and respiratory rate are not the mechanisms by which the patient is achieving adequate carbon dioxide elimination, (3) that the patient is being cared for in a setting in which continuous observation and monitoring of the airway exist, and (4) that there is skilled assistance imme-

Table 129-1   Pharmacologic Control of Pain, Agitation, and Anxiety

Drug	Dosage	Route of Administration	Onset of Action	Duration of Action
Narcotics				
Morphine	Single dose Children: 0.1-0.2 mg/kg Neonates and infants: 0.05 mg/kg Continuous infusion Children: 20 μg/kg/hr Neonates and infants: 15 μg/kg/hr Epidural <7 yr: 1 mg 8-10 yr: 1.5 mg >11 yr: 2.0 mg	IV, IM, SC	IV: 10-15 min IM: 20-30 min	4 hr
Meperidine (Demerol)	1-2 mg/kg	IV, IM, SC, PO	IV: 10 min IM: 15-20 min PO: 20 min	2-4 hr 3 hr
Fentanyl (Sublimaze)	1-5 μg/kg Continuous infusion 1-3 μg/kg/hr	IV, IM	3-5 min	30-60 min
Sufentanil (Sufenta)	0.1-0.5 μg/kg Continuous infusion 0.1-0.3 μg/kg/hr	IV	Immediate; shorter than fentanyl	30-60 min
Alfentanil (Alfenta)	1-2 μg/kg/min	IV	Immediate	11-20 min
Methadone	0.1-0.2 mg/kg	PO, IM, SC	1 hr	IM: 3-4 hr PO: 6-12 hr
Codeine	0.5-1.0 mg/kg	PO	1 hr	4-6 hr
General anesthetic and analgesic				
Ketamine (Ketalar)	5-10 mg/kg 1-2 mg/kg 1-2 mg/kg/hr	IM IV, single dose IV, continuous	3-4 min 30 sec	12-25 min 5-10 min

diately available to establish an artificial airway if sedation causes complete airway decompensation. Un-
questionably adequate sedation is indispensable for
good care of a patient on a ventilator; it relieves
anxiety, allows the patient to tolerate otherwise noxious invasion of the airway, and usually facilitates
more normal gas exchange. For certain types of patients in whom the cardiovascular reflexes associated
with airway instrumentation and manipulation can
be life threatening (i.e., patient with increased ICP,
pulmonary arterial hypertension, or severe airway
reactivity), sedation before exposure to noxious stimuli is mandatory.

PHARMACOLOGIC CONTROL OF PAIN, AGITATION, AND ANXIETY (Table 129-1)

Physicians have treated pain, agitation, and anxiety as
a single entity with fixed-dose preparations containing narcotics, antihistamines, and phenothiazines.
Although the fixed-dose preparations are used to
immobilize an uncooperative child during medical
procedures, they inadequately address the primary
component of a specific child's discomfort. One must
identify which component (pain, agitation, anxiety)
contributes most to each patient's discomfort and
choose drug therapy appropriately.

Table 129-1 Pharmacologic Control of Pain, Agitation, and Anxiety—cont'd

Drug	Dosage	Route of Administration	Onset of Action	Duration of Action
Benzodiazepines				
Diazepam (Valium)	0.1-0.2 mg/kg	PO, IV	IV: 15 min PO: 30-60 min	IV: 4-6 hr PO: 6-8 hr
Lorazepam (Ativan)	0.05-0.1 mg/kg	PO, IV, IM	IV: 15 min PO: 30-60 min	8-12 hr
Midazolam (Versed)	0.05-0.1 kg	IV, IM, PO	IV: 2-5 min IM: 20-30 min PO: 10-30 min	2 hr
Barbiturates				
Phenobarbital	2-3 mg/kg	PO, IV	IV: 5 min PO: 20-60 min	8-12 hr
Pentobarbital (Nembutal)	2-4 mg/kg	PO, IM, IV, PR	IV: <5 min IM: <20 min PO: 20-60 min PR: 30-60 min	4-6 hr

	Pentobarbital coma
	  Load: 18 mg/kg over 2 hr
	  Maintenance: 1 mg/kg/hr initial; titrate to
	    achieve drug level, 20-50 µg/ml			

Sodium thiopental (Pentothal)	4-6 mg/kg	IV	30-60 sec	5-10 min
Mephobarbital (Mebaral)	1-2 mg/kg 25-30 mg/kg	IV PR	30-60 sec 8-15 min	3-5 min 30-60 min
Hypnotic				

Chloral hydrate (Noctec)	Sedation
	  25-50 mg/kg
	Hypnotic
	  75-100 mg/kg
		PO, PR	30-60 min	6-8 hr

Once the cause of discomfort is identified, the age of the patient and the intensity and duration of the noxious stimuli must be taken into consideration to optimize drug delivery. In the newborn infant and the neonatal population it is difficult to tell when the patient is in pain. Therefore a continuous infusion of narcotic analgesic postoperatively may provide better pain relief than an as-needed dosing regimen. If pain is associated with a scheduled occurrence such as chest physiotherapy or suctioning, a scheduled dose of medication before the procedure would be appropriate. Premedication must be provided before all painful medical procedures such as central catheter or chest tube placement, bone marrow aspiration, and spinal taps. Patient-controlled anesthesia (PCA), an epidural catheter, or repeated regional blocks may be used postoperatively to administer narcotic or other analgesic medication.

Pain: Narcotics

An opioid is often the drug of choice for controlling patient pain in the PICU. Fentanyl and morphine are used most frequently in pediatric patients since support exists in the literature for dosing recommendations. In small children, newborn infants, and neonates who are unable to verbalize their pain, either scheduled administration or a continuous infusion of a narcotic will provide optimal pain relief. Epidural catheters placed for anesthesia at the time of surgery may be used postoperatively for continued administration of analgesics. The potential benefits of epidural administration of narcotics include (1) decreased total dose of narcotic, (2) use of narcotic analgesics in patients previously tolerant to parenteral narcotics, (3) improved pulmonary function, and (4) fewer side effects (primarily respiratory depression and sedation).

Mechanism of action

A specific action of narcotics occurs on the opiate receptor system located in the ventral mesencephalon, mesalimbic area, thalamus amygdala, hypothalamus, periaqueductal gray matter, spinal cord, and non-CNS organs that mimics the actions of endogenous opiate-like peptides (e.g., endorphins, enkephalins, other CNS pentapeptides). They mediate analgesia and alter emotional responses to pain, respiratory responses to pain, and vascular tone.

Effects (Table 129-2)

Cardiovascular effects. Narcotics decrease heart rate (except for an increase with meperidine). Cardiac output is minimally affected except by meperidine, which is a myocardial depressant. Histamine release, particularly with morphine, causes a decrease in systemic arterial blood pressure secondary to decreased vascular resistance.

Respiratory effects. Narcotics cause a depression that is dose related. All aspects of respiration are depressed, including rate, tidal volume, minute volume, rhythmicity, and carbon dioxide responsiveness. The respiratory rate is decreased before volume

---

ADVERSE EFFECTS OF NARCOTICS

Major hazards

Generalized respiratory depression (tidal volume, rate, rhythmicity, carbon dioxide responsiveness), including apnea, circulatory depression, hypoxia

Specific organ effects

CNS: Dysphoria, delirium, anxiety, disorientation, hallucinations, loss of consciousness, impairment of mental and physical performance, physical dependence, seizures (high-dose fentanyl); choreic movements (alfentanil)

Cardiovascular: Histamine release (flushing, whelps along course of vein, hypotension), bradycardia; tachycardia, hypertension, myocardial depression (meperidine); asystole (alfentanil); reduction of venous and arterial tone (morphine)

Respiratory: See "Major Hazards"; chest wall rigidity (seen with rapid IV administration), decreased ciliary activity

GI: Constipation, delayed gastric emptying, biliary tract spasm, nausea, emesis; increased gastric, biliary, pancreatic salivary secretions

GU: Urinary retention, urethral and vesical sphincter spasm; antidiuretic effect with oliguria

Bothersome effects

Nausea, dry mouth, orthostatic hypotension (dizziness and light-headedness), decreased potency

is decreased. Carbon dioxide responsiveness remains decreased for 3 to 4 hours after a single small or normal dose and for hours after large doses or continuous infusions. Such depression may necessitate ventilatory support and has implications for weaning a patient from respiratory support when sedatives, which are also respiratory depressants, continue to be used. High doses of morphine are associated with increased bronchial ciliary activity.

Musculoskeletal effects. Either a high dose or rapid IV bolus administration of fentanyl causes pronounced rigidity. In addition there is increased thoracic and abdominal muscle tone.

Renal effects. Narcotics have mild antidiuretic effects, which are probably related to a decrease in glomerular filtration rate caused by altered hemodynamics. ADH release is not stimulated.

Gastrointestinal effects. Narcotics cause nausea and emesis by direct stimulation of the CNS chemoreceptor trigger zone, and the nausea and vomiting are exacerbated by changes in posture. In addition an inhibition of GI tract mobility caused by an increase in smooth muscle resting tone occurs. Increases in gastric, pancreatic, biliary, and salivary secretions occur, as does an increase in biliary duct pressure.

Modification of stress responses. Stress responses are altered by narcotics and include inhibition of (1) release of ACTH, (2) release of cortisol, (3) catecholamine release due to pain since its release depends on the functional state of the sympathetic nervous system (other sources of catecholamine release caused by stress may not be inhibited), and (4) hyperglycemic response, which can be particularly abolished with administration of fentanyl.

Side effects

In standard doses the most common side effects of morphine and other narcotic analgesics are nausea, vomiting, constipation, drowsiness, and confusion. Urinary retention may occur because of increased bladder sphincter tone. Dry mouth, sweating, facial flushing, vertigo, bradycardia, palpitations, or orthostatic hypotension, hypothermia, restlessness, changes in mood, and miosis have also occurred. These effects are more common in the ambulatory patient. Because of respiratory depression and resulting hypercarbia, there may be an elevation in the

Table 129-2 Cardiovascular Effects of Common Sedatives*

Drug	Heart Rate	Systemic Arterial Blood Pressure	Cardiac Index	Systemic Vascular Resistance	Central Venous Blood Pressure	Pulmonary Artery Blood Pressure
Morphine†	→	Mild ↓	No change	→	→	Minimal →
Fentanyl	→	No change	No change	No change	No change	No change
Meperidine	←	←	→→	←	No change	Unknown
Thiopental†	←	No change to mild →	→→	←	←	No change
Benzodiazepine	Minimal change	Mild →	Mild →	Minimal change	Mild →	No change
Ketamine	↑↑	↑↑	↑↑	←	←	←
Chloral hydrate	No change to mild →	No change	No change to mild →	No change	No change	Unknown
Narcotics,† benzodiazepines, nitrous oxide, or barbituates	→	↓↓	→ to ↓↓	←	→	→

*From Kaplan J. Cardiac anesthesia. In Cardiovascular Pharmacology, vol 2. New York: Grune & Stratton, 1983.
†All effects will be increased by hypovolemia or preexisting uncompensated or poorly compensated heart disease. ↑ = increase; ↓ = decrease.

Table 129-3   Contraindications for Common Sedatives

Drug	Contraindication	Alternative
Narcotic	Apnea (relative contraindication)	Choral hydrate
	Hypovolemia	Benzodiazepine, ketamine
	Asthma (avoid morphine, meperidine)	Ketamine, fentanyl
	Hemodialysis	Avoid morphine
Ketamine	Increased intracranial pressure	Barbiturate
	Pulmonary artery hypertension	Narcotic, thorazine
	Increased intraocular pressure	Barbiturate
	Seizures (relative contraindication)	Barbiturate, benzodiazepine
	Severe systemic hypertension	Benzodiazepine, morphine
Benzodiazepine	Hepatic failure	Reduce dose; consider narcotic for which the effect can be reversed
Barbiturate	Reduced cardiac reserve	Etomidate (for anesthesia), chloral hydrate
	Porphyria	Benzodiazepine
	Asthma	Ketamine, benzodiazepine, fentanyl
Chloral hydrate	Gastric or rectal irritation	Any

Table 129-4   Special Considerations in Neonates and Premature Infants*

Drug	Difference	Modifying Action
Narcotic	Greater toxicity, particularly respiratory depression; morphine more depressant than meperidine and fentanyl	Reduce dose.
	Despite adequate plasma levels, stress responses not uniformly blunted by fentanyl	Consider supplementation with another agent.
	GI obstruction unless pain relief needed	
Ketamine	Less effective in infants <6 months of age	Choose alternative agent; if one chosen, maintain airway and control ventilation.
	Elimination half-life prolonged	
	At doses required to achieve lack of movement, apnea and respiratory depression common	
	Generalized extensor spasm; opisthotonus more common	
Benzodiazepine	Decreased elimination of drug (prolonged CNS and respiratory depression)	Choose alternative agent.
	Impaired thermoregulation	
Barbiturate	Greater penetration of blood-brain barrier	Consider using reduced dosage.
	Decreased ability to metabolize	Avoid use of long-acting agents in premature infants.
	More lethal on mg/kg basis	Use with appropriate monitoring.

* Modified from Cook DR, Marcy JH. Neonatal Anesthesia. Pasadena, Calif.: Appleton Davies, 1988.

ICP. When adequate ventilation is provided to the patient, increased ICP is not a contraindication to the use of narcotics (Tables 129-3 and 129-4). Large doses of narcotics cause respiratory depression as indicated previously. In addition larger doses may also suppress responsiveness of α-adrenergic receptors, resulting in peripheral vasodilation, reduced peripheral resistance, and inhibition of baroreceptors, leading to orthostatic hypotension, fainting, circulatory collapse, and coma (due to circulatory insufficiency). With very high narcotic levels infants and children may have convulsions.

Dosage

See below.

Anesthesia: Ketamine
Mechanism of action

Ketamine is a dissociative anesthetic with profound analgesic properties, particularly for skin, bone, muscle, and connective tissue. Ketamine can be the sole anesthetic agent for diagnostic and superficial surgical procedures when muscle relaxation is not needed. It is a poorer choice of analgesic for procedures involving visceral pain.

NARCOTIC DOSAGE

Continuous intravenous infusion

Morphine
  Load: 50 μg/kg
  Maintenance: 15 μg/kg/hr (neonates); 20 μg/kg/
    hr (newborns and children)

Fentanyl
  Load: 3-5 μg/kg
  Maintenance: 1-5 μg/kg/hr

Patient-controlled anesthesia

Morphine
  Intermittent dose: 20 μg/kg
  Lockout interval: 6 min
  Hour limit: 100 μg/kg

Epidural administration

Morphine
  0.05-0.1 mg/kg/dose*; duration of action: 8-24 hr

---

*Dose determined from adult data.

Effect

Ketamine increases heart rate and systemic arterial blood pressure, cardiac output, intracranial pressure, pulmonary arterial blood pressure, myocardial oxygen consumption, and central venous blood pressure by activation of the sympathetic nervous system and by inhibition of reuptake of norepinephrine (Table 129-2). On a tissue level, however, it is a direct myocardial depressant and to some extent an antidysrhythmic agent, particularly for epinephrine-induced dysrhythmias.

Laryngeal and pharyngeal reflexes are better preserved with ketamine than other agents, but they are not unaffected. Patients receiving ketamine have been shown to aspirate into the lungs radiographic contrast material placed both into the stomach and the posterior pharynx.

Ketamine decreases airways resistance and relaxes airway smooth muscle, making it an excellent agent for use in patients with asthma, particularly during airway instrumentation.

Side effects

In the severely hypovolemic patient whose compensation has depended on massive catecholamine output, an injection of ketamine can cause hypotension secondary to myocardial depression. The increase in myocardial oxygen consumption makes ketamine inappropriate for use in a patient with reduced myocardial reserve or coronary artery disease. Although the increase in ICP and pulmonary arterial blood pressure is not direct but related to increases in either heart rate, systemic arterial blood pressure, or cardiac output, it is not a good agent for patients with closed-head injury or pulmonary arterial hypertension.

Ketamine must be used cautiously in patients with hypovolemia to avoid depletion of catecholamine stores and must not be used without concomitant and vigorous volume replacement.

A side effect of ketamine is tremendous stimulation of production of tracheal and pharyngeal secretions, which can cause airway irritability and/or obstruction. Ketamine is never used without a sialagogue.

Like all anesthetic agents ketamine is capable of producing apnea (Table 129-4). Infants are more susceptible to respiratory depression than older children. A serious drawback to its use is the very high incidence (3% to 30%) in older children and adults of unpleasant emergent phenomena, including auditory and visual hallucinations, delirium, and agitation. Patients receiving ketamine preferably must recover in an area in which a nonstimulating atmosphere (i.e., low light, decreased sound, decreased handling) can be provided. These emergent reactions can be minimized by use of a benzodiazepine.

A fairly high incidence of extrapyramidal muscle activity, fasciculations, purposeless movement of extremities, and clonic spasms occurs when ketamine is used alone. These movements may interfere with procedures and/or examinations. Controversy exists about whether ketamine is epileptogenic and most authors believe its use is contraindicated in patients with seizure disorders (Table 129-3).

Dosage

Intravenous dosage. The fractional dose, 1 to 2 mg/kg as a bolus, will induce anesthesia rapidly, and a dissociative state will last approximately 6 to 10 minutes. Subsequent incremental doses are usually approximately 50% of the induction dose and are given at intervals of 8 to 15 minutes. Recovery occurs within 30 minutes.

Continuous infusion reduces the total dose given. It is usually given as a solution containing 1 to 2 mg/ml. An initial bolus is given to induce anesthesia; then the drug is administered at a rate of 1 to 2 mg/kg/hr.

Intramuscular dosage. The initial dose is 5 to 10 mg/kg, with induction of dissociation in 3 to 5 minutes, particularly if the deltoid muscle is used for injection. The effect generally lasts 15 to 30 minutes. If longer anesthesia is needed, an IV may be started to give either an incremental or continuous dose. Ketamine lends itself well to use for discrete procedures (as opposed to control of ventilation or treatment of anxiety). It is a potent anesthetic agent; therefore it must be administered by someone versed in its properties. Appropriate monitoring of cardiovascular and respiratory variables is mandatory during its use (airway reflex depression is possible), and it must be used in a setting in which airway support, including instrumentation, is immediately available.

Anxiety: Benzodiazepine

Decreasing anxiety is best achieved with a benzodiazepine. The main advantage of the benzodiazepines is they provide excellent amnesia. Differences between benzodiazepine agents are in duration of action, preferred route of administration, and degree of amnesia provided (Table 129-1). Some agents have active metabolites with a longer half-life ($t_{1/2}$) than the parent compound (diazepam), and accumulation of the metabolite (oxazepam) may occur with prolonged use (e.g., continuous infusion). Midazolam is the agent of choice for use as a continuous infusion since it lacks active metabolites and has a short $t_{1/2}$.

Mechanism of action

Benzodiazepines facilitate the inhibitory effect of γ-aminobutyric acid (GABA) on neuronal transmission at limbic, thalamic, hypothalamic, and spinal levels on specific receptor sites in the CNS.

Pharmacokinetics

Members of this family of drugs are metabolized by hepatic microsomal enzymes through demethylation; many metabolites are pharmacologically active and thus contribute to the potential for development of dependence and long-term side effects. Enterohepatic recirculation for orally administered doses can give rise to biphasic plasma peaks.

Cimetidine, a hepatic enzyme inhibitor, prolongs the hypnotic and other effects. Heparin displaces benzodiazepines from protein and increases the free (active) plasma fraction. Doses must be decreased with concomitant use of these drugs.

Routes

Benzodiazepines can be given orally and intravenously. Some are absorbed well intramuscularly; however, absorption of diazepam is erratic enough to preclude use of this route.

Effects

CNS effects. All degrees of CNS depression occur with administration of benzodiazepines, from hypnosis to coma secondary to actions on reticular facility and limbic systems. They reduce anxiety and aggression and are associated with profound retrograde amnesia, but benzodiazepines have no analgesic properties. They are cumulative with other CNS depressants in causing depression. All benzodiazepines are potent anticonvulsants. When used alone they have no significant cardiovascular effects but can cause myocardial depression when given in conjunction with barbiturates or narcotics.

Musculoskeletal effects. Benzodiazepines cause skeletal muscle relaxation produced by inhibition of afferent spinal pathways and potentiate neuromuscular blocking agents.

Respiratory system effects. Benzodiazepines are moderate respiratory depressants and have cumulative potentiation with other respiratory depressants. Rapid administration can cause apnea. The carbon dioxide response remains unaltered.

Toxicity and side effects

Benzodiazepines cause venous irritation, with pain, erythema, and development of thrombophlebitis, which is particularly true of diazepam, but this is not a problem with lorazepam or midazolam. They can cause myocardial depression when used in conjunction with other sedatives and narcotics. There is a great potential for abuse of these drugs with the development of tolerance.

Sedative-Hypnotics: Barbiturates

Historically, barbiturates were used to treat patient agitation. Currently their primary role is as a sedative or hypnotic for use during nonpainful procedures, when movement cannot be permitted (i.e., during MRI and CT), and as an anticonvulsant. All the barbiturate compounds are derivatives of barbituric acid and have similar side effects. They differ in their onset and duration of action (Table 129-1). The drugs decrease the excitability of both presynaptic and postsynaptic membranes. The CNS is most sensitive with standard dosing, and sedation and hypnosis precede cardiac, skeletal, or smooth muscle effects. Barbiturates have no analgesic action and may even increase the reaction to painful stimuli at subanesthetic doses. All barbiturates exhibit anticonvulsant activity, but only phenobarbital, metharbital, and mephobarbital are effective anticonvulsants in subhypnotic doses. Barbiturates have a wide range of effects on EEG tracings, and they decrease time spent in REM sleep.

Mechanism of action

Although the mechanism of action of barbiturates is unknown, it probably occurs at multiple sites in more than one way. In general there are three basic effects:

1. Facilitation or enhancement of synaptic actions of inhibitory neurotransmitters
2. Blockade of synaptic actions of excitatory neurotransmitters
3. Enhancement and/or modulation of the actions of GABA (there may be CNS target sites as well)

Metabolism

Barbiturates are metabolized by the liver, which converts the barbiturate to inactive water-soluble products excreted in the urine. The effects of the drugs, especially the shorter acting ones, depend more on distribution than metabolism. The action on any specific organ such as the brain depends more on blood flow. For organs with high blood flow (brain, lungs, heart), peak drug levels, hence drug effects, are attained very rapidly, whereas peak effect occurs more slowly for organs with low blood flow (bone, fat). After equilibration occurs between blood and high-flow organs, effects begin to be seen in other organs as the drug is redistributed. It is possible for patients to show no effects of the drug and still have significant unmetabolized drug present.

The drug is highly protein bound.

Effects (Table 129-2)

CNS effects. Barbiturates have potent effects on cerebral metabolism, with dose-related depression of metabolic oxygen consumption and cerebral blood flow (presumably secondary to autoregulation), which is a desired effect in patients with increased ICP. Depression of electrical activity with production of an isoelectric EEG occurs. There are decreased membrane excitability and impulse traffic, which provide the basis of the anticonvulsant effects. Barbiturates have no analgesic effects. They do produce the full spectrum of clinical depression from drowsiness to coma.

Cardiac effects. Barbiturates cause a decrease in myocardial contractility related to decreased bioavailability of calcium to myofibrils. Usually a compensatory (baroreceptor mediated) increase in heart rate and maintenance of cardiac output occur; however, barbiturates can cause profound decreases in cardiac output in patients with reduced reserve.

In addition there is peripheral vasodilation secondary to histamine release and decreases in CVP. These effects are most pronounced with IV administration of the short-acting barbiturates methohexital and thiopental.

Respiratory effects. A dose-related respiratory depression (decreased minute ventilation) occurs with administration of barbiturates at high IV doses. Apnea of 3 to 5 minutes' duration can occur. Respiratory depression is cumulative with administration of other respiratory depressants. Airway protective reflexes are preserved, making airway instrumentation with thiopental or methohexital alone hazardous since laryngospasm or bronchospasm will not be inhibited. The incidence of airway reflexes occurring with use of thiopental alone as a sedative or anesthetic is as follows: hiccups or cough, 5%; laryngospasm, 1%.

Musculoskeletal effects. Tremors and involuntary muscle movements occur.

Skin effects. Transient rashes related to histamine release occur.

Side effects

IV administration of barbiturates can produce severe respiratory depression, apnea, laryngospasm, coughing, and vasodilation with hypotension, especially when administered too rapidly. All barbiturates depress respiratory drive but maintain airway protective reflexes. Most barbiturates are inducers of the cytochrome P-450 enzyme system and may cause a decrease in warfarin, corticosteroid, and anticonvulsant serum levels. This induction may occur at any time from 3 days to 2 weeks after administration. Barbiturates may increase serum porphyrin and are contraindicated in patients with a history of porphyria.

Dosage (Table 129-1)

Special considerations when using these agents in neonates and premature infants are presented in Table 129-4.

ADDITIONAL READING

Anand KJS, Hickey PR. Pain and its effects in the human neonate and fetus. N Engl J Med 317:1321-1329, 1987.

• Committee on Drugs, Section on Anesthesiology. Guidelines for the elective use of conscious sedation, deep sedation, and general anesthesia in pediatric patients. Pediatrics 76:317-321, 1985.

Cousen G, Reaves JG, Stanley TA. Intravenous anesthesia and analgesia. Philadelphia: Lea & Febiger, 1988.

McGrath PJ, Urreh AM. Pain in Children and Adolescents. New York: Elsevier, 1987.

Schechter NL. Pain and pain control in children. Curr Probl Pediatr 15:1-230, 1985.

130 Paralytic Agents

Stan L. Davis

BACKGROUND AND INDICATIONS

Paralytic agents, or neuromuscular blocking agents, are among the most commonly administered drugs in the PICU. Thus it is appropriate that the discussion of these agents follows the section on sedation since only in the most unstable patient is the use of neuromuscular blockade without sedation indicated. The most common indications for neuromuscular blockade in the PICU are to facilitate tracheal intubation and mechanical ventilation or to prevent increases in oxygen consumption, intrathoracic pressure, or intracranial pressure secondary to struggling against mechanical ventilation.

Although detailed review of the physiology of the neuromuscular junction cannot be presented here, an understanding of the basic physiology is necessary for discussion of the pharmacodynamics of the neuromuscular blocking agents. The neuromuscular junction consists of the prejunctional motor nerve ending, synaptic cleft, and postjunctional membrane, which contains nicotinic cholinergic receptors (Fig. 130-1). The neurotransmitter acetylcholine is synthesized in the motor nerve terminal and stored in vesicles, which release acetylcholine into the synaptic cleft on the arrival of a nerve impulse. The acetylcholine molecules diffuse across the synaptic cleft and bind to the acetylcholine receptors, initiating a conformational change in the receptor that "opens" a potential channel formed by the receptor subunits (Fig. 130-2). The opening of this channel allows the influx of sodium and calcium ions and the efflux of potassium ions, thereby facilitating the depolarization of the motor endplate and propagation of an action potential that spreads across the skeletal muscle fibers, leading to contraction. The enzyme acetylcholinesterase is responsible for rapid hydrolysis of acetylcholine, which terminates the depolarization of the motor endplate.

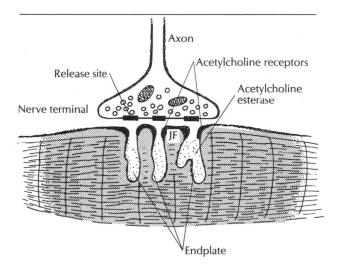

Fig. 130-1   Neuromuscular junction.

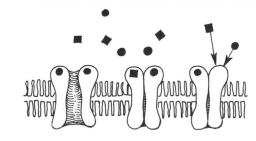

Fig. 130-2   Schematic representation of acetylcholine receptors with the ion channel in open configuration when occupied by acetylcholine molecules (circles) and closed when occupied by a neuromuscular blocking agent (squares).

921

All currently available neuromuscular blocking agents exert their activity at the site of the acetylcholine receptor. They are classified as either depolarizing (succinylcholine) or nondepolarizing (pancuronium, *d*-tubocurarine, vecuronium, atracurium) relaxants according to their effect on the motor endplate.

TECHNIQUE
Selection of Neuromuscular Blocking Agents

The selection of a neuromuscular blocking agent must be based on the needs of the patient (Table 130-1). The four variables that must be considered are time of onset, duration of action, side effects, and route of elimination for the agent chosen. This choice is not always straightforward, especially when complicated by the need for tracheal intubation without bag and mask ventilation as in the case of the patient with a full stomach. Succinylcholine remains the gold standard for a rapid-sequence intubation because of the onset of 90% neuromuscular blockade within 60 seconds. Despite a more rapid onset in children compared to adults, the nondepolarizing relaxants generally take 3 to 4 minutes to reach intubating conditions. However, if succinylcholine is contraindicated, two techniques can hasten the onset of

Table 130-1   Neuromuscular Blocking Agents

Agent	Dose	Infusion Rate	Duration of Action	Elimination	Cardiovascular Effects	Other Effects
Depolarizing						
Succinylcholine	Children: 1-1.5 mg/kg Infants: 2.0 mg/kg; IM 4 mg/kg	NA	<10 min	Plasma cholinesterase	Dysrhythmias—bradycardia, nodal rhythm, asystole	Hyperkalemia Increased intracranial and intraocular pressure
Nondepolarizing						
Pancuronium	0.1 mg/kg	NA	50-60 min	80% renal	Vagolytic—increased HR, increased MAP, increased CO	
d-Tubocurarine	0.5 mg/kg	NA	35-45 min	45% renal 10%-40% hepatic	Histamine release—decreased MAP, decreased CO	
Vecuronium	0.1 mg/kg	0.06-0.1 mg/kg/hr	25-35 min	25%-30% renal 45% + hepatic	None	
Atracurium	0.5 mg/kg	0.3-0.6 mg/kg/hr	20-30 min	Hofmann elimination and ester hydrolysis	Mild histamine release	Metabolized to laudanosine; CNS stimulation and possible seizures at high levels

NA = not applicable; HR = heart rate; MAP = mean aortic pressure; CO = cardiac output.

neuromuscular blockade with nondepolarizing agents. The technique of "priming" remains controversial, especially in pediatric patients. It involves the administration of one tenth of the normal dose of relaxant 3 to 4 minutes before giving the full dose. The inherent risks are related to the degree of weakness or respiratory distress in the patient before priming and to the fear and anxiety produced by the diplopia and dyspnea that often follow the priming dose. The second technique involves giving a relative overdose of the neuromuscular blocking agent to flood the receptors, thereby shortening the time of onset. The usual practice is to administer two times the intubation dose of a relaxant as a rapid bolus. The complications of this technique are related to the cardiovascular effects of the relaxant, which can be avoided by the use of a drug with a stable cardiovascular profile such as vecuronium.

Depolarizing Neuromuscular Blocking Agent
Succinylcholine

Succinylcholine remains the only depolarizing neuromuscular blocking agent approved for use in the United States. Succinylcholine is formed by the junction of two acetylcholine molecules and acts by binding to the acetylcholine receptor, initiating depolarization of the motor endplates in a random fashion. Neuromuscular blockade develops because the hydrolysis of succinylcholine by plasma cholinesterase (pseudocholinesterase) is much slower than the hydrolysis of acetylcholine; therefore it results in prolonged depolarization of the motor endplate. The major advantage of succinylcholine is its rapid onset of neuromuscular blockade, usually providing intubating conditions within 60 seconds after an IV dose of 1.0 to 1.5 mg/kg in children and 2.0 mg/kg in infants less than 1 year of age. In emergency situations involving a patient without venous access succinylcholine may be given intramuscularly in a dose of 4 mg/kg. The duration of action under normal circumstances is <10 minutes.

Nondepolarizing Neuromuscular Blocking Agents

In contrast to succinylcholine, the nondepolarizing neuromuscular blocking agents are large, bulky molecules that bind to one or more of the acetylcholine receptor subunits without initiating a conformational change leading to depolarization of the motor endplate. Instead, these agents block neuromuscular transmission in a competitive fashion by preventing

acetylcholine from binding to an occupied receptor (Fig. 130-2). All of these drugs contain one or more quaternary ammonium groups responsible for binding the acetylcholine receptor and either a steroidal or benzylisoquinolium nucleus, which determines the route of elimination as well as possible cardiovascular side effects.

Pancuronium

Pancuronium is a long-acting steroidal, nondepolarizing relaxant with a duration of action of 50 to 60 minutes following an intubation dose of 0.1 mg/kg. Pancuronium causes increases in heart rate, mean systemic arterial blood pressure, and cardiac output secondary to its vagolytic effect and relies on the kidney for 80% of its elimination.

d-Tubocurarine

d-Tubocurarine, also a long-acting nondepolarizing agent, produces a dose-dependent increase in plasma histamine concentration, which can result in a decrease in mean systemic arterial blood pressure. However, the significant (20%) decrease in mean systemic arterial blood pressure following an intubation dose of 0.5 mg/kg can be attenuated if the drug is injected slowly rather than as a bolus injection. d-Tubocurarine has a duration of action of 35 to 45 minutes, with both renal and hepatic elimination.

Vecuronium

Vecuronium, an analog of pancuronium, has a duration of action of 25 to 35 minutes, resulting in its classification as an intermediate-acting neuromuscular blocking agent. In addition to its shorter half-life a major advantage of vecuronium is its lack of vagolytic effects or histamine release, giving this drug very stable cardiovascular characteristics. The intubation dose of vecuronium, 0.1 mg/kg, is similar to that of pancuronium. Elimination of vecuronium is principally hepatic, and renal failure usually necessitates no change in dosage. An unexplained observation is that the clearance of vecuronium appears to increase slightly in patients with liver disease, although no mechanism has been described.

Atracurium

Atracurium is an intermediate-acting relaxant with a benzylisoquinolium ester structure responsible for its spontaneous degradation by Hofmann elimination and ester hydrolysis. Hofmann elimination is a purely chemical process that results in the molecular fragmentation of atracurium to form laudanosine and a monoquaternary acrylate. This results in a duration of action of 20 to 30 minutes, which is independent of hepatic or renal function. An intubation dose of 0.5 mg/kg atracurium induces very minimal histamine release, which becomes significant only with doses >0.6 mg/kg given rapidly.

Continuous infusions

Because of the noncumulative pharmacokinetics of vecuronium and atracurium, they are uniquely suited to administration by continuous infusion in the PICU. After the usual loading dose of either agent, a continuous infusion of 0.06 to 0.1 mg/kg/hr for vecuronium or 0.36 to 0.6 mg/kg/hr for atracurium is begun, with the infusion rate titrated to achieve the desired train-of-four ratio (see "Monitoring Neuromuscular Blockade"). On discontinuation of the infusion, recovery of neuromuscular function is both rapid and predictable, assuming that the depth of blockade has been adequately monitored.

New Neuromuscular Blocking Agents

Currently three drugs of potential interest to the intensivist are undergoing trials in humans. It is likely that all three of these new agents will be released for clinical use within the next 2 years; therefore they deserve at least brief mention. Doxacurium and pipecuronium are long-acting relaxants with almost the same pharmacokinetics as pancuronium but without the vagolytic side effects. In addition a new benzylisoquinolium relaxant, mivacurium, has been developed as the first short-acting nondepolarizing neuromuscular blocking agent. It is particularly attractive for use in the pediatric population since onset of action appears to be more rapid in children, providing intubating conditions within 60 seconds. In addition the histamine release at $2\frac{1}{2}$ times the ED_{95} dose is so minimal that no significant hypotension is observed in children. Mivacurium undergoes hydrolysis by plasma cholinesterase, with a duration of action of 15 to 20 minutes and full spontaneous recovery from a continuous infusion within 14 minutes of discontinuation.

Monitoring Neuromuscular Blockade

The ability to monitor the degree of neuromuscular blockade is extremely useful in titrating continuous infusions of neuromuscular blocking agents and in assessing the recovery of neuromuscular function after neuromuscular blockade. Two techniques cur-

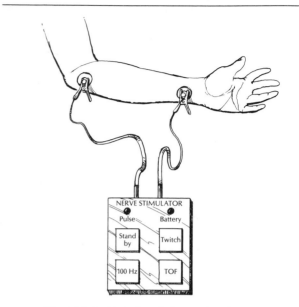

Fig. 130-3   Peripheral nerve stimulator.

rently available are mechanomyography and evoked electromyography. A simplified version of mechanomyography is discussed in this text since PICU application is easier and less expensive. A peripheral nerve stimulator is used to apply a transcutaneous electrical stimulus along the course of a peripheral nerve (Fig. 130-3). Attaching the nerve stimulator to ECG pads placed at the wrist over the ulnar nerve yields reliable results as long as the twitch response of the thumb alone is monitored. Finger twitches can sometimes represent artifact caused by direct muscle stimulation rather than stimulation of the ulnar nerve.

The most useful response to monitor in a nondepolarizing block is the train-of-four response. Train of four refers to four stimuli of equal intensity generated at a frequency of two per second. The characteristic pattern for the depression of train-of-four twitch height for depolarizing and nondepolarizing relaxants is shown in Fig. 130-4. Because of the wide margin of safety in neuromuscular transmission, the fourth twitch is not abolished until 75% blockade is achieved. In the PICU the presence of one to two twitches of the train of four provides clinically useful neuromuscular blockade (80% to 90%) and avoids the overdose of relaxant. Tetanic stimulation, a supramaximal stimulation at a frequency of 50 to 100 Hz applied for 5 seconds, is also useful in the eval-

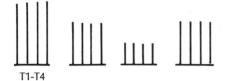

T1-T4

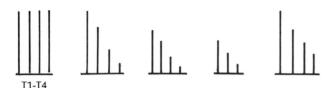

T1-T4

Fig. 130-4   Train-of-four *(TOF)* response in depolarizing block *(above)* and nondepolarizing block *(below)*.

uation of an intense neuromuscular block in the absence of a train-of-four response. The posttetanic twitch count correlates with the return of the train-of-four response.

Reversal of Neuromuscular Blockade

The pharmacologic reversal of neuromuscular blockade is achieved by increasing the concentration of acetylcholine at the neuromuscular junction, thus favoring the binding of acetylcholine rather than neuromuscular blocker to the acetylcholine receptors. This is accomplished by the administration of an acetylcholinesterase inhibitor such as neostigmine or edrophonium. The neuromuscular blockade can be too intense for pharmacologic antagonism; therefore, if recovery is not complete after an attempt at reversal, more time must be allowed rather than more antagonist given. It is also necessary to administer an anticholinergic agent before the acetylcholine stimulation of muscarinic receptors. Because of the difference in the time of onset, atropine is usually given with edrophonium and glycopyrolate with neostigmine. The usual doses used for "complete reversal" are neostigmine, 0.07 mg/kg, with glycopyrolate, 0.014 mg/kg, or edrophonium, 1 mg/kg, with atropine, 0.02 mg/kg.

RISKS AND COMPLICATIONS

There are two general areas of concern when giving neuromuscular blocking agents to patients in the PICU. The first is the effect that metabolic abnormalities or concomitant drug administration can have on the action of neuromuscular blocking agents.

Factors affecting the action of neuromuscular blocking agents in the PICU patient

Metabolic states that enhance neuromuscular blockade
    Hypothermia
    Hypokalemia (acute)
    Hypermagnesemia
Drugs that enhance neuromuscular blockade
    Aminoglycosides
    Local anesthetics
    Cardiac antidysrhythmic agents
    Furosemide
    Lithium
    Possibly the calcium antagonists
Conditions that decrease neuromuscular blockade
    Hyperkalemia
    Hemiparesis or hemiplegia (affected side shows resistance to nondepolarizing relaxants)
    Burn injuries

The second area of concern is the abnormal response of patients with neuromuscular diseases when given either depolarizing or nondepolarizing neuromuscular blocking agents. The primary concern with the nondepolarizing relaxants is the possibility of increased sensitivity to these agents, resulting in prolonged neuromuscular blockade. Increased sensitivity to nondepolarizing agents occurs in any patient with a disease that affects the prejunctional release of acetylcholine such as infant botulism or with a disease that alters receptor morphology such as myasthenia gravis. Of greater concern is the abnormal response to the depolarizing relaxant succinylcholine that occurs with a variety of neuromuscular diseases. The common pathologic event in these diseases is the proliferation of extrajunctional acetylcholine receptors, which can be present in large numbers located across the entire muscle membrane and which respond to succinylcholine by maintaining an open ion channel up to four times as long as normal receptors. Disorders that have been associated with hyperkalemic cardiac arrest after succinylcholine administration include:

Upper motor neuron lesions
Hemiparesis
Spinal cord injury
Paraplegia
Massive trauma (especially crush injuries)
Burns
Myotonias
Muscular dystrophies
Guillain-Barré syndrome

In addition the autonomic dysfunction associated with Guillain-Barré syndrome may lead to an exaggerated response to nondepolarizing agents that decrease peripheral vascular resistance or possess vagolytic properties.

The disadvantage of succinylcholine is the long list of adverse, even life-threatening side effects that may be associated with its administration. Cardiac dysrhythmias, including sinus bradycardia, nodal rhythms, ventricular ectopy, and rarely asystole are the most common adverse effects in children. These dysrhythmias are related to the ability of succinylcholine to stimulate cardiac muscarinic receptors and can be prevented by pretreatment with atropine. After the administration of succinylcholine to normal patients, an insignificant elevation in serum potassium is noted; however, life-threatening hyperkalemia can occur in patients with third-degree burns, massive trauma, upper motor neuron lesions, denervation injuries, and muscular dystrophies. This massive efflux of potassium is related to the proliferation of extra-

junctional acetylcholine receptors in these patients. The increase in extrajunctional receptors can reach significant numbers as early as 2 days after a burn or spinal cord injury and remain elevated for years. Succinylcholine also causes increases in intracranial and intraocular pressures in addition to its well-recognized association with malignant hyperthermia (see Chapter 60).

Also of concern in the PICU patient is the metabolism of atracurium to laudanosine, which with repeated doses or a continuous infusion has reached serum levels of 5 to 6 μg/ml in ICU patients studied. Laudanosine rapidly crosses the blood-brain barrier, causing CNS stimulation (as evidenced by increased EEG activity) and producing seizures in laboratory animals at high levels. Although a seizure threshold for laudanosine has not been demonstrated in humans, the levels obtained during continuous infusions are well above the seizure threshold for some animal species. Therefore the possible risk of seizures along with the CNS stimulation from laudanosine may limit the prolonged use of atracurium infusions in the PICU.

ADDITIONAL READING

Goudsouzian N, Standaert F. The infant and the myoneural junction. Anesth Analg 65:1208-1217, 1986.

Miller R, Rupp S, Fisher D, et al. Clinical pharmacology of vecuronium and atracurium. Anesthesiology 61:444-453, 1984.

Miller RD ed. Anesthesia, 2nd ed. New York: Churchill Livingstone, 1986.

Shanks C. Pharmacokinetics of the nondepolarizing relaxants applied to calculation of bolus and infusion dosage regimens. Anesthesiology 64:72-86, 1986.

Stoelting RK. Pharmacology and Physiology in Anesthetic Practice. Philadelphia: JB Lippincott, 1987.

131 Suctioning

Cindy K. Lybarger · Richard L. Vinson

INDICATIONS

Sputum is a complex fluid consisting of many substances, including mucoproteins, water, electrolytes, cellular debris, and blood. The volume, consistency, color, odor, and presence of foreign substances in the sputum may be of diagnostic value in the child with respiratory disease. An endotracheal tube acts as a foreign body and may actually increase mucous production. In addition the endotracheal tube interferes with mucociliary clearance of secretions. For these reasons suctioning is performed as a vital part of routine care for the intubated patient or the patient with a tracheostomy. Mobilization of secretions may be greatly diminished after some surgical procedures and as a result of many neurologic disorders; therefore suctioning of these patients becomes an important part of their care. Suctioning may also be indicated for the patient with an ineffective cough or with excessive or tenacious secretions.

TECHNIQUE
Endotracheal Suctioning Equipment

The ideal suctioning technique is one that removes the greatest amount of secretions with the least amount of risk to the patient. Once the need for suctioning has been determined, the following equipment is assembled:

    Adjustable vacuum regulator
    Suction canister
    Suction catheter
    Bag with manometer
    0.9% sodium chloride solution
    Water-soluble lubricant (for nasotracheal suction)
    Appropriate size mask

When suctioning the intubated patient, the appropriate size inflation bag and suction catheter must be readily available at the bedside (Table 131-1).

In general the largest catheter that can pass easily through the tube is used. The inflation bag may be connected to an inline manometer so that pressures used to ventilate the patient can be monitored. The suction apparatus must have an adjustable vacuum gauge to avoid excessive negative pressures. Maximum negative pressures are listed in Table 131-2.

Table 131-1 Recommended Catheter Sizes for Endotracheal Suctioning*

Endotracheal Tube Size	Suction Catheter Size
2.0	5
2.5	6½
3.0	6½
3.5	6½-8
4.0	8
4.5	8-10
5.0	10-12
5.5	10-12
6.0	12-14

*From Children's Medical Center of Dallas procedure manual.

Table 131-2 Maximum Negative Pressure for Airway Suctioning*

Age	Amount of Negative Pressure (cm H_2O)
Infant	60-90
Child	90-110
Older child	110-150

*From Hazinski MF. Nursing Care of the Critically Ill Child. St. Louis: CV Mosby, 1984.

Before the suctioning procedure is initiated, the equipment must be tested to ensure that it is turned on and functioning properly. An age-appropriate explanation of the procedure and what will be experienced must be given to the child before the suctioning procedure even if he apparently is unconscious.

Suctioning Technique

Aseptic technique is used to open a commercially available suction catheter package. Two gloves are used for suctioning; one remains sterile throughout the procedure, and the other protects the caregiver from contact with secretions. The sterile hand removes the catheter from the package and connects it to the suction tubing. If desired, sterile 0.9% sodium chloride solution may be instilled into the endotracheal tube with the nonsterile hand. The patient must be ventilated manually for approximately 10 breaths while he is continually assessed for tolerance of the procedure (i.e., heart rate, skin color, systemic arterial blood pressure). Generally an inspired oxygen concentration 10% higher than the patient's maintenance level is used. In selected patients, particularly those with pulmonary arterial hypertension or intracranial hypertension, an oxygen concentration of 100% is used. These groups of patients may tolerate suctioning better if premedicated with either narcotics or short-acting barbiturates. The catheter is gently inserted into the tube until resistance is felt and is then withdrawn approximately 1 mm and suction applied. The catheter is removed while continuous suction is applied while twirling the catheter. The suctioning must not last longer than 5 to 10 seconds. The patient is manually ventilated again and his tolerance of the procedure continually assessed. Two more passes of the catheter may be done, always with manual ventilation interposed between catheter insertions and suctioning. Turning the child's head to the left or right may facilitate passage of the catheter into the right and left mainstem bronchi, respectively. After the final tracheal suctioning the nares and mouth may be suctioned. Once again the child's breath sounds, vital signs, skin color, and signs of stability such as oxygen saturation or transcutaneous carbon dioxide levels if available must be assessed.

This procedure may be modified for the patient who needs relatively high ventilator settings, especially high PEEP. He may tolerate suctioning better if mechanical ventilation is resumed between passes of the suction catheter rather than if manual ventilation is attempted in between passes of the catheter. In this case the inspired oxygen concentration may be increased before suctioning to minimize the risk of hypoxemia. A special inline suctioning adapter for use on patients receiving PEEP of 6 cm H_2O or greater may be used to avoid loss of PEEP during the suctioning procedure.

The amount of suctioning needed by each patient varies. Since suctioning must be performed when necessary to ensure tube patency, assessment of the patient rather than a schedule may be used to determine need. Suctioning must be done whenever secretions are visible in the tube, when it is evident that secretions have accumulated, or when life-threatening endotracheal tube obstruction is clinically suspected.

Nasotracheal Suctioning (Without a Tube)

Nasotracheal suctioning is a means of removing excessive or thick secretions from the airways in a patient with an ineffective cough.

Explaining the procedure and the need for suctioning to the patient and/or parent is always necessary before beginning. The equipment is assembled and the oxygen flowmeter turned on to 6 to 7 L/min, although in some instances higher flows may be needed to hyperoxygenate the patient adequately. With aseptic technique the catheter package is opened, a moderate amount (5 ml or less) of water lubricant is dispensed onto a sterile part of the catheter package, and the gloves are donned. Lubricant is applied to the tip of the suction catheter.

The patient must be positioned properly, with the infant or small child in a sniffing position and the older, cooperative child in a semisitting position of approximately 45 degrees with the jaw thrust forward. The patient should breathe approximately 10 breaths of oxygen or, if necessary, should be manually ventilated with oxygen using a bag-valve-mask before insertion of the catheter. Patients with a history of pulmonary arterial hypertension must be given 100% oxygen for a minimum of 1 full minute before and after each suctioning attempt. The catheter is gently inserted into the naris on a line parallel to the patient's earlobe. If resistance is felt, the catheter should be gently twisted and the direction changed. If resistance continues, the catheter must be removed and inserted in the opposite naris. The patient must be encouraged to cough or to attempt to stimulate a cough as an attempt is made to insert the catheter into the trachea. When the trachea is entered, the patient's face will flush red and his lips will purse. When the catheter meets resistance, it should be pulled back approximately 1 mm and suction applied. The catheter is removed by applying continuous suction and twirling the catheter. Removal must occur within 5 to 10 seconds.

RISKS AND COMPLICATIONS

Complications associated with the suctioning procedure include hypoxemia, dysrhythmias, pulmonary arterial hypertension, atelectasis, mucosal damage, and bacterial growth. Hypoxemia during the suctioning procedure may occur as a result of the removal of alveolar gas, and patients who need supplemental oxygen are at greater risk for hypoxemia during the suctioning procedure. Careful monitoring of their tolerance of the procedure and performing hand ventilation immediately after each pass of the suction catheter will decrease the risk of hypoxemia. Dysrhythmias may occur as a result of hypoxemia during suctioning or as a result of vagal stimulation by the suction catheter. Atelectasis and mucosal damage can best be avoided by maintaining negative pressures within suggested guidelines (Table 131-2), withdrawing the catheter slightly before applying the suction,

and using an appropriate size suction catheter. Maintaining strict sterile technique will decrease the risk of bacterial colonization.

ADDITIONAL READING

Douglas S, Larson EL. The effect of a positive end-expiratory pressure adaptor on oxygenation during endotracheal suctioning. Heart Lung 14:396-400, 1985.

Goodnough SK. The effects of oxygen and hyperinflation on arterial oxygen tension after endotracheal suctioning. Heart Lung 14:11-17, 1985.

Gunderson LP, McPhee AJ, Donovan EF. Partially ventilated endotracheal suction. Am J Dis Child 140:462-465, 1986.

• Kleiber C, Krutzfield N, Rose EF. Acute histologic changes in the tracheobronchial tree associated with different suction catheter insertion techniques. Heart Lung 17:10-14, 1988.

Knipper JS. Minimizing the complications of tracheal suctioning. Focus AACN 13:23-26, 1986.

Riegel B, Forshee T. A review and critique of the literature on preoxygenation for endotracheal suctioning. Heart Lung 14:507-518, 1985.

• Shekleton ME, Nield M. Ineffective airway clearance related to artificial airway. Nurs Clin North Am 22:167-178, 1987.

Simbruner G, Coradello H, Fodor M, Lubec G. Effect of tracheal suction on oxygenation, circulation, and lung mechanics in newborn infants. Arch Dis Child 56:326-330, 1980.

132 Chest Physiotherapy

Becky Wade · Donna E. Badgett

INDICATIONS

Chest physiotherapy (CPT) comprises a variety of techniques used to aid in the treatment of patients with acute and chronic pulmonary diseases. These techniques may also be incorporated into the treatment of patients who need assisted or controlled ventilation. The techniques involved in CPT include postural drainage, percussion, vibration, and secretion removal. Each technique may be used alone or in any combination to meet the patient's needs.

The use of CPT is indicated in a variety of clinical conditions, including bronchiectasis, cystic fibrosis, hyaline membrane disease, pneumonia, lung abscess, bronchopulmonary dysplasia, asthma, and atelectasis. The primary goals of CPT are to aid in the mobilization of retained or excessive secretions and to improve the distribution of ventilation.

TECHNIQUE

The first step in secretion mobilization is achieved by placing the patient in the various postural drainage positions (Fig. 132-1). Gravity assists in the drainage of the vertical airways, and chest percussion is applied in an effort to shake secretions loose from the bronchial walls. Each lobe must be percussed for 1 to 2 minutes in rapid succession (approximately 100 repetitions/min). Vibrations are created by the "popping" sound of the cupped hand against the thorax. The pop also ensures that the patient is not being slapped. For maximum benefit postural drainage and percussion must be performed simultaneously.

Several factors must be considered before beginning therapy. Chest auscultation helps determine the number and degree of positions needed during each session. Positions must be modified for patients exhibiting severe or increased respiratory distress (i.e., modified or no Trendelenburg positions). Patients receiving continuous feeds must have them turned off before therapy, and any excess gastric residual must be evacuated. A 30-minute rest period between the end of CPT and the resumption of feedings is advisable. A thin cloth must be placed over the patient's skin to avoid irritation and care taken to avoid floating ribs, the sternum, spine, and other bony prominences. The patient's oxygen-enriched and/or thermal-controlled environment must not be interrupted.

Therapy begins over the affected lobe, and the majority of time is spent in this area. The entire lung must be treated prophylactically, even when not directly affected. The child is positioned on a bed or tilt-table using pillows for support. The more relaxed and comfortable the patient is, the more effective the therapy. Most infants tend to relax when held during therapy (Fig. 132-2); however, monitoring and/or support systems frequently make this impractical. Pneumatic or electric vibrators work well on small, bony, or postoperative patients; however, electric percussors must not be used on a patient who is in the oxygen-enriched environment of an Isolette.

Suctioning or coughing secretions is important throughout and after therapy since failure to do so could result in airway obstruction and/or respiratory arrest. Coughing must be encouraged after treating the patient in each position. Tussive squeeze, vibrations, and/or the tracheal-tickle maneuver is helpful when trying to induce a cough response or mobilize secretions. Tussive squeeze is performed by applying firm but gentle pressure over the draining lung field during expiration. Vibration is achieved by the therapist's stiffening and shaking his arms during the tussive squeeze maneuver to enhance its effectiveness. Expectoration can be elicited by the tracheal-tickle maneuver, which is accomplished by applying gentle

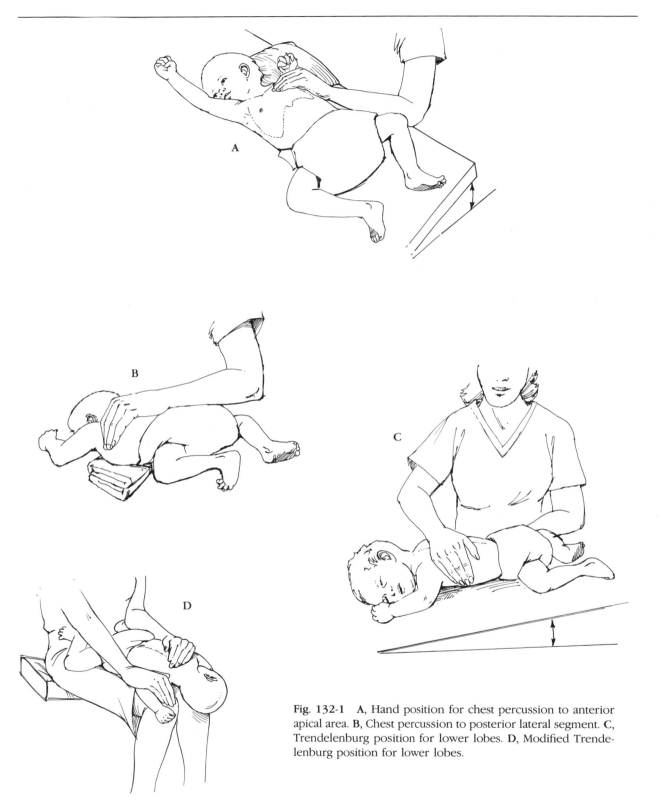

Fig. 132-1 A, Hand position for chest percussion to anterior apical area. **B,** Chest percussion to posterior lateral segment. **C,** Trendelenburg position for lower lobes. **D,** Modified Trendelenburg position for lower lobes.

pressure with the thumb on one side of the patient's trachea, followed by a quick flicking motion toward the opposite side. Patients with a suppressed gag reflex, artificial airway, or otherwise ineffective cough must be suctioned to maintain airway patency.

RISKS AND COMPLICATIONS

Patients receiving any form of CPT must be closely monitored during the procedure for symptoms of increased respiratory distress such as cyanosis, decreased level of consciousness, unstable vital signs, pain, or fatigue. Patients with increased ICP, known cardiac disease, fractured ribs, recent surgical incisions, chest tubes, gastroesophageal reflux, and traumatized internal organs require extra caution, and positioning for therapy may need modification. Head-down positions must be avoided in patients with heart disease since they may induce dysrhythmias and cyanosis. CPT must be delayed at least 1 hour after feedings to reduce the risk of vomiting and possible aspiration pneumonia.

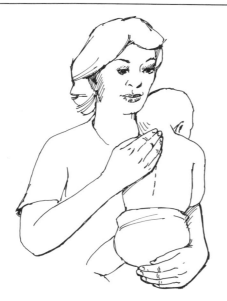

Fig. 132-2   Holding patient for chest percussion helps the infant to relax.

ADDITIONAL READING

Burgess WR, Chernick V. Respiratory Therapy in Newborn Infants and Children. New York: Thieme, 1986, pp 175-183.

Burton GG, Hodgkin JE. Respiratory Care—a Guide to Clinical Practice, 2nd ed. Philadelphia: JB Lippincott, 1984, pp 664-667.

Shapiro BA, Harison RA, Trout CA. Clinical Application of Respiratory Care. Chicago: Year Book, 1977, pp 199-209.

• Sonim NB, Schneider SN, Weng TR, Fields LJ. Pediatric Respiratory Therapy: An Introductory Text. Sarasota, Fla.: Glenn, 1974, pp 113-131.

• Young JA, Crocker D. Principles and Practice of Respiratory Therapy, 2nd ed. Chicago: Year Book, 1976, pp 399-416.

133 Inhaled Medications

Paul Lubinsky · Nick G. Anas

BACKGROUND AND INDICATIONS

Inhalation is the optimal method of delivery for many pulmonary therapeutic agents, which have proved to be better tolerated, safer, and more effective when inhaled than when administered orally or parenterally. The medications are delivered directly to the lung, resulting in a rapid onset of action and reduced side effects because of decreased dosage requirement and minimal systemic absorption. Bronchodilators are the most commonly administered inhaled medications and include agents that affect sympathetic and parasympathetic airway receptors. Other inhaled medications are mucolytics, ribavirin, steroids, antibiotics, and cromolyn sodium. The latter three are infrequently used in the PICU and are not discussed in this chapter.

MEDICATIONS
Beta-Sympathomimetics

Inhaled sympathomimetic agents that activate β_2-receptors are used commonly for the treatment of acute bronchospasm and wheezing. In addition to relaxation of bronchial smooth muscle, β-sympathomimetics inhibit mast cell degranulation, reduce mucous gland secretion, augment mucocilary clearance, and improve respiratory muscle contractility. Because these agents stimulate β_1- as well as β_2-receptors, side effects include tachycardia, dysrhythmias, vasodilation, and rarely myocardial ischemia. However, pharmacologic advances have produced agents with increased β_2 selectivity and therefore fewer side effects. Table 133-1 lists commonly inhaled sympathomimetics and compares clinically important properties.

Isoproterenol, the prototype sympathomimetic agent administered by inhalation, is potent and has a rapid onset of action. Its utility is limited by side effects and a short duration of action. The newer

agents (e.g., metaproterenol, albuterol) have a more sustained duration of action and are more β_2 selective but take longer to achieve maximal effect. From a practical point of view all are effective and safe.

Many respiratory disorders are characterized by bronchospasm that is reversed by the administration of inhaled β-sympathomimetics. They include acute severe asthma, bronchiolitis, cystic fibrosis, bronchopulmonary dysplasia, and congenital cardiac lesions with left-to-right shunting. Inhaled β-sympathomimetic agents also are indicated in the management of mucous plugging since they enhance mucociliary activity and for respiratory muscle fatigue since they augment diaphragmatic contractility.

Parasympathomimetics

Atropine and ipratropium bromide are parasympathomimetic receptor agonists that have a synergistic effect when used in combination with β-sympathomimetic agents. They are potent and selective bronchodilators whose mechanism of action is mediated through reduced levels of cyclic GMP, a metabolite that induces bronchoconstriction. Compared to β-sympathomimetics, they have a delayed onset but longer duration of action. Additionally, parasympathomimetic agents appear to be more effective in the management of bronchospasm in large airways (i.e., the first four or five generations). Both atropine and ipratropium bromide may be simultaneously delivered with inhaled β-sympathomimetic agents. The pharmacologic characteristics of the para-sympathomimetic agonists are summarized in Table 133-2.

Racemic Epinephrine

Racemic epinephrine is a preparation that contains equal amounts of dextrorotatory and levorotatory forms of epinephrine, and its activity is mediated by the stimulation of α-sympathomimetic receptors. Racemic epinephrine reduces mucosal swelling by inducing vasoconstriction and is useful in the management of conditions characterized by upper airway obstruction and inspiratory stridor (e.g., viral croup, postextubation mucosal edema, smoke inhalation, angioneurotic edema, acute laryngospasm). Racemic epinephrine may be indicated for worsening upper airway function in chronic obstructive disorders such as tracheomalacia. It has also been used during bronchoscopy to reduce mucosal edema, thus aiding in the removal of impacted foreign bodies. Racemic epinephrine (2.25% diluted to a volume of 2 ml) is administered by nebulizer in the following doses:

0-20 kg	0.25 ml
20-40 kg	0.50 ml
>40 kg	0.75 ml

Table 133-1   Commonly Used β-Sympathomimetic Agents

Agent (conc)	Dose (ml/kg) (max [ml])*	Usual Frequency in the PICU† (hr)	Relative Potency	Peak Onset of Action (min)	Duration of Action (hr)	Mechanism of Action
Isoproterenol (0.5%)	0.01-0.02 (0.5)	q 1	+ + + +	5-30	1-3	$B_1 = B_2$
Albuterol (0.5%)	0.01 (0.3)	q 2-4	+ + + +	30-60	4-6	$B_2 \gg B_1$
Terbutaline (0.1%)	0.03 (1)	q 2-4	+ + + +	5-20	4-6	$B_2 \gg B_1$
Metaproterenol (5%)	0.01 (0.3)	q 2-4	+ + +	30-60	3-5	$B_2 > B_1$
Isoetharine (1%)	0.02 (0.5)	q 2-4	+ +	15-60	1½-3	$B_2 \geq B_1$

*Doses should be rounded to the nearest 0.05 ml since the total dose is not delivered because of the vagaries of the delivery system and respiratory patterns of sick children. The total volume of the nebulized solution should be 3 to 4 ml with the 0.9% sodium chloride solution.
†Studies of continuous aerosol administration are in progress.

Table 133-2   Comparison of Nebulized Atropine and Ipratropium Bromide

	Atropine	Ipratropium*
Absorption	All mucosal surfaces	Poorly absorbed
Crosses blood-brain barrier	Yes	No
Side effects	Dry mouth Flushing Urinary retention Dyspnea, restlessness Delirium Mucociliary clearance Tachydysrhythmias at high doses	Minimal† No effect on mucociliary clearance No cardiovascular effect
Dose	0.05 mg/kg (max, 2.5 mg)	0.3 ml‡
Frequency	Every 3-4 hr	Every 3-4 hr
Peak activity	60 min	60 min
Duration	3-4 hr	4-6 hr

*Currently available only as metered-dose inhaler and for investigational use for nebulized solution.
†Side effects of ipratropium are minimal because it is poorly absorbed.
‡75 μg dose; doses in the pediatric population are not well established.

It has an immediate onset of action and may be repeated as indicated by physical examination (e.g., every 2 to 3 hours but as often as every 15 minutes). All children must be hospitalized following treatment with this agent since it has a short duration of action and does not alter the natural course of the disease.

Acetylcysteine

Acetylcysteine (Mucomyst) is an inhaled pharmacologic agent used to enhance mobilization of airway secretions. It lowers the viscosity of secretions by disrupting the sulfur bonds of the mucoproteins, resulting in greater mucociliary clearance. It is used predominately in patients with cystic fibrosis in whom viscous sputum is responsible for airway obstruction and chronic pneumonia. One to two milliliters of a 20% solution of acetylcysteine is administered in 2.5 ml of 0.9% sodium chloride solution. It must be administered in conjunction with a bronchodilator since it causes bronchospasm by irritating the airways. Acetylcysteine is administered three to four times daily, and the removal of thick secretions is enhanced by percussion and postural drainage.

Ribavirin

Ribavirin is a virustatic agent with a broad spectrum of activity against RNA and DNA viruses, with respiratory syncytial virus (RSV) infection representing the group that has been most thoroughly studied. Its indications and clinical efficacy are controversial, but ribavirin has been shown to reduce the morbidity and mortality related to RSV infections in high-risk groups (e.g., infants with congenital heart disease, immunosuppression, bronchopulmonary dysplasia, and cystic fibrosis); it also is widely used in the management of RSV bronchiolitis and pneumonia. Aerosolized administration appears to be effective against respiratory pathogens because high concentrations are achieved in airway secretions. Systemic absorption is minimal, and no significant side effects have been documented. The dose is 6 mg of ribavirin in 300 ml sterile water (20 μg/ml), which is aerosolized using a small-particle aerosol generator (SPAG) and administered via hood or face mask for 18 hours per day for 3 to 7 days. Therapy is usually instituted after confirmation of the diagnosis by either fluorescent antibody preparation or culture.

TECHNIQUE

Most inhaled medications used in the PICU are administered using a jet nebulizer (Fig. 133-1). Particles are generated by the passage of a high-velocity gas (usually oxygen) stream across a tube, creating a Bernoulli effect; the medications thus are pulled from the reservoir and become nebulized. A baffle in front of the jet stream removes the larger particles, returning them to solution for renebulization while the small particles (1 to 5 μm in diameter) are delivered to the patient's airway. Ultrasonic nebulizers use a piezoelectric crystal to generate ultrasonic sound waves that are directed at an air-liquid interface, producing a cloud of fine droplets whose diameters vary with the frequency of the sound used (e.g., the SPAG used for the administration of ribavirin). Metered-dose inhalers (MDIs) must be coordinated with the respiratory cycle, whereas nebulizers need only tidal volume breathing and are therefore the preferred method of delivery in the PICU where the patients may be uncoordinated, uncooperative, or unconscious.

The most important determinant of delivery to small airways is the particle size. Particles must be <5 μm to be able to reach the conducting airways and alveoli. The flow rates with the commonly used nebulizers must be 6 to 8 L/min to achieve adequate

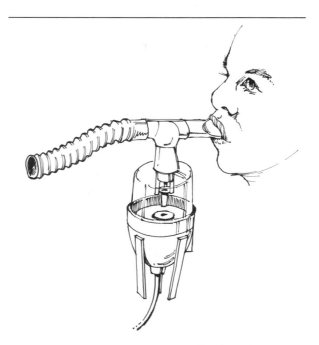

Fig. 133-1 Patient receiving aerosolized medication via jet nebulizer.

particle size. Only 10% of a measured dose is delivered to small airways due to deposition in the oropharynx and larger airways and residue in the nebulizer. The total volume in the nebulizer is 2 to 3 ml with 0.9% sodium chloride solution added as a diluent when necessary. The treatment takes 10 to 20 minutes to administer. Slow, deep inspiratory efforts provide the best delivery, but tidal volume breathing is adequate. Intermittent positive pressure breathing (IPPB) is useful only in patients with muscle weakness who cannot generate satisfactory chest wall movement, and it must not be used in patients with obstructive airways disease. If the patient is on assisted ventilation, the treatments may be given in-line in the ventilator circuit. In-line treatments are administered approximately 50 cc^3 proximal to the endotracheal tube through a side port in the ventilator tubing. They may be administered by manually coordinating a puff from a MDI with the inspiratory cycle, or the driving gas for the nebulizer may be coordinated with the ventilatory cycle so that nebulization will occur during the inspiratory phase of the respiratory cycle. Inspiratory pressures must be monitored during treatments since increased flows from the nebulizer will increase the peak inspiratory pressure and the PEEP with some ventilators.

RISKS AND COMPLICATIONS

Side effects of sympathomimetic agents most commonly result from dosage but may also result from idiosyncratic responses. Side effects of these agents involve the cardiovascular system (tachycardia, palpitations, dysrhythmias, hypertension) and CNS (anxiety, tremor, restlessness, headache, dizziness, emesis, nausea). A relative bradycardia may also occur with relief of airway obstruction. Sympathomimetic drugs also stimulate mobilization of glucose from the liver, producing hyperglycemia.

Side effects of atropine administration are listed in Table 133-2. Side effects from acetylcysteine are its unpleasant taste and tendency to produce bronchospasm, which is minimized by administering it in conjunction with a bronchodilator. Complications associated with the administration of inhaled medications (e.g., pneumothorax, bronchospasm) are minimized by avoiding the use of IPPB and by giving

constant attention to changes in the patient's vital signs and respiratory effort, which indicate an adverse response to the administered medication.

The administration of ribavirin to patients needing mechanical ventilation is associated with several problems. Flow from the aerosol generator increases the inspiratory pressure needed to deliver the desired tidal volume. Crystallization of ribavirin at the expiratory valve can result in inadvertent PEEP and lead to the development of pneumothorax or pneumopericardium. Therefore, to administer ribavirin safely to a patient on mechanical ventilation, the following recommendations must be followed: (1) place a filter in front of the expiratory valve of the ventilator circuit and place a second valve in the inspiratory line between the humidifier and the one-way valve through which the aerosol enters; (2) change the filters every 2 hours; (3) repeatedly (e.g., every 30 minutes) examine the circuit for crystal deposition; and (4) every 30 to 60 minutes, check and record the inspiratory and end-expiratory pressures being delivered to the patient.

ADDITIONAL READING

Aubier M, Vilres N, Murciano D. Effects and mechanisms of action of terbutaline on diaphragmatic contractility and fatigue. J Appl Physiol 56:922, 1984.
• Bethel RA, Irvin CG. Anticholinergic drugs and asthma. Semin Respir 8:366, 1987.
Cissik JH, Bode FR, Smith JA. Double blind crossover study of five bronchodilators: Medications and two delivery methods in stable asthma. Chest 90:489, 1986.
Davis A, Vickerson F, Worsley G, et al. Determination of a dose-response relationship for nebulized ipratropium in asthmatic children. J Pediatr 105:1002, 1984.
• Galant SP. Current status of β-adrenergic agonists in bronchial asthma. Pediatr Clin North Am 30:931, 1983.
Hall CB. Ribavirin: Beginning the blitz on respiratory viruses? Pediatr Infect Dis 4:668, 1985.
• Moren F, Newhouse MT, Dolovich MG, eds. Aerosols in Medicine. New York: Elsevier, 1985.
Wald ER, Dashefsky B, Green M. In *re* ribavirin: A case of premature adjudication. J Pediatr 112:154, 1988.
Westley RC, Cotton EK, Brooks JG. Nebulized racemic epinephrine administered by IPPB for treatment of laryngotracheobronchitis. Am J Dis Child 132:484, 1978.

134 Thoracentesis and Chest Tube Insertion

Steven R. Leonard · Hisashi Nikaidoh

BACKGROUND AND INDICATIONS
Pneumothorax

A pneumothorax is a collection of air within the pleural space, usually resulting from injury to the lung parenchyma with a subsequent air leak. In addition a hole in the chest wall may allow air to enter the pleural space because of the negative intrathoracic pressure. A pneumothorax may be surprisingly well tolerated by a patient, or it may have devastating consequences. A tension pneumothorax occurs when air can enter the pleural space but cannot escape. As the pneumothorax enlarges, it may accumulate enough pressure to cause contralateral mediastinal shift, resulting in respiratory embarrassment, decreased cardiac output, and death if not treated promptly. In pediatric patients tension pneumothorax is most likely to occur during positive pressure ventilation and must be immediately ruled out in a mechanically ventilated patient who suddenly deteriorates.

Pneumothorax is often difficult to diagnose. Indeed it may even be asymptomatic and incidentally discovered on a chest roentgenogram obtained for other reasons. Most moderate-to-large pneumothoraces, however, are accompanied by dyspnea or pleuritic chest pain. Physical examination may reveal hyperexpansion of the affected hemithorax with decreased breath sounds and hyperresonance to percussion. Contralateral shift of the mediastinum may be seen with tracheal deviation and lateral displacement of the cardiac apical impulse. Occasionally subcutaneous emphysema is present. A chest roentgenogram most effectively demonstrates the pneumothorax, and usually an anteroposterior view is sufficient. However, a supine anteroposterior radiograph may appear normal even when a significant pneumothorax is present. Additional views (e.g., up-

right inspiratory and expiratory, cross-table lateral, lateral decubitus) may be helpful. In a mechanically ventilated patient who suddenly deteriorates and has decreased breath sounds on one side of the chest, it may be necessary to decompress a tension pneumothorax with a chest tube or a large needle before a chest roentgenogram can be obtained.

A small, stable, asymptomatic pneumothorax in a spontaneously breathing patient is usually well tolerated and can be observed until it is reabsorbed. However, any symptomatic pneumothorax or a pneumothorax in a patient on positive pressure ventilation must be evacuated. This is accomplished usually by chest tube insertion; however, in a stable spontaneously breathing patient evacuation may be accomplished with thoracentesis. If this is not successful, a chest tube may be inserted.

Pleural Effusion

A pleural effusion is an abnormal collection of fluid (serum, blood, chyle, pus) in the pleural space. This space usually contains a small amount of pleural fluid, which lubricates the parietal and visceral pleural surfaces during respiration. The volume of pleural fluid is determined by an equilibrium in forces involving the colloid osmotic and hydrostatic pressures in the systemic and pulmonary capillaries and the negative intrathoracic pressure. Many disease states alter this equilibrium and cause a pleural effusion.

Pleural effusions are generally classified as transudates or exudates. Although the criteria are not absolute, some characteristics of the fluid may help to differentiate the two classes (Table 134-1). Most transudates are clear, straw-colored, odorless effusions with a specific gravity <1.016. Chemical analysis reveals normal pH, glucose level near that of serum

---

CAUSES OF PLEURAL EFFUSION

Transudates

Congestive heart failure
Cirrhosis
Renal disease
    Glomerulonephritis
    Nephrotic syndrome
Hypoalbuminemia

Exudates

Inflammatory
    Bacterial pneumonia
    Viral pneumonitis
    Tuberculosis
    Fungal diseases
    Rickettsial infection
    Parasitic infestations
Empyema
Neoplasm
    Pulmonary parenchyma
    Pleura
    Lymphatic
Sympathetic effusions
    Pancreatitis
    Intra-abdominal abscess
Postpericardiotomy syndrome
Trauma
Pulmonary embolus or infarction
Chylothorax
Collagen vascular diseases (rheumatoid arthritis)

(>60 mg/dl), and low lactate dehydrogenase (LDH) and protein levels. A cell count reveals few erythrocytes ($<100,000$/mm^3) and leukocytes (<1000/mm^3). Most of the leukocytes in transudates are lymphocytes.

Exudates may be clear, milky (chylothorax, empyema), bloody (trauma, malignancy, pulmonary embolus), or turbid (parapneumonic effusion, empyema). Most are odorless, but anaerobic empyema may have a feculent odor. The specific gravity is generally >1.016, and the fluid may be quite viscous. Acid pH usually represents an infectious process. The glucose level may be depressed (<60 mg/dl as in infectious or malignant effusions), and the lowest glucose levels are associated with rheumatoid arthritis or pleuritis. Pleural fluid usually contains elevated levels of protein (>3.0 g/dl) and LDH. The ratio of pleural fluid to serum proteins (>0.5) and the ratio of pleural fluid to serum LDH (>0.6) are helpful criteria. The leukocyte count usually exceeds 1000/mm^3 and may exceed $10,000$/mm^3 in parapneumonic effusions, empyema, sympathetic effusions, pulmonary infarction, and malignancy. A predominant lymphocytosis is usually associated with tuberculous or malignant effusion and chylothorax. Chylothorax will also have an elevated pleural fluid triglyceride level and positive Sudan fat stain test for chylomicrons.

Small pleural effusions may be asymptomatic and incidentally noted on chest roentgenograms. Even moderate effusions may not be evident when the underlying process presents with marked symptoms

---

Table 134-1   Characteristics of Pleural Effusions

	Transudate	Exudate
Appearance	Clear; straw-colored	Clear, milky, bloody, or turbid
Odor	Odorless	May be malodorous
Specific gravity	<1.016	>1.016
pH	Normal	Normal or acidic
Glucose	>60 mg/dl	<60 mg/dl
Protein level	<3.0 g/dl	>3.0 g/dl
Pleural fluid protein/serum protein	<0.5	>0.5
LDH level		
Pleural fluid LDH/serum LDH	<0.6	>0.6
Cell count		
Erythrocyte	$<100,000$/mm^3	$>100,000$/mm^3
Leukocyte	<1000/mm^3	>1000/mm^3

(e.g., pneumonia, congestive heart failure, pulmonary embolus). Most patients with a pleural effusion will have dyspnea, pleuritic chest pain, or fever, depending on the cause. The patient may have hypoexpansion of the affected hemithorax, decreased breath sounds, and dullness to percussion. Occasionally the effusion may be large enough to cause contralateral mediastinal shift. Chest radiographs (posteroanterior, lateral decubitus, cross-table lateral) will demonstrate the effusion. A supine anteroposterior view may demonstrate haziness or opacification of the hemithorax. Localization of loculated effusions is aided by sonography and computed axial tomography.

A diagnostic thoracentesis must be done for all pleural effusions of uncertain etiology. An asymptomatic transudate may be best managed by treating the underlying cause (e.g., congestive heart failure). A symptomatic effusion must be evacuated as completely as possible. If the effusion is not expected to reaccumulate, the fluid can be completely aspirated. However, if it is expected to reaccumulate (e.g., chylothorax, malignant effusion) or proves to be an empyema, it is best managed by chest tube drainage. A pleural effusion should not be completely aspirated if a chest tube is to be inserted since complete evacuation allows the lung to expand against the chest wall and injury to the lung is more likely during subsequent insertion of the chest tube.

TECHNIQUE FOR THORACENTESIS
Equipment

Equipment necessary for performing thoracentesis includes:

Thoracentesis equipment

Surgical mask and cap
Sterile gloves
Goggles
Povidone-iodine solution, 10%
Lidocaine without epinephrine, 1%
Sterile drapes
Syringes, 5 and 30 ml
Needles, 25 and 22 gauge
Collection basin
IV catheter, 20 or 18 gauge (e.g., Angiocath, Jelco)
Three-way stopcock
IV extension tubing
Culture tubes
Laboratory tubes for cell count and chemistry analysis

Procedure

The child is premedicated with morphine sulfate, 0.1 mg/kg. Children older than 1 year of age may be premedicated with a combination of meperidine, 1 mg/kg, plus promethazine hydrochloride, 0.5 mg/kg, plus chlorpromazine hydrochloride, 0.5 mg/kg. Because of the potential for respiratory depression, the child must be closely observed for several hours after the procedure (Fig. 134-1, *A*).

The patient is comfortably positioned, and adequate exposure is ensured. Infants and small children may be placed supine with a small roll under the affected hemithorax and the arm positioned superiorly. Older children may sit upright, with their arms supported on a bedside table.

The thoracentesis site is determined by correlating the physical examination (dullness to percussion, decreased tactile fremitus) with the chest roentgenogram. In the supine infant this site is generally between the midaxillary and posterior axillary lines. In the upright older child or adult thoracentesis is usually performed just below the scapular tip (near the seventh intercostal space and posterior axillary line). This site may be marked with a pen or by lightly indenting the skin with a fingernail.

Cap, mask, and sterile gloves are donned after scrubbing. Goggles may be worn if desired. The skin is widely prepared with povidone-iodine solution and is draped with sterile towels. The skin is anesthetized using a 5 ml syringe and 25-gauge needle to raise a skin wheal with 1% lidocaine. The subcutaneous tissue and chest wall (including the rib periosteum and pleura) are then anesthetized with a longer 21-gauge needle (Fig. 134-1, *B*). The needle is then advanced into the pleural space. The needle must pass over the top of the rib to avoid injury to the neurovascular bundle that is located along the inferior border of each rib. The syringe is gently aspirated to ensure that this location overlies the air or fluid collection. If no fluid or air can be aspirated, it may be necessary to relocate one intercostal space lower and repeat the process.

The IV needle is then inserted through the anesthetized tissue into the pleural space while the syringe is constantly aspirated gently and the general direction of the tract that was previously anesthetized is followed. Entrance into the pleural space is usually confirmed by a "pop" felt as the needle passes through the pleura followed by return of air or fluid into the syringe. The outer catheter is then advanced into the pleural space.

The inner needle is removed, and the 30 ml syringe with an attached three-way stopcock is placed into the catheter hub. This maneuver must be done during expiration (or positive pressure ventilation if the patient is mechanically ventilated) to prevent any air from entering the pleural space. In the brief time between removing the inner needle and attaching the stopcock, the hub must be covered by the thumb.

If this is a diagnostic thoracentesis after which a chest tube may be inserted, only enough fluid is aspirated to perform the necessary laboratory examinations. (Aspirating the pleural space until it is "dry" makes subsequent chest tube insertion more hazardous because of possible injury to the lung.) If, however, this is a therapeutic thoracentesis, all of the fluid or air is aspirated. This is facilitated by attaching the IV extension tubing to the third arm of the stopcock (Fig. 134-1, *C*). When the syringe is full, the stopcock is turned so that the fluid can be emptied through the tubing into a collection basin. The catheter position within the pleural space and the patient's position may be maneuvered to aspirate as much air or fluid as possible. However, care must be taken to prevent the catheter from kinking or slipping out of the pleural space.

When the fluid or air has been completely aspirated, the catheter is withdrawn while applying continuous suction, and a sterile dressing is applied. The pleural fluid is sent for appropriate studies. A chest radiograph must be taken immediately to assess the effectiveness of the thoracentesis and to rule out a pneumothorax.

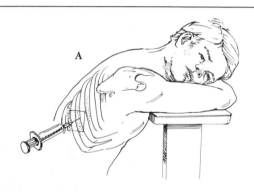

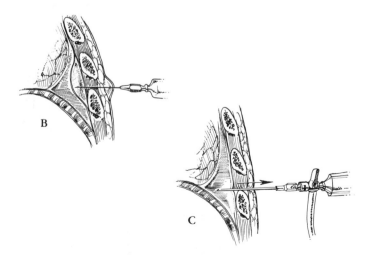

Fig 134-1   Thoracentensis. **A,** Infiltration of skin site. **B,** Infiltration of intercostal tissues and pleura. **C,** Aspiration of fluid.

TECHNIQUE FOR CHEST TUBE INSERTION
Equipment

The following equipment must be available:

Chest tube insertion equipment

Surgical mask and cap
Sterile gloves
Goggles
Povidone-iodine solution, 10%
Lidocaine without epinephrine, 1%
Sterile drapes
Syringes, 5 or 10 ml
Needles, 25 and 22 gauge
No. 15 scalpel blade
Suture for securing chest tube to skin (e.g., 2-0 silk)
Chest tube (see Table 134-2 for appropriate size)
Chest tube drainage system (e.g., Pleurevac)
Thoracostomy tray
  Hemostats
  No. 3 scalpel handle
  Sponges
  Needle holder
  Tube clamp
  Scissors

Procedure

The patient is premedicated as described previously and positioned supine with a small roll below the hemithorax; his arm is placed laterally or superiorly.

The insertion site is determined as described previously. For patient comfort a chest tube is rarely placed behind the posterior axillary line. Chest tubes placed to drain fluid are generally placed low in the chest (fifth to seventh intercostal spaces) between the midaxillary and posterior axillary lines. Lower insertion may cause injury to the diaphragm, liver, spleen, or other abdominal viscera. Chest tubes placed to evacuate a pneumothorax are generally placed high in the chest (second or third intercostal space) in the midclavicular line or the midaxillary line, thus avoiding the pectoralis muscles, which make insertion more difficult and may cause bleeding. The more lateral position is also more cosmetically acceptable.

Cap, mask, and sterile gloves are donned after scrubbing. Goggles may be worn if desired. The skin is prepared and draped as described previously. An incision is made in the skin at least one intercostal space below the interspace through which the chest tube will enter the pleural cavity. This creates a subcutaneous tunnel that helps prevent ascending infection or development of a pneumothorax during chest tube removal. A skin wheal is raised using a 25-gauge needle and lidocaine. The subcutaneous tissue, rib periosteum, chest wall muscles, and pleura are anesthetized using the longer 21-gauge needle. The needle is advanced into the pleural space and aspirated to confirm the presence of fluid or air. The needle is allowed to "walk" over the superior margin of the rib to avoid injury to the neurovascular bundle.

The appropriate-sized chest tube is selected (Table 134-2) and the length to insert determined. A clamp is placed across the tube at this level. It is important that the proximal fenestration in the tube lies within

Table 134-2 Choice of Chest Tube Size (French)

Size of Patient (kg)	Pneumothorax*	Pleural Effusion†	
		Transudate	Exudate
<3	8-10	8-10	10-12
3-8	10-12	10-12	12-16
8-15	12-16	12-16	16-20
16-40	16-20	16-20	20-28
>40	20-24	24-28	28-36

*Chest tubes inserted for a pneumothorax must be inserted high in the chest (second or third intercostal space) in the anterior or midaxillary line and directed anteriorly and superiorly.
†Chest tubes inserted for a pleural effusion must be inserted low in the chest (fifth through seventh intercostal space) in the midaxillary or posterior axillary line and directed posteriorly and inferiorly.

the pleural cavity. If necessary, the distal end of the tube is cut off.

The skin incision is made using a No. 15 scalpel blade. The incision must be just slightly longer than the diameter of the chest tube (Fig. 134-2, *A*).

The tract of the tube is dissected by inserting a hemostat through the incision and gently spreading the subcutaneous tissue and chest wall muscles, with the hemostat down to the rib over which the tube is to be placed. The hemostat is then advanced over the top of the rib, through the pleura, and into the pleural space. The pleura is spread with the hemostat. This is usually painful to the patient because it is nearly impossible to anesthetize the pleura completely with lidocaine infiltration. Entry into the pleural space is confirmed by a rush of air or fluid and by "sucking" noises during respiration (Fig. 134-2, *B*).

The tip of the chest tube is placed between the tips of a hemostat and is advanced through the tunnel into the pleural space (Fig. 134-2, *C*). The hemostat is released, the tube is advanced to the level marked by the tube clamp, and the hemostat is withdrawn. If the chest tube is being inserted for a pneumothorax, it must be positioned anteriorly and toward the apex. If it is being placed to drain fluid, it must be directed inferiorly and posteriorly.

A horizontal mattress suture of heavy silk (2-0 or 3-0) is placed through the incision as a purse-string suture, wrapped several times around the tube, and tied to secure the tube to the skin (Fig. 134-2, *D* to *F*).

The chest tube is connected to the drainage system, and the tube clamp is removed. The tubing connections are secured with tape to prevent accidental

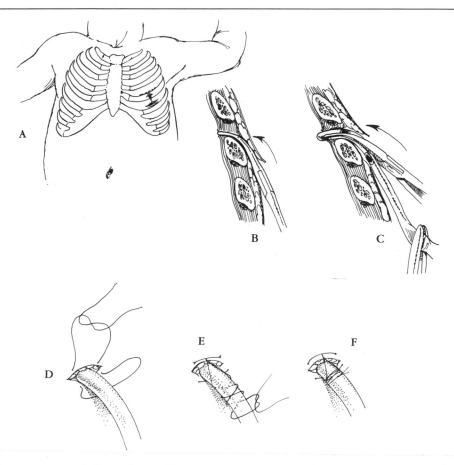

Fig 134-2   Insertion of chest tube. **A**, Skin incision. **B**, Hemostat dissection. **C**, Insertion of chest tube. **D-F**, Securing chest tube.

disconnection. Suction (-20 to -30 cm H_2O) is applied to the system.

A sterile dressing is placed around the insertion site. A small, dry dressing is adequate; using large, bulky dressings and petroleum jelly gauze is not necessary. A chest roentgenogram is obtained to confirm tube position and adequacy of drainage.

Chest Tube Care

It is seldom necessary to clamp a chest tube. Occlusion of the tube may cause a tension pneumothorax or hydrothorax. For similar reasons the tubing between the chest tube and drainage system must not become kinked. Securing the tubing to the bedsheets will prevent this and prevent the weight of the tubing from pulling on the chest tube. Chest tubes must be routinely stripped to prevent occlusion by fibrinous material or blood clot. Sterile water must be added periodically to the suction control chamber in the drainage system. As air bubbles through the chamber, water evaporates, and the level of suction will decrease.

If the patient is to be transported or transferred to another bed, the drainage system must remain below the level of the chest. The chest tube should *never* be clamped during transport.

Chest Tube Removal

The patient is premedicated if indicated. The horizontal mattress suture is untied and unwound from the chest tube. The first throw of a knot is placed in the suture (Fig. 134-3, *A*).

During a deep Valsalva maneuver (or during positive pressure ventilation if the patient is mechanically ventilated) the chest tube is *rapidly* withdrawn, and the purse-string suture is tied (Fig. 134-3, *B*). An assistant must hold pressure over the subcutaneous tract while the tube is removed and the suture is tied. A dry sterile dressing is then placed over the wound. (Using large, bulky dressings or petroleum jelly gauze is not necessary.) If there is no purse-string suture, a petroleum jelly gauze dressing is used to cover the insertion site as the chest tube is removed. It is covered with occlusive tape to prevent aspiration of air through the insertion site.

A chest roentgenogram is obtained to rule out pneumothorax.

RISKS AND COMPLICATIONS

Injury to the lung may result in bleeding or pneumothorax. Injury to the diaphragm, liver, spleen, or other abdominal viscera may occur if thoracentesis or chest tube placement is attempted too inferiorly.

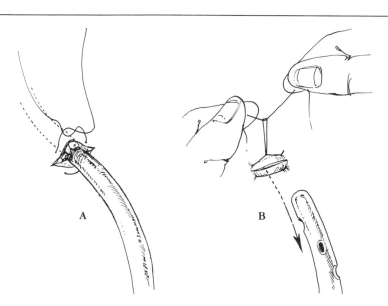

Fig 134-3   Removing the chest tube. **A**, First throw of a knot in the mattress suture. **B**, Removal of chest tube and tying purse-string suture.

Pressure of an apical chest tube on the sympathetic chain may cause temporary Horner's syndrome. Pressure of a chest tube on the aorta of a small infant may cause distal hypoperfusion.

Pleural contamination and empyema may result from breaks in sterile technique. If the proximal fenestration in the chest tube is not within the pleural cavity, persistent pneumothorax, air leak, or subcutaneous emphysema may result. Injury to the intercostal neurovascular bundle may cause bleeding.

Abnormal breast development may result from placement too near the areola in a female patient.

ADDITIONAL READING

Aschoff CR. Thoracentesis. In Mayhew HE, Rodgers LA, eds. Basic Procedures in Family Practice. New York: John Wiley, 1984, pp 136-142.

Pierson DJ. Chest tubes. In Luce JM, Pierson DJ. Critical Care Medicine. Philadelphia: WB Saunders, 1988, pp 238-246.

Rosen P, Sternbach G. Atlas of Emergency Medicine. Baltimore: Williams & Wilkins, 1983, pp 39-63.

Simon RR, Brenner BE. Procedures and Techniques in Emergency Medicine. Baltimore: Williams & Wilkins, 1982, pp 134-145.

VanWay CW, Buerk CA. Surgical Skills in Patient Care. St. Louis: CV Mosby, 1978, pp 118-127.

135 Extubation and Fiberoptic Examination

Frances C. Morriss · *Orval E. Brown* ·
Scott C. Manning · *Becky Wade*

EXTUBATION
Indications

The primary indication for the removal of an endotracheal tube is resolution of the process that necessitated its placement. If an endotracheal tube has been in place for a short period of time and the patient is relatively healthy (e.g., patient with an overdose), resolution of the primary process is all that is required before considering extubation. For the patient intubated for a long period of time other factors that might contribute to failure of extubation (i.e., need to reinstitute airway support) must be considered. Those organ systems or conditions in which preexisting or ongoing abnormalities might contribute to or increase the work of breathing must be considered. The function of the cardiovascular and respiratory systems must be as normal and as stable as possible for any particular patient; that is, the patient should be at *his* best possible function. There may be increased work of breathing after extubation, and any conditions (e.g., hypermetabolic state, anemia) that may exacerbate cardiac or respiratory work must be corrected.

There should be no acute pulmonary changes, particularly those associated with newly acquired infection and loss of lung volume. Physical examination should reveal no new findings, and secretions should be thin and clear. If an acute change has occurred, a chest roentgenogram and examination of a sputum sample for organisms and inflammatory cells may be helpful. Ventilatory support should be minimal; that is, the patient needs infrequent suctioning, a low end-expiratory pressure <2 to 3 cm H_2O, minimal or no ventilatory rate, and an FiO_2 <0.4. Respiratory support in the previous 24 hours, including increases in the frequency of bronchodilator administration, should not have been increased. A stable chemical status must be documented by either noninvasive respiratory monitoring (transcutaneous oxygen and carbon dioxide determination, oxygen saturation, or end-tidal carbon dioxide determination) or by arterial blood gas and pH determination.

Not all patients will have normal oxygenation and carbon dioxide elimination, but all must maintain stable levels of PaO_2 and $PaCO_2$ that are normal for their particular diagnosis. For example, the infant with cyanotic congenital cardiac disease will not saturate to normal levels, and the patient with chronic pulmonary disease may have a physiologic pH only because renal compensation and excretion of bicarbonate ion has balanced his inability to eliminate carbon dioxide. In patients who have needed prolonged support for respiratory failure adequate time must be allowed after that support has become minimal to assess whether fatigue will occur. This implies a period of at least 24 hours of observation. If respiratory muscle fatigue is a problem, a trial of theophylline in doses to achieve a serum level of 10 to 20 mg/ml may be tried to improve respiratory muscle, particularly diaphragmatic, function. Therapy (e.g., aerosolized bronchodilators, chest physiotherapy) must be scheduled so that the patient receives maximum benefit and yet is not exhausted at the time of extubation.

Increased cardiovascular work can contribute to a failed extubation. Patients must demonstrate an adequate cardiac output as judged by usual clinical indications (normal systemic arterial blood pressure, adequate urinary output, good capillary refill), a stable cardiac rhythm, and, if present, control of congestive heart failure. Pharmacologic augmentation of cardiac output should be minimal, and the need for diuretics, cardiac glycosides, and antihypertensives should be stable and not increasing. Even though the respiratory status may have been unchanged for some period of time, the possibility of upper airway obstruction and hypoxia after extubation exists; either of these conditions coupled with an unstable cardiovascular status such as may occur in patients after major cardiac surgery can be fatal.

CNS stability is necessary to assure good reflex protection of the airway after extubation and adequate respiratory drive and respiratory muscle function. Physical examination and observation must demonstrate absence of apnea and presence of gag and cough reflexes. Central respiratory depressants (narcotics, sedatives, tranquilizers, antihistamines) must be either discontinued or given in doses low enough to assure consciousness after extubation. All neuromuscular blocking agents must be discontinued or pharmacologically reversed to ensure adequate muscle strength to sustain breathing. For patients with primary neuromuscular disease (hypotonia, muscular dystrophies, spinal cord dysfunction, myasthenia gravis) direct evaluation of respiratory function can be useful in determining the patient's ability to sustain respiratory effort unassisted; inspiratory pressure must be >22 cm H_2O negative pressure, and vital capacity must be at least 10 to 15 cc/kg body weight. These simple tests can be repeated as needed to evaluate ongoing neuromuscular function. For comatose patients the ability to swallow and to handle oropharyngeal secretions may also need assessment. Seizures, particularly those associated previously with cyanosis or apnea, must be controlled.

Hypermetabolic states will increase oxygen consumption, placing increased demands on the cardiorespiratory system. The one most frequently seen in the PICU patient is fever; not only should the fever be controlled, but the cause identified and treated. In neonates and premature infants many abnormalities of electrolytes and glucose are associated with apnea as well as electrical dysfunction of the neuromuscular membrane; serum Na, K, Cl, PO_4, Ca, Mg, and glucose must be maintained within a normal range. For the patient who has increased fluid requirements or who is young, IV hydration with an appropriate solution must be provided for the period of time when nothing can be taken by mouth (a minimum of 8 hours). Patients with chronic disease processes, particularly those with prolonged respiratory failure, may have an inadequate caloric intake; increased caloric requirements will occur as the patient assumes more and more control of his breathing. If nutritional supplementation is inadequate, the

---

PREEXTUBATION EVALUATION

Resolution of primary process

Respiratory stability

Chest roentgenogram
Arterial blood gas and pH determination
Complete blood count
Tracheal secretion culture, Gram stain
Chest physiotherapy, bronchodilator therapy, and/
   or suctioning as needed
Benign pulmonary examination (or usual examination for a particular patient)

Cardiovascular stability

Adequate cardiac output
Stable rhythm
Minimal pharmacologic cardiac support
Adequate oxygen-carrying capacity (Hct)

Neurologic stability

Usual state of consciousness
Presence of airway protective reflexes (gag, swallow,
   cough)
Absence of apnea
Adequate control of seizures
Absence of central respiratory depressants (discontinue or decrease narcotics, tranquilizers, sedatives)
Good neuromuscular function of respiratory muscles (Consider using theophylline for fatigue and simple pulmonary function testing. Neuromuscular blockade must be absent.)

Metabolic stability

Absence of fever
Normal electrolytes and minerals (Na, K, Cl, PO_4, Mg, Ca)
Normal serum glucose
Adequate hydration
Adequate caloric intake to support work of breathing; evaluate growth chart

patient may not be able to sustain the work of breathing and thrive; this situation is particularly true in small and premature infants. Adequate weight gain as assessed by a growth chart appropriate for age is a good indication that the patient will do well without ventilatory support.

Preparation

All oral feedings should be withheld for a minimum of 4 hours before extubation. Glottic closure is incomplete immediately after extubation, predisposing the patient to aspiration of both stomach contents and oropharyngeal secretions. If reintubation is necessary, an empty stomach reduces this risk. All pain medication, muscle relaxants, and respiratory depressant drugs should be withdrawn long enough before extubation to eliminate their effects. Oxygen and suction must be available and the patient should have cardiac rhythm and oxygen saturation monitoring. A complete selection of intubation equipment, including laryngoscopes and a varied selection of endotracheal tubes, must be available at the bedside. Thiopental (4 mg/kg) and a nondepolarizing muscle relaxant must be available for possible reintubation.

Technique

The endotracheal tube and pharynx are suctioned to clear all secretions. The stomach is emptied, and if present, the NG tube is removed. Tape or other securing devices for the endotracheal tube are released, and the tube is secured manually. The patient is hyperventilated with 100% oxygen (or an appropriate Fio_2 if the patient is a premature infant) and extubated at the peak of inspiration. This induces a cough, and any secretions in the airway are expelled. Humidified oxygen is administered via a delivery system (a mask, croup tent, or face tent) that is most comfortable for the patient at a concentration that will keep his saturation >92%. The patient must be monitored carefully by the physician at the bedside for at least 10 to 15 minutes after extubation to ensure that rapid deterioration, if it occurs, can be treated promptly.

Monitoring After Extubation

The problems that most commonly necessitate reintubation are laryngeal edema, particularly in the subglottis, thick secretions obstructing the airway, fatigue resulting from the increased work of breathing, apnea, cardiovascular instability, and inadequate pulmonary function. Patients are monitored closely in the PICU for at least 24 hours after extubation. Any signs of respiratory distress or air hunger necessitate immediate reevaluation for possible reintubation. The patient is given nothing by mouth for at least 4 hours after extubation to reduce the risk of aspiration if reintubation is necessary. Sedatives or pain medications that depress respiratory drive usually are not given in the immediate postextubation period. Transcutaneous oxygen and carbon dioxide monitoring is helpful during this period.

FIBEROPTIC EXAMINATION WITH EXTUBATION
Indications

Fiberoptic nasolaryngoscopy is a safe and effective method for evaluating the larynx in infants and children. It is an invaluable tool in helping to differentiate upper airway obstruction from lower airway disease as a cause for extubation failure. This technique provides excellent noninvasive visualization of the pharynx, epiglottis, and vocal cords. Although fiberoptic examination does not visualize the subglottis well, it can give a strong indication of subglottic pathology; the trachea is not visualized. The technique is generally used in patients who have had a failed extubation and in whom upper airway problems are suspected. Other indications for fiberoptic nasolaryngoscopy include stridor, aphonia, increasing respiratory rate, deteriorating blood gas values, and high-risk factors such as prolonged intubation.

Preparation

The patient is prepared for extubation as described previously. In patients undergoing a second or third trial of extubation steroids are usually used to reduce laryngeal edema. Dexamethasone (Decadron), 0.5 mg/kg/dose for four doses, is administered. Steroid administration starts at midnight the night before extubation and is given at 6 A.M., noon, and 6 P.M. The patient is extubated early in the morning so that observation can be continued during the day. The technique of extubation is also performed as stated previously.

Technique

Immediately after extubation, if the patient's condition is stable, fiberoptic nasolaryngoscopy is performed. The patient has been previously prepared with several drops of 0.25% oxymetazoline and a few drops of 2% to 4% lidocaine in the nose. The fiberscope is inserted through the nose in patients weighing >1500 g or through the oral cavity in patients weighing <1500 g. The fiberscope is advanced through the nasal cavity or oral cavity until the epiglottis and laryngeal airway are identified. The major positive findings may include mass lesions (e.g., granulation tissue or cysts), subglottic edema, or decreased mobility or paralysis of the vocal cords. Slight bowing of the true vocal cords from the endotracheal tube is common. In patients with subglottic edema, results of the fiberoptic nasolaryngoscopy immediately after extubation may be normal because of the stenting effect of the tube. Patients developing progressive stridor, air hunger, or deteriorating blood gas values after extubation should be reexamined. The fiberscope is then withdrawn, and a racemic epinephrine treatment is given (see Chapter 133).

Patients who fail extubation are managed based on the findings of fiberoptic examination. Mass lesions are managed with microlaryngoscopy and bronchoscopy and with laser treatment if indicated. Patients with subglottic edema are managed as are patients with croup. True vocal cord paralysis may necessitate a tracheotomy if the patient's airway is inadequate.

ADDITIONAL READING

Fagraeus L. Difficult extubation following nasotracheal intubation. Anesthesiology 49:43-44, 1978.

• Fan LL, Flynn JW. Laryngoscopy in neonates and infants: Experience with the flexible fiberoptic bronchoscope. Laryngoscope 921:451-456, 1981.

Fox WW, Berman LJ, Dinwiddie R, et al. Tracheal extubation of the neonate at 2 to 3 cm H_2O continuous positive airway pressure. Pediatrics 59:257-261, 1977.

Murciano D, Auclaer MH, Pariente R, et al. A randomized control trial of theophylline in patients with severe chronic obstructive pulmonary disease. N Engl J Med 320:1521-1525, 1989.

Nussbaum E. Flexible fiberoptic bronchoscopy and laryngoscopy in infants and children. Laryngoscope 93:1033-1035, 1983.

Pransky SM, Grundfast KM. Differentiating upper from lower airway compromise in neonates. Ann Otol Rhinol Laryngol 94:509-515, 1985.

136 Tracheotomy

Orval E. Brown · Scott C. Manning · Gina Blount · Nancy L. Hatfield

The procedure of tracheotomy has been known since ancient times as a treatment for airway obstruction. An early successful tracheotomy is attributed to Asclepiades of Bithynia (circa 120-70 B.C.). In the early 1900s Chevalier Jackson introduced a systematic approach to the management of airway obstruction, including endoscopy and tracheotomy. Recent studies have revealed a changing set of indications for tracheotomy, standardization of the surgical procedure, and a systematic approach to in-hospital and home care.

INDICATIONS

Early in this century tracheotomy was performed primarily for infectious problems resulting in upper airway obstruction. In recent decades a marked shift has taken place in the indications for tracheotomy in pediatric patients. With modern hospital care many children with complex CNS, cardiac, and respiratory problems have survived. Successful management of these patients has resulted in an increased incidence of tracheotomy performed in patients without primary airway problems. The most common indication is prolonged mechanical ventilation necessitating tracheal intubation. This is seen most frequently in patients with respiratory distress syndrome, patients who have undergone cardiac and craniofacial procedures, and patients with CNS disorders. Patients with CNS disorders usually have a residual deficit after cardiac resuscitation or have had head trauma or an intracranial tumor. Patients intubated for 10 days to 2 weeks who need continued ventilatory support are candidates for tracheotomy. In older pediatric patients intubation for longer than 7 days is associated with a significant increase in laryngeal damage from intubation. Neonates tolerate intubation longer than older children, and the decision for tracheotomy in these patients is individualized and deferred for as long a period as possible. Upper air-way obstruction secondary to acquired subglottic stenosis or congenital subglottic stenosis is another major indication for tracheotomy in infants and children. Newborns with congenital laryngeal malformations or other lesions such as vocal cord paralysis, hemangioma, or cystic hygroma may also need tracheotomy.

Some patients previously treated with tracheotomy may be managed successfully with other methods. Patients with epiglottitis are treated with intubation in the operating room and then are observed for 24 to 48 hours in the PICU. Intubation has less morbidity and mortality compared to a tracheotomy in this patient population; thus tracheotomy is rarely used in the management of acute epiglottitis. Patients with viral laryngotracheobronchitis (croup) who are older than 1 year and who need airway support are intubated for 2 to 5 days. Those patients failing extubation are considered for tracheotomy. Patients with croup who are less than 1 year of age and need airway support undergo tracheotomy since the incidence of acquired subglottic stenosis is unacceptably high with intubation in this patient population.

TECHNIQUE
Location

Tracheotomy in the infant and small child is performed in the operating room under proper lighting and magnification, including the use of 2.5× loupes. In very unusual circumstances when a patient is too unstable to be transported from the PICU to the operating suite, tracheotomy may be performed in the PICU. In this instance the complete surgical team and proper instruments are brought to the patient's bedside in the PICU to provide proper support.

Securing the Airway

Patients undergoing tracheotomy are initially managed with endotracheal intubation or the airway is secured with a bronchoscope, and appropriate anesthesia is administered. Performing a tracheotomy in a young struggling infant who has been given a local anesthetic agent is a hazardous procedure and fraught with complications, particularly pneumothorax. The patient is placed in the supine position with a roll under the shoulders and with the head extended. The patient must be positioned in an absolutely straight fashion. NG tubes and esophageal stethoscopes are not placed so that a stiff tube in the esophagus cannot be mistaken for the trachea (Fig. 136-1).

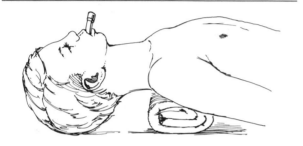

Fig. 136-1   Positioning of patient for tracheotomy.

Surgery

After routine sterile preparation the patient is draped, leaving the face and endotracheal tube or bronchoscope exposed. This exposure facilitates management of the endotracheal tube during placement of the tracheotomy tube and prevents accidental kinking and dislodgment of the tube. Since tracheotomy is a clean procedure but not a sterile one, this presents no serious break in surgical technique. The landmarks of the hyoid bone, cricoid cartilage, and sternal notch must be easily palpable.

A small transverse skin incision is made at approximately the level of the third tracheal ring (Fig. 136-2, *A*). Dissection is carried down through the subcutaneous tissue to the strap muscles, and excessive subcutaneous tissue may be excised to provide a cleaner wound. The strap muscles are separated in the midline and grasped with an Allis forceps. Midline dissection and absolute hemostasis are essential.

The thyroid isthmus and thymus gland are identified, and the thymus gland is retracted inferiorly with a vein retractor. The thyroid isthmus is dissected from the trachea using a small hemostat and is clamped, divided, and suture ligated. The cricoid cartilage and tracheal rings are identified. Two tracheal stay sutures (3-0 or 4-0 silk) are placed lateral to the incision through rings 2, 3, and 4 (Fig. 136-2, *B*). At

Fig. 136-2   **A,** Initial skin incision. **B,** Retraction sutures and tracheal incision. **C,** Insertion of tracheostomy tube.

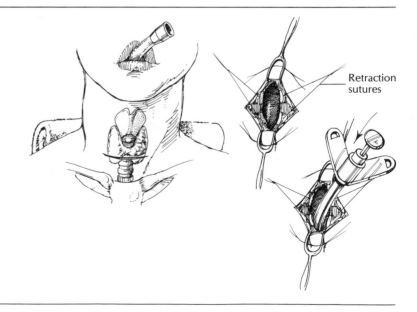

Retraction sutures

this point the previously selected proper-size trache ostomy tube is checked, and the anesthesia team is notified that the tracheotomy incision is about to be made. Coordination between surgeon and anesthesiologist is essential for smooth placement of the tracheostomy tube.

A single midline vertical incision is made at tracheal rings 3 and 4, and the wound is suctioned clear of secretions (Fig. 136-2, *B*). The endotracheal tube is withdrawn to just above the incision. The wound is opened with a small hemostat, and the tracheostomy tube is placed into the lumen (Fig. 136-2, *C*). The obturator is withdrawn, and the tracheostomy tube is connected to the anesthesia ventilator via the standard 14 mm adapter. The tracheostomy tube is secured by placement of 3-0 or 4-0 silk stay sutures through the skin and through the flanges of the tracheostomy tube. The tracheostomy ties are tied on one side of the neck, not directly posteriorly. The proper tension is reached when one finger slides easily beneath the ties. At this point, with the airway secured, the endotracheal tube may be completely removed. The shoulder roll is removed, and the previously placed stay sutures are taped to the chest using 1-inch wide paper tape. The stay sutures are separated to ensure that the right and left sides are not inadvertently crossed during an emergency.

Postoperative Care
The tube

A chest radiograph is taken with the patient on the operating table to check for tracheostomy tube tip placement above the carina and for the possibility of pneumothorax. The patient is then transported to the PICU or PARU.

The tracheal and tracheostomy tube flange stay sutures are removed 3 to 4 days after surgery. Tracheostomy ties usually are changed initially after 24 to 72 hours by the surgeon to allow adequate formation of the tracheal channel, decreasing the chance of decannulation and tracheal irritation. Specific orders about tracheostomy care for the first 72 hours must be written by the physician within the postoperative orders. After the 72-hour period routine tracheostomy care according to hospital policy is instituted.

Tracheostomy dressings are not placed immediately after the operation because they maintain a moist environment at the surgical site, increasing the opportunity for infection. The site must remain as dry as possible, a goal that may create a challenge

for the nursing staff when caring for an infant with a short neck. Maintaining a slight extension of the infant's neck and turning his head every 1 to 2 hours will assist in maintaining a dry environment. In addition changing tracheostomy dressings in the immediate postoperative period increases the risk of accidental decannulation. This can be disastrous if the wound has not matured enough to provide a patient stoma for reinsertion. Tracheostomy patients are usually observed in the PICU for 5 to 7 days postoperatively unless one-to-one nursing care can be provided elsewhere in the hospital.

Humidity/oxygen therapy

The patient's condition after surgery will dictate the type of humidity/oxygen device needed (e.g., ventilator, tracheostomy cradle). T-bar attachments to the tracheostomy tube are never used since they may inadvertently dislodge the tube from the airway. Providing continuous humidity with 0.45% sodium chloride solution or sterile water is essential since the patient's natural upper airway humidification system is bypassed. Careful regulation of humidity output will prevent excessive condensation and movement of water into the patient's trachea. Signs of excessive humidity include the need for frequent tracheal suctioning, watery and thin secretions, and increased coughing without sputum production. Overhumidification may hinder stoma healing, produce an increased growth medium for bacteria, and cause skin rashes or skin breakdown beneath the dressings or ties.

Suctioning

To assure a patent airway suctioning must be done on an as-needed basis after surgery. Initially suctioning may be needed every 10 to 15 minutes, slowly tapering to an as-needed basis as indicated by the amount and type of secretions being suctioned. Saline lavage during suctioning eases removal of dried or retained secretions and can be used in conjunction with hyperoxygenation or bagging procedures. Blood-streaked secretions are normal and are to be expected during the first 24 hours. Frank hemorrhage is a medical emergency. The amount, color, and consistency of secretions must be noted since changes could signal the beginning of infection. The use of chest physiotherapy and aerosol bronchodilator therapy may be indicated and may be started immediately after surgery.

Routine tracheostomy care

Tracheostomy care must be performed every 4 hours using one-half strength hydrogen peroxide and sterile cotton-tipped swabs. The tracheostomy site must be carefully cleansed and dried completely to prevent infection and skin breakdown. The tracheostomy ties must be changed every 24 hours or when soiled. To prevent dislodgment of the tracheostomy tube, new ties must be added before cutting the old ties. (The old ties may be cut first if a second person is available to hold the tracheostomy tube in place while new ties are applied.) The knot is tied on the side of the neck and must be snug enough that only one adult finger can fit beneath the tie comfortably. The placement of the knot can be altered from side to side with each change. If the skin underneath the ties begins to break down, a foam pad may be used to decrease irritation. The key to preventing breakdown is keeping the area clean and dry.

The initial tracheostomy tube is changed 1 week postoperatively by the surgeon. Following the initial change weekly tracheostomy tube changes are recommended. The tube may be changed as frequently as clinically indicated. If an inner cannula is used, it must be removed and cleaned with hydrogen peroxide and sterile pipe cleaners every 8 hours and rinsed in sterile water before reinsertion. It is easier on the patient if a clean inner cannula is ready for insertion before the removal of the existing cannula. Cannulae may be stored in sterile water.

It is necessary to monitor the infant's vital signs and behavior closely for signs of discomfort or inadequate oxygenation. During tracheostomy care the caregiver should assess the skin area and stoma for signs of breakdown, including rash, redness, or drainage. The nurse must also maintain the following routine equipment at the patient's bedside: suction catheters of the appropriate size for the patient, suction equipment, and a face mask of the appropriate size for the patient in case of emergency. In addition to the routine equipment already at the bedside, the following special supplies are needed: a replacement tracheostomy tube of same size, hydrogen peroxide/sterile water (equal parts), cotton-tipped swabs, tracheostomy ties, tracheostomy dressings (2 × 2 wick), and bandage scissors.

Communication

Since patients will be unable to alert caretakers to distress, pain, or other problems, they must be con-stantly observed. Patients who could speak before surgery will suffer the greatest anxiety as a result of an inability to vocalize after the tracheotomy. It is vital that these patients have some means to make contact with staff and family (e.g., bell, buzzer, writing pad and pencil, picture board). Following the acute phase of recovery the use of a fenestrated tube, tracheostomy talk, or instruction in covering the tracheostomy opening during exhalation will allow resumption of some vocal communication.

Other problems

Head position. The head position must be carefully monitored to prevent occlusion of the tracheostomy by the chin, bedding, or clothing. Erosion of the neck by tracheostomy flanges is a possibility and can be influenced by neck position. Placing a small roll under the patient's shoulders will allow a slight extension of the neck during sleep. The use of swivel adapters on the tube allows more varied positioning of ventilator tubing without a noticeable increase in dead space or tubing weight.

Tube length. Tracheostomy tubes are standard length and may be too long for some patients, primarily neonates. Shortening the tube may be necessary. Rough edges must be refinished and smoothed to prevent traumatic injury. The use of specially designed neonatal tubes is usually adequate for these patients.

Tube obstruction. In the event of acute airway obstruction from secretions, food, or foreign body aspiration, the first step is to suction the patient. If the obstruction is not relieved, the tracheostomy ties must be cut, the obstructed tube removed, and the spare tracheostomy tube inserted. Breath sounds must be auscultated to ensure proper tube placement.

Parent education. Initially parental anxiety may stem from several factors, including the loss of the child's ability to speak or make noises, cosmetic changes in the child's appearance, fear of meeting the patient's care needs, and upheaval of family routines. These fears are best addressed by early and consistent teaching. Participation by parents in daily care may begin as soon as the patient is stable. Tracheostomy teaching by the health caregivers may begin as provided in home discharge materials (see Chapter 138) and may formally begin through a physician's order. Although an order for teaching is not mandatory, it communicates the prospective plan to the entire health care team. It has also been determined that some insurance companies will reimburse the providers of specialty services involved in teaching the patient and/or family in preparation for home discharge. Suctioning, tracheostomy site care, and tie changes are good places to begin. The family needs time with staff members so their questions and concerns are fully answered. Understanding the need and reason for and possible duration of the tracheostomy will go a long way to comfort the family. Child life and social workers need to work with older patients regarding the changing body image and activity restrictions. Before the patient is discharged parents must be able to handle all phases of care, including tube changes.

Discharge. Home care equipment needs vary with each patient, and an adequate amount of time must be given to plan for and train parents on each piece of equipment. Additional qualified help for parents may be necessary. Home care representatives and social workers must be involved with parents early in the hospitalization to make arrangements.

Decannulation

Decannulation is considered when the medical process necessitating the tracheotomy tube is resolved. Patients are first evaluated via fiberoptic nasolaryngoscopy to assess vocal cord mobility (see Chapter 135). If vocal fold mobility is normal, direct laryngoscopy and bronchoscopy are performed in the operating room to assess the airway completely. The tracheostomy tube is removed and the entire airway assessed during endoscopy. If the airway is deemed adequate, the patient is admitted to the hospital for a trial of decannulation.

The patient is usually seen in the outpatient clinic where the tube is removed and the tracheal stoma is taped with a Band-Aid. The patient is carefully observed by physicians and nurses for several hours before his admission to the ward. The patient is observed overnight using an apnea monitor, and if the airway is adequate, he is discharged the next morning.

Decannulation panic is almost invariably related to an inadequate airway and necessitates a careful evaluation of the patient's airway status. It is usually not necessary to decannulate the patient in the PICU if the airway is adequate. Only very occasionally are step-down procedures such as daytime tracheostomy tube plugging or using progressively smaller tracheostomy tubes indicated.

RISKS AND COMPLICATIONS

The mortality rate of tracheotomy may range up to 50%, but if deaths from intercurrent disease are eliminated, the mortality rate from tracheotomy alone is 2% to 8%. The mortality rate in the hospital or home does not differ significantly. The rate of other reported complications ranges from 20% to 50%. Complications may be considered early (occurring in the first week) and late (occurring after 1 week). The duration of the tracheostomy has risen from an average of approximately 2 weeks when done for infectious disease to an average of 6 months because of the increased population of chronic respiratory, cardiac, and CNS patients. This increased duration of tracheostomy may give rise to an increased incidence of late complications.

Early Complications

The incidence of intraoperative complications was reported as low as 0.5% in a series from a large pediatric center where tracheotomies were performed by experienced surgeons. Meticulous anesthesia and surgical technique reduce these complications, which are primarily subcutaneous emphysema and pneumothorax. Hemorrhage from great vessels, esophageal perforation, recurrent laryngeal nerve injury, and tracheostomy tube placement in the pretracheal space should be exceedingly rare in experienced hands in major pediatric centers. Major complications encountered in the first week after the tracheotomy include accidental decannulation and mucous plugging. Mucous plugging is managed with adequate humidification and suctioning.

Early accidental decannulation. Accidental decannulation is most dangerous in the first 4 to 5 days after tracheostomy because a fistulous tract between the trachea and the skin has not yet been established and recannulation may be difficult or fatal if the tube is replaced in the subcutaneous tissue or the pretracheal space. It is for this reason that the first tracheostomy tube change is always done by the surgeon. Signs of accidental decannulation include inability to vocalize, respiratory distress, air hunger, and changes in vital signs. If the patient is on a ventilator, airway disconnect alarms will activate.

If accidental decannulation occurs, oxygen must be administered using a bag and mask technique while the patient's neck is extended using a roll placed beneath the back. This will place the trachea in approximately the same position as during the operative procedure so that the skin incision overlies the tracheal incision. The stay sutures on either side of the incision must be grasped firmly and the trachea pulled gently upward, exposing the tracheal incision (Fig. 136-2, *B*). The tracheostomy tube can then be inserted easily and ventilation resumed. A roentgenogram must be done to assure the tube is in the proper position.

Delayed Complications

The most common delayed complication is persistent tracheocutaneous fistula. This reflects a tracheostomy tube placement of long duration with an ingrowth of skin to line the fistulous track to the trachea. This complication is managed by excising or cauterizing the fistulous tract after decannulation when a stable airway is assured. Inadvertent decannulation and tube obstruction from mucous plugging are other frequent late complications. With proper hospital and home care, the rate of patient death is reported as low as 0.13 per 100 patient tracheostomy months. Careful home care management reduces the incidence and risk of these complications. Granulation tissue of the tracheostoma is a not infrequent complication, but it is easily treated with silver nitrate application to the tracheal stoma. Tracheal granulation or fibroma is treated with bronchoscopic excision or stoma revision. Subglottic and tracheal stenosis is infrequent. Innominate artery erosion is exceedingly rare with the use of flexible plastic tracheostomy tubes.

ADDITIONAL READING

Beach TP, Frank JE. Assessment of intubation in croup and epiglottitis. Ann Otol Rhinol Laryngol 91:403-406, 1982.

Black RJ, Baldwin DL, Johns AN. Tracheostomy decannulation panic in children: Fact or fiction? J Laryngol Otol 96:297-304, 1984.

Carter P, Benjamin B. Ten-year review of pediatric tracheotomy. Ann Otol Rhinol Laryngol 92:398-400, 1982.

Conner GH, Bushey MJ, Maisels MJ. Prolonged endotracheal intubation in the newborn. Ann Otol Rhinol Laryngol 59:459-461, 1980.

Downes JJ, Schreiner MS. Tracheostomy tubes and attachments in infants and children. Int Anesth Clin 23(4):37-60, 1985.

Fann LL, Flynn JW, Pathak DR. Rick factors predicting laryngeal injury in intubated neonates. Crit Care Med 11:431-433, 1983.

Gaudet PT, Peerless A, Sasaki C, et al. Pediatric tracheostomy and associated complications. Laryngoscope 88:1633-1641, 1978.

• Gerson CP, Tucker GF. Infant tracheotomy. Ann Otol Rhinol Laryngol 91:413-416, 1982.

Hawkins DB, Williams EH. Tracheostomy in infants and young children. Laryngoscope 56:331-340, 1976.

Kenna MA, Reilly JS, Stool SE. Tracheotomy in the preterm infant. Ann Otol Rhinol Laryngol 96:68-71, 1986.

Lyons AS. Medicine in Roman times. In Lyons A, Petrucelli RJ, eds. Medicine: An Illustrated History. New York: Harry N Abrams, 1978, p 232.

MacRae DL, Rae RE, Heenaman H. Pediatric tracheotomy. J Otolaryngol 13:309-311, 1984.

Mulcherjoe DK. The changing concepts of tracheostomy. J Laryngol Otol 93:899-907, 1979.

Myers EH, Stool SE, Johnson JT, eds. Tracheotomy. New York: Churchill-Livingstone, 1985.

Newlands WJ, McKerrow WS. Pediatric tracheostomy: Fifty-seven operations on fifty-three children. J Laryngol Otol 101:929-935, 1987.

Rodgens BM, Rooks JJ, Talbert JL. Pediatric tracheostomy: Long-term evaluation. J Pediatric Surg 14:258-263, 1979.

Ruben RJ, Newton L, Chambers H, et al. Home care of the pediatric patient with a tracheotomy. Ann Otol Rhinol Laryngol 91:633-640, 1982.

Swift AC, Rogers JH. The outcome of tracheostomy in children. J Laryngol Otol 101:936-939, 1987.

Teppas JJ, Herouy JH, Shermeta DW, et al. Tracheostomy in neonates and small infants: Problems and pitfalls. Surgery 89:635-639, 1988.

• Wetmore RF, Handler SD, Potsic WP. Pediatric tracheostomy: Experience during the past decade. Ann Otol Rhinol Laryngol 91:628-632, 1982.

Zulliger JJ, Garvin JP, Schuller DE, et al. Assessment of intubation in croup and epiglottitis. Ann Otol Rhinol Laryngol 91:403-406, 1982.

137 Extracorporeal Membrane Oxygenation

P. Pearl O'Rourke

BACKGROUND AND INDICATIONS

Extracorporeal membrane oxygenation (ECMO) for support of cardiopulmonary function is a direct extension of cardiopulmonary bypass (CPB) technology developed for cardiothoracic surgery. The first CPB used bubble oxygenators, which are characterized by a direct blood-gas interface. They are still used today and have the advantages of a rapid setup time and relatively low expense, but the disadvantage of the blood-gas interface is that it produces physical stress on the red blood cell (RBC), resulting in hemolysis if used for more than a few hours. The more chronic application of CPB technology (ECMO) became a possibility with the advent of membrane oxygenators, which separate the blood and gas phases with a semipermeable membrane. This protects the RBCs and prevents significant hemolysis, allowing safe extracorporeal oxygenation for longer periods of time.

Clinical reports of chronic membrane CPB for pulmonary support of patients with acute respiratory failure (ARF) were first published in the early 1970s; by 1974 bypass had been used in 150 adult ARF patients. The growing interest in the clinical application of this technology resulted in the National Institutes of Health (NIH) multicentered randomized study designed to compare the efficacy of ECMO vs. conventional mechanical ventilation in adult patients with severe ARF. The results of this study had a large impact on the future of ECMO: although ECMO could support gas exchange, there was no difference in survival rate. Further use of ECMO was discouraged.

But critics of the NIH study suggested that this study was doomed to failure because the clinical entry criteria selected patients who already had irreversible lung disease with fibrotic changes. They thought that at the time ECMO was offered to these patients, the lungs were damaged to a degree that obviated lung repair and survival. It was suggested that ECMO be reevaluated in a group of patients who clearly had reversible lung disease. Neonates with persistent pulmonary hypertension of the newborn (PPHN) were identified as such a group. In the first days of life these infants can have life-threatening ARF that generally resolves as the pulmonary vascular resistance decreases. The growing ECMO experience in these neonates has shown an improvement in patient survival and has established ECMO as a therapy for PPHN.

TECHNIQUE
Apparatus

There are two basic types of ECMO: veno-arterial (VA) and veno-veno (VV). This terminology describes the direction of blood flow; outflow is always from the venous system, whereas inflow can be into either the venous (VV) or the arterial (VA) circulation. At present VA ECMO is almost exclusively used in neonates (Fig. 137-1).

Outflow of blood in VA or VV ECMO is through a large catheter placed into the right atrium via the right internal jugular vein. A number of catheter types can be used, but to maximize venous return they are large bore (12 to 16 gauge) and tooled with multiple side holes. Blood flows by gravity from the right atrium into the ECMO circuit. To increase the venous return into the circuit the child's bed is elevated 6 to 12 inches. Because the maintenance of adequate venous flow is often the most problematic part of ECMO, proper catheter design and placement are critical.

Blood flows from the right atrium into a small reservoir or bladder (50 ml volume) in the ECMO circuit. The reservoir adds capacitance to the system

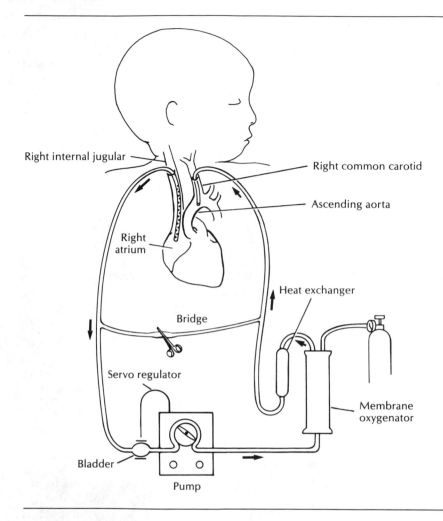

Fig. 137-1   Veno-arterial ECMO.

Right internal jugular

Right common carotid

Ascending aorta

Right atrium

Heat exchanger

Bridge

Servo regulator

Membrane oxygenator

Bladder

Pump

and safety in the event of momentary decreases in venous return. The bladder is fit with an alarm so that if there is decreased blood flow causing the bladder to collapse, the pump turns off and an audio alarm sounds.

After the bladder, the blood is actively pumped using occlusive blood pumps to minimize RBC damage. Roller pumps are most commonly used, but there is a growing interest in centrifugal pumps. Flows generated by the pump are a function of the tubing size (1/4 inch in neonates) and the number of pump head revolutions per minute.

Located immediately after the pump is the membrane oxygenator. The oxygenator is a hollow silicone rubber envelope that is rolled around a spool and placed inside a fitted silicone sleeve. Blood flows on the outside of the coiled envelope, and gas flows in a countercurrent direction inside the membrane. Oxygen and carbon dioxide diffuse through this semipermeable membrane, and carbon dioxide is flushed from the gas compartment by the gas flow. Different sizes of membranes are available (0.4, 0.8, 1.5 m²). Each one is rated for oxygen and carbon dioxide transfer and recommended blood flow rates.

Blood then goes through a heat exchanger, which regulates blood temperature to effect no net temperature loss for the patient.

Finally blood is reinfused into the patient through a single end-hole catheter (8 to 12 gauge). In VA ECMO the catheter is placed in the right common carotid artery and advanced into the ascending aorta. This site is used to return the oxygenated blood as close to the aortic root as possible to guarantee the delivery of well-oxygenated blood to the cerebral and coronary circulations. In VV ECMO blood return is through a catheter placed in the femoral vein.

The ECMO circuit is designed with a bridge that provides emergency bypass. By placing occlusive clamps on the outflow and inflow catheters and removing the bridge clamp, the child and the circuit can be effectively isolated from each other.

No particulate filter is in the system since early experience suggested the presence of a filter over many days increased thrombosis and RBC hemolysis. However, centers do use an air trap.

The volume of the entire circuit is approximately 300 to 400 ml. Before the patient is placed on ECMO, the circuit is primed with blood that is calcium and pH corrected. The circuit is heparinized to avoid clot formation and embolization to the patient; this is particularly critical in VA ECMO in which blood return has direct access to the coronary and cerebral circulations. Heparinization is monitored by activated clotting times (ACTs), which can easily be done at the bedside. ACTs are maintained in the 200 to 260 second range (normal, 90 to 120 seconds).

Procedure

When ECMO support is started, the clinician must select ECMO flow rates and gas flow through the oxygenator.

Adequate ECMO flow can be reliably assessed clinically by evaluating the arterial blood gas (ABG) values and the adequacy of perfusion. In neonates ECMO flows of approximately 300 to 400 ml/min or 100 ml/kg/min are adequate for pulmonary support. Attempts to document ECMO flow as a percent of the cardiac output (CO) have proved difficult because in a normal neonate the CO varies tremendously (120 to 300 ml/kg/min). In addition the specific neonate's CO changes with time, therapy, and resolution of the primary disease. Therefore most clinicians express ECMO as milliliters per kilogram per minute. But the percent CO supported by ECMO is estimated by evaluating the systemic arterial tracing. Because ECMO flow is nonpulsatile, if ECMO has assumed a large percent of the CO, the systemic arterial tracing should be blunted or flattened. As the ECMO flow becomes a smaller portion of the CO, the tracing will become

more pulsatile. Some clinicians suggest that a totally flattened arterial tracing correlates with ECMO flow rates >80% of the CO.

The flow and composition of gases through the membrane oxygenator are tailored to achieve adequate ABG values in the patient. Because excessive flows can cause gas embolization, there are suggested limits to maximal gas flow rates for each size membrane. During ECMO a combination of oxygen, air, and carbon dioxide is used, with the correct ratio of gases determined by a number of patient and ECMO circuit features:

Age and hence efficiency of the membrane
Size of the membrane oxygenator
Amount of ECMO flow
Patient's metabolic rate
Patient's cardiac output

Any alteration in gas composition must be immediately assessed by checking ABG values.

Management

When the patient is stable on ECMO and adequate ABG values have been documented, the conventional ventilator settings are decreased to minimize oxygen toxicity and barotrauma to the patient's lungs. Commonly used settings are FiO_2, room air; peak inspiratory pressure (PIP), 20 to 25 cm H_2O; PEEP, 0 to 5 cm H_2O; and ventilator rate, 4 to 6 breaths/min. If the ECMO flow is inadequate to sustain normal ABG values, the patient's own lungs must also participate in gas exchange, and ventilator settings are increased.

Muscle relaxants are discontinued. The patient is allowed to move but is sedated to keep the amount of spontaneous movement in a safe range. The head is maintained in the midline position to maximize venous drainage from the head.

Duration

Most clinical programs provide ECMO support for a maximum of 14 days. This decision is based on two principles: (1) the risks of ECMO increase with time and (2) if there is no improvement with the patient's own lungs within 2 weeks, the likelihood of improvement is very small. Decisions to extend ECMO beyond 14 days must be considered individually as exceptional situations.

In reality neonates with PPHN usually need ECMO for <7 to 10 days. In these children ECMO is continued until the patients' own lungs can support gas exchange with a reasonably safe amount of ventilator support. In my institution ECMO is weaned when the child can be oxygenated and ventilated with the following settings: an FiO_2 <0.30; PIP <30 cm H_2O; PEEP <5 cm H_2O; and ventilator rate <30 breaths/min.

The readiness of the patient's own lungs can be evaluated in a number of ways: radiographically, changes in compliance, and changes in ability to sustain gas exchange. The latter is assessed by determining ABG values while ventilator settings are increased and ECMO flows are weaned or by short trials off ECMO.

RISKS AND COMPLICATIONS

A number of risks and complications are associated with ECMO.

Hemorrhage. Hemorrhage is the biggest problem; heparinization is thought to be the most likely cause. Bleeding can occur in virtually any organ: the CNS, the GI tract, kidney, subcutaneous tissue, the cannulation site. Children who are started on ECMO postoperatively (e.g., after surgery for congenital diaphragmatic hernia) can also have significant blood loss at the operative site.

Although bleeding can occur anywhere, intracranial hemorrhage (ICH) is the most feared. In the case of intracranial bleeding the cause is most likely multifactorial: heparinization; ligation of the right common carotid artery that interrupts normal perfusion patterns; and disruption of the cerebral venous return with the placement of a large catheter in the right internal jugular vein, which may obstruct venous return and hence increase cerebral venous pressure.

Because the fear of ICH is so great, before any neonate is placed on ECMO, a head ultrasonogram is obtained. If there is preexisting ICH, the decision to start ECMO and heparinization must be reviewed. Some centers do not offer ECMO to a child with any preexisting ICH; other centers base ECMO inclusion or exclusion on various gradations of ICH. While the child is on ECMO, cranial ultrasonograms are obtained daily; in the event of an ICH discontinuation of ECMO support must be considered.

In an attempt to minimize hemorrhage the ACT is monitored hourly, and platelets are transfused to keep the count >80,000 to 100,000/mm³.

Embolization. The embolization of clot, air, or particulate matter is especially problematic in VA ECMO because the return of unfiltered blood into the ascending aorta produces the risk of embolization into the coronary and/or cerebral circulations. The addition of an air trap in the ECMO circuit is one attempt to decrease this risk.

Blood-membrane interaction. As blood is exposed to the membrane, there are consumption and activation of several blood products. The predictable fall in the number of platelets is one example. The possibility of activation of vasoactive plasma factors such as the prostanoid system by the blood-membrane interaction is also being studied.

Technical mishaps. ECMO is a relatively new mode of support that stretches the use of a technology that was devised for short-term cardiopulmonary support. Technical mishaps or misadventures with the entire circuit or with an individual component part are always possible and could have devastating results for the patient.

Inclusion criteria. It is important to acknowledge the risk that exists from meeting entry criteria for ECMO support. Most of these patients have already suffered some period of hypoxia and/or acidosis with potential preexisting end-organ damage.

Institutional expense. ECMO is expensive. In addition to the outlay for nondisposable and disposable equipment, personnel costs are high. Most ECMO programs require the presence of an ECMO technician at the bedside 24 hours a day; this is in addition to the nurse and other paramedical personnel required for the patient's care. In the present era of reducing hospital budgets, ECMO programs may be a resource drain.

PATIENT SELECTION

The largest single group of patients receiving ECMO support is infants with PPHN secondary to meconium aspiration syndrome, congenital diaphragmatic hernia, pneumonia, sepsis, or idiopathic causes. ECMO is presently offered only when conventional mechanical ventilation fails and the patient meets criteria for ≧80% predicted mortality (most predicted mortality is based on individual institutional chart review). The national neonatal ECMO experience has shown a survival rate of 83%: the success of ECMO correlates with the specific etiology of the PPHN. Infants with meconium aspiration syndrome have the highest survival rate (92%), whereas infants with congenital diaphragmatic hernia have lower survival rates (63%), most likely secondary to their associated pulmonary hypoplasia.

ECMO is also being used for cardiac support, most

commonly in patients who have cardiac failure after cardiothoracic surgery. The outcome of these patients correlates with the cause of their cardiac failure. Patients in whom ECMO was offered immediately after surgery because of the inability to wean from CPB have many bleeding complications and little improvement in survival. In contrast, patients who are able to wean from CPB but who have progressive cardiac failure in the hours after surgery have shown better results with ECMO support. The number of patients in these groups remains small, and more experience is needed before specific guidelines for ECMO inclusion or exclusion can be formulated.

ECMO will be extended to other patients, but the extension to patients with other diseases must be done with careful preexamination and review of the risk-benefit ratio. These patients must be selected only if they meet two basic criteria: (1) their primary disease is reversible and (2) the degree of illness is severe enough to render a poor prognosis if given standard routine therapy. These two criteria are important because in patients who have irreversible disease, ECMO may only prolong death rather than improve survival; because ECMO is such an invasive therapy, it should be used only when conventional approaches fail.

FUTURE DIRECTIONS

ECMO is an actively evolving technique, with its future doubtlessly including a number of changes in both the technology and its application. The goal of these changes is to develop safer and easier ECMO. A number of new innovations are presently being tested: heparin-bonded circuits, the use of heparinase, holo-fiber oxygenators, centrifugal blood pumps, and single-catheter VV ECMO. If any of these new innovations develop a safer ECMO system, the clinical application will rapidly expand.

At present ECMO must be viewed as an exciting new form of therapy that is invasive and carries serious risks and complications. Until its application is better defined and the technology is routine and safer, ECMO should be offered only in institutions that can adequately provide the multidisciplinary supports needed for this program.

ADDITIONAL READING

Andrews AF, Klein MD, Toomasian JM, et al. Venovenous extracorporeal membrane oxygenation in neonates with respiratory failure. J Pediatr Surg 18:339-346, 1983.

Andrews AF, Nixon CA, Cilley RE, et al. One- to three-year outcome for 14 neonatal survivors of extracorporeal membrane oxygenation. Pediatrics 78:692-698, 1986.

Bartlett RH. Extracorporeal oxygenation in neonates. Hosp Pract 139-151, 1984.

• Bartlett RH, Roloff DW, Cornell RG, et al. Extracorporeal circulation in neonatal respiratory failure: A prospective randomized study. Pediatrics 76:479-487, 1985.

• Bartlett RH, Toomasian J, Roloff D, et al. Extracorporeal membrane oxygenation (ECMO) in neonatal respiratory failure: 100 cases. Ann Surg 204:236-245, 1986.

Cilley RE, Zwischenberger JB, Andrews AF, et al. Intracranial hemorrhage during extracorporeal membrane oxygenation in neonates. Pediatrics 78:699-704, 1986.

Hill DJ, O'Brien GO, Murray JJ, et al. Prolonged extracorporeal oxygenation for acute post-traumatic respiratory failure (shock lung syndrome). N Engl J Med 634:286-292, 1972.

Krummel TM, Greenfield LG, Kirkpatrick BU, et al. Clinical use of extracorporeal membrane oxygenation in neonatal pulmonary failure. J Pediatr Surg 17:525-531, 1982.

Pyle RB, Helton WC, Johnson FW, et al. Clinical use of the membrane oxygenator. Am Surg 110:966-970, 1975.

Towne BH, Lott IT, Hicks DA, et al. Long-term follow-up of infants and children treated with extracorporeal membrane oxygenation (ECMO): A preliminary report. J Pediatr Surg 20:410-414, 1985.

Zapol WM, Snider MT, Hill JD, et al. Extracorporeal membrane oxygenation in severe acute respiratory failure: A randomized prospective study. JAMA 242:2193-2196, 1976.

138 Sending a Patient Home: Home Ventilation

*Lynn E. Rogers · Annette Musselman-Jarvis · Valerie Shasteen ·
Richard L. Vinson*

INDICATIONS

Recent advances in medical technology have made it possible to save many children who might otherwise have died from chronic lung disease. The child who needs chronic ventilator assistance poses the most complex problem on discharge from the PICU. In 1987 the Office of Technology Assessment estimated that the number of children dependent on ventilators in the United States ranged from 680 to 2000.

There are many children with conditions that may benefit from long-term chronic mechanical ventilation. Each disease, as well as each child, must be assessed to determine the feasibility of a long-term home mechanical ventilation program. The goals of long-term ventilator care should include the following: to extend life; to maintain or improve the child's quality of life; to maintain or improve the child's cardiopulmonary status; to provide an environment that will enhance individual potential; and to be cost-effective.

Guidelines are necessary, however, to ensure that physicians and allied health professionals are selecting patients who are appropriate for long-term ventilation. Many patients who are ventilator dependent may not be suitable for discharge home. The following can be used as criteria for selecting candidates to be discharged home on a ventilator: a medically stable child; patient willingness; family willingness; reliable primary caretaker; family motivation to gain skills and knowledge; reliable family support systems; financial assistance available that will support home care (e.g., private insurance, Supplemental Security Income, Medicaid); living arrangement that will allow safe home care; available local medical supervision; reliable transportation system for follow-up; and community support.

CONDITIONS FOR WHICH LONG-TERM MECHANICAL VENTILATION MAY BE APPROPRIATE

Arnold-Chiari malformation
Brain stem aneurysm
Bronchopulmonary dysplasia
Central hypoventilation syndrome (Ondine's curse)
Congenital heart disease
Cervical spinal cord injury
Cystic fibrosis
Diaphragmatic paralysis
Ellis-van Creveld syndrome
Multiple sclerosis
Muscular dystrophy
Myelodysplasia
Nemaline rod myopathy
Neonatal asphyxia
Pierre Robin syndrome
Pompe's disease
Severe head injury
Werdnig-Hoffmann disease

TECHNIQUE

The first step in developing and implementing a program for discharging ventilator-dependent children is to organize a team that will be responsible for assisting the child and family in this major undertaking. This should be a multidisciplinary team, including the following members from the hospital and the community:

Primary pulmonary physician
Clinical nurse specialist
Primary nurse from inpatient unit
Social worker
Registered respiratory therapist
Family members
Durable medical equipment vendor
Home health care agency
Physical therapist
Occupational therapist
Speech therapist
Dietician

One member, usually the clinical nurse specialist or similar individual, must act as the case manager throughout the process and as a liaison after discharge. The physician is responsible for the patient's physiologic stability and for coordination of the med-

ical plan. It is best if the patient has a primary nurse throughout hospitalization to ensure continuity in care and in the teaching process. The social worker provides support and counseling to family members who must prepare for the adjustment from hospital to home care. The respiratory therapist is responsible for teaching respiratory care and ventilator management. The physical therapist, occupational therapist, speech therapist, and dietician must be part of the process as indicated by the individual patient's needs. Participation by community agencies (home health care agency, durable medical equipment vendor, school teacher) will help facilitate a smooth transition from the hospital to home.

The process of planning discharge of a ventilator-dependent child can be divided into three major tasks: (1) parent teaching, (2) acquisition of equipment and supplies, and (3) mobilization of family and community resources.

Parent Teaching

Instructing the parents in caring for their child on a ventilator is usually the most time-consuming, yet the most important, task. At least two caregivers must be identified who will learn all aspects of the child's care. The first step is to identify the knowledge needs of the caretakers for each patient. One of the roles of the primary nurse is to assess the learning needs and abilities of the parents and/or caregivers involved and to begin the teaching process. A written education program must be prepared for each area, including measurable performance objectives, defined methodology, evaluation criteria, and documentation. Table 138-1 lists specific skills that must be taught to most families. Instruction must include demonstrations and return demonstrations, incorporating the "how to's" and "why's" of each procedure. The teaching materials must include a packet of written information and a checklist for content delivered, and the teaching process must include a return demonstration for each of the procedures the caregiver must master. Table 138-2 shows an example of a checklist for tracheostomy teaching. It is important for the health care team to encourage and support the family without intimidating or causing them apprehension or feelings of inadequacy.

The nurse and respiratory therapist must begin by allowing the parents to observe tasks involved in the care of the tracheostomy and the ventilator. At this time the parents can be encouraged to participate in

---

CRITERIA FOR DISCHARGE HOME ON MECHANICAL VENTILATION

1. Major diagnostic studies and therapeutic decisions not anticipated for at least 1 month
2. Nonpulmonary disease in major organ systems under control
3. Free of successive bouts of respiratory infection and fever
4. Acceptable arterial blood gas levels: $Paco_2$ <60 mm Hg in children with primary pulmonary disease; $Paco_2$ <45 mm Hg in children without lung disease (e.g., with neuromuscular disorders or disorders of control of breathing)
5. Fio_2 <0.40
6. Absence of life-threatening cardiac dysfunction or dysrhythmias
7. Absence of significant sustained dyspnea or severe dyspneic episodes and/or tachypnea
8. Positive trends showing on growth curve
9. Evidence of gag/cough reflex or protected airway
10. Absence of significant inhalation pneumonia
11. Psychological stability

Table 138-1   Teaching Plans Needed for the Following Skills in Home Ventilation Program

Tasks	Assessment
Ventilator function: dials, airflow, troubleshooting; include simulated problems (i.e., high- and low-pressure alarms, leaks, missing pieces, faulty valves)	Color change
	Chest excursion
	Respiratory distress
Suctioning: clean technique	Tachycardia
Changing tracheostomy tube	Tachypnea
Changing tracheostomy ties	Diaphoresis
Tracheostomy site care	Edema
Oxygen delivery	Lethargy
Aerosol treatments	Tolerance for spontaneous breathing off ventilator
Percussion, vibration	
Basic cardiopulmonary resuscitation	
Ambu bag use	
Cleaning equipment	
Gastrostomy tube care (if applicable)	
Enteral feeding (if applicable)	
Monitoring functions	
Contingency plan for equipment failure	

the child's basic daily care (i.e., playing, bathing, dressing, feeding). As family members gain skills, they can be encouraged to participate in the child's care to help build their confidence and allow health care personnel to observe and correct actions as needed. When all skills are learned, the family must assume responsibility for total care of the child with hospital personnel acting as backup only when needed. This provides a "home trial" while still in the safety of the hospital and is best accomplished if the child can be moved to a private room or a quiet corner of the PICU.

Teaching can be done by different members of the team. The important factor is that the individual with the most expertise in a particular area is the one to teach that topic. Classes should be organized according to the assessed knowledge level and potential of the learners. Topics must progress at a rate that allows adequate learning by each caretaker. Instructors should encourage questions and discussion whenever possible. Parents also need to be taught that certain reactions from the child are normal. For example, the child may become irritable with suctioning and may attempt to pull the catheter away from them. Therefore the parents need to learn how to properly restrain the child.

Acquisition of Equipment and Supplies

The first step is to identify the equipment and supplies the child will need. Having a list of all equipment and supplies for 1 month is helpful for families and also is required by most insurance companies for payment. Next the process of selecting a vendor for equipment and supplies must be done with care. Several areas must be examined: ability to supply all durable medical equipment (DME) and disposable supplies; pediatric experience; prior experience with home ventilator care; available and reliable 24-hour service by professionals; organized ongoing teaching and home supervision plan that is coordinated with inpatient program and other outpatient services; written instructions for operation and maintenance of equipment; prompt response to telephone calls regarding problems; a program of regular home visits at least monthly to check equipment and do preventive maintenance; reliable delivery of supplies; competitive pricing; direct third-party billing services; provider status with appropriate state and federal agencies; and feedback to hospital regarding problems noted in home.

To enhance understanding by families it is essential they learn about the equipment and care tasks using the exact equipment that will be used in the

Table 138-2   Checklist for Tracheostomy Teaching*

Content	Delivered Date/Instructor	Objectives	Achieved Date/Instructor
Knowledge assessment		*Parents will be able to:*	
I. Anatomy and physiology		I. Describe normal respiratory tract anatomy and physiology	
II. Need for tracheostomy		II. Describe the necessity for their child's tracheostomy	
III. Altered vocalization		III. Describe the reason for altered vocalization with a tracheostomy	
IV. Preoperative events		IV. State the purpose of preoperative events A. Blood and urine test B. Povidone-iodine bath C. Visit by anesthesiologist	
V. Events the day of surgery		V. Describe events the day of surgery A. Preoperative holding unit B. Wait during surgery C. Recovery room	
VI. Postoperative events		VI. State the purpose of postoperative events A. Heart monitor B. Frequent vital signs C. IV fluids D. Beginning oral fluids E. Vomiting F. Pain	
VII. Equipment necessary for home care		VII. Describe equipment necessary for home care	
VIII. Suctioning		VIII. Demonstrate proper suctioning technique	
IX. Changing the tracheostomy ties		IX. Demonstrate proper technique for changing tracheostomy ties	
X. Changing the tracheostomy tube		X. Demonstrate proper technique for changing the tracheostomy tube	
XI. Skin care		XI. Demonstrate appropriate skin care around the neck and stoma site	
XII. Cleaning the tracheostomy tube or inner cannula		XII. Demonstrate proper technique for cleaning the tracheostomy tube or inner cannula	
XIII. Cleaning suction catheters and connecting tubing		XIII. State the appropriate technique for cleaning suction catheters and connecting tubing	
XIV. Cleaning the suction bottle		XIV. State the appropriate technique for cleaning the suction bottle	
XV. Formula for making normal saline and sterile water solution		XV. State the appropriate formula for making normal saline and sterile water solution	
XVI. Cardiopulmonary resuscitation (CPR)		XVI. Demonstrate CPR before patient's discharge from the hospital	
XVII. Environmental considerations		XVII. State environmental considerations	
XVIII. Contacting the physician		XVIII. State when to contact the physician	
XIX. Emergency phone		XIX. State emergency phone numbers and where they are to be kept	

Handouts given: ☐ YES   ☐ NO

Additional comments: _____

*Courtesy Children's Hospital of Orange County, Calif.

home. Therefore, as soon as the patient is medically stable, all equipment must be converted to that which will be used at home. Most DME vendors are willing to do this since they recognize the benefit to the patient and family.

Mobilization of Family and Community Resources

A major issue to contend with is financial reimbursement. This can come from private insurance, state and federally funded programs, or private funds. Although many policies have provisions for payment for a child at home on a ventilator, the process of approval for such funding is long and usually requires a great deal of paperwork.

The home environment must also be evaluated and prepared for the child coming home. An early home assessment is important so that necessary changes may be made in a timely manner. The home environment must include adequate room for equipment and supplies; a proper power source; adequate number of electrical outlets (minimum of three for the ventilator, heated humidifier, and suction machine); additional outlets for feeding pumps, compressor, electric bed; close proximity of medical suppliers; fire alarm or smoke detector; power failure alarm; accessibility for patient (ramps, elevator); telephone; adequate transportation; and intercom system.

In most instances some amount of licensed nursing (LPN, RN) care is deemed necessary for safe care in the home. Care can range from 8 to 24 hours a day and depends on the child's condition, the parent's abilities, and financial reimbursement. In selecting a home health care agency the following must be considered: availability of neonatal/pediatric nurses with recent ICU experience; willingness of at least primary nurse and supervisor to spend time in the hospital becoming familiar with the child's individualized care; flexibility of hours for shifts; provisions of in-service education for home care staff; quality of feedback to physician and families; and previous record of an ethical, philosophical, family-oriented approach to quality care. It is important for families to play an active role in choosing both the

---

SAMPLE ITEMIZED LIST OF EQUIPMENT AND SUPPLIES FOR 1 MONTH OF HOME VENTILATION CARE

1. Ventilator: Portable and simple to operate with type determined by requirements of ventilation volume and Fio_2 ventilation mode; includes backup when indicated
2. Ventilation power source (battery pack/generator)
3. Ventilator circuits
4. Cascade humidifier
5. Replacement filters for ventilator (2 packages)
6. Oxygen supply
7. Manual resuscitator
8. Tracheostomy tubes (specify type and size)
9. Suction machine, nonportable
10. Suction machine, portable
11. Suction catheters (3 cases)
12. Suction connecting tubing (4)
13. Unit-dose sodium chloride 0.9%, 3 ml (360 or make own)
14. Twill tape, 1/2 inch (1 roll)
15. Tracheostomy dressing (2 boxes)
16. Sterile water: 1 L bottle (3 cases of 12 or make own)
17. Hydrogen peroxide (2 bottles)
18. Water-soluble lubricant (1 tube)
19. Cotton-tipped swabs (250)
20. Medication nebulizer
21. Hospital bed
22. Wheelchair
23. Ventilator tray

SAMPLE OF INFORMATION NEEDED BY VARIOUS INSURANCE CARRIERS FOR CONSIDERATION OF FINANCIAL REIMBURSEMENT FOR HOME VENTILATOR CARE

1. Current history and physical examination
2. Description of medical plan at home
3. List of equipment and supplies (include rental vs. purchase cost)
4. Assessed need for home nursing: amount and level of care
5. Complete nursing care plan for home
6. Hospital costs
7. Complete social assessment of child and family

CHAPTER 138 *Sending a Patient Home: Home Ventilation* **965**

home health care agency and the DME vendor. Once out of the hospital it will be the family who is primarily responsible for maintaining communication with these vendors.

Several community agencies must be contacted before a child goes home on a ventilator. The local electric, gas, and telephone companies as well as the fire department, paramedics, and nearest emergency department must be notified. Information must be supplied to them about the presence of life-sustaining equipment in use as well as measures to be taken in the event of an emergency.

Finally, after discharge has taken place, there must be an organized follow-up plan. It must include identification of primary physicians; delineation of ongoing medical plan; specification of follow-up appointment and reevaluation schedule; assessment of in-home stressors (e.g., privacy in home with nurses present 8 to 24 hours, control of child for nurturing and support while nurses provide hands-on care, home turned into a hospital); and determination of ongoing funding.

There has been much progress in the area of discharging the ventilator-dependent child home. Various centers across the country have developed sophisticated programs for this purpose. Although each is unique in its approach, all share the goal of a happy and healthy outcome for the child.

RISKS AND COMPLICATIONS

The risks and complications of having a child home on mechanical ventilation fall into three categories: (1) failure of respiratory treatment devices, (2) changes in the child's overall medical status, and (3) equipment malfunction. Respiratory treatment devices such as tracheostomy, suctioning, and oxygen administration carry risks and complications of their own and are discussed in detail in specific chapters of this book.

Changes in the child's medical status after discharge can include infection and deterioration or progression of the disease process. These changes alter the child's care in the home. It is important to teach caregivers good assessment skills in order to determine normal and abnormal findings in their child. Identification of abnormal respiratory patterns, signs of dyspnea, color changes, and alterations in behavior must be taught to caregivers before discharge. Cardiopulmonary resuscitation must also be taught before the child goes home. Caregivers need to know that being on mechanical ventilation does not eliminate the possibility of cardiopulmonary failure in their child.

Equipment malfunction is a frightening and potentially life-threatening event. Having a backup ventilator in the home is appropriate and is mandatory for children who are 24-hour dependent on mechanical ventilation. Having a generator in the home is also a good safety measure in case of power failure. This is especially important for families living in rural areas. The child must have a resuscitation bag within the immediate proximity at all times so that manual ventilation can be done if all else fails. Mechanical failure of the equipment is always a possibility, and steps must be taken to minimize this possibility. Using a reliable vendor company whose employees are knowledgeable and whose program exercises regular maintenance and turnover of equipment will ensure that equipment is functioning at an optimal level.

Prevention of potential problems is the best practice. Teaching caregivers good assessment skills will result in the early identification of important changes in the patient's condition. Being prepared both at home and while away from home is very important. At home all the necessary equipment is readily available for use; however, while the patient is away from home, this is not always true. A "package" with the following equipment must always be carried with the child wherever he goes: an extra tracheostomy tube, tracheostomy ties, scissors, suction machine, suction catheters, and a resuscitation bag. The family must also know who is the most appropriate person to call in case problems arise. A listing of all physicians, allied health professionals, and vendors must be given to the family, along with instructions on who is responsible for what areas of care. Finally, local paramedics and hospital emergency departments must be identified in case of an emergency situation.

ADDITIONAL READING

Bock RH, Lierman C, Ahmann E, et al. There's no place like home. Child Health Care 12(2):93-96, 1983.
Burr BH, Guyer B, Todres ID, et al. Home care for children on respirators. N Engl J Med 309:1319-1323, 1983.
Childress J, Diamond L, Knapper J, et al. Discharge planning to home care for the ventilator-dependent patient. Baton 1(3):1-34, 1984.
• Congress of the United States, Office of Technology Assessment. Technology-dependent children: Hospital v. home care—a technical memorandum. Washington, D.C.: US Government Printing Office, May 1987.

Frates RC, Splaingard ML, Smith EO, et al. Outcome of home mechanical ventilation in children. J Pediatr 106:850-856, 1985.

Giovannoni R. Chronic ventilator care: From hospital to home. Resp Ther 14(4):29-33, 1984.

Goldberg AI, Noah A, Fleming M, et al. Quality of care for the life-supported children who require prolonged mechanical ventilation at home. QRS 13(3):81-88, 1987.

Kopacz MA, Moriarty-Wright R. Multidisciplinary approach for the patient on a home ventilator. Heart Lung 13:255-262, 1984.

Lang A. Nursing families with an infant who requires home apnea monitoring. Issues Compr Pediatr Nurs 10(2):123-133, 1987.

Lawrence PA. Home care for ventilator-dependent children: Providing a chance to live a normal life. Dimens Crit Care Nurs 3(1):42-52, 1984.

McCarthy MF. A home discharge program for ventilator-assisted children. Pediatr Nurs 12:331-335, 380, 1986.

McCarthy S. Discharge planning for medically fragile children. Caring, November 1986, pp 38-41.

McCoy P, Votroubek W. Tucson's first homebound ventilator-dependent child, Kim Nichols. Caring, December 1986, pp 52-57.

• O'Donohue WJ, Giovannoni RM, Keens TG, et al. Long-term mechanical ventilation. Chest 90(Suppl):1S-37S, 1986.

O'Pray M. Working with families with infants with respiratory equipment in the home. Issues Compr Pediatr Nurs 12(2):113-121, 1987.

Schraeder BD. A creative approach to caring for the ventilator-dependent child. MCN 4(3):165-170, 1979.

Stelle NF, Harrison B. Technology-assisted children: Assessing discharge preparation. J Pediatr Nurs 1(3):150-157, 1986.

Tepper RS, Zander JE, Elgen H. Chronic Respiratory Problems in Infancy. Chicago: Year Book, 1986.

Votava KM, Cleveland T, Hiltunen K. Home care of the patient dependent on mechanical ventilation. Home Health Nurse 3(2):18-25, 1985.

139 Blood Product Transfusions

Naomi J. Winick

BACKGROUND AND INDICATIONS

Transfusion support has contributed to the survival and well-being of many children who have received care in the PICU. In this chapter guidelines and indications for transfusion therapy are given, the available blood components outlined, and the attendant risks discussed. In general a single laboratory value, regardless of how far it deviates from normal, cannot be used as the primary indication for transfusion. The child's primary disease and clinical condition must take precedent in determining the need for a transfusion. The primary goals in giving whole blood are to increase blood volume and increase oxygen-carrying capacity; in giving packed RBCs, to increase oxygen-carrying capacity; in giving platelets, to improve clotting that is abnormal as a result of decreased quantity or abnormal function of platelets; in giving fresh frozen plasma (FFP), to increase blood volume and replace deficient clotting factors; and in giving factor concentrates, to increase deficient clotting factors.

Whole blood and its components are obtained from local volunteer blood donor centers and/or the American Red Cross. As the volunteer donates blood, concurrent samples are drawn to test for human immunodeficiency virus (HIV) antibody, alanine aminotransferase, hepatitis B surface antigen, and hepatitis B core antibody and for performing the rapid plasma reagin test. These screening tests are designed to detect blood contaminated with HIV, hepatitis, and syphilis. In addition some centers screen for the presence of cytomegalovirus (CMV) to assure that neonates and other severely immunocompromised hosts will receive CMV-negative blood.

Blood Products
Whole blood

Whole blood is used only to replace an acute blood loss and during exchange transfusions. RBCs appropriately reconstituted with FFP, 0.9% sodium chloride solution, or plasma protein fraction can also be used for these purposes. Whole blood is procured from a donor and is anticoagulated with either acid citrate dextrose (ACD), citrate phosphate dextrose (CPD), or heparin. Whole blood loses most of its platelets within 4 hours after it is drawn, and the labile clotting factors V and VIII become markedly deficient after the blood has been stored for 48 hours. One week after blood has been drawn red cell hemolysis raises the potassium content to three times that normally found in serum, and 2,3-diphosphoglycerate (2,3-DPG) decreases, causing a shift in the oxygen dissociation curve to the left.

Packed red blood cells

A transfusion with packed RBCs is indicated for the anemic patient who needs increased tissue oxygen delivery. The diagnosis of anemia depends on the hemoglobin value and the patient's clinical condition. For example, if a child with sickle cell disease who is seen for a well child care visit has a hemoglobin level of 6 to 7 g/dl, no treatment is indicated. However, when the same child is hospitalized 2 months later with pneumonia, necessitating oxygen and ventilatory support, and his hemoglobin value is 7 g/dl, transfusion therapy may be indicated.

Packed RBCs, usually anticoagulated with CPD adenine solution, are readily available. The citrate serves as an anticoagulant, the dextrose an energy substrate, and the adenine as a substrate for 2,3-DPG, which maintains adequate intracellular levels of adenosine 5′-triphosphate (ATP). The packed cells are stored at 1° to 6° C and have a shelf life of 35 days, a hematocrit level of approximately 80%, and a hemoglobin concentration of 25 g/dl. A standard transfusion of 10 ml/kg given over 2 to 4 hours will raise a child's hemoglobin level by 2.5 to 3 g/dl and the hematocrit level by 10%. A 15 ml/kg transfusion should be considered maximal, even when the child is hemodynamically stable. The treatment of severe anemia (Hb <4 g/dl) is discussed in detail in Chapter 50.

Washed or frozen deglycerolized packed RBCs are free of most of the WBCs and plasma that normally "contaminate" standard packed RBC transfusions. Washed cells are used in patients who have had non-hemolytic transfusion reactions in the past, are chronically transfused, or may undergo bone marrow transplantation. Irradiating blood products prevents donor lymphocytes from proliferating and causing graft vs. host disease in recipients with severe defects in cell-mediated immunity.

Platelets

Platelet transfusions can be used to stop or prevent severe hemorrhage in patients with thrombocytopenia and, less commonly, platelet dysfunction. In general, without major trauma or surgery, adequate hemostasis is maintained with a platelet count of ≥50,000/mm³, assuming that platelet function is normal.

The decision to administer platelets must be based on factors in addition to the platelet count. Bleeding will be greater than that predicted by platelet number with concomitant platelet dysfunction, vascular or coagulation abnormalities, uremia, and some medications (e.g., aspirin). Hypertension, fever, trauma, and sepsis may also exacerbate bleeding in the thrombocytopenic patient. Additionally, thrombocytopenia in certain clinical situations (e.g., active bleeding, surgery, trauma, DIC, intracranial malignancies, abnormalities) necessitates more intensive platelet transfusion support and invasive diagnostic procedures or monitoring devices. Furthermore, when the patient has platelet dysfunction secondary to uremia or thrombocytopenia secondary to splenic sequestration, mechanical injury, or immune-mediated platelet destruction, the efficacy of transfused platelets will be markedly diminished. Finally, the decision to administer platelets must be made with an understanding of the attendant risks. Serious and even fatal infection can be transmitted via transfusion therapy, and patients may become sensitized to cellular antigens, forming antibodies that will later interfere with the efficacy of subsequent platelet transfusions.

After all of these data are considered, the following general recommendations are made for platelet

Table 139-1   Alternatives to Platelet Transfusion

Disorder	Therapy
Idiopathic thrombocytopenic purpura	Steroids, IV gamma globulin, splenectomy
Uremia	Desmopressin (DDAVP), cryoprecipitate, RBC transfusions to correct anemia
Epistaxis	Local pressure, nasal packs
Oral mucosal bleeding	Gelfoam, desiccated collagen preparation, topical thrombin, aminocaproic acid

transfusion support. Patients with life-threatening or clinically significant bleeding must be given platelets when thrombocytopenia of any degree or platelet dysfunction exists. Patients without significant bleeding must be given platelets under the following circumstances: (1) before major surgery if the platelet count is <50,000/mm³ or if platelet dysfunction is documented; (2) before arterial catheter placement, lumbar puncture, or minor surgical procedures if the platelet count is <20,000/mm³; (3) with fever or sepsis in a child whose platelet count is <20,000/mm³; and (4) with a platelet count of <5000/mm³ in any child whose abnormal bone marrow is not likely to recover within the next 48 hours. Adjuvant support for thrombocytopenic patients and therapies for those conditions that do not normally respond to platelet transfusions are described in Table 139-1.

Platelet products. One unit of platelets is derived from 1 unit of whole blood. Platelets are usually stored at 20° to 24° C with constant agitation for up to 5 days. Each unit will contain approximately 5.5×10^{10} platelets in a 60 to 70 ml volume. This volume can be decreased if necessary, but the process is time consuming and may interfere with platelet function. Single-donor platelets are those obtained by apheresis from a single donor. The number of platelets obtained in this fashion approximately equals those in 5 to 8 single platelet units. Single-donor platelets are more difficult to obtain and must be used within 24 hours of collection. Their use should be restricted to those patients refractory to random donor platelets or to those undergoing bone marrow transplantation when excessive antigen exposure would be harmful. HLA-matched single-donor platelets are expensive and even more difficult to obtain. They may be beneficial for patient's refractory to nonmatched single-donor platelets.

Platelet dose. One unit of platelets will theoretically increase a child's platelet count by 10,000/mm³. This increment is decreased, however, by a variety of host factors: alloimmunization, infection, or injury to the platelets during procurement, storage, or transfusion. As a general rule a minimum of 2 units of platelets must be ordered for infants, 3 for toddlers, 4 for young children, and 6 to 8 for preadolescents and adolescents. The platelets must be transfused over 30 minutes or as rapidly as volume constraints allow. A standard 170 μm blood filter must be used. Filters with a smaller pore size may filter out the platelets.

Obtaining platelet counts 1 and 24 hours after transfusion may help differentiate alloimmunization (low 1-hour platelet count) from other reasons for increased platelet consumption (1-hour count adequate, 24-hour count low). Single-donor or HLA-matched platelets may be of benefit in the alloimmunized patient, whereas increasing the number of random donor units may benefit the patient with increased platelet consumption secondary to infection or bleeding.

Fresh frozen plasma

FFP is plasma that has been separated from anticoagulated whole blood within 6 hours of donation and rapidly frozen. It is used to replace depleted clotting factors in patients with acquired bleeding disorders such as occur in liver disease or DIC. A dose of 10 to 15 ml/kg is given over 30 minutes to 2 hours every 8 to 12 hours as needed. FFP cannot be used as a source of colloid for volume replacement. Albumin or plasma protein fraction are used for this purpose since these products are less expensive and do not carry the same risk of hepatitis.

FFP must be thawed before administration and must be given within 4 hours of being thawed. No filter is necessary for FFP administration.

Factor concentrates

The use of these products is restricted to the treatment of patients with congenital deficiencies of a clotting factor. Cryoprecipitate, prepared in the blood bank, contains fibrinogen, factor VIII (approximately 75 units of factor VIII per bag), and von Willebrand factor activity. Cryoprecipitate will benefit patients with hemophilia A, von Willebrand's disease, afibrinogenemia, and rarely DIC.

Factor VIII and IX concentrates are commercially produced products containing known amounts of factor activity. Their use is restricted to patients with hemophilia and must be directed by a pediatric hematologist.

TECHNIQUE

Blood products are administered as soon as possible after they are obtained from the blood bank and must be returned to it if they will not be used for several hours to ensure properly controlled refrigeration and decrease the risk of bacterial contamination. A check system must be used to ensure that the patient's name, hospital number, and blood type are correct.

An appropriate blood filter must be used. The woven nylon clot filter (mesh size 170 μm) found in routine blood administration sets allows passage of RBC microaggregates >150 μm in size. Micropore filters (e.g., Intracept [Johnson & Johnson], Bently PFS-127, Fenwall 4C2417, and Ultipore [Pall Corporation]) can eliminate the smaller microaggregates and decrease the likelihood of respiratory distress. A double filter setup must be used for postoperative cardiac patients and for patients in whom massive transfusion is likely. Platelets come from the blood bank with a special administration set because the use of RBC filters may actually filter out the platelets. The filter used with factor VIII and factor IX concentrates is small and contained within the needle provided with the concentrate vial. FFP requires no filter.

The IV line must be flushed with 0.9% sodium chloride solution to avoid hemolysis or agglutination of the RBCs and platelets. Intermittent flushing with small volumes of 0.9% sodium chloride solution or lactated Ringer's solution may be needed to keep IV lines patent. Y tubing can be used to accommodate blood in one arm of the Y and an IV bottle in the other. An alternative method to ensure patency of the vein is to administer blood with a constant infusion pump. The rate of administration must be regulated.

A blood warmer must be used when transfusions are given to small infants or children in whom temperature control is a problem. Transfusions of ≥1 blood volume must also be warmed. Cold blood must never be given through a right atrial catheter since this may cause dysrhythmias.

Blood products opened for more than 6 hours must be considered contaminated and thus discarded. FFP must be given within 4 hours to be efficacious.

During transfusion a neonate must be watched closely for signs of hypoglycemia since he may not have adequate glycogen or glucose stores.

Blood must be administered through as large a needle as possible to avoid hemolysis, particularly at rapid rates of infusion. Access to central circulation is needed for transfusions of ≥ 1 blood volume.

RISKS AND COMPLICATIONS

Transfusion-related problems occurring within minutes to days after blood administration are usually related to fluid overload and transfusion reactions. Hemodynamically stable children will not often tolerate administration of more than 15 to 20 ml/kg of colloid-containing fluid over a few hours unless there is active bleeding. Children with any form of cardiac or pulmonary compromise and those with chronic anemia will often develop signs and symptoms of congestive heart failure, even with volumes of <10 ml/kg over 1 to 2 hours. The child's heart rate, respiratory rate, systemic arterial blood pressure, and clinical condition must be closely monitored. The transfusion must be interrupted and/or diuretics administered if volume overload becomes a problem. Additional risks and complications of excessive transfusions (≥ 1 blood volume) are discussed in Chapter 50.

Immediate transfusion reactions are most often febrile or allergic and are usually not a contraindication to continuing the transfusion. They can include temperature as high as 40° C, urticaria, angioneurotic edema, and rarely bronchospasm. Should they occur, the transfusion must be temporarily discontinued and oral acetaminophen (10 mg/kg) and oral or IV diphenhydramine (1 mg/kg) administered, depending on the severity of the reaction. After the signs and symptoms have abated, the transfusion can be resumed. These children have probably formed antibodies to antigens on transfused WBCs, platelets, or plasma proteins.

Hemolytic transfusion reactions, far less common, can be immediate or delayed (4 to 14 days after the transfusion). These reactions often follow the infusion of mismatched blood, usually resulting from clerical error. Delayed hemolysis is probably secondary to an amnestic response in the host, which

---

DIFFERENTIAL DIAGNOSIS OF HEMOLYSIS*

Destruction of recipient cells

Drugs: Penicillin, quinidine, phenylhydrazine, α-methyldopa
Congenital or acquired hemolytic anemias: G6PD, autoimmune
Infections: Mononucleosis, clostridia, malaria
Hypotonic solutions
Large hematomas
Mechanical trauma: Artificial valves, hemolytic-uremic syndrome, thrombotic thrombocytopenic purpura

Destruction of donor cells

Thermal exposure of transfused cells
Extracorporeal circulation: Cardiopulmonary bypass, dialysis
Blood infected with bacteria
Old RBCs

---

*The most significant potential complication of transfusion therapy is infection.

---

leads to antibody-mediated destruction of donor RBCs. Hemolytic reactions can be life threatening, with the patient presenting with high fever, back and abdominal pain, chills, and the passage of dark urine; jaundice and DIC may follow. The patient may have hemoglobinemia, hemoglobinuria, a positive direct Coombs' test, spherocytes on the peripheral blood smear, and a sudden anemia. Should a hemolytic reaction occur, the transfusion must be stopped immediately and the blood returned to the blood bank with a new sample of the patient's blood for recrossmatching. The child must be vigorously hydrated and given an osmotic diuretic to maintain urinary flow and avoid acute tubular necrosis. Other reasons for hemolysis must also be ruled out.

Bacterial infection. Bacterial contamination of blood products is rare. Should it occur, the recipient will develop overwhelming sepsis with fever and cardiovascular collapse, and even with aggressive therapy, survival is rare.

Posttransfusion hepatitis. This is the most common and potentially most devastating complication of transfusion therapy. Hepatitis B was once the most common type of transfusion-related hepatitis. Currently, with the exclusive use of volunteer blood donors and screening of all donor units for hepatitis B surface antigen, it accounts for <10% of the cases of posttransfusion hepatitis. Non-A, non-B (NANB) hepatitis is now most common, with a generally accepted incidence of approximately 0.5% to 1% per unit transfused. Since the diagnostic criteria for NANB are vague (ALT value ≥2.5 × the upper limit of normal on two or more occasions 1 to 6 months after a blood transfusion) and most patients have a nonicteric, asymptomatic course, it is impossible to determine precisely the risk of NANB. The risk may decrease with the exclusion of donors who have an increased ALT or antibody to the hepatitis B virus core antigen. Once diagnosed, 60% to 70% of the patients with NANB continued to have elevated serum aminotransferase levels for >1 year, with 15% to 25% developing cirrhosis, portal hypertension, and hepatic failure.

Cytomegalovirus. A member of the herpes virus group, CMV usually causes asymptomatic or mild flu-like infections in immunocompetent hosts. It is ubiquitous, with approximately 80% of healthy adults seropositive for CMV antibody. CMV is transmitted by blood and blood products with a wide variety of clinical manifestations seen in susceptible (CMV-negative) patients: hepatitis, a mononucleosis-like illness, and in severely immunocompromised patients, a life-threatening interstitial pneumonia. Neonates and other severely immunocompromised patients must receive CMV-negative blood if possible.

Human immunodeficiency virus infection. The acquisition of the AIDS virus is clearly the most publicized and highly feared risk associated with transfusion therapy. Current blood bank practices, however, have almost eliminated this route of infection with HIV. Using the "worst-case scenario," which assumes a 3% false negative rate with the enzyme-linked immunoabsorbent assay, the risk per unit of transfused blood is approximately 1:40,000.

Directed blood donation. Given the risks associated with transfusion therapy, there has been a great deal of pressure placed on health care systems to develop programs whereby patients will receive blood only from donors that have been selected by the family. Information collected to date suggests that blood drawn from directed donor populations is significantly more likely to transmit infection (hepatitis and HIV) than blood derived from anonymous volunteer blood donors. This is not surprising since volunteer units are most often drawn from repeat donors who are screened several times each year. More important, directed donor programs remove the protection of anonymity from any single donor, making it extremely difficult for a potential donor to answer questionnaires honestly and often prompting an appropriately reticent individual to donate blood.

In contrast, autologous donor programs in which patients serve as donors for themselves before elective surgery are safe, effective, and underused. Any child age 8 or older can be considered for autologous donation.

ADDITIONAL READING

Coffin C. Current issues in transfusion therapy. 2. Indications for use of blood components. Transfusion Ther 81:343-350, 1987.

• Consensus Conference. Platelet transfusion therapy. JAMA 257:1777-1780, 1987.

• Nathan DG, Oski FA, eds. Hematology of Infancy and Children. Philadelphia: WB Saunders, 1987, pp 1580-1598.

Ward J, Holmberg S, Allen J, et al. Transmission of human immunodeficiency virus (HIV) by blood transfusions screened as negative for HIV antibody. N Engl J Med 318:473-478, 1988.

Zuch T. Transfusion-transmitted AIDS reassessed. N Engl J Med 318:511-512, 1988.

140 White Blood Cell Transfusion

Richard L. Wasserman

BACKGROUND AND INDICATIONS

Granulocyte transfusion therapy continues to be a controversial modality. If, however, the key elements of granulocyte physiology are understood and the available data critically examined, the use of granulocyte transfusions in specific situations is both rational and supported. Granulocytes are crucial in the defense against most bacterial and fungal infections. They function by attaching to the surface of a microorganism, ingesting it, and killing it. This interaction at the granulocyte surface triggers a complex series of intracellular events necessary for "cidal" activity. Once sufficiently stimulated, the granulocyte is incapable of being restimulated and loses its functional ability. Contact with any surface can trigger granulocytes in this way. Early studies of WBC transfusion did not appreciate the fragile nature of functional granulocytes, and many studies used granulocytes that had inadvertently been made nonfunctional. Harvesting granulocytes using filtration techniques, storing them for more than 6 hours, and administering them through a filter all inactivate granulocytes. Studies using appropriately collected and promptly administered granulocytes have demonstrated their effectiveness in reducing mortality in the presence of life-threatening infection.

WBC transfusions are indicated for patients with life-threatening infection whose neutrophil defenses are inadequate because of reduced neutrophil numbers or abnormal function.

Neutropenia/Neutrophil Storage Pool Depletion

The most common cause of significant neutropenia is antineoplastic therapy. Patients undergoing chemotherapy for leukemia or a solid tumor often have absolute neutrophil counts $<500/mm^3$ and occasionally have no detectable neutrophils at all. Congenital neutropenia and aplastic anemia are other causes of markedly reduced neutrophil numbers.

The neutrophil storage pool is composed of those elements in the bone marrow responsible for the production of functional neutrophils. At birth the neonate's neutrophil storage pool is considerably smaller than that of an older child and may be rapidly depleted by excessive demand. The neutrophil storage pool depletion occurs in the presence of neonatal sepsis caused by any organism but is a particular feature of group B streptococcal sepsis.

Neutrophil dysfunction. Several inherited disorders of neutrophil dysfunction have been described. The most well known of these is chronic granulomatous disease, which is a deficiency of oxidative metabolism that renders the neutrophil unable to kill certain bacteria and fungi. Staphylococci, *Escherichia coli, Serratia marcescens,* and various fungal species are particular problems. Other less common disorders of granulocyte function in which cell movement, phagocytosis, and killing are defective have also been described.

The decision to use granulocyte transfusion therapy in a particular patient is based on clinical judgment. The clinical settings in which granulocyte transfusion may be an appropriate therapy are listed on p. 973.

TECHNIQUE

It is crucially important to begin mobilizing the blood transfusion service to supply granulocytes as soon as the possibility of giving WBC transfusions is considered. A minimum of 4 to 8 hours is needed to harvest granulocytes and prepare the product for administration. ABO and Rh compatibility are mandatory, but tissue typing is not necessary. A parent or other family member is often the most suitable donor for the first day's transfusion since he or she is usually readily available. A routine type and crossmatch on the child must be sent, and the donor needs to be referred to the transfusion service. It is prudent to recommend that the family recruit several potential donors immediately since a given individual may be unable to be a donor because of incompatibilities or personal health problems.

Neonates usually need a single dose of 0.5 to 1.0×10^9 granulocytes/kg of recipient body weight. Some blood banks are able to harvest this number of granulocytes from a single fresh donation of whole blood using cell separators. Older children need to receive the entire harvest from a routine granulocytopheresis. Except in neonates granulocyte transfusions must be given daily for at least 5 days. The total duration of therapy depends on the nature of the infection and the underlying defect in granulocytes. Some patients with chronic granulomatous disease have received granulocyte transfusions daily for 6 weeks or more. In the more common situation of chemotherapy-induced neutropenia, granulocyte transfusions may be discontinued when the patient's bone marrow recovers. A total neutrophil count >250/mm³ for 2 consecutive days in a patient who is recovering from infection is probably appropriate justification for discontinuing transfusion. Patients with granulocyte functional disorders are often more

---

INDICATIONS FOR WHITE BLOOD CELL TRANSFUSIONS

Neonates (up to 2 months)

Suspected sepsis *plus* an absolute neutrophil count <1500/mm³ *or* an immature/total neutrophil ratio >0.6.

Neutropenia (congenital or secondary)

Absolute neutrophil count <250/mm³ in a patient with culture-proven bacterial or fungal infection *and* an adequate response to 72 hours of broad-spectrum IV antibiotics and amphotericin B.

Neutrophil function disorder

Significant infection (usually involving head and neck, chest, or abdomen) in a patient with a known granulocyte function defect.

---

difficult to assess, and granulocyte transfusions are usually continued until there is clinical evidence of recovery and nonspecific measures of inflammation such as sedimentation rate or C-reactive protein have returned to baseline. It is seldom appropriate to give granulocyte transfusions for fewer than 5 days.

Granulocytes must be administered as soon as possible after harvest because they begin to deteriorate immediately after they leave the donor's body. Under no circumstances should granulocytes >12 hours old be administered. Since granulocytes may be activated by rough treatment, the use of peristaltic pumps or other devices that may fragment the granulocytes must be avoided. The use of syringe pumps is ideal, but in most situations no pump is necessary. The rate of administration must be rapid. Although it is unwise to push a granulocyte transfusion over a few minutes, the granulocytes cannot be allowed to set for long periods of time for the reasons mentioned previously, and 30- to 60-minute infusions are usually well tolerated. If an apparent mild transfusion reaction occurs, the rate of administration may be slowed as needed. Whether the WBC transfusion is stored in a blood bag or a syringe, it needs to be gently mixed every 10 to 15 minutes to prevent the high local concentrations of granulocytes that occur by gravity sedimentation. Mixing can be accomplished by gently squeezing the blood bag or rotating the syringe. Under no circumstances should granulocytes be passed through a filter <160 μm pore size.

RISKS AND COMPLICATIONS

The most predictable risk of granulocyte transfusion is the acquisition of non-A, non-B hepatitis. This risk is related to the total number of transfusions. Given the total unit exposure of the typical granulocyte transfusion recipient, the likelihood of developing non-A, non-B hepatitis is relatively high. The risk of other blood-borne infections is modest with a rather low risk of hepatitis B or immunodeficiency virus infection. Cytomegalovirus infection is transmitted by blood and may be a significant issue for immunocompromised neutropenic patients.

The immediate mild and severe transfusion reaction risks are similar to those for other blood products (see Chapter 139). Because damaged granulocytes release vasoactive mediators, the likelihood of a febrile or vasoactive transfusion reaction is higher with granulocytes than with other blood products;

however, the treatment is the same. Allosensitization (i.e., the production of antibodies against WBC antigens) occurs frequently with prolonged granulocyte transfusion therapy. In general this is not a major problem. Granulocyte transfusion reactions may be minimized by pretreatment with aspirin or acetaminophen, an antihistamine, or steroids.

Patients with significant pulmonary disease, particularly interstitial pneumonia or a widespread fungal pneumonitis, may experience significant deterioration of pulmonary function following granulocyte transfusion because the inflammatory cells localize to the site of the infection and create inflammation while killing the pathogens. This should not be considered a contraindication to granulocyte therapy since patients with that degree of microbial invasion are at high risk for death in the absence of granulocyte transfusion. Early reports of severe pulmonary reactions to the combination of amphotericin B and granulocyte transfusions have been refuted. Patients treated with amphotericin B for lung disease often have severe disease, and granulocyte transfusions have been shown to be no more hazardous than the pneumonia itself. Nevertheless, it is prudent to separate the granulocyte transfusion temporarily from the amphotericin.

ADDITIONAL READING

Christensen RD, Rothstein G, Anstall HB, Bybee B. Granulocyte transfusions in neonates with bacterial infection, neutropenia, and depletion of mature marrow neutrophils. Pediatrics 70:1-6, 1982.

Quie PG. The white cells: Use of granulocyte transfusions. Rev Infect Dis 9:189-193, 1987.

Winston DJ, Winston GH, Gale RP. Therapeutic granulocyte transfusions for documented infections. Ann Intern Med 97:509-515, 1982.

141 Exchange Transfusions

Daniel L. Levin

INDICATIONS

Although exchange transfusions are usually done in newborns for hyperbilirubinemia (see Chapter 73) or polycythemia (see Chapter 38), they are also used occasionally in infants and older children for other reasons. These reasons include removal of endogenous or exogenous toxic substances such as potassium, endotoxin (sepsis), sickle cells (sickle cell CNS crises), and (possibly) immunologic factors (Kawasaki's disease, neonatal myasthenia gravis). In addition exchange transfusion may be used to add components removed or altered by other therapies (e.g., dysfunctional platelets resulting in bleeding in neonates given indomethacin). Older pediatric cardiac patients may have partial exchange transfusions to decrease an excessively high hematocrit level. An exchange transfusion is a major undertaking and must be performed with the utmost of caution.

TECHNIQUE
Personnel

The exchange transfusion team comprises two physicians, one to do the exchange and one to record its progress, and a nurse to observe the patient and provide materials.

Locale

An exchange transfusion must be performed in an ICU or an operating room (in emergencies, in the delivery room) with proper lighting, heating, monitoring devices, and maintenance of sterility.

Route

In the newborn the routes for exchange transfusions, in order of preference, are:
1. Peripheral arterial catheter (out) and peripheral venous catheter or needle (in).
2. Umbilical artery and vein. This route allows isovolumetric exchange with withdrawal from

the artery and infusion into the vein. The tip of the umbilical arterial catheter must be at the level of the fourth lumbar vertebra (just cephalad to the aortic bifurcation), and the tip of the umbilical venous catheter must be cephalad to the diaphragm (in the inferior vena cava or the right atrium) (see Chapters 114 and 115 for placement).
3. Umbilical artery alone.
4. Umbilical vein with the tip of the catheter in the inferior vena cava.
5. Venous catheter introduced into the inferior or superior vena cava in the thoracic cavity via the percutaneous Seldinger technique or a cutdown. This route may be necessary in some infants, especially those with omphalitis.
6. Umbilical vein with the tip of the catheter in the portal system.

In older children the preferred routes are:
1. A systemic arterial catheter (out) and a venous catheter (in) in the superior or inferior vena cava with the catheter tip in the thoracic cavity for an isovolumetric exchange transfusion.
2. A venous catheter in the superior or inferior vena cava with the catheter tip in the thoracic cavity.

Preparation

The patient must be placed in a warm, well-lighted environment. For newborns a radiant warmer is used and all four extremities restrained. Before starting the procedure the patient's stomach contents must be aspirated, and the patient must be placed on a cardiorespiratory monitor and a pulse oximeter. In addition the emergency cart for CPR must be immediately available. The following values must be measured in all patients before the exchange transfusion: Hct and Hb, platelet count, arterial blood gas tensions and pH, heart rate, respiratory rate, serum

Na, K, Cl, and Ca, temperature, blood glucose, systemic arterial blood pressure, and CVP when available.

In newborns with hyperbilirubinemia the following must also be measured before the exchange transfusion: total serum protein, serum bilirubin (total and direct), reticulocyte count, and antibodies (Coombs' test).

In patients undergoing exchange transfusion for endogenous (e.g., ammonia) or exogenous (e.g., carbon monoxide) toxins, the blood level of the toxin must be measured before and after the procedure.

Method

In newborns with hemolytic disease donor blood that is compatible with the mother's blood must be used. For example, if the mother is ORh$^-$ and the infant ORh$^+$, ORh$^-$ blood is used so that antibodies to the Rh-positive factor that remains in the infant after the exchange will not destroy donor cells. The freshest blood possible (preferably <1 day old) must always be used. Although it is difficult to arrange in infants with thrombocytopenia (<100,000/mm^3), it is best to use fresh heparinized blood when available.

First, the blood is warmed to 35° to 37° C using a blood warmer with the appropriate tubing. A Micropore filter is used at the end of the coiled tubing. The donor unit must be agitated intermittently so that the cells do not sink, leaving RBC-poor blood at the end of the exchange. Next, the volume to be exchanged is calculated. Usually a two-volume exchange will remove 83% of the patient's RBCs. If the push-pull method is used, 5 ml is used for infants weighing <2000 g and 10 ml for infants weighing >2000 g. In older children 15 to 25 ml/kg is used.

The exchange must not be completed in <45 to 60 minutes in a vigorous patient and must be performed more slowly in a patient with unstable systemic arterial blood pressure, ventilatory status, or temperature. One milliliter of 10% calcium gluconate is administered for every 100 ml of ACD or CPD (citrated) donor blood when the serum calcium level is low (<7.5 mg/dl or ionized calcium is <4.5 mg/dl) at the beginning of the procedure. It is probably unnecessary to give calcium to infants who have a normal serum calcium level before the exchange transfusion. The patient and the monitor must always be observed for signs of distress. The exchange transfusion must be stopped if the patient's condition is unstable; if the exchange transfusion must proceed, the systemic arterial blood pressure and arterial blood gas tensions and pH must be measured after every 100 ml exchanged.

After the exchange transfusion the patient must be monitored, especially his blood glucose since hypoglycemia is common 20 to 60 minutes after the exchange transfusion if glucose is suddenly withdrawn. IV glucose must be continued until the patient is feeding again. It may be necessary to give new doses of any medications whose serum concentrations are lowered by exchange transfusions (e.g., digitalis, antibiotics, anticonvulsants). If the catheters malfunction, blood should not be forced through them. They are probably clotted, and the application of force will dislodge clots, which can have disastrous results (see Chapters 114 and 115). The catheters must be changed immediately and the exchange transfusion continued thereafter. After the exchange transfusion the following must be measured: heart rate, respiratory rate, temperature, blood glucose, systemic arterial blood pressure, arterial blood gas tensions and pH, Hct and Hb, platelet count, serum Na, K, Cl, and Ca, and the blood level of the substance exchanged (e.g., bilirubin, ammonia); a new sample must be sent for type and crossmatch and determination of blood levels of this substance continued until the postexchange transfusion trend is established.

Important points to consider for partial exchange transfusions are discussed in Chapter 38.

RISKS AND COMPLICATIONS

Patients can become hypotensive, cold, hypoglycemic, hypocalcemic, bradycardic, acidotic, hypoxic, and hypovolemic or hypervolemic during or shortly after an exchange transfusion. The possibility of transfusion reactions and the introduction of infection is always present.

Use of old (more than 4 days) or damaged (hemolyzed due to mechanical or thermal injury) RBCs may introduce a large potassium load into the patient. In small and unstable patients this can result in hyperkalemia and cardiac dysrhythmias terminating in cardiac arrest. In some infants hypernatremia, which is probably caused by excessive sodium in the donor blood, occurs after an exchange transfusion. An increased incidence of intracranial hemorrhage in infants undergoing exchange transfusions has been noted and could be due to the hypertonicity of hypernatremia.

Alternatively, a reproducible decrease in ICP during the withdrawal of blood and an increase in ICP during infusion of blood has been noted; since cerebral blood flow is directly related to systemic arterial blood pressure in infants, these rapid, alternating changes may be etiologically related to the occurrence of intracranial hemorrhage.

There is a possible but debated association between exchange transfusions and the development of necrotizing enterocolitis. When exchange transfusions are performed via the umbilical artery, necrotizing enterocolitis may be caused by emboli to the mesenteric arteries or by decreases in arterial perfusion pressure to the gut with excessively large and/or rapid withdrawal of blood. When exchange transfusions are performed using the umbilical vein with the catheter tip in the portal venous system, necrotizing enterocolitis may be caused by emboli or thrombosis and collapse of veins resulting from excessively large and/or rapid withdrawal of blood.

Aortic perforations and injuries may occur during an exchange transfusion. Exchange transfusion is a major undertaking, and these risks must be carefully considered in the decision to perform the procedure.

ADDITIONAL READING

Adamkin DH. New uses for exchange transfusion. Pediatr Clin North Am 24:599-604, 1977.

Ammann AJ, Wara DW, Dritz S, et al. Acquired immunodeficiency in an infant: Possible transmission by means of blood products. Lancet 30:956-958, 1983.

Aranda JV, Sweet AY. Alterations in blood pressure during exchange transfusion. Arch Dis Child 52:545-548, 1977.

Bada HS, Chua C, Salmon JH, et al. Changes in intracranial pressure during exchange transfusion. J Pediatr 94:129-132, 1979.

Berman B, Krieger A, Naiman JL. A new method for calculating volumes of blood required for partial exchange transfusion. J Pediatr 94:86-89, 1979.

Bjorvatn B, Bjertnaes L, Fadnes HO, et al. Meningococcal septicaemia treated with combined plasmapheresis and leucapheresis or with blood exchange. Br Med J 288:439-441, 1984.

Blanchette VS, Gray E, Hardie MJ, et al. Hyperkalemia after neonatal exchange transfusion: Risk eliminated by washing red cell concentrates. J Pediatr 105:321-324, 1984.

Brunner LS, Suddarth DS, Faries BB. Jaundice in the newborn. In Brunner LS, Suddarth DS, eds. The Lippincott Manual of Nursing Practice. Philadelphia: JB Lippincott, 1974.

Campbell N, Stewart I. Exchange transfusion in ill newborn infants using peripheral arteries and veins. J Pediatr 94:820-822, 1979.

• Charlton V, Phibbs R. Peripheral venous partial exchange transfusions for neonatal polycythemia. Clin Pediatr 22:59-60, 1983.

Chirico G, Gasparoni MC, Rondini G. Exchange transfusion for indomethacin-induced hemorrhagic complication in the neonate. J Pediatr 107:312, 1985.

Doyle PE, Eidelman AI, Lee K, et al. Exchange transfusion and hypernatremia: Possible role in intracranial hemorrhage in very-low-birth-weight infants. J Pediatr 92:548-549, 1978.

Green TP, Ferrara B, Thompson TR. Potassium removal by exchange transfusion. J Pediatr 105:507-509, 1984.

• Gregory GA, Hoffman JIE, Kitterman JA, et al. House officers manual of neonatal intensive care. San Francisco: Section of Neonatology, University of California, 1974, pp 71-75.

Hein HA, Lathrop SS. Partial exchange transfusion in term, polycythemic neonates: Absence of association with severe gastrointestinal injury. Pediatrics 80:75-78, 1987.

Hilliard J, Schreiner RL, Priest J. Hemoperitoneum associated with exchange transfusion through an umbilical arterial catheter. Am J Dis Child 133:216, 1979.

Jayabose S, Sheikh F, Mitra N. Exchange transfusion in the management of CNS crisis in sickle cell disease. Clin Pediatr 22:776-777, 1983.

Kliegman RM, Fanaroff AA. Necrotizing enterocolitis. N Engl J Med 310:1093-1102, 1984.

Malloy MH, Nichols MM. False abdominal aortic aneurysm: An unusual complication of umbilical arterial catheterization for exchange transfusion. J Pediatr 90:235-286, 1977.

Morel E, Bach JF, Briard ML, et al. Anti-acetylcholine receptor antibodies in the amniotic fluid. J Neuroimmunol 6:313-317, 1984.

Netter JC, Fries F, Carriere JP, et al. Exchange transfusion for severe Kawasaki disease. Lancet 1:452, 1984.

Oh W. Neonatal polycythemia and hyperviscosity. Pediatr Clin North Am 33:523-532, 1986.

Setzer ES, Ahmed F, Goldberg RN, et al. Exchange transfusion using washed red blood cells reconstituted with fresh-frozen plasma for treatment of severe hyperkalemia in the neonate. J Pediatr 104:443-446, 1984.

Wasserman RL. Unconventional therapies for neonatal sepsis. Pediatr Infect Dis 2:421-423, 1983.

Wiswell TE, Cornish D. Fresh frozen plasma partial exchange transfusion and necrotizing enterocolitis. Pediatrics 77:786-787, 1986.

142 Therapeutic Plasmapheresis (Plasma Exchange)

Jay D. Cook

BACKGROUND AND INDICATIONS

Abel and associates coined the term "plasmapheresis" in 1914 for a process of "plasma removal with the return of corpuscles." Although the process of plasmapheresis has been available since then, it was not until the 1960s that the process became practical with the use of continuous- and intermittent-flow centrifuges. With the manual method only 1 or 2 units of blood could be processed at a time; thus a total blood volume plasmapheresis would take 6 to 12 hours or more. With modern techniques a total volume plasmapheresis can be done in 1 to 4 hours. The theoretic basis for benefit from plasmapheresis is that the patient's blood contains a nondialyzable substance (e.g., antibody, immune complex, abnormal levels of a metabolite, exogenous toxin, unknown substance), and when it is removed by plasmapheresis, the course of a disease may be favorably affected.

Plasmapheresis, or more commonly "plasma exchange," has been used to treat many clinical conditions. This technology also allows for cytopheresis: leukocytopheresis, lymphocytopheresis, and thrombocytopheresis. In addition, by using specially designed columns, a specific plasma component may be removed and the "cleansed plasma" returned to the patient. These topics will not be discussed here.

In 1985 the AMA Panel on Therapeutic Plasmapheresis made its first assessment of the status of this technology. It divided the indications for apheresis into four groups based on the literature: (1) standard therapy, acceptable but not mandatory; (2) available evidence tends to favor efficacy if conventional therapy tried first; (3) inadequately tested at this time; and (4) no demonstrated value in controlled trials.

In general therapeutic pheresis is reserved for acute crises in patients with autoimmune disorders, autoimmune disorders refractory to conventional therapy, disorders with no other therapy, or acute crises of poisoning. In general it provides a rapid reversal of symptoms, thus stabilizing the patient so that a conventional therapy can be started.

During a therapeutic plasmapheresis 50% to 90% of the offending factor can be removed in a 1- to 4-hour period and the volume replaced with normal plasma, plasma products, inert solutions of electrolytes, or normal human albumin. Besides removing the offending substance, plasmapheresis causes a significant change in body homeostasis, which may become one of the limiting factors of the exchange. Other limiting factors are cost and venous access.

Plasma exchange is expensive: the cost of disposable equipment is $105, replacement fluids $20 to $60 a unit, and the technician's time $9 to $16 an hour. Venous access problems often mean the physician must make a clinical a judgment about the potential benefits of the pheresis vs. the hazards of maintaining a central venous catheter or the repeated trauma of femoral venous catheterization. The clinical decision to use plasma exchange for a child must be based on the balance of benefit vs. the potential untoward reactions and known complications. Two other treatment techniques (pulsed corticosteroids and pulsed gamma globulin) are as effective as plasmapheresis for acute crises in autoimmune disease and are more appropriate for children than pheresis and should be used first. Pulsed corticosteroids have been effective in treating acute graft rejections, acute glomerulonephritis, acute crises in patients with sys-

CONDITIONS PLASMA EXCHANGE HAS BEEN USED TO TREAT

Standard therapy, acceptable but not mandatory

Hyperviscosity syndrome* (older children)

Myasthenia gravis*

Idiopathic or vasculitic rapidly progressive glomerulonephritis*

Goodpasture's syndrome without anuria or pulmonary hemorrhage*

Refsum's disease

Thrombotic thrombocytopenic purpura*

Thyroid storm or thyroid hormone overdose

Overdose of certain drugs* (antilymphocyte globulin)

Severe acute polyneuropathy (Guillain-Barré syndrome)*

Available evidence tends to favor efficacy; conventional therapy tried first

Systemic lupus erythematosus, vasculitis without renal
disease*

Cryoglobulinemia*

Familial hyperlipoproteinemia type IIA*

Organ transplant rejection*

Posttransfusion purpura*

Renal failure with melanoma*

Hemophilia with factor VIIIc factor inhibitors

Cholecystitis with intractable pruritus

Inadequately tested at this time

Progressive systemic sclerosis

Raynaud's phenomenon*

Polymyositis, dermatomyositis*

Psoriatic arthritis

Juvenile rheumatoid arthritis

Chronic polyradiculoneuropathy*

Goodpasture's syndrome with anuria but no pulmonary hemorrhage*

Idiopathic thrombocytopenic purpura*

Pemphigus

Chronic hepatic failure*

Multiple sclerosis* (no demonstrated benefit)

Autoimmune hemolytic anemia*

Aplastic anemia

Cancer*

AIDS

Burn shock*

Other hyperlipidemias*

No demonstrated value in controlled trials

Psoriasis

Rheumatoid arthritis

Amyotrophic lateral sclerosis

*Conditions with which author has had personal experience.

COMPLICATIONS COMMON TO PLASMA EXCHANGE

Allergic reactions

Urticaria

Respiratory

Hemolytic

Febrile

Anaphylactic

Heparin reaction

Technical reactions

IV access

Fluid imbalance

Blood loss

Fever

   Young children on PS 400 machine

Air embolism

Hematoma

Bleeding dyscrasia from heparin (used primarily with
hypercholesterolemia)

Infections

   Immunosuppression

   Poor technique

     Poor skin preparation

     Adding medication or solutions to IV fluid im-
properly (i.e., laminar hood not used)

Metabolic reactions

Citrate toxicity

Electrolyte imbalance

   Acute: self-correcting

   Chronic: Ca, Fe

Chronic protein deficiency

   C4 deficiency

temic lupus erythematosus, and dermatomyositis. Pulsed gamma globulin has been effective in treating idiopathic and thrombotic thrombocytopenic purpura, myasthenia gravis, chronic autoimmune polyneuropathy (chronic Guillain-Barré syndrome), and dermatomyositis.

TECHNIQUE

After deciding that a patient needs pheresis, the physician must decide how frequently the procedures are needed and must ensure the adequacy of venous access.

Before starting pheresis, the plasma volume to be processed, percent of blood volume that will be extracorporeal, and fluid requirements must be calculated so that volume imbalance will not occur.

The volume of plasma to be removed is a compromise between the ideal of removing all the plasma and the practical limits. A one plasma volume pheresis will remove 50% to 60% of the plasma; one and one-half plasma volumes will remove an additional 25% to 30%, whereas a two plasma volume pheresis removes only 5% more. Thus a one and one-half plasma volume exchange is usually selected. To determine the child's plasma volume one needs to know the child's weight and hematocrit value:

$$\text{Plasma vol} = \text{Hct (plasma ml/blood ml)} \times \\ \text{Wt (kg)} \times 80 \text{ (ml blood/kg)}$$

Thus if a child weighs 23.7 kg and has a hematocrit of 43, one plasma volume would equal approximately 815 ml.

$$0.43 \times 23.7 \times 80 = 815.28 \text{ ml}$$

The hematocrit is a fraction; thus the decimal point.

Percent Extracorporeal Volume

Maintaining a constant blood volume and RBC distribution during the procedure is the most important aspect of plasmapheresis in children. Each machine needs blood to prime the system, and this volume is the extracorporeal volume. The volume of blood that can be removed safely from a child to prime the machine is ±10% of the blood volume. Blood volume from infancy until puberty is approximately 80 ml/kg. Thus the calculation for the blood volume is simple:

$$\text{Blood volume} = \text{Body weight} \times 80 \text{ ml/kg}$$

For example, if the patient weighs 23.7 kg, his blood volume is 1896 ml.

$$23.7 \text{ kg} \times 80 \text{ ml/kg} = 1896 \text{ ml}$$

Thus up to 200 ml (10% of 1896 ml) can safely be used to prime the machine. Most children who weigh 40 kg or more can be treated as safely as an adult. If the child weighs <40 kg, he may be given extra fluid by increasing the inflow at the beginning of the procedure and cutting back once he is stable. Children who weigh 15 kg or less can undergo plasma exchange safely and effectively, but depending on the machine used, nonautologous blood may be needed to prime the machine. The cell separator machine used for the procedure must be primed with a mixture of RBCs diluted with either 0.9% sodium chloride solution or fresh frozen plasma (FFP). When the procedure is completed, the blood in the extracorporeal circuit is left in the cell separator. The blood left in the machine is identical in volume to the modified whole blood mixture used in priming (i.e., 10% of the blood volume). This method can aid in correcting a patient's anemia since the priming mixture has a hematocrit of 40% to 45%.

Equipment

One machine has no significant advantage over another for plasmapheresis. The Amico 1, the IBM 2997, the Fenwal CS 3000, and the Fenwal PS 400 have all been used successfully. The first three are continuous flow systems and have the added ability to remove selected cell populations (cytopheresis). The last is a hollow-fiber membrane continuous flow machine that does not have cytopheresis capability. For small children the Fenwal PS 400, which has the smallest extracorporeal volume (i.e., less priming volume), is preferred.

Replacement Fluids

The fluids used for volume replacement in plasmapheresis are normal saline (0.9% sodium chloride solution), plasma protein fraction (PPF), albumin, and FFP.

Normal saline solution is an excellent replacement fluid and alone may be satisfactory for infrequent and/or small exchanges. Since it has no colloid osmotic pressure, it must be used in a ratio of 2:1 or 3:1 (saline solution to plasma removed) with large volume exchanges.

Normal human albumin will maintain the plasma osmotic pressure and does not transmit hepatitis or AIDS. Although albumin replaces the most plentiful blood protein, it does not replace the coagulation factors and other normal plasma proteins; long-term use may lead to specific protein deficiencies. Allergic reactions are not common.

PPF is another commercially available plasma replacement fluid. Since it is a heat-treated product, there is no risk of hepatitis or AIDS. Mild allergic reactions are common, but instances of hypotension are very rare.

FFP would seem to be the ideal replacement fluid since it is relatively cheap and has all the plasma proteins in the correct proportion. However, FFP carries the risk of transfusion-transmitted disease (hepatitis and AIDS); it must be matched for ABO compatibility; transfusion reactions are very common; and it contains extra citrate. Thus, only for thrombotic thrombocytopenic purpura and liver transplants is FFP the replacement fluid of choice because of the need for complete coagulation factors.

Anticoagulants

To prevent blood from clotting in the extracorporeal space, addition of an anticoagulant is necessary. Heparin is not the drug of choice because the whole patient becomes anticoagulated. Anticoagulate citrate dextrose, formula A (ACD-A), is most commonly used. Citrate exerts its anticoagulant effects by binding with ionized calcium, preventing the conversion of prothrombin to thrombin. Since the extracorporeal blood has no calcium reserve, anticoagulation can be achieved with a minute amount of ACD-A; since there is an adequate reserve of calcium in the body, only the extracorporeal volume of blood becomes anticoagulated. However, lowered plasma levels of calcium may result in paresthesias, muscle cramps, and cardiac irregularities. If the patient experiences significant paresthesias, cramps, or significant ECG changes, slowing the reinfusion rate or decreasing the ratio of anticoagulant to whole blood will reverse these side effects. In addition oral or IV calcium replacement (20 mg CaCl/kg, slow IV infusion) during the procedure will help alleviate these adverse effects of ACD-A. For patients with familial hypercholesterolemia, clotting problems with ACD, or previous ACD toxicity, heparin can be used safely. Heparin can be rapidly reversed at the end of the plasmapheresis by the use of protamine.

Vascular Access

Vascular access is an ever-present problem in children undergoing plasmapheresis. The minimal requirements include a 16-gauge catheter for outflow and a 19-gauge inflow catheter. The presence of previous venipunctures in the antecubital area for laboratory studies makes it impossible to insert a 16-gauge needle in either arm. Thus if plasmapheresis is contemplated, early steps must be taken to protect the site of the anticipated venipuncture. In the event of questionable venous access, the judicious use of a large-bore double-lumen central catheter is preferable to repeated trauma and wasted hours trying to start lines, especially if multiple procedures are anticipated.

Whatever access is used, it must give adequate flow to and from the cell separator. Adequate flow is defined as 20 to 60 ml/min depending on the size of the pediatric patient. Without adequate flow rates, clotting problems can, and usually do, occur as well as hemolysis from RBC destruction. The latter occurs because of unnecessary trauma to the RBCs when flow rates are <20 ml/min.

LABORATORY TESTS

Before the first procedure the following laboratory values must be determined: complete blood count, including a quantitative platelet count, PT and PTT, electrolytes, calcium, and total protein. Laboratory work after the plasma exchange must be postponed for 3 to 4 hours since electrolytes and coagulation times may be altered by the procedure for at least this long. Most of these values will return to normal within 4 to 6 hours.

MEDICATIONS

Since plasma exchange may result in a significant decrease in drug levels, the clinician must be aware that additional medications may be needed during the procedure to maintain therapeutic levels. Of particular concern are anticonvulsants, insulin, cardiotonics, vasoactive agents, and certain antibiotics. Medications should be withheld for 1 hour before and during the procedure since many are protein bound and will be removed with the patient's plasma. Some patients, particularly those with seizure disorders, may become symptomatic if medications are withheld; administration of the usual oral doses midway through and at the end of the exchange have provided a more stable course.

Special consideration must be made for giving medication intravenously. In general no medication can be added to infusing blood products since the drug may cause cell damage and lysis and thus hyperkalemia. In general this same policy must be followed for plasmapheresis. No medications can be administered directly into the outflow line, the cell separator, or the inflow lines. If medication must be given to the patient (e.g., diphenhydramine hydrochloride), it must be given via a separate line. The flow rates of the inflow line are fast enough so that slow infusions given through a port distal to the blood's entering the body have not led to any significant hemolysis.

MONITORING

Older children and adolescents can be monitored in the same way as adults; during the procedure pulse rate, systemic arterial blood pressure, temperature, mental status, and respiratory rate are checked every 10 to 15 minutes. Children 5 years or younger, particularly those less than 2 years of age, should undergo plasmapheresis in a PICU, at least for the first procedure. Continuous cardiac, systemic arterial blood pressure, and temperature monitoring must be done; the systemic arterial blood pressure must be monitored every 3 minutes during the procedure. Although it is best for the child's physician to be present at least for the first exchange, it is mandatory for the physician to be present for all plasmaphereses in children weighing 20 kg or less. Alternatively, a designated pheresis physician can be immediately accessible to the plasma exchange technician. Other signs and symptoms to observe are respirations, temperature, color, activity and movement, and (in the older child) mood swings.

RISKS AND COMPLICATIONS

The AMA Panel on Therapeutic Plasmapheresis' list of untoward effects differs slightly from my experience in performing 350 therapeutic plasmaphereses in 42 children in either autoimmune or hyperimmune states (diagnoses ranging from acute polyneuropathy [Guillain-Barré syndrome] to liver transplant rejections). Although hematomas, paresthesias secondary to citrate anticoagulation, and vasovagal reactions are the most common untoward effects, allergic reactions are the most frequent in my experience, comprising >50% of complications in my patients. All these manifestations respond well to diphenhydramine hydrochloride, 0.5 mg/kg IV. Fortunately other allergic reactions have been rare in my experience. The untoward reactions caused by poor technique are discussed below.

Blood loss occurs in either of two settings: (1) inadequate venous access accompanied by extracorporeal clot formation or (2) technical failure of disposable equipment. For a small child this blood loss can be devastating. The prudent use of central venous catheters can remedy the first situation, and the incidence of technical failure is one in every 200 exchanges.

Since the blood circulates for several minutes outside the body at room temperature, the temperature of the returning blood may be below body temperature and may lead to hypothermia. The prudent use of a blood warmer will correct this problem. The Fenwal PS 400, a hollow-fiber filtration machine, does not have a blood warmer attachment, and the hypothermia experienced by patients can be prevented by immersing the return lines in warm water. Air embolism can be fatal, and particular care must be taken to remove any air bubbles. Clinically significant hematomas are minimized by monitoring the inflow and outflow sites carefully.

Bleeding dyscrasia secondary to heparin can be avoided by monitoring the amount of heparin used carefully and reversing it at the end of the pheresis with protamine sulfate; the dose of protamine sulfate depends on the patient's actual clotting before heparinization. The ACT is reversed to the preheparinization level by using protamine. Patients with hypercholesterolemia seem to need more heparin because of increased coagulability.

Since pheresis will reduce the circulating antibodies to approximately 10% for 4 to 6 hours, the patients are very susceptible to infection. *No patient should undergo a therapeutic plasmapheresis if he has any infection.* Other preventable causes of infection resulting from poor technique are poor skin preparation or addition of medication to the pheresis solutions without the use of a laminar hood.

Untoward metabolic effects occur when the amount of citrate needed to prevent coagulation is high, causing paresthesia and cramping. Close monitoring of fluids and calculations of the amount of citrate a patient can handle will prevent this occurrence. The safe blood/citrate ratio for children

<30 kg is 18 ml of whole blood to 1 ml of ACD and 13:1 for children >30 kg.

Although there are significant electrolyte imbalances after pheresis, if fluid calculations are correct, these metabolic imbalances will be corrected within hours. Total protein, calcium, and iron must be monitored in chronic pheresis patients. Often dietary sources of these three elements must be supplemented. In addition to total protein depletion a specific protein deficiency state may occur because specific proteins may selectively not be replaced as quickly as the other blood proteins.

ADDITIONAL READING

Committee on Technical Workshops. Therapeutic Hemapheresis, A Technical Workshop. Washington, D.C.: American Association of Blood Banks, 1980.

Current status of therapeutic plasmapheresis and related techniques: Report of the AMA Panel on Therapeutic Plasmapheresis. JAMA 253:819-825, 1985.

Mac Pherson JL, Kasprisin DO. Therapeutic Hemapheresis, vols 1 and 2. Boca Raton, Fla.: CRC Press, 1985.

Robinson EAE. Potential for plasma exchange in children. Arch Dis Child 57:301-308, 1982.

The Technical Manual of the American Association of Blood Banks, 9th ed. Washington, D.C.: The Association, 1985, chap 2.

143 Pericardiocentesis

Steven R. Leonard · Hisashi Nikaidoh

BACKGROUND AND INDICATIONS

The pericardial space is normally little more than a potential space containing a small amount of serous pericardial fluid for lubrication. Many disease processes can cause pericardial effusions, and accumulation of pericardial fluid may be acute or chronic. In either event compression of cardiac chambers with impaired diastolic filling may result in decreased cardiac output (cardiac tamponade; see Chapter 40). If left untreated, death may ensue.

Pericardiocentesis is a technique for aspirating pericardial fluid for diagnostic or therapeutic purposes. Any pericardial effusion of uncertain etiology must be evaluated by microbiologic and biochemical analyses. Such diagnostic pericardiocenteses rarely must be performed on an emergency basis and can be carried out under well-controlled conditions by an experienced physician. However, cardiac tamponade may often be treated as an emergency to provide hemodynamic stabilization before the effusion can be drained more thoroughly in the operating room.

A significant pericardial effusion can be suspected by history (retrosternal pain that may be improved by leaning forward) and physical examination (dyspnea, tachycardia, pericardial friction rub, jugular venous distention, paradoxic pulse). The chest roentgenogram may demonstrate cardiomegaly with a globular heart shadow, especially when compared to previous roentgenograms. Echocardiography has become the standard for diagnosis. It is a simple, relatively inexpensive test that can be easily done at the bedside. It may provide valuable information about the size and location of the effusion.

TECHNIQUE
Equipment

The following equipment is needed:

Pericardiocentesis equipment

Surgical cap and mask
Sterile gloves
Goggles
Povidone-iodine solution, 10%
Lidocaine without epinephrine, 1%
Sterile drapes
Needles, 25 and 22 gauge
Spinal needle or IV catheter (Angiocath, Jelco) with metal hub, 20 gauge
Sterile ECG lead with alligator clip
ECG machine
Laboratory tubes for culture and chemistry analyses

Procedure

For a diagnostic pericardiocentesis the child may be premedicated with morphine sulfate, 0.1 mg/kg, or with a combination of meperidine, 1 mg/kg, plus promethazine hydrochloride, 0.5 mg/kg, plus chlorpromazine hydrochloride, 0.5 mg/kg. If pericardiocentesis is being performed for cardiac tamponade, premedication is contraindicated; such sedation may cause cardiovascular collapse. If the patient is younger than 6 to 7 years of age or uncooperative and if pericardiocentesis is not an emergency procedure for cardiac tamponade, it is probably safer to perform it in the operating room with the patient under general anesthesia.

The patient must be positioned in either a supine position or with the head of the bed slightly elevated. The ECG machine is attached for continuous monitoring of the limb leads.

The clinician dons cap, mask, and gloves after scrubbing. Goggles may be worn if desired. The patient's skin is widely prepared with povidone-iodine solution, including the anterior chest and upper abdomen. Sterile drapes are placed. Lidocaine is injected with the 25-gauge needle to raise a skin wheal in the notch just to the left of the xiphoid process where the lowest costal cartilage joins the sternum. More local anesthetic is injected into the subcutaneous tissue using the 22-gauge needle.

The sterile alligator clip is attached to the metal hub of the 20-gauge needle for use during aspiration. The other end is attached to the V lead of the ECG machine, and the machine is adjusted to monitor the precordial lead continuously (Fig. 143-1). The 30 ml syringe is attached to the needle, and the needle is inserted through the skin wheal. The needle should be held at a 45-degree angle to the skin surface and directed toward the left midscapular area (Fig. 143-2).

The needle is carefully advanced while constant gentle suction is maintained on the syringe and the ECG monitored. The needle must not be advanced beyond the point at which pericardial fluid is obtained or an injury current is noted on the ECG. If an IV catheter is being used, the external sheath can be advanced further into the pericardial cavity, the inner metal needle removed, and the syringe replaced on the hub of the outer sheath for aspiration of the fluid.

In some cases (e.g., a postoperative effusion, tuberculous effusion, traumatic hemopericardium) a bloody aspirate may be obtained. If the aspirate is bloody, the needle must not be immediately withdrawn. A portion of the fluid should be placed in a glass tube. If the blood clots, it is likely that the needle

CAUSES OF PERICARDIAL EFFUSIONS

Infectious pericarditis
Viral (coxsackie, influenza, mononucleosis)
Pyogenic (especially *Staphylococcus,* pneumococcus, *Haemophilus influenzae*)
Tuberculous

Related to systemic illnesses
Uremia
Rheumatic fever
Collagen vascular diseases
    Rheumatoid arthritis
    Systemic lupus erythematosus
    Scleroderma
Myxedema
Sarcoidosis

Related to cardiac injury
Postmyocardial infarction (Dressler's syndrome)
Postpericardiotomy syndrome

Hemopericardium
Postoperative
Trauma

Drug-induced
Procainamide
Hydralazine

Idiopathic

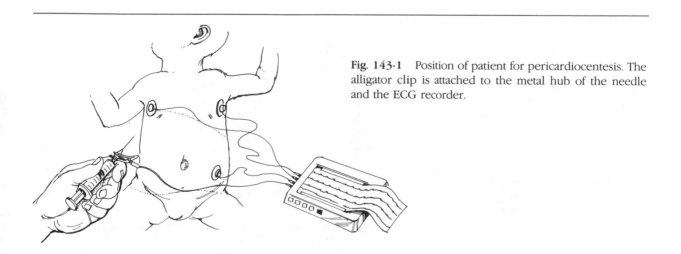

Fig. 143-1   Position of patient for pericardiocentesis. The alligator clip is attached to the metal hub of the needle and the ECG recorder.

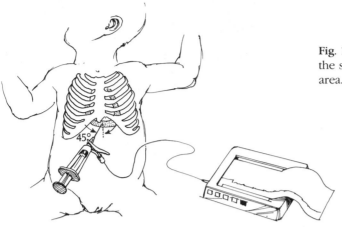

Fig. 143-2   The needle is inserted at a 45-degree angle to the skin surface and directed toward the left midscapular area.

is within a cardiac chamber. At this point it can be withdrawn and the patient monitored closely for signs of cardiac tamponade. If the blood does not clot, the fluid is probably a defibrinated clot within the pericardium, and the appropriate volume of fluid may be aspirated. Additionally, the hematocrit of the aspirated fluid may be compared to that of the patient to help differentiate intracardiac from intrapericardial blood.

If air is aspirated during pericardiocentesis for an effusion, it must be assumed that the pleural space has been entered and a pneumothorax may have resulted. If the patient's condition permits, the pericardiocentesis should be delayed and a chest roentgenogram obtained to rule out pneumothorax. Occasionally pericardiocentesis may be performed for pneumopericardium that has caused cardiac tamponade. In this case the procedure is performed as described above. When air is aspirated through the needle, the external sheath is advanced into the pericardial cavity for aspiration of the air.

Usually pericardiocentesis is done for diagnostic purposes, and it is not necessary to attempt to aspirate "dry" the pericardial cavity. Rather a sufficient volume of fluid can be obtained for the necessary analyses and the procedure terminated. If the pericardiocentesis is being performed for relief of cardiac tamponade, enough fluid should be aspirated to improve the patient's hemodynamic status until more defini-

tive drainage can be performed in the operating room.

If it is likely that continued accumulation of fluid may occur that may cause hemodynamic compromise, a guidewire may be inserted through the needle into the pericardial cavity and a soft pigtail catheter (e.g., Starszel) advanced over the wire. The catheter may then be attached to gravity drainage. Catheter placement must be confirmed with a chest roentgenogram.

RISKS AND COMPLICATIONS

Laceration of the myocardium or coronary artery may result in cardiac tamponade. Coronary artery injury may also result in myocardial infarction.

If the needle is inserted or directed too inferiorly, it may cause intra-abdominal injury, especially to the liver. If the needle is inserted or directed too laterally, it may cause bleeding from the superior epigastric vessels or injury to the lung, with subsequent pneumothorax.

The patient who has had previous cardiac surgery is at increased risk for cardiac injury because the acute margin of the heart will likely be quite adherent to the pericardium.

Attempted diagnostic pericardiocentesis in a young and/or uncooperative child may result in a cardiac injury. Such patients are best treated in the operating room under general anesthesia.

ADDITIONAL READING

Benzing G III, Kaplan S. Purulent pericarditis. Am J Dis Child 106:89, 1963.

Feldman WE. Bacterial etiology and mortality of purulent pericarditis in pediatric patients: Review of 162 cases. Am J Dis Child 133:641, 1979.

Kirsh MM, McIntosh K, Kahn DR, Sloan H. Postpericardiotomy syndromes. Ann Thorac Surg 9:158, 1970.

• Shabetai R, Fowler NO, Guntheroth WG. The hemodynamics of cardiac tamponade and constrictive pericarditis. Am J Cardiol 26:480, 1970.

Soulen RL, Lapayowker MS, Gimenez JL. Echocardiography in the diagnosis of pericardial effusion. Radiology 86:1047, 1966.

• Stewart JR, Gott VL. The use of a Seldinger wire technique for pericardiocentesis following cardiac surgery. Ann Thorac Surg 35:467, 1983.

144 Abdominal Paracentesis

William Dammert

INDICATIONS

Peritoneal tap is being quickly replaced by more sophisticated noninvasive techniques such as sonograms and CT scans. There is, however, still a role for its use in the PICU. The indications are (1) to obtain information in selected cases of ascites, peritonitis, or hemorrhage and (2) to decompress a massively distended (gas or fluid) abdomen that produces respiratory distress secondary to diaphragmatic elevation and restriction of motion.

TECHNIQUE

Position and preparation. With the patient supine, the abdomen is prepared using sterile technique; then a local anesthetic is administered. The sites most preferred are (1) the flank, (2) the anterior axillary line midway between the iliac crest and the rib margin, and (3) the midline 1 to 2 cm below the navel (after the bladder is emptied).

Equipment. A 20- or 22-gauge Intracath, a stopcock, and a syringe are needed for the procedure.

Procedure. The needle is inserted perpendicular to the abdominal wall. Once the needle is in the peritoneal cavity, it is removed and the catheter advanced. If the fluid is being sampled for diagnosis, it is sent for cultures, Gram's stain, cell count, and chemistries as needed. If the fluid is being removed to improve diaphragmatic function and thereby ventilation, an amount titrated to the patient's response is removed.

RISKS AND COMPLICATIONS

Once its tip is inside the abdomen, the needle must not be moved since this can cause organ laceration. Areas with scars from previous procedures must be avoided since there is the potential for organ fixation at the scarred site and therefore for penetration of the organ with the needle.

Vital signs must be monitored during and after the procedure, especially when large volumes of fluid are removed, since there is a potential for systemic arterial hypotension resulting from acute compartment shifts of fluid from the vascular space to the peritoneal cavity.

ADDITIONAL READING

Drapanas T, McDonald J. Peritoneal tap in abdominal trauma. Surgery 100:22, 1960.

145 Peritoneal Dialysis

Steven R. Alexander

BACKGROUND

Peritoneal dialysis was first used to treat children with acute renal failure (ARF) more than 40 years ago. Because of the intrinsic simplicity and safety of the technique and the relative ease with which it can be adapted for use in patients of any age or body size, peritoneal dialysis is still widely considered to be the acute dialytic treatment of choice for pediatric patients. The development of continuous ambulatory peritoneal dialysis (CAPD) in 1976 has resulted in an equally important role for peritoneal dialysis in the maintenance of infants and children who have end-stage renal disease (ESRD). During the last decade CAPD and its mechanized cousin, continuous cycling peritoneal dialysis (CCPD), have become the chronic dialytic modalities of choice in many pediatric ESRD programs in the United States and Canada. Thus, for those involved in the care of critically ill children who suffer from either acute or chronic renal failure, a knowledge of peritoneal dialysis has never been more important than it is today.

History of Peritoneal Dialysis in Children

The peritoneal cavity has been used to treat critically ill pediatric patients for at least 70 years. In 1918 Blackfan and Maxcy described the successful treatment of severely dehydrated infants using intraperitoneal saline solution injections, a technique that is still used in rural areas of some developing countries. The first description of peritoneal dialysis as a potential therapy for uremia is attributed to Ganter, a German physiologist, who in 1923 reported that the intermittent intraperitoneal infusion and drainage of a saline solution resulted in improvement in the condition of guinea pigs made uremic by ureteral ligation. Clinical application of these observations was routinely unsuccessful before 1946 when Fine and associates first described a technique they called con-

tinuous peritoneal lavage. These methods were adopted in 1949 by Swan and Gordon in Denver, who used a system of continuous peritoneal lavage to treat three acutely anuric children, 9 months, 3 years, and 8 years of age. Two rigid operating room suction tips covered by metal sheaths with multiple perforations were surgically implanted, one into the upper abdomen, the other into the pelvis. Large volumes of dialysate (average: 33 L/day) flowed continuously by gravity from 20 L carboys into the peritoneal cavity and were drained by water suction. Dialysate temperature was regulated by varying the number of 60 watt light bulbs in a box placed over the inflow fluid path. The two older children regained normal renal function after 9 and 12 days of therapy; the infant was sustained for 28 days before she succumbed to obscure complications.

During the 1950s the development of disposable nylon catheters and commercially prepared dialysis solutions made intermittent peritoneal dialysis (IPD) a practical short-term treatment for ARF. Successful adaptation of this technique for use in pediatric patients was reported in 1961 and 1962 by groups in Indianapolis and Memphis who also documented the effectiveness of IPD as a treatment for certain poisonings (boric acid and salicylate) common at that time in infants and small children. The use of IPD rapidly gained popularity during the 1960s when this simple technique was refined to such an extent that many of the manual IPD procedures that are used today to treat children with ARF differ little from those used 20 years ago.

Because the manual IPD technique required reinsertion of the dialysis catheter for each treatment, prolonged use of IPD in children with chronic renal failure was unacceptable. By the early 1970s the availability of permanent peritoneal catheters and automated dialysate delivery systems made IPD a reasonable alternative to chronic hemodialysis for children with ESRD. However, enthusiasm for chronic IPD among pediatric nephrologists was never great. Long-term IPD had most of the undesirable features of chronic hemodialysis (e.g., severe dietary restrictions, fluid limitations, prolonged immobility during treatments, complex machinery requiring extensive nursing or parental supervision), yet IPD failed to provide the single great advantage offered by hemodialysis: efficiency. The inherent inefficiency of the peritoneal membrane as a dialysis system mandated a minimum of 40 hours of IPD per week, compared to the 12 hours per week required for maintenance hemodialysis.

A new era in the use of peritoneal dialysis in children was heralded in 1976 when Popovich and Moncrief described what they at first called a "novel portable-wearable equilibrium (peritoneal dialysis) technique," a technique now known as CAPD. The concept was simple yet ingenious. The efficiency of any dialysis method is determined by the flow rates of blood and dialysate, the permeability of the dialysis membrane, the composition of the dialysate, and the time on dialysis. Unable to materially alter peritoneal blood flow rates or membrane permeability characteristics and knowing that automated dialysate delivery systems had achieved maximum dialysate flow rates above which peritoneal solute transfer did not increase, Popovich and Moncrief devised a method (CAPD) that kept the dialysate in contact with the peritoneal membrane essentially 24 hours per day, 7 days per week, thereby maximizing time on dialysis.

CAPD uses a Silastic peritoneal catheter permanently implanted in the abdominal wall to which is attached a disposable plastic bag containing a single dialysis exchange. The dialysate in the bag is infused by gravity flow into the peritoneal cavity, and then the empty bag and transfer tubing are folded and carried in a pocket while the patient goes about normal daily activities, during which time dialysis is also occurring continuously. After 4 to 6 hours the dialysate is drained into the empty bag, and that bag is removed, discarded, and replaced by a bag of fresh dialysate, which is infused to begin the cycle again.

CAPD was first used in a child in 1978 in Toronto. Pediatric nephrologists throughout North America and western Europe soon recognized the potential advantages offered by CAPD to their young patients, perhaps because peritoneal dialysis as a treatment

for ARF was a familiar modality. CAPD combined the simplicity and safety of acute peritoneal dialysis with a number of desirable chronic dialysis features: near steady-state biochemical and fluid control, no dysequilibrium syndrome, minimal dietary restrictions, freedom from painful dialysis needle punctures, improved control of hypertension, and a reduced requirement for blood transfusions. Even more important, CAPD allowed children of all ages to receive dialysis routinely in their homes and thus to have more normal childhoods. Finally, with CAPD it became possible to offer treatment to very young infants with ESRD, a patient group previously considered unsuitable for chronic renal replacement therapy.

Recently the manual CAPD exchange procedure has been replaced for many pediatric patients by CCPD, an automated technique that uses a cycling machine preset to deliver a prescribed volume of dialysate at regular intervals throughout the night as the child sleeps. During the day the child keeps at least a portion of an exchange in place within the peritoneal cavity, thereby maintaining most of the physiologic advantages of continuous peritoneal dialysis. Although either CAPD or CCPD can be used successfully in most children, CCPD offers added convenience for parents and less interference with the child's daily activities. Both of these continuous peritoneal dialysis techniques have made contributions to the modern treatment of children with ARF.

Anatomy and Physiology

The peritoneal cavity functions as a dialysis system when solutes and fluid are exchanged between the peritoneal capillary blood and the dialysis solution that bathes the surface of the peritoneal membrane. The peritoneal membrane is the largest serous membrane of the body. It covers the viscera, forms the visceral mesentery that connects loops of bowel (the visceral peritoneum), and reflects over and covers the inner surface of the abdominal wall (the parietal peritoneum). Because it is continuous, this membrane forms a closed space that normally contains a small amount of serous fluid secreted by the mesothelial cells that line its surface. When additional fluid is instilled, the peritoneal space expands, distending the abdominal wall. Most children can tolerate intraperitoneal volumes of up to 45 ml/kg body weight without discomfort; most adults can comfortably accept 2 L or more of intraperitoneal fluid.

A thin layer of mesothelial cells covers the surface

of the peritoneal membrane, beneath which lies an interstitium containing extracellular fluid, connective tissue fibers, blood vessels, and lymphatics. On the undersurface of the diaphragm the peritoneal membrane is pocked by direct openings to large lymphatic channels (lacunae) through which intraperitoneal fluid is pumped unidirectionally out of the peritoneal cavity during respiration. (This is the route taken by red blood cells when fetal intraperitoneal transfusions were used to treat erythroblastosis fetalis.) Except for this direct route into the lymphatic lacunae, fluid and solute exchange during peritoneal dialysis takes place across the semipermeable peritoneal membrane, driven by the diffusion of solutes whose concentrations in peritoneal capillary blood and dialysate are different (diffusive transport) and by osmosis. When solutes are transferred as a result of osmotic fluid shifts independent of concentration gradients, the process is termed convective transport. In peritoneal dialysis, as in hemodialysis, both diffusive and convective transport are important mechanisms by which the blood is cleared of accumulated solutes.

For a substance to pass from the blood into the peritoneal cavity it must traverse the capillary endothelium, the interstitium, and the mesothelial cell layers. Resistance to the movement of molecules will be encountered at each of these structures and at the mesothelial cell interface with the peritoneal cavity where stagnant fluid films can further restrict mass transfer. The major path for solute and water movement across the endothelium and the mesothelium is thought to be via intercellular gaps, whereas the interstitium is thought to contain channels or pores through which diffusion must take place. The hydration state of the interstitium may influence the rate of mass transfer since fewer interstitial channels are available when the peritoneal membrane becomes dehydrated.

Molecular size, charge, and steric configuration are important determinants of the rates at which substances can overcome the resistance to movement across the peritoneal membrane. Fig. 145-1 shows solute concentration-time profiles for urea, creatinine, inulin, and protein during a typical long-dwell exchange. After 2 hours dialysate urea concentration is nearly 90% equilibrated with plasma. This fact allows ready determination of dialysate urea clearance rates during prolonged-dwell peritoneal dialysis. Peritoneal urea clearance may be calculated using the standard clearance formula:

$$Cu = \frac{Du \times V}{Pu}$$

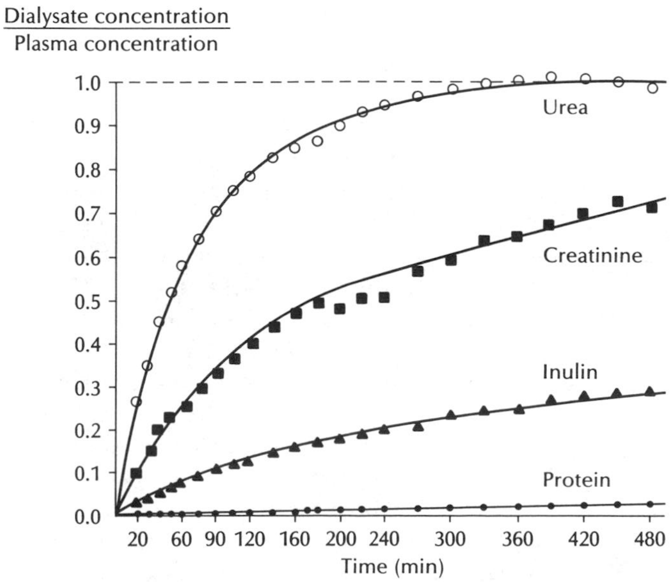

Dialysate concentration
Plasma concentration

Fig. 145-1   Solute concentration-time profiles for a typical prolonged-dwell exchange in CAPD. Note that by 4 hours dialysate urea concentration has fully equilibrated with plasma urea concentration and dialysate creatinine concentration is approximately 60% of plasma creatinine concentration. (Reproduced with permission from Popovich RP, Moncrief JW, Nolph KD, et al. Continuous ambulatory peritoneal dialysis. Ann Intern Med 88:449-456, 1978.)

where Cu is the peritoneal urea clearance rate, Du is dialysate urea concentration, Pu is plasma urea concentration (BUN), and V is the volume of dialysate drained from the patient per unit of time. When exchanges exceed 2 hours in duration, Du and Pu approach equality, and urea clearance becomes simply V, the total dialysate drain volume per unit time. With shorter exchanges, however, clearance can be determined only when the concentrations of urea in blood and drained dialysate are measured directly.

The dialysate creatinine concentration-time profile (Fig. 145-1) may also be used to obtain a rapid (although imprecise) estimate of the small-solute transport capabilities of the peritoneal membrane in an individual patient. If after a 4-hour dwell period the dialysate creatinine concentration has risen to at least 50% of the serum creatinine concentration, small-solute dialysis is likely to be successful in this patient.

Anatomic studies have shown that the surface area of the peritoneum is directly proportional to the body surface area in both children and adults. Thus relative to body mass, the surface area of the child's peritoneum is greater than that of the adult, and this property might be reflected in an increased ability to transfer solutes and water across the peritoneum of younger patients. Not all of the peritoneal membrane participates equally in mass transfer, with major exchange sites thought to be located in mesentery, omentum, intestinal serosa, and parietal peritoneum. The larger total peritoneal surface area of young individuals does not necessarily mean that the *effective* peritoneal surface area is concomitantly increased. Unfortunately there have been few studies of peritoneal mass transfer kinetics in pediatric subjects, and the available data are, for the most part, sparse and inconclusive.

Several clinically important observations in pediatric patients have been confirmed by experimental studies. In peritoneal dialysis the removal of fluid from the blood to the dialysate (a process known as ultrafiltration) occurs primarily because of the greater osmotic pressure exerted by the dialysate as a result of its high dextrose concentration (1.5 to 4.25 g of hydrated dextrose/dl in dialysate vs. 0.1 g glucose/dl of blood). During the course of a dialysis exchange the main osmotic driving force for ultrafiltration is attenuated by the constant diffusion of dextrose out of the dialysate into the blood. The peritoneum of infants and young children allows the passage of dextrose at a more rapid rate than in older children and adults. Ultrafiltration is often difficult in infants when long-dwell exchanges are used, probably because the infant rapidly absorbs dextrose from the dialysate, resulting in a rapid decline in the osmolar gradient between blood and dialysate. Thus higher dialysate dextrose concentrations and shorter dwell times are frequently used in infants to offset this problem. That these maneuvers are neither always necessary nor consistently successful suggests that other factors such as direct lymphatic absorption of dialysate via subdiaphragmatic lacunae may also be important in some infants. Recent studies have suggested that subdiaphragmatic lymphatic absorption of dialysate is greater in children than in adults.

It has also been shown that protein (predominantly albumin) is lost into the dialysate more rapidly in pediatric patients. These losses can average 0.3 g/kg/day or more and may be much greater during episodes of peritonitis. Nutritional support of the child receiving a prolonged course of peritoneal dialysis should take into account the absorption of sufficient dialysate dextrose to provide up to 8 to 10 kcal/kg/day (depending on dialysate dextrose concentration used and exchange rate), along with the loss of 0.3 to 0.5 g of protein/kg/day into the dialysate. It may be helpful in the individual child to measure peritoneal dextrose and protein exchange directly.

INDICATIONS AND CONTRAINDICATIONS

Peritoneal dialysis can be an effective treatment for infants and children suffering from acute or chronic renal failure, from intoxication with certain dialyzable poisons, from severe hypernatremia due to NaCl poisoning, or from one of a small group of congenital metabolic disorders. For children with acute renal failure the choice among the available renal replacement therapies (hemodialysis, peritoneal dialysis, continuous arteriovenous hemofiltration [CAVH], exchange transfusion) must take into account the degree of expertise and experience of the facility, as well as the patient's size and clinical condition. For example, life-threatening degrees of hyperkalemia and acidosis are most rapidly and effectively corrected using hemodialysis, but in some centers peritoneal dialysis may be preferred, especially in smaller patients, because of the speed with which peritoneal dialysis can be instituted in those centers and/or the relative lack of pediatric experience among the hemodialysis nursing staff. Some centers prefer to use exchange transfusion to treat neonates with life-threatening hyperkalemia, perhaps because an exchange transfusion is a familiar procedure that can be accomplished quickly in most newborn ICUs. Hemodynamically unstable patients tolerate hemodialysis poorly; such patients may be more safely treated with peritoneal dialysis or CAVH. Hemodialysis and hemoperfusion (see Chapters 146 and 147) are the preferred therapies for poisonings, but peritoneal dialysis is an acceptable alternative for children too small to receive hemodialysis at the facility in which they are being treated and too unstable for transfer to a pediatric hemodialysis center.

Peritoneal dialysis has emerged as the most effective supportive treatment for infants with congenital hyperammonemic coma caused by a urea cycle defect. Congenital urea cycle enzymopathies are characterized by a reduced capacity to synthesize urea, which leads to accumulation of ammonia and other nitrogenous urea precursors. Severely affected neonates develop vomiting, lethargy, seizures, and coma within the first few days of life. The CNS symptomatology is thought to be largely due to the effects of the elevated blood ammonium concentration. Thus emergency treatment is aimed at rapid and sustained removal of accumulating ammonium.

Hemodialysis is the most efficient method for removal of ammonium, but treatments with hemodialysis must be limited to several hours, whereas endogenous ammonium production in these babies is persistent early in the course of treatment. Peritoneal dialysis can be continued indefinitely, providing time during which the diagnosis of the specific urea cycle defect can be made. Studies have also shown peritoneal dialysis is superior to exchange transfusion in these infants, largely because rebound hyperammonemia, which usually follows either exchange transfusion or hemodialysis, is avoided. Peritoneal dialysis removes 10 times more nitrogen as glutamine, glutamate, and alanine than as ammonium, and this continuous removal of the major precursors of ammonium accounts in part for the success of peritoneal dialysis in this setting.

Peritoneal dialysis has also been useful in the acute management of transient hyperammonemia of the newborn, maple syrup urine disease, proprionic acidemia, and congenital lactic acidosis. Many other serious afflictions of infants and children have been treated in the past with peritoneal dialysis without

much success. They include hyaline membrane disease, hyperbilirubinemia, Reye's syndrome, and hepatic coma.

There are few absolute contraindications to peritoneal dialysis in pediatric patients, most of which result from the absence of an adequate or intact peritoneal cavity. A patient's size or age is not a consideration, the technique having been successfully adapted for use in very premature newborns weighing as little as 500 g. Neonates with omphalocele, diaphragmatic hernia, or gastroschisis cannot be treated with peritoneal dialysis. Recent abdominal surgery is only a relative contraindication as long as there are no draining abdominal wounds. Children with vesicostomies and other urinary diversions, bilateral polycystic kidneys, colostomies, gastrostomies, prune-belly syndrome, and recent bowel surgery have all been successfully treated with peritoneal dialysis in my center and others. I routinely use peritoneal dialysis to treat ARF and severe acute rejection episodes associated with renal transplantation as long as the allograft has been placed in an extraperitoneal location. Extensive intra-abdominal adhesions may prevent successful peritoneal dialysis in some patients. Minor adhesions may be surgically lysed to create a continuous peritoneal cavity, but when many adhesions must be destroyed, the procedure is followed by prolonged intraperitoneal hemorrhage and only minimally effective peritoneal mass transfer once the bleeding finally ceases. The presence of a ventriculoperitoneal shunt in hydrocephalic children and the presence of severe cellulitis of the abdominal wall are additional relative contraindications to peritoneal dialysis in children.

TECHNIQUE
Catheters

Nephrologists have traditionally relied on percutaneously placed "temporary" polyethylene catheters for acute peritoneal dialysis. Recently there has been a trend in many pediatric centers in favor of surgical placement of "permanent" Tenckhoff silicone rubber catheters for acute dialysis. The choice remains somewhat arbitrary, reflecting local practice rather than any systematic comparison of the relative merits of the two quite different approaches to acute peritoneal access.

Surgical placement of a Tenckhoff catheter for ARF has the obvious advantages of assurance of good immediate function and almost indefinite catheter life span. These advantages must be weighed in the individual patient against the risks and delays associated with an operative procedure necessitating the use of general anesthesia. For unstable infants surgical catheter placement at the bedside is accomplished rapidly in most PICUs.

Temporary catheters

The most widely used percutaneous catheter is the Trocath (Quinton Instruments, Seattle, Wash.), which comes in adult and pediatric sizes. For small infants weighing <2.5 kg, a standard 14-gauge polyethylene IV catheter may be used, although the pediatric Trocath has been used successfully in infants weighing as little as 800 g. For these tiny babies the fenestrated distal segment of the Trocath is trimmed to a length of only 2 cm to ensure that all fenestrations remain within the peritoneal cavity after insertion.

I have recently had good luck in several infants weighing <1000 g using the Starzl "pigtail" catheter (Starzl Chest Drainage Set; Cook Instrument Co., Bloomington, Ind.) designed for continuous gravity drainage of pleural effusions. This 5 F catheter ends in a small curl, the inner side of which has multiple perforations. The infant's peritoneal cavity is first filled with fluid using a 23-gauge steel needle. With the use of a modification of the Seldinger technique, a guidewire is inserted at a shallow angle through an entry point that is at the level of and 2 to 3 cm lateral to the umbilicus. The pigtail catheter is straightened as it is passed over the guidewire into the peritoneal cavity, where it resumes its curled configuration as the guidewire is withdrawn. Thus the catheter's curl is allowed to come to rest in the midline, anterior to the abdominal contents and flat against the underside of the anterior abdominal wall. During placement the catheter can be easily palpated through the thin abdominal wall of these tiny babies. To function well the curl must remain superficial, avoiding entanglement in loops of bowel. Although my smallest patient successfully treated with the pigtail catheter weighed only 450 g, more experience with this device will be necessary before it can be recommended over the 14-gauge IV catheters used for peritoneal access in such babies in the past.

Percutaneous temporary catheter placement technique. Percutaneous placement of a temporary peritoneal catheter in a pediatric patient is a simple procedure. However, great care and attention to detail must be exercised, for it is, after all, a technique requiring the forceful penetration of the abdomen with a sharpened steel rod. The incidence of intraperitoneal hemorrhage at the time of percutaneous catheter insertion has been reported to be as high as 5% in pediatric patients. The following guidelines are applicable to most pediatric and adult patients.

1. The bladder must be emptied with a straight urinary catheter, which is removed after successful placement of the peritoneal catheter to reduce the risk of urinary tract infection.

2. Adequate sedation of older infants and children is necessary. Adults may be instructed to perform the Valsalva maneuver at the moment of trocar insertion, but rarely are children able to cooperate to this degree. Children old enough to describe it remember percutaneous catheter placement while they were under local anesthesia alone as a terrifying and painful experience. In conscious children standard doses of meperidine and hydroxyzine hydrochloride are used for preoperative sedation. Good sedation may increase the intraperitoneal priming volume needed to safely perforate the now-relaxed child's peritoneum. Careful attention must be given to cardiorespiratory status throughout the procedure to prevent respiratory embarrassment caused by a large priming volume. In a PICU setting continuous heart rate and blood pressure monitoring and oximetry are appropriate.

3. The skin of the lower abdomen is scrubbed with a surgical skin cleaner such as chlorhexidine, followed by the application of an appropriate antiseptic such as povidone-iodine.

4. A local anesthetic is injected at a point in the midline that is two thirds of the distance up from the symphysis to the umbilicus.

5. Using good sterile techniques (with gown, mask, gloves) the clinician selects a 16-gauge polyethylene over-the-needle catheter (e.g., Intracath; Deseret Medical, Inc., Sandy, Utah) for infusion of dialysate to distend the abdomen. Smaller steel needles (18 to 21 gauge) may be used without polyethylene catheters, but inflow is slower and subcutaneous infusion may be unrecognized for some time. The Intracath is first attached to the dialysate inflow line and inserted below the skin surface; an assistant then opens the clamp on the inflow line. If the drip chamber in the inflow line is watched, dialysate can be seen to pass drop by drop into the subcutaneous tissue. The Intracath is next advanced until a steady stream of dialysate is observed in the drip chamber,

demonstrating free flow of dialysate into the peritoneal cavity. The Intracath is then advanced a bit farther, the inflow line momentarily detached while the steel needle is withdrawn, the line reattached, and the remaining plastic catheter advanced until it is well within the peritoneal cavity. At least 30 ml/kg of *warmed* dialysate is infused while close attention is given to the vital signs of the child. Neonates may need additional ventilatory and/or circulatory support at this stage. When adequately filled, the abdomen will be fully distended and the abdominal wall taut enough to provide firm resistance to insertion of the dialysis catheter and trocar. A priming volume of up to 50 ml/kg may be needed, with the usual limit in each case determined by the point at which respiratory fluctuations in the inflow stream become apparent.

6. After the catheter is removed, a small stab wound is made with a No. 11 blade at the site of the puncture, taking care not to enter the peritoneum.

7. The dialysis catheter is trimmed if necessary for smaller infants. The ideal intraperitoneal catheter length is 1 cm less than the distance from xiphoid to umbilicus; this length ensures that the first fenestrations will remain at least 3 cm inside the peritoneal cavity. Generally, short catheters perform better than long ones. The cut edges of the catheter must be beveled with iris scissors.

8. The dialysis catheter and trocar are inserted using steady pressure and a rotating motion directed at right angles to the plane of the abdominal wall at the insertion site. Considerable force may be needed to puncture the peritoneum; if the abdominal wall can be depressed substantially without penetrating the peritoneum, additional distending fluid is needed. Once the peritoneum has been penetrated, the trocar and catheter are directed toward the right or left lower quadrant, and the catheter is advanced as the trocar is withdrawn.

9. When good in-and-out flow of dialysate has been demonstrated, the extra-abdominal portion of the catheter is trimmed so that only 4 to 6 cm extends above the abdominal wall. The catheter is secured with a silk purse-string suture and water-resistant tape.

10. Should the initial in-and-out exchanges yield cloudy or persistently bloody returned fluid or result in the appearance of diarrhea or polyuria (the high dextrose concentration of dialysate quickly resolves any question about the origin of the diarrhea or poly-

uria), the catheter must be removed and replaced, either percutaneously or surgically. Poor catheter drainage is a much more frequently encountered problem at this stage and is usually due to omental envelopment or obstruction of the temporary catheter. When poor drainage occurs it is probably best to replace the temporary catheter with a surgically placed chronic catheter.

11. Initial exchange volumes are usually 20 to 30 ml/kg, with a gradual increase to 40 to 50 ml/kg over the first 24 hours of dialysis when a percutaneously placed catheter is used. When surgically placed catheters are used, a smaller exchange volume (15 to 20 ml/kg) is necessary during the initial 24 hours of dialysis to reduce the likelihood of dialysate leakage at the insertion site (see below).

Permanent peritoneal catheters

Most of the permanent peritoneal catheters used in children are made of Silastic rubber to which has been bonded at least one circumferential "cuff" made of Dacron felt, which is used to fix the catheter in the subcutaneous tissue. The two most popular designs for chronic use are the Tenckhoff (either straight or curled) and the Toronto Western Hospital. Both are available in an assortment of sizes from several manufacturers. No clearly superior pediatric catheter design has emerged, and controversy continues over the relative advantages of using one or two cuffs, the optimum length of the subcutaneous tunnel, and the choice of surgical placement procedures.

Any permanent catheter may be used to treat either acute or chronic renal failure, although most surgeons prefer to minimize the scope of the operation in the acute setting and therefore prefer to place either straight or curled single-cuff Tenckhoff catheters for acute dialysis. These catheters are also easiest to remove, although their removal requires a second (although minor) surgical procedure.

Surgical technique. Successful catheter placement is probably more a function of the level of experience and commitment of the surgical team than the choice of catheter design or placement technique. The catheter placement procedure described below was developed at The Oregon Health Sciences University by Edward S. Tank, M.D., in collaboration with the author; the procedure is depicted in Fig. 145-2. A modified adult size, curled, one-cuff Tenckhoff catheter is used in all children weighing >5 kg. By special

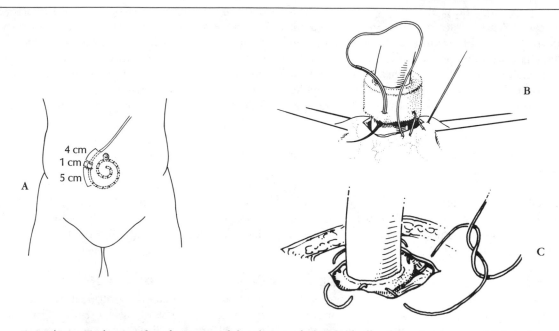

Fig. 145-2 Technique for placement of the short-curled Tenckhoff catheter in a young child. **A,** A 4 cm subcutaneous tunnel is shown directed medially. The 1 cm cuff is depicted sutured at the point of entry into the peritoneal cavity. Catheter fenestrations begin 5 cm below the cuff as the catheter begins to curl. **B,** Attachment of the base of the cuff to the peritoneal membrane with a nonabsorbable purse-string suture. **C,** Closure of the anterior rectus sheath, incorporating the top of the cuff in another purse-string suture. (From Alexander SR, Tank ES, Corneil AT. Five years' experience with CAPD/CCPD catheters in infants and children. In Fine RN, Sclearer K, Mebls O, eds. CAPD in Children. Heidelberg: Springer-Verlag, 1985, pp 179-190.)

request the cuff is glued by the manufacturer (Quinton Instrument Company, Seattle, Wash.) at a point 5 cm above the first fenestrations in the curl (Fig. 145-2, *A*). This short cuff-to-fenestration distance results in a catheter that begins curling almost immediately on entry into the peritoneal cavity and that cannot migrate.

The catheter entry site and the course of the subcutaneous tunnel are chosen preoperatively, avoiding old surgical scars when possible. Children with vesicostomies or colostomies may need long subcutaneous tunnels to locate the exit site as far from the stoma as possible.

The operative procedure begins with a 2 to 4 cm incision made horizontally over the midportion of the rectus muscle near the level of the umbilicus. The anterior rectus sheath is incised and the rectus muscle separated bluntly. The peritoneum is exposed, fixed by two temporary sutures, and then incised. Digital examination assures that no bowel is adherent to the peritoneum at the entry site. If omentum is found to lie below the incision, the small patch of omental tissue that is readily available through the incision is carefully ligated and excised, thus clearing a path for the catheter. This "porthole" omentectomy may not be necessary in many infants and smaller children.

The short, curled catheter is soaked in saline solution to wet the Dacron cuff and then is threaded over a lubricated catheter guide, which straightens the curl. Care is taken to notice the direction in which the catheter will begin to curl when it is pushed off the guide. Catheter and guide are introduced through the incision, and the tip is passed just beneath the anterior abdominal wall to a point in the midline several centimeters below the umbilicus. While the guide is held in position, the catheter is gently eased off the guide and into the peritoneal cavity until the cuff reaches the level of the peritoneal incision. As the catheter slides off the guide, it will resume the curled configuration. Care must be taken to ensure that the curl lies flat beneath the abdominal wall in a plane that is anterior to the abdominal contents. When the curl is otherwise directed, it can become entangled with omentum or loops of bowel as it slides off the guide.

The peritoneum is closed around the catheter with a purse-string of nonabsorbable suture. The suture may be passed through the substance of the base of the cuff in several places (Fig. 145-2, *B*). When secured, this suture pulls a collar of peritoneum around the base of the cuff, creating a nearly watertight seal and anchoring the catheter in position. In infants and other patients with little subcutaneous tissue, a similar purse-string suture may be used to close the anterior rectus sheath and fix it to the upper aspect of the cuff as shown in Fig. 145-2, *C*.

At this point approximately 15 ml/kg of dialysate or 0.9% sodium chloride solution is infused and drained immediately. If the closure is watertight and dialysate flows briskly out of the peritoneal cavity, the catheter is believed to be in good functional position. If outflow is not brisk, the catheter must be removed and repositioned. Catheters that drain poorly in the operating room never improve with use and must be revised.

A short subcutaneous tunnel is created next, with care taken to make a skin aperture that is small and fits snugly around the catheter. A 4 mm skin biopsy punch will create an ideal skin exit aperture. The direction of the tunnel may be toward or away from the midline.

Specialized Dialysis Equipment

Most of the peritoneal dialysis equipment used to treat children is readily available. The automated cyclers designed for pediatric CCPD that provide exchange volumes as small as 100 ml have become standard equipment in children's hospitals with active dialysis programs. These cyclers can be cumbersome in the PICU setting in which space at the bedside is often severely limited. However, a cycler will save a PICU nurse as much as 5 to 10 minutes per exchange in comparison to a manual peritoneal dialysis system. When the cycler is also maintained by the dialysis program nursing staff, the PICU nurse

need only be trained to respond to the cycler's simple alarms in the same way that parents are taught to troubleshoot these user-friendly machines in the home.

Manual peritoneal dialysis systems are still frequently used in most newborn and pediatric ICUs. When the exchange volume is small, placement of a volumetric measuring device (e.g., Volutrol, Buretrol) in the infusion circuit facilitates monitoring of delivered dialysate volumes. Drained volumes may be measured in several ways. When the expected volume is <120 ml, a second Volutrol is placed in the outflow circuit for direct measurement of drained volumes. In this arrangement the dialysate drain line is attached to a 14-gauge needle that perforates the medicine port on the top of the outflow Volutrol, which is taped upright to the side of the infant's warmer near the floor. For patients with larger drain volumes the dialysate drain line can be attached to a large waste dialysate bag, which is placed on an infant scale. The increase in weight of the waste bag after each exchange represents that exchange's drained volume (assuming 1 g equals 1 ml). The measuring device used with urinary catheters may also be modified to serve as the peritoneal dialysate outflow receptacle. In all of these systems the patient must be approximately 36 inches above the drained dialysate receptacle. Shorter outflow fluid paths may not generate sufficient negative pressure to ensure complete drainage of the peritoneal cavity.

Standard peritoneal dialysis Y-tubing used in adults may be used in most children as long as a volumetric measuring device is placed in the inflow circuit to measure delivered volumes. For infants whose exchange volumes are <200 ml, adult Y-tubing sets have too much dead space. In this situation a peritoneal dialysis circuit can be patched together using IV extension tubing and a three-way stopcock. A complete and disposable peritoneal dialysis tubing circuit designed for use in infants is now available (Gesco Dialy-nate Set; Gesco International, San Antonio, Tex.).

There is also a manual system known as the "octopus" for children whose exchange volumes match the volumes in the commercially available CAPD dialysate bags (i.e. 250, 500, 750, 1000, 1500, 2000 ml). The octopus consists of a multiple-pronged manifold and tubing set used for cycler dialysis. Five-prong and 12-prong sets are available. Each day the dialysis nurse attaches all of that day's exchange bags in a single procedure, leaving the fresh dialysate bags hanging from an IV pole at the bedside. Individual exchanges are then performed by the PICU or floor nurse, who simply opens and closes clamps on the tubing leading first from the patient to an empty drain bag, then from a fresh dialysate bag to the patient. Entry into the system fluid path is thus restricted to the dialysis nursing staff. The octopus system may be of benefit when PICU and floor nursing staffs are unfamiliar with the CAPD exchange procedure and automated cyclers are unavailable.

Dialysate must always be warmed to body temperature before it is infused. Adults may only complain of discomfort during the inflow of dialysate that is at room temperature, but in the infant cool dialysate rapidly lowers core body temperature and can result in an acute hypotensive episode. Dialysate may be warmed with water-filled heating pads wrapped around the bag of fresh dialysate or with blood-transfusion warming coils placed in the inflow circuit. Microwave heating may be used to warm single-exchange bags but is impractical when more than one exchange is to be drawn from the same bag and risks severe thermal injury to the peritoneum if not done with great care.

Choice of Dialysate

Dialysate is available from a growing number of manufacturers in three standard dextrose concentrations: 1.5, 2.5, and 4.25 g/dl. Since the dialysate dextrose concentration is the most important determinant of the rate of ultrafiltration, the choice of 1.5%, 2.5%, or 4.25% dialysate will be determined by clinical con-

siderations such as the fluid status of the patient and the residual urinary output. Acute dialysis is begun with the 2.5% solution to obtain better ultrafiltration at the outset when fluid overload is common and the patient is relatively hypertonic as a result of a high BUN concentration. Some infants with renal failure secondary to obstructive uropathy or congenital dysplasia will have large residual urinary outputs and must be treated with 1.5% solution to avoid dehydration. The 1.5% solution may also provide adequate ultrafiltration in some oliguric adolescents whose peritoneal membranes function more like those of adults, for whom 1.5% solutions is standard. However, the majority of acutely oliguric pediatric patients will need 2.5% solutions to remove enough fluid to allow room for adequate nutrition (IV or PO), transfusions, and other therapies. The most hypertonic dialysate (4.25%) is reserved for patients who are severely fluid overloaded or who have demonstrated problems with ultrafiltration. Hyperglycemia, hypotension, hypernatremia, and hyponatremia are common complications when 4.25% solutions are used for more than a few exchanges, especially in small infants.

Most commercially available dialysate contains 132 mEq/L of sodium, along with calcium and magnesium as additional cations and chloride and lactate as anions. Early observations of stable pediatric CAPD patients suggested that prolonged use of dialysate containing only 35 mEq/L of lactate resulted in subnormal serum bicarbonate levels. Thus most pediatric nephrologists prefer dialysate that contains at least 45 mEq/L of lactate for chronic use. Older for-

Table 145-1   Peritoneal Dialysis Solution Containing Bicarbonate*

	ml	Na+ (mEq)	Cl- (mEq)	Mg++ (mEq)	SO4= (mEq)	HCO3- (mEq)	Hydrous Dextrose (g)
NaCl (0.45%)	896.0	69	69				
NaCl (2.5 mEq/ml)	12.0	30	30				
NaHCO3 (1.0 mEq/ml)	40.0	40				40	
MgSO4 (10%)	1.8			1.5	1.5		
D50W	50.0						25
	999.8	139	99	1.5	1.5	40	25

Calculated osmolality = 423 mOsm/kg H2O.
*Modified from Nash MA, Russo JC. Neonatal lactic acidosis and renal failure: The role of peritoneal dialysis. J Pediatr 91:101-105, 1977.

mulations that contained higher concentrations of sodium and in which acetate was used as the buffer are no longer recommended.

Some critically ill infants are unable to tolerate the lactate that is absorbed from commercial dialysis solutions. Such babies are often hypoxic and hypotensive, and they usually have an ongoing metabolic acidosis in part due to accumulation of endogenous lactic acid. These babies may be treated with a dialysate that has been reformulated to contain bicarbonate in place of lactate. A typical bicarbonate-containing dialysate formula is shown in Table 145-1. Note that calcium must be given intravenously when bicarbonate-containing dialysate is used. It is also wise to measure the sodium content of each new batch of these "homemade" dialysates before they are put into use; errors in formulation can lead to the rapid development of serious degrees of either hyponatremia or hypernatremia.

Dialysate additives

Heparin. Heparin sulfate at a concentration of 500 units/L is routinely added to peritoneal dialysate during the initial 24 hours following catheter placement (either surgical or percutaneous) and during episodes of peritonitis. Addition of heparin to prevent the formation of thick fibrin strands clearly visible in the drained dialysate occasionally will be needed on a routine basis. In vitro studies have shown that higher doses of heparin are no more effective in preventing fibrin formation. The 500 units/L heparin dose has not been found to cause systemic heparinization.

Antibiotics. Many parenteral antibiotics may be added directly to dialysate, as shown in Table 145-2 and discussed in the section "Peritonitis." A first-generation cephalosporin (e.g., cephalothin [Keflin], 250 mg/L) is routinely added as prophylaxis during the first 24 hours following catheter placement. Further prophylactic antibiotic use is not recommended. In general the intraperitoneal route must not be used to deliver antibiotics to a patient with serious infection (other than peritonitis) unless adequate absorption can be confirmed by following antibiotic blood levels.

Potassium. Children receiving protracted courses of peritoneal dialysis for ARF may become hypokalemic because of the severe restrictions on potassium intake during initial stabilization and the steady removal of potassium by dialysis. When the serum po-

tassium concentration falls below 4.0 mEq/L, KCl may be added to the dialysate at the desired serum concentration (i.e., 4 mEq/L). Although this is not effective therapy for hypokalemia, it minimizes further peritoneal losses of potassium. Higher dialysate potassium concentrations (e.g., 20 mEq/L) have been found to cause pain and may cause sclerosis of the peritoneal membrane.

Amino acids. Parenteral amino acid preparations may be added to dialysate as a nutritional supplement. Depending on the preparation used, a child will absorb up to 85% of the amino acids delivered in dialysate when a concentration of 1 g amino acids/dl of dialysate is used. Sodium lactate must also be added to counter the dilutional effects of the amino acid solution volume on the dialysate sodium and lactate concentrations. Additional dextrose is not needed since the amino acids exert a potent osmotic effect. Intraperitoneal amino acids may be used to supplement IV TPN regimens when ultrafiltration is insufficient to allow adequate IV TPN volumes. The use of intraperitoneal amino acids in children with ARF has not been carefully studied. An amino acid preparation that contains only the essential amino acids (plus histidine) should be used when the BUN is >50 mg/dl.

Bicarbonate. With a properly placed catheter and in the absence of peritonitis, peritoneal dialysis should be a painless procedure. Rarely a patient will be especially sensitive to the highly acidic dialysate solutions. The addition of sodium bicarbonate, 10 mEq to each liter of dialysate, may be helpful.

Peritoneal Dialysis Prescription

The initial peritoneal dialysis prescription for the child with ARF must reflect the clinical status of the child and the immediate goals of dialytic therapy. In the severely uremic child frequent exchanges are often needed for the first 24 to 48 hours to remove accumulated solutes and excess fluid and to correct acidosis and hypertension. The treatment is begun with 2.5% dextrose solutions containing heparin and a first-generation cephalosporin.

Exchange volumes used in children routinely range from 35 to 45 ml/kg, although smaller volumes (e.g., 15 to 20 ml/kg) must be used during the initial 24 to 48 hours after surgical catheter placement to reduce the risk of dialysate leakage. In the most acute situation the prescribed exchange volume is infused over 5 minutes, allowed to dwell for 15 to 20 minutes,

Table 145-2 Antibiotic Dosing Guidelines for the Treatment of Peritonitis in Pediatric Patients Receiving Continuous Peritoneal Dialysis*

| | Half-Life (H) | | | Dose‡ | | |
| | | | | Initial | | Maintenance |
	Normal	ESRD	CAPD	mg/kg	mg/L of Dialysate	mg/L of Dialysate
Aminoglycosides						
Amikacin†	1.6	39	ND	5.0-7.5 IV/IP	—	6-7.5
Gentamicin†	2.2	53	32	1.5-1.7 IV/IP	—	4-6
Netilmicin†	2.1	42	ND	1.5-2.0 IV/IP	—	4-6
Tobramycin†	2.5	58	36	1.5-1.7 IV/IP	—	4-6
Cephalosporins						
Cefamandole	1.0	10	8.0	—	500	ND
Cefazolin	2.2	28	27	—	250-500	125-250
Cefoperazone	1.8	2.3	2.2	—	1000	500
Cefotaxime	0.9	2.5	2.4	—	1000	250
Cefoxitin	0.8	20	15	—	500	100
Ceftazidime	1.8	26	16	—	500	125
Ceftizoxime	1.6	28	11	—	500	125
Ceftriaxone	8.0	15	13	—	500	ND
Cefuroxime	1.3	18	15	—	750	250
Cephalothin	0.2	3.7	ND	—	1000	250
Moxalactam	2.2	20	16	—	500	ND
Cephradine	0.9	12	ND	—	250	125-250
Cephalexin	0.8	19	9	12.5 PO	—	12.5 mg/kg/dose q 8 hr PO
Penicillins						
Ampicillin	1.2	15	ND	—	250	50
Azlocillin	0.9	5.1	ND	—	250	250
Ticarcillin	1.2	15	ND	75 IV	—	75 mg/kg/dose q 12 hr IV

ESRD = creatinine clearance <10 ml/min/1.73 m², patient not on dialysis; NA = not applicable; ND = no data; IV = intravenous; PO = oral; IP = intraperitoneal.
*Modified for pediatric patients from recommendations in Keane WF, Everett ED, Fine RN, et al. CAPD-related peritonitis management and antibiotic therapy recommendations. Peritoneal Dial Bull 7:55-68, 1987.
†Monitoring by frequent serum drug levels recommended.
‡The route of administration is intraperitoneal unless otherwise stated.
These data should only be used as initial guidelines. Individualized dosing is recommended when possible. Initial IP doses are based on a 2- to 4-hour dwell, single exchange.
The pharmacokinetic data and dosing recommendations presented here are based on published lierature reviewed through January 1987 and personal experience. Those dosage recommendations that differ from product labeling are based on more recent experience. There is no evidence that mixing different antibiotics in dialysis fluid (except for aminoglycosides and penicillins) is deleterious for the drugs or patients. Do not use the same syringe to mix antibiotics.

Table 145-2 Antibiotic Dosing Guidelines for the Treatment of Peritonitis in Pediatric Patients Receiving Continuous Peritoneal Dialysis—cont'd

| | Half-Life (H) | | | Dose | | |
| | | | | Initial | | Maintenance |
	Normal	ESRD	CAPD	mg/kg	mg/L of Dialysate	mg/L of Dialysate
Vancomycin and others						
Vancomycin†	6.9	161	83	15 IP/IV	—	25.30
Clindamycin	2.8	2.8	ND	—	150	150
Erythromycin	2.1	4.0	ND	—	150	75
Metronidazole	7.9	7.7	11	7.5 PO/IV	—	ND
Rifampin	4	8	ND	10 PO	—	5-10 mg/kg/dose q 12 hr PO
Trimethoprim/sulfamethoxazole	14/10	33/13	34/14	4/20 PO/IP	—	20-40/100-200
Antifungal						
Amphotericin B	360	360	ND	0.25 IV	—	0.5-1.0 mg/kg/dose q 24 hr IV
Flucytosine†	4.2	115	ND	12.5 PO/IP	—	12.5 mg/kg/dose q 12 hr PO *or* 50-100 mg/L IP
Ketoconazole	2	1.8	2.4	2-5 PO	—	2-5 mg/kg/dose q 12 hr PO
Miconazole	24	25	ND	—	50	50

and drained for 5 to 10 minutes. More than two complete exchanges per hour are technically feasible but are rarely worthwhile since with higher exchange rates a greater portion of each hour becomes devoted to filling and draining the peritoneal cavity.

Once the child has been stabilized, if a permanent catheter is in place, peritoneal dialysis may be continued indefinitely while awaiting the return of renal function. By gradually extending dwell periods while increasing exchange volumes, a typical maintenance CAPD or CCPD regimen (e.g., for CAPD: 35 to 45 ml/kg per exchange, four to five exchanges per day; for CCPD: similar exchange volumes, five nightly 2-

hour exchanges with a sixth left in place during the day) may be reached in a few days. Familiarity with these continuous, prolonged-dwell peritoneal dialysis techniques used to maintain children with ESRD has led to adoption of similar methods as the standard approach to acute peritoneal dialysis. After an appropriate period of frequent exchanges to correct fluid and electrolyte disturbances and lower the BUN, the near steady-state biochemical and fluid control achievable with continuous peritoneal dialysis regimens may be of particular benefit to critically ill children. There have been no controlled comparisons of CAPD/CCPD vs. traditional IPD in this setting.

RISKS AND COMPLICATIONS
Peritonitis

The most frequent complication of peritoneal dialysis is peritonitis. Sixty-five percent of children treated with CAPD or CCPD will have had at least one episode of peritonitis before they have completed the first 12 months of therapy. The data on peritonitis in the acute setting are not as consistent, but in several large series the incidence of peritonitis was found to be directly proportional to time on dialysis. Early observations revealed a dramatic increase in the incidence of peritonitis when temporary catheters were left in place for more than 72 hours. Improved methods for handling dialysate exchanges in the PICU may have reduced infection risks to the point that a well-functioning temporary catheter may occasionally be used for longer periods, but most authors believe that a temporary catheter left in place for more than 5 days invites infection. Despite the frequency with which peritonitis is encountered, most authorities warn against the use of prophylactic antibiotics and urge instead meticulous technique and a high degree of vigilance.

Peritonitis usually presents with cloudy peritoneal effluent in a febrile child who may also have abdominal pain and tenderness. The peritoneal effluent will usually contain >100 WBCs/mm^3, >50% of which are polymorphonuclear cells. A Gram stain of a centrifuged specimen of the cloudy fluid will demonstrate organisms in only 25% of cases that eventually show positive peritoneal fluid cultures. Blood cultures are almost never positive in the ambulatory patient. It is widely held that most episodes of peritonitis are due to inoculation of the peritoneal dialysis fluid during the exchange procedure or to local seeding from infections of the catheter tunnel or skin exit site. The bacteriology of peritonitis lends support to this view of its pathogenesis. The most frequently cultured pathogens are *Staphylococcus epidermidis* and *S. aureus*, although gram-negative organisms and *Candida* sp together account for up to 30% of peritonitis episodes in children treated with CAPD or CCPD. The child in the PICU may be more likely than the ambulatory peritoneal dialysis patient to acquire peritonitis via the hematogenous route. In newly septic patients it should not be surprising that the offending organism may be cultured from both blood and peritoneal fluid when clinical evidence of peritonitis is also present.

When any of the signs and symptoms of peritonitis are present, a sample of the peritoneal effluent is obtained for cell count (with differential), Gram's stain, and culture. Blood cultures must also be obtained in the PICU patient, although they will rarely be positive. Intraperitoneal antibiotic therapy is begun immediately and continued for 7 to 10 days. Most authorities currently recommend the empiric use of a first-generation cephalosporin in combination with an aminoglycoside until bacteriologic identification of the organism and its antimicrobial sensitivities are known. Table 145-2 contains current recommendations on the intraperitonal use of some of the antibiotics commonly used to treat peritonitis.

Critically ill children may be at increased risk to acquire either fungal (including *Candida*) or fecal peritonitis. Fecal peritonitis occurs when the integrity of the bowel mucosa has been interrupted; it is most often seen in adults as a consequence of diverticulitis, a distinctly uncommon condition in children. Critically ill children may have areas of bowel ischemia that are predisposed to perforation, especially when oral feedings are instituted. There is no evidence to suggest that peritoneal dialysis makes perforation more likely in these children, but it does make the clinical presentation more dramatic. Fecal peritonitis is usually heralded by peritoneal effluent which contains thick mucus that is soon replaced by obvious fecal material in the drainage from subsequent exchanges. Following surgical exploration and either bowel resection or repair, peritoneal dialysis may be continued in most patients using smaller exchange volumes and appropriate intraperitoneal antibiotics.

Candida peritonitis is a particularly vexing complication that occurs most often in children who are receiving or have recently received broad-spectrum antibiotics. Thus the PICU patient may be at increased risk. Many treatment strategies have been proposed, none of which has gained universal acceptance. Early attempts to clear these infections using intraperitoneal amphotericin B while leaving the peritoneal catheter in place have largely been abandoned. Amphotericin B appears to be a potent peritoneal sclerosing agent, and recurrence of *Candida* peritonitis is common when the peritoneal catheter is left in situ during treatment. Most centers now routinely remove the catheter and give amphotericin B intravenously, meaning that most patients must be supported by hemodialysis for the 2 to 3 weeks needed to clear the infection. During the period off peritoneal dialysis, the inflamed peritoneal cavity remains unrinsed by dialysate, which usually leads to extensive adhesion formation. Peritoneal transport function is often severely diminished after an episode of *Candida* peritonitis, preventing further treatment with peritoneal dialysis.

Candida peritonitis is particulary difficult to manage in small infants for whom alternative dialysis therapy may be unavailable. I have recently had limited success with the following strategy, which is not presented as a definitive approach, but which may be helpful to others forced to grapple with this infection in small infants. When *Candida* peritonitis is diagnosed, the infant is begun on IV amphotericin B and oral 5-fluorocytosine (5FC). After 24 to 48 hours of aggressive dialysis the peritoneal catheter is removed and the infant's renal failure managed conservatively for several days, hopefully long enough to obtain results of antibiotic sensitivity tests on the organism. A new peritoneal catheter is then surgically placed at a site distant from the original catheter entry site. Therapy is continued for another 3 weeks with two drugs to which the yeast is sensitive, one of which must be amphotericin B. When 5FC is used, blood levels must be closely followed to avoid potentially overwhelming bone-marrow toxicity. If the patient is unable to receive oral 5FC, the parenteral preparation may be obtained from the manufacturer on a compassionate-release basis. (Although available for years in Europe and Canada, parenteral 5FC has not received FDA approval.) Parenteral 5FC may be given intraperitoneally.

Fluid and Electrolyte Abnormalities

Potentially serious derangements of fluid and electrolyte homeostasis have resulted from the use of peritoneal dialysis in pediatric patients, especially small infants. Almost all can be anticipated and avoided with careful monitoring and appropriate adjustment of therapy. Frequent laboratory studies are needed during stabilization with acute peritoneal dialysis. Once initial stabilization has been accomplished, the use of a continuous prolonged-dwell regimen such as CAPD will reduce the likelihood and the severity of most of the complications listed below.

Hypovolemia. Hypovolemia can occur when ultrafiltration is too aggressive and is most often seen with prolonged use of 4.25% solutions. Ultrafiltration will continue even as the child becomes progressively more dehydrated, there being no mechanism short of hypovolemic shock by which

the peritoneum can retard ultrafiltration driven by the osmolar gradient between dialysate and blood. Careful attention to the amount of fluid removed by each exchange and frequent weighing of the patient is sufficient to avoid this complication, even when 4.25% solutions are used. Patients must always be weighed "empty" at the end of a drain cycle. Ultrafiltration can be modulated by adjusting dialysate dextrose concentration and the length of exchange cycles, with shorter dwell periods associated with increased net ultrafiltration. Even in relatively unstable patients treated with continuous peritoneal dialysis, it is usually possible to find a cycle length and dialysate dextrose concentration that yields a steady and predictable 24-hour rate of ultrafiltration, thus simplifying fluid management.

Hypervolemia. Hypervolemia resulting from inadequate ultrafiltration may occur when the dialysis regimen is not adjusted for any substantial increase in fluid administration such as with transfusions of blood products. Occasionally an exchange will result in a "positive" balance (i.e., less than the infused volume is returned). This is usually due to mechanical factors interfering with complete drainage of the peritoneal cavity and will be corrected by a large drain volume with the next exchange. Occasionally infants will absorb dialysate, especially if prolonged dwell periods and the 1.5% solution are used.

Hyponatremia. Hyponatremia often develops in infants receiving standard IV fluids (e.g., 0.22% saline solution) or being fed commercial formulas or breast milk, all of which provide inadequate sodium to replace peritoneal sodium losses caused by ultrafiltration. Ultrafiltrate and serum sodium concentrations are equal unless very rapid exchanges are being performed (see below). Daily dialysate sodium losses can be estimated by multiplying the 24-hour ultrafiltrate volume times the serum sodium concentration. Appropriate adjustments in IV fluid sodium concentration (usually at least 0.45% saline solution is needed) can then be made, or additional sodium can be provided in the infant's formula.

Hypernatremia. Hypernatremia is rarely a direct consequence of peritoneal dialysis unless an error has been made in the formulation of a batch of homemade dialysate (similar concern must be raised in the hyponatremic patient receiving dialysate that was not commercially manufactured). When frequent exchanges are used to produce large ultrafiltrate volumes, mild hypernatremia can be seen. This is due to sieving effects during the convective transport of sodium across the peritoneal membrane whereby net water movement is always slightly faster than sodium transport.

Hyperglycemia. Hyperglycemia is frequently seen during the early stages of acute peritoneal dialysis when rapid exchange rates and high dialysate dextrose concentrations combine to deliver large amounts of dextrose to the infant. Critically ill patients unable to efficiently metabolize the absorbed carbohydrate may quickly develop blood glucose levels >300 mg/dl. The most effective approach to this problem is to reduce the dialysate dextrose concentration and the exchange rate, but that is not always possible. Some patients may respond to the addition of small amounts of insulin to the dialysate (1 unit of regular insulin/4 g of dialysate dextrose). When making this calculation, it must be remembered that the concentration of dextrose listed on the dialysate container reflects by convention the weight per volume of *hydrated* dextrose. The measured dextrose concentration of "1.5%" dialysate is actually 1.30 g/dl and that of "4.25%" is 3.86 g/dl. Intraperitoneally administered insulin is absorbed directly into the portal circulation, which may be physiologically advantageous.

Hypoproteinemia. Hypoproteinemia is commonly seen in patients on prolonged courses of peritoneal dialysis and is caused by the steady loss of protein into the dialysate. Additional protein must be provided in the form of nutritional supplements (either IV or PO) to offset these losses. In the previously poorly nourished patient serum albumin levels may fall to <2.5 g/dl after only a few days of peritoneal dialysis; IV albumin supplementation may be necessary to maintain an adequate plasma colloid osmotic pressure.

Hypokalemia. Hypokalemia develops in most children treated with peritoneal dialysis for more than a few days. When serum potassium levels fall to <4.0 mEq/L, further decline can be slowed by adding KCl to the dialysate at the desired serum concentration (i.e., 4 mEq/L). Additional IV or PO potassium will be needed to correct the potassium deficit when serum levels fall below 3.5 mEq/L.

Hypophosphatemia. Hypophosphatemia is a late complication that develops slowly and is readily treated by increasing parenteral or oral phosphate intake. Phosphate removal by peritoneal dialysis is relatively inefficient, and little supplementation is needed to bring serum levels back within normal ranges. Temporary discontinuation of oral antacids (which are also phosphate binders) may be sufficient to correct mild hypophosphatemia in PICU patients who are receiving the phosphate binders as prophylaxis against peptic ulcer disease.

Miscellaneous Complications

Dialysate leakage. Reflux of small amounts of hypertonic dialysate into the subcutaneous tissue around the catheter tunnel can result in large accumulations of subcutaneous fluid as tissue fluids are drawn to the hypertonic dialysate by osmosis. If the leak is small, it will seal, and the subcutaneous fluid collection will be reabsorbed slowly over a few days. When dialysate leaks directly out of the exit site, the problem can be more serious. Small leaks may seal if peritoneal dialysis can be suspended for 24 hours and then resumed with smaller exchange volumes. Large leaks necessitate catheter revision. In small infants with thin abdominal walls it is often impossible to avoid or repair a small dialysate leak.

Catheter exit site infection. Minor irritation at the catheter exit site caused in part by the trauma of catheter manipulation may lead to local cellulitis. When inflammation extends at least 1 cm from the exit wound and/or purulent material collects around the catheter, aggressive systemic antibiotic therapy is needed to prevent progression to a tunnel infection and to reduce the risk of peritonitis. Most of these infections are due to staphylococci, but cultures are needed, especially in the PICU setting in which unusual pathogens may be encountered.

Peritoneal eosinophilia. Cloudy peritoneal fluid that contains primarily eosinophils is an alarming, but benign condition that may occur soon after catheter placement. It is not a true peritonitis since no causative organism can be isolated. It is assumed to be due to a local hypersensitivity response to various chemical stimuli and has been observed with use of intraperitoneal antibiotics in patients who are allergic to these drugs. The condition is without symptoms and usually resolves in a few days without therapy.

Poor catheter drainage. This frustrating situation has many causes, few of which are amenable to easy resolution. If fluid flows freely into the peritoneal cavity but drains slowly or not at all, the catheter has probably become wrapped in omentum, which floats away during infusion and then is drawn back into the catheter during the drain cycle. When long catheters are placed in infants, the tip may migrate against the posterior wall of the peritoneum, which can obstruct outflow. Fibrin clots can form within the catheter lumen. It is often helpful to obtain a three-dimensional view of the catheter's position using flat plate and cross-table lateral films of the abdomen. If the catheter appears to be in good position on the roentgenogram, it may be possible to dislodge an obstruction by forcefully injecting a small amount of dilute contrast media during fluoroscopy. Usually these efforts are in vain, and surgical revision is needed.

Painful dialysis. Optimum peritoneal dialysis is painless. Pain during dialysate inflow may be due to a jet stream of dialysate striking the same area repeatedly. This type of pain is easily resolved by slowing the rate of infusion. Cramping pain during the dwell cycle may be due to intolerance of the acid pH of the dialysate or to dialysate that is too hot or too cold. Pain occurring near the end of a drain cycle is probably caused when peritoneal tissues are drawn into the catheter and resolves when the next exchange is infused. Shoulder pain caused by diaphragmatic irritation may occur in children sitting upright who have had air infused into the peritoneal cavity when dialysate tubing was incompletely purged. The air is eventually absorbed. Finally, painful dialysis may be the first evidence of peritonitis.

Bloody peritoneal fluid. Blood may appear in the dialysate of patients with coagulopathies such as DIC. It may also be the result of minor trauma to the peritoneal membrane at the catheter entry site. In ambulatory female patients bloody fluid is most often seen during menstruation or ovulation. On rare occasions bloody dialysate reflects true intraperitoneal hemorrhage, necessitating surgical intervention. Erosion by the catheter through a small artery on the surface of the bowel has been reported.

Respiratory compromise. In patients who already have some degree of respiratory compromise the use of typical exchange volumes may elevate the diaphragm and cause further respiratory compromise. In such a case smaller, more frequently cycled exchanges should be used.

ADDITIONAL READING

Abbad FCB, Ploos van Amstel SLB. Continuous ambulatory peritoneal dialysis in small children with acute renal failure. Proc Eur Dial Transplant Assoc 19:607-613, 1982.

Alexander SR. Peritoneal dialysis in children. In KD Nolph, ed. Peritoneal Dialysis, 3rd ed. Norwell, Mass.: Kluwer, 1989, pp 343-364.

• Alexander SR, Tank ES, Corneil AT. Five years' experience with CAPD/CCPD catheters in infants and children. In Fine RN, Scharer K, Mehls O, eds. CAPD in Children. New York: Springer-Verlag, 1985, pp 179-190.

Blackfan KD, Maxcy KF. The intraperitoneal injection of saline solution. Am J Dis Child 15:19-28, 1918.

Chan JCM. Acute renal failure in children: Principles of management. Clin Pediatr 13:686-695, 1974.

Donn SM, Swartz RD, Thoene JG. Comparison of exchange transfusion, peritoneal dialysis and hemodialysis for the treatment of hyperammonemia in an anuric newborn infant. J Pediatr 95:67-70, 1979.

El-Dahr S, Gomez RA, Campbell FG, et al. Rapid correction of acute salt poisoning by peritoneal dialysis. Pediatr Nephrol 1:602-604, 1987.

Feinstein EI, Chesney RW, Zelikovic I. Peritonitis in childhood renal disease. Am J Nephrol 8:147-165, 1988.

• Fine RN, Salusky IB, Ettinger RB. The therapeutic approach to the infant, child, and adolescent with end-stage renal disease. Pediatr Clin North Am 34:789-802, 1987.

Fine RN, Salusky IB, Hall T, et al. Peritonitis in children undergoing continuous ambulatory peritoneal dialysis. Pediatrics 71:806-809, 1983.

Gruskin AB, Alexander SR, Baluarte HJ, et al. Issues in pediatric dialysis. Am J Kidney Dis 7:306-311, 1986.

Hogg RJ, Coln D, Chang J, et al. The Toronto Western Hospital catheter in a pediatric dialysis program. Am J Kidney Dis 3:219-233, 1983.

Keane WF, Everett ED, Fine RN, et al. CAPD related peritonitis management and antibiotic therapy recommendations. Peritoneal Dial Bull 7:55-68, 1987.

Morgenstern BZ, Baluarte H. Peritoneal dialysis kinetics in children. In Fine RN, ed. Chronic Ambulatory Peritoneal Dialysis (CAPD) and Chronic Cycling Peritoneal Dialysis (CCPD) in Children. Boston: Martinus Nijhoff, 1987, pp 47-62.

Steele BT, Vigneaux A, Blatz S, et al. Acute peritoneal dialysis in infants weighing <1500 g. J Pediatr 110:126-129, 1987.

Swan H, Gordon HH. Peritoneal lavage in the treatment of anuria in children. Pediatrics 4:586-595, 1949.

Von Lilien T, Salusky IB, Boechat I, et al. Five years' experience with continuous ambulatory or continuous cycling peritoneal dialysis in children. J Pediatr 111:513-518, 1987.

146 Hemodialysis

Billy S. Arant, Jr.

BACKGROUND AND INDICATIONS

Hemodialysis is a treatment used in the intensive care setting primarily to augment or replace renal excretory function. In general almost any water-soluble substance in the extracellular fluid of a patient that is not protein or tissue bound can be removed rapidly by hemodialysis. When hemodialysis is combined with charcoal hemoperfusion, certain drugs and toxins can be removed from the body even more rapidly than by hemodialysis alone. When the appropriate equipment and trained personnel are available, hemodialysis may be initiated as soon as vascular access to the circulation can be established. Dialyzers, blood lines, and vascular catheters of many different sizes must be stocked; emergency delivery of the appropriate equipment can delay treatment for up to 24 hours, for unless the hospital has a chronic hemodialysis facility for children, neither the equipment nor the personnel will be available for other than adult-sized patients (>40 kg body weight).

Principles of Hemodialysis

Any technique for effecting hemodialysis is an adaptation of or improvement on the simple experiment of immersing a cellophane bag filled with whole blood into a bath of a balanced electrolyte solution similar to interstitial fluid. Water-soluble solutes move across the semipermeable cellophane membrane and down concentration gradients. If the concentration of a substance such as sodium is the same on both sides of the membrane, the concentration of the substance will not change no matter how long the two solutions are exposed to each other. Alternatively, small molecules can be removed from or added to the blood by lowering or raising its concentration in the electrolyte solution. The steeper the concentration gradient, the more efficient is the removal of the targeted substance from the blood. Frequent changing of the bath maintains the concentration difference at a maximum. Larger molecules such as proteins, substances bound to protein, blood cells, and bacteria cannot cross the membrane; thus the bath does not have to remain sterile.

Water moves across the membrane according to pressure and osmotic gradients. By increasing the pressure within the bag (positive pressure), water can be forced through the pores of the membrane into the bathing solution very much like Starling's forces effect movement of plasma water across capillary walls. Moreover, water can be pulled from the bag if a vacuum is created on the outside of the bag (negative pressure). Finally, osmotic movement of water from the blood can be achieved by raising the concentration of an osmotically active molecule such as glucose in the bath (dialysate). Other factors such as the temperature of the solutions, the membrane surface area, the rate of blood flow across the membrane, and the permeability of the membrane will influence the efficiency of osmosis and diffusion.

Modern equipment designs incorporate features that facilitate efficient hemodialysis treatment. Most dialysis machines manufactured recently can provide up to 1000 ml/min of dialysate delivered with a constant osmolarity at body temperature, effect a wide range of positive and negative pressures within the system for water removal (ultrafiltration), detect air in the column of blood, monitor the volume of fluid removed from the blood as it passes through the dialyzer, and detect the presence of hemoglobin within the dialysate to foretell membrane rupture. The water supply for hemodialysis must be deionized to protect the patient against any variation in the mineral content of the dialysate and must be treated by reverse osmosis to remove coliform bacteria since these organisms can gain access to the blood should a membrane leak occur.

TECHNIQUE
Acute Hemodialysis
Access

Access must be established to the circulation (see Chapter 114). This can be accomplished with the usual percutaneous techniques for either single- or double-lumen subclavian or femoral catheters ($\geq$gauge F 6). Because of the large volume of blood removed from and returned to the patient rapidly during hemodialysis, the tip of the subclavian catheter must be at the level of the right atrium and that of the femoral catheter within the inferior vena cava. Alternatively, two vascular catheters from different access sites can be used, and one may be an arterial catheter.

Calculating extracorporeal blood volume

The volume of blood that can be removed from the circulation over a short period of time is approximately 10% of the circulating blood volume. In the 70 kg adult whose blood volume is approximately 5 L, 500 ml can be withdrawn gradually without producing any hemodynamic change. This is the basis for 1 unit of whole blood having a volume of 400 to 500 ml and is an obvious reason for routinely excluding children and small adults as blood donors. The volume needed to fill completely the tubing and artificial kidney (priming volume) used for hemodialysis in adults is 250 to 400 ml, which will not produce hemodynamic change in patients weighing >40 kg whose blood volumes are at least 3000 ml (75 ml/kg). Equipment with a smaller priming volume is available for treating smaller patients. When one calculates the volume of blood that can be outside the patient's body at any given moment during hemodialysis (extracorporal blood volume = 75 ml/kg $\times$ 0.10), the blood-filled tubing and the artificial kidney are selected for priming volumes that correspond most closely to the patient's extracorporeal blood volume. The smallest volume for currently marketed equipment that can provide effective hemodialysis treatment is 68 ml, which equals the extracorporeal blood volume of a patient weighing 10 kg. Smaller patients or larger dialyzers mean that the system must be primed with blood for each hemodialysis treatment.

Determining rate of blood flow through artificial kidney

There are several criteria for deciding the appropriate rate at which the patient's blood must be pumped through the artificial kidney. First, blood cannot be removed from the patient at a rate faster than it can be returned since to do so would mean that the extracorporeal volume would gradually increase during hemodialysis and produce hemodynamic alterations in the patient. Second, each artificial kidney has specific membrane characteristics that, according to the blood flow through the kidney, determine the clearance rate of a substance. For every membrane and artificial kidney model there is an upper limit of blood flow rate for solute removal. In general the minimum blood flow that provides a clearance rate of urea or creatinine of 2 to 3 ml/min/kg body weight is satisfactory. Third, the desired rate of blood flow may not be possible in every patient when mechanical obstruction interferes with blood entering the catheter or when the volume of blood entering the blood-filled tubing causes reductions in cardiac output and effective arterial blood volume. All calculations of extracorporeal volume may be accurate, but the cardiovascular hemodynamics in any one patient may necessitate using a higher blood volume to fill vascular beds that will not vasoconstrict sufficiently to maintain systemic arterial blood pressure and peripheral perfusion. The rate of blood flow may have to be adjusted initially or even frequently throughout the treatment to match the dialyzer to the patient. Antihypertensive drugs must not be administered before or during hemodialysis other than in unusual circumstances to avoid systemic arterial hypotension during a time when 10% of the blood volume is removed from the circulation.

Ultrafiltration

The amount of fluid removed from the blood during its transit through the artificial kidney is determined by the blood flow rate, the pressure created within the confines of the membrane by the volume of blood, and the resistance within the system to blood flow. When the artificial kidney has a rigid outside wall, a vacuum or negative pressure can be generated to extract fluid across the semipermeable membrane. The sum of positive pressure within the system and the negative pressure around the membrane is referred to as the transmembrane pressure. The specifications for every dialyzer state the volume of ultrafiltrate per millimeter of mercury of transmembrane pressure. To remove 400 ml of fluid from a patient during a 4-hour hemodialysis treatment a transmembrane pressure to effect an ultrafiltration rate of 100 ml per hour would be applied.

Anticoagulation

Blood in the extracorporeal circulation will clot without the addition of an anticoagulant. There are two different approaches to anticoagulating patients during hemodialysis. The first is heparinization to prolong the activated clotting time (ACT) by 50% to 100% of a baseline value, which will vary among patients. Each patient, therefore, must be treated individually. The heparin may be administered as an initial bolus of 50 units/kg body weight followed either by a continuous infusion of heparin in sodium chloride solution to deliver 25% of the initial dose every hour or by intermittent bolus administration of heparin when ACT falls to <1½ times greater than the pretreatment value.

For patients who have had recent surgery or vascular trauma in whom anticoagulation may risk bleeding complications, regional heparinization can be used. By this technique heparin is infused into the arterial blood catheter (into blood being conducted from the patient to the dialyzer) in an amount to prolong the ACT 1½- to 2-fold, but protamine is infused into the venous blood catheter (into blood conducted from dialyzer to patient) to counteract the heparin so that the clotting time of the blood while it is in the patient remains nearly normal. The ratio of heparin to protamine is 1.3:1. More important, the responses of patients may be quite different so that anticoagulant administration to the patient must be monitored frequently in case the dose must be modified. Heparin is metabolized within 4 to 6 hours in most patients, but if bleeding is a concern, protamine can be administered at the end of a hemodialysis treatment to render the ACT closer to the pretreatment value measured in the patient.

Charcoal Hemoperfusion

A cartridge containing activated charcoal can be interposed in blood-filled tubing so that the patient's blood has direct contact with the charcoal. This technique is based on the same principle as placing charcoal in the gastrointestinal tract after toxin or drug ingestion. A filter traps any charcoal particles that may escape the cartridge. When hemodialysis is not required, the filter can be used, but a blood pump is necessary to force the blood through the cartridge. Moreover, the cartridge must be prepared with heparinized sodium chloride solution, and heparin requirements for anticoagulation during the procedure are greater than for hemodialysis alone.

Monitoring

Cardiovascular status. Systemic arterial blood pressure and heart rate must be monitored frequently, depending on the previous stability of the patient, to detect unexpected trends suggestive of fluid overload or depletion.

Body weight. Although ultrafiltration may be estimated by monitoring devices built into the equipment, the readout may be inaccurate. Moreover, systemic arterial blood pressure changes may be due to changes in blood volume or peripheral vascular resistance. A constant readout of body weight accomplished with a bed or chair scale will monitor changes in body water accurately.

Hematocrit. A change in hematocrit level may reflect hemoconcentration as fluid is removed or hemodilution as fluid is administered in excess of that removed by dialysis ultrafiltration or hemolysis. Hematocrit must be measured at the outset, once during the procedure, and at the end of hemodialysis.

Activated clotting time. Anticoagulation therapy can be determined as adequate and not excessive only by serial measurements of clotting time. Measurements are obtained usually before heparin is administered, 30 minutes after heparin is first given, and at 30- to 60-minute intervals during dialysis to facilitate adjustments in the dose of heparin.

Body temperature. Body temperature must be recorded hourly or when the patient complains of being unusually warm or cold.

Dialysate osmolarity. A sample of dialysate must be tested hourly to be certain that the solution is being mixed appropriately by the equipment.

Electrolytes. Serum electrolyte concentrations as well as calcium and phosphorous concentrations, must be measured immediately before and at the completion of dialysis to detect unexpected changes produced by the treatment. Many derangements can be corrected during hemodialysis by altering the concentrations of the substances in the dialysate or by infusing them into the large volume of blood circulating through the dialyzer.

RISKS AND COMPLICATIONS

Hemorrhagic hypotension. Vascular catheters for infusions and hemodynamic monitoring are familiar to critical care personnel. When these same catheters are used for hemodialysis, not only will 10% or more of the circulating blood volume be outside the body at any given moment, but a membrane rupture, a loosened connection, or a break in the blood-filled tubing connected to the dialyzer can result in life-threatening hemorrhage at any moment. Trained personnel stay on constant alert for this kind of emergency. The appropriate response to this event would be to clamp both blood-filled tubings between the patient and the site of blood loss, then stop the blood pump.

Circulatory shock. Although the patient may tolerate hemodialysis for several hours without apparent hemodynamic instability, a sudden drop in systemic arterial blood pressure either because of a decrease in peripheral vascular resistance or too rapid ultrafiltration may be observed at any time. Treatment is by blood volume expansion. This problem is more common in patients with impaired cardiac output who tolerate even small changes in blood volume poorly.

Tissue ischemia. Patients with occlusive vascular disease who depend on a minimum systemic arterial blood pressure to perfuse tissues may experience angina, claudication, or altered consciousness during hemodialysis.

Air embolism. The high rate of blood flow through the extracorporeal circulation facilitates rapid entry of air into the patient's venous circulation. Bubble detectors in the venous catheter will, when functioning properly, occlude blood return to the patient. The time of greatest risk for air embolism occurs after completion of the hemodialysis treatment and during the time when blood in the tubing is being returned to the patient. Should air escape detection or enter the patient's venous circulation, the patient should be placed with the left shoulder in a dependent position in an effort to trap the air in the right atrium. Other treatment includes oxygen administration and cardiac monitoring. An echocardiogram may be helpful in identifying the presence of air in the heart.

Hemolysis. When RBCs are exposed to sudden changes in plasma osmolarity, lysis may occur. All solutions administered in large volumes during dialysis must be isotonic to plasma. When the proportioning system that mixes dialysate concentrate with the water malfunctions and changes in the osmolarity of the dialysate escape detection by the monitoring device, sudden shifts in plasma electrolytes and osmolarity can occur with consequent lysis of RBCs, electrolyte derangements, free hemoglobin in plasma, anemia, and changes in brain water, causing altered states of consciousness and even sudden death.

Changes in body temperature. During hemodialysis the patient's blood is exposed to dialysate in a volume ratio of approximately 1:5. If the dialysate is not maintained at body temperature, hypothermia or hyperthermia can develop rapidly. When this goes unnoticed, death may occur. Altering the temperature of the dialysate can be used as a means of altering the patient's temperature during treatment instead of administering antipyretics or using warming/cooling blankets. If the patient is febrile, adjustments in the temperature of the dialysate can help to restore body temperature to a more satisfactory value.

ADDITIONAL READING

Nevins TE, Mauer SM. Infant hemodialysis. In Fine RN, Gruskin AB, eds. End Stage Renal Disease in Children. Philadelphia: WB Saunders, 1984, pp 39-53.

Papadopoulou ZL, Novello AC, Calcagno PL. Hemoperfusion in therapeutic medicine. In Fine RN, Gruskin AB, eds. End Stage Renal Disease in Children. Philadelphia: WB Saunders, 1984, pp 77-84.

Potter DE. Hemodialysis in children with ESRD: Technical aspects. In Fine RN, Gruskin AB, eds. End Stage Renal Disease in Children. Philadelphia: WB Saunders, 1984, pp 30-38.

147 Hemoperfusion

Steven R. Alexander

BACKGROUND

Hemoperfusion is a blood purification technique that is designed to remove toxic substances from the circulation by pumping the blood in an extracorporeal circuit directly through a cartridge packed with a highly adsorbent material such as activated charcoal or resin. Since there is no semipermeable membrane involved in the process, hemoperfusion efficiently removes many highly protein-bound and lipid-soluble compounds that do not cross dialysis or hemofiltration membranes. Thus hemoperfusion has been used most successfully as an adjunct in the management of severely intoxicated children who have ingested a potentially lethal amount of certain drugs and poisons such as theophylline, glutethimide, and paraquat that are not as effectively removed by hemodialysis.

Hemoperfusion has also been used in the treatment of severe hepatic encephalopathy. However, effectiveness in treating hepatic encephalopathy has not been convincingly demonstrated despite more than a decade of clinical experience. Efforts to find a role for hemoperfusion in the treatment of renal failure have been even less rewarding. In contrast to dialysis, hemoperfusion does not remove urea or water and cannot control blood electrolyte composition. Hemoperfusion was once combined with hemodialysis to treat patients with chronic renal failure in the hope that the more efficient removal of "middle molecules" possible with hemoperfusion would result in fewer uremic symptoms. These regimens have largely been abandoned. Hemoperfusion may eventually find a role in deferoxamine chelation therapy, which is used to treat chronic aluminum toxicity in hemodialysis patients, but at present few dialysis centers are using hemoperfusion in this manner.

One promising application of hemoperfusion technology currently under investigation is the de-velopment of specific immunoadsorbents designed to selectively remove potentially pathogenic immune complexes from the circulation (e.g., anti-DNA antibody complexes in patients with severe SLE). Another line of research still in its early stages is the development of aggressive blood purification regimens that use sequential hemoperfusion treatments along with plasma exchange and hemodialysis/hemofiltration in the treatment of multiple organ system failure.

In 1990, however, the use of hemoperfusion in most pediatric centers is limited to the treatment of selected cases of severe drug overdose or poisoning and the occasional heroic treatment of a child who has suffered acute hepatic failure in an effort to support that child until a suitable liver transplant donor can be found. Thus hemoperfusion is used infrequently in most PICUs, and few pediatric nephrologists have much personal experience with the technique. Published experience in children is also limited and largely confined to case reports and small series. Fortunately the principles governing the safe and effective use of hemoperfusion in children are relatively straightforward, and the technical skills and much of the equipment needed to perform pediatric hemoperfusion are almost the same as those used in pediatric hemodialysis. Recent improvements in hemoperfusion adsorbent devices, including the development of smaller cartridges suitable for use in infants and young children, have made the technique both safer and easier to perform. Pediatric nephrologists and dialysis nurses who may be unfamiliar with hemoperfusion, but who routinely perform hemodialysis in children, should not be discouraged by inexperience from attempting hemoperfusion in a child who needs it. With appropriate attention to detail and awareness of the ways in which hemoperfusion differs from hemodialysis, successful hemoperfusion is readily achieved by accomplished pediatric hemodialysis teams who may have little or no prior hemoperfusion experience.

Development of Hemoperfusion

The medicinal use of sorbents, especially charcoal, is an ancient practice. Both Egyptian and Chinese physicians were prescribing charcoal at least 15 centuries before the birth of Christ. Hippocrates used wood charcoal to treat epilepsy, vertigo, and anthrax. Eighteenth-century physicians applied charcoal to gangrenous ulcers to remove foul odors and recommended a suspension of charcoal and water as a mouthwash.

German chemists discovered the phenomenon of adsorption during the 1770s when they observed that gases exposed to charcoal were removed by it from the atmosphere. The French discovery that charcoal could decolorize many liquids led to the extensive use of charcoal in the cane and beet sugar industries in Europe in the early 1800s. The Industrial Revolution fueled the search for better decolorizing charcoals, yielding charcoals made from bone, blood, peat, paper mill waste, coconut shells, fruit pits, corncobs, fish, and many other materials. It was during this period that the first studies of charcoal as a poison antidote were performed. In 1831, after observing that charcoal prevented the death of animals given arsenic or strychnine, Touery, a Parisian pharmacist, survived a potentially lethal dose of strychnine mixed with charcoal in a demonstration before the French Academy of Medicine. Responding to a public outcry in 1850 over the alleged addition of strychnine to certain English pale ales, Graham and Hofman demonstrated that charcoal could be used by health authorities to extract and detect strychnine in ale.

During the following 75 years the effectiveness of charcoal as an antidote for a wide variety of poisons was clearly established. Discovery of the chemical process of "activation" in 1900 greatly enhanced the adsorptive capacity and thus the efficacy of charcoal as an antidote. During the early 1900s U.S. physicians also prescribed charcoal for a wide variety of intestinal disorders, including dyspepsia, flatulence, fetid breath, and worms in children.

In 1948 Muirhead and Reid introduced the concept of hemoperfusion to clinical medicine when they demonstrated in vitro that sorbents had the capacity to remove toxins directly from the blood. Their work was clinically relevant only because by 1944

Kolf had developed the extracorporeal circulation methods necessary to perform hemodialysis safely. During the next 10 years Schreiner and other dialysis pioneers explored the use of resins and other sorbents that could be included as part of the extracorporeal hemodialysis circuit. Poor biocompatibility and little effectiveness in controlling uremia made the use of sorbents seem much less promising than dialysis during the early development of these two techniques. In 1964 Yatzidis began a series of in vitro and in vivo experiments that demonstrated the effectiveness of charcoal hemoperfusion in the treatment of severe barbiturate poisoning. In 1965 Yatzidis performed a demonstration as dramatic (if not as personally hazardous) as Tourery's 130 years earlier when he successfully treated two patients in barbiturate coma. Both patients abruptly regained consciousness during hemoperfusion.

It soon became apparent, however, that these early hemoperfusion systems were associated with a variety of potentially serious adverse effects. Charcoal and synthetic resins are not biocompatible substances. Hemolysis, platelet depletion, and pyrogenic reactions frequently resulted from blood passing over the hemoperfusion column, and studies in animals demonstrated extensive microembolization of charcoal particles to the lungs and other organs. These problems were widely known among nephrologists during this period, many of whom doubted that hemoperfusion could be made a safe procedure. Some of these same doubts may persist among clinicians who are aware of the early failures and unfamiliar with the advances in hemoperfusion adsorbent technology that have occurred since 1969.

In 1969 Chang discovered how to "microencapsulate" activated charcoal particles in a biocompatible coating of collodion-albumin and thereby established hemoperfusion as a viable therapeutic modality. Subsequent improvements in coating materials have further enhanced biocompatibility and essentially eliminated microembolization. Another line of research has led to the development of safe nonionic synthetic adsorbent resins that have advantages over charcoal in the removal of certain substances and could potentially lead to "designer" adsorbents directed at specific classes of toxic substances.

Until recently clinical use of hemoperfusion in children was limited by the large priming volumes needed by the available cartridges. Cartridges with priming volumes as low as 50 ml are now readily available, and these devices, along with improvements in temporary vascular access techniques and catheters designed for pediatric use, have removed most of the technical obstacles to more widespread use of hemoperfusion in children.

Indications in Poisoning and Drug Overdose

Following the implementation of the Poison Prevention Packaging Act of 1970 there was a dramatic decline in the incidence of accidental ingestions by young children. Between 1974 and 1981 ingestions of aspirin, acetaminophen, oven cleaners, lighter fluids, and antifreeze by children less than 5 years of age decreased from 2.9/1000 to <2.0/1000. Deaths from accidental aspirin ingestion by young children decreased by 67% between 1970 and 1978 and have declined even further during the 1980s.

Yet, as aspirin has declined as a frequent intoxicant of children, other dangerous drugs have become more important. Accidental or intentional ingestions of hazardous substances still account for >100,000 emergency department visits by pediatric patients each year. Fortunately the vast majority of these ingestions do not result in serious morbidity, and mortality rates are low, with <1% of hospitalized poisoned patients dying as a result of intoxications. This low overall mortality rate obscures the fact that >100 poisoned children (<14 years of age) die each year, and another 500-plus fatal poisonings occur among adolescents and young adults (15 to 24 years of age). It is in this group of severely poisoned children and adolescents that techniques capable of rapid removal of the poison from the blood (e.g., hemodialysis, hemoperfusion) can be most beneficial.

The decision to use dialysis or hemoperfusion to remove a toxic substance from the circulation of a child is often difficult. The observation that many severely poisoned patients have survived with only meticulous supportive care in the PICU reduces the perceived imperative for direct blood purification in the minds of many clinicians. Serious concerns (both real and exaggerated) about the risks associated with extracorporeal blood purification procedures, when combined with the lack of clear guidelines on when these procedures are most likely to offer substantial benefits, may lead to a general reluctance to use dialysis or hemoperfusion in all but the most gravely ill patients and may delay the institution of such therapy beyond the time when rapid drug removal is

likely to be most beneficial (i.e., before irreversible injury has occurred).

Clinical considerations that may be helpful in deciding when to use either hemodialysis or hemoperfusion as an adjunct in the management of severely poisoned patients are as follows:

1. Intoxication with a drug or poison that can be removed by hemodialysis or hemoperfusion at a rate exceeding the patient's current endogenous liver or kidney excretion rate
2. Progressive deterioration despite optimal supportive therapy
3. Severe intoxication with impairment of midbrain function as manifested by apnea, hypotension, or hypothermia
4. The presence of impaired function of the organ(s) normally responsible for excretion of the drug
5. Intoxication with agents that are metabolized to more toxic substances (e.g., ethylene glycol to oxalic acid) or that have delayed effects (e.g., paraquat, *Amanita phalloides*)
6. The presence of complications that are the consequences of coma (e.g., aspiration pneumonia) or the presence of underlying conditions that predispose to and/or increase the risks associated with prolonged coma (e.g., chronic lung disease, septicemia)
7. Blood level in a range associated with high mortality rate (see text)
8. Ingestion of a potentially lethal dose (see text)

Of greatest importance in the individual patient is determining the rate of clinical deterioration despite maximal supportive care. Guidelines based on blood levels of certain drugs have been proposed but are difficult to interpret. For example, hemoperfusion has been recommended for patients with theophylline intoxication at plasma levels ranging from 30 to 100 mg/dl, depending on the reference consulted. It is also questionable to base a decision primarily on estimates of the total ingested amount, especially when the patient is a small child for whom such estimates are notoriously unreliable. When poisonings by more than a single agent are involved, hemoperfusion must be considered at lower blood levels and estimated ingested amounts.

With the possible exception of theophylline ingestion, in which plasma levels >100 mg/dl are generally considered sufficient indication for hemoperfusion regardless of the clinical status of the patient, most centers will consider hemoperfusion only in severely encephalopathic, comatose patients. The duration of coma is inversely correlated with intact neurologic survival in studies of poisoned patients, and hemoperfusion may indeed shorten the period of coma in many of these patients. Earlier use of hemoperfusion in patients with less severe encephalopathies may be warranted now that the technique itself is easier and safer to perform. Earlier use of hemoperfusion to *prevent* rather than just treat worsening encephalopathy has been suggested, but systematic evaluation of such an approach has not been done. In 1990 the decision to use hemoperfusion in an individual case is still largely a clinical judgment made with few generally accepted objective criteria.

The preceding discussion presumes that the drug or poison involved can be removed by hemoperfusion. Drugs that have been reported as removed by hemoperfusion based on data compiled and summarized by Winchester during the past decade are listed on p. 1014. The absence of a specific compound from the list may only indicate that the results of attempts to remove that particular compound by hemoperfusion have not been reported.

Some of the compounds listed are also removed by hemodialysis. Several general considerations are helpful when choosing between the two therapies.

Water-soluble drugs that diffuse rapidly across the dialysis membrane (e.g., lithium, bromide, ethanol, methanol) are best removed by hemodialysis. If a drug is equally well removed by both therapies, hemodialysis is usually preferred since the problem of cartridge saturation is avoided. Hemodialysis also allows treatment of any coexisting acid-base disturbances (e.g., salicylate intoxication). When renal failure is present, hemodialysis should be used alone (e.g., in ethylene glycol intoxication) or in combination with hemoperfusion when hemodialysis alone will not adequately remove the poison (e.g., paraquat). The choice of hemoperfusion over hemodialysis is usually made when the drug is highly protein bound or lipid soluble, as reflected in Table 147-1, which contains data on comparative plasma extraction ratios for several commonly encountered intoxicants. Hemoperfusion is more effective at removal of lipid-soluble drugs such as glutethimide, along with barbiturates and nonbarbiturate hypnotics, sedatives, and tranquilizers.

Indications in Hepatic Encephalopathy

Although the use of hemoperfusion for severe hepatic failure was first described by Chang in 1972, effectiveness in treating this condition has yet to be convincingly demonstrated. Early enthusiastic reports of improved survival among patients with stage

Table 147-1   Plasma Drug Extraction Ratios With Hemodialysis and Charcoal or Resin Hemoperfusion*

Drug	Hemodialysis	Charcoal Hemoperfusion	XAD-4 Resin Hemoperfusion
Acetylsalicylic acid	0.5	0.5	—
Amobarbital	0.3	0.3	0.9
Digoxin	0.2	0.3-0.6	0.4
Ethchlorvynol	0.2	0.7	1.0
Glutethimide	0.2	0.65	0.8
Methaqualone	0.1	0.4-1.0	1.0
Paraquat	0.5	0.6	—
Pentobarbital	—	0.5	0.85
Phenobarbital	0.3	0.5	0.85
Theophylline	0.5	0.7	0.75

*Extraction ratio $= \dfrac{\text{(Inlet concentration)} - \text{(Outlet concentration)}}{\text{Inlet concentration}}$

Calculated for blood flow rate of 200 ml/min at the midpoint of the procedure (see Chang, 1982, in Additional Reading).

IV hepatic coma treated with hemoperfusion compared to patients treated with conservative management alone have not been consistently confirmed. Very little pediatric experience with hemoperfusion in this setting has been reported.

Early efforts to improve survival with hemoperfusion focused on providing artificial liver support during the often prolonged period needed for the patient to recover from acute liver failure. Outcome in both treated and conservatively managed groups was poor (13% to 30% survival). The uniformly high mortality rates associated with stage IV hepatic encephalopathy have led to the use of orthoptic liver transplantation to treat these children and to renewed

---

DRUGS AND POISONS REMOVED BY HEMOPERFUSION

Alcohols

Ethanol*
Isopropanol*
Methanol*

Analgesics

Acetaminophen
Acetylsalicylic acid and other
    salicylates*
Codeine
Phenylbutazone
Propoxyphene†

Antidepressants

Amitriptyline†
Amphetamine
Clomipramine†
Doxepin†
Imipramine†
Nortriptyline†

Antimicrobials

Ampicillin
Chloramphenicol
Clindamycin
Erythromycin
Gentamicin
Isoniazid
Penicillins
Quinine

Barbiturates

Amobarbital
Pentobarbital
Phenobarbital
Secobarbital
Thiopental
Many others

Cardiovascular agents

Digitoxin
Digoxin
Procainamide
Quinidine

*Nonbarbiturate hypnotics, sedatives,
and tranquilizers*

Carbromal
Chloral hydrate
Chlordiazepoxide†
Chlorpromazine†
Diazepam†
Ethchlorvynol
Glutethimide
Meprobamate
Methaqualone
Methsuximide
Methyprylon
Oxazepam†
Pentenamide
Promethazine

*Herbicides, insecticides,
animal/plant toxins*

Amanita phalloides toxin
Camphor
Chlordane
Chlorinated insecticides
Dimethoate
Demeton-S-methyl sulfoxide
Nitrostigmine
Organophosphates
Paraquat
Parathion
Polychlorinated biphenyls

Solvents/gases

Carbon tetrachloride
Ethylene oxide
Trichloroethanol

Miscellaneous

Aminophylline
Angiotensin
Diphenhydramine
Dopamine
Epinephrine
Heparin
Methotrexate
Norepinephrine
Oxalic acid
Paraldehyde
Phenytoin
Phenols
Podophyllin
Theophylline
Thyroid hormone

---

*Hemodialysis preferred (see text).

†Highly tissue bound (large V_d) and/or highly protein bound with low free fraction in plasma. Repeated/prolonged treatment may be necessary; posttreatment rebound is common.

interest in hemoperfusion as a component of artificial liver support during the time needed to find a suitable liver donor. Treatment strategies using hemoperfusion while awaiting liver transplantation can only be considered highly experimental at this point.

There is understandable controversy over the use of hemoperfusion in this setting. Not only are there no generally accepted indications for attempting a trial of hemoperfusion in a child with severe hepatic encephalopathy, but most investigators cannot even agree on how often and for how long hemoperfusion must be performed in such patients. Unlike acute renal failure, in which abnormalities in readily measured solutes (e.g., urea, creatinine) provide guidance for renal replacement therapy, there is little agreement on how to monitor hemoperfusion therapy in patients with acute liver failure. Most pediatric nephrologists share a similar, if not uniform, concept of what constitutes "adequate" renal replacement therapy. The adequacy of artificial liver replacement therapies (e.g., hemoperfusion) will remain largely conjectural until it is known which toxic metabolites accumulating in the circulation must be followed to assess effectiveness of therapy.

Patients with liver failure are often difficult to treat with hemoperfusion. Many of these patients already have severe coagulopathies and low platelet counts. The additional thrombocytopenia induced by the hemoperfusion treatment can precipitate active bleeding. Generous use of platelet and clotting factor transfusions are usually needed to perform hemoperfusion safely in these patients. Hypotension during hemoperfusion is also encountered more frequently in these patients, especially during the first few minutes of therapy as endogenous and exogenous catecholamines and other pressor substances are removed from the circulation by the cartridge. It is wise to have additional volume expanders and premixed pressor infusions (e.g., epinephrine) available for immediate use at the start of each hemoperfusion treatment in such patients.

TECHNIQUE
Charcoal
Adsorption by activated charcoal

Adsorbent materials used in hemoperfusion are highly porous and have a tremendous surface area. A typical activated charcoal used for hemoperfusion has a surface area of >1000 m^2/g. This extensive surface area is achieved when a carbonaceous ma-

terial undergoes pyrolysis followed by a stage of controlled oxidation. This latter stage is what is meant by "activation" of the charcoal. Most carbonaceous materials can be converted into charcoal, and the final properties of the charcoal will reflect the source material. For example, coconut shells yield a strong, dense charcoal, which is highly resistant to mechanical abrasion. All charcoals contain many impurities, depending on the source material; none is pure carbon. However, some manufacturers prefer to use the term "activated carbon" when the source material is not of animal or vegetable origin (e.g., petroleum-based "carbons").

Pyrolysis of the source material is achieved by heating it to temperatures of 600° to 900° C in the absence of air. Incorporation of metallic chlorides in this first mixture greatly increases the porosity of the resulting charcoal. Oxidation ("activation") is then carried out using steam (or carbon dioxide) injected and maintained at high temperatures. The oxidizing gas selectively erodes the internal surfaces of the tiny charcoal particles, developing an extensive internal network of communicating pores, which have diameters ranging from <10 to >500 Å, depending on the source material and the specifics of the activation step.

When activated charcoal is bathed in a liquid such as plasma, molecules diffuse first through the large surface pores and then, if the molecules are small enough, through the internal network of micropores in which adsorption to the charcoal's surface eventually takes place. Although the intermolecular forces involved in the chemical process of adsorption appear relatively weak, the total surface area of the charcoal that is actively participating in the process is so extensive that many molecules become "trapped" in the charcoal's micropores and effectively bound to its surface. Charcoal successfully competes with plasma proteins for many highly protein-bound drugs; those few molecules that are not protein bound are continually adsorbed to the charcoal, thereby removing them from the circulation and freeing additional molecules from their transport proteins as the binding reaction equilibrium shifts to replace the free drug removed from the plasma by the charcoal. Adsorption is reversible, but "desorption" is always much slower than adsorption unless the charcoal is rinsed in a nonaqueous solvent. Even then, some solutes are essentially impossible to remove from the charcoal.

The rate of adsorption of a given substance is influenced by such factors as temperature, pH, and the presence of other competing solutes. Sorbents are always much more efficient at removing a specific compound from a simple solution in vitro than when that same compound is dissolved in plasma in which it must compete for pore space in the charcoal with many other plasma solutes. Inorganic compounds display a wide range of adsorbability, with strongly dissociated salts like sodium chloride and potassium nitrate not at all adsorbed and weakly dissociated solutes like mercuric chloride very well adsorbed. Organic substances are more readily adsorbed than inorganic substances, and among organic compounds the lower the solubility in water, the better the compound is adsorbed. Bigger molecules and molecules with branched rather than straight chains are adsorbed better. The obvious limit to these maxims is reached when the molecular sizes become so large that a significant number of the smaller, inner pores become inaccessible to the larger molecules.

Once all of the accessible pores have been occupied by either the toxic compound or a competing solute, no further adsorption is possible, and the charcoal must be replaced. This tendency to become "saturated" over time is an important feature of hemoperfusion and limits the effectiveness of any single treatment to the time required to saturate the cartridge.

Polymers used to coat activated charcoal

A variety of polymer coatings have been developed in an effort to increase the safety of the hemoperfusion system by increasing biocompatibility and limiting the risk of charcoal microembolization. Currently available systems employ such coating materials as cellulose nitrate (Hemokart; Erika), cellulose acetate (Adsorba; Gambro), acrylic hydrogel (Hemacol; Warner-Lambert), heparin-hydrogels (Biocompatible; Clark), and many others. In all of these systems the presence of the coating may inhibit the rate of adsorption of toxic substances, which must first diffuse through the coating material before reaching the charcoal. For compounds of low molecular weight the decrease in adsorption seen with coated vs. uncoated charcoal is minimal, but for large molecules slowed diffusion through the polymeric coating may become the adsorption rate-limiting step.

Although all coatings increase biocompatibility and reduce microembolization, only the heparin-hydrogel developed by Clark purports to prevent clotting of the cartridge. Clark maintains that its cartridges simply will not clot and that the heparin-hydrogel is also less destructive to platelets than other coatings. No comparative data are available to support or refute these claims. Unfortunately patients treated with the Clark system must still be heparinized since thrombosis of the vascular access and blood tubing may still occur.

Uncoated charcoal systems have also been developed. The most widely used of these devices is the fixed-bed charcoal system (B-D Hemodetoxifier) in which carefully washed activated charcoal granules are fixed along a thin layer of polyethylene, which is then rolled into a tube.

Monionic resins

At least one clinically useful adsorbent device does not use charcoal. The uncharged polystyrene resin, Amberlite XAD-4 (XR-004; Extracorporeal Medical Specialties), has specific adsorptive attraction for lipid-soluble solutes. Removal of lipid-soluble drugs such as glutethimide and methaqualone is more efficient with XAD-4 resin hemoperfusion than with activated charcoal. Whether this difference is clinically important is not clear from the available information.

Technical Considerations
Vascular access

Hemoperfusion relies on the same vascular access as hemodialysis (i.e., an arteriovenous shunt or a double-lumen central venous hemodialysis catheter). Single-needle hemodialysis devices, which both withdraw and return blood via the same catheter lumen, are not recommended for use in hemoperfusion as a result of the loss of efficiency caused by the unavoidable recirculation of blood within the single-lumen portion of the circuit. If the child is too small to tolerate a double-lumen dialysis catheter, a second large venous access for return of treated blood can be attempted.

The hemoperfusion circuit

Standard hemodialysis blood lines and the blood pumps on hemodialysis machines are used for hemoperfusion. A typical extracorporeal circuit is

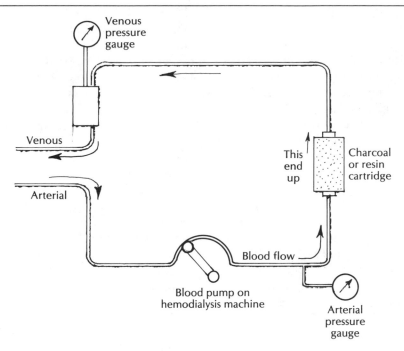

Fig. 147-1   Schematic diagram of a typical extracorporeal circuit used for hemoperfusion. Note that the cartridge is mounted upright on the hemodialysis machine and that blood flows in an "antigravity" direction.

shown in Fig. 147-1. The choice of blood lines (adult to infant) and the size of the hemoperfusion cartridge are determined by the size of the child. The total volume of the extracorporeal circuit, including the cartridge, should not exceed 10% of the child's estimated circulating blood volume (i.e., 8 ml/kg). If using a cartridge that is larger than recommended cannot be avoided, the system must be rinsed with heparinized saline solution as usual and then primed with packed RBCs that have been resuspended in an appropriate volume of saline solution or plasma. The addition of heparin to the blood prime (at least 500 units/300 ml) may help prevent clotting during the initial perfusion of the circuit.

Blood is pumped from the patient in an antigravity direction through the hemoperfusion device (Fig. 147-1) at blood flow rates of 2 to 4 ml/kg/min. Maximum blood flow rates in larger children and adolescents need not exceed 100 ml/min to achieve good results, and rapid flow rates (i.e., >150 ml/min)

are not recommended. Careful attention must be paid to the pressures measured in the circuit before and after the cartridge. An increasing arteriovenous pressure differential is probably due to clotting within the cartridge. When this occurs, the procedure must be terminated at once since increased pressures can cause particulate embolization from the cartridge.

Preparation of the hemoperfusion cartridge

Most cartridges are sterilized by the manufacturer and thus have a limited shelf life. Hemoperfusion is performed infrequently in even the busiest PICUs, which makes maintenance of a large supply of presterilized pediatric-size hemoperfusion cartridges impractical for most centers. One can stock unsterilized cartridges (Clark) that have a shelf life of many years. The Clark cartridge must be very carefully sterilized before use. It can only be steam autoclaved at no more than 250° F for no more than 30 minutes. The rapid drying cycle available on many steam autoclaves must *not* be used since to do so will result in cracking.

All hemoperfusion cartridges must be rinsed before use with heparinized saline solution (5000 units heparin/L) to remove microparticulate matter. Most manufacturers recommend at least a 2 L rinse, the last half of which is performed at high flow rates (300 ml/min). Some cartridges must also have a final rinse with a 5% dextrose solution to reduce the risk of hypoglycemia during treatment. The system must also be pressure tested to 300 mm Hg and discarded if a leak is detected at high pressure.

Heparinization

Patients must be heparinized as for hemodialysis with a loading dose of 100 units/kg and additional heparin as needed to keep the postcartridge blood activated clotting time (ACT) two times normal. A continuous heparin infusion (5 to 20 units/kg/hr) following the loading dose may make the target ACT easier to maintain. Patients with severe coagulopathies whose ACT is already greater than twice normal do not need heparin initially but may need it later during therapy. The ACT must be monitored closely throughout treatment since heparin is efficiently removed by hemoperfusion. The ACT must be measured at intervals no greater than the time needed for the passage of one blood volume through the circuit (e.g., for a child weighing 20 kg receiving hemoperfusion at a blood flow rate of 3 ml/kg/min, the ACT must be measured at least every 26.7 minutes [see below]). Thrombocytopenic patients may suffer a further decline in platelet count during hemoperfusion, resulting in reduced heparin requirements.

Monitoring during hemoperfusion

The following must be monitored during hemoperfusion.
1. ACT in postcartridge blood every 20 to 30 minutes
2. Blood sugar by Dextrostix every 30 minutes
3. Ionized calcium every hour
4. Platelet count every hour
5. Blood pressure frequently (preferably continuously), especially in patients receiving infusions of pressors
6. Drug levels drawn before and after the cartridge every hour to assess degree of charcoal saturation and need for a new cartridge

Duration of therapy

Most hemoperfusion treatments are arbitrarily 3 to 4 hours in length. When drug levels can be followed, treatment can be tailored to the needs of the individual patient and the rate at which the charcoal becomes saturated with the drug. Continuous treatments lasting many hours are possible as long as the cartridges are replaced appropriately. Toxic substances with large volumes of distribution may be effectively cleared from the circulation after 2 or 3 hours of hemoperfusion, only to rebound to former toxic levels a short time after treatment is discontinued as tissue stores of the substance are released into the circulation. A pattern of sequential treatments, each lasting several hours and separated by an equilibration period of variable length, may be an effective strategy in such situations. Every effort must be made to resume hemoperfusion *before* blood levels rebound to life-threatening levels.

Simultaneous hemoperfusion and hemodialysis

Patients needing dialysis for renal failure who also need hemoperfusion (e.g., in poisonings with lipid-soluble and other agents poorly removed by dialysis) may have both procedures performed simultaneously. The hemodialysis membrane is placed in the arterial limb of the extracorporeal hemoperfusion circuit so that blood from the patient first undergoes dialysis and then passes through the hemoperfusion cartridge (Fig. 147-2). Such a system necessitates a large extracorporeal blood volume, and additional heparin may be needed to prevent clotting of the dialyzer. Close monitoring of the ACT is necessary.

Choice of a hemoperfusion cartridge

Table 147-2 lists some of the hemoperfusion systems that are available in pediatric sizes in the United States. Many others are available in Europe and Japan. The choice of one system over another is difficult since no controlled comparative studies of the in vivo performance of the various brands have been published. In our center practical considerations have led to the selection of the Clark system. The long shelf life of the unsterilized Clark cartridges allows maintenance of a supply of all three sizes without fear that the infrequent and unpredictable need for hemoperfusion in the PICU will result in discarding of expensive outdated presterilized cartridges.

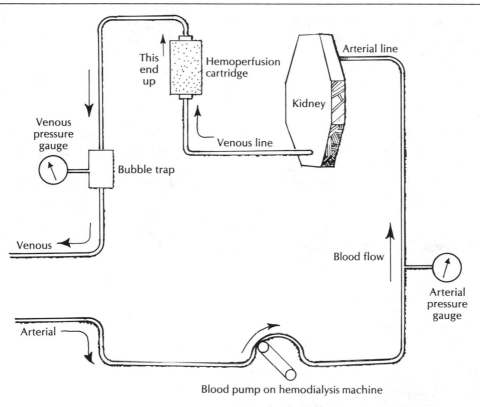

Fig. 147-2   Schematic diagram of the extracorporeal circuit used when hemoperfusion is performed simultaneously with hemodialysis (see text for details).

Table 147-2   Some Hemoperfusion Cartridges Available in Pediatric Sizes

Manufacturer	Brand	Priming Volumes (ml)	Charcoal Content (g)
Gambro	Adsorba	140	150
		260	300
Erika	Hemokart	66	60
		85	85
		155	155
Clark	Biocompatible hemoperfusion systems	50	50
		100	100
		250	350

RISKS AND COMPLICATIONS

Thrombocytopenia. Thrombocytopenia remains the most frequent complication of both charcoal and resin hemoperfusion, although the development of more biocompatible hemoperfusion systems has greatly reduced its severity. Studies in both children and adults suggest that platelet counts may fall to approximately 60% of pretreatment values during a 3-hour hemoperfusion treatment. The observed reduction in platelet count is only rarely associated with clinically important bleeding, and pretreatment values are usually recovered within 24 to 48 hours after a single treatment in a patient who does not have an ongoing consumptive coagulopathy.

When hemoperfusion is used in the management of patients with severe hepatic failure and/or DIC with associated platelet activation, thrombocytopenia may be more severe. Activated platelets are more readily consumed by the cartridge and more easily damaged by passage through the hemoperfusion circuit, a process that increases removal of damaged platelets from the circulation by the reticuloendothelial system.

Severely thrombocytopenic patients (platelet count <50,000/mm³) in need of hemoperfusion optimally should receive a platelet transfusion before treatment. However, in the absence of active bleeding hemoperfusion may be instituted emergently in such patients when clinical circumstances mandate rapid blood purification. Platelets may be given as soon as they become available or may be reserved for transfusion at the completion of the hemoperfusion treatment.

Hypocalcemia. Although calcium is readily adsorbed by activated charcoal, symptomatic hypocalcemia during hemoperfusion is uncommon. Frequent measurements of serum ionized calcium levels during treatment along with appropriate calcium supplementation as needed should prevent this complication.

Hypoglycemia. Simple sugars are also readily adsorbed during hemoperfusion. Some manufacturers recommend rinsing the cartridge with a 5% dextrose solution to reduce the risk of hypoglycemia during treatment. Pediatric patients need to have a continuous source of IV dextrose during hemoperfusion, along with frequent Dextrostix testing. If IV access is a problem, the dextrose infusion can be piggybacked into the postcartridge hemoperfusion blood line.

Hypothermia. Some infants will become hypothermic during hemoperfusion as the blood in the extracorporeal circuit cools to room temperature. A radiant warmer or heating mattress may be used to maintain stable body temperature. Radiant heating of the hemoperfusion cartridge itself is not recommended since temperatures in the cartridge cannot be controlled. Wrapping the cartridge in a water-filled heating pad maintained at 37° C may be helpful when other methods for maintaining the infant's temperature are unsuccessful.

Hypotension. Hemodynamically unstable patients may experience a precipitous drop in systemic arterial blood pressure shortly after hemoperfusion is begun. Patients receiving infusions of pressors are at particular risk since these agents are adsorbed by the charcoal. Endogenous catecholamines are also removed from the circulation during hemoperfusion, as are cortisol, angiotensin, aldosterone, and thyroxine. Systemic blood pressure must be monitored closely in all patients, and appropriate adjustments in pressor infusion rates can be made. Marginally hypovolemic patients will become frankly hypotensive in this setting unless given adequate plasma volume expansion.

A combination of volume expansion and increased pressor infusion rates usually results in prompt stabilization of the systemic arterial blood pressure at acceptable levels. As hemoperfusion progresses, blood pressure often becomes easier to maintain on steadily decreasing pressor infusion rates as a result of saturation of the cartridge. Another period of instability and hypotension can be expected in these patients each time a new cartridge is placed in the circuit.

Miscellaneous complications. Leukopenia, fibrinogenopenia, anemia, and charcoal microembolization have largely disappeared as complications since the development of biocompatible coated adsorbents. Complications associated with central venous access, including hemorrhage, thrombosis, embolic disorders, and infection, must be considered. Patients with renal insufficiency and/or major disturbances of fluid and electrolyte metabolism will not benefit from and may actually worsen during hemoperfusion. These patients should be treated with a combination of hemoperfusion and hemodialysis if hemodialysis alone is inadequate.

ADDITIONAL READING

Chang TMS. Hemoperfusion in 1981. Contrib Nephrol 29:11-22, 1982.

Chang TMS. Hemoperfusion, exchange transfusion, cross circulation, liver perfusion, hormones and immobilized enzymes. In Brunner G, Schmidt FW, eds. Artificial Liver Support. Berlin: Springer-Verlag, 1981, pp 26-133.

Cooney DO. Activated Charcoal: Antidotal and Other Medical Uses. New York: Marcel Dekker, 1980.

Gelfand MC. Hemoperfusion in toxic ingestions and hepatic encephalopathy: Have the expectations been achieved? Contrib Nephrol 29:101-113, 1982.

Hirasawa H, Odaka M, Sugai T, et al. Prognostic value of serum osmolal gap in patients with multiple organ failure treated with hemopurification. Artif Organs 12:382-387, 1988.

• Papadopoulou ZL, Novello AC. The use of hemoperfusion in children: Past, present and future. Pediatr Clin North Am 29:1039-1052, 1982.

Winchester JF. Use of dialysis and hemoperfusion in treatment of poisoning. In Daugidas JT, Ing TS, eds. Handbook of Dialysis. Boston: Little Brown, 1988, pp 437-448.

• Winchester JF. Active methods for detoxification: Oral sorbents, forced diuresis, hemoperfusion and hemodialysis. In Haddad LM, Winchester JF, eds. Clinical Management of Poisoning and Drug Overdose. Philadelphia: WB Saunders, 1983, pp 154-169.

Winchester JF, Gelfand MC, Krepshield JH, et al. Dialysis and hemoperfusion of poisons and drugs: Update. Trans Am Soc Artif Intern Organs 23:762-784, 1977.

Yau Y, Yao-Ting Y, Ji-Chang S, et al. A new DNA immune adsorbent for hemoperfusion in SLE therapy: A clinical trial. Artif Organs 12:444-448, 1988.

148 Continuous Arteriovenous Hemofiltration

Steven R. Alexander

BACKGROUND

The most recent addition to the renal replacement therapy arsenal is continuous arteriovenous hemofiltration (CAVH), a promising new approach to the treatment of acute renal failure that offers several advantages over traditional dialysis modalities when used in critically ill, unstable patients. The simplicity and inherent logic of the CAVH system is striking: a small filter, which is highly permeable to water and small solutes but impermeable to plasma proteins and the formed elements of the blood, is placed in a low-resistance extracorporeal circuit connecting a large artery and vein. Blood is pumped through the CAVH circuit by the heart, with the patient's arterial-to-venous pressure gradient providing sufficient perfusion pressure to drive the CAVH system. As the blood perfuses the "hemofilter," an ultrafiltrate of plasma is removed in a manner analogous to glomerular ultrafiltration. The ultrafiltrate is concurrently replaced using a fluid with an electrolyte composition that is either similar to that of normal plasma or specifically designed to correct electrolyte abnormalities present in the individual patient. A portion of the ultrafiltrate volume can be replaced with total parenteral nutrition (TPN) solutions, and in patients with fluid overload a portion of the ultrafiltrate volume is simply not replaced, resulting in predictable and *controllable* negative fluid balance.

The most notable characteristic of CAVH is that it provides *continuous* renal replacement therapy, thus allowing removal of solutes and modification of the volume and composition of the extracellular fluid to occur evenly over time. Unstable patients, who are often intolerant of the abrupt fluid and solute changes that accompany standard hemodialysis treatments, can usually be treated safely with CAVH. The preci-

sion and stability with which water and electrolyte balance can be maintained using CAVH is unmatched by any of the alternative dialysis therapies; even continuous peritoneal dialysis (see Chapter 145) does not allow the physician to *control* the ultrafiltration rate as can be done in CAVH, and only with CAVH can electrolytes be removed or added to the patient independently of changes in the volume of total body water. The CAVH technique is simple. It can be initiated rapidly in the PICU setting and does not require complex equipment or the presence of a dialysis nurse.

All of these features have made CAVH a particularly attractive therapy for the critically ill pediatric patient whose condition has been further compromised by renal failure. Unfortunately, although there is substantial and rapidly proliferating literature on the use of CAVH in adults, reported experience with CAVH in children is sparse. The first description of successful CAVH in a pediatric patient appeared in 1985, and to date published pediatric experience totals fewer than 50 patients. Thus the CAVH guidelines and suggestions offered in this chapter necessarily reflect to a large degree the author's personal experience, which encompasses approximately 45 infants and children treated with CAVH since 1985. The specific techniques described here are primarily those currently used at Children's Medical Center of Dallas, many of which are certain to be modified as our experience with this new modality grows. Moreover, the indications offered in this chapter for the use of CAVH in children must be considered tentative at best. Much more experience will be needed before clinical settings can be identified in which CAVH would be preferred over hemodialysis or peritoneal dialysis. Although it appears CAVH has an important role to play in the PICU, that role is still evolving and has yet to be clearly defined.

Development of CAVH

The origins of CAVH can be traced to the early days of the development of chronic hemodialysis. In the mid-1960s Henderson and his associates described a renal replacement therapy that relied solely on the process of ultrafiltration, using membranes that were much more permeable to water and small solutes than the usual hemodialysis membranes. The technique was termed "diafiltration" and later, more appropriately, "hemofiltration."

Henderson showed that by pumping blood at high flow rates through an extracorporeal circuit that contains a highly permeable filter, large volumes of an ultrafiltrate of plasma can be generated. This "uremic" ultrafiltrate can be replaced concurrently with fluid that has an electrolyte composition similar to that of normal plasma. Hemofiltration is thus technically similar to hemodialysis: both modalities require vascular access, an extracorporeal circuit, a semipermeable membrane, and a blood pump. There are, however, differences between the two modalities in the manner in which solutes are removed from the blood.

During any renal replacement therapy there are two transport mechanisms that can be involved in the transfer of solutes across a semipermeable membrane: *diffusion* and *convection*. Diffusive transport is driven by the solute concentration gradients that exist between blood and dialysate. Solute molecules are transferred across the membrane in the direction of the lower solute concentration and at a rate inversely proportional to their molecular weight. For example, during peritoneal dialysis urea diffuses across the peritoneal membrane from blood to dialysate while dextrose diffuses from dialysate to blood. Convective transport occurs when a solute molecule is swept through the membrane by a moving stream of solvent, a process that is also called "solvent drag." Convective transport is independent of any solute concentration gradient that might be present across the membrane; only the direction and force (or rate) of transmembrane solvent flux are important determinants of convective transport.

During hemodialysis solute movement across the dialysis membrane from blood to dialysate is primarily the result of diffusive transport. Convective transport also occurs during hemodialysis when fluid is removed from the blood, but convection accounts for only a small fraction of the total solute removed during a hemodialysis treatment (see Chapter 146). During hemofiltration, since no dialysate is used, diffusive transport cannot occur. Solute transfer is entirely dependent on convective transport. The relative inefficiency with which solutes are removed from the blood by convective transport alone is one of the most distinctive features of hemofiltration.

Henderson proposed hemofiltration as an alternative to chronic hemodialysis. To be an effective chronic treatment for uremia, hemofiltration must generate a very large volume of ultrafiltrate (e.g., 25 to 50 L per treatment for the average adult with end-stage renal disease [ESRD] who receives 3-hour hemofiltration treatments three times per week). All but approximately 2 of the nearly 50 L of ultrafiltrate generated during a single hemofiltration treatment must be continuously and accurately replaced with a sterile, pyrogen-free replacement fluid. The replacement fluid is costly, and as a result, hemofiltration is substantially more expensive than hemodialysis. High costs and the technical problems involved in precise measurement and rapid replacement of very large volumes of ultrafiltrate stifled interest in hemofiltration as a chronic renal replacement therapy in all but a few ESRD centers.

Several early investigators noted that hemofiltration had at least one potentially important advantage over hemodialysis: when chronic hemodialysis patients were converted to treatment with chronic hemofiltration, they consistently experienced a marked reduction in the number of episodes of symptomatic hypotension occurring during treatments. In 1976 Bergstrom and associates reported that unstable hemodialysis patients (with either acute or chronic renal failure) tolerated fluid removal better if ultrafiltration alone were performed before the initiation of standard diffusion hemodialysis. Henderson and others had originally suggested that hemofiltration might be a safe method with which to remove fluid from unstable, oliguric patients who had acute congestive heart failure. Thus the stage was set for CAVH to emerge as a modified hemofiltration technique that was especially well suited for use in critically ill, unstable patients.

The conceptualization of CAVH as a treatment for acute renal failure was the work of Peter Kramer, a nephrologist in Göttingen, West Germany, who was familiar with the use of intermittent pumped hemofiltration in patients with acute and chronic renal failure. The story is told by one of Dr. Kramer's former students that in May 1977, as Kramer was preparing to perform a 3-hour pumped hemofiltration treatment on an unstable adult ICU patient, one of the vascular access catheters intended for the femoral vein was inadvertently placed in the femoral artery. Seizing the moment, Kramer placed the second catheter in the contralateral femoral vein and connected the hemofilter between the arterial and venous blood lines. To his delight Kramer observed that the patient's cardiac function alone was a sufficient driving force to produce large volumes of ultrafiltrate from this simple "arteriovenous" hemofiltration circuit. By allowing the circuit to operate continuously 24 hours per day, Kramer demonstrated that his "CAVH" system could generate enough ultrafiltrate to serve as a complete renal replacement therapy in anuric adults. He also showed that the CAVH system could be safely and successfully maintained in continuous operation for many days. (One of Kramer's early patients received 38 days of CAVH, eventually recovering normal renal function.)

It is a sad footnote to the history of CAVH that Dr. Kramer died suddenly in 1984 before he could fully appreciate the impact his contributions would have on the management of acute renal failure in patients of all ages throughout the world.

INDICATIONS

The clinical indications for CAVH in pediatric patients have not been clearly defined. In general CAVH can be an effective renal replacement therapy in the following clinical settings: (1) acute renal failure; (2) diuretic-resistant fluid overload resulting from poor cardiac output, with or without renal failure; (3) electrolyte or acid-base disturbances; and (4) unstable chronic renal failure patients who cannot be treated with hemodialysis or peritoneal dialysis. Most patients with acute renal failure can be successfully treated using either hemodialysis or peritoneal dialysis. However, patients with multiple organ system failure are often intolerant of standard dialysis therapies because of hemodynamic instability. These patients are usually hypercatabolic and need large volumes of TPN and other parenteral fluids. It is in these patients that CAVH may become the treatment of choice.

CAVH may also be preferred in patients with fluid overload and hemodynamic instability who are re-

Table 148-1   Hemodynamic Response to Fluid Removal With Different Renal Replacement Therapies

	Acetate Hemodialysis	Bicarbonate Hemodialysis	CAVH
Cardiac output	↓	↓	↑↑
Peripheral resistance	↓↓	↑→	↓
Blood pressure	↓↓	→	↑

↓ = decrease; ↑ = increase; → = no change.

fractory to diuretics because of poor cardiac output. Fluid removal by hemodialysis is poorly tolerated by these patients, and peritoneal dialysis may be ineffective because of inadequate perfusion of the peritoneum. Neonates and other small infants who have these problems may do particularly well when treated with CAVH.

It is unclear why CAVH is so well tolerated by hemodynamically unstable patients. The hemodynamic response to fluid removal with different renal replacement therapies is summarized in Table 148-1. Note that cardiac output falls during fluid removal by hemodialysis but not during CAVH. Peripheral resistance also falls during hemodialysis when acetate is used as the buffer, often resulting in marked hypotension. Hemodialysis with bicarbonate buffer produces a stable to slightly increased peripheral resistance and a more stable systemic arterial blood pressure. During CAVH peripheral resistance decreases, whereas cardiac output increases; the net result is usually an *increase* in systemic arterial blood pressure as a result of an overall improvement in myocardial function. Peripheral vasodilation and afterload reduction may explain, in part, the improvement in cardiac function seen in patients treated with CAVH. Other possible explanations include the removal of cardiotoxic factors from the circulation such as myocardial depressant factor or endotoxins.

Some pediatric patients seem to be particularly well suited for CAVH. These include:

1. Infants and small children with congestive heart failure who also have diuretic-unresponsive oliguria despite inotropic support
2. Neonates with fluid overload who can be dif-

ficult to treat with the use of peritoneal dialysis because of poor perfusion of the peritoneal membrane

3. Oliguric patients requiring large volumes of TPN or other fluids (e.g., blood products in patients with DIC), perhaps because fluid removal is adjusted concurrently with fluid administration during CAVH
4. Patients with combined renal and hepatic failure, both before and after liver transplantation
5. Hemodynamically unstable children following cardiac surgery
6. Patients receiving prolonged extracorporeal membrane oxygenation (ECMO) who develop renal insufficiency or fluid-electrolyte disturbances or high TPN requirements
7. Patients maintained on cardiopulmonary bypass for prolonged periods during cardiac surgery
8. Patients with septic shock

CONTRAINDICATIONS

Active bleeding is a relative contraindication to CAVH, especially if peritoneal dialysis can be performed. A recent CNS hemorrhage that might be extended by heparinization is also a relative contraindication unless alternative anticoagulation methods are used. The presence of a severe coagulopathy should not be considered a contraindication to CAVH. Such patients usually do not need heparinization, and CAVH can be remarkably successful in patients whose coagulopathy keeps their filters from clotting. These patients are at increased risk for local bleeding during placement of the arterial access.

CAVH must *not* be considered as emergency treatment for life-threatening hyperkalemia. Potassium removal by CAVH is slow compared to potassium removal with hemodialysis or even peritoneal dialysis. However, if the hyperkalemic patient is not a candidate for dialysis or tolerates it poorly, CAVH may be attempted using one of the techniques designed

Table 148-2   Renal Replacement Therapies in Acute Renal Failure

Modality	Goals	Solute Transport	Uremia Control	Tolerance by Unstable Patient
Hemodialysis (HD)	Complete renal replacement therapy (RRT)	Diffusion and convection	Excellent	Poor
Peritoneal dialysis (PD)	Complete RRT	Diffusion and convection	Good	Fair to good
Isolated ultrafiltration	Isotonic plasma volume contraction often before HD in unstable patient	Convection	Inadequate	Good
Slow continuous ultrafiltration (SCUF)	Continuous removal of plasma water and solutes without replacement	Convection	Poor	Excellent
Continuous arteriovenous hemofiltration (CAVH)	Continuous removal of uremic plasma water replaced with balanced electrolyte solution	Convection	Good only when large volumes replaced	Excellent
Continuous arteriovenous hemodiafiltration (CAVHD)	Combines CAVH and HD without blood pumps	Convection and diffusion	Good to excellent	Excellent

to increase solute clearances (i.e., CAVHD or high-flow pre-dilution, described later in this chapter).

TECHNIQUE
Definitions

As with most new therapies, the advent of CAVH has been accompanied by a plethora of esoteric terms, most of which have limited utility. There are at least three basic configurations to the clinical application of continuous hemofiltration (without blood pumps)

that are listed in Table 148-2: continuous arteriovenous hemofiltration (CAVH); slow continuous ultrafiltration (SCUF); and continuous arteriovenous hemodiafiltration (CAVHD). Selected characteristics of hemodialysis, peritoneal dialysis, and isolated ultrafiltration are also included in Table 148-2 for comparison with the hemofiltration techniques.

CAVH as designed by Kramer is intended to be a complete renal replacement therapy, requiring large volumes of ultrafiltrate and replacement fluid. The

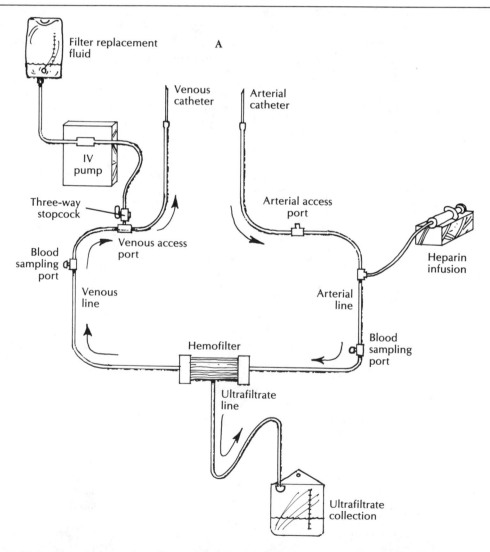

Fig. 148-1   Commonly used configurations for continuous hemofiltration. **A,** CAVH. **B,** SCUF. (Courtesy Amicon Division, W.R. Grace & Co., Danvers, Mass.)

basic components of the CAVH circuit are shown in Fig. 148-1, *A*. SCUF is the process that uses continuous hemofiltration only to remove excess fluid such as in the patient with diuretic-unresponsive oliguria (with or without uremia). The circuit used for SCUF is the same as for CAVH except that no replacement fluid is administered (Fig. 148-1, *B*). The process that allows dialysate to flow through the ultrafiltrate compartment of the hemofilter, thereby increasing solute removal by the addition of diffusive transport, is

CAVHD; the CAVHD circuit is diagrammed in Fig. 148-1, *C*.

It is also possible to perform hemofiltration without arterial access, using a blood pump. When performed continuously using relatively slow blood flow rates, this procedure is called continuous venovenous hemofiltration (CVVH). Much of the inherent simplicity and convenience of CAVH is lost when CVVH is used. Moreover, in our center the continuous operation of an extracorporeal blood pump in

B

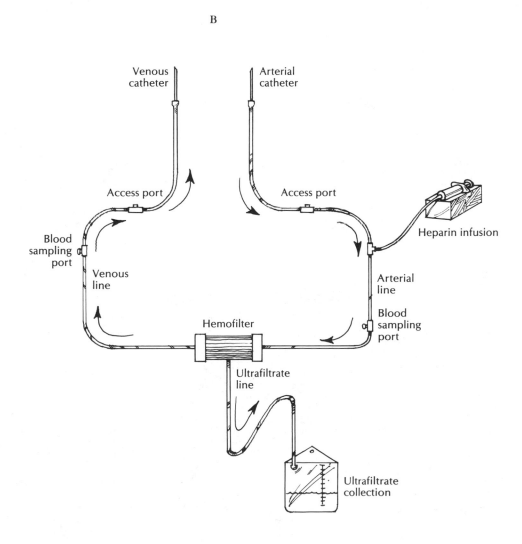

Continued.

the PICU would require the continuous presence of a hemodialysis nurse, resulting in a staffing nightmare for our dialysis program. For this reason we have not used CVVH.

However, there may be a role for an initial period of pump-assisted CAVH in infants and small children who have severe systemic hypotension caused at least

in part by congestive heart failure. Initially blood pressure in these infants may not be adequate to drive the CAVH system without blood pump assistance. After several hours of pump-assisted CAVH or SCUF, cardiac function may improve sufficiently to allow the use of standard CAVH. The pump-assisted CAVH circuit is diagrammed in Fig. 148-1, *D*.

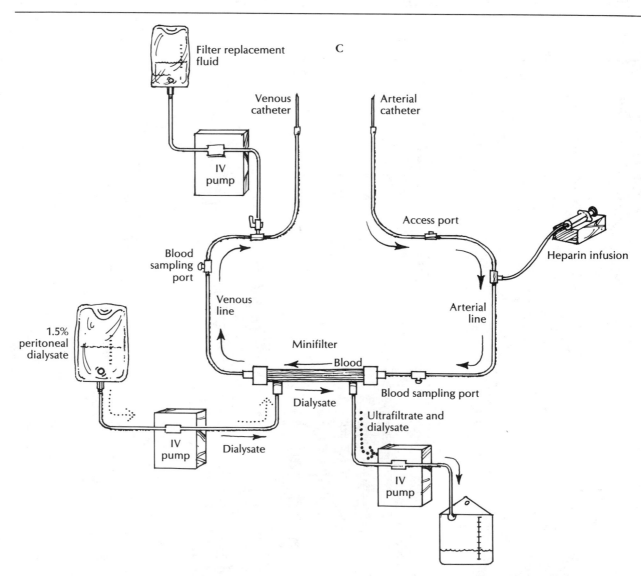

Fig. 148-1, cont'd **C**, CAVHD. **D**, Pump-assisted CAVH. Diagrams of tubing sets and hemofilters shown in *A, B,* and *D* are modeled after the Amicon D-10. *C* shows the Amicon Minifilter and tubing set.

Basic Concepts

CAVH extracorporeal circuit

The standard CAVH system (Fig. 148-1, *A*) consists of (1) arterial and venous access; (2) arterial and venous blood tubing containing multiple ports for blood sampling and attachment of the replacement fluid line; (3) a hemofilter; (4) a heparin administration line attached to the arterial blood tubing; and (5) an ultrafiltrate line leading from the hemofilter to a collection device. Blood flowing from the arterial access catheter is joined by a continuous heparin infusion before it passes through the hollow fibers of the hemofilter. As the anticoagulated blood perfuses the filter, an ultrafiltrate is formed and is collected in the

D

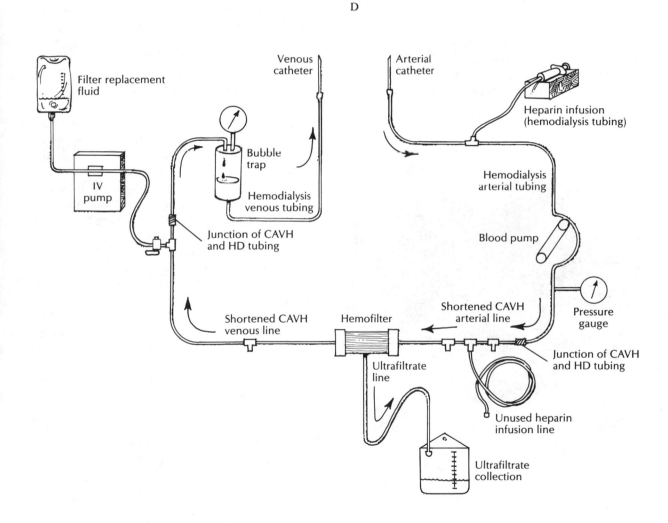

space within the filter that surrounds the hollow fibers. The ultrafiltrate flows out through the ultrafiltrate line and down to a collection device positioned 30 to 40 cm below the filter. In Fig. 148-1, *A*, replacement fluid is shown being administered into the venous line, but it can be administered through the access port on either the arterial (pre-dilution) or the venous (post-dilution) side of the filter.

CAVH membranes

The CAVH membrane is shown in Fig. 148-2. It is a composite structure consisting of (1) an inner thin layer adjacent to the blood path, which contains pores of equal diameter and length and which is surrounded by (2) a supporting superstructure (an "exoskeleton"), which provides mechanical integrity without restricting the passage of water or any solutes small enough to pass first through the pores of the

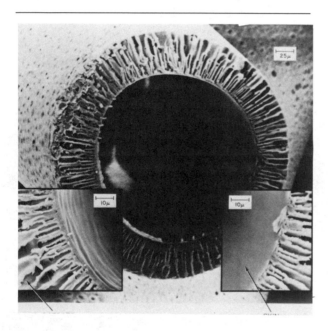

Fig. 148-2 Scanning electron micrograph showing a transection of a typical hollow-fiber hemofiltration membrane. Inner diameter equals 200 μm. Inset shows the inner thin layer, pockmarked by pores of equal diameter and length. Note the ever-increasing diameters of the channels that traverse the outer superstructure of the membrane. (From Lysaght M, Boggs D. Transport in continuous arteriovenous hemofiltration and slow continuous ultrafiltration. In Paganani EP, ed. Acute Continuous Renal Replacement Therapy. Boston: Kluwer, 1986, pp 43-50.)

inner layer. The hemofiltration membrane superstructure is responsible for the membrane's high permeability to water. Unlike hemodialysis membranes, which contain long interconnecting pores of different sizes that extend throughout the full thickness of the membrane, resulting in high resistance to fluid flow, the hemofiltration membrane superstructure consists of channels of ever-increasing diameter that offer little resistance to fluid flow. CAVH membranes from different manufacturers may have different pore sizes, but all of the pores in any one membrane tend to be of similar size. Most hemofiltration membranes offer no impediment to transport of solutes with molecular mass <500 to 1000 daltons (e.g., urea, creatinine, uric acid, sodium, potassium, ionized calcium, almost all drugs not bound to plasma proteins), and all CAVH membranes are impermeable to albumin and other solutes with molecular mass >50,000 daltons.

Several different synthetic materials have been developed for use in hemofiltration membranes (e.g., polysulfone, polyacrylonitrile, polyamide). Fortunately all of these materials are much more biocompatible than the materials currently used in hemodialysis membranes (e.g., cupruphan, cellulose acetate). For example, complement activation, which is common during hemodialysis (see Chapter 146), does not occur during hemofiltration. Similarly, leukopenia, which occurs early during hemodialysis treatments and may be associated with hypoxemia, is not encountered during hemofiltration. Thrombocytopenia and hemolysis also are not seen during CAVH. The high degree of biocompatibility demonstrated by hemofiltration membranes is an obviously essential feature of a treatment that requires that the membrane remain in constant contact with the blood for very prolonged periods (days to weeks).

Factors governing ultrafiltration in CAVH

The ultrafiltration rate (Qf) in CAVH is a function of the surface area of the membrane participating in ultrafiltration (Ap), the permeability coefficient of the membrane to water (k), and the transmembrane pressure gradient (TMP):

$$Qf = (Ap) \times (k) \times (TMP)$$

As in the glomerular capillary, for ultrafiltration to occur in CAVH or SCUF there must be a transmembrane pressure gradient (the filtration pressure) that favors movement of water from the blood to the opposite side of the membrane. The filtration pressure is primarily determined by the net sum of three pressures: (1) the positive hydraulic pressure of the blood; (2) the negative hydrostatic pressure exerted by the ultrafiltrate column; and (3) the oncotic pressure within the filter fibers. This relationship can be approximated by the following equation:

$$TMP = \frac{(Pi + Po)}{2} + (Pf) - \frac{(\pi i + \pi o)}{2}$$

where TMP is the filtration pressure or transmembrane pressure gradient; Pi is the hydraulic pressure of the blood at the inlet of the filter; Po is the hydraulic pressure of the blood at the outlet of the filter; Pf is the negative hydrostatic pressure exerted by the ultrafiltrate column; πi is the oncotic pressure at the inlet of the filter; and πo is the oncotic pressure at the outlet of the filter.

A more rigorous calculation of TMP is beyond the scope of this text.

The relationship between oncotic, hydraulic, and hydrostatic pressures is extremely important in CAVH. Although the same forces are theoretically involved in determining TMP during standard hemodialysis, additional positive or negative pressure can be mechanically applied to the hemodialysis circuit to maintain the net TMP favoring ultrafiltration as high as 300 to 400 mm Hg. Plasma protein concentration and the resulting oncotic pressure that opposes ultrafiltration during hemodialysis is inconsequential in comparison to the mechanically applied TMP and thus may be ignored.

Not so with CAVH, where the net TMP favoring ultrafiltration may be only 10 to 20 mm Hg. Several factors are at work to keep the TMP low during CAVH. Hydraulic pressure reaching the filter (Pi) is much less than the patient's systemic arterial pressure, primarily due to pressure loss that occurs when blood flows through the arterial access catheter. Hydraulic pressure continues to fall throughout the length of the arterial limb of the circuit. The length and internal diameter of the arterial tubing are important determinants of hydraulic pressure loss, with short, large-bore tubing minimizing pressure losses. Additional hydraulic pressure loss occurs within the filter fibers, depending, in part, on the resistance to flow inherent in the design of each filter. Currently available CAVH filters and tubing are designed to minimize hydraulic pressure losses; thus, if pressure loss occurs in the arterial limb of the circuit, it is almost always the consequence of inadequate, kinked, or thrombosed

arterial access. The insertion of a three-way stopcock or any other flow-restricting device into the arterial limb of the circuit will also have an undesirable effect on Pi.

The negative hydrostatic pressure (Pf) generated by the weight of the column of ultrafiltrate is determined by the height of the filter above the collection device according to the formula:

$$Pf \text{ (in mm Hg)} = [\text{Height (in cm)}] \times (0.74)$$

When the height of the filter is 40 cm above the collection device (a typical bedside configuration), Pf is approximately 30 mm Hg. This additional 30 mm Hg favoring ultrafiltration that is provided by the Pf is critically important to the production of ultrafiltrate during CAVH, where hydraulic pressures reaching the filter inlet (Pi) are often relatively low. For example, in a typical CAVH circuit Pi often falls to only 20 to 30 mm Hg, even when the patient's mean systemic arterial pressure is 90 mm Hg or more. In children, who often have mean systemic arterial pressures below 60 mm Hg, the total of the pressure favoring ultrafiltration (Pi + Pf) rarely exceeds 50 mm Hg at its highest point at the filter inlet. Hydraulic pressure continues to fall as the blood encounters the resistance of the filter. By the time the filter outlet is reached, Pf is usually the predominant pressure favoring ultrafiltration.

Ultrafiltration is opposed by the oncotic pressure within the filter fibers, which is a function of plasma protein concentration. Oncotic pressure can be estimated using the formula:

$$\text{Oncotic pressure (in mm Hg)} = [(2.1) \times (c) + [(0.16) \times (c^2)] + [(0.009) \times (c^3)]$$

where c is the total serum protein concentration in g/dl.

When total serum protein concentration is between 6 and 8 g/dl, the oncotic pressure at the filter inlet (πi) ranges between 20 and 35 mm Hg. At this point Pi + Pf is greater than πi, and ultrafiltration occurs. However, as blood perfuses the filter, ultrafiltrate is removed, and the plasma protein concentration and its corresponding oncotic pressure increase accordingly. A point of "filtration pressure equilibrium" is reached in most hemofilters when the rising oncotic pressure (πe) equals the sum of the falling hydraulic pressure (Pe) and the stable hydrostatic pressure: $\pi e = Pe + Pf$. When filtration pressure equilibrium is reached, ultrafiltration abruptly ceases.

The filter blood flow rate (QB) is also a critical factor in the development of filtration pressure equilibrium. The rate at which the oncotic pressure rises is determined by the filtration fraction (FF), which is that fraction of plasma water removed by ultrafiltration. For any given filtration pressure FF is determined by the QB. When QB is high, FF remains low, oncotic pressure rises slowly, and filtration pressure equilibrium is reached slowly, if at all. When QB is low, FF is increased and with it the oncotic pressure. Filtration pressure equilibrium is reached earlier in the filter, resulting in a decrease in the ultrafiltration rate and predisposing the filter to clotting. These concepts as defined by Bosch and Ronco and others are presented schematically in Fig. 148-3.

Consideration of the factors responsible for filtration pressure equilibrium is particularly important when CAVH is attempted in pediatric patients who often have low systemic (hydraulic) pressures and low filter blood flow rates. The hemofilters used in adults contain hollow fibers that are long enough to allow the development of filtration pressure equilibrium at some point in the filter. This point occurs particularly early when one of these "long" adult filters is used in a hypotensive child who has a low QB (Fig. 148-3). In this setting a relatively large segment of the filter becomes unavailable for ultrafiltration. The blood beyond the filtration pressure equilibrium point is characterized by a higher Hct value, higher protein concentration, and higher viscosity. The movement of highly viscous blood through a long segment of the filter not used for filtration leads to increased resistance to blood flow within the filter and a further drop in hydraulic pressure. Eventually a vicious cycle develops, which ultimately results in clotting of the filter.

The problems associated with filtration pressure equilibrium in pediatric CAVH have led us to the almost exclusive use of two hemofilters, the Amicon Minifilter and the Amicon D-10, which are designed to minimize the effects of these problems. We have also routinely administered filter replacement fluid on the arterial side of the filter (i.e., pre-dilution mode) to keep oncotic pressure low. These maneuvers are discussed in detail later in this chapter.

Filter blood flow (QB)

It is apparent from the preceding discussion that adequate QB is a prerequisite to successful CAVH. QB is determined primarily by the mean arterial pressure of the patient, the arterial vascular access site (e.g., femoral artery, umbilical artery, arteriovenous shunt, fistula), and the internal diameter, configuration (tapered vs. straight), and length of the arterial access catheter. QB is also influenced by blood viscosity (Hct and protein concentration), the length and internal diameter of the hemofilter tubing, the patency of the hemofilter blood pathways (i.e., how many of the filter's hollow fibers have clotted or are obstructed by entrapment of air), and the backflow pressure in the venous limb of the circuit, which is determined by the resistance generated by the venous access catheter and the patient's venous pressure. Maximum QB yields maximum Qf.

Blood flow at the filter inlet (QB) can be easily estimated by obtaining simultaneous blood samples for Hct determination from the sampling ports located on the arterial [(Hct)inlet] and venous [(Hct)-

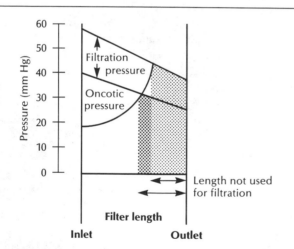

Fig. 148-3 Schematic representation of filtration pressure equilibrium. Two different filtration pressures are shown. The shaded areas represent the filter length not used for ultrafiltration because of filtration pressure equilibrium. At the lower filtration pressure filtration pressure equilibrium occurs nearer the filter inlet, resulting in an increase in the length not available for ultrafiltration. (Modified from Bosch JP, Ronco C. Continuous arteriovenous hemofiltration [CAVH] and other continuous replacement therapies: Operational characteristics and clinical use. In Maher JF, ed. Replacement of Renal Function by Dialysis, 3rd ed. Boston: Kluwer, 1989, pp 347-359.)

outlet] lines (Fig. 148-1, *A*) while measuring the spontaneous ultrafiltration rate (Qf) from a timed volumetric collection (in ml/min):

$$QB = \frac{(Qf) \times [(Hct)outlet]}{[(Hct)outlet] - [(Hct)inlet]}$$

Plasma flow at the filter inlet (QP) is calculated from the QB and the Hct value at the inlet:

$$QP = (QB) - (RBC\ mass)$$

where the RBC mass at the inlet equals

$$\frac{(QB) \times [(Hct)inlet]}{100}$$

and where (Hct)inlet is expressed as a percentage.

Filtration fraction

The FF is an important indicator of the efficiency of the CAVH system, reflecting that fraction of plasma water that is being removed by ultrafiltration. The FF can be calculated from the following formulas:

$$FF(\%) = \frac{Qf}{QP} \times 100$$

$$FF(\%) = (1) - \frac{(Pro)inlet}{(Pro)outlet} \times 100$$

where Qf is the ultrafiltration rate (ml/min); QP is the plasma flow rate at the inlet (ml/min); and (Pro) is the blood total protein concentration (g/dl) measured at the arterial ([Pro]inlet) and venous ([Pro]outlet) sampling ports.

The optimum FF is one that is high enough to provide an adequate ultrafiltration rate to meet the solute and fluid removal needs of the individual patient but not so high that it leads to increased blood viscosity, increased oncotic pressure, an earlier filtration pressure equilibrium point, and consequent filter clotting. When conditions will allow, the FF should probably be kept near 30%. A higher FF is possible and may be unavoidable when blood pressure and QB are low, but such high FFs are usually associated with frequent clotting of the filter.

Composition of the ultrafiltrate

The ultrafiltrate formed during CAVH has essentially the same small-solute composition as plasma water. Representative plasma and ultrafiltrate concentrations for several solutes reported by Kaplan and others are listed in Table 148-3. Note that there is a small but detectable difference in the handling of cations and anions resulting from the Gibbs-Donnan

Table 148-3 Concentrations of Selected Solutes in Ultrafiltrate and Plasma During CAVH With Corresponding Sieving Coefficients*

Solute	Ultrafiltrate Concentration	Plasma Concentration	Sieving Coefficient
Sodium (mEq/L)	135.3	136.2	0.993
Potassium (mEq/L)	4.05	4.11	0.985
Chloride (mEq/L)	103.7	99.3	1.046
CO_2 (mEq/L)	22.13	19.78	1.124
BUN (mg/dl)	82.9	79.1	1.048
Creatinine (mg/dl)	6.63	6.5	1.020
Uric acid (mg/dl)	7.54	7.35	1.016
Phosphorus (mg/dl)	4.15	3.94	1.044
Glucose (mg/dl)	173.0	164.5	1.043
Total proteins (g/dl)	0.13	6.21	0.021
Albumin (g/dl)	0.02	2.65	0.008
Calcium (mg/dl)	5.12	8.08	0.637
Total bilirubin (mg/dl)	0.44	12.1	0.030
Direct bilirubin (mg/dl)	0.26	7.35	0.030
CPK (IU/L)	66.5	80.9	0.676
Magnesium (mEq/L)	1.53	1.74	0.879

*Reproduced with permission from Kaplan AA, Longnecker RI, Folkert VW. Continuous arteriovenous hemofiltration: A report of 6 months experience. Ann Intern Med 100:358-367, 1984.

effect created by the acccumulation of anionic proteins on the plasma side of the membrane, which tends to retard passage of cations and encourage passage of anions. These effects are not clinically important. It is important to note the lower ultrafiltrate concentration of calcium, which results from protein binding of a portion of total plasma calcium. Ultrafiltrate calcium concentration is then a reasonable approximation of plasma ionized calcium concentration.

Solute clearance and sieving coefficients

CAVH relies entirely on convective transport for clearance of solutes from the blood. In the absence of a gradient for diffusion the ratio between ultrafiltrate and plasma concentrations of a given solute is called the sieving coefficient (S):

$$S = \frac{\text{Concentration of x in ultrafiltrate } [(x)Uf]}{\text{Concentration of x in plasma } [(x)plasma]}$$

Sieving coefficients are also given for the solutes listed in Table 148-3. When S is known for a given solute, the concentration of the solute in the ultrafiltrate [(x)UF] will be simply:

$$(x)UF = (S) \times (x)plasma$$

Therefore solute clearance (Cx) in CAVH can be calculated as follows:

$$Cx = \frac{[(x)Uf] \times (Qf)}{[(x)plasma]}$$
$$= (S) \times (Qf)$$

Since S for most small solutes is approximately 1 (Table 148-3), the clearance of these solutes closely approximates the ultrafiltration rate, Qf. For example, urea clearance [C(urea)] obtained with CAVH is simply

$$C(urea) = Qf$$

Technical Considerations
Vascular access

In no other extracorporeal therapy is the quality of the vascular access as critical to the success of the procedure as it is in CAVH. Achieving adequate arterial access in infants and young children can be particularly difficult. Four types of access are commonly used for CAVH in pediatric patients:

1. Percutaneous or surgical cannulation of a major artery and vein

2. Placement of a Scribner arteriovenous shunt, usually in a lower extremity
3. Use of an existing arteriovenous fistula or graft for arterial access, with venous return via another site
4. Possibly use of the umbilical artery and vein in newborns (up to approximately 5 days of age)

Successful CAVH in infants and children has been reported using the umbilical, radial, brachial, dorsalis pedis, and femoral arteries. It has been our experience that in most infants and small children the femoral artery is the only vessel large enough to accept safely a catheter of sufficient size to provide adequate blood flow.

The femoral and external jugular veins are most often used during CAVH for venous return. Long central venous catheters are poorly suited for CAVH because the resistance to flow encountered in these catheters is usually high enough to severely retard blood flow through the circuit.

Catheters of several different designs and sizes have been used in pediatric CAVH patients with varying success rates. When systemic arterial blood pressure and flow are high, almost any standard vascular access catheter will be adequate. It is in the hypotensive patient that catheter and access site characteristics must be optimized. The following general observations and suggestions may be helpful:

1. Short, large-bore catheters provide the best blood flow and least hydraulic pressure loss.
2. The catheter should not be so large that it completely occludes the femoral or brachial artery since collateral circulation to the extremity may be inadequate.
3. Most infants weighing at least 4 kg will tolerate a No. 5 F catheter in the femoral vessels. Femoral access in smaller infants probably should not exceed 4 F.
4. When possible, using the femoral artery and vein on the same side should be avoided. When this cannot be avoided, the leg may become cyanotic, a condition that should be tolerated for only the 24 to 48 hours of initital stabilization during which alternative venous access (e.g., jugular or subclavian veins) should be attempted.
5. Using long, tortuous central venous lines for CAVH venous return should be avoided; the resistance in these lines is too high to permit adequate QB.

6. When placing an arterial catheter using the Seldinger technique, the arterial puncture wound must not be dilated as a separate step in the procedure. A catheter that can be placed over and inserted simultaneously with the dilator should be used. The catheter is then the largest structure that has invaded the wall of the artery; leakage around the arterial access catheter is thereby minimized.

7. Femoral access may be difficult to maintain in the infant or young child who is not comatose or paralyzed. Simply flexing the leg at the hip can partially obstruct blood flow in many catheters and result in filter clotting. Femoral access in alert, older children is tolerable without paralysis or restraints but requires prolonged immobility and heavy sedation.

8. In the neonate (up to approximately 5 days of age) access via the umbilical vessels may be attempted, using catheters no smaller than 5 F. The arterial catheter tip must reside below the level of the renal arteries to reduce the risk of thromboembolic injury to the already injured kidneys. Care must be taken that the venous catheter tip resides in the vena cava, not in a hepatic vein.

Short, over-the-dilator catheters suitable for femoral artery and vein access in small infants are available from several manufacturers in 4 and 5 F sizes. Blood flow rates through these catheters can be unpredictable despite an adequate systemic arterial blood pressure. In vitro studies by Jenkins, Kuhn, and Funk have documented the variability of maximum flow rates observed when catheters of the same nominal size are used. This occurs because the size ("5 F") reflects only the *outer* diameter of the catheter, which is carefully controlled by the manufacturer. The *inner* diameter of the catheter, which is the critical determinant of blood flow, can vary substantially, not only between 5 F catheters made by different manufacturers, but between different batches of 5 F catheters made by the same manufacturer.

The device currently preferred in our center for percutaneous femoral access in patients weighing >7 kg is a No. 6 F catheter sheath. We originally used No. 5 F catheters inserted through a 6 F femoral sheath because the sheath was the only small device we could find that was inserted over a dilator. It soon became obvious that the internal 5 F catheter was

superfluous and that much better blood flow was obtained from the sheath alone. The 6 F sheath designed for use with a 5 F pulmonary artery catheter makes an almost ideal CAVH catheter. It is available in a complete kit (Percutaneous Sheath Introducer Kit, 6 F internal diameter sheath; Arrow International, Reading, Pa.). The sheath is relatively short and has an untapered tip and a thin wall, which accounts for its only slightly larger outer diameter. It is designed for prolonged use and can be anchored firmly with sutures at the skin puncture site. A side port adapter is available in the same kit, offering an important advantage when it is difficult to anchor the sheath (e.g., in edematous infants with deep femoral creases). During filter replacement procedures the new filter tubing can be attached to the side port adapter without disturbing the sheath itself, thereby reducing the risk of dislodging the access. The 90-degree turn in the blood path created by the addition of the side port adapter to the sheath apparently does not diminish blood flow in the circuit. In fact, blood flow is so good through the 6 F sheath that we have not found it necessary to use a larger size, regardless of the size of the patient (up to at least 50 kg).

The only significant drawback to the use of the 6 F sheath is the relative ease with which it becomes crimped when the hip is flexed. Very brief periods of hip flexion can result in dramatic reduction in filter blood flow and a clotted filter. A more flexible sheath would be ideal as long as increased flexibility was not achieved at the expense of substantially increased wall thickness.

For older children and adolescents who are not comatose or paralyzed, we prefer to use a Scribner shunt in a distal extremity. Others have had success with percutaneous or surgical placement of 5 F or 16-gauge catheters in the radial or brachial artery.

Choice of a hemofilter for pediatric patients

Several of the currently available hemofilters that have been used in children are listed in Table 148-4. Specifications and in vitro performance data on the newest pediatric hemofilter, the Amicon Minifilter-Plus, are included in Table 148-4, although clinical experience with this hemofilter is limited at this time. An adult size filter, the Amicon Diafilter D-20, is also listed for comparison. All of the filters in Table 148-4 use the hollow-fiber design. As in hemodialsyn, it is also possible to build a hemofilter for CAVH that has the parallel plate membrane configuration. To

Table 148-4 Some of the Hemofilters Available for Use in Pediatric Patients

	Amicon Minifilter	Amicon Minifilter-Plus	Gambro FH22	Amicon D-10	Amicon D-20
Fiber diameter (μm)	1100	570	215	200	200
Fiber length (cm)	10	12.7	11.5	9.5	12.5
No. of fibers	50 (?)	350	2100	6000	5000
Surface area (m²)	0.015	0.08	0.16	0.20	0.4
Filter volume (cc)	6	15	11	25	38
Tubing volume (cc)	6	?	?	7*-36	7*-30
Typical achievable Qf† (ml/min)	0.5-1.5	1-6	2-5	5-12	>15

*Lower tubing volumes obtained by cutting out dead space and splicing cut tubing together.
†Qf = ultrafiltration rate at QB = 20 ml/min to 100 ml/min; Hct = 30%; data supplied by manufacturers.

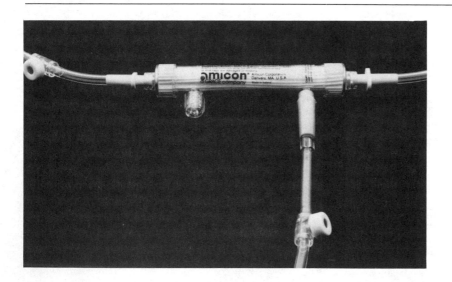

Fig. 148-4 The Amicon Minifilter. (Courtesy Amicon Division, W.R. Grace & Co., Danvers, Mass.)

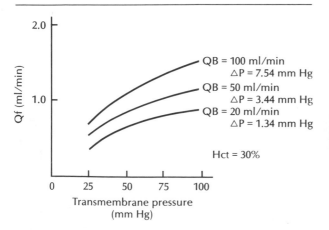

Fig. 148-5 Ultrafiltration rate (Qf) in ml/min achieved with the Minifilter at varying transmembrane pressures (TMP) and at blood flow rates (QB) that equal 20, 50, and 100 ml/min and Hct of 30%. Based on in vitro data provided by the manufacturer.

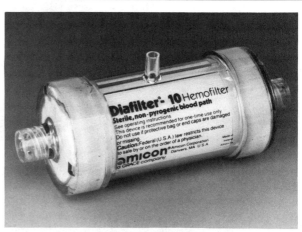

Fig. 148-6 The Amicon Diafilter D-10 hemofilter. (Courtesy of Amicon Division, W.R. Grace & Co., Danvers, Mass.)

date the available parallel plate hemofilters are too large for practical use in small pediatric patients.

No controlled studies have compared hemofilters in pediatric patients. For reasons given below, we now prefer to use either the Amicon Minifilter (in infants weighing <5 kg) or the Amicon D-10 (in *all* other pediatric patients, including adolescents weighing as much as 50 kg). There are obviously many other filters available (especially in Europe and Japan) that might perform as well in young children. Limiting the following discussion to the Amicon Minifilter and the D-10 merely reflects our largest clinical experience.

As with all extracorporeal therapies in children, the total volume of the filter and blood lines should not exceed 10% of the child's estimated blood volume (i.e., approximately 8 ml/kg). The total extracorporeal circuit volume of the Amicon Minifilter (tubing plus filter) is only 12 ml. The D-10 filter itself needs approximately 25 ml, to which must be added approximately 36 ml to fill the tubing. Tubing sets for the D-10 can be shortened by cutting out segments of unnecessary tubing and splicing the cut ends with connectors provided with the D-10 kit. When this is done, the tubing volume can be greatly reduced. A shorter D-10 tubing set with 20 ml total volume is now available.

The Amicon Minifilter. The Minifilter is shown in Fig. 148-4. An early prototype of this tiny filter was originally constructed solely for use in hemodialysis research; placement of this prototype hemofilter in a dialysis circuit allowed convenient sampling of the plasma ultrafiltrate during dialysis. In response to the urgent need for a CAVH device suitable for use in small infants, the manufacturer agreed to release the prototype Minifilter on a compassionate basis while development of the Minifilter was underway. Early work with this prototype led to the development of a much-improved Minifilter, which has now become widely available.

Ronco's elegant studies have defined the operational characteristics of the Minifilter, which are intended to make this device safe and effective in small infants. The hollow fibers are large bore and relatively short, thereby ensuring minimal resistance to blood flow. Membrane surface area (A) is small (0.025 m²), and FF rarely exceeds 10%. Thus, despite the low blood flow rates and systemic arterial blood pressures encountered in small infants, filtration pressure equilibrium is never achieved, and the risk of clotting the filter is minimal. Another consequence of the low FF and small A is the low ultrafiltration rates that can be achieved with the Minifilter, as can be seen in Fig. 148-5. Note that even when QB equals 100 ml/min (which is almost never seen during CAVH in infants), Qf remains <1.5 ml/min at TMP as high as 50 mm Hg.

Low Qf was considered an important safety feature when the Minifilter was designed; a higher Qf could increase the risk of rapid volume depletion and shock if ultrafiltration were not adequately restricted. Unfortunately the low achievable Qf also limits the achievable urea clearance. In severely catabolic infants CAVH with the Minifilter may not keep pace with urea generation, resulting in an unacceptably high BUN and the need to abandon CAVH for an alternative dialysis modality. Such infants may now be treated with CAVHD, as is described below.

The Diafilter D-10. The primary advantages of the D-10 (Fig. 148-6) are its short fiber length and large surface area (0.2 m²). Achievable Qf is quite high, even at relatively low QB and blood pressures (Fig. 148-7). Even when systolic blood pressure is only 60 mm Hg, a Qf of 5 to 7 ml/min or more is often possible with the D-10. The high Qf provided by the D-10 is desirable because it is accompanied by an equally high solute clearance rate. However, to use the D-10 safely in small patients, *Qf must be carefully controlled at all times.* We have found it convenient to "down-regulate" Qf by attaching the D-10 ultrafiltrate line to the inlet port on a volumetric IV fluid infusion pump. By setting the pump at the desired Qf, only the desired volume of ultrafiltrate is re-

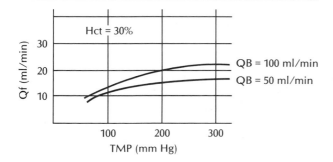

Fig. 148-7 Ultrafiltration rates (Qf) obtained with the D-10 hemofilter at varying transmembrane pressures (TMP) and at blood flow rates (QB) of 50 and 100 ml/min. Hct equals 30%. Based on in vitro data provided by the manufacturer.

moved each hour. Fluid calculations are simplified, and nursing time is reduced as long as the desired Qf does not exceed the capacity of the filter to produce ultrafiltrate. Since maximum Qf may decline as a filter "ages" (i.e., becomes partially occluded) or as a result of decreasing systemic arterial blood pressure, it is important to monitor Qf closely, even when a volumetric pump is used on the ultrafiltrate line.

Filter replacement fluid

The composition of the filter replacement fluid (FRF) must reflect the needs of the individual patient. There are no commercially available CAVH fluids in the United States. We have used a modification of the "University of Michigan formula," as shown on p. 1039. Four 1 L bags are prepared by the pharmacy to be hung simultaneously and are attached to a five-pronged tubing manifold normally used for automated (cycler) peritoneal dialysis (Baxter/Travenol 5C4426). As long as the bags are hung at the same level above the manifold and are filled equally, they each will contribute 25% of the final FRF that reaches the patient. The goal is to provide a physiologic solution to replace plasma water. The use of the cycler tubing manifold allows delivery of calcium and magnesium in the same final solution with bicarbonate without the precipitation that would occur if these solutes were combined in the same bag. The brief period of mixing that occurs within the final tubing segment on the way to the patient is too short to allow precipitation to take place.

Occasionally a patient will need super-physiologic concentrations of bicarbonate in the FRF to correct severe metabolic acidosis. This is easily achieved, as shown on p. 1039. When the high bicarbonate formula is used, care must be taken to avoid overcorrection, resulting in metabolic alkalosis.

Potassium is usually excluded from the initial FRF formula in patients with renal failure. Eventually most patients need some potassium supplementation. We prefer to give potassium (and phosphate) as part of the TPN solution. When this route cannot keep pace with the patient's needs, potassium salts may be added to the FRF solutions. It is safer, although less convenient, to add a physiologic concentration of potassium (e.g., 4 mEq/L of KCl or K phosphate) to *each* of the four FRF bags. If 16 mEq of KCl were added to a single bag and if that bag were hung higher than the others or lines from the others became occluded, serious hyperkalemia could develop with ter-

rifying rapidity. For related reasons hypokalemia should never be treated by using KCl in the FRF at final concentrations >4 mEq/L. In pediatric patients the power of the CAVH system to rapidly and inexorably remake the extracellular fluid in the image of the FRF must be respected.

Many adults are successfully treated with CAVH using lactated Ringer's solution as the FRF. It has the advantage of convenience and reduced cost and eliminates the worry about a pharmacy error in formulation of one of the Michigan bags, a problem that has resulted in development of hyponatremia in two of our patients. Bosch and others have reported that the high lactate administration rates that are needed when Ringer's solution is used as FRF have been well tolerated by their adult patients. No controlled studies have been done comparing the two FRF methods (Michigan formula vs. Ringer's solution) in either adults or children. We believe that the Michigan solution may be preferable in critically ill pediatric patients, especially those who have hepatic dysfunction, but we have not examined this question systematically.

Anticoagulation of the CAVH circuit

The need to anticoagulate the CAVH circuit can present substantial risks in some patients. Heparinization must be accomplished with great caution, with the heparin dose tightly controlled by close monitoring of the activated clotting time (ACT). Patients with coagulopathies may not need any heparin beyond that used to prime the filter. Often these patients need increasing heparin doses as their coagulopathy improves.

If a patient's ACT is >200 seconds before treatment, we do not use heparin until the ACT spontaneously improves and a filter clots. Often these events occur simultaneously. For patients who do not have a coagulopathy, a loading dose of heparin similar to that used in hemodialysis must be given (e.g., 20 to 50 units/kg). This dose is best given at least 3 to 5 minutes before the CAVH circuit is connected to ensure that the filter does not clot when it is first perfused. Additional heparin is given as a continuous infusion into the arterial limb of the CAVH circuit. We begin at an infusion rate of 5 units/kg/hr and then adjust the rate until the ACT of the blood drawn from the venous limb of the circuit (post-filter) is 1½ times baseline. It is usually possible to find a heparin infusion rate that keeps the post-filter ACT equal to

1½ times baseline without increasing the arterial (pre-heparin) ACT more than 5% to 10% above baseline, thereby anticoagulating the filter without severely anticoagulating the patient.

Such "tight" heparinization necessitates close monitoring of both the arterial (pre-heparin) and venous (post-filter) ACT and undoubtedly results in reduced average filter life. However, this seems a reasonable price to pay for minimizing the risk of bleeding complications. Unlike hemodialysis in which the bleeding risk resulting from heparinization is confined to a few hours each day during and for a short time after dialysis treatments, CAVH requires *continuous* heparinization and thus presents a much greater bleeding risk. Despite our best efforts, bleeding continues to occur in up to 15% of those heparinized CAVH patients who are at a high risk for

bleeding (e.g., postoperative patients or those with prior ischemic tissue injury undergoing necrosis).

Alternatives to standard heparinization are currently being developed. We have found that the use of high flow rates of FRF infused into the arterial limb of the circuit ("high-flow pre-dilution") reduces heparin requirements, probably by diluting clotting factors, improving the mixing of heparin with the blood, and decreasing blood viscosity and protein concentration before the blood reaches the filter. Studies are under way in our center to confirm these observations. A low molecular weight heparin with high affinity for antithrombin III yet with little effect on PTT, which can also be completely removed in the ultrafiltrate, is undergoing clinical trials in Europe. New membrane materials are being developed that contain heparin molecules bound to the surface in

---

FILTER RELACEMENT FLUID (FRF) FORMULATIONS*

Physiologic FRF

Bag No. 1: 1000 ml 0.9% NaCl + 7.5 ml 10% CaCl$_2$ (10.35 mEq Ca)
Bag No. 2: 1000 ml 0.9% NaCl + 1.6 ml 50% MgSO$_4$ (6.4 mEq Mg)
Bag No. 3: 1000 ml 0.9% NaCl
Bag No. 4: 900 ml sterile H$_2$O + 100 ml NaHCO$_3$ (100 mEq NaHCO$_3$) + 10 ml D$_{50}$W (5 g dextrose)
Final FRF composition: Na = 140 mEq/L
Cl = 120 mEq/L
HCO$_3$ = 25 mEq/L
Ca = 2.6 mEq/L
Mg = 1.6 mEq/L
Dextrose = 124 mg/dl
K = 0

FRF with additional bicarbonate

Bag No. 1: 1000 ml 0.9% NaCl + 7.5 ml 10% CaCl$_2$
Bag No. 2: 1000 ml 0.9% NaCl + 1.6 ml 50% MgSO$_4$
Bag No. 3: 850 ml sterile water + 150 ml NaHCO$_3$ (150 mEq NaHCO$_3$)
Bag No. 4: 900 ml sterile water + 100 ml NaHCO$_3$ (100 mEq NaHCO$_3$) + 10 ml D$_{50}$W (5 g dextrose)
Final FRF Composition: Na = 139 mEq/L
Cl = 82 mEq/L
HCO$_3$ = 62 mEq/L
Ca = 2.6 mEq/L
Mg = 1.6 mEq/L
Dextrose = 124 mg/dl
K = 0

*Modified from the University of Michigan FRF.

contact with the blood. Analogues of PGI_2 that can produce anticoagulation without the potent vasodilatory and hypotensive effects that now characterize the use of PGI_2 are being evaluated.

Regional heparinization of the CAVH circuit using protamine to reverse the heparin has been reported in adults, but there are no reports of this technique being used in children. Regional anticoagulation using sodium citrate may be more promising, using a modification of the technique developed for citrate hemodialysis. We have used citrate anticoagulation during CAVH with moderate success in two patients who had each recently suffered a major hemorrhagic episode in the early postoperative period. Citrate anticoagulates blood by binding available calcium ions; this effect must be reversed by a constant calcium infusion before the blood is returned to the patient. Citrate anticoagulation of the D-10 hemofilter was achieved in our two patients using an infusion of hypertonic trisodium citrate into the arterial limb of the circuit (appropriate modifications of the FRF were made to avoid hypernatremia). A 10% calcium chloride solution was infused into the venous limb of the circuit. Average filter life span in these two patients was the same with citrate anticoagulation as we usually observe in patients treated with tight heparinization (i.e., 12 to 24 hours per filter); however, both citrate-treated patients developed hypercalcemia, hypercitratemia, and metabolic alkalosis as consequences of the difficulties we encountered in titrating citrate and calcium infusion rates to reflect the fluctuations in QB seen in these two highly unstable patients. More experience with citrate anticoagulation will be needed before this method can be recommended as an alternative to standard CAVH heparinization.

Replacement of drugs removed by CAVH

The continuous nature of CAVH has raised concerns about the loss into the ultrafiltrate of a substantial amount of circulating pharmacologic agents. Several approaches to the adjustments of drug therapy needed during CAVH have been proposed, but none is entirely satisfactory.

Perhaps the simplest method uses the familiar and readily available tables prepared by Bennett and associates that provide dosage adjustments for many drugs used in patients with reduced renal function. Bennett's tables offer dosing regimens for most commonly used drugs when the patient's glomerular fil-

tration rate (GFR) is known or can be approximated. To use this approach in CAVH the GFR is simply the Qf in ml/min/1.73 m^2 plus any residual renal clearance. For drugs with wide therapeutic windows (e.g., penicillins, cephalosporins) it is usually sufficient to adjust CAVH dosage regimens based on Bennett's tables and the CAVH GFR.

For drugs with narrow therapeutic windows a more rigorous approach is needed. When drug levels are available and the volume of distribution (V_d) of the drug is known, it is not necessary to know the rate of removal by CAVH to adjust the dosing regimen. Golper has described this method for tobramicin as follows:

$$\text{Loading dose} = [(\text{Desired peak}) - (\text{Current level})] \times V_d \times \text{Weight}$$
$$= 6 \text{ mg/L} \times 0.23 \times 10 \text{ kg}$$
$$= 13.8 \text{ mg}$$

where $V_d = 0.23$ L/kg; desired peak level $= 6$ mg/L; and current level $= 0$.

$$\text{Maintenance dose} = [(6-2)] \times 0.23 \times 10 \text{ kg}$$
$$= 9.2 \text{ mg}$$

where desired peak $= 6$ mg/L and current trough $= 2$ mg/L.

The Golper method gives no information on how long it will take to reach the desired trough level, and it assumes that frequent drug levels will be obtained to monitor therapy. This method also assumes that the V_d is known and remains constant.

More complex methods for drug dosing during CAVH are based on attempts to estimate and predict the amount of drug removed over time. The amount of any drug appearing in the ultrafiltrate at any moment is determined by the concentration of the drug in plasma and the sieving coefficient (S) for that drug specific to the hemofilter being used. Most drugs are well below 500 to 1000 daltons in size and so can be considered to pass freely through the pores of all of the CAVH membranes currently in use. Thus only that fraction of the total plasma concentration of a drug that is bound to protein will be restricted by the membrane. S for different drugs is related to the degree of protein binding of each drug.

Golper and associates have used readily available data on protein binding of different drugs obtained in normal subjects in an attempt to predict S for a number of commonly used agents. Unfortunately protein binding can be highly unpredictable, especially in patients who are critically ill. When S has been measured in patients treated with CAVH, it has been, at best, only a rough approximation of the predicted S based on protein-binding data. Direct measurement of S is still the only reliable way to determine this coefficient. Sieving coefficients that have been directly measured for a number of commonly used agents are listed in Table 148-5.

In the steady state drug removal by CAVH can be expressed as follows:

Amount of drug X removed =

$$(UF) \times (Sx) \times \frac{[(X)t_0 + (X)t_1]}{2}$$

Table 148-5 Measured Sieving Coefficients (S)* and Volumes of Distribution (V_d)† for Selected Drugs in CAVH

Drug	S ($x \pm$ SEM)	N (measurements of S performed)	V_d (L/kg)
Amikacin	0.88 ± 0.03	8	0.22-0.29
Amphotericin	0.40	1	4.0
Ampicillin	0.69 ± 0.21	4	0.17-0.31
Cefoperazone	0.27	1	—
Cefotaxime	0.51 ± 0.01	2	—
Ceftriaxone	0.71	1	—
Cefapirin	1.70 ± 0.49	2	0.15-0.50
Clindamycin	0.98	1	0.61-1.14
Cyclosporin	0.00	2	—
Digoxin	0.96 ± 0.06	12	5.1-7.4
Erythromycin	0.37	1	0.5-0.7
Gentamicin	0.81 ± 0.02	13	0.23-0.26
Metronidazole	0.86 ± 0.03	4	0.6-0.8
Mezlocillin	0.68 ± 0.11	4	—
N-Acetyl pro-cainamide	0.92 ± 0.02	9	—
Nafcillin	0.54 ± 0.12	4	0.28-0.70
Oxacillin	0.02	1	0.19-0.41
Phenobarbital	0.86 ± 0.01	2	0.7-1.0
Phenytoin	0.45 ± 0.06	14	0.5-0.7
Procainamide	0.86 ± 0.02	9	2.2
Streptomycin	0.30	1	—
Theophylline	0.85 ± 0.01	2	0.3-0.7
Tobramycin	0.78 ± 0.06	6	0.22-0.25
Vancomycin	0.76 ± 0.06	11	0.47-0.84

*Compiled from data reported in the references cited at the end of this chapter and from unreported measurements by the author.
†Compiled from the references cited at the end of this chapter.

where (UF) = volume of ultrafiltrate produced during time t_0 to t_1; (Sx) = sieving coefficient for drug X; $(X)t_0$ = plasma concentration of X at time t_0; and $(X)t_1$ = plasma concentration of X at time t_1.

Although helpful conceptually, this formulation oversimplifies the pharmacokinetics involved. A more rigorous treatment of this question necessitates the use of more complex mathematics and is beyond the scope of this text.

Much more work must be done to better understand the pharmacologic aspects of CAVH and to develop convenient models for drug dosing during treatment. Ideally these models would allow dosing based on Qf, S, and V_d when only the loading dose is known and blood levels cannot be determined easily (which is the situation encountered for many drugs used in the PICU). In addition the effects of CAVH on infusions of inotropes and other agents commonly used in PICU patients have not been defined.

Recommendations for Performing CAVH in Pediatric Patients
CAVH circuit

Fig. 148-8 shows our current configuration for pre-dilution, ultrafiltration-controlled CAVH using the Amicon D-10 filter, femoral artery and vein access, and the modified Michigan formula FRF. The FRF infusion is shown in the pre-dilution mode. The circuit begins at the femoral artery access catheter, with a No. 6 F sheath with sidearm adapter in place. To this is attached a hemodialysis Y-connector (Argon No. 501301), and to the outer arm of the Y is attached the arterial limb of the CAVH tubing. We use the large-bore three-way stopcock (red) that is supplied with the D-10 tubing to connect the tubing to the Y-connector (unless QB is very low, in which case all potential sources of resistance, including the red stopcock, must be eliminated). The circuit ends at the femoral vein access catheter in the opposite groin, which has a similar Y-connector and three-way stopcock (blue) attachment to the venous limb of the CAVH tubing.

The bypass. A short bypass tubing segment connects the arterial and venous limbs of the circuit. The bypass does not come with the D-10 tubing set. To construct the bypass we use a 6-inch pressure tubing segment from an American Edwards pressure monitoring kit (Catalog No. 51-41MK035) and a double male Luer adapter (Cobe No. 90-184-000) to connect the inner arms of the arterial and venous Y-connectors. Pressure tubing was chosen because it was available in our PICU (this item was not used to monitor pressures and could be saved in a sterile package for use with CAVH) and because one end of the tubing segment came attached to a three-way stopcock. (Any IV extension tubing and three-way stopcock can be used instead of the pressure tubing segment.) The bypass is filled with heparinized saline solution, which must be flushed periodically. The stopcock in the bypass circuit provides access for flushing.

We use the bypass circuit whenever a filter clots

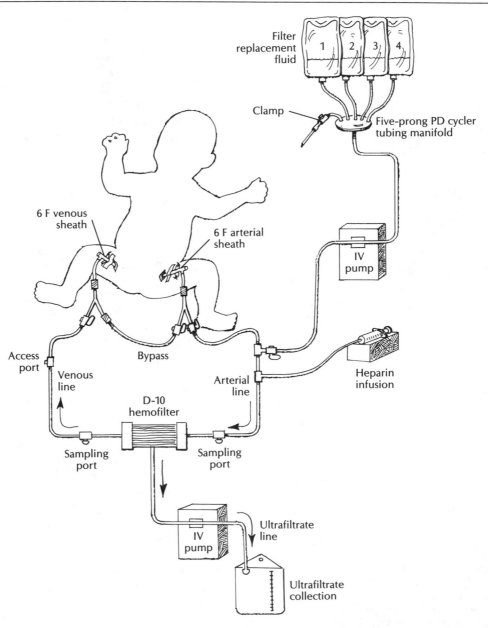

Fig. 148-8   Configuration of the CAVH circuit used most often in our center. The bypass circuit is described in detail in the text. Note that FRF is infused in a pre-dilution mode and Qf is controlled.

and must be changed. As soon as clotting is noted in the filter and/or its tubing, the outer arms of the Y-connectors are clamped, and the bypass circuit is opened. Blood is allowed to circulate through the bypass during the filter replacement procedure, thereby preventing thrombosis of the vascular access catheters. The bypass circuit must be carefully aspirated and flushed at least twice daily with heparinized bacteriostatic saline solution to remove the small clots that can form in the stagnant backwash of the inner arms of the Y-connectors.

D-10 hemofilter. The D-10 hemofilter is either placed on the patient's bed or attached, using a hemodialyzer clamp, to an IV pole at the bedside at the level of the bed surface. The hemofilter must be tilted at a 30- to 60-degree angle, venous end up, to create a small air bubble trap in the top corner of the venous end of the filter blood compartment. The filter must be in full view at all times. It is easy to lose the filter among the clutter of the PICU bed, a situation that can be minimized by keeping the filter on a small white towel on which nothing else is placed.

Heparin infusion line. The heparin infusion line comes built into the arterial limb of the D-10 tubing. The heparin solution is prepared with 0.9% sodium chloride at a heparin concentration of 0.5 to 1.0 unit/kg/ml. At this concentration the heparin infusion will usually be operating at a minimum of 5 to 10 ml/hr. More concentrated heparin solutions and slower infusion rates may be used with the Minifilter, but a specialized pump (e.g., Harvard pump) is needed to avoid intermittent heparin administration at such slow infusion rates. When heparin is given in small volumes, it may not adequately mix with the blood before reaching the hemofilter.

Ultrafiltrate line. The ultrafiltrate line leaving the hemofilter is intended to be inserted into any closed container. Special devices are available that continuously monitor the spontaneous Qf by weighing the ultrafiltrate. Digital readout allows the nurse to see quickly the volume of ultrafiltrate formed during the previous time period (usually every 15 to 30 minutes) and to adjust the FRF infusion rate accordingly.

We prefer to *control* Qf rather than just monitor it. Controlled Qf is achieved by attaching the ultrafiltrate line to the inlet port of a volumetric IV infusion pump. After the yellow cap has been cut off, the ultrafiltrate line, a double male Luer adapter connects the ultrafiltrate line to a short IV tubing extension set that is inserted into the inlet port of the IV infusion pump. The pump's air detector must be "blinded" to

the presence of air bubbles in the line by wrapping the tubing segment that passes over the air detector's photoelectronic cell with tape. The desired Qf is set as the hourly infusion rate for the pump, and the "volume delivered" setting can be used to alert the nurse to a period of inadequate ultrafiltration. As a filter begins to age, it will no longer deliver the desired Qf. At such times bubbles will appear in the ultrafiltrate line, and the actual delivered ultrafiltrate volume will be less than desired, which could lead to fluid overload if high FRF infusion rates are being used. Thus, even though the pump is ostensibly controlling Qf, the delivered ultrafiltrate volume must be measured each hour. When delivered Qf begins to be less than prescribed Qf, either the prescribed Qf must be reduced to an amount the filter can deliver or the filter must be replaced.

Available IV infusion pumps are not ideal for CAVH ultrafiltration control because all operate discontinuously. Short bursts of negative pressure quickly fill the small chamber in the pump's tubing cassette, regardless of the prescribed infusion rate; the rate at which the chamber is emptied is modulated by the pump's infusion rate setting. When the chamber is filling, high pressures can be generated in the ultrafiltrate circuit. Fortunately, hemofilter membranes are capable of withstanding pressures of ≥ 500 mm Hg and have not ruptured at maximum pump settings (999 ml/hr). The intermittent application of negative pressure to the filter results in short periods of maximum Qf alternating with longer periods during which Qf equals 0 as the pump chamber is emptied. A continuous pump is needed that can deliver volumes with the accuracy of the discontinuous volumetric pumps currently available.

Filter replacement fluid: Pre-dilution

In Fig. 148-8 the four bags of FRF are connected to the infusion pump by a five-pronged peritoneal dialysis cycler tubing manifold. The FRF infusion line is attached in the pre-dilution mode to a three-way stopcock that has been connected to the arterial limb of the CAVH circuit at the T-connector, which is built into the CAVH tubing. A similar arrangement on the venous limb would allow FRF to be infused in the post-dilution mode.

Initiating CAVH

1. At least two filters and tubing sets must be primed with heparinized 0.9% sodium chloride solution (5000 units heparin/L) according to the manu-

facturer's instructions. Each filter requires a 2 L prime to remove air trapped in the hollow fibers. It takes approximately 30 minutes to prime a filter. The IV set used to deliver the sodium chloride prime cannot be a "microdrip" system; microdrip systems (e.g., Volutrol) do not deliver fluid fast enough to purge the CAVH system of air.

2. Gently tapping the filter with a rubber mallet will help dislodge air bubbles during priming. Air entrapped in a hollow fiber retards blood flow and promotes thrombosis. The best rubber mallets are owned by cardiopulmonary bypass technicians who use them for the same purpose. The filter must not be tapped with a hard object such as a hemostat; the filter will crack.

3. If the heparinized 0.9% sodium chloride priming solution is warmed to 37° C in a microwave, air is more easily purged during filter priming. The solution must not be heated beyond 37° C.

4. Primed filters may be kept refrigerated for 48 hours before use. We keep at least two primed filters on hand in a small refrigerator reserved for this purpose whenever a patient is being treated with CAVH. Although this practice wastes two filters per patient, we believe that the ability to replace a clotted filter quickly is more important to the welfare of the patient.

5. Refrigerated filters must be allowed to warm to room temperature before use. A rapid rinse with sodium chloride solution that has been warmed to 37° C may be used to warm the filter.

6. Arterial and venous access catheters can usually be placed during the time needed to prime the first two filters.

7. Baseline ACT, PT, PTT, platelet count, electrolytes, BUN, creatinine, ionized calcium, phosphorus, magnesium, total serum protein, glucose, and CBC values must be obtained.

8. Specific FRF solutions are ordered according to the individual patient's condition. The Michigan formula provides either a physiologic solution containing 25 mEq/L of bicarbonate or a higher bicarbonate solution if metabolic acidosis is severe. Potassium must not be ordered in the FRF solutions unless the serum potassium level is already <3 mEq/L.

9. The baseline ACT and other clotting studies are used to determine whether initial heparinization will be needed. If baseline ACT is <200 seconds and bleeding risks in this patient are not excep-

tional, an IV loading dose of heparin (20 to 50 units/kg) is administered approximately 5 minutes before the CAVH circuit is connected.

10. All pumps and equipment must be arranged at the bedside. If high-flow pre-dilution is to be used, FRF solution bags must be warmed to 37° C and kept warm with water-filled warming pads (K^D pads).

11. Samples from the appropriate FRF solution bags must be sent for measurement of the sodium concentration (see discussion of hypernatremia and hyponatremia in sections on "Risks and Complications").

12. The CAVH tubing circuit Y-connectors are attached to the arterial and venous access catheters using sterile technique. The main circuit remains clamped; the bypass circuit is opened to protect the access catheters.

13. The heparin infusion is attached to the heparin line and the starting heparin infusion rate is determined by the baseline ACT. A starting rate of 5 units/kg/hr is often adequate.

14. The CAVH circuit is unclamped and opened, arterial limb first. The ultrafiltrate line remains clamped, and the bypass circuit is clamped.

15. The flow of blood through the circuit must be carefully observed. By timing the passage of the leading edge of the blood through the circuit, an estimate of QB can be obtained. For the D-10 the time needed to perfuse the circuit completely reflects the time needed for 61 ml of blood to traverse the circuit. For example, if blood reaches the venous access catheter in 30 seconds, QB can be estimated as 122 ml/min.

16. The heparin infusion is started as soon as blood begins to perfuse the CAVH circuit.

17. The circuit must be inspected for air bubbles and preparations made to aspirate air through the sampling ports using a 50 ml syringe and an 18-gauge needle. If large air bubbles occur, the circuit must be clamped. It is usually possible to aspirate most of the air via one of the sampling ports without clamping the circuit. Small air bubbles will be trapped in the filter and pose little threat to the patient, although filter function will be proportionately diminished. It is best to assign one person the task of aspirating air bubbles whenever a new circuit is placed into service.

18. All connections must be examined for leaks. The bypass circuit is aspirated and flushed with heparinized, bacteriostatic sodium chloride solution.

The bypass circuit is kept closed with clamps on both ends during operation of the main CAVH circuit.

19. The clamps are opened on the ultrafiltrate line.

20. The spontaneous Qf is measured by carefully collecting the ultrafiltrate that is produced in the first 5 to 10 minutes of filter operation. The collection device may be any container, but it should be held near the floor, allowing full extension of the ultrafiltrate line.

21. Near the end of the 5- to 10-minute spontaneous Qf measurement, blood samples are drawn simultaneously from the arterial and venous sampling ports to be sent for Hct determination.

22. The ultrafiltrate line is clamped and connected to the Qf control pump. Small patients treated with the D-10 may not tolerate more than 5 minutes of spontaneous Qf without marked volume depletion.

23. The desired Qf is determined by using the measured spontaneous Qf as an initial upper limit. Maximum Qf gives maximum clearance of solutes and correction of electrolyte and fluid disturbances. The desired Qf is set on the ultrafiltration pump. Controlled Qf is not begun until the FRF infusion is also ready to be started.

24. FRF solution bags are spiked with prongs from the five-prong cycler manifold using appropriate technique. The manifold line is connected to the FRF infusion pump and the line from the infusion pump to the stopcock on the T-connector in the arterial tubing segment for the pre-dilution FRF mode (Fig. 148-8). All four FRF bags must contain equal volumes and hang freely at the same height above the manifold.

25. The pre-dilution FRF infusion rate (QPD) is set. The desired QPD = (controlled Qf) − [(TPN rate) + (any desired hourly patient volume loss)].

26. QB and QP are calculated using spontaneous Qf and measured arterial and venous Hct values. QPD should not be greater than QP regardless of spontaneous Qf. When QPD exceeds QP, solute clearance becomes progressively less efficient as the filter removes more FRF than plasma ultrafiltrate.

27. ACT is obtained every 30 minutes from both limbs of the circuit (pre-heparin infusion and post-filter).

28. The heparin infusion is adjusted to keep venous (post-filter) ACT approximately 1½ times base-

line (never >200 seconds) and arterial (pre-heparin) ACT no more than approximately 10% above baseline.

29. Actual Qf is monitored hourly and compared to desired Qf. If actual measured Qf is less than desired, Qf and QPD are reduced accordingly. Qf and QPD should be considered to operate in tandem. Changes in Qf and QPD must be of equal magnitude to maintain the same fluid balance. One pump is never changed without an equivalent change in the other pump unless a different fluid balance state is desired.

30. Serum chemistries are monitored frequently during the first 24 to 48 hours of CAVH and at least every 8 hours thereafter.

31. The patient is weighed before and every 24 hours after starting CAVH.

32. Daily surveillance blood cultures are obtained from the CAVH circuit.

RISKS AND COMPLICATIONS
Clotting of the Filter

The most frequent CAVH complication is clotting of the filter. The factors predisposing the filter to clotting have been discussed earlier. They include systemic hypotension; low filter blood flow; high resistance anywhere in the circuit, especially in the arterial or venous access; high FF; long filter fibers with early development of filtration pressure equilibrium; air pockets within the filter fibers; momentary crimping of the access catheter or kinks in the filter tubing; and inadequate anticoagulation. Of the factors listed, inadequate anticoagulation is probably encountered least often.

The average filter life span varies widely among patients and may also change as conditions change in the individual patient. An average filter life of approximately 12 hours is a reasonable goal. When filters clot more frequently, the overall effectiveness of CAVH becomes questionable. When a filter clots, the patient experiences a significant loss of blood equal to the volume in the filter and tubing, and renal replacement therapy is suspended until a new filter can be obtained. Thromboembolic and infectious complications are more likely to occur in patients with frequent filter clotting.

Much of this chapter has been devoted to techniques designed to minimize the risk of filter clotting. Unfortunately pediatric patients are especially susceptible to this problem for reasons that have been discussed.

Inadequate Solute Clearance

Hypercatabolic patients may need solute clearance rates in excess of those possible with standard CAVH. The use of the D-10 hemofilter in small patients usually provides sufficient urea clearance to offset high urea generation rates. For example, in a 10 kg infant a urea clearance of 5 ml/min is readily obtained using the D-10 filter. This results in a daily urea clearance of 7.2 L, which is identical to that which would be obtained with 4 hours/day of hemodialysis at a standard hemodialysis urea clearance rate of 3 ml/kg/min of treatment.

When additional small solute removal is needed, the use of *high-flow pre-dilution* may be helpful. Kaplan first observed that urea clearance was increased when the FRF was infused into the arterial limb of the filter tubing. In this configuration FRF is used to lower the plasma protein concentration and thus decrease the oncotic pressure within the filter fibers. Filtration pressure equilibrium occurs later, resulting in an increase in the area of the membrane participating in solute clearance. Dilution of clotting factors also helps by reducing the rate at which filter fibers become occluded by thrombi.

High-flow pre-dilution may have an additional beneficial effect on urea clearance. Kaplan has suggested that when pre-dilution is used, the dilution of the plasma allows urea to diffuse out of the RBCs before reaching the membrane. Pre-dilution CAVH might be effectively removing urea from both intra- and extracellular urea pools. Studies are under way in our center and others to examine this hypothesis.

When high-flow pre-dilution is used, the FRF rate and the Qf must be carefully chosen to avoid disturbances in fluid balance. One practical approach to selecting the QPD is based on the spontaneous Qf measured when a new filter is placed in line. The initial QPD is equal to the spontaneous Qf minus the desired negative fluid balance for TPN and/or volume depletion. Spontaneous Qf is measured by collecting the ultrafiltrate formed during the first 5 to 10 minutes of CAVH by gravity drainage alone before connecting the ultrafiltrate line to its pump. For example, in a patient receiving TPN at 50 ml/hr who needs to lose 50 ml/hr to correct fluid overload, a measured spontaneous Qf of 750 ml/hr would result in an initial QPD of 650 ml/hr (=11 ml/min). From that point onward, any change in Qf must prompt an equivalent change in QPD to maintain the same fluid balance. For example, if Qf falls to 500 ml/hr as a result of aging of the filter, QPD must be reduced to 400 ml/hr. Once the desired "dry weight" is achieved and further volume depletion is unnecessary, QPD in this patient would thereafter be equal to Qf minus 50 ml/hr.

The limits of QPD are determined by the maximum Qf achievable with the hemofilter being used. When the Minifilter is used, maximum Qf is <1.5 ml/min, which makes high-flow pre-dilution impossible. Fortunately the Minifilter's clearances of urea and other solutes can be increased by the use of CAVHD. There are two ultrafiltrate ports on the Minifilter (Fig. 148-4), one of which remains capped during standard CAVH or SCUF. To perform CAVHD, peritoneal dialysate is infused into one of the ultrafiltrate ports and collected, along with the formed ultrafiltrate from the other port. Early CAVHD techniques devised by Ronco used gravity to drip peritoneal dialysate (1.5% dextrose) through the Minifilter at 1 to 3 ml/min. The optimum dialysate flow rate for CAVHD has not been determined.

We have used CAVHD with controlled Qf as follows (Fig. 148-1, *C*):

1. Peritoneal dialysate (1.5% or 2.5% dextrose) is pumped into the Minifilter ultrafiltrate compartment at a flow rate (QD) of from 100 to 300 ml/hr, depending on clinical requirements. Dialysate flow is in the opposite direction to blood flow.
2. The ultrafiltrate line is attached to a second pump, which is set at (QD + desired Qf) ml/hr.
3. Desired Qf (ml/hr) equals TPN rate plus desired hourly fluid loss plus FRF rate.

Bleeding Caused by Excessive Heparin

"Tight" heparinization as described above is recommended to reduce the risk of this complication. No heparin is needed when baseline ACT is >200 seconds.

Air Embolism

The CAVH circuit provokes anxiety among hemodialysis nurses because it contains no air detection system. Air entering the circuit at any point can be transferred directly to the patient's central venous circulation. Usually the amount is small, but vigilance is necessary to keep the circuit purged of any large collections of air. When a blood pump is used (Fig. 148-1, *D*), an air detection system must be added to the circuit.

Thromboembolism

Clots in the circuit can also pass directly into the venous circulation. The presence of thrombi in the filter can be detected by simple inspection. Occasionally these clots can be removed by flushing the filter. With the circuit bypass open and the main circuit of the UF line clamped, 100 to 200 ml of heparinized 0.9% saline solution is forcefully injected through any available arterial limb access port and drained through a venous limb access port.

Hypovolemia and Hypervolemia

Maintaining fluid balance during CAVH is simple; total intake should equal total output. If errors are made in selecting FRF flow rates, fluid volume status can change rapidly, especially in infants. Patients receiving high-flow pre-dilution are at particular risk for hypervolemia if a falling Qf goes unnoticed. All patients receiving CAVH need hourly monitoring of Qf and fluid balance by the PICU nurse. We recommend a thorough review of fluid balance by the responsible physician every 8 to 12 hours. Frequent weights are also necessary.

Hypernatremia and Hyponatremia

Errors in preparation of the Michigan FRF solutions can cause rapid development of severe disorders of serum sodium concentration. The sodium concentration of the final solution reaching the patient should always be 135 to 145 mEq/L. We routinely measure the sodium concentration in all solutions that are made by more than simply adding calcium or magnesium to 0.9% sodium chloride solution. For example, sodium concentration is routinely measured on a sample from bag No. 4 (see p. 1039) each time a new set of FRF bags is prepared by the pharmacy. If 0.9% sodium chloride solution is used in all four bags, the patient's serum sodium concentration will rapidly approach 154 mEq/L.

Hyponatremia may also develop if relatively large volumes of hypotonic TPN are infused. Sodium balance during CAVH is as straightforward as fluid balance: for every 100 ml of TPN infused, 100 ml of plasma water will be removed. If the TPN contains only 4 mEq of sodium/dl and plasma sodium concentration equals 14 mEq/dl, a negative sodium balance of 10 mEq is achieved with every 100 ml of ultrafiltrate formed. This is a prime example of the power of CAVH to change electrolyte concentration while keeping the volume of total body water constant.

Depletion of Other Electrolytes, Minerals, and Water-Soluble Vitamins

Many important substances are lost into the ultrafiltrate. Adequate replacement is thought to be accomplished by the use of complete TPN solutions that contain vitamins and trace elements in addition to major electrolytes and amino acids. Systematic balance studies have not been done to test this presumption. All patients undergoing CAVH should also be receiving the maximum tolerable TPN.

Anemia

Frequent clotting of the filter results in substantial blood loss incurred with each filter exchange. When transfusions are needed, they may be administered through the venous limb of the CAVH circuit. To avoid further depletion of the Hct level when a new filter and its tubing are placed in service, it is possible to prime the CAVH circuit with packed RBCs resuspended in 0.9% sodium chloride solution; however, we have found this adds unnecessary complexity to the filter priming procedure. Instead, we prefer to administer a transfusion of packed RBCs when the new filter is attached. Qf is increased by an amount equal to the volume of the packed RBC transfusion. More rapid transfusion is possible with CAVH because volume status remains constant; plasma water is being exchanged milliliter for milliliter with a solution of packed RBCs that has <50% of its volume as plasma. This is another example of the way CAVH can adjust the composition of the patient's fluids (this time the Hct) while maintaining a constant fluid volume.

Hypothermia

Small infants may become hypothermic when blood perfusing the CAVH circuit is allowed to cool to room temperature. If heating blankets and radiant warmers cannot maintain the infant's temperature, a heating pad must be placed beneath the hemofilter. The hemofilter should not be wrapped in a heating pad since this will prevent the frequent inspection for clot formation that is an essential component of CAVH maintenance.

Infection

The CAVH circuit offers many opportunities for invading organisms to enter the central circulation. Only meticulous nursing technique can keep the risk of contamination at an acceptable level. Sterile technique begins with the priming of the filter and extends to every event that requires entering or interrupting the circuit for any reason. Catheter exit site care must be aggressive and uncompromising; our protocols are based on those used to care for percutaneous hemodialysis catheter exit sites.

ADDITIONAL READING

Bennett WM, Aronoff GR, Morrison G, et al. Drug prescribing in renal failure: Dosing guidelines for adults. Am J Kidney Dis 3:155-193, 1983.

• Bosch JP, Ronco C. Continuous arteriovenous hemofiltration (CAVH) and other continuous replacement therapies: Operational characteristics and clinical use. In JF Maher, ed. Replacement of Renal Function by Dialysis, 3rd ed. Boston: Kluwer, 1989, pp 347-359.

• Golper TA. Continuous arteriovenous hemofiltration in acute renal failure. Am J Kidney Dis 6:373-386, 1985.

Heiss KF, Pettit B, Hirschi RB, et al. Renal insufficiency and volume overload in neonatal ECMO managed by continuous ultrafiltration. Trans Am Soc Artif Intern Organs 33:557-560, 1987.

Henderson LW. Hemofiltration. Kidney 20:25-30, 1987.

Jenkins RD, Kuhn RJ, Funk JE. Clinical implications of catheter variability on neonatal continuous arteriovenous hemofiltration (CAVH). Trans Am Soc Artif Intern Organs 11:108-111, 1988.

Kaplan AA, Longnecker RE, Folkert VW. Continuous arteriovenous hemofiltration: A report of 6 months experience. Ann Intern Med 100:358-367, 1984.

Kramer P, Kaufhold G, Grone HJ, et al. Management of anuric intensive care patients with arteriovenous hemofiltration. Int J Artif Organs 3:225-230, 1980.

Leone MR, Jenkins RD, Golper TA, et al. Early experience with continuous arteriovenous hemofiltration in critically ill pediatric patients. Crit Care Med 14:1058-1063, 1986.

• Lieberman KV. Continuous arteriovenous hemofiltration in children. Pediatr Nephrol 1:330-338, 1987.

Lieberman KV, Nardil H, Bosch JP. Treatment of acute renal failure in an infant using continuous arteriovenous hemofiltration. J Pediatr 106:646-649, 1985.

Lysaght M, Boggs D. Transport in continuous arteriovenous hemofiltration and slow continuous ultrafiltration. In Paganini EP, ed. Acute Continuous Renal Replacement Therapy. Boston: Kluwer, 1986, pp 43-50.

Ronco C. Continuous arteriovenous hemofiltration in infants. In Paganini EP, ed. Acute Continuous Renal Replacement Therapy. Boston: Kluwer, 1986, pp 201-246.

Ronco C, Brendolan A, Bragantini L, et al. Treatment of acute renal failure in newborns by continuous arteriovenous hemofiltration. Kidney Int 29:908-915, 1986.

Stannat S, Bahlmann J, Kressling D, et al. Complement activation during hemodialysis: Comparison of polysulfone and cuprophan membranes. Contrib Nephrol 46:102-108, 1985.

149 Total Parenteral Nutrition

Charles E. Mize · Stephanie Allen

INDICATIONS

Total parenteral nutrition (TPN) can be a major adjunct in homeostatic control of metabolic fluid, electrolyte, caloric, and nitrogen needs. It can be used in medical or surgical patients and, if initiated presurgically for metabolic regulation or aggressive nutrition, can be continued throughout the actual surgical procedure.

To meet each child's nutritional needs, a nutrition support team can be an extremely effective vehicle to help implement ongoing decisions. Usually the team consists of members from the following services: medical, surgical, nursing, dietary, pharmacy, social work, physical therapy, and child life therapy.

TECHNIQUE
TPN Assessment

It is important to evaluate the child's metabolic and underlying nutrition status before initiating TPN. Infections, cardiorespiratory stress, and acute and chronic starvation will all affect the prospective calculations and metabolic responses to parenteral therapy. The child is assessed periodically throughout therapy to establish a metabolic rate matched to

Table 149-1   Construction of Optimal Nutrition Support: Nutritional Metabolism Variables, Evaluation Tools, and Professional Expertise

Variable	Tool	Professional Contact
Metabolic rate	Nitrogen balance Resting energy expenditure	Physician Respiratory technician
Current nutritional status	Anthropometric measurements	Therapeutic dietician
Vitamin, mineral, trace element deficiency	Laboratory values	Physician/nurse
Route of administration	Length of TPN therapy: short-term (e.g., <2 wk with peripheral line) vs. long-term (>2 wk with central line)	Physician/surgeon/nurse
Nutrient-drug compatibilities/interactions	Visualization of tubing for precipitation Monitoring daily TPN and coupled medication orders	Nurse Pharmacist
Volume and composition of fluid	Input and output record (per shift) Weight gain Presence of edema	Physician Physician/nurse Physician/nurse
Psychosocial needs	Developmental assessment Financial/emotional support Physical/feeding assessment	Child life therapist Social worker Physical therapist Speech pathologist

TOTAL PARENTERAL NUTRITION

PHYSICIAN CALCULATION   Body weight _____ Kg   Date _____

Calories Desired   *Volume & Protein*

Lipid _____ g/kg/d _____ g _____ Cal/d (g × 11)

Glucose _____ g/kg/d _____ g _____ Cal/d (g × 3.4)   Volume _____ ml/kg/d _____ ml/d

        Total _____ Cal/d

        Total ÷ kg _____ Cal/kg/d   Amino acid (AA) _____ g/kg/d _____ g/d

Submit order to pharmacy by 10:00 A.M. if solution is to be used on this date

PHARMACY FORMULATION   Time first bottle needed _____   Rate of infusion _____ ml/hr

	Reference Solutions		Bottle # _____	Bottle # _____	Bottle # _____
Check box to order reference solutions:	*Starter* ☐	*Full* ☐	*(Number bottles sequentially)*		
Final bottle volume	500 ml	500 ml	_____ ml	_____ ml	_____ ml
Amino acids					
As 10% amino acid _____ (Name)	8.5 g	14.0 g	_____ g	_____ g	_____ g
As _____ (Other)	_____ g	_____ g	_____ g	_____ g	_____ g
Glucose					
As 50% glucose monohydrate	62.5 g	110.0 g	_____ g	_____ g	_____ g
As 70% glucose monohydrate	_____ g	_____ g	_____ g	_____ g	_____ g
Additives (pediatric recommended)					
Sodium (3-8 mEq/kg/24 hr): Total	12.5 mEq	12.5 mEq	_____ mEq	_____ mEq	_____ mEq
As sodium chloride	12.5 mEq	12.5 mEq	_____ mEq	_____ mEq	_____ mEq
As sodium acetate	_____ mEq	_____ mEq	_____ mEq	_____ mEq	_____ mEq
Potassium (2-4 mEq/kg/24 hr): Total	10.4 mEq	10.6 mEq	_____ mEq	_____ mEq	_____ mEq
As potassium chloride	6 mEq	4 mEq	_____ mEq	_____ mEq	_____ mEq
As potassium acetate	_____ mEq	_____ mEq	_____ mEq	_____ mEq	_____ mEq
*Phosphate (1-2 mmol/kg/24 hr): Total	3 mmol	4.5 mmol	_____ mmol	_____ mmol	_____ mmol
As potassium phosphate	3 mmol	4.5 mmol	_____ mmol	_____ mmol	_____ mmol
As sodium phosphate	_____ mmol	_____ mmol	_____ mmol	_____ mmol	_____ mmol
*Calcium (1-2 mEq/kg/24 hr)					
As calcium gluconate	4 mEq	6 mEq	_____ mEq	_____ mEq	_____ mEq
Magnesium (1-3 mEq/kg/24 hr)					
As magnesium sulfate	8 mEq	8 mEq	_____ mEq	_____ mEq	_____ mEq
Trace elements					
As zinc (150-300 µg/kg/24 hr)	500 µg	500 µg	_____ µg	_____ µg	_____ µg
As manganese (5-10 µg/kg/24 hr)	25 µg	25 µg	_____ µg	_____ µg	_____ µg
As copper (15-30 µg/kg/24 hr)	80 µg	80 µg	_____ µg	_____ µg	_____ µg
As chromium (0.2-0.4 µg/kg/24 hr)	1.0 µg	1.0 µg	_____ µg	_____ µg	_____ µg
As selenium	_____ µg	_____ µg	_____ µg	_____ µg	_____ µg
As iron	_____ µg	_____ µg	_____ µg	_____ µg	_____ µg
Multivitamin infusion—Pediatric (5 ml/day)	5 ml	5 ml	_____ ml	_____ ml	_____ ml
Heparin _____	500 units	500 units	_____ units	_____ units	_____ units
Other _____	_____	_____	_____	_____	_____
Other _____ Insulin regular _____	_____	_____	_____	_____	_____
Sterile water	q.s. ml	q.s. ml	_____ ml	_____ ml	_____ ml
Lipid (triglyceride emulsion)					
As 10% soybean or safflower base	_____ ml	_____ ml	_____ ml	_____ ml	_____ ml
As 20% soybean or safflower base	_____ ml	_____ ml	_____ ml	_____ ml	_____ ml
Final glucose concentration	12.5%	22.0%	_____ %	_____ %	_____ %
Nonprotein caloric density	0.43 cal/ml	0.75 cal/ml	_____ cal/ml	_____ cal/ml	_____ cal/ml

*Do not exceed 15 mEq calcium/L and 10 mmol phosphorus/L in any bottle without nutrition or pharmacy consultation.

Physician signature _____   Signature R.N. _____

Fig. 149-1 TPN work sheet.

caloric needs; current nutritional status; coexisting vitamin, mineral, or trace element deficiencies; adequacy of route of administration (central catheter or peripheral vein); nutrient-drug compatibilities/interactions; optimal volume of all types of fluid regulation per shift and per day; and psychosocial needs.

Table 149-1 describes the best tools to use for this evaluation and suggests which professional discipline

(or nutrition support team member, if available) would be the best resource for each assessment.

Composition of TPN Solutions

A well-balanced TPN formulation comprises all the elements suggested in Fig. 149-1. They are designed around needs that start at baseline estimates of the levels suggested in Table 149-2. For such formula-

Table 149-2   Estimated Daily TPN Needs for Metabolic Maintenance, Growth, and Tissue Repair of Infants*

Protein	1.5-4.5 g/kg	Vitamins	
Calories	120-200/kg	A	600 µg
Water	120-180 ml/kg	B_1	0.5-5 mg
Sodium	3-8 mEq/kg	B_2	0.5-2 mg
Potassium	2-4 mEq/kg	B_6	0.5-2 mg
Chloride	2-4 mEq/kg	B_{12}	1 µg
Calcium	1-2 mEq/kg	C	75-100 µg
Phosphorus	1-3 mmol/kg	D	10-15 µg
Magnesium	1-3 mEq/kg	E	3-5 mg
Zinc	150-300 µg/kg	K	50-100 µg
Copper	20 µg/kg	Folic acid	35-50 µg
Chromium	200 ng/kg	Niacin	10-30 mg
Manganese	2-10 µg/kg	Biotin	50-300 µg
Selenium	1-2 µg/kg	Pantothenate	5-10 mg
		Essential fatty acid	0.5-1.0 g/kg

*Reproduced by permission from Mize CE, Teitell BC. In Levin DL, Morriss FC, Moore GC, eds. A Practical Guide to Pediatric Intensive Care, 2nd ed. St. Louis: CV Mosby, 1984.

Table 149-3   Concentrations of Amino Acids and Electrolytes in Selected Solutions

Solution	Total Amino Acid (g/dl)	Osmolarity (mOsm/L)	pH	Electrolytes				
				Na (mEq/L)	K (mEq/L)	Cl (mEq/L)	Acetate (mEq/L)	P (mmol/L)
Aminosyn II, 10%	10	873	5-6.5	45.3			71.8	
Aminosyn-HBC, 7%	7	665	5.2	7		40	72	
Aminosyn-PF, 7%	7	586	5.4	3.4			32.5	
Aminosyn-RF, 5.2%	5.2	475	5.2		5.4		105	
FreAmine III, 10%	10	950	6.5	10		<3	89	10
FreAmine HBC, 6.9%	6.9	620	6.5	10		<3	57	
HepatAmine, 8%	8	785	6.5	10		<3	62	10
NephrAmine, 5.4%	5.4	435	6.5	5		<3	44	
Novamine, 15%	15	1388	5.2-6				151	
ProcalAmine, 3% with glycerine 3%	3	735	6.8	35	24	41	47	3.5
RenAmine, 6.5%	6.5	600	6.0			31	60	
Travasol, 10%	10	1000	6.0			40	87	
TrophAmine, 6%	6	525	5.5	5		<3	56	
TrophAmine, 10%	10	875	5.5	5		<3		

Table 149-4   Products of Substrate Oxidation

	Product Formed			
	Carbon Dioxide		Metabolic Water	
Reaction	mmol per Gram of Substrate	mmol per Substrate Calorie	Gram per Gram of Substrate	Gram per Substrate Calorie
Glucose to CO_2 and H_2O	33.3	8.9	0.60	0.16
C-18 triglyceride to CO_2 and H_2O	64.5	6.8	1.06	0.11
Glucose to C-18 fatty acid	11.1	3.0	0.16	0.04

tions, a variety of commercial amino acid products exist (examples are shown in Table 149-3) and can be chosen best in consultation with the pharmacist.

Glucose is predominantly chosen for a carbohydrate source, although glycerol in some formulations can be used adequately if sufficient quantities can be given for a given patient goal. Not all desired vitamins are available in parenteral form, particularly in optimal concentrations, and small enteral intake may be necessary even on a nothing by mouth regimen. Iron may be given when needed parenterally. Heparin used at 1 to 3 units/ml final concentration normally will not affect hemostasis.

Parenteral lipid can be given separately or as a part of a combined amino acid–glucose–lipid (3-in-1) mixture. The latter is used less in small or low birthweight infants because of their propensity for relatively sluggish triglyceride clearance, which often necessitates using lower lipid dosage and more frequent adjustments of continuous infusion rates than in older patients. Continuous lipid infusion is used most often for pediatric patients. Only 50% to 60% of long-chain triglyceride fatty acids of commercial lipid preparations are essential fatty acids (EFA), which is an important consideration when calculating EFA and vitamin E needs (see Chapter 74).

The amount of water delivered to the tissues that is derived from complete oxidation of glucose or fatty acid may become important when net water balance is critical. This metabolic water can be calculated from the amount of infused substrate (Table 149-4), and must be added to the other free water received to arrive at a total potential tissue water load. An important modification of metabolic conversion occurs, however, if glucose is given in such high amounts that it exceeds oxidative needs and is con-

verted to fat, rather than being completely combusted; in this case the net metabolic water is much less. A guideline for estimating total metabolic water from complete glucose oxidation (the most common source of this water at the substrate levels clinically infused) is shown in Table 149-5. This same complete oxidative process leads to CO_2 net formation (Table 149-4) and may contribute significantly to CO_2 levels in conditions of pulmonary insufficiency (see below). Switching partially to lipid when possible may reduce this CO_2 burden moderately.

Procedure

Consultation. Either individual consultations are requested or the nutrition support team is consulted; written recommendations must be completed in the chart. Pre-TPN laboratory work is drawn and the results analyzed. The initial minimal laboratory tests must provide values for the following: Ca, albumin, hemogram, ALT (SGPT), PO_4, Na, BUN, creatinine, bicarbonate, total serum protein, Cl, Mg, NH_3, K, and bilirubin (D/T). If results of each of the tests were not obtained within the 24 hours before starting TPN, they *should* optimally be drawn within the *24* hours *before* starting TPN (either peripheral or central). If these tests are not obtained within that period, they should be drawn at the time of starting TPN. (Additional studies may be necessary, depending on the patient's clinical status.)

The route of TPN administration is decided and an appropriate access device placed. This step must be given thorough consideration for optimal restitution outcome.

The site. Peripheral devices must be assessed every hour by the nursing staff to prevent infiltration that can result in tissue necrosis. Sites must be main-

Table 149-5   Water of Oxidation of Glucose

Glucose Solution	Metabolic Water Increment Produced by Complete Oxidation (ml H_2O/ml glucose solution)
D_{10}	0.055
D_{12-15}	0.068
D_{20}	0.109
D_{22}	0.120
D_{30}	0.164
D_{40}	0.218

tained by using occlusive dressings that are themselves changed every 72 hours. If long-term therapy is anticipated (e.g., >2 weeks), a central venous catheter must be considered and, if used, maintained according to strict aseptic protocol. The advantages of a tunneled Silastic catheter placement must be weighed against surgical risks when choosing a central venous access device. If a polyurethane or polyethylene device is placed, careful radiographic evaluation of catheter tip location is recommended because of the increased risk of vessel, pleural, or atrial perforation. Implantable devices are currently available in titanium as well as plastic (best for magnetic resonance imaging visualization) and may be chosen when intermittent access is warranted. Sites must be visualized at tri-weekly dressing changes using an appropriate aqueous antiseptic (e.g., povidone-iodine, Hibiclens) and an occlusive barrier such as sterile tape or transparent dressing.

Orders. TPN fluid orders are written by the physician, specifying composition and rate changes on a daily basis. Fig. 149-1 is an example of specified TPN fluid orders. It is important to anticipate total fluid intake when starting additional IV medications to prevent fluid overload.

Additionally, if only one administration site is available for TPN and the use of incompatible medications dictate stopping the TPN for defined intervals, the pharmacist can aid in calculating net solution preparation volume, stock solution concentrations for optimal nutrient densities in the TPN solution, and the need for possibly more than one TPN formulation in each shift or day period to accommodate drug, fluid, and nutrient constraints.

Pumps. Infusion pumps are needed for all TPN administration to ensure accurate delivery. The pump must meet the following specifications for pediatric use: activation of a continuous low infusion during an audible flow alarm; occlusion alarm; in-line air detector; in-line (0.22 μm) filter; Luer-Lok connections; minimal number of connections (preferably none) between fluid bag and IV device; and rate-setting safety feature to assure that rates are not changed by the patient or unauthorized ancillary personnel. NOTE: The key concept of an infusion system, with compatible Y-tubing for lipid infusion, is to maintain a closed system.

Tubing. TPN solutions and tubing must be changed every 24 hours, and blunt hemostats (without "teeth") must be used during either tubing changes to clamp the extension tubing connected to the peripheral or central device or during changes of the central line itself. All air must be purged from the new system before it is connected to the patient, and strict aseptic technique must be maintained when the system is open to air (e.g., gloves and masks must be worn when disconnecting tubing, and ostomy secretions avoided in the area of tubing connections). A 30-second scrub with aqueous antiseptic oxidant (e.g., povidone-iodine) is necessary before the tubing is separated, and all connections must be taped to prevent accidental disconnection.

Increasing glucose infusion. When introducing a child to a higher glucose concentration, rates are progressively increased by increments that will allow a gradual approach to a planned maintenance fluid rate. Every urinary void (or every 4 hours in patients with indwelling catheters) must be tested for sugar and the rate of TPN decreased accordingly if glucosuria is present. A standard nursing protocol and physician's orders must be instituted for assessment of glucosuria by paper tape glucose indicators (e.g., Testape, Chemstrip). The extent of urinary glucose will most often reflect the blood sugar. If urinary glucose is 1+, the physician must be notified; if 2+, a blood glucose estimate by Chemstrip is obtained and the physician notified if >120 mg/dl; if ≥3+, the blood glucose is determined by the chemical laboratory immediately, the glucose infusion rate is adjusted downward pending laboratory results, and the physician is notified for further action.

Generally on day 1 a plan to infuse 80 calories/kg/day and 1.5 to 2.5 g amino acids/kg/day is initiated. Any glucose concentration of more than 12.5% must be infused through either a percutaneous longline (subclavian or antecubital approach) or a central venous catheter whose tip is within 2 cm of the junction of the right atrium and superior vena cava, thus avoiding increased risk for superior vena cava syndrome. This is also an optimal site for avoiding caval or atrial perforation. By adjusting the input rate of the TPN fluid to 300 to 500 mg glucose/kg/hr and increasing the rate gradually (by 25% increments every 15 minutes), the desired fluid volume maintenance rate may be attained.

If TPN is abruptly stopped for any reason (peripheral vein infiltration, central vein thrombosis, sudden catheter removal), the serum glucose level must be monitored and the same glucose load (i.e., in mg/kg/hr) infused via an alternate route in order to prevent hypoglycemia. This may necessitate a rate increase with a solution containing a decreased glucose concentration. Medications must also be infused in a similar glucose-containing solution if at all possible while the TPN is temporarily stopped; otherwise an alternate infusion for glucose should be available for use during medication periods.

Medications. Confirm with the pharmacy which medications are compatible with the TPN to prevent deleterious drug-nutrient interactions. When medi-

cations are infused simultaneously with the TPN through a medication line, the lipid infusion must be halted temporarily to observe the tubing for any visible precipitate. To prevent fluid overload, use of a syringe pump system is recommended. Use of a protective needle device into the existing tubing to prevent needle dislodgment, binding, or breaking is helpful in active patients and/or patients who are transported frequently.

MONITORING

Once a patient is started on TPN, specific indices must be monitored to assess clinical progress and to prevent any complications if possible. Often the underlying illness dictates the stability and need for more or less frequent measurements. It is advisable to establish some type of routine system that can be altered to meet each patient's needs. Parenteral nutrition is generally continued until at least 70% (optimally 90%) of optimal nutrition is being given enterally, but monitoring generally is continued until TPN is stopped. Table 149-6 is a summary of one type of routine monitoring system.

Table 149-6 Monitoring Variables for Pediatric TPN Patients

Variable	Suggested Frequency
Intake and output	Hourly
Vital signs	Every shift
Weight	Daily
Anthropometrics	Bimonthly
Head circumference (infants)	Daily
Urinary glucose	Every void or twice a shift if patient is catheterized
Laboratory studies	
Monday (fingerstick): CBC, K, phosphorus	Weekly
Thursday (venipuncture): Na, K, Cl, bicarbonate, NH₃, bilirubin (conjugated and total), ALT, Ca, BUN, creatinine, phosphorus, prealbumin, albumin	Weekly
Triglyceride	Daily until tolerance is established
Blood cultures (peripheral and central line) and urine cultures	Indicated for temperature >38.5° C (axillary)
Serum glucose	If glycosuria >120 mg/dl and for abrupt cessation of TPN
Access check	Hourly
Developmental testing	
Infant	Every 2-3 months
Child	Annually

RISKS AND COMPLICATIONS
Infections

The most significant complication of TPN therapy is systemic sepsis. Early signs and symptoms include unexplained temperature elevation, glucosuria, hyperglycemia, and/or unexplained weight gain. Later symptoms include lethargy, feeding difficulty (if feeding), hypoglycemia, and hypothermia.

Prophylactic antibiotics must be considered for a patient receiving TPN who begins displaying any of these symptoms, until all cultures are reported at 24 and 48 hours. Infection does not always necessitate catheter removal, which depends on the organism, patient response to antibiotics, and/or the presence of negative blood culture once antibiotics are discontinued. For patients with multilumen catheters it has been suggested that antibiotic doses be infused through all ports of the catheter to sterilize the line and prevent future seeding of the infection. It is important to recognize, differentiate, and track catheter-related sepsis vs. catheter-source sepsis. Catheter-related sepsis is defined as the presence of positive blood cultures with a source other than the catheter identified as the etiologic agent. Catheter-source sepsis is defined as the presence of positive blood cultures with the catheter identified as the etiologic agent because no other source is identified. Infection control expertise can be a valuable tool in prevention of infectious episodes; once trends are recognized, staff members can be educated on ways to prevent future nosocomial infection (see Chapters 41 and 114).

Thorough assessment and treatment of local catheter site infections often prevent systemic sepsis. Thorough assessment necessitates changing from triweekly dressing changes to scrupulous daily dressing changes to assess the site response to local or systemic antibiotic therapy.

Mechanical Risks

Mechanical complications usually become more significant the longer a patient is on TPN. These complications usually involve the equipment (pump, tubing) used to deliver TPN, vehicles for monitoring the patient during therapy (inability to withdraw the blood from the central line), and/or the access device itself. Table 149-7 summarizes the complications, possible causes, and treatment for mechanical problems. A knowledgeable certified nursing staff can be invaluable to the success of administering TPN and preventing mechanical complications. However, once these complications occur, a system must be organized to handle them 24 hours a day, usually necessitating some kind of on-call system for the nutrition support team nurse.

Metabolic Complications

As compared to infections and mechanical complications, the less frequent issues of metabolic complications encompass hyperglycemia, nitrogen intolerance, hypertriglyceridemia, hypophosphatemia and/or hypokalemia, and vitamin or trace mineral deficiency or excess.

Hyperglycemia is associated with either relative peripheral insulin resistance or possibly too rapid advancement of TPN that contains high glucose concentrations. Reducing infusion rates or using exogenous insulin (compatible with all TPN aqueous solutions) usually can control this problem; use insulin:glucose ratios (insulin units:grams glucose) from 1:4 to 1:20 through a separate insulin solution infusion.

Nitrogen intolerance is associated with genetic metabolic disorders (Chapter 17) or insufficient hepatic processing of IV amino acids. The latter may be expressed as mild hyperammonemia or developing cholestasis. Reduced nitrogen infusion may be prudent temporarily. Covering infusion lines with aluminum foil to reduce light-activated cholestatic derivatives in TPN formulations may help reduce the risk of cholestasis. The use of taurine-containing solutions has been suggested, but its long-term efficacy is yet unproved. Nonetheless it may be necessary to remove all amino acids from the TPN solution and give the amino acid or protein requirements enterally in small liquid volume amounts that can be tolerated by the patient. Oral feeds generally ameliorate cholestasis. Balanced amino acid solutions should always be used unless extraordinary disease circumstances exist.

Hypertriglyceridemia is associated with metabolic inhibition of glyceride clearance, insufficient endothelial lipoprotein lipase activity (that may also be cachetin-inhibited in the presence of severe infection or tumor growth), or renal insufficiency. Pulmonary oxygenation and leukocyte function have been reported to be compromised in association with decreased lipid clearance; decreasing, if not stopping,

Table 149-7   Mechanical Complications of TPN

Complication	Possible Cause	Treatment
Pumps		
Activation of pump flow reduction signal or indicator	Air in line; sudden movement of drop counting device	Remove air (hang new solution) and reset pump
Activation of occlusion signal or indicator	Kink in tubing or occluded central line	Untwist tubing; decide whether occlusion is result of precipitant or thrombosis (each listed below); in meantime establish another route for glucose infusion
Tubing		
Hole in tubing or cracked hub	Use of metal hemostats with teeth	Use only smooth hemostats designated for TPN/central line use
	Toddler teething on tube	Keep tubing out of reach or protect with oxygen therapy tubing over IV tubing
Cracked in-line filter	Trauma to filter	Change tubing immediately; protect tubing when putting side rails up and during transport
Peripheral infiltration	Catheter dislodgment	Elevate extremity
Central venous catheter		
Partial occlusion (thrombosis)	Frequent blood drawing	Administer fibrinolytic therapy (urokinase, streptokinase)
	Slow infusion rates	Increase rate or use heparin lock
	Inadequate heparinization technique	Revise technique
Partial occlusion (precipitant)	Incompatible medication; slow infusion rate	Give slow 0.9% sodium chloride solution as drip
Total occlusion (thrombosis)	Pump malfunction; failure to open catheter after clamping	Administer fibrinolytic therapy; use long-line catheter threaded into central line to infuse the agent
Total occlusion (precipitant)	Same as partial occlusion	Use guidewire catheter clearance of precipitant, HCl/heparin installation to dissolve precipitant; replace catheter
Broken/severed catheter	Trauma; sequalae to occlusion; catheter defects	Perform blunt needle repair or permanent repair, depending on catheter type; may necessitate catheter replacement
Perforation pneumothorax (myocardial perforation, potentially fatal complication)	Catheter dislodgment	Remove catheter under surgical visualization; evacuate chest
Air embolism (consider always with unexplained dysrhythmias; uncommon but potentially fatal complication)	Air in line related to complications of catheter insertion; infusions allowed to run dry; breakage of catheter; disrupted connections	Immediately inspect line for break; aspirate line immediately, clamp line, then flood air entry line site with fluid (prevent further air entrainment); place patient in left Trendelenburg position; provide oxygen; perform resuscitation
Superior vena cava syndrome	Too fast flow rate for too small vessel; too high glucose concentration	Elevate patient's head; decrease flow rate and/or glucose concentration of fluid

the rate of infusion until plasma triglycerides normalize is invariably mandatory.

Hypophosphatemia and/or hypokalemia is associated with excessive body fluid mineral loss or with rapid nutritional restitution and rapid new tissue growth. Documenting the site and extent of losses will aid decisions about replacement in the form of enteral or parenteral inorganic phosphate salts (sodium phosphate or potassium phosphate).

Vitamin or trace mineral deficiency or excess are associated with underzealous or overzealous use of parenteral preparations. Body fluid measurements and/or net input-output balances when possible are necessary for making proper readjustments.

Developmental Considerations

An important and real problem for the PICU patient receiving TPN is that of acquired developmental delay. Studies document that neonates on long-term TPN do not progress normally and show diverse delays, the greatest in developed language and gross motor skills. Language delays may be linked to the observed feeding difficulties that occur when oral intake is reintroduced after a long NPO period, the length of which appears to be proportionately related to the appearance of the feeding difficulty. To counter such difficulties the infant must be allowed to use and develop oral actions, even if this does not provide significant nutritional intake, in order to minimize the risk for extraordinary oral sensitization. Suggested steps include the following:

1. Allow ingestion through a nipple of 5 ml of sterile water (even if infant is otherwise NPO) every 3 to 4 hours to maintain a normal suck/swallow pattern.
2. Cycle TPN when possible (e.g., 12 hours on TPN, 12 hours off TPN) to assess potential improvement of appetite with offered oral sucking during the off hours.
3. Provide an appropriate pacifier to at least maintain a suck reflex, even while not allowing much swallowing (except saliva).
4. Encourage hand-mouth stimulation.
5. Stroke the mouth and buccal cavity during the NPO period, using textured items (e.g., washcloth, soft rubber toys) to attempt prevention of oral sensitization.

Refusal to eat may necessitate further investigation for additional problems (see Chapter 150).

The extent of illness, maturity, and degree of constancy in developmental stimulation may contribute to the additionally observed motor skill delays. Sequential testing (e.g., Denver or Bayley tests) can direct a plan by child life, physical therapy, primary nursing, and family or foster caretakers to appropriate developmental motor stimulation. Once delays are documented, activities must be initiated at the infant's measured developmental level to plan progress in motor activities at which the child can succeed. A firm schedule for each infant (e.g., Nursing Kardex/daily bedside action plan) addresses attention by all care providers (including laboratory technicians, respiratory therapists) to issues such as controlled naps, feeding times/intervals, and stimulation consistency for progress in infant learning, which can be enhanced if not actually exaggerated when the infant is exposed to conditions with which he can progressively cope.

ADDITIONAL READING

Allen S, Harper K. Developmental delays in infants on long-term TPN. Nutr Support Serv 3(4):42-43, 1983.

• Allen S, Orr M, Wagner Y, Mize C, Teitell B. Pediatric Nursing Syllabus for Total Parenteral Nutrition. Dallas: Children's Medical Center, 1984.

Curnow A, Adower J, Behrens E, Toomey J, Georgeson K. Urokinase therapy for Silastic catheter-induced intravascular thrombi in infants. Arch Surg 120:1237-1247, 1985.

Feurer I, Mullen TL. Bedside measurement of resting energy expenditure and respiratory quotient via indirect calorimetry. Nutr Clin Prac 3:4333-4349, 1986.

Kerner J, ed. Manual of Pediatric Nutrition. New York: John Wiley, 1983.

Lebenthal E, ed. Total Parenteral Nutrition. New York: Raven Press, 1986.

Mulvihill S, Fonkalsund E. Complications of superior versus inferior vena cava occlusion in infants receiving central total parenteral nutrition. J Pediatr Surg 19:752-757, 1984.

Nauna R, Suskind R. Parenteral nutrition in the pediatric patient. In Rombeau TL, Caldwell MD, eds. Parenteral Nutrition: Clinical Nutrition, vol 2. Philadelphia: WB Saunders, 1986.

Orr M, Allen S. Optimal oral experiences for infants on long-term total parenteral nutrition. Nutr Clin Prac 1:208-295, 1986.

• Pereira GR, Glassman M. Parenteral nutrition in the neonate. In Rombeau TL, Calwell MD, eds. Parental Nutrition: Clinical Nutrition, vol. 2. Philadelphia: WB Saunders, 1986, pp 702-720.

Prince A, Heller B, Levy J, Heird W. Management of fever in patients with central vein catheters. Pediatr Infect Dis 5:20-24, 1986.

Robinson L, Wright B. Central venous catheter occlusion caused by body-heat–mediated calcium-phosphate precipitate. Am J Hosp Pharm 39:120-121, 1982.

Roslyn J, Berquist W, Pitt H, Man L, Kangarloo H, DenBisten L, Amest M. Increased risk of gallstones in children receiving total parenteral nutrition. Pediatrics 71:784-789, 1983.

Sruita A, Skeda K, Nagaski A, Hayashida Y, Kaniko T, Hamano Y, Nakato M, Fung K. Follow-up studies of children treated with a long-term intravenous nutrition (IVN) during the neonatal period. J Pediatr Surg 17:37-41, 1982.

150 Total Enteral Nutrition

Charles E. Mize · Cynthia Cunningham ·
Mary Orr-McDonald

BACKGROUND AND INDICATIONS

Total enteral nutrition (TEN) must be used when the child cannot or will not take adequate oral feedings and when the GI tract is functional. Factors that may contribute to the inability to feed orally include prematurity, respiratory distress, easy fatigability, comatose or semicomatose state, gastroesophageal reflux, selective paralysis, and nonspecific anorexia. Any child unable to consume adequate nutrients orally for >2 days needs to be considered for specialized enteral support. This support may include specially prepared formulas and/or bolus or continuous tube feedings into selected portions of the GI tract. Possible contraindications to the use of enteral feeds include ileus (although controlled jejunostomy feeds may be helpful), risk of aspiration, or necrotizing enterocolitis.

Nutrient Requirements

The recommended dietary allowances (RDA) are used as guidelines for enteral nutrition. The RDA (Table 150-1) are estimated to exceed the requirements (except energy) of most healthy individuals and therefore ensure that the needs of most of the population are met. The RDA cover only healthy individuals and may not meet the requirements for children affected by disease states or medications.

Formula Selection

Breast milk, infant formulas, and enteral feedings are listed in Table 150-2. The feedings may be selected to meet individual medical or physiologic requirements. If given in sufficient quantity to meet energy needs, the breast milk or formulas will usually provide adequate vitamins and minerals. Breast milk may be obtained from manual or pump expression; if it

will be used within 24 hours, it should be kept refrigerated. If it will not be used within 24 hours, it must be frozen, but it must not be kept more than 4 months. Freezing inactivates leukocytes but preserves many desirable immunologic properties. Breast-fed infants must have vitamin D, iron, and fluoride supplementation.

Tube feedings designed for adults are often used for children more than 1 year of age. Because the volume of formula consumed by a child is less than that of an adult, vitamin and mineral intake may be inadequate. Individual evaluation of nutritional adequacy is therefore necessary.

Drug-Nutrient Interactions

Compromised infants who are in the PICU and receiving diverse drugs may be candidates for altered drug effects not only from drug-drug altered metabolic or therapeutic interactions, but from modest to sometimes larger effects of nutrients or enteral feeds that may modify rate of entry to the tissues (e.g., through the GI tract or via tissue metabolism). The effects are primarily those of pharmacokinetic alterations or drug half-life changes rather than from a change in drug metabolite efficacy. Such changes may only be effected if a well-balanced diet is not used (e.g., with use of a ketogenic diet or predominantly carbohydrate-rich diet). Nonetheless, drug-induced altered nutrient utilization can occur, especially with enteral feeds, in several ways: (1) induced malabsorption, (2) promotion of larger than normal urinary losses of small molecular weight nutrients, (3) specific drug inhibition of nutrient uptake, or (4) impaired nutrient conversion or metabolism to active compounds. Of these, the use of enteral laxatives or antibiotics that often decrease nutrient absorption necessitates particular attention in the PICU. Oil-based (in contrast to glycerol-based) materials will inhibit absorption of fat-soluble vitamins and lipids. Broad-based antibiotics that may be retained in the intestinal lumen (e.g., neomycin) will diminish absorption of lipid, nitrogen, and several macrominer-

als (K, Ca, Fe). Diuretics are notorious for causing urinary hyperexcretion of several macrominerals and some microminerals, as do corticoids and aminoglycoside antibiotics. The magnitude of such losses or malabsorptive effects must be estimated for compen-

Table 150-1 Food and Nutrition Board, National Academy of Sciences–National Research Council Recommended Dietary Allowances,[a] revised 1989 (Designed for the maintenance of good nutrition of practically all healthy people in the United States)

Category	Age (yr) or Condition	Weight[b] kg	Weight[b] lb	Height[b] cm	Height[b] in	Protein (g)	Fat-Soluble Vitamins Vitamin A (μg RE)[c]	Fat-Soluble Vitamins Vitamin D (μg)[d]	Fat-Soluble Vitamins Vitamin E (mg α-TE)[e]	Fat-Soluble Vitamins Vitamin K (μg)
Infants	0.0-0.5	6	13	60	24	13	375	7.5	3	5
	0.5-1.0	9	20	71	28	14	375	10	4	10
Children	1-3	13	29	90	35	16	400	10	6	15
	4-6	20	44	112	44	24	500	10	7	20
	7-10	28	62	132	52	28	700	10	7	30
Males	11-14	45	99	157	62	45	1000	10	10	45
	15-18	66	145	176	69	59	1000	10	10	65
	19-24	72	160	177	70	58	1000	10	10	70
	25-50	79	174	176	70	63	1000	5	10	80
	51+	77	170	173	68	63	1000	5	10	80
Females	11-14	46	101	157	62	46	800	10	8	45
	15-18	55	120	163	64	44	800	10	8	55
	19-24	58	128	164	65	46	800	10	8	60
	25-50	63	138	163	64	50	800	5	8	65
	51+	65	143	160	63	50	800	5	8	65
Pregnant						60	800	10	10	65
Lactating	1st 6 mo					65	1300	10	12	65
	2nd 6 mo					62	1200	10	11	65

[a]The allowances, expressed as average daily intakes over time, are intended to provide for individual variations among most normal persons as they live in the United States under usual environmental stresses. Diets should be based on a variety of common foods in order to provide other nutrients for which human requirements have been less well defined.

[b]Weights and heights of reference adults are actual medians for the U.S. population of the designated age, as reported by NHANES II. The median weights and heights of those under 19 years of age were taken from Hamill PVV, Drizd TA, Johnson CL, Reed RB, Rache AF, Moore WM. Physical growth: National Center for Health Statistics percentile. Am J Clin Nutr 32:607-629, 1979. The use of these figures does not imply that the height-to-weight ratios are ideal.

sation attempts if the drug is continued. It is likely in PICU care that drug-induced nutrient effects will most often surface when the patient's nutrition is marginal before drug use is initiated or when the patient's disease process actively predisposes to hy-permetabolism and/or potential deficiency states during drug therapy. Actual drug or nutrient concentrations in blood or tissue sites must ultimately be measured to ensure a desired final concentration at that site.

Text continued on p. 1075.

Water-Soluble Vitamins							Minerals						
Vita-min C (mg)	Thia-min (mg)	Ribo-flavin (mg)	Niacin (mg NE)ᶠ	Vita-min B₆ (mg)	Folate (μg)	Vita-min B₁₂ (μg)	Cal-cium (mg)	Phos-pho-rus (mg)	Magne-sium (mg)	Iron (mg)	Zinc (mg)	Iodine (μg)	Sele-nium (μg)
30	0.3	0.4	5	0.3	25	0.3	400	300	40	6	5	40	10
35	0.4	0.5	6	0.6	35	0.5	600	500	60	10	5	50	15
40	0.7	0.8	9	1.0	50	0.7	800	800	80	10	10	70	20
45	0.9	1.1	12	1.1	75	1.0	800	800	120	10	10	90	20
45	1.0	1.2	13	1.4	100	1.4	800	800	170	10	10	120	30
50	1.3	1.5	17	1.7	150	2.0	1200	1200	270	12	15	150	40
60	1.5	1.8	20	2.0	200	2.0	1200	1200	400	12	15	150	50
60	1.5	1.7	19	2.0	200	2.0	1200	1200	350	10	15	150	70
60	1.5	1.7	19	2.0	200	2.0	800	800	350	10	15	150	70
60	1.2	1.4	15	2.0	200	2.0	800	800	350	10	15	150	70
50	1.1	1.3	15	1.4	150	2.0	1200	1200	280	15	12	150	45
60	1.1	1.3	15	1.5	180	2.0	1200	1200	300	15	12	150	50
60	1.1	1.3	15	1.6	180	2.0	1200	1200	280	15	12	150	55
60	1.1	1.3	15	1.6	180	2.0	800	800	280	15	12	150	55
60	1.0	1.2	13	1.6	180	2.0	800	800	280	10	12	150	55
70	1.5	1.6	17	2.2	400	2.2	1200	1200	320	30	15	175	65
95	1.6	1.8	20	2.1	280	2.6	1200	1200	355	15	19	200	75
90	1.6	1.7	20	2.1	260	2.6	1200	1200	340	15	16	200	75

ᶜRetinol equivalents. 1 retinol equivalent = 1 μg retinol or 6 μg β-carotene.
ᵈAs cholecalciferol. 10 μg cholecalciferol = 400 IU of vitamin D.
ᵉα-Tocopherol equivalents. 1 mg *d*-α-tocopherol = 1 α-TE.
ᶠ1 NE (niacin equivalent) is equal to 1 mg of niacin or 60 mg of dietary tryptophan.

Table 150-2 Infant Formulas and Tube Feedings*

Product	100 ml				Composition (% g/100 g)			mEq/100 ml			mg/100 ml			Osmolality	Comments
	kcal	CHO (g)	Fat (g)	PRO (g)	Carbohydrate	Fat	Protein	Na	K	Cl	Ca	P	Fe	mOsm/kg H₂O	
Casein (feeding normal full-term infants or sick infants without special nutritional requirements)															
Enfamil 20 with iron (Mead Johnson)	68	7.0	3.8	1.5	Lactose	Coconut (55) Soy (45) Soy lecithin Mono- and di-glycerides	Whey (60) Casein (40)	0.8	1.9	1.2	47	32	1.3	300	
Gerber baby formula with iron (Gerber)	68	7.3	3.7	1.5	Lactose	Soy (60) Coconut (40)	Casein (82) Whey (18)	1.0	1.9	1.3	51	39	1.2		The powder contains corn (60) and coconut (40) oil
Similac PM 60/40 (Ross)	68	6.9	3.8	1.5	Lactose (Citrate)	Corn (50) Coconut (50) Mono- and di-glycerides	Demineralized whey (60) Casein (40)	0.7	1.5	1.1	38	19	0.15	280	Ready-to-feed contains soy and coconut oil
Similac 20 with iron (Ross)	68	7.2	3.6	1.5	Lactose (Citrate)	Soy (60) Coconut (40) Soy lecithin	Casein (82) Whey (18)	0.8	1.9	1.3	51	39	1.2	300	The powder contains coconut (50) and corn (50) oil
SMA (Wyeth)	67	7.2	3.6	1.5	Lactose (Citrate)	Oleo (33) Coconut (27) Safflower (25) Soy (15) Soy lecithin <1	Reduced mineral whey (60) Casein (40)	0.7	1.4	1.1	42	28	1.2	300	Nucleotides added
Cow milk†	63	4.8	3.4	3.4	Lactose	Cow butterfat	Casein (82) Whey (18)	2.2	4.0		123	96	0.05	N/A	For use after 1 yr
Goat milk†	71	4.6	4.3	3.7	Lactose	Goat butterfat	Goat milk	2.2	5.4		138	114	0.05	N/A	Folacin and vitamin D deficient unless added
Human milk† (mature)	71	7.2	4.6	1.1	Lactose	Human butterfat	Whey (60) Casein (40)	0.7	1.4		34	14	0.03	N/A	Composition varies with stage of lactation

Soy (feeding for infants intolerant to casein or lactose)

Isomil (Ross)	68	6.8	3.7	1.8	Corn syrup solids (56) Sucrose (44) (Citrate)	Soy (60) Coconut (40) Mono- and di-glycerides Soy lecithin	Soy isolate	1.3	1.9	1.2	71	51	1.2	240	
Isomil SF (Ross)	68	6.9	3.7	1.8	Glucose polymers (Citrate)	Soy (60) Coconut (40) Mono- and di-glycerides Soy lecithin	Soy isolate	1.3	1.9	1.2	71	51	1.2	150	
I-Soyalac (Loma Linda)	69	6.9	3.7	2.1	Sucrose Tapioca Dextrin (Citrate)	Soy Soy lecithin	Soy isolate	1.2	2.0	1.5	69	48	1.3	270	
Nursoy (Wyeth)	67	6.9	3.6	2.1	Sucrose (98) Citrate (2)	Oleo (33) Coconut (27) Safflower (25) Soy (15) Soy lecithin <1	Soy isolate	0.9	1.8	1.1	60	42	1.2	296	
Prosobee (Mead Johnson)	68	6.8	3.6	2.0	Corn syrup solids (Citrate)	Coconut (55) Soy (45) Soy lecithin Mono- and di-glycerides	Soy isolate	1.1	2.1	1.6	64	50	1.3	200	The powder contains coconut (55) and corn (45) oil
RCF (Ross)	41	<1	3.6	2.0		Soy (60) Coconut (40)	Soy isolate	1.3	1.8	1.2	70	50	0.1	74	Carbohydrate to be added

Incomplete infant feedings for special purposes

Provimin (Ross)	10	tr	tr	2.4	Citrate	Coconut	Casein L-Amino acids	1.7	2.8	2.1	79	56	0.7		No selenium or chromium; fat and CHO to be added 1 Tbsp = 7 g
S-29 (Wyeth)	67	9.8	2.2	1.7	Lactose (Citrate)	Oleo (33) Coconut (27) Safflower (25) Soy (15) Soy lecithin <1	Reduced mineral whey	0.05	0.8	0.06	16	19	1.3	359	Deficient minerals (insufficient for growth) 1 Tbsp = 10 g

CHO = carbohydrate; PRO = protein; MCT = medium-chain triglycerides.

*From Cunningham C, Mize CE. Infant Formulas and Tube Feedings, 4th ed. Columbus, Ohio: Ross Laboratories.

†Agricultural Handbook No. 8-1. Washington, D.C.: U.S. Department of Agriculture, Agricultural Research Center, revised November 1976.

Continued.

Table 150-2 Infant Formulas and Tube Feedings—cont'd

Product	100 ml				Composition (%) g/100 g			mEq/100 ml			mg/100 ml			Osmolality	Comments
	kcal	CHO (g)	Fat (g)	PRO (g)	Carbohydrate	Fat	Protein	Na	K	Cl	Ca	P	Fe	mOsm/kg H₂O	

Casein hydrolysates (for infants requiring low molecular weight peptides or amino acids)

Product	kcal	CHO (g)	Fat (g)	PRO (g)	Carbohydrate	Fat	Protein	Na	K	Cl	Ca	P	Fe	mOsm/kg H₂O	Comments
Alimentum (Ross)	68	6.9	3.8	1.9	Sucrose (67) Modified tapioca starch (33) (Citrate)	MCT (56) Safflower (44) Soy	Hydrolyzed casein	1.3	2.0	1.5	71	51	1.2	370	
Nutramigen (Mead Johnson)	68	9.1	2.7	1.9	Corn syrup solids (83) Modified cornstarch (17)	Corn oil	Hydrolyzed casein	1.4	1.9	1.6	64	42	1.3	320	
Pregestimil (Mead Johnson)	68	7.0	3.6	1.9	Corn syrup solids (59) Cornstarch (20) Dextrose (19) Citrate (2)	MCT (60) Corn (20) Safflower (20) Soy lecithin	Hydrolyzed casein	1.1	1.9	1.6	64	42	1.3	350	

Premature (for rapidly growing premature infants until reaching about 1800 g)

Product	kcal	CHO (g)	Fat (g)	PRO (g)	Carbohydrate	Fat	Protein	Na	K	Cl	Ca	P	Fe	mOsm/kg H₂O	Comments
Enfamil Premature 24 with iron (Mead Johnson)	81	8.9	4.1	2.4	Corn syrup solids (60) Lactose (40) (Citrate)	Soy (40) MCT (40) Coconut (20) Mono- and diglycerides	Whey (60) Casein (40)	1.4	2.1	1.9	133	67	1.5	300	
Enfamil human milk fortifier (Mead Johnson)	3.5	0.68	0.0	0.18	Corn syrup solids (75) Lactose (25)		Whey (60) Casein (40)	0.08	0.10	0.12	23	11	0	—	To be mixed with human milk; not intended as sole source of nutrients Values are for 1 packet (0.95 g/packet)
Similac Natural Care (Ross)	81	8.6	4.4	2.2	Lactose (50) Glucose polymers (50) (Citrate)	MCT (50) Soy (30) Coconut (20) Mono- and diglycerides Soy lecithin	Cow milk whey	1.5	2.7	1.9	171	85	0.3	300	To be mixed with human milk; not intended as sole source of nutrients
Similac Special Care 24 with iron (Ross)	81	8.6	4.4	2.2	Lactose Glucose polymers (Citrate)	MCT Soy Coconut Mono- and diglycerides	Cow milk whey	1.5	2.7	1.9	146	73	1.5	300	

(Wyeth)

Product					Carbohydrate	Fat	Protein							mOsm	Comments
(Wyeth)					(50) Lactose (50) (Citrate)	Safflower (25) Oleo (20) Soy (18) MCT (10) Soy lecithin (<1)	Casein (40)							280	

Electrolyte solutions

Product					Carbohydrate	Fat	Protein							mOsm	Comments
Lytren (Mead Johnson)	10	2.0	0	0	Dextrose (78) Citrate (22)			5.0	2.5	4.5	0	0	0	0	220
Pedialyte (Ross)	10	2.5	0	0	Dextrose (81) Citrate (19)			4.5	2.0	3.5	0	0	0	0	250
Rehydrolyte (Ross)	10	2.5	0	0	Dextrose (81) Citrate (19)			7.5	2.0	6.5	0	0	0	0	305

1 kcal/ml (adult products for normal nutritional needs; if used for children <6 yr, consult registered dietitian for nutritional adequacy)

Product					Carbohydrate	Fat	Protein							mOsm	Comments
Attain (Sherwood)	100	12	4.0	4.0	Maltodextrin (99) (Citrate) (1)	Corn (96) Soy lecithin (4)	Casein	3.0	2.9	3.0	63	63	0	1.1	300	
Ensure (Ross)	106	14.5	3.7	3.7	Corn syrup (70) Sucrose (30) (Citrate)	Corn Soy lecithin	Casein (88) Soy isolate (12)	3.7	4.0	3.7	53	53	0	1.0	470	
Ensure HN (Ross)	106	14.1	3.6	4.4	Corn syrup (60) Sucrose (40) (Citrate)	Corn Soy	Casein (89) Soy isolate (11)	3.5	4.0	3.7	76	76	0	1.4	470	
Instant Breakfast	106	13.5	3.1	5.7	Sucrose Corn syrup solids Lactose	Cow butterfat	Casein Whey	4.2	5.5	N/A	185	154	0	1.7	694	Values are for 1 envelope and 8 oz whole cow milk; figures given for vanilla (figures vary according to flavors)
Isocal (Mead Johnson)	106	13.3	4.4	3.4	Maltodextrins (Citrate)	Soy (75) MCT (20) Lecithin (5)	Casein (80) Soy isolate (20)	2.3	3.4	3.0	63	53	0	1.0	300	
Isocal HN (Mead Johnson)	106	12.4	4.5	4.4	Maltodextrins (Citrate)	Soy (54) MCT (43) Polyglyceride fatty acid esters (3)	Casein (78) Soy isolate (22)	4.0	4.1	4.1	85	85	0	1.5	300	
Isosource (Sandoz)	120	16.6	4.2	4.3	Maltodextrin (Citrate)	MCT (50) Canola (50) Soy lecithin	Casein Soy isolate	3.1	4.3	3.2	68	68	0	1.2	390	

Continued.

Table 150-2 Infant Formulas and Tube Feedings—cont'd

Product	100 ml				Composition (%) g/100 g			mEq/100 ml			mg/100 ml			Osmolality	Comments
	kcal	CHO (g)	Fat (g)	PRO (g)	Carbohydrate	Fat	Protein	Na	K	Cl	Ca	P	Fe	mOsm/kg H₂O	
1 kcal/ml—cont'd															
Isosource HN (Sandoz)	120	15.6	4.2	5.3	Maltodextrin (Citrate)	MCT (50) Canola (50) Soy lecithin	Casein Soy isolate	3.1	4.3	3.2	68	68	1.2	390	
Osmolite (Ross)	106	14.5	3.9	3.7	Hydrolyzed cornstarch (Citrate)	MCT (50) Corn (40) Soy (10) Soy lecithin	Casein (88) Soy isolate (12)	2.8	2.6	2.4	53	53	0.9	300	
Osmolite HN (Ross)	106	14.1	3.7	4.4	Hydrolyzed cornstarch (Citrate)	MCT (50) Corn (40) Soy (10) Soy lecithin	Casein Soy isolate (12)	4.0	4.0	4.1	76	76	1.4	300	
Resource (Sandoz)	106	14.5	3.7	3.7	Maltodextrin Sucrose (Citrate)	Corn Lecithin	Casein Soy isolate	3.0	3.0	2.8	55	55	1.0	430	
Sustacal (Mead Johnson)	100	14.0	2.3	6.1	Sucrose (71) Corn syrup (29) (Citrate)	Partially hydrogenated soy (98) 18:2 (37) 18:3 (2) Lecithin (2)	Casein (80) Soy isolate (20)	4.1	5.4	4.2	101	93	1.7	620	Chocolate, 700 mOsm/kg
Special purpose (incomplete feeding)															
Aminaid (McGaw)	196	36.6	4.6	1.9	Maltodextrin (65) Sucrose (35)	Partially hydrogenated soy oil (98) Lecithin (2) Mono- and diglycerides (<1)	Essential L-amino acids	<1.5		0	0	0	0	700	No vitamins; deficient minerals; histidine-enriched; useful in renal failure
Citrotein (Sandoz)	66	12.0	0.2	4.1	Sucrose Maltodextrins (Citrate)	Partially hydrogenated soy Mono- and diglycerides	Egg white	3.1	1.8	2.7	106	106	3.8	480	
Portagen (Mead Johnson)	68	7.8	3.3	2.4	Corn syrup solids (73) Sucrose (25) Lactose (2) (Citrate)	MCT (86) Corn (12) Lecithin (2)	Casein	1.6	2.2	1.6	64	48	1.3	220	Available in powder only
Ross SLD (Ross)	70	13.7	<0.1	3.8	Sucrose (65) Hydrolyzed cornstarch (35)		Egg white	3.6	3.3	2.8	70	70	1.3	545	Useful in supplementing clear fluids

Comply (Sherwood)	150	18.0	6.0	6.0	Hydrolyzed cornstarch (99) (Citrate) (1)	Corn (95) Soy lecithin (5)	Casein	4.8	4.7	4.8	100	100	1.8	410
Ensure Plus (Ross)	150	20.0	5.3	5.5	Corn syrup (77) Sucrose (23) (Citrate)	Corn Soy lecithin	Casein Soy isolate	4.6	5.0	5.6	70	70	1.3	690
Ensure Plus HN (Ross)	150	20.0	5.0	6.3	Hydrolyzed cornstarch (78) Sucrose (22)	Corn Soy lecithin	Casein Soy isolate (11)	5.1	4.6	4.5	106	106	1.9	650
Pulmocare (Ross)	150	10.6	9.2	6.3	Sucrose (54) Hydrolyzed cornstarch (46) (Citrate)	Corn Soy lecithin	Casein	5.7	4.4	4.8	105	105	1.9	490
Resource Plus (Sandoz)	150	20.0	5.3	5.5	Maltodextrin Sucrose (Citrate)	Corn Lecithin	Casein Soy isolate	3.9	4.5	4.5	63	63	1.4	600
Sustacal HC (Mead Johnson)	150	19.0	5.8	6.1	Corn syrup solids (72) Sucrose (28) (Citrate)	Corn (94) Lecithin (6)	Casein	3.6	3.8	3.6	85	85	1.5	650
Traumacal (Mead Johnson)	150	14.3	6.8	8.3	Corn syrup (68) Sucrose (31) (Citrate) (1)	Soy (64) MCT (32) Lecithin (4)	Casein	5.1	3.6	4.5	75	75	0.9	490

Isocal HCN (Mead Johnson)	200	20.0	10.2	7.5	Corn syrup (99) (Citrate) (<1)	Soy (69) MCT (27) Lecithin (4)	Casein	3.5	4.3	3.4	100	100	1.8	690
Magnacal (Sherwood)	200	25.0	8.0	7.0	Maltodextrin Sucrose (Citrate)	Partially hydrogenated soy (95) Soy lecithin (2) Mono- and di-glyceride (3)	Casein	4.4	3.2	2.7	100	100	1.8	590
Two Cal HN (Ross)	200	21.7	9.1	8.4	Hydrolyzed cornstarch (87) Sucrose (13) (Citrate)	Corn (80) MCT (20) Soy lecithin	Casein	5.7	6.3	4.7	105	105	1.9	690

Continued.

Table 150-2 Infant Formulas and Tube Feedings—cont'd

Product	100 ml			Composition (%) g/100 g				mEq/100 ml			mg/100 ml			Osmolality	Comments
	kcal	CHO (g)	Fat (g)	PRO (g)	Carbohydrate	Fat	Protein	Na	K	Cl	Ca	P	Fe	mOsm/kg H₂O	

Pediatric feeding (for normal nutritional needs of children 1-6 yr)

Product	kcal	CHO (g)	Fat (g)	PRO (g)	Carbohydrate	Fat	Protein	Na	K	Cl	Ca	P	Fe	mOsm/kg H₂O	Comments
Pediasure (Ross)	100	11.0	5.0	3.0	Hydrolyzed cornstarch Sucrose (Citrate)	Safflower (50) Soy (30) MCT (20) Mono- and diglycerides Soy lecithin	Casein (82) Whey (18)	1.7	3.4	2.9	97	80	1.4	<310	For age 1-6 yr

Feedings with fiber (dietary fiber contains both soluble and insoluble fiber and is the undigested portion of the fiber)

Product	kcal	CHO (g)	Fat (g)	PRO (g)	Carbohydrate	Fat	Protein	Na	K	Cl	Ca	P	Fe	mOsm/kg H₂O	Comments
Enrich (Ross)	110	16.0	3.7	4.0	Hydrolyzed cornstarch (58) Sucrose (32) Soy polysaccharide (10)	Corn Soy lecithin	Casein (87) Soy isolate (13)	3.6	4.3	4.0	71	71	1.3	480	1.4 g dietary fiber/ 100 ml
Glucerna (Ross)	100	9.4	5.6	4.2	Hydrolyzed cornstarch (53) Soy polysaccharide (25) Fructose (21) (Citrate) (14)	Safflower Soy Soy lecithin	Casein	4.0	4.0	4.1	70	70	1.3	375	1.4 g dietary fiber/ 100 ml
Jevity (Ross)	106	15.2	3.7	4.4	Hydrolyzed cornstarch (86) Soy polysaccharide (14) (Citrate) (14)	MCT (50) Corn (40) Soy (10) Soy lecithin	Casein	4.0	3.7	4.0	91	76	1.4	310	1.4 g dietary fiber/ 100 ml
Profiber (Sherwood)	100	13.2	4.0	4.0	Hydrolyzed cornstarch (90) Soy fiber (9) (Citrate) (1)	Corn (95) Soy lecithin (5)	Casein	3.2	3.2	3.4	67	67	1.2	300	1.2 g dietary fiber/ 100 ml
Sustacal with fiber (Mead Johnson)	106	14.0	3.5	4.6	Maltodextrin (51) Sucrose (49) Soy polysaccharide (Citrate)	Corn (94) Lecithin (3) Mono- and diglycerides (3)	Casein (80) Soy isolate (20)	3.1	3.6	4.0	85	70	1.3	480	0.6 g dietary fiber/ 100 ml

Product					Carbohydrate source	Fat source	Protein source								
Ultracal (Mead Johnson)	104	12.1	4.5	4.3	Maltodextrin (97); Oat and soy fiber (Citrate) (3)	Soy (60); MCT (40); Mono- and diglycerides (<1); Soy lecithin (<1)	Casein	4.0	3.0	4.0	83	83	1.5	310	1.4 g dietary fiber/100 ml
Blenderized															
Compleat (Sandoz)	107	12.8	4.3	4.3	Maltodextrin; Vegetables; Fruits; Lactose (Citrate)	Corn; Mono- and diglycerides	Beef; Casein; Whey	5.6	3.6	3.2	68	120	1.2	450	
Compleat modified (Sandoz)	107	14.1	3.7	4.3	Maltodextrin; Vegetables; Fruits (Citrate)	Corn; Mono- and diglycerides	Beef; Casein	4.3	3.6	3.2	68	92	1.2	300	
Vitaneed (Sherwood)	100	12.8	4.0	4.0	Maltodextrin; Vegetables; Fruits; Soy fiber (Citrate)	Corn (94); Soy lecithin (6)	Beef; Casein	3.0	3.2	2.8	67	67	1.2	300	
Elemental and partially elemental (complete feeding useful for limited digestion/absorption)															
Criticare HN (Mead Johnson)	106	22.0	0.5	3.8	Maltodextrin (92); Modified cornstarch (6) (Citrate) (2)	Safflower (77); Soy (12); Mono- and diglycerides (<1); Polyglycerol fatty acid esters (10)	Hydrolyzed casein (97); Amino acids (3)	2.7	3.4	3.0	53	53	1.0	650	
Pepti 2000 (Sherwood)	100	19.0	1.0	4.0	Maltodextrin	MCT; Corn	Hydrolyzed lactalbumin	3.0	3.0	3.0	63	63	1.1	490	
Reabilan (O'Brien)	100	13.2	3.9	3.2	Dextrin maltose (80); Tapioca (20)	MCT (40); Primrose (23); Soy (16); Soy lecithin (13); Mono- and distearate (8)	Casein and whey Hydrolysate >92; Amino acids (8)	3.0	3.2	5.6	50	50	1.0	350	
Reabilan HN (O'Brien)	133	15.8	5.2	5.8	Dextrin maltose (80); Tapioca (20)	MCT (40); Primrose (23); Soy (16); Soy lecithin (13); Mono- and distearate (8)	Casein and whey hydrolysate (92); Amino acids (8)	4.3	4.2	7.0	45	50	1.9	490	

Continued.

Table 150-2 Infant Formulas and Tube Feedings—cont'd

Product	100 ml				Composition (%) g/100 g			mEq/100 ml			mg/100 ml			Osmolality	Comments
	kcal	CHO (g)	Fat (g)	PRO (g)	Carbohydrate	Fat	Protein	Na	K	Cl	Ca	P	Fe	mOsm/kg H₂O	

Elemental and partially elemental—cont'd

Product	kcal	CHO (g)	Fat (g)	PRO (g)	Carbohydrate	Fat	Protein	Na	K	Cl	Ca	P	Fe	mOsm/kg H₂O	Comments
Tolerex (Norwich Eaton)	100	22.6	0.1	1.7	Glucose oligosaccharides Citrate Glycerol	Safflower	L-Amino acids	2.0	3.0	2.7	56	56	1.0	550	Glutamine added; calculated protein factor equiv. = 0.83
Vital High Nitrogen (Ross)	100	18.5	1.1	4.2	Hydrolyzed cornstarch (83) Sucrose (17) Lactose <1 (Citrate)	Safflower (55) MCT (45) Soy lecithin Mono- and di-glycerides	Partially hydrolyzed whey, meat, and soy (87) Essential amino acids (13)	2.5	3.6	2.9	67	67	1.2	500	
Vivonex TEN (Norwich Eaton)	100	20.6	0.3	3.2	Maltodextrin Modified starch Glycerol (Citrate)	Safflower	L-Amino acids	2.0	2.0	2.3	50	50	0.9	630	Glutamine added; calculated protein factor equiv. = 0.83

Carbohydrate

Product	kcal	CHO (g)	Fat (g)	PRO (g)	Carbohydrate	Fat	Protein	Na	K	Cl	Ca	P	Fe	mOsm/kg H₂O	Comments
Cornstarch (Argo)	350	83	Trace	0	Polysaccharides										1 Tbsp powder = 10 g
Corn syrup (Karo)	287	74	0	0	Polysaccharides (48) Glucose (26) Maltose (13) Trisaccharide (11) Fructose (2)			6.5		6.5	46	16	4.1		1 Tbsp = 20 g
Moducal (Mead Johnson)	380	95			Maltodextrin			3.0	0.13	4.8					1 Tbsp = 8 g powder; 8% solution = 69 mOsm/kg H₂O
Polycose (Ross)	380	94			Hydrolyzed cornstarch: G1-7 (59) G8-12 (9) G13-25 (11) >25 (2)			<4.8	<0.3	<6.3	<30	<5			Liquid solution contains 2.0 cal/ml; 1 Tbsp powder = 6.0 g

Product (manufacturer)	kcal	CHO	Fat	Protein	CHO source	Fat source	Protein source							Comments
Sumacal (Sherwood)	380	95			Maltodextrin			4.3	<1	<1	5.9	<1	<1	
Protein														
Casec (Mead Johnson)	370	0	2	88		Cow butterfat	Casein	6.5		0.3	1600	800		1 Tbsp powder = 4.7 g
Promod (Ross)	424	<10	9	75	Lactose	Cow butterfat, Soy lecithin	Whey	<9.8	<25.0		<667	<502		1 Tbsp powder = 4 g; 1 scoop powder = 6.6 g
Propac (Sherwood)	395	6	8	75	Lactose	Lecithin	Whey	9.8	12.8	1.4	350	300		1 Tbsp powder = 4 g
Fat														
Corn oil	900	0	100			Corn oil								
Microlipid (Sherwood)	450/100 ml		50/100 ml			Safflower (98), Soy lecithin (<1), Polyglycerides (2)								mOsm/kg H$_2$O = 60
MCT (Mead Johnson)	830	0	100			<C8 (6), C8 (67), C10 (23), >C10 (4)								
Defined formulations only for special metabolic indications														
HIS 1 (Mead Johnson)	270	17	0	51	Sucrose	0	L-Amino acids	47	59	47	2400	1860	34	No histidine; 1 Tbsp powder = 10 g
HIS 2 (Mead Johnson)	300	7	0	67	Sucrose	0	L-Amino acids	28	34	28	1310	1010	15	No histidine; 1 Tbsp powder = 10 g
HOM 1 (Mead Johnson)	280	18	0	52	Sucrose	0	L-Amino acids	47	59	46	2400	1860	34	No methionine; 1 Tbsp powder = 10 g
HOM 2 (Mead Johnson)	300	5	0	69	Sucrose	0	L-Amino acids	28	34	28	1310	1010	15	No methionine; 1 Tbsp powder = 10 g
Lofenalac (Mead Johnson)	462	60	18	15	Corn syrup solids (82), Tapioca (16), (Citrates) 2	Corn	Hydrolyzed casein (93), L-Amino acids (7)	9.5	12.0	9.0	430	320	8.6	Deficient in phenylalanine; tyrosine enriched; 1 Tbsp powder = 9.6 g
Low methionine diet (3200K) (Mead Johnson)	518	51	28	15.5	Corn syrup solids	Coconut (55), Corn (45)	Soy isolate	8.0	16.1	12.1	480	380	9.7	Low methionine

Continued.

Table 150-2 Infant Formulas and Tube Feedings—cont'd

Defined formulations only for special metabolic indications—cont'd

Product	100 ml				Composition (%) g/100 g			mEq/100 ml			mg/100 ml			Osmolality	Comments
	kcal	CHO (g)	Fat (g)	PRO (g)	Carbohydrate	Fat	Protein	Na	K	Cl	Ca	P	Fe	mOsm/kg H_2O	
LYS 1 (Mead Johnson)	280	23	0	48	Sucrose		L-Amino acids	47	59	46	2400	1860	34		No lysine 1 Tbsp powder = 9.0 g
LYS 2 (Mead Johnson)	300	12	0	64	Sucrose		L-Amino acids	28	34	28	1310	1010	15		No lysine 1 Tbsp powder = 9.0 g
Maxamaid MSUD (Ross)	350	62	<1	25	Sucrose Hydrolyzed cornstarch (Citrate)		L Amino acids	25	21	13	810	810	12		No isoleucine, no leucine, no valine 1 Tbsp powder = 10 g
Maxamaid XMET (Ross)	350	62	<1	25	Sucrose Hydrolyzed cornstarch (Citrate)		L-Amino acids	25	21	13	810	810	12		No methionine 1 Tbsp powder = 10 g
Maxamaid Xmet, Thre, Val, Isoleu (Ross)	350	62	<1	25	Sucrose Hydrolyzed cornstarch (Citrate)		L-Amino acids	25	21	13	810	810	12		No methionine, no threonine, no valine, low isoleucine 1 Tbsp powder = 10 g
Maxamaid XP (Ross)	350	62	<1	25	Sucrose Hydrolyzed cornstarch (Citrate)		L-Amino acids	25	21	13	810	810	12		No phenylalanine 1 Tbsp powder = 10 g
Maximaid Xphen, Tyr (Ross)	350	62	<1	25	Sucrose Hydrolyzed cornstarch (Citrate)		L-Amino acids	25	21	13	810	810	12		No phenylalanine, no tyrosine 1 Tbsp powder = 10 g
Maximum MSUD (Ross)	340	45	<1	39	Sucrose Hydrolyzed cornstarch (Citrate)	Soy Lecithin	L-Amino acids	24	18	16	670	670	23.5		No isoleucine, no leucine, no valine 1 Tbsp powder = 10 g
Maximum XP (Ross)	340	45	<1	39	Sucrose Hydrolyzed cornstarch (Citrate)	Soy Lecithin	L-Amino acids	24	18	16	670	670	23.5		No phenylalanine 1 Tbsp powder = 10 g

Product					Carbohydrate source	Fat source	Protein source							Comments
MSUD diet powder (Mead Johnson)	473	63	20	9.9	Corn syrup solids (84) Modified tapioca (16)	Corn	L-Amino acids	8.0	12.5	10.4	490	270	8.9	No leucine, no isoleucine, no valine / 1 Tbsp powder = 12.5 g
MSUD 1 (Mead Johnson)	280	29	0	41	Sucrose		L-Amino acids	47	59	46	2400	1860	34	No leucine, no isoleucine, no valine / 1 Tbsp powder = 10 g
MSUD 2 (Mead Johnson)	310	22	0	54	Sucrose		L-Amino acids	28	34	28	1310	1010	15	No branched-chain amino acids / 1 Tbsp powder = 10 g
OS 1 (Mead Johnson)	280	29	0	42	Sucrose		L-Amino acids	47	59	46	2400	1860	34	No valine, no threonine, no methionine; ≤100 mg isoleucine/100 g / 1 Tbsp powder = 10 g
OS 2 (Mead Johnson)	300	20	0	56	Sucrose		L-Amino acids	28	34	28	1310	1010	15	No valine, no threonine, no methionine; ≤150 mg isoleucine/100 g / 1 Tbsp powder = 10 g
Phenyl-Free (Mead Johnson)	410	66	6.8	20	Sucrose (64) Corn syrup solids (18) Modified tapioca (18)	Corn (66) Coconut (28) Lecithin (6)	L-Amino acids	18	35	26	510	510	12.2	No phenylalanine, tyrosine enriched / 1 Tbsp powder = 9.9 g
PKU 1 (Mead Johnson)	280	19	0	50	Sucrose		L-Amino acids	47	59	46	2400	1860	34	No phenylalanine, tyrosine enriched / 1 Tbsp powder = 10 g
PKU 2 (Mead Johnson)	300	7	0	67	Sucrose		L-Amino acids	28	34	28	1310	1010	15	No phenylalanine, tyrosine enriched / 1 Tbsp powder = 10 g
PKU 3 (Mead Johnson)	290	3	0	68	Sucrose		L-Amino acids	28	34	28	1310	1010	21	No phenylalanine, tyrosine enriched / 1 Tbsp powder = 10g

Continued.

Table 150-2 Infant Formulas and Tube Feedings—cont'd

Defined formulations only for special metabolic indications—cont'd

Product	100 ml				Composition (%) g/100 g			mEq/100 ml			mg/100 ml			Osmolality	Comments
	kcal	CHO (g)	Fat (g)	PRO (g)	Carbohydrate	Fat	Protein	Na	K	Cl	Ca	P	Fe	mOsm/kg H₂O	
Protein free diet (Mead Johnson) (80056)	486	72	22	0	Corn syrup solids (85) Modified tapioca (15)	Corn		3.7	8.7	3.8	540	300	11		Deficient in sodium, potassium, and chloride / 1 Tbsp powder = 12 g
TYR I (Mead Johnson)	270	21	0	47	Sucrose		L-Amino acids	47	59	46	2400	1860	34		No phenylalanine, no tyrosine / 1 Tbsp powder = 10 g
TYR 2 (Mead Johnson)	300	12	0	63	Sucrose		L-Amino acids	28	34	28	1310	1010	15		No phenylalanine, no tyrosine / 1 Tbsp powder = 10 g
UCD 1 (Mead Johnson)	260	8	0	56	Sucrose		Essential L-amino acids	55	72	55	2800	2200	40		Histidine, cystine, and tyrosine added / 1 Tbsp powder = 10 g
UCD 2 (Mead Johnson)	290	6	0	67	Sucrose		Essential L-amino acids	28	34	28	1310	1010	15		Histidine added / 1 Tbsp powder = 10 g
3200AB (low Phe/Tyr) (Mead Johnson)	462	60	18	15	Glucose polymers (82) Tapioca (16) (Citrates) 2	Corn	Hydrolyzed casein (97) L-Amino acids (3)	10	12	9	430	320	8.6		Deficient in phenylalanine and tyrosine / 1 Tbsp powder = 9.6 g
Mono- and disaccharide-free powder 3232A (Mead Johnson)	517	33	33	22	Tapioca Starch	MCT (85) Corn (14) Soy lecithin (1)	Hydrolyzed casein (97) L-Amino acids (3)	15	22	19	740	490	14.8		Carbohydrate to be added

TECHNIQUE
Selecting a Nasoenteric Feeding Tube

Tube size. Tubes for small infants are usually No. 5 or No. 6 F. For older children and adolescents a No. 8 F is generally used. Blenderized formula or viscous tube feedings usually need a larger bore tube.

Tube type. A large variety of enteral feeding tubes is available. The limited number of comparative studies have not conclusively demonstrated the most desirable features. Table 150-3 summarizes the general types of nasoenteric tubes available and the advantages and disadvantages of each. More studies are needed to identify the most appropriate tubes for PICU patients. Direct gastrostomy tubes, usually of larger internal bore diameter, are generally of latex rubber and without weighted ends or stylets (e.g., Foley or mushroom style urinary catheters). Nasoenteric tubes may in turn be threaded through the gastrostomy tubes (with distal openings) for placement in the upper small bowel as needed.

Insertion of Nasoenteral Tubes

Orogastric tube insertion. Since infants are obligatory nose breathers, it may be preferable to pass the feeding tube through the mouth rather than the nares. Insertion through the mouth may decrease distress and help stimulate sucking. Since orogastric tubes are difficult to secure, they are usually inserted just before the feeding and removed after the feeding is completed.

Nasogastric tube insertion. Indwelling gastric tubes are usually placed through the nose. The length of the tube for insertion may be estimated by measuring from the tip of the nose to the earlobe and then to the tip of the xiphoid process. However, this measurement merely provides an estimate, and the placement must be verified. Bedside verification can be done by one of two methods: (1) aspiration of gastric contents and measurement of the pH, which should be <5, or (2) injection of a small amount (3 to 5 ml) of air while simultaneously listening with a stethoscope placed over the stomach. If the tube is properly positioned, sounds of gurgling will be auscultated. Although both of these methods offer strong evidence of appropriate tube position, radiographic confirmation is the best method for verifying tube placement.

Intubated or sedated patients who have a styleted tube inserted are at risk for inadvertent tube placement in the trachea or pleural space. Radiographic confirmation of placement is recommended for these patients. In addition a tube design that pre-

---

Table 150-3   Nasoenteric Feeding Tubes

	Advantages	Disadvantages
Polyvinylchloride (PVC) non-weighted, nonstyleted tubes	Less expensive Probable decreased risk of perforation during insertion No stylet needed for insertion or re-positioning	May stiffen with long-term use, leading to increased risk of perforation Less comfortable than soft tubes Increased incidence of nonelective extubation
Nonweighted polyurethane or silicone tubes	More comfortable than PVC tubes Water-activated lubricant (on most tubes) facilitates insertion and removal Improved flow rate of fiber-containing formulas (over PVC)	Usually needs stylet for insertion Increased risk of perforation during insertion Repositioning necessitates complete removal of tube to stylet
Weighted polyurethane or silicone tubes with stylet	Weight may facilitate passage into duodenum or jejunum* Weight may decrease accidental tube dislodgment* Easier insertion in intubated patients See other advantages listed under nonweighted polyurethane tubes	Nasoduodenal or nasojejunal placement may dictate fluoroscopic visualization or administration of metoclopramide More expensive See other disadvantages listed under non-weighted polyurethane tubes

*Not well supported by clinical evidence.

vents the stylet tip from passing beyond the tip of the tube or out of a side portal must be selected. Any time that it must be repositioned, the tube must be completely removed from the patient before reinserting the stylet.

After the tube is placed, it must be secured to the cheek. In most cases the tube must not be secured to the forehead or nose because of possible obstruc-

tion or erosion of the nares. Tube placement can be alternated between nares with each insertion to minimize irritation or erosion of mucosa. The nasal mucosa must be carefully inspected at least two to three times daily for evidence of any irritation. For active infants or toddlers the tube may also be taped behind the ear and down the back to help prevent accidental removal.

Table 150-4   Comparison of Sites of Tube Placement

Type	Indications	Advantages	Disadvantages	Contraindications
Nasogastric	Inadequate oral intake Continuous drip feedings Nocturnal feedings Premature infants (inadequate suck/swallow) Refusal to eat	Promotes normal hormonal and digestive processes Easy to insert	Increased risk of aspiration pneumonia Increased risk of tube dislodgment May obstruct nares May damage nasal mucosa Bypasses oral cavity; high risk of feeding and oral-motor problems	No gag reflex Gastric obstruction Intractable vomiting Gastroesophageal reflux
Gastrostomy	Ineffective sucking and swallowing reflexes Oropharyngeal, tracheal, esophageal anomalies Long-term coma Esophageal injury Long-term enteral feeds (not manageable with nasogastric feeds)	Improved stability of tube Prevents need for repeated reinsertion of tube	Risk of exit site infection Requires surgical placement or percutaneous insertion via endoscope Bypasses oral cavity; high risk of feeding and oral-motor problems	—
Transpyloric	Children at risk for aspiration pneumonia, including those with gastroesophageal reflux, gastric outlet obstruction, intractable vomiting, intubation	Decreased risk of dislodgment	May necessitate continuous infusion via a pump Placement may necessitate fluoroscopic visualization or use of metoclopramide (metoclopramide may cause dumping syndrome) Bypasses oral cavity	—

Site of Placement

Sites of tube placement must be carefully considered according to accessible anatomy, projected length of controlled feeding, and support resources for tube maintenance. Key issues are summarized in Table 150-4.

Selecting an Enteral Feeding Pump

Continuous enteral feedings must be administered with a pump. Historically IV infusion pumps have been used for the administration of continuous drip feedings, but recently more sophisticated enteral pumps have been developed for use with pediatric populations. The advantages of using enteral pumps include decreased expense, decreased risk of accidental connection of enteral tubing to an IV infusion, and simpler pump operation. The disadvantages of enteral pumps may include diminished accuracy and fewer alarms to alert nurses of impending problems. The desired features for a pediatric enteral feeding pump include (1) 10% or better accuracy; (2) ability to make rate changes in 1 ml/hr increments; (3) inclusion of the following alarms: *flow/occlusion* to indicate if tubing is empty or obstructed, *low battery,* and *pump malfunction;* and (4) visual digital display of volume infused.

Delivery of Enteral Feeds

Tube feedings must be delivered at *room temperature.* Unless contraindicated, patients receiving tube feedings can be given small amounts of additional water.

Intermittent bolus feedings. These feedings are the preferred method of administration for (1) long-term use with good tolerance of feeding and (2) transition from constant infusion. Delivery must be slow, allowing 15 to 30 minutes per feeding, and must not be forced with the plunger of the syringe. Feedings must be followed by water (room temperature) to flush the tube. Regurgitation may be prevented by allowing the patient to remain in a sitting position 30 minutes after feeding. If the child's condition permits, he can be burped after the feeding.

Constant infusion. The method of administration for a constant infusion is pump controlled, which reduces the incidence of gastric retention, diarrhea, and vomiting and allows accurate control of infusion rate. Gravity drip is not recommended. The pump apparatus typically includes a bag or bottle for the formula. To decrease the risk of bacterial contami-

nation, the volume of formula in the bag must not exceed the amount to be infused over 8 hours for ready-to-feed formulas or the amount to be infused over 4 hours for prepared formulas that need refrigeration. Rate of administration is individualized to meet varying age, disease process, and nutrient requirements. Administration is begun at 1 to 2 ml/kg/hr and advanced as tolerated.

Concentration of Enteral Feeds

The concentration of initial feedings must never be greater than isotonic concentration (300 mOsm/kg water). With nasogastric and gastric tubes, the volume and concentration of the formula are *not* increased at the same time. With jejunal tubes, the full volume of the formula is reached before the concentration is advanced since more concentrated jejunostomy feedings are not well tolerated. If unusual circumstances necessitate use of a hypertonic solution, very gradual increases are necessary.

RISKS AND COMPLICATIONS
Common Risks

Common problems that occur during TEN in the PICU include diarrhea, abdominal distention, and/or perceived abdominal discomfort as well as feeding tube occlusions and gastric retention of enteral feeds. A problem-solving summary is shown in Table 150-5 that can gauge initial action pending more definitive workup of underlying medical processes or mechanical disruptions.

Prevention and Treatment of Feeding Problems

Infants receiving prolonged enteral tube feedings or parenteral nutrition without the opportunity for simultaneous oral feedings may develop a marked aversion to any oral activities and may suffer delays in the acquisition of language and gross motor skills. Infants who do not experience the normal progressive development of sucking and swallowing and who do not experience normal hunger and satiation cycles are at high risk for feeding problems. Specific types of patients at risk include (1) infants who need surgical intervention to the GI tract; (2) premature infants (<34 weeks of age); (3) infants receiving TPN or enteral tube feedings longer than 1 month; (4) infants who lack strong parental involvement in daily care or consistent primary nursing; and (5) infants who experience unpleasant sensations associated with feedings such as respiratory distress, cramping, or emesis.

Early identification of infants at risk allows prompt intervention, which may help to prevent or ameliorate feeding difficulties. Appropriate interventions are (1) thorough assessment of the child's feeding history and skills by a multidisciplinary team; (2) encouragement of daily parental involvement and primary nursing; (3) routine cuddling of child in the "en-face" feeding position; (4) if the infant is on an NPO regimen or on tube feeds, providing oral stimulation, including tactile stimulation, oral massage, and use of a pacifier, during tube feedings; and (5) oral feedings introduced as early as possible, even

Table 150-5 Problem Solving

Problem	Possible Cause(s)	Intervention
Diarrhea or abdominal cramping	Formula delivered too rapidly	Decrease rate of delivery
	Hypertonic formula	Change to a formula with lower osmolarity if appropriate
		Decrease rate and volume delivered and give continuously
		Increase rate as tolerated
	Hypertonic medication delivered by enteral route	Eliminate additions of medications to formula if possible or dilute them well
	Bacterial contamination of formula or administration set	Evaluate methods of formula preparation and delivery
		Formulas can hang at room temperature for no more than 4 to 8 hr
	Formula too cold	Allow formula to come to room temperature before administering
	Mucosal atrophy	Malnourished patients may benefit from total parenteral nutrition until nutritional status is improved and enteral feedings can gradually be introduced
	Substrate intolerance (especially lactose)	Substitute formula without suspected substrate
	Hypoalbuminemia with resultant edema of GI mucosa	Decrease rate and/or concentration of feeding
Repeated occlusion of tube	Failure to irrigate feeding tube regularly	Irrigate feeding tube (usually with water) at least every 8 hr if feeding is given continuously or after each feeding if given intermittently
	Administration of medication via feeding tube	Some medications coagulate the enteral feed or occlude the tube; physical compatibility must be established before administering any medication via tube
		Flush tube with water after administration of any medication
Gastric retention of formula	High osmolarity of formula	Use formula with lower osmolarity and avoid hyperosmolar medications if possible
	High fat (especially long-chain) content	Reduce fat content of formula (substituting carbohydrate calories) if appropriate
	Calorie-dense formula	Consider formula change
	Underlying disease state contributing to gastric retention	Consider transpyloric feedings
		Position child in upright or right-side-down position after feeds

small volumes (3 to 5 ml), which help the infant develop coordinated sucking and swallowing.

If the child develops feeding problems, he needs to be evaluated by a speech pathologist, occupational therapist, or another specialist trained in the treatment of oral-motor dysfunction. A comprehensive plan including daily oral stimulation by a consistent caretaker must be developed to treat the feeding problem.

ADDITIONAL READING

Bohnker BK, Artman LE, Hoskins WJ. Narrow bore nasogastric feeding tube complications. Nutr Clin Prac 2:203-209, 1987.

Committee on Dietary Allowances. National Academy of Science: Recommended Daily Dietary Allowances, 9th ed. Washington, D.C.: The Academy, 1980.

Fagerman KE, Lysen LK. Enteral feeding tubes: A comparison and history. Nutr Supp Serv 7 (9):10-14, 1987.

Forbes GB, Woodruff CW, eds. Pediatric Nutrition Handbook. Elk Grove Village, Ill.: American Academy of Pediatrics, 1985.

Heird WC, Cooper A. Nutrition in infants and children. In Shils ME, Young VR, eds. Modern Nutrition in Health and Diseases. Philadelphia: Lea & Febiger, 1988, pp 944-961.

• Kennedy-Caldwell C, Caldwell MD. Pediatric enteral nutrition. In Rombeau JL, Caldwell MD, eds. Enteral and Tube Feeding. Philadelphia: WB Saunders, 1984, pp 434-479.

Kleinman RE. Standard and specialized enteric feeding practices in nutrition. In Walker WA, Watkins JB, eds. Nutrition in Pediatrics. Boston: Little Brown, 1985, pp 847-854.

Koehane PP, Attrill H, Silk DB. Clinical indications for weighted feeding tubes. Clin Nutr 2:25-26, 1983.

Linder MC. Nonnutritive components of foodstuffs: Endogenous or added. In Linder MC, ed. Nutritional Biochemistry and Metabolism. New York: Elsevier, 1985, pp 221-238.

Moore MC, Green HL. Tube feeding of infants and children. Pediatr Clin North Am 32:401-417, 1985.

• Orr MJ, Allen SS. Optimal oral experiences for infants on long-term total parenteral nutrition. Nutr Clin Prac 1:288-295, 1986.

Powers DE, Moore AD. Food Medication Interactions, 5th ed. Phoenix: F-M1 Publishing, 1986.

Queen PM, Wilson SE. Growth and nutrient requirements of infants. In Grand RJ, Sutphen JL, Dietz WH, eds. Pediatric Nutrition: Theory and Practice. Boston: Butterworth, 1987, pp 327-349.

Rees LG, Attrill H, Quin D, Silk DB. Improved design of nasogastric feeding tubes. Clin Nutr 5:203-207, 1986.

Robbins S, Thorp JW, Wadsworth C. Tube Feeding of Infants and Children. Washington, D.C.: American Society of Parenteral and Enteral Nutrition, 1984.

Roe DA. Risk factors in drug-induced nutritional deficiencies. In Roe DA, Campbell TC, eds. Drugs and Nutrients: The Interactive Effects. New York: Marcel Dekker, 1984, pp 505-523.

Walker WA, Hendricks KM. Manual of Pediatric Nutrition. Philadelphia: WB Saunders, 1985.

Ward J. Evaluation of enteral feeding pumps for pediatric use. J Pediatr Nurs 1:133-136, 1986.

151 Medical Imaging in the PICU

Thomas Smith

BACKGROUND AND INDICATIONS

The beginning of medical imaging in the PICU dates back to the use of a portable roentgenographic unit at the bedside. It was used to obtain a chest roentgenogram, an abdominal roentgenogram, a skull roentgenogram, or an extremity film in a patient who was acutely or desperately ill and in no condition to be moved to the radiology department. Unfortunately this meant using one of the poorest pieces of diagnostic equipment, the small portable roentgenographic machine, to obtain critical information about the sickest patients. Although obtaining a portable radiograph of the chest or abdomen is still the most common examination, technical improvements have been made that have resulted in better images from much better machines (Fig. 151-1). The new portable units are smaller, more compact, more powerful, more easily moved (or even self-propelled by battery power), and unfortunately much more expensive.

The development of a mobile C-arm has taken medical radiographic imaging a quantum leap further in the PICU. Currently, fluoroscopy (with or without video recording) can be performed at the bedside and is frequently used for monitoring of catheter placements. Visualization of injections of contrast and localization of foreign bodies are also possible (Fig. 151-2). Availability varies, but in some institutions this unit is most used in the trauma center where readily available timely images may be of critical importance. In many hospitals such a unit is usually used in the radiology department during the day for special or invasive procedures but is available for use in the operating room, emergency department, or PICU when needed. A technologist trained in its use is also always available. Physically these units are slightly larger, standing approximately 6 feet high, 3 feet wide, and 6 feet long, than the standard portable

roentgenographic unit. They fit in hospital elevators and operate on any 115-volt, 20-ampere electrical outlet, requiring no additional x-ray shielding beyond that used for regular portable roentgenographic units.

Other imaging modalities in addition to the basic radiograph have resulted from the recent rapid growth in electronics and the development of computer technology. Not only are many new means of diagnosis available, but several are portable and can be performed at the bedside. These newer imaging techniques include real-time and Doppler ultrasonography, the use of radionuclides, single photon emission tomography (SPECT), positron emission tomography (PET), computed tomography (CT), and magnetic resonance imaging (MRI).

ULTRASONOGRAPHY

One of the biggest and most significant developments has been the evolution and improvement of the real-time ultrasound machine. Ultrasonography is well established as the primary imaging modality in the evaluation of the infant brain for evidence of structural defects or the presence of abnormal areas such as hemorrhage or for determination of the status of the ventricular system. The use of ultrasonography in the abdomen as an affordable screening procedure requiring no radiation and providing cross-sectional images is well known and accepted. In the small infant the status of the kidneys can be readily determined, and an obstructive process such as marked hydronephrosis secondary to ureter-pelvic junction obstruction or posterior urethral valves can be easily diagnosed. Adrenal hemorrhage, abdominal tumors such as neuroblastoma or Wilms', pyloric stenosis, duodenal atresia, or even intussusception are all conditions that can be diagnosed by ultrasonography.

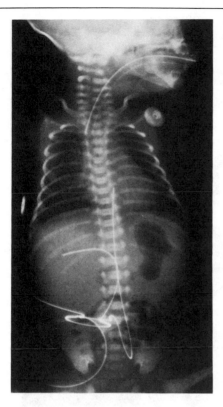

Fig. 151-1 Radiograph obtained by a portable unit of a premature infant with mild respiratory distress syndrome and unacceptable position of the umbilical venous catheter in the right lobe of the liver. The umbilical arterial catheter and the endotracheal tube are properly positioned.

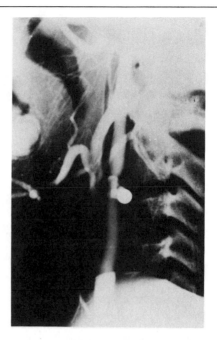

Fig. 151-2 A single lateral angiogram demonstrates a foreign body (CO_2 pellet) that has just nicked the internal carotid artery at the level of C2-3 in a teenage boy.

Although patency of the aorta and inferior vena cava can be determined by real-time ultrasound (Fig. 151-3), Doppler ultrasound is emerging as the noninvasive diagnostic procedure of choice in the evaluation of circulatory abnormalities. It has been extended in utero to evaluation of the fetus and the umbilical vessels and postnatally to the major abdominal vessels, especially the portal and renal vessels in conjunction with the inferior vena cava and the aorta. This noninvasive procedure may prove to be the examination of choice when questions are raised about the patency of or the flow pattern in any major vessel, particularly when angiography may be technically difficult or the status of the patient may be precarious and a contraindication to transport from the PICU to a remote angiography suite.

It is of critical importance to realize that both real-time and Doppler ultrasound are highly operator dependent. An ultrasound machine can be compared to a violin because both require a highly trained, talented specialist to produce diagnostic images or beautiful music, respectively, whereas in untrained or poorly skilled hands the same equipment may produce inadequate, nondiagnostic images or only noise.

The most frequently requested ultrasound studies at Stony Brook are to determine the status of neonatal heads, particularly after traumatic deliveries or seizure-type activity to ascertain the presence of intracranial hemorrhage or some focal abnormality. Next in frequency are abdominal studies carried out to evaluate the liver, spleen, adrenal glands, pancreas, or kidneys or the status of the major vessels for a variety of clinical situations ranging from trauma to major organs to evaluation of a possible abdominal mass. Acutely ill patients, particularly those on ventilators, may be difficult to transport, so often the ultrasound studies are performed at the bedside us-

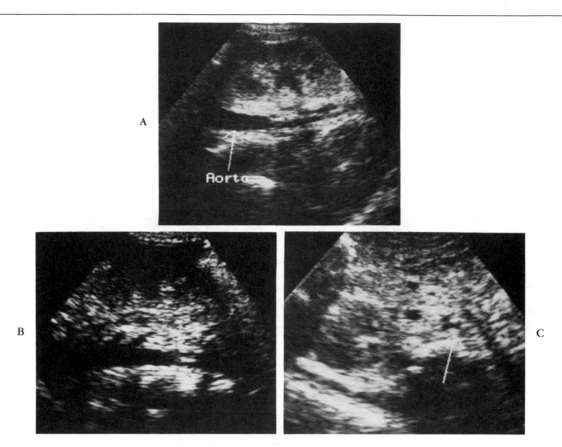

Fig. 151-3   Real-time ultrasound images. **A**, The abdominal aorta, longitudinally, contains an umbilical aortic catheter. **B** and **C**, Longitudinal and transverse ultrasound studies confirm the presence of a clot within the aorta actually obstructing the left renal artery after removal of the aortic catheter.

ing more sophisticated and compact equipment, which has benefited greatly from recent advances in both electronics and computer technology.

NUCLEAR MEDICINE

Another area of imaging that has become more important is that of nuclear medicine, which comprises radionuclide isotope administration followed by localization in one area or organ system with the subsequent emission of gamma rays that can be detected by a scintillation device or gamma camera. Technologic advances, especially the computer, currently enable us to improve on previous image quality plus

carry out dynamic assessment of isotope appearance or accumulation of radioactivity in a target organ. Portable gamma cameras are available for bedside use, but more often than not the patients are moved to the equipment rather than the reverse. Most mobile cameras are large, heavy, expensive, and not easily movable. Even units containing their own power supply are difficult to get on and off elevators, a jarring process to these sensitive pieces of electronic equipment. The most often requested emergency nuclear studies are performed to determine CNS flow or brain death (Fig. 151-4) or to evaluate renal flow and function, particularly after a transplant.

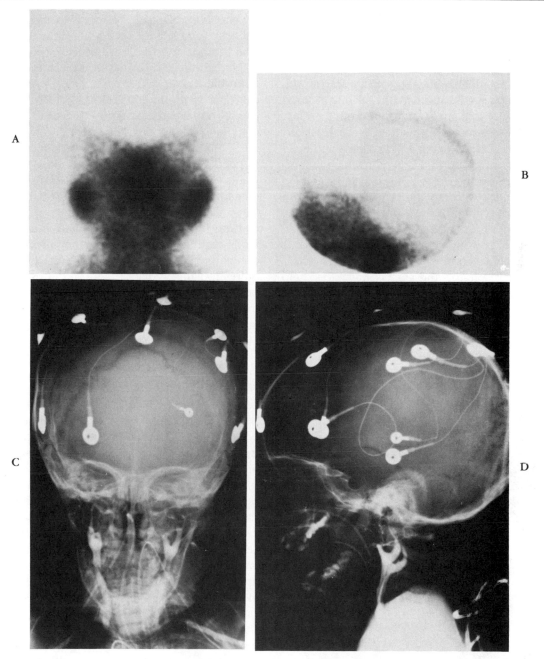

Fig. 151-4   **A** and **B**, Anteroposterior and lateral portable nuclear medicine images show lack of flow of isotope into the skull because of marked elevation of intracranial pressure. **C** and **D**, Anteroposterior and lateral angiograms confirm the nuclear isotope findings of brain death.

PATIENT TRANSPORT

The problem of transporting PICU patients raises several critical care questions and relates directly to the several more complicated imaging modalities for which bringing the equipment to the child is not an option. This problem applies specifically to CT, MRI, and angiography and will eventually include PET and SPECT. Who accompanies the patient from the PICU to one of these remote destinations is usually determined by the severity of the child's illness and need for ventilatory support. In a facility in which numerous transports are necessary, a designated transport nurse may assist with moving critical patients from place to place within, or even outside, the hospital. This person is also available to monitor and provide any necessary nursing support while the patient is having a diagnostic procedure such as CT or nuclear scan. Often a respiratory therapist is available to help manage ongoing ventilatory problems, hand ventilating ventilator-dependent patients by bag-valve-tube if necessary while they are not using the stationary mechanical equipment. Frequently, however, the PICU nurse or the physician (house officer, attending pediatrician, anesthesiologist) may be needed to accompany a particularly ill or unstable patient. Each case must be considered on an individual basis, and special scheduling must be arranged with the imaging facility to provide prompt and efficient handling of such critical patients.

Problems are unique to the specific imaging modality, as exemplified by MRI for which transfer to a special nonmagnetic cradle is necessary and metal equipment cannot be taken into the room containing the scanner without disastrous consequences for the magnet. Ventilatory support and close observation within the magnet are difficult, and the required scanning times are much longer than those necessary for CT studies. Since CT can be performed more easily and quickly, is less expensive, and is usually more readily available as an emergency procedure, it is done more frequently than MRI, even though CT requires ionizing radiation and MRI does not. Ninety percent of emergency CT scans are of the head and frequently involve PICU patients either on the way to or from the PICU and/or the operating room (Fig. 151-5).

RECENT ADVANCES

Having readily available image processing in the PICU or close by has become a topic of increasing interest recently as the number of seriously ill, traumatized, postoperative, and PICU patients has increased. Primary care physicians are demanding prompt and better service from ancillary supportive services, including the medical imaging department. The radiology department has responded by providing automated daylight cassette loading, unloading, and film processing systems in the PICU in an attempt to improve service, decrease turnaround time, cut costs, and increase productivity. Newer film-screen combinations are being used, including rare-earth screens to provide sharper, faster images (radiographs) with less radiation exposure.

Specialized personnel with extra training and interest are able to provide better images with fewer repeats, processes that waste valuable time and film, not to mention the discomfort and problems created for the patient. Close supervision of the technologist by the radiologist promotes better care, better images, and better staff morale. Knowing a good diagnostic image can be obtained by competent staff members with a minimum of hassle at any time of the day or night in a matter of only a few minutes is

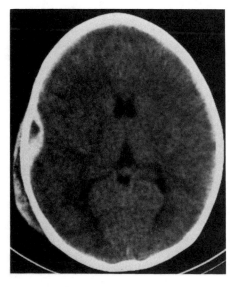

Fig. 151-5 A single CT image without contrast shows a right cephalhematoma and a right subdural hematoma in a 3-year-old child who fell.

of tremendous importance to the responsible physician in the PICU. It is the proper end result of a cooperative effort involving numerous health care professionals.

Several methods of making appropriate images available to the PICU are available. One useful system is that of an automated display view-box, which holds the most recent images of interest for each patient in the PICU. Immediately adjacent to this viewer is a cabinet for storage of the patient's film folder in which formal, typed reports and all previous images are kept. With a large viewer it is possible to find, for example, the images for the patient in bed No. 1 on panel No. 1. Film rounds can take place with the attending physician and the house staff as a part of clinical work rounds or at a separate mutually convenient time with the attending physician. The films are therefore always available, and any new films are placed appropriately on the viewer by the technologist when completed. The radiologist may review the films and render a report at the viewer at any time, but in my experience the early afternoon has proved to be best time since the majority of new films and portable studies are obtained in the morning and work rounds are usually completed. The dictated reports may then be typed and finished reports placed in the patient's folder as soon as they are reviewed and signed.

With the new digital image systems further changes are anticipated, not only in displaying the various images, but also in the process of reviewing, reporting, and distributing the transcribed reports by computer directly to the patient's record and film folder. Recording and storage of medical images on large disks will make them retrievable by computer from a remote terminal such as one located in the PICU and reduce considerably some of the problems now encountered with "finding" films from multiple imaging areas. The need for transcriptionists will be eliminated by voice-activated computers that will convert spoken reports into laser-printed reports. These reports can be transmitted electronically from computer to computer within the hospital or from the medical imaging department to any place a report is desired. These systems are in place at the moment in several pioneering departments; the technology is being further developed and refined. Predictably, as modernization progresses, these changes are going to be widely distributed. Everyone is going to hear much more about computers, digital images, image manipulation and transfer, and data management, particularly in the PICU.

Abbreviations

AA	ascorbic acid	APGAR	appearance, pulse, grimace, activity, respiration	Ba	barium		
A-aDo$_2$	alveolar-arterial oxygen content difference			BAL	British anti-Lewisite (dimercaprol); bronchoalveolar lavage		
ABG	arterial blood gas	aPTT	activated partial thromboplastin time				
ABO	ABO blood types			BCAA	branched-chain amino acids		
ACD	acid citrate dextrose	AR	ascorbate reductase	Be	beryllium		
ACD-A	anticoagulant citrate dextrose, formula A	Ara-C	cytosine arabinoside	Bi	bismuth		
		ARDS	adult respiratory distress syndrome	BMR	basal metabolism rate		
ACE	angiotensin-converting enzyme	ARF	acute respiratory failure; acute renal failure	BPD	bronchopulmonary dysplasia		
ACT	activated clotting time			BSA	body surface area		
ACTH	adrenocorticotropic hormone	As	arsenic	BUN	blood urea nitrogen		
ADH	antidiuretic hormone	ASAIO	American Society for Artificial Internal Organs				
ADP	adenosine diphosphate	ASD	atrial septal defect	C$_{dyn}$	dynamic compliance		
		ASGS	acquired subglottic stenosis	C$_{H_2O}$	free-water clearance		
AFB	acid-fast bacillus						
AG	abdominal girth	ASHBEAMS	American Society of Hospital Based Emergency Air Medical Service	C$_x$	solute clearance		
AIDS	acquired immunodeficiency syndrome			CA	alveolar compliance		
Al	aluminum	AST	aspartate transaminase	Ca	calcium		
ALG	antilymphocyte globulin	ATG	antithymocyte globulin	cAMP	adenosine 3',5'-cyclic phosphate		
ALT	alanine transaminase	ATN	acute tubular necrosis	CaEDTA	calcium ethylenediaminetetraacetic acid		
ALTE	apparent life-threatening events	ATP	adenosine 5'-triphosphate	Cao$_2$	arterial oxygen content		
AMP	adenosine monophosphate	ATPase	adenosine triphosphatase	CAPD	continuous ambulatory peritoneal dialysis		
AMV	assisted mechanical ventilation	Au	gold	CAVC	common atrioventricular canal		
APACHE	Acute Physiology and Chronic Health Evaluation	a-vDo$_2$	arterial-venous oxygen content difference	CAVH	continuous arteriovenous hemofiltration		
APCC	activated prothrombin concentrate complex	AZA	azathioprine	CAVHD	continuous arteriovenous hemodiafiltration		
		AZT	azidothymidine (zidovudine)				

CBC	complete blood count	CPD	citrate phosphate dextrose; continuous peritoneal dialysis
CBF	cerebral blood flow		
CBG	capillary blood gas	CPK	creatine phosphokinase
CCHD	cyanotic congenital heart disease	CPP	cerebral perfusion pressure
Cco_2	capillary oxygen content	CPR	cardiopulmonary resuscitation
CCPD	continuous cycling peritoneal dialysis	CPT	chest physiotherapy
Cd	cadmium	Cr	chromium; renal clearance
CDC	Centers for Disease Control		
CDI	central diabetes insipidus	CRF	corticotropin releasing factor
CDP	continuous distending pressure	CRP	c-reactive protein
		CSF	cerebrospinal fluid
Ch	hepatic clearance	CT	computed tomography
CI	cardiac index		
CIMS	clinical information management systems	Cu	copper
		CVC	central venous catheter
C_L	lung compliance	$C\bar{v}o_2$	mixed venous oxygen content
Cl	clearance		
Cl_p	plasma clearance	CVP	central venous blood pressure
Cl_t	total clearance		
CMV	cytomegalovirus; controlled mechanical ventilation	CVVH	continuous venovenous hemofiltration
CN^-	free cyanide groups; cyanide anion	CXR	chest roentgenogram
		CyA	cyclosporine A
CO	cardiac output; carbon monoxide	D	dextrose; dose administered
CO_2	carbon dioxide	DA	ductus arteriosus
Co_2	oxygen content of blood	DBP	diastolic blood pressure
Co	cobalt		
COHb	carboxyhemoglobin	DDAVP	desmopressin complex
COWS	cold opposite, warm same	delta T (ΔT)	temperature difference
Cp	plasma concentration	DIC	disseminated intravascular coagulation
Cp_{ss}	steady-state plasma concentration	DKA	diabetic ketoacidosis
CPAP	continuous positive airway pressure	D_L	conductance of alveolar capillary membrane
CPB	cardiopulmonary bypass	dl	deciliter
DME	durable medical equipment		
DMPS	2,3-dimercapto-α-propanesulfonic acid		
DNA	deoxyribonucleic acid		
Do_2	oxygen delivery		
DOCA	aqueous deoxycorticosterone acetate		
DOT	Department of Transportation		
1,3-DPG	1,3-diphosphoglycerate		
2,3-DPG	2,3-diphosphoglycerate		
DRGs	diagnosis-related groups		
DST	donor-specific blood transfusion		
DTPA	diethylenetriaminepentaacetic acid		
DTRs	deep tendon reflexes		
D_5W	5% dextrose in water		
$D_{10}W$	10% dextrose in water		
$D_{25}W$	25% dextrose in water		
$D_{50}W$	50% dextrose in water		
e^-	electron		
EABV	effective arterial blood volume		
EACA	epsilon aminocaproic acid		
EBV	estimated blood volume; Epstein-Barr virus		
ECF	extracellular fluid		
ECMO	extracorporeal membrane oxygenation		
EDTA	ethylenediaminetetraacetic acid; European Dialysis & Transplant Association		
EFA	essential fatty acids		

ELAMs	endothelial-leuko-cyte-adhesion mol-ecules	FRC	functional residual capacity	HBsAg	hepatitis B surface antigen
ELISA	enzyme-linked im-munosorbent assay	FRF	filter replacement fluid	HBV	hepatitis B virus
EMP	Embden-Meyerhof pathway	FSP	fibrin split product	HC	heel-crown
		FVC	forced vital capac-ity	H_2CO_3	carbonic acid
EMS	Emergency Medi-cal Services			HCO_3^-	bicarbonate
ESR	erythrocyte sedi-mentation rate	GABA	γ-aminobutyric acid	Hct	hematocrit
ESRD	end-stage renal disease	GBS	Guillain-Barré syn-drome	HFJ	high-frequency jet (ventilation)
$etCo_2$	end-tidal carbon dioxide	GCS	Glasgow Coma Scale	HFO	high-frequency os-cillatory ventilation
ETT	endotracheal tube	GER	gastroesophageal reflux	HFV	high-frequency ventilation
F	bioavailability fac-tor	GFR	glomerular filtra-tion rate	Hg	mercury
				Hib	*Haemophilus in-fluenzae* type b
FAA	Federal Aviation Agency	GGT	gamma glutamyl transferase	HIV	human immuno-deficiency virus
FAD/FADH	oxidized/reduced flavin adenine di-nucleotide	GH	growth hormone	HIV-ab	human immuno-deficiency virus antibody
		GI	gastrointestinal	HLA	human leukocyte antigen; histocom-patibility antigens
5FC	5-fluorocytosine	GM-CSF	granulocyte mac-rophage–colony-stimulating factor		
FCC	Federal Communi-cations Commis-sion	GMP	guanine mono-phosphate	HMD	hyaline membrane disease
FDPs	fibrin degradation products	G3P	glyceraldehyde-3-phosphate	HMS	hexose monophos-phate shunt
FE_{Na}	fractional excre-tion of sodium	G6P	glucose-6-phos-phate	H_2O	water
				HPLC	high-pressure liq-uid chromatogra-phy
Fe	iron	GPD	glyceraldehyde phosphate dehy-drogenase		
Fe^{+2}	divalent ferrous state			HR	heart rate
Fe^{+3}	trivalent ferric state	G6PD	glucose-6-phos-phate dehydroge-nase	HSP	Henoch-Schönlein purpura
				HSV	herpes simplex vi-rus
FEV_1	forced expiratory volume in 1 sec-ond	GSH	reduced glutathi-one	HUS	hemolytic-uremic syndrome
FF	filtration fraction	GSHR	glutathione reduc-tase	ICF	intracellular fluid
FFP	fresh frozen plasma	GSSG	oxidized glutathi-one	ICN	intensive care nursery
FGS	focal glomerulo-sclerosis			ICP	intracranial pres-sure
FHF	fulminant hepatic failure	H	hydrogen ion	I:E	inspiratory/expira-tory ratio
		H_1, H_2	histamine recep-tors		
Fio_2	fraction of inspired oxygen	Hb	hemoglobin	IgA	immunoglobulin A
		HBIG	hepatitis B im-mune globulin	IgG	immunoglobulin G
FO	foramen ovale			IgM	immunoglobulin M
FOC	frontal-occipital head circumfer-ence	HBsAb	hepatitis B surface antibody	IL-1	interleukin-1
				IL-2	interleukin-2
				IM	intramuscular

IMV	intermittent mandatory ventilation	LIC	localized intravascular coagulation	MRI	magnetic resonance imaging
IP	intraperitoneal	LL(+)	possible electrode labels	MRSA	methicillin-resistant *Staphylococcus aureus*
IPD	intermittent peritoneal dialysis	LMB	leukomethylene blue		
IPPB	intermittent positive pressure breathing	LPA	latex particle agglutination	MUGA	multigated nuclear scan
ITP	idiopathic thrombocytopenic purpura	LPS	lipopolysaccharides	Na	sodium
		LRD	live, related donor	NAC	*N*-acetylcysteine
IVC	inferior vena cava	LTC$_4$	leukotriene C$_4$	NaCl	sodium chloride
IVH	intraventricular hemorrhage	LVH	left ventricular hypertrophy	NAD	nicotinamide adenine dinucleotide
IVP	intravenous push			NAD-MHR	NAD-methemoglobin reductase
IVRT	isovolemic relaxation time	MAI	*Mycobacterium avium-intracellulare*	NAD/NADH	oxidized/reduced nicotinamide adenine dinucleotide
IWL	insensible water loss	MALG	Minnesota antilymphocyte globulin	NADP/NADPH	oxidized-reduced nicotinamide adenine dinucleotide phosphate
		MAO	monoamine oxidase		
JCAH	Joint Commission on Accreditation of Hospitals	MAP	mean arterial blood pressure; mean airway pressure	NaHCO$_3$	sodium bicarbonate
JCAHO	Joint Commission on Accreditation of Healthcare Organizations			NANB	non-A, non-B
		MBC	minimum bactericidal concentration	NaN$_2$O$_2$	sodium nitrite
		MCL	modified chest lead	NaOH	sodium hydroxide
JET	junctional ectopic tachycardia	MCT	medium-chain triglyceride	NAPRTCS	North American Pediatric Renal Transplant Cooperative Study
K	potassium	MCV	mean corpuscular volume	NaSCN	sodium thiocyanate
K$_{el}$	elimination constant	MDI	metered dose inhaler	NaSSO$_4$	sodium thiosulfate
K$_t$	respiratory time constants	Mg	magnesium	NBT	nitroblue tetrazolium
KUB	kidney, ureters, and bladder	MH	malignant hyperthermia	NDI	nephrogenic diabetes insipidus
LAD	left axis deviation	MHAUS	Malignant Hyperthermia Association of the United States	NEC	necrotizing enterocolitis
LAN	local area network			NG	nasogastric
LAP	left atrial blood pressure	MHC	major histocompatibility complex	NH$_4$	ammonium
LAV	lymphadenopathy-associated virus	MIC	minimum inhibitory concentration	Ni	nickel
				NIH	National Institutes of Health
LBW	low birthweight	MLC	mixed lymphocyte culture	NMS	neuroleptic malignant syndrome
LD	loading dose				
LDH	lactate dehydrogenase	Mn	manganese	NPO	nothing by mouth
LES	lower esophageal sphincter	MOSF	multiple organ system failure	O$_2^-$	superoxide molecule
LFT	liver function test	mOsm	milliosmole	OAA	oxidized ascorbic acid
Li	lithium	MPAP	mean pulmonary arterial blood pressure		

OKT3 — orthoclone T3 antibody

OPO — organ procurement organization

P_{es} — esophageal pressure

P_{50} — hemoglobin molecule 50% saturated

P_{tp} — transpulmonary pressure

PA — pulmonary artery; plasminogen activator

P_A — alveolar gas pressure

P_{ACO_2} — alveolar carbon dioxide tension

P_{aCO_2} — arterial carbon dioxide tension

PAF — platelet activating factor

PAH — pulmonary arterial hypertension

P_{AH_2O} — alveolar water pressure

PALS — pediatric advanced life support

P_{AN_2} — alveolar nitrogen tension

P_{AO_2} — alveolar oxygen tension

P_{aO_2} — arterial oxygen tension

PAoP — pulmonary arterial occlusion pressure

PAP — pulmonary arterial blood pressure

PARU — postanesthesia recovery unit

Paw — airway pressure

P_B — barometric pressure

Pb — lead

PBS — peripheral blood smear

P_C — pulmonary capillary gas pressure

PCA — patient-controlled anesthesia

PCC — prothrombin complex concentrate

P_{CO_2} — carbon dioxide tension

PCP — phencyclidine; *Pneumocystis carinii* pneumonia

PCWP — pulmonary capillary wedge pressure

PD — potential difference; peritoneal dialysis

PDA — patent ductus arteriosus

PE — pericardial effusion

PEEP — positive end-expiratory pressure

PET — positron emission tomography

P_{etCO_2} — end-tidal carbon dioxide

PFL — perfluorochemical

PFO — patent foramen ovale

PGE_1 — prostaglandin E_1

6PGD — 6-phosphogluconate dehydrogenase

$PGF_{2\alpha}$ — prostaglandin F_2 alpha

PGI_2 — prostacylin

pH — hydrogen ion concentration

PHA — phytohemagglutinin

P_{H_2O} — water vapor pressure

PHT — mitral pressure half-time

PICU — pediatric intensive care unit

P_{iO_2} — partial pressure of inspired oxygen

PIP — peak inspiratory pressure

PIV — peripheral intravenous source

PLEDS — paroxysmal lateral epileptiform discharges

PMN — polymorphonuclear leukocytes

P_{N_2} — nitrogen tension

PO — by mouth

PO_4 — phosphate

P_{O_2} — oxygen tension

PPF — plasma protein fraction

PPHN — persistent pulmonary hypertension of the newborn

PRA — percent recirculating antibodies; panel-reactive antibody

PRISM — Pediatric Risk of Mortality

PRN — as needed

PSI — Physiologic Stability Index

PT — prothrombin time

Pt — platinum

P_{tcCO_2} — transcutaneous carbon dioxide tension

P_{tcO_2} — transcutaneous oxygen tension

P_{tcO_2}/P_{aO_2} — transcutaneous-to-arterial oxygen tension index

PT/PTT — prothrombin time/partial thromboplastin time

PTT — partial thromboplastin time

PVC — premature ventricular contractions

$P_{\bar{v}CO_2}$ — venous carbon dioxide tension

$P_{\bar{v}O_2}$ — venous oxygen tension

PVR — pulmonary vascular resistance

PVRI — pulmonary vascular resistance index

PW — pulsed wave

PWP — pulmonary wedge pressure

QB — filter blood flow

Qf — ultrafiltration rate

qid — four times per day

QP — plasma flow

QPD — pre-dilution filter replacement fluid infusion rate

$\dot{Q}s$ — shunt flow

$\dot{Q}s/\dot{Q}t$	shunt fraction	S_2	second heart sound	$S\bar{v}o_2$	mixed venous oxygen saturation
$\dot{Q}_T$	total flow	S_3	third heart sound	SVR	systemic vascular resistance
R	respiratory exchange quotient (difference)	S_{osm}	serum osmolality	SVRI	systemic vascular resistance index
		Sao_2	oxygen saturation		
		SAP	systemic artery blood pressure	T	time
R_{exp}	expiratory resistance	SAP:PAP	systemic/pulmonary arterial blood pressure ratio	T_b	body temperature
				T_e	environmental temperature
R_{trs}	total respiratory system resistance	Sb	antimony		
RAD	right axis deviation			$t_{1/2}$	half life
RAH	right atrial hypertrophy	SBP	systemic blood pressure; spontaneous bacterial peritonitis	T_3	triiodothyronine
				T_4	levothyroxine
RAP	right atrial blood pressure			tc	core temperature
Raw	airways resistance	SC	subcutaneous	$tcco_2$	transcutaneous carbon dioxide
RC	airway time constants	SCID	severe combined immunodeficiency disease		
				tco_2	transcutaneous oxygen
RDA	recommended dietary allowances	SCUF	slow continuous ultrafiltration	TDM	therapeutic drug monitoring
REM	rapid eye movement	SD	standard deviation	TE	time for expiration
		Se	selenium	TEN	total enteral nutrition
RES	reticuloendothelial system	SEB	staphylococcal enterotoxin B		
RFI	renal failure index	SI	stroke index	THAM	tris-hydroxymethyl-aminomethane
Rh	Rhesus factor	SIADH	syndrome of inappropriate secretion of antidiuretic hormone	TI	time for inspiration
RIJ	right internal jugular vein			Ti	titanium
RNA	ribonucleic acid			TISS	Therapeutic Intervention Scoring System
R5P	ribulose-5-phosphate	SIDS	sudden infant death syndrome		
RR	respiratory rate	SIMV	synchronized intermittent mandatory ventilation	Tl	thallium
RRT	renal replacement therapy			TMP	transmembrane pressure gradient
RSV	respiratory syncytial virus	SL	sublingual	TMP/SMX	trimethoprim/sulfamethoxazole
		SLE	systemic lupus erythematosus		
RVEDP	right ventricular end-diastolic pressure	Sn	tin	TNF	tumor necrosis factor
		SPAG	small-particle aerosol generator	TPA	tissue plasminogen activator
RVEDV	right ventricular end-diastolic volume	SPECT	single photon emission tomography	TPN	total parenteral nutrition
RVH	right ventricular hypertrophy	SU	shoulder-umbilicus	TSH	thyroid-stimulating hormone
RVP	right ventricular blood pressure	SVC	superior vena cava		
		SVC-RA	superior vena cava–right atrium (junction)	TSP	total serum protein
RVSTI	right ventricular systolic time intervals			TSS	toxic shock syndrome
Rx	treatment	SVC-RPA	superior vena cava–right pulmonary artery	TSST-1	toxic shock syndrome toxin-1
S	sieving coefficient; sulfur	SVCS	superior vena cava syndrome	TT	thrombin time

TTP	thrombotic thrombocytopenic purpura	V	vanadium	VEC	vascular endothelial cell
TxA_2	thromboxane A_2	V_d	volume of distribution	VI	ventilatory index
		V_{gas}	gas flow	$\dot{V}_{O_2}$	oxygen consumption
U	uranium	V_i	initial volume		
U_{osm}	urine osmolality	V_t	tissue volume	$\dot{V}/\dot{Q}$	ventilation/perfusion ratio
UNOS	United Network for Organ Sharing	VA	venoarterial		
		V_A	alveolar ventilation	VSD	ventricular septal defect
UO	urinary output	$\dot{V}_{CO_2}$	carbon dioxide production	V_T	tidal volume
USCPSC	United States Consumer Product Safety Commission	VCUG	voiding cystourethrogram	VV	veno-veno
		V_D	physiologic dead space	vWF	von Willebrand factor
USRDS	United States Renal Data System	VDRL	Venereal Disease Research Laboratories	VZIG	varicella zoster immunoglobin
UTI	urinary tract infection			VZV	varicella zoster virus
UUN	urine urea nitrogen	V_D/V_T	percent dead space ventilation	Zn	zinc
UVC	umbilical vein catheterization	V_E	minute ventilation		

Index